(S)3333953

DAVIS'S

Comprehensive Manual of

Laboratory
and
Diagnostic Tests

with Nursing Implications

EIGHTH EDITION

DAVIS'S

Comprehensive Manual of

Laboratory
and
Diagnostic Tests

with Nursing Implications

EIGHTH EDITION

Anne M. Van Leeuwen

Mickey Lynn Bladh

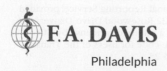

F.A. DAVIS

Philadelphia

F. A. Davis Company
1915 Arch Street
Philadelphia, PA 19103
www.fadavis.com

Printed in the United States of America

Last digit indicates print number: 10 9 8 7 6 5 4 3 2 1

Publisher: Lisa B. Houck
Art and Design Manager: Carolyn O'Brien
Senior Content Project Manager: Julia Curcio
*Davis*Plus *Project Manager:* Sandra Glennie

As new scientific information becomes available through basic and clinical research, recommended treatments and drug therapies undergo changes. The authors and publisher have done everything possible to make this book accurate, up to date, and in accord with accepted standards at the time of publication. The authors, editors, and publisher are not responsible for errors or omissions or for consequences from application of the book, and make no warranty, expressed or implied, in regard to the contents of the book. Any practice described in this book should be applied by the reader in accordance with professional standards of care used in regard to the unique circumstances that may apply in each situation. The reader is advised always to check product information (package inserts) for changes and new information regarding dose and contraindications before administering any drug. Caution is especially urged when using new or infrequently ordered drugs.

Library of Congress Cataloging-in-Publication Data

Names: Van Leeuwen, Anne M., author. | Bladh, Mickey Lynn, author.
Title: Davis's comprehensive handbook of laboratory & diagnostic tests with nursing implications / Anne M. Van Leeuwen, Mickey Lynn Bladh.
Other titles: Davis's comprehensive handbook of laboratory and diagnostic tests with nursing implications | Comprehensive handbook of laboratory & diagnostic tests with nursing implications .| Comprehensive handbook of laboratory and diagnostic tests with nursing implications
Description: Eighth edition. | Philadelphia: F.A. Davis Company, [2019] | Includes index.
Identifiers: LCCN 2018041971 (print) | LCCN 2018042955 (ebook) | ISBN 9780803694484 | ISBN 9780803674950 (hard cover)
Subjects: | MESH: Clinical Laboratory Techniques | Nursing Diagnosis—methods | Handbooks | Nurses' Instruction
Classification: LCC RB38.2 (ebook) | LCC RB38.2 (print) | NLM QY 39 | DDC 616.07/5—dc23
LC record available at https://lccn.loc.gov/2018041971

Dedication

Inspiration springs from Passion.... Passion is born from unconstrained love, commitment, and a vision no one else can own.

Lynda—my best friend and an extraordinarily gifted nurse—thank you, I could not have done this without your love, strong support, and belief in me. My gratitude to Mom, Dad, Adele, Gram ... all my family and friends, for I am truly blessed by your humor and faith. A huge hug for my daughters, Sarah and Margaret—I love you very much. To my puppies, Maggie, Taylor, and Emma, for their endless and unconditional love. Many thanks to my friend and wonderful coauthor Mickey; to all the folks at F.A. Davis, especially Rob and Julia for their guidance, support, and great ideas. And, very special thanks to Lisa Houck, publisher, for her friendship, excellent direction, and unwavering encouragement.

Anne M. Van Leeuwen, MA, BS, MT (ASCP)
Medical Laboratory Scientist & Independent Author
Phoenix Arizona

An eternity of searching would never have provided me with a man more loving and supportive than my husband, Eric. He is the sunshine in my soul, and I will be forever grateful for the blessing of his presence in my life. I am grateful to my five children, Eric, Anni, Phillip, Mari, and Melissa, for the privilege of being their mom; always remember that you are limited only by your imagination and willingness to try. To my darling grandchildren, watching you grow up always reminds me of the joy of discovery. Life is a gift and the trick is not to focus on its troubles but to enjoy the ride, remember to dance in the rain. To Anne, a forever friend who saw in me the potential to spread my wings, thanks for your patience and guidance, and thanks to Lynda for the miracle of finding me. Thanks to those at F. A. Davis for your kind support. Lastly, to my late beloved parents, thanks with hugs and kisses.

Mickey L. Bladh, RN, MSN
Nurse Educator & Author
Hacienda Heights California

We are so grateful to all the people who have helped us make this book possible. We thank our readers for allowing us this important opportunity to touch their lives. Our goal has always been to assist each individual to find a way to blend emotional and intellectual intelligence into a competent and compassionate approach to patient care. We are also thankful for our association with the F.A. Davis Company. We value and appreciate the efforts of all the people associated with F.A. Davis because without their hard work this publication could not succeed. We recognize all the wonderful people in leadership, the editors, freelance consultants, designers, IT gurus, and digital applications developers, as well as those in sales & marketing, distribution, and finance. We have a deep appreciation for the Davis Educational Consultants. They are tasked with being our voice. Their exceptional ability to communicate is what actually brings our book to the market. We would like to give special acknowledgment to the outstanding publishing professionals who were our core support team throughout the development of this edition:

Lisa Houck, *Publisher*
Robert Allen, *Manager, Content Architecture*
Julia Curcio, *Senior Content Project Manager*
Cynthia Naughton, *Production Manager, Digital Content*
Sandra Glennie, *Project Manager, DavisPlus*
Carolyn O'Brien, *Art & Design Manager*
Jaclyn White, *Senior Marketing Manager*
Bob Butler, *Production Manager*

Why This Book Will Help You Be a Better Nurse: The Intersection of Nursing Care and Lab/Dx Testing

We hear every day from students and instructors that they want a laboratory and diagnostic test reference that will help them "connect the dots"—that will show them how to integrate laboratory and diagnostic test results into safe, compassionate, and effective nursing care. We have revised the eighth edition of the Handbook not only to be the comprehensive reference it was originally designed to be but also to provide improvements that more effectively answer that need.

Additional objectives for this 8th edition include the following:

- **Creation of a more portable product** by decreasing its overall size while making sure that each study stands on its own without repeating too much information.
- **Renaming studies for wider recognition** and faster location or to create broader topics for specific studies with multiple modes of analysis (e.g., Chlamydia Testing, rather than Chlamydia Group Antibody, IgG and IgM).
- **Combination of like studies under a single title** to make them easier to find and to conserve space (e.g., CT, MRI, iron, hepatitis, therapeutic drug monitoring studies). We address over 600 tests under 325 individual titles.
- **Development of a more efficient design** that places the "need to know" information at the beginning of each study.
- **Making the content more "visible"** to the reader by presenting information in shorter statements, smaller paragraphs, and as tables and bulleted lists.

We have also restored more than 80 mini-studies to full coverage in the book.

WHAT'S NEW IN THE 8TH EDITION?
- The *Common Use* heading has been replaced with *Rationale*, a more nurse-centered term used to summarize why a test is ordered.
- We moved information about patient preparation to the top of each study. Likewise, we shifted the Critical Findings section to immediately follow Normal Findings.
- We expanded the Overview to provide the study type (e.g., blood, urine, MRI, CT) and body systems related to the study.
- We included the explanation of the procedural portion of each study in Teaching the Patient What to Expect. The information explains in patient-friendly language why the health-care provider has ordered the test and provides the information a nurse would need to:
  - Describe the procedure's common use
  - Describe how the procedure is conducted
  - Describe where the procedure is conducted
  - Answer questions
  - Provide reassurance
- We reorganized the nursing implications section under three main headings:
  1. Before the Study: Planning and Implementation
  2. After the Study: Potential Nursing Actions and Patient/Family Teaching
  3. Follow-Up, Evaluation, and Desired Outcomes

- We kept disease-related nutritional recommendations and cancer screening guidelines but limited the detailed information to a study commonly used to diagnose the condition, so there are now six main studies with detailed guidelines (atherosclerotic cardiovascular disease [ASCVD], diabetes, breast CA, prostate CA, colon CA, cervical CA); we added a reference to the relevant main study in the related studies.
- We created a student checklist that condenses the main nurse-centered information in one place, organized by phase (pretest, intratest, and posttest). The checklist is located in the back of the book.
- We added Maternal Markers, a new study that covers the process of maternal genetic screening, current evidence-based recommendations, determination of carrier status, first- and second-trimester screening (triple screen, quad screen, penta screen), cell-free fetal DNA testing, genetic diagnostic and confirmatory tests, calculated prenatal screen risks, and a table that summarizes the types of screening tests. We put the tests together so as to present them as a process, which their combination truly is, rather than as a number of individual bits of information.
- We brought back the summary reference tables for Laboratory and Diagnostic critical findings.
- We have included new or updated information on:
  - Genetic and genomic implications for health maintenance
  - Molecular testing, companion diagnostics, and precision medicine
  - Pediatric and older adult considerations
  - Specific contraindications and corresponding rationales
  - Specific nursing problems, associated patient signs and symptoms, and potential nursing interactions
  - Specific complications with corresponding rationales and potential interventions
  - Patient education, including references to Web sites for information related to specific health conditions or disease management guidelines
  - Centers for Disease Control and Prevention (CDC) guidelines regarding lead exposure
  - Current terminology, such as *acute kidney injury* (vs. acute kidney damage), *chronic kidney disease* (vs. chronic kidney damage), *benign prostatic hyperplasia* (vs. benign prostatic hypertrophy), *biliary cholangitis* (vs. biliary cirrhosis), *chronic obstructive pulmonary disease (COPD)* (vs. emphysema), *heart failure* (vs. congestive heart failure), *precision diagnostics* (vs. precision or personalized medicine)
  - Recommendations for defining the presence of sepsis and septic shock, including clinical guidelines to facilitate more rapid identification of patients at risk
  - American College of Obstetricians and Gynecologists recommendations regarding genetic screening, genetic diagnostic testing, and cell-free fetal DNA testing
  - Expected post-study outcomes are expressed in statements that provide follow-up instructions or explanations and which reflect the collaborative nature of nurse-to-patient/family interactions in achieving specific desired outcomes

Evidence-based practice is reflected throughout in:

- Suggestions for patient teaching that reflect changes in standards of care, particularly with respect to current guidelines for cancer screening
- The most current CDC guidelines for communicable infections such as syphilis, tuberculosis, and HIV
- The most current guidelines for the prevention of cardiovascular disease developed by the American College of Cardiology and the American Heart Association in conjunction with members of the National Heart, Lung, and Blood Institute's ATP IV Expert Panel
- Best practices for preventing surgical site infections
- Best practice for addressing the need to obtain informed/written consent

Critical Findings sections include:

- A simple statement that reinforces the role of the nurse in providing timely notification and documentation of critical values
- Conventional and SI units
- Commonly reported adult, pediatric, and neonatal values

WHAT'S NEW ONLINE?

Davis*Plus*

The following additional information is available at the Davis*Plus* Web site (http://davispl.us/vanleeuwen8):

- Fast Find: Lab & Dx. Purchasers have access to the searchable library of studies for all the studies included in the text.
- Adopters will have access to a searchable, digital version of the print edition via VitalSource.

Preface

Laboratory and diagnostic testing. The words themselves often conjure up cold and impersonal images of needles, specimens lined up in collection containers, and high-tech electronic equipment. But they do not stand alone. They are tied to, bound with, and tell of health or disease in the blood and tissue of a person. Laboratory and diagnostic studies augment the health-care provider's assessment of the quality of an individual's physical being. Test results guide the plans and interventions geared toward strengthening life's quality and endurance. Beyond the pounding noise of the MRI, the cold steel of the x-ray table, the sting of the needle, the invasive collection of fluids and tissue, and the probing and inspection is the gathering of evidence that supports the health-care provider's ability to discern the course of a disease and the progression of its treatment. Laboratory and diagnostic data must be viewed with thought and compassion, however, as well as with microscopes and machines. We must remember that behind the specimen and test result is the person from whom it came, a person who is someone's son, daughter, mother, father, husband, wife, or friend.

This book is written to help health-care providers in their understanding and interpretation of laboratory and diagnostic procedures and their outcomes. Just as important, it is dedicated to all health-care professionals who experience the wonders in the science of laboratory and diagnostic testing, performed and interpreted in a caring and efficient manner.

The authors continue to enhance and update four main areas in this new edition: organization of the content, pathophysiology that affects test results, patient safety, and patient/family education with expected patient outcomes.

Organization of the content: Time is a precious commodity. The content in the 8th edition has been significantly revised to put the "need to know" information at the top of each study, in the order we imagine readers might prioritize what they need to know. Portability is another important feature of a comprehensive reference book. To that end, repetitive content from the individual studies has been consolidated in the:

- Laboratory/Diagnostic Procedural Checklist for Students
- Appendix A: Patient Preparation and Specimen Collection
- Appendix B: Laboratory Critical Findings
- Appendix C: Diagnostic Critical Findings

The summarized reference tables for critical findings are available in this print edition and online. Also, closely related studies have been combined under a single title to further reduce the size of the book without affecting the number of studies included in the book.

Pathophysiology that affects test results: The Potential Diagnosis section includes explanations of increased or decreased laboratory values to assist in associating pathophysiology with study findings. The authors present a range of age-specific reference normal laboratory values for the neonatal, pediatric, adult, and older adult populations. It should be mentioned that standardized information for the complexity of neonatal, pediatric, and older adult populations is difficult to document. Studies to establish normal ranges for neonates and pediatric patients are limited in number—it is understandable that parents would be reluctant to have their children participate in such studies, especially those involving blood tests. Neonates and pediatric patients are not "little adults," as so often has been said. Their organ systems are not fully developed and continue to mature over time, which can change the definition of a "normal" finding, incrementally, over time. Evaluating laboratory findings in older adults is also a challenging task. Older adults often have complex health situations. Laboratory values may be increased or decreased in older adults due to the sole or combined effects of malnutrition, alcohol use, medications, and the presence of multiple chronic or acute diseases with or without muted symptoms.

Patient safety: The authors appreciate that nurses are the strongest patient advocates with a huge responsibility to protect the safety of their patients, and we have observed student nurses in clinical settings being interviewed by facility accreditation inspectors, so we have updated reminders for a variety of safety topics. Examples include information related to positive patient identification; hand-off communication of critical information; proper timing of diagnostic procedures; rescheduling of specimen collection for therapeutic drug monitoring; use of evidence-based practices for prevention of surgical site infections; descriptions of study related complications and how to avoid them; the nurse's role in the process of obtaining an informed written patient consent before providing care, treatment, or services; information regarding the move to track or limit exposure to radiation from imaging studies for adults; and the Image Gently campaign for pediatric patients who undergo diagnostic studies that utilize radiation.

Patient/family education with expected patient outcomes: The fourth area of emphasis coaches the nurse in providing patient education and provides examples for the nurse to anticipate and respond to a patient's questions or concerns. Elements of this area include describing the purpose of the procedure, study-specific patient preparation, addressing concerns about pain, understanding potential nursing problems in conjunction with the implications of the test results, and potential treatment considerations with related patient/family education, describing postprocedural care and expected patient outcomes. Related Web sites for patient education are included throughout the book to provide additional educational resources for the patient and the nurse.

Laboratory and diagnostic studies are essential components of a complete patient assessment. Examined in conjunction with an individual's history and physical examination, laboratory studies and diagnostic data provide clues about health status. Nurses are increasingly expected to integrate an understanding of laboratory and diagnostic procedures and expected outcomes in assessment, planning, implementation, and evaluation of nursing care. The data help develop and support nursing diagnoses, interventions, and outcomes.

Nurses may interface with laboratory and diagnostic testing on several levels, including:

- Interacting with patients and families of patients undergoing diagnostic tests or procedures, and providing pretest, intratest, and posttest information and support
- Maintaining quality control to prevent or eliminate problems that may interfere with the accuracy and reliability of test results
- Providing education and emotional support at the point of care
- Ensuring completion of testing in a timely and accurate manner

- Collaborating with other health-care professionals in interpreting findings as they relate to planning and implementing total patient care
- Communicating significant alterations in test outcomes to appropriate health-care team members
- Coordinating interdisciplinary efforts

Whether the nurse's role at each level is direct or indirect, the underlying responsibility to the patient, family, and community remains the same.

The authors hope that the changes and additions made to the book will reward users with an expanded understanding of and appreciation for the place laboratory and diagnostic testing holds in the provision of high-quality nursing care and will make it easy for instructors to integrate this important content in their curricula. The authors would like to thank all the users of the previous editions for helping us identify what they like about this book as well as what might improve its value to them. We want to continue this dialogue. As writers, it is our desire to capture the interest of our readers, to provide essential information, and to continue to improve the presentation of the material in the book and ancillary products. We encourage our readers to provide feedback to the Davis Web site and to the publisher's sales professionals. Your feedback helps us modify the material—to change with your changing needs.

ASSUMPTIONS

- The authors recognize that preferences for the use of specific medical terminology may vary by institution. Much of the terminology used in this Handbook is sourced from *Taber's Cyclopedic Medical Dictionary.*
- The definition, implementation, and interpretation of national guidelines for the treatment of various medical conditions changes as new information and new technology emerge. The publication of updated information may at times be contentious among the professional institutions that offer either support or dissent for the proposed changes. This can cause confusion when a patient asks questions about how his or her condition will be identified and managed. The authors believe that the most important discussion about health care occurs between the patient and his or her health-care provider(s). Although the individual studies may point out various screening tests used to identify a disease, the authors often refer the reader to Web sites maintained by nationally recognized authorities on specific topics that reflect the most current information and recommendations for screening, diagnosis, and treatment.
- Most institutions have established policies, protocols, and interdisciplinary teams that provide for efficient and effective patient care within the appropriate scope of practice. It is not our intention that the actual duties a nurse may perform be misunderstood by way of misinterpreted inferences in writing style, but the information prepared by the authors considers that specific limitations are understood by the licensed professionals and other team members involved in patient care activities and that the desired outcomes are achieved by order of the appropriate health-care provider.

Reviewers

Nell Britton MSN, RN, CNE
Nursing Faculty
Trident Technical College Nursing Division
Charleston South Carolina

Cheryl Cassis MSN, RN
Professor of Nursing
Belmont Technical College
St. Clairsville Ohio

Pamela Ellis RN, MSHCA, MSN
Nursing Faculty
Mohave Community College
Bullhead City Arizona

Stephanie Franks MSN, RN
Professor of Nursing
St. Louis Community College–Meramec
St. Louis Missouri

Linda Lott MSN
AD Nursing Instructor
Itawamba Community College
Fulton Mississippi

Martha Olson RN, BSN, MS
Nursing Associate Professor
Iowa Lakes Community College
Emmetsburg Iowa

Barbara Thompson RN, BScN, MScN
Professor of Nursing
Sault College
Sault Ste. Marie Ontario

Edward C. Walton MS, APN-C, NP-C
Assistant Professor of Nursing
Richard Stockton College of New Jersey
Galloway New Jersey

Jean Ann Wilson RN, BSN
Coordinator Norton Annex
Colby Community College
Norton Kansas

Contents

Contents

Acetylcholine Receptor Antibody

SYNONYM/ACRONYM: AChR, AChR-binding antibody, AChR-blocking antibody, and AChR-modulating antibody.

RATIONALE: To assist in confirming the diagnosis of myasthenia gravis (MG).

PATIENT PREPARATION: There are no food, fluid, activity, or medication restrictions unless by medical direction.

NORMAL FINDINGS: (Method: Radioimmunoassay) AChR-binding antibody: Less than 0.4 nmol/L; AChR-blocking antibody: Less than 25% blocking; and AChR-modulating antibody: Less than 30% modulating.

CRITICAL FINDINGS AND POTENTIAL INTERVENTIONS: N/A

OVERVIEW: (**Study type:** Blood collected in a red-top tube; **related body system:** Musculoskeletal system.) MG is an acquired autoimmune disorder that can occur at any age. Its exact cause is unknown. It seems to strike women between ages 20 and 40 yr; men appear to be affected later in life than women. It can affect any voluntary muscle, but muscles that control eye and eyelid movement, facial movement, and swallowing are most frequently affected. Antibodies may not be detected in the first 6 to 12 mo after the first appearance of symptoms. Normally, when impulses travel down a nerve, the nerve ending releases a neurotransmitter called *acetylcholine* (ACh), which binds to receptor sites in the neuromuscular junction, eventually resulting in muscle contraction. There are three types of AChR autoantibodies: AChR-binding antibodies render ACh unavailable for muscle receptor sites, resulting in muscle weakness; AChR-blocking antibodies impair or prevent ACh from attaching to receptor sites on the muscle membrane, resulting in poor muscle contraction; and AChR-modulating antibodies destroy AChR sites, interfering with neuromuscular transmission.

Testing for AChR-binding antibody is the most often requested of the three antibodies. There are two other types of autoantibodies, but they are rarely absent when binding antibody is detected. Antibodies to AChR sites are present in 90% of patients with generalized MG and in 55% to 70% of patients who either have ocular forms of MG or are in remission. Approximately 10% to 15% of people with confirmed MG do not demonstrate detectable levels of AChR-binding, AChR-blocking, or AChR-modulating antibodies. Secondary testing is performed, in these cases, for anti-MuSK (muscle-specific receptor tyrosine kinase) antibody, which is produced in 40% to 70% of the remaining 15% who have MG but test negative for AChR autoantibodies. MG is a common complication associated with thymoma. Remission after thymectomy is associated with a progressive decrease in antibody level. Other markers used in the study of MG include striational muscle antibodies, thyroglobulin, human leukocyte antigen (HLA)-B8, and HLA-DR3. A diagnosis of MG should be based on abnormal findings from two different diagnostic tests. These tests include the AChR antibody

A

assay, anti-MuSK antibody assay, edrophonium chloride test, repetitive nerve stimulation, and single-fiber electromyography (see EMG study for more detailed information). Prior to the edrophonium chloride test, the patient receives an injection of edrophonium chloride or Tensilon, a medication that temporarily blocks the degradation of acetylcholine. An MG-positive finding is indicated by normal measurable neuromuscular transmissions that dissipate as the effects of the injection wear off. Repetitive nerve stimulation testing involves sending small pulses of electricity, over and over, to specific muscles to measure a decreased response due to muscle weakening.

INDICATIONS
- Confirm the presence but not the severity of MG.
- Detect subclinical MG in the presence of thymoma.
- Monitor the effectiveness of immunosuppressive therapy for MG.
- Monitor the remission stage of MG.

INTERFERING FACTORS
Factors that may alter the results of the study
- Drugs and other substances that may increase AChR levels include penicillamine (long-term use may cause a reversible syndrome that produces clinical, serological, and electrophysiological findings indistinguishable from MG).
- Biological false-positive results may be associated with amyotrophic lateral sclerosis, autoimmune hepatitis, Lambert-Eaton myasthenic syndrome, primary biliary cholangitis, and encephalomyeloneuropathies associated with cancer of the lung. MG patients may also produce autoantibodies, such as antinuclear antibody and

rheumatoid factor, not primarily associated with MG that demonstrate measurable reactivity.
- Immunosuppressive therapy may be recommended for treatment of MG; administration of immunosuppressive drug prior to testing may cause negative test results.
- Recent radioactive scans or radiation within 1 wk of the test can interfere with test results when radioimmunoassay is the test method.

POTENTIAL MEDICAL DIAGNOSIS: CLINICAL SIGNIFICANCE OF RESULTS
Increased in
- Autoimmune liver disease
- Generalized MG *(Defective transmission of nerve impulses to muscles evidenced by muscle weakness. It occurs when normal communication between the nerve and muscle is interrupted at the neuromuscular junction.)*
- Lambert-Eaton myasthenic syndrome
- Primary lung cancer
- Thymoma associated with MG *(It is believed that miscommunication in the thymus gland directed at developing immune cells may trigger the development of autoantibodies responsible for MG.)*

Decreased in
- Postthymectomy *(The thymus gland produces the T lymphocytes responsible for the innate cell mediated immunity directed at cells in the body that have been infected by bacteria, viruses, parasites, fungi, or protozoans. T lymphocytes are also associated with an adaptive immune surveillance, identification, and destruction function directed at cells that have been invaded by precancerous and cancerous cells. Removal of the thymus gland is strongly associated with a decrease in AChR antibody levels.)*

NURSING IMPLICATIONS

POTENTIAL NURSING PROBLEMS: ASSESSMENT & NURSING DIAGNOSIS

Problems	Signs and Symptoms
Airway *(related to increasing weakness, paralysis)*	Difficulty swallowing, aspiration, cyanosis, anxiety, hypoxemia
Mobility *(related to weakness, tremors, spasticity)*	Unsteady gait, lack of coordination, difficult purposeful movement, inadequate range of motion
Nutrition *(related to spasticity, altered level of consciousness, paresis, increasing weakness, paralysis)*	Difficulty chewing, swallowing food; weight loss
Self-care *(related to spasticity, altered level of consciousness, paresis, increasing weakness, paralysis)*	Difficulty fastening clothing and performing personal hygiene, inability to maintain appropriate appearance, difficulty with independent mobility, declining physical function
Urination *(related to neurogenic bladder, spastic bladder; associated with disease process)*	Urinary retention, urinary frequency, urinary urgency, pain and abdominal distention, urinary dribbling

BEFORE THE STUDY: PLANNING AND IMPLEMENTATION

Teaching the Patient What to Expect

▶ Inform the patient that the test is used to identify antibodies responsible for decreased neuromuscular transmission and associated muscle weakness.

▶ Explain that a blood sample is needed for the test.

AFTER THE STUDY: POTENTIAL NURSING ACTIONS

Avoiding Complications

▶ Explain the importance of stating any prior reactions, complications, or family history of complications experienced with general anesthesia or cholinesterase inhibitors. Succinylcholine-sensitive patients may not metabolize anesthetics quickly, resulting in prolonged or unrecoverable apnea. If thymectomy is considered, the surgeon should be aware of this potential complication.

Treatment Considerations

▶ If a diagnosis of MG is made, a computed tomography (CT) scan of the chest should be ordered to rule out thymoma.

▶ Airway: Teach techniques to evaluate swallowing effectiveness to prevent aspiration risk from muscle weakness that causes difficulty chewing and swallowing.

▶ Comfort/Mobility: Keep the immediate environment cool to decrease aggravating MG symptoms; use passive or active range of motion to decrease muscle tightness; administer analgesics, tranquilizers, antispasmodics, and neuropathic pain medication, as ordered.

▶ Self-Care: Reinforce self-care techniques as taught by occupational therapy; ensure the patient has adequate time to perform self-care; encourage use of assistive devices to maintain independence; assess ability to perform activities of daily living (ADLs); provide care assistance appropriate to degree of disability while maintaining as much independence as possible.

▶ Therapeutic Management: Administer medications as ordered and exactly at the prescribed times: ACh inhibitors,

A

analgesics, tranquilizers, antispasmodics, and neuropathic pain medication. Some medications are most effective when given 30 to 60 min before meals to facilitate chewing and swallowing.

▶ Urination: Assess amount of fluid intake, as it may be necessary to limit fluids to control incontinence; assess risk of urinary tract infection with limiting oral intake; begin bladder training program; teach catheterization techniques to family and patient self-catheterization.

Safety Considerations
▶ Airway: Teach the patient and family that the safest position for eating and drinking is with the head of the bed elevated in order to decrease choking risk. Teach the family how to recognize choking signs and what to do if the patient begins choking.

▶ Mobility: Assess gait, muscle strength, weakness and coordination, physical endurance, and level of fatigue; assess ability to perform independent ADLs; assess ability for safe, independent movement. Teach family to place self-care items within the patient's reach to promote as much independence in care as possible and to decrease injury risk.

Nutritional Considerations
▶ Assess for signs and symptoms of malnutrition or dehydration. Discuss meal plans, such as diets that offer soft solid foods or thick liquids, as provided by registered dietitian or speech pathology consultant. Reinforce the importance of giving medications at the exact times recommended and in relation to meal times.

Follow-Up, Evaluation, and Desired Outcomes
▶ Acknowledges contact information provided for speech pathology services, emotional support with counseling services, or the Myasthenia Gravis Foundation of America (www.myasthenia.org) and the Muscular Dystrophy Association (www.mdausa.org)
▶ Recognizes the importance of adherence to recommended physical therapy including performance of range-of-motion activities, and acceptance of the physical limitations related to the disease process.

Adrenal Gland Scan

SYNONYM/ACRONYM: Adrenal scintiscan, adrenal scintigraphy, metaiodobenzylguanidine or MIBG scan.

RATIONALE: To assist in the diagnosis of adrenal gland tumors (adrenocortical cancer, adenomas, neuroblastomas, and pheochromocytomas).

PATIENT PREPARATION: There are no food, fluid, or activity restrictions unless by medical direction. A number of medications may interfere with MIBG radionuclide uptake, most commonly ACE inhibitors, amiodarone, antihypertensives (reserpine, guanethidine, labetalol), calcium channel blockers, decongestants (ephedrine, phenylephrine, phenylproanolamine, pseudoephedrine), opioids, sympathomimetics (amphetamines, cocaine, epinephrine, methamphetamine, norepinephrine), and tricyclic antidepressants. These medications may be ordered to be withheld by medical direction prior to the scan. No procedures using barium contrast medium should be scheduled before this procedure. Protocols may vary among facilities.

A

NORMAL FINDINGS
• No evidence of tumors
• Normal bilateral uptake of radionuclide and secretory function of adrenal cortex.

CRITICAL FINDINGS AND POTENTIAL INTERVENTIONS: N/A

OVERVIEW: (Study type: Nuclear scan; related body system: Endocrine system.) This study, which has largely been replaced by CT, MRI, SPECT/CT, and PET/CT studies, is used to detect the presence and location of adrenal pheochromocytomas. Measurement of 24-hr urine specimens for catecholamines (epinephrine and norepinephrine) and metanephrines (principle catecholamine metabolites: homovanillic acid and vanillylmandelic acid) is often used in conjunction with diagnostic studies in the investigation of adrenal tumors; urinary levels would be elevated in the presence of adrenergic tumors. Plasma catecholamines and metanephrines may also be evaluated.

A single adrenal gland is located above each kidney and consists of two parts. The outer cortex is where the adrenal hormones, including cortisol and aldosterone, are produced. The cortex is also where the majority of adrenal tumors are identified, most of which are benign. The inner part of the adrenal gland is called the *medulla* and is where the neurohormones epinephrine and norepinephrine are produced. Tumors in the medulla are relatively rare and include neuroblastomas and pheochromocytomas, tumors that arise from catecholamine-producing chromaffin cells. Pheochromocytomas and paragangliomas can also develop from extra-adrenal chromaffin cells that are usually located in the abdomen. Adrenal imaging can be used in combination with other diagnostic tools, such as biopsy, x-ray, and ultrasound. There are a number of radionuclides that may be used in neuroendocrine scintiscans such as the MIBG scan (metaiodobenzylguanidine labelled with I-123 or I-131), NP-59 scan (iodomethyl-19-norcholesterol), and octreotide scan (In-111 labelled pentetreotide). The radionuclides are synthetic analogs of naturally occurring substances in the body known to selectively bind to receptor sites on the tumor cells, visualizing areas of concern in primary or metastatic locations. MIBG is an analog of norepinephrine, NP-59 is a cholesterol analog, and octreotide is an analog of somatostatin. The uptake of the radionuclide occurs gradually over time, and imaging is performed within 24 to 48 hr of radionuclide injection and continued daily for 3 to 5 days. The imaging equipment can be a simple gamma camera that produces two-dimensional images; single-photon emission computed tomography (SPECT) imaging taken by a gamma camera that rotates around the body to produce a three-dimensional image; or a combination of technologies such as SPECT-CT, which combines three-dimensional images taken with standard CT imaging equipment followed by imaging provided by a rotating

SPECT camera system. Imaging can reveal increased uptake, unilateral or bilateral uptake, or absence of uptake in the detection of pathological processes. Following prescanning treatment with corticosteroids, suppression studies can also be done to differentiate the presence of tumor from hyperplasia of the glands. MBIG is used therapeutically, at higher doses, to treat adrenal cancer. Nuclear imaging studies are also used to evaluate the effectiveness of therapeutic interventions.

INDICATIONS

- Aid in locating adrenergic tumors *(rare catecholamine-producing tumors such as pheochromocytoma)*.
- Determine adrenal suppressibility with prescan administration of corticosteroid to diagnose and localize adrenal adenoma, aldosteronomas, androgen excess, and low-renin hypertension.
- Differentiate between asymmetric hyperplasia and asymmetry from aldosteronism with dexamethasone suppression test.

INTERFERING FACTORS

Contraindications

✷ Patients who are pregnant or suspected of being pregnant, unless the potential benefits of a procedure using radiation far outweigh the risk of radiation exposure to the fetus and mother.

✷ Conditions associated with adverse reactions to contrast medium (e.g., asthma, food allergies, or allergy to contrast medium). Although patients are asked specifically if they have a known allergy to iodine or shellfish, it has been well established that the reaction is not to iodine; an actual iodine allergy would be problematic because iodine is required for the production of thyroid hormones. In the case of shellfish, the reaction is to a muscle protein called tropomyosin; in the case of iodinated contrast medium, the reaction is to the noniodinated part of the contrast molecule. Patients with a known hypersensitivity to the medium may benefit from premedication with corticosteroids and diphenhydramine; the use of nonionic contrast or an alternative noncontrast imaging study, if available, may be considered for patients who have severe asthma or who have experienced moderate to severe reactions to ionic contrast medium.

Factors that may alter the results of the study
- Barium procedures should be scheduled after the MIBG scan; residual barium may produce misleading artifacts on subsequent imaging.

Other considerations
Perform all adrenal blood studies before doing this test.

POTENTIAL MEDICAL DIAGNOSIS: CLINICAL SIGNIFICANCE OF RESULTS

Abnormal findings related to
The radioactive tracer will accumulate in abnormal tissue, and "hot spots" will identify specific areas of concern.

- Adrenal gland suppression
- Adrenal infarction
- Benign adrenal tumor
- Ganglioneuroblastoma
- Ganglioneuroma
- Hyperplasia
- Medullary thyroid cancer
- Neuroblastoma
- Paraganglioma
- Pheochromocytoma

NURSING IMPLICATIONS

BEFORE THE STUDY: PLANNING AND IMPLEMENTATION

Teaching the Patient What to Expect

▶ Inform the patient this procedure can visualize and assess the function of the adrenal gland, which is located near the kidney.

▶ Pregnancy is a general contraindication to procedures involving radiation. Explain to the female patient that she will be asked the date of her last menstrual period. Pregnancy testing may be performed to determine the possibility of pregnancy before exposure to radiation.

▶ Review the procedure with the patient. Address concerns about pain and explain that on day 1 there may be moments of discomfort or pain experienced when the IV line is inserted for injection of the radionuclide.

▶ Explain that a separate IV line may be inserted to allow infusion of other fluids such as saline, anesthetics, sedatives, medications used in the procedure, or emergency medications if required; some discomfort may be experienced.

▶ Explain that the procedure takes approximately 60 min and is usually performed in a nuclear medicine department by a health-care provider (HCP) and staff who specialize in this procedure. Scanning usually involves a prolonged schedule over a period of days; images are taken on days 1, 2, and 3. Each image takes 20 min, and total imaging time is 1 to 2 hr per day.

▶ Reassure the patient that the radionuclide poses no radioactive hazard and rarely produces adverse effects.

▶ Jewelry and other metallic objects will need to be removed from the area to be examined each time the patient comes for a scan, on days 1, 2, and 3.

▶ Baseline vital signs and neurological status will be recorded prior to each scan. Protocols may vary among facilities.

Potential Nursing Actions

◈ *Make sure a written and informed consent has been signed prior to the procedure and before administering any medications.*

Safety Considerations

▶ Administer saturated solution of potassium iodide (SSKI or Lugol iodine solution) 24 hr before the study to prevent thyroid and gastric uptake of the free radioactive iodine; the solution is usually added to another liquid (e.g., orange juice) and administered orally. Protocols may vary among facilities.

AFTER THE STUDY: POTENTIAL NURSING ACTIONS

Avoiding Complications

▶ Establishing an IV site and injection of radionuclides are invasive procedures. Complications are rare but do include risk for allergic reaction *(related to contrast medium)*, hematoma *(related to blood leakage into the tissue following needle insertion)*, bleeding from the puncture site *(related to a bleeding disorder or the effects of natural products and medications with known anticoagulant, antiplatelet, or thrombolytic properties)*, or infection *(which might occur if bacteria from the skin surface is introduced at the puncture site)*. Monitor the patient for complications related to the procedure (e.g., allergic reaction, anaphylaxis, bronchospasm). Immediately report symptoms such as fast heart rate, difficulty breathing, skin rash, itching, or chest pain to the appropriate HCP. Observe/assess the needle/catheter insertion site for bleeding, inflammation, or hematoma formation.

Treatment Considerations

▶ Inform the patient that radionuclide is eliminated from the body within 6 to 24 hr. Unless contraindicated, advise the patient to drink increased amounts of fluids for 24 to 48 hr to eliminate the radionuclide from the body and to take prescribed antihypertensive and diuretic medications. Monitor fluid (water) and electrolytes, heart rate, blood pressure, and daily weight.

◗ Instruct the patient in the care and assessment of the injection site and to apply cold compresses to the puncture site as needed to reduce discomfort or edema.

Safety Considerations
◗ Breastfeeding patients should consult with the requesting HCP regarding alternative testing that does not involve radiation. In general, if a woman who is breastfeeding must have a nuclear scan, she should not breastfeed the infant for 72 hr after the scan, until the radionuclide has been eliminated. She should be instructed to express the milk in order to prevent cessation of milk production; the milk can be stored and used after the 3-day period.
◗ Refer to organizational policy for additional precautions that may include instructions on handwashing, toilet flushing, limited contact with others, and other aspects of nuclear medicine safety.

Nutritional Considerations
◗ Teach the patient to eat a low-sodium diet and a diet high in fiber to enhance bowel motility, decrease gastrointestinal bleed risk; teach patient also to increase calcium and vitamin D intake with diet and supplements as appropriate.

Follow-Up, Evaluation, and Desired Outcomes
◗ Understands the information provided on the relationship between injury risk, altered cortisol levels, and adrenal disease.
◗ Acknowledges contact information provided for the American Cancer Society (www.cancer.org).
◗ Understands the necessity of taking SSKI (120 mg/day) for 14 days after the injection of the radionuclide. The iodine solution continues to block uptake of the radioactive iodine by the thyroid gland while the radionuclide is being excreted from the body.

Adrenocorticotropic Hormone
(and Challenge Tests)

SYNONYM/ACRONYM: Corticotropin, ACTH.

RATIONALE: To assist in the investigation of adrenocortical dysfunction using ACTH and cortisol levels in diagnosing disorders such as Addison disease, Cushing disease, and Cushing syndrome.

PATIENT PREPARATION: There are no food or fluid restrictions unless by medical direction. Drugs that enhance steroid metabolism may be withheld by medical direction before metyrapone stimulation testing. Instruct the patient to refrain from smoking, avoid alcohol use, avoid strenuous exercise for 12 hr before the test, and remain in bed or at rest for 1 hr immediately before the test. Samples should be collected at the same time of day, between 0600 and 0800.

Procedure	Indications	Medication Administered, Adult Dosage	Recommended Collection Times
ACTH stimulation, rapid test	Suspect adrenal insufficiency (Addison disease) or congenital adrenal hyperplasia	1 mcg (low-dose physiological protocol) cosyntropin intramuscular (IM) or IV; 250 mcg (standard pharmacological protocol) cosyntropin IM or IV	Three cortisol levels: Baseline immediately before bolus, 30 min after bolus, and 60 min (optional) after bolus. Baseline and 30-min levels are adequate for accurate diagnosis using either dosage; low-dose protocol sensitivity is most accurate for 30-min level only.
Corticotropin-releasing hormone (CRH) stimulation	Differential diagnosis between ACTH-dependent conditions such as Cushing disease (pituitary source) or Cushing syndrome (ectopic source) and ACTH-independent conditions such as Cushing syndrome (adrenal source)	IV dose of 1 mcg/kg human CRH	Eight cortisol and eight ACTH levels: Baseline collected 15 min before injection, 0 min before injection, and then 5, 15, 30, 60, 120, and 180 min after injection
Dexamethasone suppression (overnight)	Differential diagnosis between ACTH-dependent conditions such as Cushing disease (pituitary source) or Cushing syndrome (ectopic source) and ACTH-independent conditions such as Cushing syndrome (adrenal source)	Oral dose of 1 mg dexamethasone (Decadron) at 2300	Cortisol level at 0800 on the morning after the dexamethasone dose
Metyrapone stimulation (overnight)	Suspect hypothalamic/pituitary disease such as adrenal insufficiency, ACTH-dependent conditions such as Cushing disease (pituitary source) or Cushing syndrome (ectopic source), and ACTH-independent conditions such as Cushing syndrome (adrenal source)	Oral dose of 30 mg/kg metyrapone with snack at 2400	Cortisol, 11-deoxycortisol, and ACTH at 0800 on the morning after the metyrapone dose

NORMAL FINDINGS: Method: Immunochemiluminescent assay for ACTH and cortisol; high-performance liquid chromatography tandem mass spectrometry (LC-MS/MS) for 11-deoxycortisol.

ACTH

Age	Conventional Units	SI Units (Conventional Units × 0.22)
Cord blood	50–570 pg/mL	11–125 pmol/L
Newborn	10–185 pg/mL	2–41 pmol/L
1 wk–9 yr	5–46 pg/mL	1.1–10.1 pmol/L
10–18 yr	6–55 pg/mL	1.3–12.1 pmol/L
19 yr–Adult		
Male supine (specimen collected in morning)	7–69 pg/mL	1.5–15.2 pmol/L
Female supine (specimen collected in morning)	6–58 pg/mL	1.3–12.8 pmol/L

Values may be unchanged or slightly elevated in healthy older adults. Long-term use of corticosteroids, to treat arthritis and autoimmune diseases, may suppress secretion of ACTH.

ACTH Challenge Tests

ACTH (Cosyntropin) Stimulated, Rapid Test	Conventional Units	SI Units (Conventional Units × 27.6)
Baseline	Cortisol greater than 5 mcg/dL	Greater than 138 nmol/L
30- or 60-min response	Cortisol 18–20 mcg/dL or incremental increase of 7 mcg/dL over baseline value	497–552 nmol/L or incremental increase of 193.2 nmol/L over baseline value

Corticotropin-Releasing Hormone Stimulated	Conventional Units	SI Units (Conventional Units × 27.6)
	Cortisol peaks at greater than 20 mcg/dL within 30–60 min	Greater than 552 nmol/L
		SI Units (Conventional Units × 0.22)
	ACTH increases twofold to fourfold within 30–60 min	Twofold to fourfold increase within 30–60 min

Dexamethasone Suppressed Overnight Test	Conventional Units	SI Units (Conventional Units × 27.6)
	Cortisol less than 1.8 mcg/dL next day	Less than 49.7 nmol/L

Metyrapone Stimulated Overnight Test	Conventional Units	SI Units (Conventional Units × 27.6)
	Cortisol less than 3 mcg/dL next day	Less than 83 nmol/L
		SI Units (Conventional Units × 0.22)
	ACTH greater than 75 pg/mL	Greater than 16.5 pmol/L
		SI Units (Conventional Units × 28.9)
	11-deoxycortisol greater than 7 mcg/dL	Greater than 202 nmol/L

CRITICAL FINDINGS AND POTENTIAL INTERVENTIONS: N/A

OVERVIEW: (**Study type:** Blood collected in a prechilled lavender-top [EDTA] tube for ACTH and from a prechilled red-top tube for cortisol and 11-deoxycortisol; **related body system:** Endocrine system.) Gold-, tiger-, and green-top (heparin) tubes are also acceptable for cortisol, but care must be taken to use the same type of collection container for serial measurements. Alternatively, specimens can be collected in a prechilled heparinized plastic syringe and carefully transferred into the appropriate tube types by gentle injection to avoid hemolysis. Immediately transport specimen, tightly capped and in an ice slurry, to the laboratory. Hypothalamic-releasing factor stimulates the release of ACTH from the anterior pituitary gland. ACTH stimulates adrenal cortex secretion of glucocorticoids, androgens, and, to a lesser degree, mineralocorticoids. Cortisol is the major glucocorticoid secreted by the adrenal cortex. ACTH and cortisol test results are evaluated together because a change in one normally causes a change in the other. ACTH secretion is stimulated by insulin, metyrapone, and vasopressin. It is decreased by dexamethasone. Cortisol excess from any source is termed *Cushing syndrome.* Cortisol excess resulting from ACTH excess produced by the pituitary is termed *Cushing disease.* ACTH levels exhibit a diurnal variation, peaking between 0600 and 0800 and reaching the lowest point between 1800 and 2300. Evening levels are generally one-half to two-thirds lower than morning levels. Cortisol levels also vary diurnally, with the peak values occurring between 0600 and 0800 and reaching the lowest levels between 2000 and 2400. Specimens are typically collected at 0800 and 1600. This pattern may be reversed in individuals who sleep during daytime hours and are active during nighttime hours. Salivary cortisol levels are known to parallel blood levels and can be used to screen for Cushing disease and Cushing syndrome.

INDICATIONS
- Determine adequacy of replacement therapy in congenital adrenal hyperplasia.
- Determine adrenocortical dysfunction.
- Differentiate between increased ACTH release with decreased cortisol levels and decreased ACTH release with increased cortisol levels.

INTERFERING FACTORS
Contraindications

❖ The metyrapone stimulation test is contraindicated in patients with suspected adrenal insufficiency because it may induce an acute adrenal crisis, a life-threatening condition, in patients whose adrenal function is already compromised.

Factors that may alter the results of the study
- Drugs and other substances that may increase ACTH levels include insulin, metoclopramide, metyrapone, mifepristone (RU 486), spironolactone, and vasopressin.
- Drugs and other substances that may decrease ACTH levels include corticosteroids (e.g., dexamethasone) and pravastatin.

- Excessive physical activity can produce elevated levels.
- Test results are affected by the time the test is done because ACTH levels vary diurnally, with the highest values occurring between 0600 and 0800 and the lowest values occurring at night.

❖ Rapid clearance of metyrapone, resulting in falsely increased cortisol levels, may occur if the patient is taking drugs that enhance steroid metabolism (e.g., phenytoin, rifampin, phenobarbital, mitotane, and corticosteroids). The requesting health-care provider (HCP) should be consulted prior to a metyrapone stimulation test regarding a decision to withhold these medications.

Other considerations

❖ Metyrapone may cause gastrointestinal distress and/or confusion. Administer oral dose of metyrapone with milk and snack.

POTENTIAL MEDICAL DIAGNOSIS: CLINICAL SIGNIFICANCE OF RESULTS

ACTH Result
Because ACTH and cortisol secretion exhibit diurnal variation with values being highest in the morning, a lack of change in values from morning to evening is clinically significant. Decreased concentrations of hormones secreted by the pituitary gland and its target organs are observed in hypopituitarism. In primary adrenal insufficiency (Addison disease), because of adrenal gland destruction by tumor, infectious process, or immune reaction, ACTH levels are elevated, while cortisol levels are decreased. Both ACTH and cortisol levels are decreased in secondary adrenal insufficiency (i.e., secondary to pituitary insufficiency). Excess ACTH can be produced ectopically by various lung cancers such as oat-cell cancer and large-cell cancer of the lung and by benign bronchial carcinoid tumor.

Challenge Tests and Results

The **ACTH (cosyntropin) stimulated rapid test** *directly evaluates adrenal gland function and indirectly evaluates pituitary gland and hypothalamus function. Cosyntropin is a synthetic form of ACTH. A baseline cortisol level is collected before the injection of cosyntropin. Specimens are subsequently collected at 30- and 60-min intervals. If the adrenal glands function normally, cortisol levels rise significantly after administration of cosyntropin.*

The CRH stimulation test works as well as the dexamethasone suppression test (DST) in distinguishing Cushing disease from conditions in which ACTH is secreted ectopically (e.g., tumors not located in the pituitary gland that secrete ACTH). Patients with pituitary tumors tend to respond to CRH stimulation, whereas those with ectopic tumors do not. Patients with adrenal insufficiency demonstrate one of three patterns depending on the underlying cause:

- *Primary adrenal insufficiency— high baseline ACTH (in response to IV-administered ACTH) and low cortisol levels pre- and post-IV ACTH.*
- *Secondary adrenal insufficiency (pituitary)—low baseline ACTH that does not respond to ACTH stimulation. Cortisol levels do not increase after stimulation.*
- *Tertiary adrenal insufficiency (hypothalamic)—low baseline ACTH with an exaggerated and prolonged response to stimulation. Cortisol levels usually do not reach 20 mcg/dL (SI = 552 nmol/L).*

*(The **DST** is useful in differentiating the causes of increased cortisol levels. Dexamethasone is a synthetic glucocorticoid that is significantly more potent than cortisol. It works by negative feedback. It suppresses the release of ACTH in patients with a normal hypothalamus. A cortisol level less than 1.8 mcg/dL [SI = 49.7 nmol/L] usually excludes Cushing syndrome. With the DST, a baseline morning cortisol level is collected, and the patient is given a 1-mg dose of dexamethasone at bedtime. A second specimen is collected the following morning. If cortisol levels have not been suppressed, adrenal adenoma is suspected. The DST also produces abnormal results in the presence of certain psychiatric illnesses [e.g., endogenous depression]).*

*The **metyrapone stimulation test** is used to distinguish corticotropin-dependent causes (pituitary Cushing disease and ectopic Cushing disease) from corticotropin-independent causes (e.g., cancer of the lung or thyroid) of increased cortisol levels. Metyrapone inhibits the conversion of 11-deoxycortisol to cortisol. Cortisol levels should decrease to less than 3 mcg/dL if normal pituitary stimulation by ACTH occurs after an oral dose of metyrapone. Specimen collection and administration of the medication are performed as with the overnight dexamethasone test.*

Increased in

Overproduction of ACTH can occur as a direct result of either disease (e.g., primary or ectopic tumor that secretes ACTH) or stimulation by physical or emotional stress, or it can be an indirect response to abnormalities in the complex feedback mechanisms involving the pituitary gland, hypothalamus, or adrenal glands.

ACTH Increased in

- **Addison disease** (*primary adrenocortical hypofunction*)
- **Carcinoid syndrome**
- **Congenital adrenal hyperplasia**
- **Cushing disease** (*pituitary-dependent adrenal hyperplasia*)
- **Cushing syndrome** (*ectopic secretion of ACTH*)
- **Depression**
- **Ectopic ACTH-producing tumors**

A

- Menstruation
- Nelson syndrome *(ACTH-producing pituitary tumors)*
- Pregnancy
- Sepsis
- Septic shock
- Type 2 diabetes

Decreased in
Secondary adrenal insufficiency due to hypopituitarism (inadequate production

by the pituitary) can result in decreased levels of ACTH. Conditions that result in overproduction or availability of high levels of cortisol can also result in decreased levels of ACTH.*

ACTH Decreased in
- Adrenal adenoma
- Adrenal cancer
- Cushing syndrome
- Exogenous steroid therapy

Summary of the Relationship Between Cortisol and ACTH Levels in Conditions Affecting the Adrenal and Pituitary Glands

Disease	Cortisol Level	ACTH Level
Addison disease (adrenal insufficiency)	Decreased	Increased
Cushing disease (pituitary adenoma)	Increased	Increased
Cushing syndrome related to ectopic source of ACTH	Increased	Increased
Cushing syndrome (ACTH independent; adrenal cancer or adenoma)	Increased	Decreased
Congenital adrenal hyperplasia	Decreased	Increased

NURSING IMPLICATIONS

POTENTIAL NURSING PROBLEMS: ASSESSMENT & NURSING DIAGNOSIS

Problems	Signs and Symptoms
Fluid volume (water) *(related to retention of sodium and water secondary to cortisol excess)*	Weight gain, hypertension, tachycardia, edema, jugular vein distention, shortness of breath, abnormal blood gas results
Infection risk *(related to impaired immune response secondary to elevated cortisol level, collagen tissue loss, catabolism of peripheral tissues)*	Delayed wound healing, inhibited collagen formation, impaired blood flow to edematous tissues, symptoms of infection (temperature, increased heart rate, increased blood pressure, shaking, chills, mottled skin, lethargy, fatigue, swelling, edema, pain, localized pressure, diaphoresis, night sweats, confusion, vomiting, nausea, headache)
Injury risk *(related to poor wound healing, decreased bone density, capillary fragility)*	Easy bruising, blood in stool, skin breakdown, fracture, poor wound healing, thin skin
Mobility *(related to change in muscle and bone structure secondary to excess cortisol)*	Fatigue, muscle weakness, porous bones with fracture risk

A

Teaching the Patient What to Expect

▶ Inform the patient this test can assist in evaluating the amount of hormone produced by the pituitary gland located at the base of the brain.

▶ Explain that a blood sample is needed for the test, samples are obtained at specific times to determine high and low levels of ACTH, and more than one sample may be necessary to ensure accurate results.

▶ As appropriate, instruct the patient to report any postadministration reaction to metyrapone.

Potential Nursing Actions

▶ Weigh patient and report weight to the pharmacy for accurate dosing of ordered metyrapone; may be 30 mg/kg body weight to a maximum of 3 grams total or per protocol.

Avoiding Complications

▶ Observe/assess the patient who has been administered metyrapone for signs and symptoms of an acute adrenal (addisonian) crisis, which may include abdominal pain, anxiety, bone marrow depression, coma, confusion, decreased white blood cell count (WBC), dehydration, dizziness, sudden and significant fatigue or weakness, headache, hypotension, loss of consciousness, nausea and vomiting, excessively increased perspiration of the face and hands, shock, tachycardia, tachypnea. Potential interventions include immediate corticosteroid replacement (IV or IM), airway protection and maintenance, administration of dextrose for hypoglycemia, correction of electrolyte imbalance, and rehydration with IV fluids.

Treatment Considerations

▶ Fluid volume: Monitor intake and output; assess for symptoms of fluid overload (shortness of breath, tachycardia, hypertension, positive jugular vein distention, edema). Monitor fluid and electrolytes for imbalance (potassium, sodium). Monitor heart rate, blood pressure, daily weight. Low-sodium diet. Administer prescribed medications (antihypertensive, diuretics).

▶ Infection risk: Decrease environmental exposure by placing the patient in a private room or isolation, as appropriate; monitor and trend vital signs (heart rate, temperature, blood pressure) and laboratory values that would indicate an infection (WBC, CRP); promote good hygiene and assist as needed; administer prescribed medications (antibiotics, antipyretics) and IV fluids; use cooling measures; encourage oral fluids; obtain ordered cultures; encourage lightweight clothing and bedding.

▶ Injury risk: Assess for bruising; assess stool for occult blood; assess for skin breakdown; assess wound for healing progress; facilitate ordered bone density screening.

Safety Considerations

▶ Discuss adherence to the HCP's request to wear a medic alert bracelet indicating adrenal insufficiency and steroid use.

▶ Mobility: Assist with activity; assist patient to meet activities of daily living; assess the severity of mobility limitations; implement the use of assistive devices as needed to prevent fall risk or injury.

Follow-Up, Evaluation, and Desired Outcomes

▶ Acknowledges contact information provided for the Cushing's Support and Research Foundation (https://csrf.net).

▶ Understands that the results of this procedure may require additional testing to evaluate or monitor disease progression or necessary change in therapy. If a diagnosis of Cushing disease is made, pituitary computed tomography (CT) or magnetic resonance imaging (MRI) may be indicated prior to surgery. If a diagnosis of ectopic corticotropin syndrome is made, abdominal CT or MRI may be indicated prior to surgery.

A

▶ Agrees to adhere to the HCP's request to increase oral fluid intake with a diet high in sodium and low in potassium (Addison disease).

▶ Adheres to the prescribed administration of steroids and understands the necessity of altering the medication regime during times of illness and stress.

Alanine Aminotransferase

SYNONYM/ACRONYM: ALT.

RATIONALE: To assess liver function related to liver disease and/or damage.

PATIENT PREPARATION: There are no food, fluid, activity, or medication restrictions unless by medical direction.

NORMAL FINDINGS: Method: Spectrophotometry.

Age	Conventional and SI Units
Newborn	7–41 units/L
Child, Adult	
Male	19–36 units/L
Female	24–36 units/L
Greater than 90 yr	
Male	6–38 units/L
Female	5–24 units/L

Values may be slightly elevated in older adults due to the effects of medications and the presence of multiple chronic or acute diseases with or without muted symptoms.

CRITICAL FINDINGS AND POTENTIAL INTERVENTIONS: N/A

OVERVIEW: (**Study type:** Blood collected in a gold-, red-, red/gray-, or green-top [heparin] tube; **related body system:** Digestive system.) ALT is an enzyme produced by the liver. The highest concentration of ALT is found in liver cells; moderate amounts are found in kidney cells; and smaller amounts are found in heart, pancreas, spleen, skeletal muscle, and red blood cells. When liver damage occurs, serum levels of ALT may increase as much as 50 times normal, making this a sensitive test for evaluating liver function. ALT is part of a group of tests known as LFTs, or liver function tests, used to evaluate liver function: ALT; albumin; alkaline phosphatase; aspartate aminotransferase (AST); bilirubin, direct; bilirubin, total; and protein, total.

INDICATIONS

• Compare serially with AST levels to track the course of liver disease.
• Monitor liver damage resulting from hepatotoxic drugs.
• Monitor response to treatment of liver disease, with tissue repair indicated by gradually declining levels.

INTERFERING FACTORS
Factors that may alter the results of the study

- Drugs and other substances that may increase ALT levels by causing cholestasis include anabolic steroids, dapsone, estrogens, ethionamide, oral contraceptives, sulfonylureas, and zidovudine.
- Drugs and other substances that may increase ALT levels by causing hepatocellular damage include acetaminophen (toxic), acetylsalicylic acid, anticonvulsants, asparaginase, cephalosporins, chloramphenicol, clofibrate, cytarabine, danazol, enflurane, erythromycin, ethambutol, ethionamide, ethotoin, florantyrone, foscarnet, gentamicin, gold salts, halothane, ibufenac, indomethacin, interleukin-2, isoniazid, lincomycin, low-molecular-weight heparin, metahexamide, metaxalone, methoxsalen, methyldopa, naproxen, nitrofurans, oral contraceptives, probenecid, procainamide, and tetracyclines.
- Drugs and other substances that may decrease ALT levels include cyclosporine, interferons, metronidazole (affects enzymatic test methods), and ursodiol.

POTENTIAL MEDICAL DIAGNOSIS: CLINICAL SIGNIFICANCE OF RESULTS
Increased in
Related to release of ALT from damaged liver, kidney, heart, pancreas, red blood cells, or skeletal muscle cells.

- Acute pancreatitis
- AIDS *(related to hepatitis B co-infection)*
- Biliary tract obstruction
- Burns (severe)
- Chronic alcohol misuse
- Cirrhosis
- Fatty liver
- HELLP syndrome of pregnancy (hemolysis, elevated liver enzymes, low platelet count)
- Hepatic cancer
- Hepatitis
- Infectious mononucleosis
- Muscle injury from intramuscular injections, trauma, infection, and seizures (recent)
- Muscular dystrophy
- Myocardial infarction
- Myositis
- Pancreatitis
- Pre-eclampsia
- Shock (severe)

Decreased in
- Pyridoxal phosphate deficiency *(related to a deficiency of pyridoxal phosphate that results in decreased production of ALT)*

NURSING IMPLICATIONS

POTENTIAL NURSING PROBLEMS: ASSESSMENT & NURSING DIAGNOSIS

Problems	Signs and Symptoms
Fluid volume (water) **Deficit:** *(related to vomiting, decreased intake, compromised kidney function, overly aggressive diuresis)*	**Deficit:** Decreased urinary output, fatigue, sunken eyes, dark urine, decreased blood pressure, increased heart rate, and altered mental status

(table continues on page 18)

A

Problems	Signs and Symptoms
Excess: Fluid overload, abdominal ascites *(overload related to overly aggressive fluid resuscitation; ascites related to hypoalbumenia, imbalanced aldosterone, altered [low] serum osmotic pressure)*	**Excess:** Fluid resuscitation—edema, shortness of breath, rales, rhonchi, and diluted laboratory values Abdominal ascites—increasing abdominal girth Fluid resuscitation and abdominal ascites—increased weight
Gastrointestinal (GI) problems *(related to altered motility, irritation of the GI tract, taste alterations, pancreatic and gastric secretions)*	Nausea, vomiting, abdominal distention, unexplained weight loss, steatorrhea, diarrhea, visible abdominal distention, ascites, diminished or absent bowel sounds
Insufficient nutrition *(related to metabolic imbalances, excess alcohol use, anorexia)*	Increased liver function tests; hyperglycemia with polyuria, weight loss, weakness, nausea, vomiting; hypocalcemia with confusion, intestinal cramping, diarrhea; hypertriglyceridemia; altered thiamine with weakness, confusion
Pain *(related to organ inflammation and surrounding tissues, excessive alcohol intake, infection)*	Emotional symptoms of distress, crying, agitation, facial grimace, moaning, verbalization of pain, rocking motions, irritability, disturbed sleep, diaphoresis, altered blood pressure and heart rate, nausea, vomiting, self-report of pain, upper abdominal and gastric pain after eating fatty foods or alcohol intake with acute pancreatic disease, pain that may be decreased or absent in chronic pancreatic disease

BEFORE THE STUDY: PLANNING AND IMPLEMENTATION

Teaching the Patient What to Expect

▶ Inform the patient this test can assist with evaluation of liver function and help identify liver disease.
▶ Explain that a blood sample is needed for the test.

AFTER THE STUDY: POTENTIAL NURSING ACTIONS

Avoiding Complications
▶ The patient with cirrhosis should be carefully observed for the development of ascites, in which case fluid and electrolyte balance requires strict attention.

Treatment Considerations
▶ Fluid Volume Deficit: Collaborate with health-care provider (HCP) regarding administration of IV fluids to support optimal hydration. Monitor laboratory values that reflect alterations in fluid status: potassium, BUN, Cr, calcium, Hgb, and Hct. Administer replacement electrolytes, as ordered, to manage underlying cause of fluid alteration; monitor urine characteristics and respiratory status. Trend vital signs

and daily weight, and perform strict intake and output.

◗ Fluid Volume Overload: Measure abdominal girth and trend size. Monitor and trend laboratory values: albumin, protein, and globulin. Assess for dehydration and increase fluids if present (fluid shifts from intravascular to extravascular can result in concerns related to hydration status). Administer ordered diuretics. Trend vital signs and daily weight, and perform strict intake and output.

◗ GI Problems: Perform nasogastric intubation to remove gastric secretions and decrease pancreatic secretions, which may result in autodigestion. Monitor nasogastric tube for patency and amount of drainage, and assess bowel sounds frequently. Measure abdominal girth to monitor degree of abdominal distention.

◗ Pain: Collaborate with the patient and HCP to identify the best pain management modality. Refrain from activities that may increase pain. Apply heat or cold to the best effect in managing pain, and monitor pain severity.

Nutritional Considerations

◗ Increased ALT levels may be associated with liver disease. In general, patients should be encouraged to eat a well-balanced diet that includes foods high in fiber.

Dietary recommendations will vary depending on the condition and its severity. For example, a soft foods diet is recommended if esophageal varices develop, fat substitutes are recommended if bile duct disease is diagnosed, and salt intake should be limited if ascites develop.

◗ Administer ordered enteral or parenteral nutrition; monitor laboratory values (albumin, protein, potassium) and collaborate with HCP on replacement strategies; correlate laboratory values with IV fluid infusion, and collaborate with the HCP and pharmacist to adjust to patient needs; ensure adequate pain control, and monitor vital signs for alterations associated with metabolic imbalances.

Follow-Up, Evaluation, and Desired Outcomes

◗ Acknowledges contact information provided for the Centers for Disease Control and Prevention (www.cdc .gov/diseasesconditions)

◗ Understands information regarding causative factors of pancreatitis and liver disease, the disease process, and proactive lifestyle changes to better manage health.

◗ Accepts the importance of adhering to the medication regimen as prescribed to limit pancreatic secretions and decrease pain.

Albumin and Albumin/Globulin Ratio

SYNONYM/ACRONYM: Alb, A/G ratio.

RATIONALE: To assess liver or kidney function and nutritional status.

PATIENT PREPARATION: There are no food, fluid, activity, or medication restrictions unless by medical direction.

NORMAL FINDINGS: (Method: Spectrophotometry) Normally, the A/G ratio is greater than 1.

Age	Conventional Units	SI Units (Conventional Units × 10)
Newborn	2.6–3.6 g/dL	26–36 g/L
Child	3.4–5.2 g/dL	34–42 g/L
Adult	3.7–5.1 g/dL	37–51 g/L
Older Adult	3.2–4.6 g/dL	32–46 g/L
Greater than 90 yr	2.9–4.5 g/dL	29–45 g/L

Albumin levels are affected by posture. Results from specimens collected in an upright posture are higher than results from specimens collected in a supine position.

CRITICAL FINDINGS AND POTENTIAL INTERVENTIONS: N/A

OVERVIEW: (**Study type:** Blood collected in a gold-, red-, red/gray-, or green-top [heparin] tube; **related body system:** Digestive and Urinary systems.) Most of the body's total protein is a combination of albumin and globulins. Albumin, the protein present in the highest concentrations, is the main transport protein in the body for hormones, therapeutic drugs, calcium, magnesium, heme, and waste products such as bilirubin. Albumin also significantly affects plasma oncotic pressure, which regulates the distribution of body fluid between blood vessels, tissues, and cells. Albumin is synthesized in the liver. Low levels of albumin may be the result of either inadequate intake, inadequate production, or excessive loss. Albumin levels are more useful as an indicator of chronic deficiency than of short-term deficiency. Hypoalbuminemia or low serum albumin, a level less than 3.4 g/dL (SI = 34 g/L), can stem from many causes and may be a useful predictor of mortality. Normally, albumin is not excreted in urine. However, in cases of kidney injury or disease, some albumin may be lost due to decreased kidney function, as seen in nephrotic syndrome, and in pregnant women with preeclampsia and eclampsia.

The A/G ratio is useful in the evaluation of liver and kidney disease. The ratio is calculated using the following formula:

albumin/(total protein − albumin)

where globulin is the difference between the total protein value and the albumin value. For example, with a total protein of 7 g/dL and albumin of 4 g/dL, the A/G ratio is calculated as 4/(7 − 4) or 4/3 = 1.33. A reversal in the ratio, where globulin exceeds albumin (i.e., ratio less than 1), is clinically significant.

INDICATIONS
• Assess nutritional status of hospitalized patients, especially older adult patients.
• Evaluate chronic illness.
• Evaluate liver disease.

INTERFERING FACTORS
Factors that may alter the results of the study
• Drugs and other substances that may increase albumin levels include carbamazepine, furosemide, phenobarbital, and prednisolone.
• Drugs and other substances that may decrease albumin levels include acetaminophen (poisoning), amiodarone, asparaginase, dextran, estrogens, ibuprofen, interleukin-2, methotrexate, methyldopa, niacin, nitrofurantoin, oral

contraceptives, phenytoin, prednisone, and valproic acid.

Other considerations
- Availability of administered drugs is affected by variations in albumin levels.

POTENTIAL MEDICAL DIAGNOSIS: CLINICAL SIGNIFICANCE OF RESULTS

Increased in
Any condition that results in a decrease of plasma water (e.g., dehydration); look for increase in Hgb and Hct. Decreases in the volume of intravascular liquid automatically result in concentration of the components present in the remaining liquid, as reflected by an elevated albumin level.
- Hyperinfusion of albumin

Decreased in
- *Insufficient intake:*
  Malabsorption *(related to lack of amino acids available for protein synthesis)*
  Malnutrition *(related to insufficient dietary source of amino acids required for protein synthesis)*
- *Decreased synthesis by the liver:*
  Acute and chronic liver disease (e.g., alcohol misuse, cirrhosis, hepatitis) *(evidenced by a decrease in normal liver function; the liver is the body's site of protein synthesis)*
  Genetic analbuminemia *(related to genetic inability of the liver to synthesize albumin)*
- *Inflammation and chronic diseases result in production of acute-phase reactant and other globulin proteins; the increase in globulins causes a corresponding relative decrease in albumin:*
  Amyloidosis
  Bacterial infections
  Monoclonal gammopathies (e.g., multiple myeloma, Waldenström macroglobulinemia)
  Parasitic infestations
  Peptic ulcer
  Prolonged immobilization
  Rheumatic diseases

Severe skin disease
Tumor
- *Increased loss over body surface:*
  Burns *(evidenced by loss of interstitial fluid albumin)*
  Enteropathies (e.g., gluten sensitivity, Crohn disease, ulcerative colitis, Whipple disease) *(evidenced by sensitivity to ingested substances or related to inadequate absorption from intestinal loss)*
  Fistula (gastrointestinal or lymphatic) *(related to loss of sequestered albumin from general circulation)*
  Hemorrhage *(related to fluid loss)*
  Kidney disease *(related to loss from damaged renal tubules)*
  Pre-eclampsia *(evidenced by excessive renal loss)*
  Rapid hydration or overhydration *(evidenced by dilution effect)*
  Repeated thoracentesis or paracentesis *(related to removal of albumin in accumulated third-space fluid)*
- *Increased catabolism:*
  Cushing disease *(related to excessive cortisol induced protein metabolism)*
  Heart failure *(evidenced by dilution effect)*
  Thyroid dysfunction *(related to overproduction of albumin-binding thyroid hormones)*
- *Increased blood volume (hypervolemia):*
  Pre-eclampsia *(related to fluid retention)*
  Pregnancy *(evidenced by increased circulatory volume from placenta and fetus)*

NURSING IMPLICATIONS

BEFORE THE STUDY: PLANNING AND IMPLEMENTATION

Teaching the Patient What to Expect
▶ Inform the patient this test can assist with evaluation of liver and kidney function as well as chronic disease.
▶ Explain that a blood sample is needed for the test.

A

Potential Nursing Actions
◗ Assess for signs of edema or ascites; measure abdominal girth and trend.

Safety Considerations
◗ To prevent development of toxic drug concentrations, patients receiving therapeutic drug treatments should have their drug levels monitored when levels of the transport protein albumin are decreased.

AFTER THE STUDY: POTENTIAL NURSING ACTIONS

Nutritional Considerations
◗ Dietary recommendations may be indicated and will vary depending on the condition and its severity.
◗ Monitor protein, potassium, and albumin levels; consider small frequent meals; administer ordered antiemetics.

Aldolase

SYNONYM/ACRONYM: ALD.

RATIONALE: To assist in the diagnosis of muscle-wasting diseases such as muscular dystrophy or other diseases that cause muscle and cellular damage, such as hepatitis and cirrhosis of the liver.

PATIENT PREPARATION: There are no food, fluid, activity, or medication restrictions unless by medical direction.

NORMAL FINDINGS: Method: Spectrophotometry.

Age	Conventional and SI Units
Newborn	6–32 units/L
Child	3.4–8.8 units/L
Adult	Less than 8.1 units/L

CRITICAL FINDINGS AND POTENTIAL INTERVENTIONS: N/A

OVERVIEW: (**Study type:** Blood collected in a gold-, red-, or red/gray-top tube; **related body system:** Musculoskeletal system.) ALD, an enzyme found throughout muscles, organs, and red blood cells (RBCs) in the body, catalyzes the breakdown of glucose to lactate. When trauma or disease causes cellular breakdown of these muscles or organs, large amounts of ALD are released into the blood and can be used to identify or mark the progress of disease. This test is not commonly requested because measurement of liver enzymes such as aspartate aminotransferase and alanine aminotransferase and skeletal muscle markers such as creatine kinase (CK), in addition to other diagnostic tests such as muscle biopsy and genetic testing, is generally sufficient to provide the necessary information. ALD is elevated in some cases of skeletal muscle disease in the presence of normal CK levels.

INDICATIONS
- Assist in the diagnosis of Duchenne muscular dystrophy.
- Differentiate neuromuscular disorders, such as dermatomyositis, muscular dystrophy, and polymyositis, from neurological disorders, such as multiple sclerosis, myasthenia gravis, and polio.

INTERFERING FACTORS
Factors that may alter the results of the study
- Hemolysis falsely increases aldolase values

POTENTIAL MEDICAL DIAGNOSIS: CLINICAL SIGNIFICANCE OF RESULTS
Increased in
ALD is released from any damaged cell in which it is stored, so diseases of skeletal muscle, cardiac muscle, pancreas, RBCs, and liver that cause cellular destruction demonstrate elevated ALD levels.

- Cancer (lung, breast, and genitourinary tract and metastasis to liver)
- Dermatomyositis
- Duchenne muscular dystrophy
- Hepatitis (acute viral or toxic)
- Limb girdle muscular dystrophy
- Myocardial infarction
- Pancreatitis (acute)
- Polymyositis
- Severe crush injuries
- Tetanus
- Trichinosis *(related to myositis)*

Decreased in
- Hereditary fructose intolerance *(evidenced by hereditary deficiency of the aldolase B enzyme)*
- *Late stages of muscle-wasting diseases in which muscle mass has significantly diminished*

NURSING IMPLICATIONS

BEFORE THE STUDY: PLANNING AND IMPLEMENTATION

Teaching the Patient What to Expect
- Inform the patient this test can assist with identification of liver, organ, and muscle damage.
- Explain that a blood sample is needed for the test.

AFTER THE STUDY: POTENTIAL NURSING ACTIONS

Avoiding Complications
- Explain the importance of preventing contractures and permanent loss of elasticity or shortening of muscles or joints through the daily performance of range-of-motion and stretching exercises. Discuss the balance between daily exercise and energy management.
- Teach the patient and family to make frequent assessments for skin breakdown from prolonged sitting. Suggest that additional comfort and prevention of skin breakdown can be accomplished by the use of a special mattress or bed.
- In situations where the patient is unable to move without assistance, describe how proper body alignment in the bed or chair can be maintained by the use of blanket rolls, sandbags, or pillows.

Treatment Considerations
- Explain and demonstrate the implementation of incentive spirometry and diaphragmatic breathing exercises to maintain adequate gas exchange related to weakened respiratory muscles.
- Monitor daily weight for weight gain or loss.
- Recommend the use of support stockings to promote venous return by application of pressure on the veins and elevation of the lower extremities to decrease pedal edema for patients in a seated position for long periods of time. Explain that stockings should not

be used if there are any skin lesions or areas of gangrene and should be removed and replaced with clean dry stockings at least twice daily.

Safety Considerations
♦ Assist the family in evaluating safety issues in the home, such as stairs and carpeting (impairs mobility of crutches, wheelchairs, and other equipment). Recommend the use of rubber-soled shoes to help prevent slipping. Teach the proper way to safely transfer the patient.
♦ Assist the family in evaluating accessibility of the home environment by considering ramps, widened doorways, and living space on ground floor.
♦ Decrease aspiration risk by teaching techniques to evaluate swallowing effectiveness related to muscle weakness.

Nutritional Considerations
♦ Discuss the importance of good nutrition. Explain that obesity may become an issue as activity levels decline or when the patient is in a wheelchair most of the day. Describe a low-calorie, high-protein diet, and explain that the diet should help prevent additional weight gain, which puts further strain on already weakened muscles.

♦ Select foods appropriate to deteriorating swallowing functions to prevent aspiration.
♦ Lack of mobility may cause constipation, which can be managed by increasing dietary fiber, encouraging intake of fluids, and using stool softeners.

Follow-Up, Evaluation, and Desired Outcomes
♦ Acknowledges contact information provided for the Muscular Dystrophy Association (www.mda.org). The Centers for Disease Control and Prevention has funded Parent Project Muscular Dystrophy to establish the National Task Force for the Early Identification of Neuromuscular Disorders (www.childmuscleweakness.org).
♦ Confirms adequacy of home pain management strategies to facilitate maximum functional status with appropriate use of assistive devices and adequacy of individualized fall risk interventions.
♦ Agrees to participate in a support group for individuals with a diagnosis of muscular disease to express their concerns and fears regarding the genetic disease transmission, progressive nature, and long-term effects on the family.

Aldosterone

SYNONYM/ACRONYM: N/A

RATIONALE: To assist in the evaluation of hypertension and diagnosis of primary hyperaldosteronism disorders such as Conn syndrome and Addison disease.

PATIENT PREPARATION: There are no fluid restrictions unless by medical direction. The required position, supine/lying down or upright/sitting up, must be maintained for 2 hr before specimen collection. The patient may be prescribed a normal-sodium diet (1 to 2 g of sodium per day) 2 to 4 wk before the test. Under medical direction, the patient should avoid diuretics, antihypertensive drugs and herbals, and cyclic progestogens and estrogens for 2 to 4 wk before the test. The patient should also be advised to avoid consuming any products derived from or that contain licorice root for 2 wk before the test. Protocols may vary among facilities.

NORMAL FINDINGS: Method: Chemiluminescent Immunoassay.

Age	Conventional Units	SI Units (Conventional Units × 0.0277)
Newborn	5–102 ng/dL	0.14–2.82 nmol/L
1–3 wks	6–180 ng/dL	0.17–5 nmol/L
1 mo–2 yr	7–99 ng/dL	0.19–2.7 nmol/L
3–14 yr	4–30 ng/dL	0.11–0.83 nmol/L
15 yr–adult	31 ng/dL or less	0.86 nmol/L or less
Supine	3–16 ng/dL	0.08–0.44 nmol/L
Upright (sitting for at least 2 hr)	4–30 ng/dL	0.11–0.83 nmol/L
Older adult	Levels decline with age	

These values reflect a normal sodium diet. Values for a low-sodium diet are three to five times higher. Blood levels fluctuate with dehydration and fluid overload.

CRITICAL FINDINGS AND POTENTIAL INTERVENTIONS: N/A

OVERVIEW: (Study type: Blood collected in a gold-, red-, red/gray-, green- [heparin], or lavender-top [EDTA] tube; related body system: Endocrine and Urinary systems.) Aldosterone is a mineralocorticoid secreted by the zona glomerulosa of the adrenal cortex and is regulated by the renin-angiotensin system. Changes in renal blood flow trigger or suppress release of renin from the glomeruli. The presence of circulating renin stimulates the liver to produce angiotensin I. Angiotensin I is converted by the lungs and kidneys into angiotensin II, a potent trigger for the release of aldosterone. Aldosterone and the renin-angiotensin system work together to regulate sodium and potassium levels. Aldosterone acts to increase sodium reabsorption in the renal tubules. This results in excretion of potassium, increased water retention, increased blood volume, and increased blood pressure. This test is of little diagnostic value in differentiating primary and secondary aldosteronism unless plasma renin activity is measured simultaneously (see study titled "Renin"). A variety of factors influence serum aldosterone levels, including sodium intake, certain medications, and activity. Secretion of aldosterone is also affected by adrenocorticotropic hormone (ACTH), a pituitary hormone that primarily stimulates secretion of glucocorticoids and minimally affects secretion of mineralocorticosteroids. Patients with serum potassium less than 3.6 mEq/L and 24-hr urine potassium greater than 40 mEq/L fit the general criteria to test for aldosteronism. Renin activity, measured in ng/mL/hr, is low in primary aldosteronism and high in secondary aldosteronism.

Computed tomography can miss adrenal adenomas; therefore, measurement of the aldosterone/renin ratio (ARR) from an adrenal venous sampling technique

A

is the gold standard to distinguish between adrenal cortex adenoma (a benign unilateral hyperplasia that can be surgically corrected) and bilateral hyperplasia (treated medically with aldosterone antagonists). Specimens are obtained by an experienced health-care provider (HCP), customarily a radiologist, using an imaging-guided catheter inserted into the adrenal veins to collect blood for analysis. Specimen labels must include time of collection, patient position (upright or supine), and exact source of specimen (left versus right) in addition to the corresponding patient demographics and date. A normal ARR is less than 25. Ratios greater than 20 obtained after a screening test may indicate the need for further evaluation with a challenge study such as a sodium-loading protocol. A captopril protocol can be substituted for patients who may not tolerate the sodium-loading protocol. An ARR between 25 and 40 is suggestive of primary hyperaldosteronism, a condition most commonly identified in patients ages 30 to 50 years; some criteria require both an elevated ratio and an aldosterone level that exceeds 15 ng/dL. An ARR greater than 50 is significant. The ratio is markedly increased in both unilateral and bilateral hyperaldosteronism. Unilateral hyperplasia is associated with an increase in the ARR from samples obtained on the side of the tumor relative to the values measured from the other side; there is little difference between the ratios obtained from both sides in patients with bilateral hyperplasia.

INDICATIONS

- Evaluate hypertension of unknown cause, especially with hypokalemia not induced by diuretics.
- Investigate suspected hyperaldosteronism (Conn's syndrome), *as indicated by elevated levels.*
- Investigate suspected hypoaldosteronism, as indicated by decreased levels.

INTERFERING FACTORS

Factors that may alter the results of the study

- Drugs and other substances that may increase aldosterone levels include amiloride, ammonium chloride, angiotensin, angiotensin II, dobutamine, dopamine, endralazine, fenoldopam, hydralazine, hydrochlorothiazide, laxatives (misuse), metoclopramide, nifedipine, opiates, potassium, spironolactone, and zacopride.
- Drugs and other substances that may decrease aldosterone levels include atenolol, captopril, carvedilol, cilazapril, enalapril, fadrozole, glycyrrhiza (licorice), ibopamine, indomethacin, lisinopril, nicardipine, NSAIDs, perindopril, ranitidine, saline, sinorphan, and verapamil. Prolonged heparin therapy also decreases aldosterone levels.
- Diet can significantly affect results. A low-sodium diet can increase serum aldosterone, whereas a high-sodium diet can decrease levels. Decreased serum sodium and elevated serum potassium increase aldosterone secretion. Elevated serum sodium and decreased serum potassium suppress aldosterone secretion.
- Upright body posture, stress, strenuous exercise, and late pregnancy can lead to increased levels.
- Ingestion of large amounts of licorice can result in symptoms also

associated with hyperaldosteronism; most candy contains very little real licorice. Licorice inhibits short-chain dehydrogenase/reductase enzymes. These enzymes normally prevent cortisol from binding to aldosterone receptor sites in the kidney. In the absence of these enzymes, cortisol acts on the kidney and triggers the same effects as aldosterone, which include increased potassium excretion, sodium retention, and water retention. Aldosterone levels are not affected by licorice ingestion, but the simultaneous measurements of electrolytes may provide misleading results.

POTENTIAL MEDICAL DIAGNOSIS: CLINICAL SIGNIFICANCE OF RESULTS
Increased in

Increased With Decreased Renin Levels
Primary hyperaldosteronism (evidenced by overproduction related to abnormal adrenal gland function)
- Adenomas (Conn syndrome)
- Bilateral hyperplasia of the aldosterone-secreting zona glomerulosa cells

Increased With Increased Renin Levels
Secondary hyperaldosteronism (related to conditions that increase renin levels, which then stimulate aldosterone secretion)
- Bartter syndrome *(related to excessive loss of potassium by the kidneys, leading to release of renin and subsequent release of aldosterone)*
- Chronic obstructive pulmonary disease
- Cirrhosis with ascites formation *(related to diluted concentration of sodium by increased blood volume)*
- Diuretic misuse *(related to direct stimulation of aldosterone secretion)*

- Heart failure *(related to diluted concentration of sodium by increased blood volume)*
- Hypovolemia *(secondary to hemorrhage and transudation)*
- Laxative misuse *(related to direct stimulation of aldosterone secretion)*
- Nephrotic syndrome *(related to excessive renal protein loss, development of decreased oncotic pressure, fluid retention, and diluted concentration of sodium)*
- Starvation (after 10 days) *(related to diluted concentration of sodium by development of edema)*
- Thermal stress *(related to direct stimulation of aldosterone secretion)*
- Toxemia of pregnancy *(related to diluted concentration of sodium by increased blood volume evidenced by edema; placental corticotropin-releasing hormone stimulates production of maternal adrenal hormones that can also contribute to edema)*

Decreased in

Without Hypertension
- Addison disease *(related to lack of function in the adrenal cortex)*
- Hypoaldosteronism *(secondary to renin deficiency)*
- Isolated aldosterone deficiency

With Hypertension
- Acute alcohol intoxication *(related to toxic effects of alcohol on adrenal gland function and therefore secretion of aldosterone)*
- Diabetes *(related to impaired conversion of prorenin to renin by damaged kidneys, resulting in decreased aldosterone)*
- Excess secretion of deoxycorticosterone *(related to suppression of ACTH production by cortisol, which in turn affects aldosterone secretion)*

A

- Turner syndrome (25% of cases) *(related to congenital adrenal hyperplasia resulting in underproduction* *of aldosterone and overproduction of androgens)*

NURSING IMPLICATIONS

POTENTIAL NURSING PROBLEMS: ASSESSMENT & NURSING DIAGNOSIS

Problems	Signs and Symptoms
Increased Aldosterone: Altered electrolytes *(hypokalemia, hypernautremia secondary to hyperaldosteronism)*	Hypokalemia—weakness, fatigue, drowsiness, muscle cramps, cognitive changes Hypernatremia—confusion, agitation, muscle twitching, seizures, tremors
Increased Aldosterone: Fluid volume overload *(related to hypervolemia associated with excessive production of aldosterone; hypernatremia and excessive water reabsorption)*	Shortness of breath, peripheral edema, increased work of breathing, weight gain, hypertension
Decreased Aldosterone: Mobility *(related to dizziness, fatigue, weakness secondary to adrenal insufficiency and decreased cortisol levels)*	Weakness, wasting, pain in muscles and joints, decreased endurance, activity intolerance, difficult purposeful movement, reluctance to attempt to engage in activity
Decreased Aldosterone: Tissue perfusion *(related to inadequate fluid volume, decreased cortisol levels)*	Hypotension, dizziness, cool extremities, pallor, capillary refill greater than 3 sec in fingers and toes, weak pedal pulses, altered level of consciousness, altered sensation, urinary output less than 30 mL/hr

BEFORE THE STUDY: PLANNING AND IMPLEMENTATION

Teaching the Patient What to Expect

▶ Inform the patient this test evaluates dehydration and can assist in identification of the causes of muscle weakness or high blood pressure.

▶ Explain that a blood sample is needed for the test. Inform the patient that multiple specimens may be required. As appropriate, explain that blood specimens may be collected directly from the left and right adrenal veins by a radiologist via catheterization and takes approximately 1 hr.

▶ Inform the patient that the required position, supine/lying down or upright/sitting up, must be maintained for 2 hr before specimen collection. If a supine specimen is requested on an inpatient, the specimen should be collected early in the morning before rising.

Potential Nursing Actions

▶ Fluid Volume: Trend laboratory values that reflect alterations in fluid status; potassium, BUN, Cr, calcium, Hgb and Hct, and sodium. Manage underlying cause of fluid alteration; collaborate with HCP to adjust oral and IV fluids to provide optimal hydration status.

AFTER THE STUDY: POTENTIAL NURSING ACTIONS

Avoiding Complications

▶ Monitor blood pressure; assess for dizziness; assess extremities for skin temperature, color, warmth; assess capillary refill; assess pedal pulses; monitor for numbness, tingling, hyperesthesia, hypoesthesia; monitor for deep venous thrombosis; carefully use heat and cold on affected areas; use foot cradle to keep pressure off of affected body parts.

Treatment Considerations

▶ Altered Electrolytes: Collaborate with HCP to administer ordered electrolyte replacement therapy and trend associated laboratory results. Monitor for ongoing symptoms of electrolyte disturbance (hypokalemia, hypernatremia).

Safety Considerations

▶ Mobility: Muscle atrophy can make safe mobility a concern. Provide assistance with mobility and teach the safe use of assistive devices; allow sufficient time to perform tasks without being rushed.

Nutritional Considerations

▶ Aldosterone levels are involved in the regulation of body fluid volume. Educate patients about the importance of proper water balance. Tap water may also contain other nutrients. Water-softening systems replace minerals (e.g., calcium, magnesium, iron) with sodium, so caution should be used if a low-sodium diet is prescribed.

▶ Because aldosterone levels affect sodium levels, adjustments to dietary sodium may need to be implemented. Educate patients with low sodium levels that the major source of dietary sodium is table salt. Many foods, such as milk and other dairy products, are also good sources of dietary sodium. Most other dietary sodium is available through consumption of processed foods; some examples are baking mixes (pancakes, muffins), sauces (barbecue), butter, canned soups and sauces, dry soup mixes, frozen or microwave meals, ketchup, pickles, and snack foods (potato chips, pretzels). Patients who need to follow low-sodium diets should avoid beverages such as colas, ginger ale, Gatorade, lemon-lime sodas, and root beer. Many over-the-counter medications, including antacids, laxatives, analgesics, sedatives, and antitussives, contain significant amounts of sodium. The best advice is to emphasize the importance of reading all food, beverage, and medicine labels. Potassium is present in all plant and animal cells, making dietary replacement simple. An HCP or a nutritionist should be consulted before considering the use of salt substitutes. Fruits, vegetables (artichokes, avocados, bananas, cantaloupe, dried fruits, kiwi, mango, milk, dried beans, nuts, oranges, peaches, pears, pomegranate, potatoes, prunes, pumpkin, spinach, sunflower seeds, Swiss chard, tomatoes, and winter squash), and meats are rich in potassium.

Follow-Up, Evaluation, and Desired Outcomes

▶ Demonstrates self-care techniques as taught by occupational therapy and self-reflects on emotional response to limited mobility.

▶ Accepts the necessity of using assistive devices to maintain independence and of determining if there is any interference with the ability to engage in activities of daily living (e.g., difficulty fastening clothing, performing personal hygiene; inability to maintain appropriate appearance).

▶ Acknowledges the need to notify the HCP of any signs and symptoms of dehydration or fluid overload related to elevated aldosterone levels or compromised sodium regulatory mechanisms.

▶ Understands to report any gastric distress or dark stools associated with prescribed medication use and the importance of adhering to the medication regime with the understanding that sudden cessation is dangerous.

A

Alkaline Phosphatase and Isoenzymes

SYNONYM/ACRONYM: Alk Phos, ALP and fractionation, heat-stable ALP.

RATIONALE: To assist in the diagnosis of liver and bone disease.

PATIENT PREPARATION: There are no food, fluid, activity, or medication restrictions unless by medical direction.

NORMAL FINDINGS: Method: Spectrophotometry for total alkaline phosphatase, inhibition/electrophoresis for fractionation.

Age/Gender	Total ALP Conventional and SI Units	Bone Fraction Conventional and SI Units	Liver Fraction Conventional and SI Units
Newborn			
Male	75–375 units/L	NA	NA
Female	65–350 units/L	NA	NA
1–8 yr			
Male	70–364 units/L	50–319 units/L	Less than 8–76 units/L
Female	73–378 units/L	56–300 units/L	Less than 8–53 units/L
9–12 yr			
Male	112–476 units/L	78–339 units/L	Less than 8–81 units/L
Female	98–448 units/L	78–353 units/L	Less than 8–62 units/L
13–14 yr			
Male	112–476 units/L	78–389 units/L	Less than 8–48 units/L
Female	56–350 units/L	28–252 units/L	Less than 8–50 units/L
15 yr			
Male	70–378 units/L	48–311 units/L	Less than 8–39 units/L
Female	42–168 units/L	20–115 units/L	Less than 8–53 units/L
16 yr			
Male	70–378 units/L	48–311 units/L	Less than 8–39 units/L
Female	28–126 units/L	14–87 units/L	Less than 8–50 units/L
17 yr			
Male	56–238 units/L	34–190 units/L	Less than 8–39 units/L
Female	28–126 units/L	17–84 units/L	Less than 8–53 units/L
Adult			
Male	35–142 units/L	11–73 units/L	0–93 units/L
Female	25–125 units/L	11–73 units/L	0–93 units/L

ALP levels vary by age and gender; values in children are higher than in adults because of the level of bone growth and development. Values may be slightly elevated in older adults.

CRITICAL FINDINGS AND POTENTIAL INTERVENTIONS: N/A

OVERVIEW: (Study type: Blood collected in a gold-, red-, red/gray-, or green-top [heparin] tube; related body system: Digestive and Musculoskeletal systems.) ALP is an enzyme found in the liver;

in Kupffer cells lining the biliary tract; and in bones, intestines, and placenta. Additional sources of ALP include the proximal tubules of the kidneys, pulmonary alveolar cells, germ cells, vascular bed, lactating mammary glands, and granulocytes of circulating blood. ALP is referred to as alkaline because it functions optimally at a pH of 9.

There are a number of isoenzymes of ALP. Elevations in two main ALP isoenzymes, however, are of clinical significance and are used to identify the source of increased ALP levels: ALP_1 of liver origin and ALP_2 of bone origin. Measurement of bone-specific ALP is also used as an indicator of increased bone turnover and estrogen deficiency in postmenopausal women.

INDICATIONS
- Evaluate signs and symptoms of various disorders associated with elevated ALP levels, such as biliary obstruction, hepatobiliary disease, and bone disease, including malignant processes.
- Differentiate obstructive hepatobiliary tract disorders from hepatocellular disease; greater elevations of ALP are seen in the former.
- Determine effects of kidney disease on bone metabolism.
- Determine bone growth or destruction in children with abnormal growth patterns.

INTERFERING FACTORS
Factors that may alter the results of the study
- Drugs and other substances that may increase ALP levels by causing cholestasis *related to diseases of the liver, bile duct, or pancreas that result in impaired flow of bile*

include anabolic steroids, erythromycin, ethionamide, gold salts, imipramine, interleukin-2, isocarboxazid, nitrofurans, oral contraceptives, phenothiazines, sulfonamides, and tolbutamide.
- Drugs and other substances that may increase ALP levels by causing hepatocellular damage include acetaminophen (toxic), amiodarone, anticonvulsants, arsenicals, asparaginase, bromocriptine, captopril, cephalosporins, chloramphenicol, enflurane, ethionamide, foscarnet, gentamicin, indomethacin, lincomycin, methyldopa, naproxen, nitrofurans, probenecid, procainamide, progesterone, ranitidine, tobramycin, tolcapone, and verapamil.
- Drugs and other substances that may cause an overall decrease in ALP levels include alendronate, azathioprine, calcitriol, clofibrate, estrogens with estrogen replacement therapy, and ursodiol.
- Hemolyzed specimens may cause falsely elevated results.
- Elevations of ALP may occur if the patient is nonfasting, usually 2 to 4 hr after a fatty meal.
- Young children may have increased ALP levels during growth spurts.

POTENTIAL MEDICAL DIAGNOSIS: CLINICAL SIGNIFICANCE OF RESULTS
Increased in
Related to release of alkaline phosphatase from damaged bone, biliary tract, and liver cells.

- Liver disease:
  Biliary atresia
  Biliary obstruction, intra- or extra- (acute cholecystitis, cholelithiasis, intrahepatic cholestasis of pregnancy, primary biliary cholangitis)
  Cancer
  Cirrhosis
  Diabetes (diabetic hepatic lipidosis)

A

Granulomatous or infiltrative liver
diseases (sarcoidosis, amyloidosis,
tuberculosis)
Hepatitis
Infectious mononucleosis
• **Bone disease:**
Healing fractures
Metabolic bone diseases (rickets,
osteomalacia)
Metastatic tumors in bone
Osteogenic sarcoma
Osteoporosis
Paget disease (osteitis deformans)
• **Other conditions:**
Advanced pregnancy *(related to additional
sources: placental tissue and new fetal
bone growth; marked decline is seen with
placental insufficiency and imminent fetal
demise)*
Cancer of the breast, colon, gallbladder,
lung, or pancreas
Familial hyperphosphatemia
Heart failure
HELLP syndrome of pregnancy (hemoly-
sis, elevated liver enzymes, low platelet
count)
Hyperparathyroidism
Perforated bowel
Pneumonia
Pulmonary and myocardial infarctions
Pulmonary embolism
Ulcerative colitis

Decreased in
• Anemia (severe)
• Celiac disease
• Folic acid deficiency
• HIV-1 infection
• Hypervitaminosis D
• Hypophosphatasia *(related to
insufficient phosphorus source
for ALP production; congenital
and rare)*
• Hypothyroidism (characteristic
in infantile and juvenile cases)
• Nutritional deficiency of zinc
or magnesium
• Pernicious anemia
• Scurvy *(related to vitamin C
deficiency)*
• Whipple disease
• Zollinger-Ellison syndrome

NURSING IMPLICATIONS

BEFORE THE STUDY: PLANNING AND IMPLEMENTATION

Teaching the Patient What to Expect
◗ Inform the patient this test can assist with determining the presence of liver or bone disease.
◗ Explain that a blood sample is needed for the test.

AFTER THE STUDY: POTENTIAL NURSING ACTIONS

Avoiding Complications
◗ The patient with cirrhosis should be observed for development of ascites, which requires strict attention to fluid and electrolyte balance.

Treatment Considerations
◗ Monitor and trend vital signs. Administer ordered parenteral fluids with strict intake and output and daily weight. Monitor urine color, and if not NPO, encourage the intake of oral fluids. Trend laboratory studies associated with hydration (BUN and Cr), and potassium loss due to nasogastric suction.
◗ Administration of ordered NSAIDs, opi-oids, and antiemetics. Maintain ordered NPO status. Position on the side with knees bent toward the chest. Adequate anxiety management can facilitate comfort care.

Safety Considerations
◗ Consider fall precaution interventions that can limit injury risk to those with progressive compromised bone stabil-ity or liver function.

Nutritional Considerations
◗ Increased ALP levels may be associ-ated with liver disease. In general, patients should be encouraged to eat a well-balanced diet that includes foods high in fiber. Dietary recommendations will vary depending on the condition and its severity. For example, a soft foods diet is recommended if esopha-geal varices develop, fat substitutes are recommended if bile duct disease is diagnosed, or salt intake should be limited if ascites develop.

Allergen-Specific Immunoglobulin E

SYNONYM/ACRONYM: Allergen profile, ImmunoCAP specific immunoglobulin E (IgE).

RATIONALE: To assist in identifying environmental and occupational allergens responsible for causing allergic reactions.

PATIENT PREPARATION: There are no food, fluid, activity, or medication restrictions unless by medical direction.

NORMAL FINDINGS: Method: Immunoassay or fluorescence enzyme immunoassay (FEIA).

Immunoassay and ImmunoCAP Scoring Guide (FEIA)	Conventional and SI Units Allergen-Specific IgE
Specific IgE Allergen Antibody Level	kU/L
Absent or undetectable allergy	Less than 0.35
Low allergy	0.35–0.7
Moderate allergy	0.71–3.5
High allergy	3.51–17.5
Very high allergy	17.6–50
Very high allergy	51–100
Very high allergy	Greater than 100

CRITICAL FINDINGS AND POTENTIAL INTERVENTIONS: N/A

OVERVIEW: (**Study type:** Blood collected in a gold-, red-, or red/gray-top tube; **related body system:** Immune system.) Allergen-specific IgE is generally requested for groups of allergens commonly known to incite an allergic response in the affected individual. The test is based on the use of an anti-IgE reagent to detect IgE in the patient's serum, produced in response to specific allergens. The panels include allergens such as animal dander, antibiotics, dust, foods, grasses, insects, latex, mites, molds, trees, venom, and weeds. Immunoassay methods are alternatives to skin test anergy and provocation procedures, which can be inconvenient, painful, and potentially hazardous to patients. Traditional immunoassay and ImmunoCAP FEIA are technologies that have been developed to have minimal interference from nonspecific binding to total IgE versus allergen-specific IgE.

A nasal smear can be examined for the presence of eosinophils to screen for allergic conditions. Either a single smear or smears of nasal secretions from each side of the nose should be submitted, at room temperature, for Hansel staining and evaluation. Normal findings vary by laboratory, but generally, greater than 10% to 15% is considered eosinophilia, or increased presence of eosinophils.

A

INDICATIONS

- Evaluate patients who refuse to submit to skin testing or who have generalized dermatitis or other dermatopathic conditions.
- Monitor response to desensitization procedures.
- Test for allergens when skin testing is inappropriate, such as in infants or when there is a known history of allergic reaction to skin testing.
- Test for specific allergic sensitivity before initiating immunotherapy or desensitization shots.
- Test for specific allergic sensitivity when skin testing is unreliable *(patients taking long-acting antihistamines may have false-negative skin test)*.
- Test for suspected latex allergy.

INTERFERING FACTORS

Factors that may alter the results of the study
- Results may be invalid for patients already taking local or systemic corticosteroids.

POTENTIAL MEDICAL DIAGNOSIS: CLINICAL SIGNIFICANCE OF RESULTS

- Different scoring systems are used in the interpretation of results.

Increased in
Related to production of IgE, the antibody that primarily responds to conditions that stimulate an allergic response

- Allergic rhinitis (Hay Fever)
- Anaphylaxis
- Asthma (exogenous)
- *Echinococcus* infection
- Eczema
- Hookworm infection
- Latex allergy
- Schistosomiasis
- Visceral larva migrans

Decreased in
- Asthma (endogenous)
- Pregnancy

NURSING IMPLICATIONS

BEFORE THE STUDY: PLANNING AND IMPLEMENTATION

Teaching the Patient What to Expect
- Inform the patient this test can assist in identification of causal factors related to allergic reaction.
- Explain that a blood sample is needed for the test.

AFTER THE STUDY: POTENTIAL NURSING ACTIONS

Avoiding Complications
- Remind the patient of the importance of avoiding triggers and of adhering to the recommended therapy, even if signs and symptoms disappear. Lifestyle adjustments may be necessary depending on the specific allergens identified.
- Explain how to identify exposure to allergen sources (e.g., latex) to assist in reduction or elimination of continued exposure.
- Teach the patient to recognize the signs and symptoms of an allergic reaction, especially anaphylaxis.
- Anticipate the need for intubation for a compromised airway.
- Anticipate the need for alternative oxygen therapy such as heliox-a helium-oxygen mixture.
- Administer ordered medications: steroids, anticholinergics, β_2-adrenergic agonist; pace activities to conserve energy; monitor oxygen saturation to maintain SpO_2 of 90% or greater (confirm with therapist).

Treatment Considerations
- Administer allergy treatment if ordered. As appropriate, educate the patient/caregiver in the proper technique for administering his or her own treatments (eyedrops, inhalers, nasal sprays, oral medications, or shots) as well as safe handling and maintenance of treatment materials.
- Note secretion color, consistency, and amount.
- Observe for cyanosis (blue tinge to lips, tongue, mouth, nailbeds), and trend pulse oximetry and arterial blood gas results.

▶ Position the patient to facilitate breathing with head elevated 30 to 45 degrees.

▶ Monitor fatigue and work of breathing; encourage slow, deep breaths.

Safety Considerations

▶ Suggest the patient wear an allergy-specific (e.g., peanuts, penicillin) medic alert bracelet in the case of severe allergy/allergies.

Nutritional Considerations

▶ Recommend consultation with a registered dietitian if food allergies are present.

Follow-Up, Evaluation, and Desired Outcomes

▶ Acknowledges the necessity of adhering to medication regimen and avoiding allergen triggers.

▶ Accepts that prompt treatment should be sought if allergen exposure triggers a respiratory response requiring immediate intervention (wheezing, nasal flare, increased work of breathing, use of accessory muscles, cyanosis), as a respiratory response can quickly become life threatening.

Alpha₁-Antitrypsin and Alpha₁-Antitrypsin Phenotyping

SYNONYM/ACRONYM: α_1-antitrypsin: A₁AT, α_1-AT, AAT; α_1-antitrypsin phenotyping: A₁AT phenotype, α_1-AT phenotype, AAT phenotype, Pi phenotype.

RATIONALE: To assist in the identification of chronic obstructive pulmonary disease (COPD) and liver disease associated with α_1-antitrypsin (α_1-AT) deficiency.

PATIENT PREPARATION: There are no food, fluid, or activity restrictions unless by medical direction. Oral contraceptives should be withheld 24 hr before the specimen is collected, although this restriction should first be confirmed with the health-care provider (HCP) ordering the test.

NORMAL FINDINGS: Method: Rate nephelometry for α_1-AT, isoelectric focusing/high-resolution electrophoresis for α_1-AT phenotyping.

α_1-Antitrypsin

Age	Conventional Units	SI Units (Conventional Units × 0.01)
Newborn	124–348 mg/dL	1.24–3.48 g/L
Child	110–279 mg/dL	1.1–2.79 g/L
Adult	126–226 mg/dL	1.26–2.26 g/L

α_1-Antitrypsin Phenotyping

There are three major protease inhibitor phenotypes:

- MM—Normal
- SS—Intermediate; heterozygous
- ZZ—Markedly abnormal; homozygous

A

The total level of measurable α_1-AT varies with genotype. The effects of α_1-AT deficiency depend on the patient's personal habits but are most severe in patients who smoke tobacco.

CRITICAL FINDINGS AND POTENTIAL INTERVENTIONS: N/A

OVERVIEW: (Study type: Blood collected in a gold-, red-, red/gray-, or lavender-top [EDTA] tube; related body system: Digestive and Respiratory systems.) α_1-AT is the main glycoprotein produced by the liver. Its inhibitory function is directed against proteolytic enzymes, such as trypsin, elastin, and plasmin, released by alveolar macrophages and bacteria. In the absence of α_1-AT, functional tissue is destroyed by proteolytic enzymes and replaced with excessive connective tissue. COPD develops at an earlier age in α_1-AT–deficient patients with COPD than in other patients with COPD. α_1-AT deficiency is passed on as an autosomal recessive trait. Inherited deficiencies are associated early in life with development of lung and liver disorders. In the pediatric population, the ZZ phenotype usually presents as liver disease, cholestasis, and cirrhosis. Greater than 80% of ZZ-deficient individuals ultimately develop chronic lung or liver disease. It is important to identify inherited deficiencies early in life. Typically, α_1-AT–deficient patients have circulating levels less than 50 mg/dL (0.5 g/L). Patients who have α_1-AT values less than 100 mg/dL (1 g/L) should be phenotyped. Elevated levels are found in normal individuals when an inflammatory process, such as rheumatoid arthritis, bacterial infection, tumor or vasculitis, is present. Decreased levels are found in affected patients with COPD and in children with cirrhosis of the liver. Deficiency of this enzyme is the most common cause of liver disease in the pediatric population. Decreased α_1-AT levels also may be elevated into the normal range in patients who are heterozygous α_1-AT–deficient during concurrent infection, pregnancy, estrogen therapy, steroid therapy, cancer, and postoperative periods. Patients who are homozygous α_1-AT–deficient do not show such an elevation. Knowledge of genetics assists the nurse in identifying patients and family members who may benefit from additional education, risk assessment, and counseling. Genetics is the study and identification of genes, genetic mutations, and inheritance. For example, genetics provides some insight into the likelihood of inheriting a medical condition such as a deficiency of α_1-AT.

INDICATIONS
- Assist in establishing a diagnosis of COPD.
- Assist in establishing a diagnosis of liver disease.
- Detect hereditary absence or deficiency of α_1-AT.

INTERFERING FACTORS
Factors that may alter the results of the study
- Drugs and other substances that may increase serum α_1-AT levels include aminocaproic acid, estrogen therapy, oral contraceptives (high-dose preparations),

streptokinase, tamoxifen, and typhoid vaccine
- Rheumatoid factor causes false-positive elevations.

Other considerations
- α_1-AT is an acute-phase reactant protein, and any inflammatory process elevates levels. If a serum C-reactive protein is performed simultaneously and is positive, the patient should be retested for α_1-AT in 10 to 14 days.

POTENTIAL MEDICAL DIAGNOSIS: CLINICAL SIGNIFICANCE OF RESULTS

Increased in
- Acute and chronic inflammatory conditions *(related to rapid, non-specific response to inflammation)*
- Cancers *(related to rapid, nonspecific response to inflammation)*
- Estrogen therapy
- Postoperative recovery *(related to rapid, nonspecific response to inflammation or stress)*
- Pregnancy *(related to rapid, nonspecific response to stress)*
- Steroid therapy
- Stress (extreme physical) *(related to rapid, nonspecific response to stress)*

Decreased in
- COPD *(related to malnutrition and evidenced by decreased protein synthesis)*
- Homozygous α_1-AT–deficient patients *(related to decreased protein synthesis)*
- Liver disease (severe) *(related to decreased protein synthesis)*
- Liver cirrhosis (infant or child) *(related to decreased protein synthesis)*
- Malnutrition *(related to insufficient protein intake)*
- Nephrotic syndrome *(related to increased protein loss from diminished renal function)*

NURSING IMPLICATIONS

BEFORE THE STUDY: PLANNING AND IMPLEMENTATION

Teaching the Patient What to Expect
- Inform the patient this test can assist in identifying lung and liver disease.
- Explain that a blood sample is needed for the test.

AFTER THE STUDY: POTENTIAL NURSING ACTIONS

Avoiding Complications
- Assess for fluid retention, as it can lead to pulmonary edema.
- Discuss the ramifications of abnormal findings with the patient to facilitate protection of the lungs (e.g., avoid contact with persons who have respiratory or other infections; avoid the use of tobacco; avoid areas having highly polluted air; and avoid work environments with hazards such as fumes, dust, and other respiratory pollutants).

Treatment Considerations
- Instruct the patient to resume usual medication as directed by the HCP.
- Monitor respiratory rate and effort based on assessment of patient condition. Assess lung sounds frequently. Monitor for secretions and suction as necessary. Consider use of pulse oximetry to monitor oxygen saturation, and administer ordered oxygen. Elevate the head of the bed 30 degrees. Monitor IV fluids, avoid aggressive fluid resuscitation, and observe for abdominal ascites.

Nutritional Considerations
- Malnutrition is commonly seen in α_1-AT–deficient patients who have severe respiratory disease for many reasons, including fatigue, lack of appetite, and gastrointestinal distress. Research has estimated that the daily caloric intake required for respiration in patients with COPD is 10 times higher than that required in healthy individuals. Inadequate nutrition can result in hypophosphatemia, especially

A

in respirator-dependent patients. During periods of starvation, phosphorus leaves the intracellular space and moves outside the tissue, resulting in dangerously decreased phosphorus levels. Adequate intake of vitamins A and C is important to prevent pulmonary infection and to decrease the extent of lung tissue damage. The importance of following the prescribed diet should be stressed to the patient and caregiver.

▶ Water balance must be closely monitored in α_1-AT–deficient patients with COPD.

▶ Document food intake with possible calorie count; assess barriers to eating; consider using a food diary; monitor continued alcohol use, as it is a barrier to adequate nutrition; daily weight; dietary consult with assessment of cultural food selections; administer multivitamin as prescribed; parenteral and enteral nutrition as needed; assess liver function tests (alanine aminotransferase, alkaline phosphatase, aspartate aminotransferase), glucose, protein, albumin, bilirubin, folic acid, thiamine, electrolytes.

Follow-Up, Evaluation, and Desired Outcomes

▶ Acknowledges the importance of smoking cessation to overall health management.

▶ Understands the necessity to keep scheduled laboratory appointments to monitor liver function and disease progress.

▶ Maintains specific home oxygen therapy to manage ineffective gas exchange.

▶ Successfully demonstrates diaphragmatic breathing and pursed-lip breathing to enhance breathing patterns as appropriate.

▶ Because decreased α_1-AT can be an inherited disorder, it may be appropriate to recommend resources for genetic counseling if levels less than 100 mg/dL (1 g/L) are reported. Patient is aware that α_1-AT phenotype testing can be performed on family members to determine the homozygous or heterozygous nature of the deficiency.

Alveolar/Arterial Gradient and Arterial/ Alveolar Oxygen Ratio

SYNONYM/ACRONYM: Alveolar-arterial difference, A/a gradient, a/A ratio.

RATIONALE: To assist in assessing oxygen delivery and diagnosing causes of hypoxemia, such as pulmonary edema, acute respiratory distress syndrome, and pulmonary fibrosis.

PATIENT PREPARATION: There are no food, fluid, activity, or medication restrictions unless by medical direction. Indicate the type of oxygen, mode of oxygen delivery, and delivery rate as part of the test requisition process. Wait 30 min after a change in type or mode of oxygen delivery or rate for specimen collection.

NORMAL FINDINGS: Method: Selective electrodes that measure Po_2 and Pco_2.

Alveolar/arterial gradient	Less than 10 mm Hg at rest (room air); 20–30 mm Hg at maximum exercise activity (room air)
Arterial/alveolar oxygen ratio	Greater than 0.75 (75%)

Values normally increase with increasing age (see study titled "Blood Gases").

CRITICAL FINDINGS AND POTENTIAL INTERVENTIONS: N/A

OVERVIEW: (Study type: Blood (arterial) collected in a heparinized syringe; **related body system:** Respiratory system.) It is important that no room air be introduced into the collection container because the gases in the room and in the sample will begin equilibrating immediately. The end of the syringe must be stoppered immediately after the needle is withdrawn from the puncture site; follow the facility's safety protocol regarding sharps. Apply a pressure dressing over the puncture site. Samples should be mixed by gentle rolling of the syringe between the hands to ensure proper mixing of the heparin with the sample, which will prevent the formation of small clots leading to rejection of the sample. The tightly capped sample should be placed in an ice slurry immediately after collection. Information on the specimen label should be protected from water in the ice slurry by first placing the specimen in a protective plastic bag. Promptly transport the specimen to the laboratory for processing and analysis. A test of the ability of oxygen to diffuse from the alveoli into the lungs is of use when assessing a patient's level of oxygenation. This test can help identify the cause of hypoxemia (low oxygen levels in the blood) and intrapulmonary shunting that might result from one of the following three situations: ventilated alveoli without perfusion, unventilated alveoli with perfusion, or collapse of alveoli and associated blood vessels. Information regarding the alveolar/arterial (A/a) gradient can be estimated indirectly using the partial pressure of oxygen (Po_2) (obtained from blood gas analysis) in a mathematical formula:

A/a gradient = Po_2 in alveolar air (estimated from the alveolar gas equation) − Po_2 in arterial blood (measured from a blood gas).

An estimate of alveolar Po_2 is accomplished by subtracting the water vapor pressure from the barometric pressure, multiplying the resulting pressure by the fraction of inspired oxygen (Fio_2; percentage of oxygen the patient is breathing), and subtracting this result from 1.25 times the arterial partial pressure of carbon dioxide (Pco_2). The gradient is obtained by subtracting the patient's arterial Po_2 from the calculated alveolar Po_2:

Alveolar Po_2 = [(barometric pressure − water vapor pressure) × Fio_2] − [1.25 × Pco_2].

The a/A ratio reflects the percentage of alveolar Po_2 that is contained in arterial Po_2. It is calculated by dividing the arterial Po_2 by the alveolar Po_2:

a/A = Pa o_2 /PA o_2.

The A/a gradient increases as the concentration of oxygen the patient inspires increases. If the gradient is abnormally high, either there is a problem with the ability of oxygen to pass across the alveolar membrane or oxygenated blood is being mixed with non-oxygenated blood. The a/A ratio is not dependent on Fio_2; it does not increase with a corresponding increase in inhaled oxygen. For patients on a mechanical ventilator with a changing Fio_2, the a/A ratio can be used to determine if oxygen diffusion is improving.

INDICATIONS
- Assess intrapulmonary or coronary artery shunting.
- Assist in identifying the cause of hypoxemia.

INTERFERING FACTORS
Contraindications
Arterial puncture in any of the following circumstances:

⬥ Inadequate circulation *as evidenced by an abnormal (negative) Allen test or the absence of a radial artery pulse.*

⬥ Significant or uncontrolled bleeding disorder, *as the procedure may cause excessive bleeding;* caution should be used when performing an arterial puncture on patients receiving anticoagulant therapy or thrombolytic medications.

⬥ Infection at the puncture site *carries the potential for introducing bacteria from the skin surface into the bloodstream.*

⬥ Congenital or acquired abnormalities of the skin or blood vessels in the area of the anticipated puncture site such as arteriovenous fistulas, burns, tumors, vascular grafts.

Factors that may alter the results of the study
- Specimens should be collected before administration of oxygen therapy or antihistamines.
- The patient's temperature should be noted and reported to the laboratory if significantly elevated or depressed so that measured values can be corrected to actual body temperature.
- Exposure of sample to room air affects test results.
- Prompt and proper specimen processing, storage, and analysis are important to achieve accurate results. Specimens should always be transported to the laboratory as quickly as possible after collection.

Delay in transport of the sample or transportation without ice may affect test results.

POTENTIAL MEDICAL DIAGNOSIS: CLINICAL SIGNIFICANCE OF RESULTS
Increased in
- Acute respiratory distress syndrome (ARDS) *(related to thickened edematous alveoli)*
- Atelectasis *(related to mixing oxygenated and unoxygenated blood)*
- Arterial-venous shunts *(related to mixing oxygenated and unoxygenated blood)*
- Bronchospasm *(related to decrease in the diameter of the airway)*
- Chronic obstructive pulmonary disease *(related to decrease in the elasticity of lung tissue)*
- Congenital cardiac septal defects *(related to mixing oxygenated and unoxygenated blood)*
- Underventilated alveoli *(related to mucus plugs)*
- Pneumothorax *(related to collapsed lung, shunted air, and subsequent decrease in arterial oxygen levels)*
- Pulmonary edema *(related to thickened edematous alveoli)*
- Pulmonary embolus *(related to obstruction of blood flow to alveoli)*
- Pulmonary fibrosis *(related to thickened edematous alveoli)*

NURSING IMPLICATIONS

BEFORE THE STUDY: PLANNING AND IMPLEMENTATION

Teaching the Patient What to Expect
▸ Inform the patient this test can help to assess respiratory status and identify the cause of the respiratory problems.
▸ Explain that an arterial blood sample is needed for the test and advise rest for 30 min before specimen collection.
▸ Address concerns about pain, and explain that an arterial puncture may

be painful. The site may be anesthetized with 1% to 2% lidocaine before puncture.

- Inform the patient that specimen collection usually takes 10 to 15 min.

Potential Nursing Actions
- Ensure an ice slurry is prepared and available for specimen transport.
- If the sample is to be collected by radial artery puncture, perform an Allen test before puncture to ensure that the patient has adequate collateral circulation to the hand. The modified Allen test is described in the study titled "Blood Gases."

Safety Considerations
- The person collecting the specimen should be notified beforehand if the patient is receiving anticoagulant therapy or taking aspirin or other natural products that may prolong bleeding from the puncture site.

AFTER THE STUDY: POTENTIAL NURSING ACTIONS

Avoiding Complications
- Samples for A/a gradient evaluation are obtained by arterial puncture, which carries a risk of bleeding, especially in patients with bleeding disorders

or who are taking medications for a bleeding disorder. Apply pressure to the puncture site for at least 5 min in the unanticoagulated patient and for at least 15 min in a patient receiving anticoagulant therapy. Observe/assess puncture site for bleeding or hematoma formation. Apply pressure bandage.

Treatment Considerations
- Consider respiratory and oxygenation assessment, including respiratory rate, rhythm, work of breathing, cyanotic evaluation, and pulse oximetry to monitor oxygen status.

Safety Considerations
- Institute bleeding precautions for patients who are on coagulation therapy.

Nutritional Considerations
- Nutritional status may be compromised for those patients with poor respiratory status.

Follow-Up, Evaluation, and Desired Outcomes
- Demonstrates how to use controlled breathing to improve breathing patterns.
- Acknowledges the importance of continuous oxygen to support homeostasis.

Alzheimer Disease Markers

SYNONYM/ACRONYM: CSF tau protein and β-amyloid-42, AD, APP, PS-1, PS-2, Apo E4.

RATIONALE: To assist in diagnosing Alzheimer disease and monitoring the effectiveness of therapy.

PATIENT PREPARATION: There are no food, fluid, activity, or medication restrictions unless by medical direction.

NORMAL FINDINGS: (Method: Enzyme-linked immunosorbent assay) Simultaneous tau protein and β-amyloid-42 measurements in cerebrospinal fluid (CSF) are used in conjunction with detection of apolipoprotein E4 alleles (restriction fragment length polymorphism) and identification of mutations in the β-amyloid precursor protein (APP), presenilin 1 (PS-1), and presenilin 2 (PS-2) genes (polymerase chain reaction and DNA sequencing) as biochemical and genetic markers of Alzheimer disease (AD). Scientific studies indicate that a combination of elevated tau protein and decreased β-amyloid-42 protein levels are consistent with the presence of AD. The testing laboratory should be consulted for interpretation of results.

CRITICAL FINDINGS AND POTENTIAL INTERVENTIONS: N/A

OVERVIEW: (Study type: Cerebrospinal fluid [CSF] collected in a plain plastic conical tube for tau protein and β-amyloid-42 and blood collected in a full lavender-top tube for apolipoprotein E4 [ApoE4] genotyping, β-amyloid precursor protein, presenilin 1, and presenilin 2; related body system: Nervous system.) Late-onset AD is the most common cause of dementia in the older adult population. AD is a disorder of the central nervous system (CNS) that results in progressive and profound memory loss followed by loss of cognitive abilities and death. It may follow years of progressive formation of β-amyloid plaques and brain tangles, or it may appear as an early-onset form of the disease. Two recognized pathological features of AD are neurofibrillary tangles and amyloid plaques found in the brain. Abnormal amounts of the phosphorylated microtubule-associated tau protein are the main component of the classic neurofibrillary tangles found in patients with AD. Tau protein concentration is believed to reflect the number of neurofibrillary tangles and may be an indication of the severity of the disease. β-Amyloid-42 is a free-floating protein normally present in CSF. It is believed to accumulate in the CNS of patients with AD, causing the formation of amyloid plaques on brain tissue. The result is that these patients have lower CSF values than age-matched healthy control participants. The study of genetic markers of AD has led to an association between an inherited autosomal dominant mutation in the APP, PS-1, and PS-2 genes and overproduction of amyloid proteins. Mutations in these genes are believed to be responsible for some cases of early-onset AD. An association also exists between a gene that codes for the production of ApoE4 and development of late-onset AD. Diagnosis of AD includes a thorough physical examination, a complete medical history, neurological examination, tests of mental status, blood tests, and brain imaging procedures. For additional information refer to the study titled, "Positron Emission Tomography, Various Sites (brain)." Lumbar puncture is performed as a sterile procedure with the use of a spinal needle to capture a spinal fluid specimen for analysis. Needle size is important because the smaller the bevel, the more time it takes to collect a sufficient volume of fluid; usually, a 22-gauge needle is used. Once the needle has been properly placed, the stylet is removed, allowing CSF to drip from the needle. A stopcock and manometer are attached to the hub of the needle to measure initial CSF pressure. Normal pressure for an adult in the lateral recumbent position is 60 to 200 mm H_2O. After the CSF has been removed, the puncture site is cleansed with an antiseptic solution and direct pressure is applied with dry gauze to stop bleeding or CSF leakage.

INDICATIONS
- Assist in establishing a diagnosis of AD.
- Monitor the effectiveness of AD therapy.

INTERFERING FACTORS
Contraindications

✦ Patients with infection present at the needle insertion site.

✦ Patients with degenerative joint disease or coagulation defects.

✦ Patients with increased intracranial pressure *because overly rapid removal of CSF can result in herniation.*

Factors that may alter the results of the study

- CSF pressure may be elevated if the patient is anxious, holding his or her breath, tensing muscles, or flexing the knees too firmly against the abdomen. If the initial pressure is elevated, the health-care provider (HCP) may perform a Queckenstedt test, which would be performed by the application of pressure to the jugular vein for about 10 sec. CSF pressure usually rises in response to the occlusion, then rapidly returns to normal within 10 sec after the pressure is released. A sluggish response may indicate CSF obstruction.
- Some patients with AD may have normal levels of tau protein because of an insufficient number of neurofibrillary tangles.

POTENTIAL MEDICAL DIAGNOSIS: CLINICAL SIGNIFICANCE OF RESULTS
Increased in

Tau protein is increased in AD.

Presence of ApoE4 alleles is a genetic risk factor for AD.

Identification of mutations in the APP, PS-1, and PS-2 genes is associated with forms of AD.

Decreased in

β-Amyloid-42 is decreased in up to 50% of healthy control participants.

- β-Amyloid-42 is decreased in AD *(related to accumulation in the brain with a corresponding decrease in CSF).*
- β-Amyloid-42 is decreased in Creutzfeldt-Jakob disease.

NURSING IMPLICATIONS

BEFORE THE STUDY: PLANNING AND IMPLEMENTATION

Teaching the Patient What to Expect

▶ Inform the patient this test can assist in diagnosing AD and/or evaluating the effectiveness of medication used to treat AD.

▶ Advise that a blood sample and CSF specimen are needed for the test. The blood sample will be collected by venipuncture and CSF specimen by lumbar puncture.

▶ Address concerns about pain, and explain that there may be some discomfort during both the venipuncture and lumbar puncture.

▶ Inform the patient/caregiver that the CSF specimen collection will be performed by an HCP trained to perform the procedure and takes approximately 20 min. The procedure for lumbar puncture is described in the study titled "Cerebrospinal Fluid Analysis."

▶ Once the procedure is completed, observe/assess the puncture site for bleeding, CSF leakage, or hematoma formation; cover the site with gauze; and secure the gauze with an adhesive bandage. It is possible that there may be a postprocedure headache.

▶ Specimens should be promptly transported to the laboratory for processing and analysis.

Potential Nursing Actions

✦ *Make sure a written and informed consent has been signed prior to the procedure and before administering any medications.*

A

‣ Assess the patient's ability to maintain required position and provide assistance as needed.

AFTER THE STUDY: POTENTIAL NURSING ACTIONS

Avoiding Complications

‣ Headache is a common minor complication experienced after lumbar puncture and is caused by leakage of the spinal fluid from around the puncture site, *probably related to the tear in the dura after the needle has been withdrawn.* On a rare occasion, the headache may require treatment with an epidural blood patch in which an anesthesiologist or pain management specialist injects a small amount of the patient's blood into the epidural space of the puncture site. The blood patch forms a clot and seals the puncture site to prevent further leakage of CSF and provides relief within 30 minutes. Other complications include lower back pain after the procedure, bleeding near the puncture site, or brainstem herniation due to increased intracranial pressure. Observe/assess the puncture site for leakage, and frequently monitor body signs, such as temperature and blood pressure.

Treatment Considerations

‣ After the procedure, position the patient flat, on either the back or the abdomen, although some HCPs allow 30 degrees of elevation. Maintain this position for 8 hr. Changing position is acceptable as long as the body remains horizontal.
‣ Observe/assess the patient for neurological changes, such as altered level of consciousness, change in pupils, reports of tingling or numbness, and irritability.
‣ Monitor vital signs and neurologic status every 15 min for 1 hr, then every 2 hr for 4 hr, and as ordered after lumbar puncture. Take the temperature every 4 hr for 24 hr. Compare with baseline values. Protocols may vary among facilities.

‣ To prevent or relieve headache due to lumbar puncture, administer ordered or permitted caffeinated fluids to replace lost CSF. Advise the patient that headache may begin within a few hours up to 2 days after the procedure and may be associated with dizziness, nausea, and vomiting. The length of time for the headache to resolve varies considerably.
‣ Alzheimer is a progressive disease that decreases patients' ability to provide self-care. Observe the ability to feed, dress, bathe, and toilet themselves.

Safety Considerations

‣ Alzheimer results in progressive cognitive deficits that place the patient at risk for injury related to wandering and inability to note unsafe conditions or follow directions. Ensure the patient is able to follow postprocedure instructions, or provide assistance to do so. Ongoing memory loss can result in the inability to safely manage medications, resulting in over- or underdosing self; secure medications to prevent the patient from self-dosing.

Nutritional Considerations

‣ Alzheimer patients may forget to eat and drink. Monitor weight and intake and output.
‣ Assistance may be required to follow postprocedure hydration recommendations.

Follow-Up, Evaluation, and Desired Outcomes

‣ Acknowledges contact information provided for the Alzheimer's Association (www.alz.org)
‣ Agrees to seek assistance to manage anxiety related to test results, perceived loss of independence, and fear of shortened life expectancy.
‣ Acknowledges the necessity to discuss decisions that may be necessary when considering future placement in a secure facility for medical management and treatment.
‣ Accepts that there will be increasing emotional liability (mood swings, anger, depression, aggression) as cognitive function declines.

Amino Acid Screen, Blood and Urine

A

RATIONALE: To assist in diagnosing congenital metabolic disorders in infants, typically homocystinuria, maple syrup urine disease, phenylketonuria (PKU), and tyrosinuria.

PATIENT PREPARATION: Instruct the caregiver/patient that a 12-hr fast is required prior to the procedure, as protein intake may alter results. If the patient is a neonate, most state regulations require screening specimens to be collected between 24 and 48 hr after birth to allow sufficient time after protein intake for abnormal metabolites to be detected. As appropriate, provide the required urine collection container and specimen collection instructions.

NORMAL FINDINGS: (Method: Liquid chromatography/mass spectrometry) There are numerous amino acids. Values vary, and the testing laboratory should be consulted for corresponding ranges.

CRITICAL FINDINGS AND POTENTIAL INTERVENTIONS: N/A

OVERVIEW: (Study type: Blood collected in a green-top [heparin] tube *or* urine from a random or timed specimen collected in a clean plastic collection container with hydrochloric acid as a preservative; related body system: Digestive, Reproductive, and Urinary systems.) Amino acids are required for the production of proteins, enzymes, coenzymes, hormones, nucleic acids used to form DNA, pigments such as Hgb, and neurotransmitters. All 50 states have a newborn screening program. Tests included in the screening profile vary among the states. Properly collected blood spot cards contain sufficient sample to perform both screening and confirmatory testing. Confirmatory testing for specific aminoacidopathies is generally performed on infants after an initial blood screening test with abnormal results. Confirmatory testing can include fatty acid oxidation probe tests on skin samples, enzyme uptake testing of skin or muscle tissue samples, enzyme assays of blood samples, DNA testing, gas chromatography/mass spectrometry, and tandem mass spectrometry. Testing for common genetically transferred conditions can be performed on either or both prospective parents by blood tests, skin tests, or DNA testing. DNA testing can also be performed on the fetus, in utero, through the collection of fetal cells by amniocentesis or chorionic villus sampling. Genetics is the study and identification of genes, genetic mutations, and inheritance. For example, genetics provides some insight into the likelihood of inheriting a medical condition such as an aminoacidopathy. Knowledge of genetics assists in identifying those who may benefit from additional education, risk assessment, and counseling. Further information regarding inheritance of genes can be found in the study titled "Genetic Testing." Counseling and written, informed consent are recommended and sometimes required before genetic testing. Certain congenital enzyme deficiencies interfere with normal amino acid metabolism and cause excessive accumulation of or deficiencies in amino acid levels. The major genetic disorders include PKU, tyrosinuria, and alcaptonuria, a defect in the phenylalanine-tyrosine conversion pathway. Accumulation of phenylalanine in infants lacking the enzyme phenylalanine hydroxylase results in progressive intellectual disabilities. Renal aminoaciduria is also associated with conditions marked by defective tubular reabsorption from congenital disorders, such as hereditary fructose intolerance, cystinuria, and Hartnup disease. Early diagnosis and treatment of certain aminoacidopathies can prevent intellectual disabilities, reduced growth rates, and various unexplained symptoms. In most cases when plasma levels are elevated, urine levels are also elevated. Amino acid quantitation from plasma specimens is more informative, less variable, and less prone to analytic interference than from urine specimens. Urine specimens may be required to assist in the identification of disorders involving defective renal transport in which elevated levels are manifested only in the urine. Values are age dependent.

INDICATIONS

- Assist in the detection of noninherited disorders evidenced by elevated amino acid levels.
- Detect congenital errors of amino acid metabolism.

INTERFERING FACTORS
Factors that may alter the results of the study

Blood

- Drugs and other substances that may increase plasma amino acid levels include amino acids, bismuth salts, glucocorticoids, levarterenol, and 11-oxysteroids.
- Drugs and other substances that may decrease plasma amino acid levels include diethylstilbestrol, epinephrine, insulin, and progesterone.

Newborn Blood

- Blood specimens for newborn screening that are collected after transfusion may produce invalid results.
- Blood specimens for newborn screening that are collected earlier than 24 hr after the first feeding *(false-negative results related to insufficient time after feeding for the abnormal metabolites to accumulate)* or from neonates receiving total parenteral nutrition *(false-negative results if circulating levels of the amino acids are increased above the detectable limit of the test)* may produce invalid results.
- Blood specimens for newborn screening that are improperly applied to the filter paper circles may produce invalid results.
- Touching blood spots after collection on the filter paper card may contaminate the sample and produce invalid results.
- When collecting blood samples for newborn screening, it is important to apply each blood drop to the correct side of the filter paper card and to fill each circle with a single application of blood. Overfilling or underfilling the circles will cause the specimen

A

card to be rejected by the testing facility. Newborn screening cards should be allowed to air dry for several hours on a level, nonabsorbent, unenclosed area. If multiple patients are tested, cards must not be stacked. State regulations usually require the specimen cards to be submitted within 24 hr of collection.

Urine
- Drugs and other substances that may increase urine amino acid levels include acetylsalicylic acid, bismuth, cisplatin, corticotropin, hydrocortisone, insulin, streptozocin, tetracycline, triamcinolone, and valproic acid; numerous drugs and other substances may affect the test method and falsely increase urine amino acid levels.
- Drugs and other substances that may decrease urine amino acid levels include insulin.
- Dilute urine (specific gravity less than 1.01) should be rejected for analysis.

Other considerations
- Amino acids exhibit a strong circadian rhythm; values are highest in the afternoon and lowest in the morning. Protein intake does not influence diurnal variation but significantly affects absolute concentrations.

POTENTIAL MEDICAL DIAGNOSIS: CLINICAL SIGNIFICANCE OF RESULTS

Blood
Increased in
Increased amino acid accumulation (total amino acids) occurs when a specific enzyme deficiency prevents its catabolism, with liver disease, or when there is impaired clearance by the kidneys:

- Acute kidney injury *(related to impaired clearance)*

- Aminoacidopathies *(usually related to an inherited disorder; specific amino acids are implicated)*
- Burns *(related to increased protein turnover)*
- Chronic kidney disease *(related to impaired clearance)*
- Diabetes *(related to gluconeogenesis in which protein is broken down as a means to generate glucose)*
- Fructose intolerance *(related to hereditary enzyme deficiency)*
- Malabsorption *(related to lack of transport and opportunity for catabolism)*
- Reye syndrome *(related to liver damage)*
- Severe liver damage *(related to decreased production of amino acids by the liver)*
- Shock *(related to increased protein turnover from tissue death and decreased deamination due to impaired liver function)*

Decreased in
Decreased (total amino acids) in conditions that result in increased renal excretion or insufficient protein intake or synthesis:

- Adrenocortical hyperfunction *(related to excess cortisol, which assists in conversion of amino acids into glucose)*
- Carcinoid syndrome *(related to increased consumption of amino acids, especially tryptophan, to form serotonin)*
- Fever *(related to increased consumption)*
- Glomerulonephritis *(related to increased renal excretion)*
- Hartnup disease *(related to increased renal excretion)*
- Huntington chorea *(related to increased consumption due to muscle tremors; possible insufficient intake)*
- Malnutrition *(related to insufficient intake)*

A

- Nephrotic syndrome *(related to increased renal excretion)*
- Pancreatitis (acute) *(related to increased consumption as part of the inflammatory process and increased ureagenesis)*
- Polycystic kidney disease *(related to increased renal excretion)*
- Rheumatoid arthritis *(related to insufficient intake evidenced by lack of appetite)*

Urine
Increased in

Increased amino acid accumulation (total amino acids) occurs when a specific enzyme deficiency prevents its catabolism or when there is impaired clearance by the kidneys:

- Primary causes *(inherited):*
  Aminoaciduria (specific)
  Cystinosis *(may be masked because of decreased glomerular filtration rate, so values may be in normal range)*
  Fanconi syndrome
  Fructose intolerance
  Galactosemia
  Hartnup disease
  Lactose intolerance
  Lowe syndrome
  Maple syrup urine disease
  Tyrosinemia type I
  Tyrosinosis
  Wilson disease
- Secondary causes *(noninherited):*
  Acute leukemia
  Chronic kidney disease *(reduced glomerular filtration rate)*
  Diabetic ketoacidosis
  Epilepsy *(transient increase related to disturbed renal function during grand mal seizure)*
  Folic acid deficiency
  Hyperparathyroidism
  Liver necrosis and cirrhosis
  Multiple myeloma
  Muscular dystrophy (progressive)
  Osteomalacia *(secondary to parathyroid hormone excess)*
  Pernicious anemia

Thalassemia major
Vitamin deficiency *(B, C, and D; vitamin D–deficiency rickets, vitamin D–resistant rickets)*
Viral hepatitis *(related to the degree of hepatic involvement)*

Decreased in: N/A

NURSING IMPLICATIONS

BEFORE THE STUDY: PLANNING AND IMPLEMENTATION

Teaching the Patient What to Expect
- Education regarding newborn screening should begin during the prenatal period and be reinforced at the time of preadmission testing.
- Inform the parent/caregiver this test can assist in identification of inborn infant disorders.
- Explain that a blood or urine sample is needed for the test; specimens from neonates are collected by heelstick and applied to filter paper spots on the birth state's specific screening program card.

Potential Nursing Actions
- Provide, if available, an educational brochure to the parents.
- Validate that the requesting health-care provider (HCP) has explained the newborn screening process to the parents before discharge.

AFTER THE STUDY: POTENTIAL NURSING ACTIONS

Avoiding Complications
- Strict adherence to each individual's specified treatment regime will provide the best chance for diagnostic improvement.

Treatment Considerations
- Confer with the family to identify any history of amino acid disorders.
- Advise that the HCP will contact the family/patient to provide treatment options for the specific identified condition.

Nutritional Considerations

● Amino acids are classified as essential (i.e., must be present simultaneously in sufficient quantities), conditionally or acquired essential (i.e., under certain stressful conditions, they become essential), and nonessential (i.e., can be produced by the body, when needed, if diet does not provide them).

● Essential amino acids include lysine, threonine, histidine, isoleucine, methionine, phenylalanine, tryptophan, and valine.

● Conditionally essential amino acids include cysteine, tyrosine, arginine, citrulline, taurine, and carnitine.

● Nonessential amino acids include alanine, glutamic acid, aspartic acid, glycine, serine, proline, glutamine, and asparagine. A high intake of specific amino acids can cause other amino acids to become essential.

Follow-Up, Evaluation, and Desired Outcomes

● Understands information provided regarding access to genetic or other counseling services. Acknowledges contact information provided for the March of Dimes (www.marchofdimes.com), National Library of Medicine (https://medlineplus.gov/newborn-screening.html), general information (http://newbornscreening.info/Parents/facts.html), or state department of health newborn screening program. There are numerous support groups and informational Web sites for specific conditions, including the Fatty Oxidation Disorders (FOD) Family Support Group (www.fodsupport.org), Organic Acidemia Association (www.oaanews.org), and the United Mitochondrial Disease Foundation (www.umdf.org).

● Agrees to attend support groups with other parents of children having a similar diagnosis.

Ammonia

SYNONYM/ACRONYM: NH_3.

RATIONALE: To assist in diagnosing liver disease such as hepatitis and cirrhosis and evaluating the effectiveness of treatment modalities. Also used to assist in diagnosing infant Reye syndrome.

PATIENT PREPARATION: There are no food, fluid, activity, or medication restrictions unless by medical direction.

NORMAL FINDINGS: Method: Enzymatic.

Age	Conventional Units	SI Units (Conventional Units × 0.587)
Newborn	170–340 mcg/dL	100–200 micromol/L
10 d–24 mo	70–135 mcg/dL	41–79 micromol/L
25 mo–adult	15–60 mcg/dL	9–35 micromol/L

CRITICAL FINDINGS AND POTENTIAL INTERVENTIONS: N/A

A

OVERVIEW: (**Study type:** Blood collected in completely filled lavender- [EDTA] or green-top [Na or Li heparin] tube; related body system: Digestive system.) Specimen should be transported tightly capped and in an ice slurry. Blood ammonia (NH_3) comes from two sources: deamination of amino acids during protein metabolism and degradation of proteins by colon bacteria. The liver converts ammonia in the portal blood to urea, which is excreted by the kidneys. When liver function is severely compromised, especially in situations in which decreased hepatocellular function is combined with impaired portal blood flow, ammonia levels rise. Congenital enzyme defects that prevent the breakdown of ammonia or conditions that affect the ability of the kidneys to excrete ammonia can also result in increased blood levels. Ammonia is potentially toxic to the central nervous system and may result in encephalopathy or coma if toxic levels are reached.

INDICATIONS
- Evaluate advanced liver disease or other disorders associated with altered serum ammonia levels.
- Identify impending hepatic encephalopathy with known liver disease.
- Monitor the effectiveness of treatment for hepatic encephalopathy, indicated by declining levels.
- Monitor patients receiving hyperalimentation therapy.

INTERFERING FACTORS
Factors that may alter the results of the study
- Drugs and other substances that may increase ammonia levels include asparaginase, chlorothiazide, chlorthalidone, fibrin hydrolysate, furosemide, isoniazid, levoglutamide, mercurial diuretics, oral resins, thiazides, and valproic acid.
- Drugs/organisms and other substances that may decrease ammonia levels include diphenhydramine, kanamycin, monoamine oxidase inhibitors, neomycin, tetracycline, and *Lactobacillus acidophilus*.
- Cigarette smoking increases ammonia levels.
- Hemolysis falsely increases ammonia levels because intracellular ammonia levels are three times higher than plasma.
- Prompt and proper specimen processing, storage, and analysis are important to achieve accurate results. The specimen should be collected on ice; the collection tube should be filled completely and then kept tightly stoppered. Ammonia increases rapidly in the collected specimen, so analysis should be performed within 20 min of collection.

POTENTIAL MEDICAL DIAGNOSIS: CLINICAL SIGNIFICANCE OF RESULTS
Increased in
- Gastrointestinal hemorrhage *(related to decreased blood volume, which prevents ammonia from reaching the liver to be metabolized)*
- Genitourinary tract infection with distention and stasis *(related to decreased renal excretion; levels accumulate in the blood)*
- Hepatic coma *(related to insufficient functioning liver cells to metabolize ammonia; levels accumulate in the blood)*
- Inborn enzyme deficiency *(evidenced by inability to metabolize ammonia)*

- Liver failure, late cirrhosis *(related to insufficient functioning liver cells to metabolize ammonia)*
- Reye syndrome *(related to insufficient functioning liver cells to metabolize ammonia)*

- Total parenteral nutrition *(related to ammonia generated from protein metabolism)*

Decreased in: N/A

NURSING IMPLICATIONS

POTENTIAL NURSING PROBLEMS: ASSESSMENT & NURSING DIAGNOSIS

Problems	Signs and Symptoms
Bleeding *(related to altered levels of clotting factors, portal hypertension, esophageal bleeding)*	Altered level of consciousness, hypotension, increased heart rate, decreased Hgb and Hct, capillary refill greater than 3 sec, cool extremities
Confusion *(related to an alteration in fluid and electrolytes, hepatic disease and encephalopathy, acute alcohol consumption, hepatic metabolic insufficiency)*	Disorganized thinking; restlessness; irritability; altered concentration and attention span; changeable mental function over the day; hallucinations; inability to follow directions; disoriented to person, place, time, and purpose; inappropriate affect
Nutrition *(related to excess alcohol intake, insufficient eating habits, altered liver function)*	Known inadequate caloric intake, weight loss, muscle wasting in arms and legs, stool that is pale or gray-colored, skin that is flaky with loss of elasticity
Skin *(related to jaundice and elevated bilirubin levels, excessive scratching)*	Jaundiced skin and sclera, dry skin, itching skin, damage to skin associated with scratching

BEFORE THE STUDY: PLANNING AND IMPLEMENTATION

Teaching the Patient What to Expect

▶ Inform the patient this test can assist with the evaluation of liver function related to processing protein waste. May be used to assist in diagnosis of Reye syndrome in infants.
▶ Explain that a blood sample is needed for the test.

AFTER THE STUDY: POTENTIAL NURSING ACTIONS

Avoiding Complications

▶ Skin: Apply lotion to keep the skin moisturized, avoid alkaline soaps, discourage scratching, apply mittens if patient is unable to follow direction to avoid scratching, administer antihistamines as ordered.

Treatment Considerations

▶ Bleeding: Increase frequency of vital sign assessment with variances in results, monitor for vital sign trends, administer blood or blood products as ordered, administer stool softeners as needed, encourage intake of foods rich in vitamin K, avoid foods that may irritate esophagus.
▶ Dietary and fluid restrictions may be required; diuretics may be ordered.

A

The patient should be frequently monitored for weight gain, intake and output, and abdominal girth.

Safety Considerations

▶ Confusion: Treat the medical condition; correlate confusion with the need to reverse altered electrolytes; evaluate medications; prevent falls and injury through use of postural support, bed alarm, or the appropriate use of restraints; consider pharmacological interventions; track accurate intake and output to assess fluid status; monitor blood ammonia level; determine last alcohol use; assess for symptoms of hepatic encephalopathy such as confusion, sleep disturbances, incoherence; protect the patient from physical harm; administer lactulose as prescribed.

Nutritional Considerations

▶ Document food intake with possible calorie count; assess barriers to eating; consider using a food diary; monitor continued alcohol use, as it is a barrier to adequate protein nutrition; monitor glucose levels; monitor daily weight; perform dietary consult with assessment of cultural food selections. Teach the patient that small, frequent meals throughout the day can increase overall caloric intake and improve nutritional status.

▶ Increased ammonia levels may be associated with liver disease. In general, patients should be encouraged to eat a well-balanced diet that includes foods high in fiber. Dietary recommendations will vary depending on the condition and its severity. For example, recommend a diet of soft foods if esophageal varices develop or limitations on salt intake if ascites develop.

Follow-Up, Evaluation, and Desired Outcomes

▶ Accepts the necessity of accurate self-administration of lactulose to reduce absorption of ammonia; decreased blood ammonia level will help prevent hepatic encephalopathy.

▶ Acknowledges the importance of making food selections that are appropriate for the degree of liver disease (high protein and high carbohydrate can support nutrition until liver disease prohibits these food selections).

▶ Understands that scratching can damage the skin and precipitate an infection.

Amniotic Fluid Analysis and L/S Ratio

SYNONYM/ACRONYM: N/A

RATIONALE: To assist in identification of fetal gender, genetic disorders such as hemophilia and sickle cell anemia, chromosomal disorders such as Down syndrome, anatomical abnormalities such as spina bifida, alloimmune hemolytic disease of the newborn (HDN), and hereditary metabolic disorders such as cystic fibrosis. To assess for preterm infant fetal lung maturity to assist in evaluating for potential diagnosis of respiratory distress syndrome (RDS).

PATIENT PREPARATION: There are no food, fluid, activity, or medication restrictions unless by medical direction.

NORMAL FINDINGS: Method: Macroscopic observation of fluid for color and appearance, immunochemiluminometric assay (ICMA) for α_1-fetoprotein, electrophoresis for acetylcholinesterase, spectrophotometry for Cr, bilirubin, and chromatography for lecithin/sphingomyelin (L/S) ratio and phosphatidylglycerol, tissue culture for chromosome analysis, dipstick for leukocyte esterase, and automated cell counter for white blood cell count and lamellar bodies.

Test	Reference Value
Color	Colorless to pale yellow
Appearance	Clear
α_1-Fetoprotein (AFP)	Less than 2 MoM
Acetylcholinesterase	Absent
Cr	1.8–4 mg/dL at term (159.1–353.6 micromol/L) (SI Units = Conventional Units × 88.4)
Bilirubin	Less than 0.075 mg/dL in early pregnancy (Less than 1.28 micromol/L) (SI Units = Conventional Units × 17.1)
	Less than 0.025 mg/dL at term (Less than 0.428 micromol/L) (SI Units = Conventional Units × 17.1)
Bilirubin ΔOD_{450}	Less than 0.05 ΔOD in early to mid-pregnancy (approximately 14–27 weeks, using the Queenan curve when gestational age is less than 27 weeks)
	Less than 0.06 ΔOD in late pregnancy (approximately 28–36 weeks, using the Liley Chart when gestational age is equal to or greater than 27 weeks)
	Less than 0.03 ΔOD at term (approximately 37–40 weeks, using the Liley Chart when gestational age is equal to or greater than 27 weeks)
L/S ratio	
Mature (nondiabetic)	Greater than 2:1 in the presence of phosphatidyl glycerol
Borderline	1.5 to 1.9:1
Immature	Less than 1.5:1
Phosphatidylglycerol	Present at term
Chromosome analysis	Normal karyotype
White blood cell count	None seen
Leukocyte esterase	Negative
Lamellar bodies	Findings and interpretive ranges vary depending on the type of instrument used

MoM = Multiples of the median.

CRITICAL FINDINGS AND POTENTIAL INTERVENTIONS
• An L/S ratio less than 1.5:1 is predictive of RDS at the time of delivery.

Timely notification to the requesting health-care provider (HCP) of any critical findings and related symptoms is a role expectation of the professional nurse. A listing of these findings varies among facilities.

Infants known to be at risk for RDS can be treated with surfactant by intratracheal administration at birth.

A

OVERVIEW: (Study type: Body fluid, amniotic fluid collected in a clean amber glass or plastic container; related body system: Reproductive system.) Amniotic fluid is formed in the membranous sac that surrounds the fetus. The total volume of fluid at term is 500 to 2,500 mL. In amniocentesis, fluid is obtained by ultrasound-guided needle aspiration from the amniotic sac. This procedure is generally performed between 14 and 16 weeks' gestation for accurate interpretation of test results, but it also can be done between 26 and 35 weeks' gestation if fetal distress is suspected. Fluid is tested to identify fetal genetic and neural tube defects, infection, renal malfunction, lung maturity, and hemolytic diseases of the newborn. Examples of genetic defects commonly tested for and identifiable from a sample of amniotic fluid include sickle cell anemia, cystic fibrosis, and inborn errors of metabolism. Available rapid tests can be used to differentiate between amniotic fluid and other body fluids in a vaginal specimen collection. Nitrazine paper impregnated with an indicator dye will produce a color change indicative of vaginal pH. Normal vaginal pH is acidic (4.5–6), and the color of the paper will not change. Amniotic fluid has an alkaline pH (7.1–7.3), and the paper will turn blue. False-positive results occur in the presence of semen, blood, alkaline urine, vaginal infection, or antibiotic treatment. Amniotic fluid crystallization, or fern test, is the observation of a fern pattern when fluid air dries on a glass slide. The fern pattern is from the protein and sodium chloride content of the amniotic fluid. False-positive results occur in the presence of blood, urine, or cervical mucus. Both tests can produce false-negative results when a small amount of fluid is leaked. Result reliability is significantly diminished with the passage of time (greater than 24 hr). AmniSure is an immunoassay performed using a vaginal swab sample. This rapid test detects placental alpha microglobulin-1 (PAMG-1) protein, found in high concentrations in amniotic fluid. AmniSure does not have the high frequency of false-positive and false-negative results found with the pH and fern tests.

RDS is the most common problem encountered in the care of premature infants. RDS, also called *hyaline membrane disease,* results from a deficiency of phospholipid lung surfactants. The phospholipids in surfactant are produced by specialized alveolar cells and stored in granular lamellar bodies in the lung. In normally developed lungs, surfactant coats the surface of the alveoli. Surfactant reduces the surface tension of the alveolar wall during breathing. When there is an insufficient quantity of surfactant, the alveoli are unable to expand normally, and gas exchange is inhibited. Amniocentesis, a procedure by which fluid is removed from the amniotic sac, is used to assess fetal lung maturity.

Lecithin is the primary surfactant phospholipid, and it is a stabilizing factor for the alveoli. It is produced at a low but constant rate until the 35th wk of gestation, after which its production sharply increases. Sphingomyelin, another phospholipid component of surfactant, is also produced at a constant rate after the 26th wk of gestation. Before the 35th wk, the L/S ratio is usually less than 1.6:1. The ratio increases to 2 or greater when the rate of lecithin production increases after the 35th wk of gestation. Other phospholipids, such as phosphatidyl glycerol (PG) and phosphatidyl inositol (PI), increase over time in amniotic fluid as well. The presence of PG indicates that the fetus is within 2 to 6 wk of lung maturity (i.e., at full term). Simultaneous measurement of PG with the L/S ratio improves diagnostic accuracy. Production of phospholipid surfactant is delayed in mothers with diabetes. Therefore, caution must be used when interpreting the results obtained from a patient who is diabetic, and a higher ratio is expected to predict maturity.

HDN, also called erythroblastosis fetalis, is a condition that occurs after red blood cells (RBCs) from an Rh negative mother become sensitized by fetal RBCs from an Rh positive baby. Rh sensitization of the mother can result from a miscarriage, trauma such as a fall or blow to the abdominal area, after an invasive prenatal test (such as amniocentesis), or when the placenta detaches during birth. The mother's immune system recognizes the baby's RBCs as foreign and makes antibodies that cause the fetal RBCs to hemolyze. Bilirubin is a breakdown product of Hgb, the oxygen carrying protein in RBCs. Bilirubin measurements from amniotic fluid are used to screen for hemolysis in high risk situations, sometimes serial measurements are required to monitor elevated measurements or therapeutic interventions such as administration of RhIG, fetal transfusions, or a decision to deliver the baby.

Testing for common genetically transferred conditions can be performed on either or both prospective parents by blood tests, skin tests, or DNA testing. DNA testing can also be performed on the fetus, in utero, through the collection of fetal cells by amniocentesis or chorionic villus sampling. Genetics is the study and identification of genes, genetic mutations, and inheritance. For example, genetics provides some insight into the likelihood of inheriting a medical condition such as cystic fibrosis or of errors of amino acid metabolism. Knowledge of genetics assists in identifying those who may benefit from additional education, risk assessment, and counseling. Further information regarding inheritance of genes can be found in the study titled "Genetic Testing." Counseling and written, informed consent are recommended and sometimes required before genetic testing.

INDICATIONS

- Assist in the diagnosis of (in utero) metabolic disorders, such as cystic fibrosis, or errors of lipid, carbohydrate, or amino acid metabolism.
- Assist in the evaluation of fetal lung maturity when preterm delivery is being considered.
- Detect infection secondary to ruptured membranes.
- Detect fetal ventral wall defects.

A

- Determine the optimal time for obstetric intervention in cases of threatened fetal survival caused by stresses related to maternal diabetes, toxemia, hemolytic diseases of the newborn, or postmaturity.
- Determine fetal gender when the mother is a known carrier of a sex-linked abnormal gene that could be transmitted to male offspring, such as hemophilia or Duchenne muscular dystrophy.
- Determine the presence of fetal distress in late-stage pregnancy.
- Evaluate fetus in families with a history of genetic disorders, such as Down syndrome, Tay-Sachs disease, chromosome or enzyme anomalies, or inherited hemoglobinopathies.
- Evaluate fetus in mothers of advanced maternal age (some of the aforementioned tests are routinely requested in mothers age 35 and older).
- Evaluate fetus in mothers with a history of miscarriage or stillbirth.
- Evaluate known or suspected hemolytic disease involving the fetus in an Rh-sensitized pregnancy, indicated by rising bilirubin levels, especially after the 30th wk of gestation.
- Evaluate suspected neural tube defects, such as spina bifida or myelomeningocele, as indicated by elevated α_1-fetoprotein (see study titled "Maternal Markers" for information related to triple-marker testing).
- Identify fetuses at risk of developing RDS.

INTERFERING FACTORS
Contraindications

⬧ Women with a history of premature labor, incompetent cervix, or in the presence of placenta previa or abruptio placentae. There is some risk to having an amniocentesis performed, and the risk should be weighed against the need to obtain the desired diagnostic information. A small percentage (0.5%) of patients have experienced complications including premature rupture of membranes (PROM), premature labor, spontaneous abortion, and stillbirth.

Factors that may alter the results of the study

- Bilirubin may be falsely elevated if maternal Hgb or meconium is present in the sample; fetal acidosis may also lead to falsely elevated bilirubin levels.
- Bilirubin may be falsely decreased if the sample is exposed to light or if amniotic fluid volume is excessive.
- Maternal serum Cr should be measured simultaneously for comparison with amniotic fluid Cr for proper interpretation. Even in circumstances in which the maternal serum value is normal, the results of the amniotic fluid Cr may be misleading. A high fluid Cr value in the fetus of a mother who is diabetic may reflect the increased muscle mass of a larger fetus. If the fetus is big, the Cr may be high, and the fetus still may have immature kidneys.
- Contamination of the sample with blood or meconium or complications in pregnancy may yield inaccurate L/S ratios; fetal blood falsely elevates the L/S ratio.
- α_1-Fetoprotein and acetylcholinesterase may be falsely elevated if the sample is contaminated with fetal blood.
- Karyotyping cannot be performed under the following conditions: (1) failure to promptly deliver samples for chromosomal analysis to the laboratory performing the test or (2) improper incubation of the sample, which causes cell death.

A

POTENTIAL MEDICAL DIAGNOSIS: CLINICAL SIGNIFICANCE OF RESULTS

- Yellow, green, red, or brown fluid *indicates the presence of bilirubin, blood (fetal or maternal), or meconium, which indicate fetal distress or death, hemolytic disease, or growth retardation.*

- Elevated bilirubin levels *indicate fetal hemolytic disease or intestinal obstruction. Measurement of bilirubin usually is not performed before 20 to 24 weeks' gestation because no action can be taken before then. The severity of hemolytic disease is graded by optical density (OD) zones. A trend of increasing values with serial measurements may indicate the need for intrauterine transfusion or early delivery, depending on the fetal age. After 32 to 33 weeks' gestation, early delivery is preferred over intrauterine transfusion because early delivery is more effective in providing the required care to the neonate.*

- Cr concentration greater than 2 mg/dL (greater than 176.8 micromol/L) (SI Units = Conventional Units × 88.4) *indicates fetal maturity (at 36–37 wk) if maternal Cr is also within the expected range. This value should be interpreted in conjunction with other parameters evaluated in amniotic fluid and especially with the L/S ratio because normal lung development depends on normal kidney development.*

- An L/S ratio less than 2:1 and absence of phosphatidylglycerol at term *indicate fetal lung immaturity and possible respiratory distress syndrome. Other conditions that decrease production of surfactants include advanced maternal age, multiple gestation, and polyhydramnios. Conditions that may increase production of surfactant include hypertension, intrauterine growth retardation, malnutrition, maternal diabetes, placenta previa, placental infarction, and premature rupture of the membranes. The expected L/S ratio for the fetus of a mother who is diabetic is higher (3.5:1).*

- *Lamellar bodies are specialized alveolar cells in which lung surfactant is stored.* They are approximately the size of platelets. Their presence in sufficient quantities is an indicator of fetal lung maturity. Amniotic fluid lamellar body counts less than 15,000/microL are suggestive of immature lung development and predictive for increased risk of developing RDS; counts greater than 50,000/microL are predictive of mature lung development.

- Elevated AFP levels and presence of acetylcholinesterase may indicate a neural tube defect (see study titled "Maternal Markers") *related to leakage from the open spinal cord into the amniotic fluid.* Elevation of AFP and/or acetylcholinesterase is also indicative of ventral wall defects. The presence of AFP and acetylcholinesterase in amniotic fluid is abnormal; however, the test is not a sensitive marker for neural tube defects; false-positive results can be caused by contamination of the sample with fetal blood, which normally contains measurable levels of AFP and acetylcholinesterase. Abnormal results can be confirmed by testing the amniotic fluid for the presence of fetal Hgb (Hgb F). If Hgb F is detected, then the specimen is likely contaminated with fetal blood and the results are unreliable.

A

- Abnormal karyotype *indicates genetic abnormality (e.g., Tay-Sachs disease, intellectual disability, chromosome or enzyme anomalies, and inherited hemoglobinopathies).* (See study titled "Chromosome Analysis, Blood.")
- Elevated white blood cell count and positive leukocyte esterase *are indicators of infection.*

NURSING IMPLICATIONS

POTENTIAL NURSING PROBLEMS: ASSESSMENT & NURSING DIAGNOSIS

Problems	Signs and Symptoms
Fear *(related to fetal imperfections secondary to developmental abnormality)*	Anxiety; restlessness; sleeplessness; increased tension; continuous questioning; increased blood pressure, heart rate, respiratory rate
Knowledge *(related to insufficient information associated with diagnosed developmental abnormality, lack of familiarity or understanding with disease and treatment)*	Lack of interest or questions, multiple questions, anxiety related to disease and management, stating inaccurate information, frustration, confusion
Spirituality *(related to anxiety associated with fetal developmental abnormality, unexpected life changes)*	Anger; stated feelings of lack of peace or serenity, alienation from others, hopelessness; request to meet with spiritual leader

BEFORE THE STUDY: PLANNING AND IMPLEMENTATION

Teaching the Patient What to Expect

- Explain that this procedure can assist in evaluation of fetal well-being.
- Explain that an amniotic fluid sample is needed for the test. Address concerns about pain, and explain there may be some discomfort during the amniocentesis.
- Amniocentesis is performed by an HCP specializing in this procedure and usually takes approximately 20 to 30 min to complete.
- Partial disrobing will be required with removal of clothes below the waist before being assisted to a supine position on the examination table with the abdomen exposed.
- Proper positioning may require that the head or legs be raised slightly

to promote comfort and to relax the abdominal muscles. A pillow or rolled blanket may be placed under the right side to prevent hypertension caused by great-vessel compression with a large uterus.

- Maternal and fetal baseline vital signs will be recorded. Maternal and fetal vital signs and uterine contractions should be monitored throughout the procedure. Fetal vital signs will be monitored using ultrasound. Protocols may vary among facilities.
- Ultrasound will be used to assess the position of the amniotic fluid, fetus, and placenta.
- Sterile technique is used during the procedure after cleaning the suprapubic area with an antiseptic solution and protecting the site with sterile drapes.
- A local anesthetic is injected prior to amniocentesis and may cause a

stinging sensation. A sensation of pressure may be experienced when a spinal needle is inserted through the abdominal and uterine walls. Explain how to use focused and controlled breathing for relaxation during the procedure.

▶ After the procedure, slight pressure is applied to the site after the fluid is collected and the needle is withdrawn. If there is no evidence of bleeding or other drainage, a sterile adhesive bandage is applied to the site.

Potential Nursing Actions

▶ Verify maternal Rh type results. If Rh-negative, check for prior sensitization. Assess for a family history of genetic disorders. Record the date of the last menstrual period and determine the pregnancy weeks' gestation and expected delivery date.

✦ *Make sure a written and informed consent has been signed prior to the procedure and before administering any medications.*

▶ Instruct patients less than 20 weeks' gestation to drink extra fluids 1 hr before the test and to refrain from urination. A full bladder raises the uterus up and out of the way for easier visualization during the ultrasound procedure.

▶ Instruct patients 20 weeks' gestation or more to void before the test. An empty bladder is less likely to be accidentally punctured during specimen collection.

▶ As required, assemble the necessary equipment, including an amniocentesis tray with solution for skin preparation, local anesthetic, 10- or 20-mL syringe, needles of various sizes (including a 22-gauge, 5-in. spinal needle), sterile drapes, sterile gloves, and foil-covered or amber-colored specimen collection containers. Extra needles should be available for replacement in the event of needle contamination.

AFTER THE STUDY: POTENTIAL NURSING ACTIONS

Avoiding Complications

▶ Hemorrhage or infection can occur following amniocentesis. Instruct the patient to observe for and report excessive bleeding, redness of skin, fever, or chills. Maternal Rh sensitization can result from fetal red blood cells (RBCs) mixing with blood of an Rh-negative mother carrying an Rh-positive fetus. RhIG or RhoGAM may be administered after amniocentesis to Rh-negative mothers to prevent formation of Rh antibodies. Monitor the patient for complications related to the procedure (e.g., premature labor, infection, leakage of amniotic fluid). The patient should report moderate to severe abdominal pain or cramps, change in fetal activity, increased or prolonged leaking of amniotic fluid from abdominal needle site, vaginal bleeding that is heavier than spotting, and chills or fever. Observe/assess the amniocentesis site for bleeding, inflammation, or hematoma formation per facility protocol.

Treatment Considerations

▶ Compare fetal heart rate and maternal life signs (i.e., heart rate, blood pressure, pulse, and respiration) with baseline values and closely monitor every 15 min for 30 to 60 min after the amniocentesis procedure or per facility protocol.

▶ Administer, as ordered, standard RhIG or RhoGAM dose to maternal Rh-negative patients to prevent maternal Rh sensitization should the fetus be Rh-positive.

▶ Instruct the patient to rest until all symptoms have disappeared before resuming normal levels of activity.

▶ Explain that the patient can expect mild cramping, leakage of small amounts of amniotic fluid, and vaginal spotting for up to 2 days following the procedure.

Follow-Up, Evaluation, and Desired Outcomes

▶ Acknowledges contact information provided for counseling related to pregnancy termination and genetic counseling or access to support groups in relation to diagnosed developmental disability if a chromosomal abnormality is determined.

▶ Describes the care and lifestyle changes necessary to support healthy development of the disabled infant.

▶ Understands instruction provided for the administration of medications and the importance of consulting with the HCP or pharmacist to understand the potential significant adverse effects and systemic reactions.

♦ Accepts that normal results do not guarantee a healthy fetus. Provide a nonjudgmental, nonthreatening atmosphere for discussing the risks and difficulties of delivering and raising a developmentally challenged infant as well as for exploring other options (termination of pregnancy or adoption). It is also important to discuss problems the mother and father may experience (guilt, depression, anger) if fetal abnormalities are detected.

Amylase

SYNONYM/ACRONYM: N/A

RATIONALE: To assist in diagnosis and evaluation of the treatment modalities used for pancreatitis.

PATIENT PREPARATION: There are no food, fluid, activity, or medication restrictions unless by medical direction.

NORMAL FINDINGS: Method: Enzymatic.

Age	Conventional and SI Units
Newborn–6 mo	0–30 units/L
Child	11–90 units/L
Adult–older adult	100–300 units/L

Values may be slightly elevated in pregnancy and in older adults due to the effects of medications and the presence of multiple chronic or acute diseases with or without muted symptoms.

CRITICAL FINDINGS AND POTENTIAL INTERVENTIONS: N/A

OVERVIEW: (**Study type:** Blood collected in a gold-, red-, red/gray-, or green-top [heparin] tube; **related body system:** Digestive system.) Amylase is a digestive enzyme mainly secreted into the acinar cells of the pancreas and by the parotid glands. Pancreatic amylase is secreted into the pancreatic common bile ducts and then into the duodenum where it assists in the digestion of carbohydrates by splitting starch into disaccharides. Amylase is a sensitive indicator of pancreatic acinar cell damage and pancreatic obstruction.

Newborns and children up to age 2 yr have little measurable serum amylase. In the early years of life, most of this enzyme is produced by the salivary glands. Amylase can be separated into pancreatic (P_1, P_2, P_3) and salivary (S_1, S_2, S_3) isoenzymes. Isoenzyme patterns are useful in identifying the organ source. Requests for amylase isoenzymes are rare because of the expense of the procedure and limited clinical utility of the result. Isoenzyme analysis is primarily used to assess decreasing pancreatic function in children 5 yr and older who have been diagnosed with cystic fibrosis and who may be candidates for enzyme replacement. Cyst fluid amylase levels with isoenzyme analysis is useful in differentiating pancreatic tumor (low enzyme concentration) and pseudocysts (high enzyme concentration). Lipase is usually ordered in conjunction with amylase because lipase is more sensitive and specific to conditions affecting pancreatic function.

INDICATIONS

- Assist in the diagnosis of early acute pancreatitis; serum amylase begins to rise within 6 to 24 hr after onset and returns to normal in 2 to 7 days.
- Assist in the diagnosis of macroamylasemia, a disorder seen in alcohol misuse, malabsorption syndrome, and other digestive problems.
- Assist in the diagnosis of pancreatic duct obstruction, which causes serum amylase levels to remain elevated.
- Detect blunt trauma or inadvertent surgical trauma to the pancreas.
- Differentiate between acute pancreatitis and other causes of abdominal pain that require surgery.

INTERFERING FACTORS

Factors that may alter the results of the study
- Drugs and other substances that may increase amylase levels include acetaminophen, aminosalicylic acid, amoxapine, asparaginase, aspirin, azathioprine, bethanechol, calcitriol, chlorthalidone, cholinergics, clozapine, codeine, corticosteroids, corticotropin, desipramine, dexamethasone, diazoxide, ethyl alcohol, felbamate, fentanyl, fluvastatin, glucocorticoids, hydantoin derivatives, hydrochlorothiazide, hydroflumethiazide, meperidine, mercaptopurine, methacholine, methyclothiazide, methyldopa, metolazone, minocycline, morphine, nitrofurantoin, opium alkaloids, pegaspargase, pentazocine, potassium iodide, prednisone, procyclidine, tetracycline, thiazide diuretics, valproic acid, zalcitabine, and zidovudine.
- Drugs and other substances that may decrease amylase levels include anabolic steroids, citrates, fluorides, and glucose.
- Elevated amylase levels frequently occur (75% of the time) after endoscopic retrograde cholangiopancreatography.

POTENTIAL MEDICAL DIAGNOSIS: CLINICAL SIGNIFICANCE OF RESULTS
Increased in
Amylase is released from any damaged cell in which it is stored, so conditions that affect the pancreas and parotid glands and cause cellular destruction demonstrate elevated amylase levels.

- Acute appendicitis *(related to enzyme release from damaged pancreatic tissue)*
- Administration of some drugs (e.g., morphine) is known to increase amylase levels *(related to increased biliary tract pressure as evidenced by effect of narcotic analgesic drugs)*
- Afferent loop syndrome *(related to impaired pancreatic duct flow)*
- Aortic aneurysm *(elevated amylase levels following rupture are associated with a poor prognosis; both S and P subtypes have been identified following rupture. The causes for elevation are mixed and difficult to state as a generalization)*
- Abdominal trauma *(related to release of enzyme from damaged pancreatic tissue)*

- Alcohol misuse *(related to increased secretion; salivary origin most likely)*
- Biliary tract disease *(related to impaired pancreatic duct flow)*
- Burns and traumatic shock
- Cancer of the head of the pancreas (advanced) *(related to enzyme release from damaged pancreatic tissue)*
- Chronic kidney disease *(related to decreased renal excretion as evidenced by accumulation in blood)*
- Common bile duct obstruction, common bile duct stones *(related to impaired pancreatic duct flow)*
- Diabetic ketoacidosis *(related to increased secretion; salivary origin most likely)*
- Duodenal obstruction *(accumulation in the blood as evidenced by leakage from the gut)*
- Ectopic pregnancy *(related to ectopic enzyme production by the fallopian tubes)*
- Extrapancreatic tumors (especially esophagus, lung, ovary)
- Gastric resection *(accumulation in the blood as evidenced by leakage from the gut)*
- Hyperlipidemias (etiology is unclear, but there is a distinct association with amylasemia)
- Hyperparathyroidism (etiology is unclear, but there is a distinct association with amylasemia)
- Intestinal infarction *(related to impaired pancreatic duct flow)*
- Intestinal obstruction *(related to impaired pancreatic duct flow)*
- Macroamylasemia *(related to decreased ability of renal glomeruli to filter large molecules as evidenced by accumulation in the blood)*
- Mumps *(related to increased secretion from inflamed tissue; salivary origin most likely)*
- Pancreatic ascites *(related to release of pancreatic fluid into the abdomen and subsequent absorption into the circulation)*
- Pancreatic cyst and pseudocyst *(related to release of pancreatic fluid into the abdomen and subsequent absorption into the circulation)*
- Pancreatitis *(related to enzyme release from damaged pancreatic tissue)*
- Parotitis *(related to increased secretion from inflamed tissue; salivary origin most likely)*
- Perforated peptic ulcer whether the pancreas is involved or not *(related to enzyme release from damaged pancreatic tissue; involvement of the pancreas may be unnoticed upon gross examination yet be present as indicated by elevated enzyme levels)*
- Peritonitis *(accumulation in the blood as evidenced by leakage from the gut)*
- Postoperative period *(related to complications of the surgical procedure)*
- Pregnancy *(related to increased secretion; salivary origin most likely related to hyperemesis or hyperlipidemia induced pancreatitis related to increased estrogen levels)*
- Some tumors of the lung and ovaries *(related to ectopic enzyme production)*
- Tumor of the pancreas or adjacent area *(related to release of enzyme from damaged pancreatic tissue)*

Decreased in
- Hepatic disease (severe) *(may be due to lack of amino acid production necessary for enzyme manufacture)*
- Pancreatectomy
- Pancreatic insufficiency
- Toxemia of pregnancy

NURSING IMPLICATIONS

A

POTENTIAL NURSING PROBLEMS: ASSESSMENT & NURSING DIAGNOSIS

Problems	Signs and Symptoms
Fluid volume (water) *(related to vomiting, decreased oral intake, diaphoresis, NPO with NGT, overly aggressive fluid resuscitation, compromised kidney function, overly aggressive diuresis)*	**Deficit:** Decreased urinary output, fatigue, sunken eyes, dark urine, decreased blood pressure, increased heart rate, and altered mental status **Excess:** Edema, shortness of breath, increased weight, ascites, rales, rhonchi, and decreased laboratory values *(related to dilutional effect of excess fluid)*
Gas exchange *(related to accumulation of pleural fluid, atelectasis, ventilation perfusion mismatch, altered oxygen supply)*	Irregular breathing pattern, use of accessory muscles, altered chest excursion, adventitious breath sounds (crackles, rhonchi, wheezes, diminished breath sounds), copious secretions, signs of hypoxia
Nutrition *(related to altered pancreatic function, excessive alcohol intake, insufficient eating habits, altered pancreatic or liver function)*	Inadequate caloric intake, weight loss, muscle wasting in arms and legs, stool that is pale or gray-colored, skin that is flaky with loss of elasticity
Pain *(related to pancreatic inflammation and surrounding tissues, excessive alcohol intake, infection)*	Emotional symptoms of distress, crying, agitation, facial grimace, moaning, verbalization of pain, rocking motions, irritability, disturbed sleep, diaphoresis, altered blood pressure and heart rate, nausea, vomiting, self-report of upper abdominal and gastric pain after eating fatty foods or alcohol intake with acute pancreatic disease; pain may be decreased or absent in chronic pancreatic disease

BEFORE THE STUDY: PLANNING AND IMPLEMENTATION

Teaching the Patient What to Expect

▶ Inform the patient this test can assist in evaluating pancreatic health and/or the effectiveness of medical treatment for pancreatitis.

▶ Explain that a blood sample is needed for the test.

AFTER THE STUDY: POTENTIAL NURSING ACTIONS

Treatment Considerations

▶ Fluid Volume: Explain symptoms of fluid overload and deficit, including principles of proper hydration. Teach how to measure intake and output and record results accurately.

▶ Gas Exchange: Explain incentive spirometer use with deep cough to maintain open airways and move secretions interfering with adequate oxygenation. As appropriate, explain how to accurately self-administer oxygen.

Nutritional Considerations

- Vitamin B$_{12}$ may be ordered for parenteral administration to patients with decreased levels, if their disease prevents adequate oral absorption.
- A progressive diet including; clear liquid diet, low-fat, high-carbohydrate, may begin after the return of bowel sounds. Small, frequent meals

and dietary alterations are recommended in the case of gastrointestinal disorders.

Follow-Up, Evaluation, and Desired Outcomes

- Understands the link between alcohol use and disease process and that increased amylase levels may be associated with gastrointestinal disease and/or alcoholism.
- Agrees to avoid alcohol and to seek appropriate counseling.

Angiography, Various Sites
(Abdomen, Adrenal, Carotid, Kidneys, Lungs)

SYNONYM/ACRONYM: Angiogram, arteriography.

RATIONALE: To visualize and assess internal organs/structures for abnormal or absent anatomical features, abscess, aneurysm, cancer or other masses, infection, or presence of disease.

PATIENT PREPARATION: There are no activity restrictions unless by medical direction. Instruct the patient to fast and restrict fluids for 8 hr, or as ordered, prior to the procedure. Fasting may be ordered as a precaution against aspiration related to possible nausea and vomiting. The American Society of Anesthesiologists has fasting guidelines for risk levels according to patient status. More information can be located at www.asahq.org.

Note: If iodinated contrast medium is scheduled to be used in patients receiving metformin or drugs containing metformin for type 2 diabetes, the drug may be discontinued on the day of the test and continue to be withheld for 48 hr after the test. Regarding the patient's risk for bleeding, the patient should be instructed to avoid taking natural products and medications with known anticoagulant, antiplatelet, or thrombolytic properties or to reduce dosage, as ordered, prior to the procedure. Number of days to withhold medication is dependent on the type of anticoagulant. Note the last time and dose of medication taken. Patients on beta blockers before the surgical procedure should be instructed to take their medication as ordered during the perioperative period. Protocols may vary among facilities.

NORMAL FINDINGS

- Normal structure, function, and patency of organ vessels
- Contrast medium normally circulates throughout area of inquiry symmetrically and without interruption.

- No evidence of obstruction, variations in number and size of vessels and organs, malformations, cysts, or tumors

CRITICAL FINDINGS AND POTENTIAL INTERVENTIONS
- Abdominal abscess
- Abdominal aneurysm
- Pulmonary embolism
- Stroke
- Adrenal disease

Timely notification to the requesting health-care provider (HCP) of any critical findings and related symptoms is a role expectation of the professional nurse. A listing of these findings varies among facilities.

OVERVIEW: (Study type: X-ray, special/contrast; related body system: Circulatory, Digestive, Endocrine, Respiratory, Urinary systems.) Angiography provides x-ray visualization of organs and associated branches of the vasculature and organ parenchyma. A digital image is taken prior to injection of the contrast and then again after the contrast has been injected through a catheter, which has been inserted into an artery (arteriography) or vein (venography). Fluoroscopy is used to guide catheter placement, and angiograms (high-speed x-ray images) provide images of the organ and associated vessels of interest that are displayed on a monitor and are recorded for future viewing and evaluation. The x-ray equipment is mounted on a C-shaped arm with the x-ray device beneath the table on which the patient lies. Over the patient is an image intensifier that receives the x-rays after they pass through the patient. Digital subtraction angiography (DSA) is a computerized method of removing from the image undesired structures, such as bone, from the surrounding area of interest. By subtracting the preinjection image from the postinjection image, a higher-quality, unobstructed image can be created. Patterns of circulation, organ function, and changes in vessel wall appearance can be viewed to help diagnose the presence of vascular abnormalities, aneurysm, tumor, trauma, or lesions. The catheter used to administer the contrast medium to confirm the diagnosis of organ lesions may be used to deliver chemotherapeutic drugs or different types of materials administered to stop bleeding. Catheters with attached inflatable balloons for angioplasty and wire mesh stents are used to widen areas of stenosis and to keep vessels open, frequently replacing surgery. Embolotherapy can also be accomplished through the same catheter when the site of bleeding or extravasation is located. Angiography is also valuable because other imaging studies cannot always visualize a tumor, especially if it is small. Angiography is one of the definitive tests for organ disease and may be used to evaluate chronic disease and organ failure, treat arterial stenosis, differentiate a vascular cyst from hypervascular cancers, and evaluate the effectiveness of medical or surgical treatment.

In addition to its other indications, adrenal angiography is used to accomplish adrenal venous sampling which can be very challenging. Blood samples may be taken from the vein of each gland and the distal portion of the vena cava to assess cortisol and adrenocorticotropic hormone (ACTH) levels. The information is used to assist in determining a diagnosis of ACTH-independent Cushing syndrome (benign or malignant adrenal growth that secretes cortisol) or primary hyperaldosteronism (excessive adrenal gland production of aldosterone). The gold standard for distinguishing between a cortisol-secreting tumor and unilateral or bilateral adrenal hyperplasia is considered to be measurement of aldosterone/cortisol ratios taken from a series of samples during adrenal angiography. Cortisol levels will be elevated if related to Cushing syndrome. A ratio of greater than 4:1 is indicative of unilateral hyperplasia. Ratios between each gland are similar and usually less than 3:1 in the presence of bilateral hyperplasia. Obtaining the correct diagnosis from the angiogram is important because treatment for adrenal adenoma and unilateral adrenal hyperplasia is surgical removal of the affected adrenal gland, whereas bilateral adrenal hypertrophy is treated medically.

Carotid angiography evaluates blood vessels in the neck carrying arterial blood to the brain and is accomplished by the injection of contrast material into the carotid artery through a catheter that has been initially inserted into the femoral artery.

Pulmonary angiograms are requested less frequently in favor of CT pulmonary angiograms, which are less invasive, faster, have fewer complications, and are of similar quality.

INDICATIONS

General

- Allow infusion of thrombolytic drugs into an occluded artery.
- Assist with angioplasty, atherectomy, or stent placement.
- Assist with the collection of blood and tissue samples for laboratory analysis.
- Detect and evaluate tumors before surgery or embolization, *evidenced by arterial supply, extent of venous invasion, and tumor vascularity.*
- Detect arterial occlusion, *evidenced by a transection of the affected artery caused by trauma or a penetrating injury.*
- Detect arterial or venous stenosis, *evidenced by vessel dilation, collateral vessels, or increased vascular pressure.*
- Detect absence of an organ or associated structure; arteriovenous fistula, aneurysms, congenital defects; emboli in vessels, or thrombosis.
- Differentiate between tumors and cysts.
- Evaluate chronic organ disease.
- Evaluate the vascular system of prospective organ donors before surgery.
- Evaluate organ transplantation for function or organ rejection.
- Evaluate placement of a shunt or stent.

Abdominal

- Detect peripheral arterial disease (PAD).

Adrenal

- Detect adrenal hyperplasia.

- Evaluate medical therapy or surgery of the adrenal glands.
- Identify pheochromocytoma.

Carotid
- Assess risk of stroke.
- Determine the need for further treatment.
- Evaluate the degree of carotid artery blockage.

Lungs
- Detect anomalous pulmonary venous drainage and vascular changes associated with chronic obstructive pulmonary disease, blebs, and bullae.
- Determine the cause of recurrent or severe hemoptysis.
- Evaluate pulmonary circulation.
- Hemodynamic measurements during pulmonary angiography can assist in the diagnosis of pulmonary hypertension and cor pulmonale.

INTERFERING FACTORS
Contraindications
⬥ Patients who are pregnant or suspected of being pregnant, unless the potential benefits of a procedure using radiation far outweigh the risk of radiation exposure to the fetus and mother.

⬥ Conditions associated with adverse reactions to contrast medium (e.g., asthma, food allergies, or allergy to contrast medium). Although patients are asked specifically if they have a known allergy to iodine or shellfish (shellfish contain high levels of iodine), it has been well established that the reaction is not to iodine; an actual iodine allergy would be problematic because iodine is required for the production of thyroid hormones. In the case of shellfish, the reaction is to a muscle protein called *tropomyosin*; in the case of iodinated contrast medium, the reaction is to the noniodinated part of the contrast molecule. Patients with a known hypersensitivity to the medium may benefit from premedication with corticosteroids and diphenhydramine; the use of nonionic contrast or an alternative noncontrast imaging study, if available, may be considered for patients who have severe asthma or who have experienced moderate to severe reactions to ionic contrast medium.

⬥ Conditions associated with preexisting renal insufficiency (e.g., chronic kidney disease, single kidney transplant, nephrectomy, diabetes, multiple myeloma, treatment with aminoglycosides and NSAIDs) *because iodinated contrast is nephrotoxic.*

⬥ Patients who are chronically dehydrated before the test, especially older adults and patients whose health is already compromised, *because of their risk of contrast-induced acute kidney injury.*

⬥ Patients with pheochromocytoma, *because iodinated contrast may cause a hypertensive crisis.*

⬥ Patients with bleeding disorders or receiving anticoagulant therapy, *because the puncture site may not stop bleeding.*

Factors that may alter the results of the study
- Gas or feces in the gastrointestinal (GI) tract resulting from inadequate cleansing or failure to restrict food intake before the study.
- Retained barium from a previous radiological procedure; barium studies should be performed more than 4 days before angiography.
- Metallic objects (e.g., jewelry, body rings) within the examination field, which may inhibit organ visualization and cause unclear images.
- Inability of the patient to cooperate or remain still during the procedure, because movement can produce blurred or otherwise unclear images.

POTENTIAL MEDICAL DIAGNOSIS: CLINICAL SIGNIFICANCE OF RESULTS

Abnormal findings related to

General
- Abscess or inflammation, *as seen by edema in the area of the vessel*
- Aneurysms, *visualized by a bulging in a vessel*
- Arteriovenous fistula or other abnormalities
- Cancer
- Congenital anomalies
- Cysts visualized by areas with a halo of contrast surrounding them or tumors, *indicated by areas of increased density due to the vascularity which collects the contrast*
- Trauma causing tears or other disruption, *indicated by blood outside the vessel*
- Vascular blockage, stenosis, dysplasia, or organ infarction, *indicated by a narrowing or blocked artery*

Abdomen
- PAD

Adrenal
- Adrenal adenoma
- Bilateral adrenal hyperplasia
- Pheochromocytoma

Carotid
- Increased stroke risk *related to occluded carotid artery*

Kidneys
- Intrarenal hematoma

Lungs
- Bleeding caused by tuberculosis, bronchiectasis, sarcoidosis, or aspergilloma
- Pulmonary embolism (PE) acute or chronic, *visualized as an area of interrupted opacity in the pulmonary artery*
- Pulmonary sequestration

NURSING IMPLICATIONS

POTENTIAL NURSING PROBLEMS: ASSESSMENT & NURSING DIAGNOSIS

Problems	Signs and Symptoms
Abdomen: Inadequate cardiac output *(related to dissection, rupture)*	Altered level of consciousness; hypotension; increased, potentially thready pulse; delayed capillary refill; diminished peripheral pulses; cool skin; restlessness; anxiety
Abdomen: Inadequate tissue perfusion *(related to dissection, rupture, trauma, stricture, occlusion)*	Elevated blood pressure, pulsing abdominal mass, elevated heart rate, self-report of severe abdominal pain that radiates to the flank, possible pain in the back and groin
Abdomen: Pain *(related to diminished perfusion, rupture, dissection, trauma, stricture, occlusion)*	Self-report of severe abdominal pain that radiates to the flank, possible pain in the back and groin, agitation, restlessness, crying, stoicism
Adrenal: Body image *(related to altered androgen production, cortisol excess, altered protein metabolism, altered body fat distribution)*	Abnormal hair growth, muscle and bone matrix wasting, moon-shaped face, obesity located in the trunk of the body, presence of a cervicodorsal lump, verbalization of negative feelings about body image, social withdrawal

Problems	Signs and Symptoms
Adrenal: Fluid overload *(related to water retention associated with excess cortisol)*	Shortness of breath, tachycardia, hypertension, positive jugular vein distention, edema, electrolyte imbalance (potassium, sodium)
Carotid: Inadequate tissue perfusion *(related to blockage, hemorrhage, mass, edema, infection, plaque, atrophy, abscess, cyst, tumor)*	Diminished or altered level of consciousness, expressive or receptive aphasia, loss of sensory functionality, slurred speech, difficulty swallowing, difficulty in completing a learned activity or in recognizing familiar objects (apraxia, agnosia), motor function deficits, spatial neglect, facial droop and/or varying degrees of flaccid extremities, pain, fever
Kidneys: Infection *(related to obstruction, aneurysm, inflammation, cyst, anomaly, structural abnormality, abscess, inflammation, trauma, injury)*	Positive culture, chills, elevated temperature, elevated white blood cell count, flank pain, hematuria, urinary frequency
Kidneys: Pain *(related to infection, inflammation, obstruction, anomaly, structural abnormality, bleeding, infection, trauma)*	Self-report of pain; facial grimace; crying; restlessness; diaphoresis; nausea; vomiting; guarding; social withdrawal; elevated blood pressure, heart rate, respiratory rate; pallor
Lungs: Breathing *(related to fear, anxiety, pain, insufficient oxygenation, inflammation, infection, mass, embolus)*	Shortness of breath; skin that is cool, clammy, and cyanotic; anxiety; chest pain; decreased oxygenation; abnormal blood gas; increased work of breathing (use of accessory muscles); increased respiratory rate
Lungs: Inadequate gas exchange *(related to obstruction, mass, infection, bleeding, embolus, tumor inflammation)*	Difficulty breathing, shortness of breath (dyspnea), chest pain (pleuritic), diminished oxygenation, cyanosis, increased heart rate, increased respiratory rate, restlessness, anxiety, fear, adventitious breath sounds (rales, crackles), sense of impending death and doom, hemoptysis, abnormal arterial blood gas
Lungs: Pain *(related to embolus, mass, inflammation, infection, malformations, tumor)*	Self-report of pain, increased respiratory rate, increased heart rate, fear, anxiety, restlessness, crying, moaning

BEFORE THE STUDY: PLANNING AND IMPLEMENTATION

Teaching the Patient What to Expect
- Inform the patient this procedure can assist in assessing internal organs and other anatomical areas of interest.

- Explain that prior to the procedure, laboratory testing may be required to determine the possibility of bleeding risk (coagulation testing) or to assess for impaired kidney function (Cr level and estimated glomerular filtration rate) if use of iodinated contrast medium is anticipated.

‣ Pregnancy is a general contraindication to procedures involving radiation. Explain to the female patient that she will be asked the date of her last menstrual period. Pregnancy testing may be performed to determine the possibility of pregnancy before exposure to radiation.

‣ Explain that reducing health-care-associated infections is an important patient safety goal, and a number of different safety practices will be implemented during their procedure. Advise the patient that hair in the area near the catheter insertion site may be clipped or shaved and the area cleaned with an antiseptic solution to cleanse bacteria from the skin in order to reduce the risk for infection. *Note:* The World Health Organization, Centers for Disease Control and Prevention, and Association of periOperative Registered Nurses recommend that hair not be removed at all unless it interferes with the incision site or other aspects of the procedure because hair removal by any means is associated with increased infection rates. When hair removal is necessary, facilities must use a protocol that is based on scientific literature or the endorsement of a professional organization. Clipping immediately before the procedure and in a location outside the procedure area is preferred to shaving with a razor. Shaving creates a break in skin integrity and provides a way for bacteria on the skin to enter the incision site.

‣ Review the procedure with the patient. Address concerns about pain and explain that there may be moments of discomfort or pain experienced when the IV line or catheter is inserted to allow infusion of fluids such as saline, anesthetics, sedatives, contrast medium, medications used in the procedure, or emergency medications.

‣ Explain that contrast medium will be injected, by catheter, at a separate site from the IV line.

‣ Advise that a burning and flushing sensation may be felt throughout the body during injection of the contrast medium, and the patient may experience an urge to cough, flushing, nausea, or a salty or metallic taste.

‣ Advise the patient that the procedure is usually performed in a radiology or vascular suite by an HCP and takes approximately 30 to 60 min.

‣ Instruct the patient to remove jewelry and other metallic objects from the area of examination.

‣ Baseline vital signs will be recorded and monitored throughout the procedure. Protocols may vary among facilities.

‣ Explain that electrocardiographic electrodes will be placed for cardiac monitoring to establish a baseline rhythm and identify any ventricular dysrhythmias.

‣ Explain that peripheral pulses will be marked with a pen before the venography, allowing for a quicker and more consistent assessment of the pulses after the procedure.

‣ Positioning for this procedure is in the supine position on an examination table. The selected area will be cleansed and covered with a sterile drape.

‣ A local anesthetic will be injected at the site, and a small incision is made or a needle inserted under fluoroscopy.

‣ Once contrast medium is injected, a rapid series of images is taken during and after the filling of the vessels to be examined. Delayed images may be taken to examine the vessels after a time and to monitor the venous phase of the procedure.

‣ Advise the patient that he or she will be instructed to inhale deeply and hold his or her breath while the x-ray images are taken, and then instructed to exhale.

‣ Advise taking slow, deep breaths if nausea occurs during the procedure. An ordered antiemetic drug can be administered as needed. An emesis basin can be ready for use.

‣ Explain to the patient that he or she will be monitored for complications related to the procedure (e.g., allergic reaction, anaphylaxis, bronchospasm).

‣ Explain that once the study is completed, the needle or catheter is removed, and a pressure dressing is applied over the puncture site.

A

Potential Nursing Actions

✦ *Make sure a written and informed consent has been signed prior to the procedure and before administering any medications.*

▶ Glucagon or an anticholinergic drug may be given to stabilize movement of the stomach muscles; peristaltic contractions (motion) may alter study findings.

▶ If iodinated contrast medium is scheduled to be used in patients receiving metformin or drugs containing metformin for type 2 diabetes, the drug may be discontinued on the day of the test and continue to be withheld for 48 hr after the test. Protocols may vary among facilities.

Safety Considerations

▶ Anticoagulants, aspirin, and other salicylates should be discontinued by medical direction for the appropriate number of days prior to a procedure if bleeding is a potential complication.

AFTER THE STUDY: POTENTIAL NURSING ACTIONS

Avoiding Complications

▶ Establishing an IV site and injection of contrast medium are invasive procedures. Complications are rare but include risk for allergic reaction *(related to contrast reaction),* bleeding from the puncture site *(related to a bleeding disorder or the effects of natural products and medications with known anticoagulant, antiplatelet, or thrombolytic properties; postprocedural bleeding from the site is rare because at the conclusion of the procedure a resorbable device, composed of non-latex-containing arterial anchor, collagen plug, and suture, is deployed to seal the puncture site),* blood clot formation *(related to thrombus formation on the tip of the catheter sheath surface or in the lumen of the catheter; the use of a heparinized saline flush during the procedure decreases the risk of emboli),* hematoma *(related to blood leakage into the tissue following needle insertion),* infection *(which might occur if bacteria from the skin surface is introduced at the puncture site),* tissue damage *(related to extravasation or leaking of contrast into the tissues during injection),* nerve injury or damage to a nearby organ *(which might occur if the catheter strikes a nerve or perforates an organ),* or nephrotoxicity *(a deterioration of renal function associated with contrast administration).* Monitor the patient for complications related to the procedure (e.g., allergic reaction, anaphylaxis, bronchospasm, infection, injury). Immediately report symptoms such as difficulty breathing, chest pain, fever, hyperpnea, hypertension, nausea, palpitations, pruritus, rash, tachycardia, urticaria, or vomiting to the appropriate HCP. Observe/assess the needle/catheter insertion site for bleeding, inflammation, or hematoma formation. Administer ordered antihistamines or prophylactic steroids if the patient has an allergic reaction. Assess extremities for signs of ischemia or absence of distal pulse caused by a catheter-induced thrombus.

▶ Some system-specific adverse effects are abdomen (GI) *(nausea, vomiting, diarrhea, cramping),* adrenal *(hypertension associated with pheochromocytoma),* brain *(headache, confusion, dizziness, seizure),* kidney *(oliguria, hypertension, contrast induced nephropathy),* lung (respiratory) *(laryngeal edema, bronchospasm, pulmonary edema).*

Treatment Considerations

▶ Instruct the patient to resume usual diet, fluids, medications, or activity, as directed by the HCP. Kidney function should be assessed before metformin is resumed.

▶ Monitor vital signs and neurological status every 15 min for 1 hr, then every 2 hr for 4 hr, then as ordered by the HCP or per facility protocol. Take temperature every 4 hr for 24 hr or per facility protocol.

▶ Monitor peripheral pulses as well as changes in the color or temperature of the skin around the insertion site that may be indicative of bleeding.

A

▶ Maintain bedrest in the supine position *to prevent stress on the puncture site* for 2 to 6 hr depending on the location of the insertion site.

▶ Monitor intake and output and renal status at least every 8 hr. Compare with baseline values. Protocols may vary among facilities.

▶ Provide IV fluid to support blood pressure (rapid rate as appropriate) or blood transfusion as ordered.

▶ Other general postprocedural assessments are as follows: Assess pain character, location, duration, intensity; use an easily understood pain-rating scale; place in a position of comfort; administer ordered medications; consider alternative measures for pain management (imagery, relaxation, music, etc.); assess and trend vital signs; facilitate a calm, quiet environment; encourage oral fluids if not contraindicated; administer ordered parenteral fluids; monitor voiding patterns (urgency, frequency, incontinence) and for the presence of hematuria; strain urine; monitor and trend laboratory and diagnostic studies.

Safety Considerations

▶ Advise diabetic patients to avoid all medications containing metformin for 48 hr following a procedure with iodinated contrast. Iodinated contrast can temporarily impair kidney function, and failure to withhold metformin may indirectly result in drug-induced lactic acidosis, a dangerous and sometimes fatal adverse effect of metformin (related to renal impairment that does not support sufficient excretion of metformin).

Follow-Up, Evaluation, and Desired Outcomes

▶ Understands the importance of maintaining bedrest for 4 to 6 hr after the procedure or as ordered and of applying cold compresses to the puncture site as needed to reduce discomfort or edema.

▶ Verbalizes how to correctly assess the site for bleeding, hematoma formation,

bile leakage, and inflammation and how to provide site care.

▶ Acknowledges the importance of adhering to the therapy regimen. States significant adverse effects associated with the prescribed medication and the option for literature review provided by a pharmacist.

▶ Acknowledges contact information provided for the Legs for Life (www .legsforlife.org).

Abdomen

▶ Acknowledges the importance of managing hypertension to decrease bleeding risk.

▶ Verbalizes the signs and symptoms of transfusion reaction.

Adrenal

▶ Discusses end-of-life options as appropriate to the prognosis.

▶ Agrees that adequate rest and adherence to the recommended therapeutic regime is key to the patient's overall health.

Carotid

▶ States the importance of adhering to follow-up diagnostic and laboratory studies necessary to monitor health status and the effectiveness of treatment modalities.

Kidney

▶ Describes dietary and lifestyle changes that will facilitate renal health.

▶ Acknowledges the importance of completing the prescribed antibiotic regime.

▶ Demonstrates the correct technique to measure and record intake and output.

Lung

▶ Discusses the importance of remaining on bedrest to prevent oxygen desaturation with activity. Discusses the importance of keeping oxygen in use, as ordered.

▶ Correctly states the reportable signs of bleeding (bleeding gums, black tarry stools, blood in urine, hematoma) if started on thrombolytics.

Angiotensin Converting Enzyme

A

SYNONYM/ACRONYM: Angiotensin I–converting enzyme (ACE).

RATIONALE: To assist in diagnosing, evaluating treatment, and monitoring the progression of sarcoidosis, a granulomatous disease that primarily affects the lungs.

PATIENT PREPARATION: There are no food, fluid, or medication restrictions unless by medical direction.

NORMAL FINDINGS: Method: Spectrophotometry.

Age	Conventional Units	SI Units (Conventional Units × 16.667)
Newborn–child	5–83 units/L	83–1,383 nKat/L
Adult	12–68 units/L	200–1,133 nKat/L

CRITICAL FINDINGS AND POTENTIAL INTERVENTIONS: N/A

OVERVIEW: (**Study type:** Blood collected in a gold-, red-, or red/gray-top tube; **related body system:** Circulatory, Endocrine, Respiratory systems.) Production of angiotensin-converting enzyme (ACE) occurs mainly in the epithelial cells of the pulmonary bed. ACE levels are used primarily in the evaluation of active sarcoidosis, a granulomatous disease that can affect many organs, including the lungs. Sarcoidosis is identified more frequently in females than in males, most often between 20 and 40 years of age, and is 10 to 15 times more common in people of African descent than in Caucasians. Other ethnic groups prone to develop sarcoidosis include individuals of Scandinavian, German, Irish, or Puerto Rican descent. Serial levels are useful in correlating the therapeutic response to corticosteroid treatment.

Increasing ACE levels with positive gallium scans in sarcoidosis patients receiving steroids indicate a poor response to therapy. Monitoring ACE levels may also have some utility in assessing the risk of pulmonary damage in affected patients receiving antineoplastic drugs. Thyroid hormones may play a role in regulating ACE levels. Decreased levels have been noted in patients with clinical hypothyroidism and anorexia nervosa, whereas increased levels have been noted in patients with hyperthyroidism. Elevations of serum ACE have been reported in 20% to 30% of patients with abnormal α_1-antitrypsin variants. ACE levels are sometimes ordered on cerebrospinal fluid to evaluate patients with neurosarcoidosis. Results must be interpreted with care because of the nonspecificity of increased

A

and decreased ACE levels, especially in the pediatric population among whom normal values run higher than in other age groups.

Conversion of angiotensin I to angiotensin II by ACE helps regulate arterial blood pressure, and for this reason, ACE levels are used to evaluate hypertension. Angiotensin II stimulates the adrenal cortex to produce aldosterone. Aldosterone is a hormone that helps the kidneys maintain water balance by retaining sodium and promoting the excretion of potassium. (See studies titled "Aldosterone" and "Renin.")

INDICATIONS

- Assist in establishing a diagnosis of sarcoidosis.
- Assist in the evaluation of Gaucher disease.
- Assist in the treatment of sarcoidosis.
- Evaluate hypertension.
- Evaluate the severity and activity of sarcoidosis.

INTERFERING FACTORS

Factors that may alter the results of the study

- Drugs and other substances that may increase serum ACE levels include nicardipine.
- Drugs and other substances that may decrease serum ACE levels include benazepril, captopril, cilazapril, enalapril, fosinopril, lisinopril, nicardipine, pentopril, perindopril, prednisone (some patients), propranolol, quinapril, ramipril, and trandolapril.
- Prompt and proper specimen processing, storage, and analysis

are important to achieve accurate results. Failure to freeze sample if not tested immediately may cause falsely decreased values because ACE degrades rapidly.

POTENTIAL MEDICAL DIAGNOSIS: CLINICAL SIGNIFICANCE OF RESULTS
Increased in

- Bronchitis (acute and chronic) *(related to release of ACE from damaged pulmonary tissue)*
- Connective tissue disease *(related to release of ACE from scarred and damaged pulmonary tissue)*
- Gaucher disease *(related to release of ACE from damaged pulmonary tissue; Gaucher disease is due to the hereditary deficiency of an enzyme that results in accumulation of a fatty substance that damages pulmonary tissue)*
- Hansen disease (leprosy)
- Histoplasmosis and other fungal diseases
- Hyperthyroidism (untreated) *(related to possible involvement of thyroid hormones in regulation of ACE)*
- Pulmonary fibrosis *(related to release of ACE from damaged pulmonary tissue)*
- Rheumatoid arthritis *(related to development of interstitial lung disease, pulmonary fibrosis, and release of ACE from damaged pulmonary tissue)*
- Sarcoidosis *(related to release of ACE from damaged pulmonary tissue)*

Decreased in

- Advanced pulmonary cancer *(related to lack of functional cells to produce ACE)*

- The period following corticosteroid therapy for sarcoidosis
(*evidenced by cessation of effective
therapy*)

NURSING IMPLICATIONS

BEFORE THE STUDY: PLANNING AND IMPLEMENTATION

Teaching the Patient What to Expect

▶ Inform the patient this test can assist in identifying various health problems.

▶ Explain that a blood sample is needed for the test.

Potential Nursing Actions

▶ Review the patient's personal health record and confirm the patient's age, as this study is rarely performed on patients under the age of 20.

AFTER THE STUDY: POTENTIAL NURSING ACTIONS

Avoiding Complications

▶ Explain the increased risk for infection to patients who will be receiving long-term corticosteroid treatment, and review ways to avoid illness. Teach patients the signs and symptoms of steroid withdrawal so they will be aware of changes that will occur as their body reacts to decreasing levels of steroid medication.

Treatment Considerations

▶ For patients who have diabetes and are on corticosteroid therapy, explain the importance of frequent glucose monitoring.

▶ Demonstrate the use of oxygen, as needed.

Nutritional Considerations

▶ Educate patients regarding access to nutritional counseling services. Stress the importance of a nutritious diet with adequate amounts of fluid. ACE levels affect the regulation of fluid balance and electrolytes. Dietary adjustment may be considered if sodium allowances need to be regulated. Educate patients with low sodium levels that the major source of dietary sodium is found in table salt. Many foods, such as milk and other dairy products, are also good sources of dietary sodium. Most other dietary sodium is available through consumption of processed foods. Patients who need to follow low-sodium diets should be advised to avoid beverages such as colas, ginger ale, Gatorade, lemon-lime sodas, and root beer. Many over-the-counter medications, including antacids, laxatives, analgesics, sedatives, and antitussives, contain significant amounts of sodium. The best advice is to emphasize the importance of reading all food, beverage, and medicine labels. A health-care provider or registered dietitian should be consulted before considering the use of salt substitutes.

Follow-Up, Evaluation, and Desired Outcomes

▶ Acknowledges contact information provided for the U.S. Department of Agriculture's resource for nutrition (www.choosemyplate.gov).

▶ Understands the increased risk for infection while receiving long-term corticosteroid treatment and states ways to avoid illness.

▶ Demonstrates the correct use of oxygen, as needed.

A

Antiactin Antibody (Smooth Muscle) and Antimitochondrial M2 Antibody

SYNONYM/ACRONYM: Antiactin antibody, ASMA; mitochondrial M2 antibody, M2 antibody, AMA.

RATIONALE: To assist in the differential diagnosis of chronic liver disease, typically biliary cholangitis.

PATIENT PREPARATION: There are no food, fluid, activity, or medication restrictions unless by medical direction.

NORMAL FINDINGS: Method: Immunoassay, enzyme-linked immunosorbent (ELISA).

Actin smooth muscle antibody, IgG

Negative	Less than 20 units
Weak positive	20–30 units
Positive	Greater than 30 units

Mitochondrial M2 antibody, IgG

Negative	Less than 20 units
Weak positive	20.1–24.9 units
Positive	Greater than 25 units

CRITICAL FINDINGS AND POTENTIAL INTERVENTIONS: N/A

OVERVIEW: (**Study type:** Blood collected in a red-top tube; **related body system:** Digestive and Immune systems.) Primary biliary cholangitis (PBC), formerly called primary biliary cirrhosis, is a disease in which the small bile ducts of the liver are destroyed by an inflammatory process. Antimitochondrial antibodies are found in 90% of patients with PBC. Mitochondrial M2 antibody has a higher degree of specificity than any of the other three types of detectable mitochondrial antibodies (M1, M5, M6) for PBC. PBC is identified most frequently in women ages 35 to 60. Testing is useful in the differential diagnosis of chronic liver disease because antimitochondrial antibodies are rarely detected in extrahepatic biliary obstruction, various forms of hepatitis, and cirrhosis. Antismooth muscle antibodies are autoantibodies found in high titers in the sera of patients with autoimmune diseases of the liver and bile duct. Smooth muscle antibodies are directed against the F-actin subunits present in all smooth muscle fibers and are therefore not organ specific. Simultaneous testing for antimitochondrial antibodies can be useful in the differential diagnosis of chronic liver disease.

INDICATIONS

Actin smooth muscle antibodies (ASMA)
• Differential diagnosis of liver disease.

Mitochondrial M2 antibodies (AMA)
• Assist in the diagnosis of PBC.
• Assist in the differential diagnosis of chronic liver disease.

INTERFERING FACTORS
Factors that may alter the results of the study
• Drugs and other substances that may increase mitochondrial M2 (AMA) levels include labetalol *(related to liver damage).*
• Drugs and other substances that may decrease mitochondrial M2 (AMA) levels include cyclosporine and ursodiol.

POTENTIAL MEDICAL DIAGNOSIS: CLINICAL SIGNIFICANCE OF RESULTS
Increased in
The exact cause of PBC is unknown. There is a high degree of correlation between the presence of ASMA and AMA with PBC, and PBC therefore is thought to be an autoimmune disease. The antibodies have been identified in the sera of patients with other autoimmune diseases.

ASMA
• Autoimmune hepatitis
• Chronic active viral hepatitis
• Infectious mononucleosis
• PBC
• Primary sclerosing cholangitis

AMA
• Hepatitis (alcohol misuse, viral)
• PBC

• Rheumatoid arthritis (occasionally)
• Systemic lupus erythematosus (occasionally)
• Thyroid disease (occasionally)

Decreased in: N/A

NURSING IMPLICATIONS

BEFORE THE STUDY: PLANNING AND IMPLEMENTATION

Teaching the Patient What to Expect
▶ Inform the patient this test can assist in the diagnosis of liver disease.
▶ Explain that a blood sample is needed for the test.

Potential Nursing Actions
▶ Assess and trend liver enzymes (ALT, AST, ALKP, GGT) and ammonia.

AFTER THE STUDY: POTENTIAL NURSING ACTIONS

Avoiding Complications
▶ Observe the cirrhotic patient carefully for the development of ascites; if ascites develops, pay strict attention to fluid and electrolyte balance. Measure and trend abdominal girth to evaluate the extent of ascites and fluid retention.

Treatment Considerations
▶ Increase frequency of vital signs and trend; administer blood or blood products as ordered; administer stool softeners as needed; encourage intake of foods rich in vitamin K; avoid foods that may irritate esophagus.
▶ Suggest the use of eye drops and throat lozenges to alleviate symptoms associated with dry eyes and lack of moisture in the mucous membranes of the mouth and throat.
▶ Apply lotion to keep the skin moisturized; avoid alkaline soaps; discourage scratching; apply mittens if patient is not able to follow direction to avoid scratching; administer antihistamines as ordered.

A

A

Safety Considerations

▶ Loss of bone density can lead to osteoporosis and increased fall risk. Increased physical activity can stimulate osteoblast activity and improve bone growth. Avoid risky activities that can lead to fracture. Ensure a safe environment in both the clinical and home setting to decrease fall injury risk. Teach the patient specific measures than can decrease fall risk (use of assistive devices, postural support devices, removal of items that can cause tripping). Use fall precautions and restraints if necessary. Consider pharmacological interventions for confused patients.

Nutritional Considerations

▶ The presence of antimitochondrial or antismooth muscle antibodies may be associated with liver disease. In general, patients should be encouraged to eat a well balanced diet that includes foods high in fiber. Dietary recommendations will vary depending on the condition and its severity. For example, recommend a diet of soft foods if esophageal varices develop, fat substitutes for bile duct disease, or limitations on salt intake if ascites develop.

▶ Document food intake with possible calorie count; assess barriers to eating; consider using a food diary; monitor continued alcohol use, as it is a barrier to adequate protein nutrition; monitor glucose levels; dietary consult with assessment of cultural food selections.

Follow-Up, Evaluation, and Desired Outcomes

▶ States understanding of the importance of eating small, frequent meals throughout the day to increase overall caloric intake and improve nutritional status.

▶ Acknowledges that scratching can damage the skin and precipitate an infection.

▶ Understands that adherence to taking lactulose can decrease blood ammonia level and help prevent hepatic encephalopathy.

Anticardiolipin Antibody, Immunoglobulin A, Immunoglobulin G, and Immunoglobulin M

SYNONYM/ACRONYM: Antiphospholipid antibody, lupus anticoagulant, LA, ACA.

RATIONALE: To detect the presence of antiphospholipid antibodies, which can lead to the development of blood vessel problems and complications including stroke, heart attack, and miscarriage.

PATIENT PREPARATION: There are no food, fluid, activity, or medication restrictions unless by medical direction.

NORMAL FINDINGS: Method: Immunoassay, enzyme-linked immunosorbent assay (ELISA).

IgA (APL = 1 unit IgA phospholipid)	IgG (GPL = 1 unit IgG phospholipid)	IgM (MPL = 1 unit IgM phospholipid)
Negative: 0–11 APL	Negative: 0–14 GPL	Negative: 0–12 MPL
Indeterminate: 12–19 APL	Indeterminate: 15–19 GPL	Indeterminate: 13–19 MPL

IgA (APL = 1 unit IgA phospholipid)	IgG (GPL = 1 unit IgG phospholipid)	IgM (MPL = 1 unit IgM phospholipid)
Low-medium positive: 20–80 APL Positive: Greater than 80 APL	Low-medium positive: 20–80 GPL Positive: Greater than 80 GPL	Low-medium positive: 20–80 MPL Greater than 80 MPL

CRITICAL FINDINGS AND POTENTIAL INTERVENTIONS: N/A

OVERVIEW: (Study type: Blood collected in a red-top tube; related body system: Circulatory, Immune, and Reproductive systems.) Anticardiolipin (ACA) is one of several identified antiphospholipid antibodies. ACAs are of IgG, IgM, and IgA subtypes, which react with proteins in the blood that are bound to phospholipid and interfere with normal blood vessel function. The two primary types of problems they cause are narrowing and irregularity of the blood vessels and blood clots in the blood vessels. ACAs are found in individuals with lupus erythematosus, lupus-related conditions, infectious diseases, drug reactions, and sometimes fetal loss. ACAs are often found in association with lupus anticoagulant. Increased antiphospholipid antibody levels have been found in pregnant women with lupus who have had miscarriages. β_2 Glycoprotein 1, or apolipoprotein H, is an important facilitator in the binding of antiphospholipid antibodies such as ACA. A normal level of β_2 glycoprotein 1 is 19 units or less when measured by ELISA. β_2 Glycoprotein 1 measurements are considered to be more specific than ACA because they do not demonstrate nonspecific reactivity as do ACA in sera of patients with syphilis

or other infectious diseases. The combination of noninflammatory thrombosis of blood vessels, low platelet count, and history of miscarriage is termed *antiphospholipid antibody syndrome.* It is documented as present if at least one of the clinical and one of the laboratory criteria are met.

Clinical criteria
- Vascular thrombosis: One or more events of arterial, venous, or small vessel thrombosis confirmed by histopathology or imaging studies.
- Pregnancy morbidity defined as either one or more unexplained deaths of a morphologically normal fetus at or beyond the 10th wk of gestation; one or more premature births of a morphologically normal neonate before the 34th wk of gestation due to eclampsia or severe pre-eclampsia; or three or more unexplained consecutive spontaneous abortions before the 10th wk of gestation, where maternal and paternal abnormalities have been excluded.

Laboratory criteria (all measured by a standardized ELISA, according to recommended procedures)
- ACA IgG or IgM detectable at greater than 40 units on two or more occasions at least 12 wk apart.

A

- Lupus anticoagulant (LA) detectable on two or more occasions at least 12 wk apart.
- Anti-β_2 glycoprotein 1 antibody, IgG, or IgM detectable on two or more occasions at least 12 wk apart.

INDICATIONS
- Assist in the diagnosis of antiphospholipid antibody syndrome.

INTERFERING FACTORS
Factors that may alter the results of the study
- Drugs and other substances that may increase anticardiolipin antibody levels include chlorpromazine, hydralazine, penicillin, procainamide, phenytoin, and quinidine.

Other considerations
- Cardiolipin antibody is partially cross-reactive with syphilis reagin antibody and lupus anticoagulant. False-positive rapid plasma reagin results may occur.

POTENTIAL MEDICAL DIAGNOSIS: CLINICAL SIGNIFICANCE OF RESULTS
Increased in
Although ACAs are observed in specific diseases, the exact mechanism of these antibodies in disease is unclear. In fact, the production of ACA can be induced by bacterial, treponemal, and viral infections. Development of ACA under this circumstance is transient and not associated with an increased risk of antiphospholipid antibody syndrome. Patients who initially demonstrate positive ACA levels should be retested after 6 to 8 wk to rule out transient antibodies that are usually of no clinical significance.

- Antiphospholipid antibody syndrome
- Chorea
- Drug reactions
- Epilepsy
- Infectious diseases
- Mitral valve endocarditis
- Patients with lupus-like symptoms (often antinuclear antibody–negative)
- Placental infarction
- Recurrent fetal loss (strong association with two or more occurrences)
- Recurrent venous and arterial thromboses
- Stroke (in adults under the age of 50 years)
- Systemic lupus erythematosus (SLE)

Decreased in: N/A

NURSING IMPLICATIONS

BEFORE THE STUDY: PLANNING AND IMPLEMENTATION

Teaching the Patient What to Expect
- Inform the patient this test can assist in evaluating the amount of potentially harmful circulating antibodies.
- Explain that a blood sample is needed for the test.

AFTER THE STUDY: POTENTIAL NURSING ACTIONS

Treatment Considerations
- Allow the patient to talk about his or her feelings by listening with caring and concern.
- Assess the patient's level of active participation in the provision of self-care associated with the activities of daily living.

Follow-Up, Evaluation, and Desired Outcomes
- Acknowledges contact information provided for the Lupus Foundation of America (www.lupus.org).
- Seeks a support system or spiritual leader to relieve emotional distress associated with loss of potential child or loss of function secondary to disease process.

Anticyclic Citrullinated Peptide Antibody

A

SYNONYM/ACRONYM: Anti-CCP antibodies, ACPA.

RATIONALE: To assist in diagnosing and monitoring rheumatoid arthritis.

PATIENT PREPARATION: There are no food, fluid, activity, or medication restrictions unless by medical direction.

NORMAL FINDINGS: IgG Ab (Method: Immunoassay, enzyme-linked immunosorbent assay [ELISA]).

Negative	Less than 20 units
Weak positive	20–39 units
Moderate positive	40–59 units
Strong positive	60 units or greater

CRITICAL FINDINGS AND POTENTIAL INTERVENTIONS: N/A

OVERVIEW: (**Study type:** Blood collected in a gold-, red-, or red/gray-top tube; **related body system:** Immune and Musculoskeletal systems.) Rheumatoid arthritis (RA) is a chronic, systemic autoimmune disease that damages the joints. Inflammation caused by autoimmune responses can affect other organs and body systems. The American Academy of Rheumatology's current criteria focuses on earlier classification of newly presenting patients who have at least one swollen joint unrelated to another condition. The criteria include four determinants based on patient history and clinical findings:

1. Joint involvement (number and size of joints involved)
2. Serological test results (rheumatoid factor [RF] and/or anticitrullinated protein antibody [ACPA])
3. Indications of acute inflammation (C-reactive protein [CRP] and/or erythrocyte sedimentation rate [ESR])
4. Duration of symptoms (weeks)

Each determinant includes specific criteria with assigned values (e.g., duration of symptoms less than 6 wk = 0, duration of symptoms equal to or greater than 6 wk = 1). The scores from each determinant are added together. A score of 6 of 10 or greater for the score-based algorithm defines the presence of RA. Patients with longstanding RA, whose condition is inactive, or whose prior history would have satisfied the previous classification criteria by having four of seven findings—morning stiffness, arthritis of three or more joint areas, arthritis of hand joints, symmetric arthritis, rheumatoid nodules, abnormal amounts of rheumatoid factor, and radiographic changes—should remain classified as having RA. The ACR favors the consideration of classification criteria rather than endorsement of *diagnostic* criteria for RA because of the difficulty in establishing a consistent set of criteria. The study of RA is complex, and it is believed that multiple genes may be involved in the manifestation of RA. The diagnosis of RA is made on an individual basis by considering the ACR's classification criteria, in the presence of additional information unique to the patient and his or her genetic predisposition, lifestyle, and environment.

Scientific research has revealed an unusual peptide conversion from arginine to citrulline that results in formation of antibodies whose presence provides the basis for this test. Studies show that detection of antibodies formed against citrullinated peptides is specific and sensitive in detecting RA in both early and established disease. Anti-CCP assays have 96% specificity and 78% sensitivity for RA, compared to the traditional IgM RF marker with a specificity of 60% to 80% and sensitivity of 75% to 80% for RA. Anti-CCP antibodies are being used as a marker for erosive disease in RA, and the antibodies have been detected in healthy patients years before the onset of RA symptoms and diagnosed disease. Some studies have shown that as many as 40% of patients seronegative for RF are anti-CCP positive. The combined presence of RF and anti-CCP has a 99.5% specificity for RA. Women are two to three times more likely than men to develop RA. Although RA is most likely to affect people ages 35 to 50, it can affect all ages.

INDICATIONS
- Assist in the diagnosis of RA in both symptomatic and asymptomatic individuals.
- Assist in the identification of erosive disease in RA.
- Assist in the diagnostic prediction of RA development in undifferentiated arthritis.

INTERFERING FACTORS: N/A

POTENTIAL MEDICAL DIAGNOSIS: CLINICAL SIGNIFICANCE OF RESULTS
Increased in
- RA *(The immune system produces antibodies that attack the joint tissues. Inflammation of the synovium, membrane that lines the joint, begins a process called **synovitis**. If untreated, the synovitis can expand beyond the joint tissue to surrounding ligaments, tissues, nerves, and blood vessels.)*

Decreased in: N/A

NURSING IMPLICATIONS

POTENTIAL NURSING PROBLEMS: ASSESSMENT & NURSING DIAGNOSIS

Problems	Signs and Symptoms
Mobility *(related to inflammation, joint stiffness, pain, joint deformity, muscle weakness)*	Inability to meet physical demands associated with activities of daily living, ineffective range of motion, pain
Pain *(related to progressive joint degeneration, inflammation)*	Self-report of pain or discomfort, elevated heart rate and blood pressure, facial grimace, crying, moaning, diaphoresis, nausea, restlessness, irritability, guarding of affected joints

Problems	Signs and Symptoms
Self-care deficit *(related to loss of mobility, pain, inflammation, joint stiffness or deformity)*	Unable to complete activities of daily living without assistance (eating, bathing, dressing, toileting)

BEFORE THE STUDY: PLANNING AND IMPLEMENTATION

Teaching the Patient What to Expect

▶ Inform the patient this test can assist in identifying the cause of joint inflammation.

▶ Explain that a blood sample is needed for the test.

Potential Nursing Actions

▶ Assess the flexibility of affected joints to determine any barriers to blood draw.

AFTER THE STUDY: POTENTIAL NURSING ACTIONS

Treatment Considerations

▶ Mobility: Facilitate the use of assistive devices and assist in maintaining body alignment. Administer ordered medications (analgesics, steroids), facilitate physical therapy, and encourage ambulation.

▶ Pain: Assess pain character, location, duration, and intensity. Use an easily understood pain rating scale. Place in a position of comfort and administer ordered analgesics. Consider alternative measures for pain management (imagery, relaxation, music, etc.) and evaluate response and readjust pain management strategies.

▶ Self-Care: Assess self-care deficits, and identify and encourage areas where the patient can provide own care. Evaluate the family's ability to assist with self-care needs. Home health evaluation can determine environmental safety. Provide assistive devices to help with self-care.

Safety Considerations

▶ Recognizes the importance of using assistive devices to prevent falls and injury due to limited mobility.

Follow-Up, Evaluation, and Desired Outcomes

▶ Acknowledges contact information provided for the American College of Rheumatology (www.rheumatology .org) or the Arthritis Foundation (www .arthritis.org).

▶ Recognizes the importance of physical activity, physical therapy, and occupational therapy toward maintaining functionality and independent lifestyle. Demonstrates how to perform therapeutic exercises and verbalizes the importance of maintaining an exercise regime.

▶ Family states the importance of providing assistance only as necessary in order to maintain functional status.

▶ Seeks emotional support for chronic pain resulting from joint inflammation, impaired mobility, muscular deformity, and perceived loss of independence.

▶ Adheres to medication regime. Treatment with disease-modifying antirheumatic drugs and biological response modifiers may take as long as 2 to 3 mo to demonstrate their effects.

Antidiuretic Hormone

SYNONYM/ACRONYM: Vasopressin, arginine vasopressin hormone, ADH.

RATIONALE: To evaluate disorders that affect urine concentration related to fluctuations of ADH secretion, such as diabetes insipidus.

PATIENT PREPARATION: There are no food, fluid, or medication restrictions unless by medical direction. The patient should be encouraged to be calm and in a sitting position for specimen collection.

NORMAL FINDINGS: Method: Radioimmunoassay.

Age	Antidiuretic Hormone*	SI Units (Conventional Units × 0.923)
Newborn	Less than 1.5 pg/mL	Less than 1.4 pmol/L
Child (normally hydrated)	0.5–1.7 pg/mL	Less than 0.5–1.6 pmol/L
Adult (normally hydrated)	1–5 pg/mL	0.9–4.6 pmol/L

*Conventional units.

Recommendation
This test should be ordered and interpreted with results of a serum osmolality.

Serum Osmolality*	Antidiuretic Hormone	SI Units (Conventional Units × 0.923)
270–280 mOsm/kg	Less than 1.5 pg/mL	Less than 1.4 pmol/L
280–285 mOsm/kg	Less than 2.5 pg/mL	Less than 2.3 pmol/L
285–290 mOsm/kg	1–5 pg/mL	0.9–4.6 pmol/L
290–295 mOsm/kg	2–7 pg/mL	1.8–6.5 pmol/L
295–300 mOsm/kg	4–12 pg/mL	3.7–11.1 pmol/L

*Conventional units.

CRITICAL FINDINGS AND POTENTIAL INTERVENTIONS
Effective treatment of the syndrome of inappropriate antidiuretic hormone production (SIADH) depends on identifying and resolving the cause of increased ADH production. Signs and symptoms of SIADH are the same as those for hyponatremia, including irritability, tremors, muscle spasms, convulsions, and neurological changes. The patient has enough sodium, but it is diluted in excess retained water.

OVERVIEW: (**Study type:** Blood collected in a prechilled lavender-top [EDTA] tube; **related body system:** Endocrine system.) Instructions regarding appropriate handling and transport of the specimen should be obtained from the testing facility prior to specimen collection. ADH is formed by the hypothalamus and stored in the posterior pituitary gland. ADH is important in the regulation of water reabsorption and is released in response to increased serum osmolality or decreased blood volume. ADH secretion exhibits diurnal variation; the highest levels occur at night, which helps prevent the need for urination during the night. When the hormone is active, water is reabsorbed by the kidneys into the circulating plasma instead of being excreted, and small amounts of concentrated urine are produced; in its absence, large amounts of dilute urine are produced. Although a 1% change in serum osmolality stimulates ADH secretion, blood volume must decrease by approximately 10% for ADH secretion to be induced. Psychogenic stimuli, such as stress, pain, and anxiety, may also stimulate ADH release, but the mechanism is unclear. The ADH suppression, or water load, test is used in the differential diagnosis of SIADH from other causes related to sodium imbalances (e.g., adrenal insufficiency, excessive loss of sodium) or conditions that result in the development of edema (e.g., heart failure, myxedema, nephrosis). The suppression test is performed over a 6-hr period, in the fasting state, by administration of water at the initiation of the test (20 mL/kg of body weight to a maximum of 1,500 mL) followed by hourly measurements of serum and urine osmolality. The idea of osmolality being increased or decreased can be confusing in disease states because blood and urine levels vary in response to each other's compensatory mechanisms in maintaining water balance. Normal serum osmolality is 275 to 295 mOsm/kg; urine osmolality is 250 to 900 mOsm/kg; and the normal ratio of serum osmolality to urine osmolality is 1:3. Urine and serum values should be evaluated together. Normally we associate low values with small concentrations and high values with large concentrations. In the case of SIADH, urine osmolality values decrease in response to an abnormal increase in ADH secretion, telling the kidneys to retain water, concentrate the urine, and dilute the blood volume. A smaller urine osmolality number indicates highly concentrated urine, and a larger number indicates more dilute urine. Patients with SIADH excrete none or a very small amount of the water and have a more concentrated urine that measures a higher urine osmolality than expected if ADH was being properly suppressed (greater than 100 mOsm/kg, is an indication of the kidneys' inability to dilute the urine), whereas patients with an imbalance of sodium or significant edema excrete some water and have a relatively more dilute or decreased urine osmolality than patients with SIADH (less than 300 mOsm/kg). Patients should be closely monitored and educated regarding the signs and symptoms of water intoxication, a potential complication of the suppression test.

INDICATIONS
- Assist in the diagnosis of known or suspected malignancy associated with SIADH, such as oat cell lung cancer, thymoma, lymphoma, leukemia, pancreatic cancer, prostate gland cancer, and intestinal cancer; elevated ADH levels indicate the presence of this syndrome.
- Assist in the diagnosis of known or suspected pulmonary conditions associated with SIADH, such as tuberculosis, pneumonia, and positive-pressure mechanical ventilation.
- Detect central nervous system trauma, surgery, or disease that may lead to impaired ADH secretion.
- Differentiate neurogenic (central) diabetes insipidus from nephrogenic diabetes insipidus by decreased ADH levels in neurogenic diabetes insipidus or elevated levels in nephrogenic diabetes insipidus if normal feedback mechanisms are intact.

A

• Evaluate polyuria or altered serum osmolality to identify possible alterations in ADH secretion as the cause.

INTERFERING FACTORS
Factors that may alter the results of the study
• Drugs and other substances that may increase ADH levels include cisplatin, ether, furosemide, hydrochlorothiazide, lithium, methyclothiazide, and polythiazide.
• Drugs and other substances that may decrease ADH levels include chlorpromazine, clonidine, ethanol, and phenytoin.
• Recent radioactive scans or radiation within 1 wk before the test can interfere with test results when radioimmunoassay is the test method.
• ADH exhibits diurnal variation, with highest levels of secretion occurring at night; first morning collection is recommended.
• ADH secretion is also affected by posture, with higher levels measured while upright.

POTENTIAL MEDICAL DIAGNOSIS: CLINICAL SIGNIFICANCE OF RESULTS
Increased in
• Acute intermittent porphyria *(speculated to be related to the release of ADH from damaged cells in the hypothalamus and effect of hypovolemia; the mechanisms are unclear)*
• Brain tumor *(related to ADH production from the tumor or release from damaged cells in an adjacent affected area)*
• Disorders involving the central nervous system, thyroid gland, and adrenal gland *(numerous conditions influence the release of ADH)*
• Ectopic production *(related to ADH production from a systemic tumor)*

• Guillain-Barré syndrome *(relationship to SIADH is unclear)*
• Hypovolemia *(potent instigator of ADH release)*
• Nephrogenic diabetes insipidus *(related to lack of renal system response to ADH stimulation; evidenced by increased secretion of ADH)*
• Pain, stress, or exercise *(all are potent instigators of ADH release)*
• Pneumonia *(related to SIADH)*
• Pulmonary tuberculosis *(related to SIADH)*
• SIADH *(numerous conditions influence the release of ADH)*
• Tuberculous meningitis *(related to SIADH)*

Decreased in
Decreased production or secretion of ADH in response to changes in blood volume or pressure.

• Hypervolemia *(related to increased blood volume, which inhibits secretion of ADH)*
• Nephrotic syndrome *(related to destruction of pituitary cells that secrete ADH)*
• Pituitary (central) diabetes insipidus *(related to destruction of pituitary cells that secrete ADH)*
• Pituitary surgery *(related to destruction or removal of pituitary cells that secrete ADH)*
• Psychogenic polydipsia *(evidenced by decreased osmolality, which inhibits secretion of ADH)*

NURSING IMPLICATIONS

BEFORE THE STUDY: PLANNING AND IMPLEMENTATION

Teaching the Patient What to Expect
▶ Inform the patient this test can assist in providing information about effective urine concentration.

▶ Explain that a blood sample is needed for the test.

AFTER THE STUDY: POTENTIAL NURSING ACTIONS

Avoiding Complications

▶ Observe the patient for signs and symptoms of hyponatremia and fluid retention. Frequently monitor level of consciousness, input and output, vital signs, weight, and results of other laboratory values to include sodium, urine specific gravity, and osmolality.

Treatment Considerations

▶ Inform the patient, as appropriate, that treatment for fluid retention may include diuretic therapy and fluid restriction to successfully eliminate the excess water. Teach the patient about managing fluid restrictions. Ideally, the patient should be in a quiet environment with as little environmental stimulation as possible.

Nutritional Considerations

▶ Add dietary sodium to assist in reversal of hyponatremia as appropriate.

▶ Review specific fluid limitations for those at risk for fluid overload.

Antifungal Antibody

SYNONYM/ACRONYM: Antifungal antibodies.

RATIONALE: To assist in the diagnosis of fungal infections.

PATIENT PREPARATION: There are no food, fluid, activity, or medication restrictions unless by medical direction.

NORMAL FINDINGS: (Method: Complement fixation, immunodiffusion, serologic testing) Negative or no antibody detected.

CRITICAL FINDINGS AND POTENTIAL INTERVENTIONS

• Lists of specific organisms may vary among facilities; specific organisms are required to be reported to local, state, and national departments of health.

Timely notification to the requesting health-care provider (HCP) of any critical findings and related symptoms is a role expectation of the professional nurse. A listing of these findings varies among facilities.

OVERVIEW: (Study type: Blood collected in a red-top tube; related body system: Immune and Integumentary systems.) Fungi, organisms that normally live in soil, can be introduced into humans through the accidental inhalation of spores or inoculation of spores into tissue through trauma. Yeast are classified as a single-celled fungus. Individuals most susceptible to fungal infections are usually debilitated by chronic disease, are receiving prolonged antibiotic therapy, or have impaired immune systems. Fungal diseases may be classified according to the involved tissue type. Dermatophytoses involve superficial and cutaneous tissue. There are also subcutaneous and systemic mycoses. Systemic fungal infections, especially those caused by fluconazole-resistant fungi, can be life threatening. Identification of the infectious agent and effective therapeutic treatment can be more time sensitive than what is required for the natural course of growth by culture. Fungal antibody testing is used to assist in the diagnosis of fungal infections. Fungal cultures are noted to be slow growing, which causes delays in identification and selection of treatment modalities. Rapid, direct testing platforms are not yet widely available, but molecular-based blood assays are being developed and approved for use in clinical situations. For example, the T2Candida panel employs a combination of molecular technology (DNA amplification) with magnetic resonance technology to identify five common yeast species from a single blood sample in 3 to 5 hr. DNA sequencing of the internal transcribed spacer region of fungal ribosomal ribonucleic acid is another method used to provide relatively rapid identification of many fungi at the genus and species level.

INDICATIONS

- Identify organisms responsible for nail infections or abnormalities.
- Identify organisms responsible for skin eruptions, drainage, or other evidence of infection.
- Identify organisms responsible for systemic infection and sepsis.

INTERFERING FACTORS

Factors that may alter the results of the study

- Prompt and proper specimen processing, storage, and analysis are important to achieve accurate results.

POTENTIAL MEDICAL DIAGNOSIS: CLINICAL SIGNIFICANCE OF RESULTS

Positive findings in

- *Aspergillus spp.*
- *Blastomyces dermatitidis*

- *Candida albicans*
- *Coccidioides immitis*
- *Cryptococcus neoformans*
- *Histoplasma capsulatum*

NURSING IMPLICATIONS

BEFORE THE STUDY: PLANNING AND IMPLEMENTATION

Teaching the Patient What to Expect

▶ Inform the patient that positive results can indicate fungal infection; negative results do not rule out a fungal infection, as some antibody titers diminish or disappear altogether 1 to 4 wk after infection has occurred.

▶ Explain that a blood sample is needed for the test. Inform the patient that several tests may be necessary to confirm diagnosis.

Potential Nursing Actions

▶ If possible, ensure that ordered cultures have been collected prior to beginning antibiotic therapy.

AFTER THE STUDY: POTENTIAL NURSING ACTIONS

Avoiding Complications

▶ Encourage the patient or caregiver to seek early diagnosis and treatment for repeat candida infections and evaluation for other causes of symptoms.

Treatment Considerations

▶ The use of cotton underwear can decrease the risk of candida fungal infection. Monitor and trend laboratory studies; perform white blood cell count and fungal culture. Administer ordered antibiotics, increase oral fluid intake as appropriate, administer ordered parenteral fluids, and monitor and trend temperature.

▶ Assess pain character, location, duration, and intensity. Use an easily understood pain rating scale. Place in a position of comfort, and administer ordered medications. Consider alternate measures for pain management (imagery, relaxation, music, etc.). Assess and trend vital signs.

Follow-Up, Evaluation, and Desired Outcomes
▶ Acknowledges that untreated infection can be passed to a sex partner.

▶ Aware that long-term use of broad spectrum antibiotics or corticosteriods can place one at risk for development of a candida fungal infection.

A

Antigliadin Antibody (Immunoglobulin G and Immunoglobulin A), Antiendomysial Antibody (Immunoglobulin A), and Antitissue Transglutaminase Antibody (Immunoglobulin A)

SYNONYM/ACRONYM: Endomysial antibodies (EMA), gliadin deamidated peptide (IgG and IgA) antibodies, tTG.

RATIONALE: To assist in the diagnosis and monitoring of gluten-sensitive enteropathies that may damage intestinal mucosa.

PATIENT PREPARATION: There are no food, fluid, activity, or medication restrictions unless by medical direction.

NORMAL FINDINGS: Method: Enzyme linked immunosorbent assay (ELISA) for gliadin antibody and tissue transglutaminase antibody; indirect immunofluorescence for endomysial antibodies.

	Conventional Units
IgA and IgG gliadin antibody	Less than 20 units
Tissue transglutaminase antibody	Less than 20 units
Endomysial antibodies	Negative

CRITICAL FINDINGS AND POTENTIAL INTERVENTIONS: N/A

OVERVIEW: (Study type: Blood collected in a red-top tube; **related body system:** Digestive and Immune systems. Some molecular test methods utilize samples of saliva or buccal swabs [cells collected from the inside lining of the cheek].) Gliadin is a water-soluble protein found in the gluten of wheat, rye, oats, and barley. The intestinal mucosa of certain individuals does not digest gluten, allowing a toxic buildup of gliadin and intestinal inflammation. The inflammatory response interferes with intestinal absorption of nutrients and damages the intestinal mucosa. In severe cases, intestinal mucosa can be lost. Immunoglobulin G (IgG) and immunoglobulin A (IgA) gliadin antibodies are detectable in the serum of patients with gluten-sensitive enteropathy. Endomysial antibodies and tissue transglutaminase (tTG) antibody are two other serological tests commonly used

A

to investigate gluten-sensitive enteropathies. Gliadin IgA tests are the most sensitive for celiac disease (CD). However, it is also recognized that a significant percentage of patients with CD are also IgA deficient, meaning false-negative IgA results may be misleading in some cases. Estimates of up to 98% of individuals susceptible to CD carry either the DQ2 or DQ8 HLA cell surface receptors, which initiate formation of antibodies to gliadin. While it appears there is a strong association between CD and these gene markers, up to 40% of individuals without CD also carry the DQ2 or DQ8 markers. Molecular testing is available to establish the absence or presence of these susceptibility markers. CD is an inherited condition with significant impact on quality of life for the affected individual. Genetics is the study and identification of genes, genetic mutations, and inheritance. For example, genetics provides some insight into the likelihood of inheriting a medical condition such as CD. Knowledge of genetics assists in identifying those who may benefit from additional education, risk assessment, and counseling. Further information regarding inheritance of genes can be found in the study titled "Genetic Testing." Counseling and written, informed consent are recommended and sometimes required before genetic testing. Serological markers are useful in disease monitoring because research has established a relationship between amount of gluten in the diet and degree of intestinal damage as reflected by the level of detectable antibodies. CD shares an association with a number of other conditions, such as type 1 diabetes, Down syndrome, and Turner syndrome.

INDICATIONS

- Assist in the diagnosis of asymptomatic gluten-sensitive enteropathy in some patients with dermatitis herpetiformis.
- Assist in the diagnosis of gluten-sensitive enteropathies.
- Assist in the diagnosis of nontropical sprue.
- Monitor dietary adherence of patients with gluten-sensitive enteropathies.

INTERFERING FACTORS

Factors that may alter the results of the study

- Conditions other than gluten-sensitive enteropathy can result in elevated antibody levels without corresponding histological evidence. These conditions include Crohn disease, postinfection malabsorption, and food protein intolerance.

Other considerations

- A negative IgA gliadin result, especially with a positive IgG gliadin result in an untreated patient, does not rule out active gluten-sensitive enteropathy.

POTENTIAL MEDICAL DIAGNOSIS: CLINICAL SIGNIFICANCE OF RESULTS

Increased in

Evidenced by the combination of detectable gliadin or endomysial antibodies and improvement with a gluten-free diet.

- Asymptomatic gluten-sensitive enteropathy
- Celiac disease
- Dermatitis herpetiformis (*etiology of this skin manifestation is unknown, but there is an*

association related to gluten-sensitive enteropathy)
- Nontropical sprue

Decreased in
- IgA deficiency *(related to an inability to produce IgA and*

evidenced by decreased IgA levels and false-negative IgA gliadin tests)
- Children under the age of 18 mo *(related to immature immune system and low production of IgA)*

NURSING IMPLICATIONS

POTENTIAL NURSING PROBLEMS: ASSESSMENT & NURSING DIAGNOSIS

Problems	Signs and Symptoms
Fatigue *(related to chronic anemia and lack of nutrients secondary to gastrointestinal malabsorption)*	Decreased concentration, increased physical complaints, unable to restore energy with sleep, reports being tired, unable to maintain normal routine
Nutrition *(related to inability to digest gluten rich foods, damaged intuitional villi, malabsorption)*	Pale skin, weight loss, abdominal pain, diarrhea, gas, acid reflux, bloating, constipation

BEFORE THE STUDY: PLANNING AND IMPLEMENTATION

Teaching the Patient What to Expect
▶ Inform the patient this test can assist with evaluating the ability to digest gluten foods such as wheat, rye, and oats.
▶ Explain that a blood sample is needed for the test.

Potential Nursing Actions
▶ Inquire regarding the presence of a first-degree relative with celiac disease or other gluten digestive disorder. A first-degree relative is a parent, child, or sibling.

AFTER THE STUDY: POTENTIAL NURSING ACTIONS

Treatment Considerations
▶ Fatigue: Pace activities to preserve energy stores. Rate fatigue on a numeric scale to trend degree of fatigue over time. Identify what aggravates and decreases fatigue. Assess for related emotional factors such as depression. Evaluate current diet choices to assess for gluten ingestion in relation to fatigue, and monitor for

physiologic factors such as anemia. Monitor Hgb and Hct.

Nutritional Considerations
▶ Encourage the patient with abnormal findings to consult with a registered dietitian to plan a gluten-free diet. This dietary planning is complex because patients are often malnourished and have other related nutritional problems.
▶ Advise strict avoidance of foods containing gluten as even incidental amounts such as crumbs can cause bowel damage.

Follow-Up, Evaluation, and Desired Outcomes
▶ Acknowledges contact information provided for the Celiac Disease Foundation (https://celiac.org) or GI Kids (www.gikids.org/content/3/en/celiac-disease).
▶ Recognizes importance of adhering to the therapeutic regime designed by the health-care provider, as nonadherence can result in long-term problems such as infertility, miscarriage, central nervous system disorders, and neurological symptoms.

A

Antiglomerular Basement Membrane Antibody

SYNONYM/ACRONYM: Goodpasture antibody, anti-GBM.

RATIONALE: To assist in differentiating Goodpasture syndrome (an autoimmune disease) from renal dysfunction.

PATIENT PREPARATION: There are no food, fluid, activity, or medication restrictions unless by medical direction.

NORMAL FINDINGS: (Method: Enzyme immunoassay) Less than 20 units/mL = negative.

CRITICAL FINDINGS AND POTENTIAL INTERVENTIONS: N/A

OVERVIEW: (Study type: Blood collected in a gold-, red-, or red/gray-top tube; **related body system:** Immune, Respiratory, Urinary systems. Lung or kidney tissue also may be submitted for testing. Refer to related biopsy studies for specimen-collection instructions.) Glomerulonephritis, or inflammation of the kidney, is initiated by an immune response, usually to an infection. It can be classified as either antibody-mediated or cell-mediated glomerulonephritis. Goodpasture syndrome is a rare hypersensitivity condition characterized by the presence of circulating antiglomerular basement membrane (anti-GBM) antibodies in the blood and the deposition of immunoglobulin and complement in renal basement membrane tissue. Severe and progressive glomerulonephritis can lead to the development of pulmonary hemorrhage and idiopathic pulmonary hemosiderosis. The presence of anti-GBM antibodies can also be demonstrated in renal biopsy tissue cells of affected patients. Autoantibodies may also be directed to act against lung tissue in Goodpasture syndrome.

INDICATIONS
• Differentiate glomerulonephritis caused by anti-GBM from glomerulonephritis from other causes.
• Monitor therapy for glomerulonephritis caused by anti-GBM.

INTERFERING FACTORS: N/A

POTENTIAL MEDICAL DIAGNOSIS: CLINICAL SIGNIFICANCE OF RESULTS
Increased in
• Glomerulonephritis *(of autoimmune origin as evidenced by the presence of anti-GBM antibodies)*
• Goodpasture syndrome *(related to nephritis of autoimmune origin)*
• Idiopathic pulmonary hemosiderosis

Decreased in: N/A

A

NURSING IMPLICATIONS

BEFORE THE STUDY: PLANNING AND IMPLEMENTATION

Teaching the Patient What to Expect

▶ Inform the patient this test can assist in diagnosing a disease that can affect the kidneys or lungs.

▶ Explain that a blood sample is needed for the test.

AFTER THE STUDY: POTENTIAL NURSING ACTIONS

Follow-Up, Evaluation, and Desired Outcomes

▶ Adherence to therapeutic regimen.

Antineutrophil Cytoplasmic Antibody (P-ANCA, C-ANCA)

SYNONYM/ACRONYM: Cytoplasmic antineutrophil cytoplasmic antibody (c-ANCA), perinuclear antineutrophil cytoplasmic antibody (p-ANCA).

RATIONALE: To assist in diagnosing and monitoring the effectiveness of therapeutic interventions for Wegener syndrome.

PATIENT PREPARATION: There are no food, fluid, activity, or medication restrictions unless by medical direction.

NORMAL FINDINGS: (Method: Indirect immunofluorescence) Negative.

CRITICAL FINDINGS AND POTENTIAL INTERVENTIONS: N/A

OVERVIEW: (**Study type:** Blood collected in a red-top tube; **related body system:** Circulatory, Digestive, Immune, Respiratory, Urinary systems.) Antineutrophil cytoplasmic autoantibodies (ANCA) are associated with vasculitis and glomerulonephritis. There are two types of cytoplasmic neutrophil antibodies, identified by their cellular staining characteristics. c-ANCA (cytoplasmic) is specific for proteinase 3 in neutrophils and monocytes and is found in the sera of patients with Wegener granulomatosis (WG). Wegener syndrome includes granulomatous inflammation of the upper and lower respiratory tract and vasculitis. Systemic necrotizing vasculitis is an inflammation of the blood vessels. p-ANCA (perinuclear) is specific for myeloperoxidase, elastase, and lactoferrin, as well as other enzymes in neutrophils. p-ANCA is present in the sera of patients with pauci-immune necrotizing glomerulonephritis. Diagnosis of WG is difficult because the signs and symptoms are seen in many other diseases. Other than the ANCA blood test, tissue biopsy is the definitive test with presence of granuloma being the positive finding.

INDICATIONS

- Assist in the diagnosis of WG and its variants.
- Differential diagnosis of ulcerative colitis.
- Distinguish between biliary cholangitis and sclerosing cholangitis.
- Distinguish between vasculitic disease and the effects of therapy.

INTERFERING FACTORS: N/A

POTENTIAL MEDICAL DIAGNOSIS: CLINICAL SIGNIFICANCE OF RESULTS

Increased in

The exact mechanism by which ANCA are developed is unknown. One theory suggests colonization with bacteria capable of expressing microbial superantigens. It is thought that the superantigens may stimulate a strong cellular autoimmune response in genetically susceptible individuals. Another theory suggests the immune system may be stimulated by an accumulation of the antigenic targets of ANCA due to ineffective destruction of old neutrophils or ineffective removal of neutrophil cell fragments containing proteinase, myeloperoxidase, elastase, lactoferrin, or other proteins.

- c-ANCA
  WG and its variants
- p-ANCA
  Alveolar hemorrhage
  Angiitis and polyangiitis
  Autoimmune liver disease
  Capillaritis
  Churg-Strauss syndrome
  Crescentic glomerulonephritis
  Felty syndrome
  Glomerulonephritis
  Inflammatory bowel disease
  Kawasaki disease
  Leukocytoclastic skin vasculitis
  Microscopic polyarteritis
  Rheumatoid arthritis
  Vasculitis

Decreased in: N/A

NURSING IMPLICATIONS

BEFORE THE STUDY: PLANNING AND IMPLEMENTATION

Teaching the Patient What to Expect
- Inform the patient this test can assist in identifying the cause of inflammatory activity.
- Explain that a blood sample is needed for the test.

Potential Nursing Actions
- The patient should be assessed for signs and symptoms related to renal *(related to presence of hematuria or RBC casts)*; respiratory *(related to cough, dyspnea, and/or abnormal chest x-ray showing nodules or infiltrates)*; cutaneous *(related to skin lesions)*; musculoskeletal *(related to painful or arthritic joints)*; and ear, nose, and throat *(related to chronic sinusitis, chronic otitis media, hearing loss, oral ulcers, and/or abnormal nasal discharge)*, as these sites are most commonly involved in WG.

AFTER THE STUDY: POTENTIAL NURSING ACTIONS

Avoiding Complications
- Ensure adequate oxygenation with a saturation greater than 92% for patients with a compromised respiratory status. Adequate oxygenation will support body function.

Treatment Considerations
- The main goal for treatment of WG is reducing inflammation within the blood vessels in order to prevent further damage to associated sites (kidneys and lungs) and to decrease risk for other complications (eyes, ears, skin, joints). Treatment often includes a combination of immune system suppressants, which may include corticosteroids *(initially administered in high doses to reduce inflammation and then gradually tapered down)*, antibiotics *(related to infections that arise in immunosuppressed patients)*, and cytotoxic drugs *(related to immune system suppression)*.

▶ Assess for infection by monitoring and tending laboratory studies: BUN, Cr, WBC count, Hgb, Hct, electrolytes, and urine cultures. Monitor for results of complementary diagnostic studies: KUB, CT, MRI, and IVP. Administer ordered antibiotics; increase oral fluid intake as appropriate; administer ordered parenteral fluids; monitor and trend temperature.

▶ Assess respiratory status to establish a baseline: rate, rhythm, depth, and work of breathing. Administer ordered oxygen and evaluate effectiveness with pulse oximetry. Elevate the head of the bed to facilitate breathing, monitor and trend arterial blood gas results, assess for cyanosis, and administer ordered steroids and other medications.

Antinuclear Antibody, Anti-DNA Antibody, Anticentromere Antibody, Antiextractable Nuclear Antigen Antibody, Anti-Jo Antibody, and Antiscleroderma Antibody

SYNONYM/ACRONYM: Antinuclear antibodies (ANA), anti-DNA (anti-ds DNA), antiextractable nuclear antigens (anti-ENA, ribonucleoprotein [RNP], Smith [Sm], SS-A/Ro, SS-B/La), anti-Jo (antihistidyl transfer RNA [tRNA] synthase), and antiscleroderma (progressive systemic sclerosis [PSS] antibody, Scl-70 antibody, topoisomerase I antibody).

RATIONALE: To diagnose multiple systemic autoimmune disorders; primarily used for diagnosing systemic lupus erythematosus (SLE).

PATIENT PREPARATION: There are no food, fluid, activity, or medication restrictions unless by medical direction.

NORMAL FINDINGS: Method: Indirect fluorescent antibody for ANA and anticentromere; Immunoassay multiplex flow for anti-DNA, anti-ENA, anti-Scl-70, and anti-Jo-1.

ANA and anticentromere: Titer of 1:40 or less. Anti-ENA, anti-Jo-1, and anti-Scl-70: Negative. Reference ranges for anti-DNA, anti-ENA, anti-Scl-70, and anti-Jo-1 vary widely due to differences in methods, and the testing laboratory should be consulted directly.

Anti-DNA

Negative	Less than 5 international units
Indeterminate	5–9 international units
Positive	Greater than 9 international units

CRITICAL FINDINGS AND POTENTIAL INTERVENTIONS: N/A

A

OVERVIEW: (Study type: Blood collected in a red-top tube; related body system: Immune and Musculoskeletal systems.) ANA are autoantibodies mainly located in the nucleus of affected cells. The presence of ANA indicates SLE, related collagen vascular diseases, and immune complex diseases. Antibodies against cellular DNA are strongly associated with SLE. Anticentromere antibodies are a subset of ANA. Their presence is strongly associated with CREST syndrome (*c*alcinosis, *R*aynaud phenomenon, *e*sophageal dysfunction, *s*clerodactyly, and *t*elangiectasia). Women are much more likely than men to be diagnosed with SLE. Jo-1 is an autoantibody found in the sera of some ANA-positive patients. Compared to the presence of other autoantibodies, the presence of Jo-1 suggests a more aggressive course and a higher risk of mortality. The clinical effects of this autoantibody include acute onset fever, dry and crackled skin on the hands, Raynaud phenomenon, and arthritis. The extractable nuclear antigens (ENAs) include ribonucleoprotein (RNP), Smith (Sm), SS-A/Ro, and SS-B/La antigens. ENAs and antibodies to them are found in various combinations in individuals with combinations of overlapping rheumatologic symptoms.

The American College of Rheumatology (ACR)'s current classification includes a list of 11 criteria associated with a diagnosis of SLE. The patient should have four or more of these to establish suspicion of lupus. The symptoms do not have to manifest at the same time; they can present serially or simultaneously during any timeframe in which they are being evaluated.

ACR Classification criteria
- Positive ANA in the absence of a drug known to induce lupus
- Discoid rash (red raised patches)
- Hematological disorder (hemolytic anemia with reticulosis, leukopenia less than $4 \times 10^3/$microL or $4 \times 10^9/L$; lymphopenia less than $1.5 \times 10^3/$microL or $1.5 \times 10^9/L$, where the leukopenia or lymphopenia occurs on more than two occasions; and thrombocytopenia less than $100 \times 10^3/$microL or $100 \times 10^9/L$, where the thrombocytopenia occurs in the absence of drugs known to cause it)
- Immunological disorder (evidenced by abnormal anti-DNA antibody titer, positive anti-Sm antibody, or positive anti-phospholipid antibodies [as demonstrated by an abnormal anti-cardiolipin antibody level, positive lupus anticoagulant study, or false-positive serological syphilis test], known to be positive for at least 6 mo and confirmed to be falsely positive by a negative *Treponema pallidum* immobilization or fluorescent treponemal antibody testing [FTA-ABS])
- Malar rash (rash over the cheeks, sometimes described as a butterfly rash)
- Neurological disorder (seizures or psychosis in the absence of drugs or metabolic disturbances known to cause these effects)
- Nonerosive arthritis involving two or more peripheral joints (as affected by effusion, swelling, and/or tenderness)
- Oral ulcers

- Photosensitivity (exposure resulting in development of or increase in skin rash)
- Renal disorder (evidenced by urine findings: protein greater than either 3+ or 0.5 g/day *or* presence of cellular casts)
- Serositis (pleuritis: history of pleuritic pain, audible rubbing on exam, or evidence of effusion in pleural fluid) *or* pericarditis: ECG, audible rubbing, or evidence of effusion in pericardial fluid)

The ACR favors the consideration of classification criteria rather than endorsement of *diagnostic* criteria for SLE because of the difficulty in establishing a consistent set of criteria. SLE is a disease whose cause is complex, is influenced by numerous factors, and may only intermittently display previously documented signs and symptoms. The diagnosis of SLE is made for patients on an individual basis by considering the ACR's classification criteria in the presence of additional information unique to the patient and to his or her lifestyle and environment.

INDICATIONS

- Assist in the diagnosis and evaluation of SLE.
- Assist in the diagnosis and evaluation of suspected immune disorders, such as rheumatoid arthritis, systemic sclerosis, polymyositis, Raynaud syndrome, scleroderma, Sjögren syndrome, and mixed connective tissue disease.
- Assist in the diagnosis and evaluation of idiopathic inflammatory myopathies.

INTERFERING FACTORS

Factors that may alter the results of the study

- Drugs and other substances that may cause positive ANA results include acebutolol (diabetics), acetazolamide, anticonvulsants (increases with concomitant administration of multiple antiepileptic drugs), carbamazepine, chlorpromazine, ethosuximide, gemfibrozil, hydralazine, isoniazid, methyldopa, nitrofurantoin, penicillins, phenytoin, primidone, procainamide, quinidine, and trimethadione.

Other considerations

- A patient can have lupus and test ANA-negative.

POTENTIAL MEDICAL DIAGNOSIS: CLINICAL SIGNIFICANCE OF RESULTS

ANA Pattern*	Associated Antibody	Associated Condition
Rim and/or homogeneous	Double-stranded DNA	SLE
	Single- or double-stranded DNA	
Homogeneous	Histones	SLE
Speckled	Sm (Smith) antibody	SLE, mixed connective tissue disease, Raynaud scleroderma, Sjögren syndrome
	RNP	Mixed connective tissue disease, various rheumatoid conditions
	SS-B/La, SS-A/Ro	Various rheumatoid conditions

(table continues on page 98)

A

ANA Pattern*	Associated Antibody	Associated Condition
Diffuse speckled with positive mitotic figures	Centromere	PSS with CREST, Raynaud syndrome
Nucleolar	Nucleolar, RNP	Scleroderma, CREST

*ANA patterns are helpful in that certain conditions are frequently associated with specific patterns.

Increased in
- Anti-Jo-1 *is associated with dermatomyositis, idiopathic inflammatory myopathies, and polymyositis.*
- ANA *is associated with drug-induced lupus erythematosus.*
- ANA *is associated with lupoid hepatitis.*
- ANA *is associated with mixed connective tissue disease.*
- ANA *is associated with polymyositis.*
- ANA *is associated with progressive systemic sclerosis.*
- ANA *is associated with Raynaud syndrome.*
- ANA *is associated with rheumatoid arthritis.*
- ANA *is associated with Sjögren syndrome.*
- ANA and anti-DNA *are associated with SLE.*
- Anti-RNP *is associated with mixed connective tissue disease.*

- Anti-Scl 70 *is associated with progressive systemic sclerosis and scleroderma.*
- Anti-SS-A and anti-SS-B *are helpful in antinuclear antibody (ANA)–negative cases of SLE.*
- Anti-SS-A/ANA–positive, anti-SS-B–negative patients *are likely to have nephritis.*
- Anti-SS-A/anti-SS-B–positive sera *are found in patients with neonatal lupus.*
- Anti-SS-A–positive patients *may also have antibodies associated with antiphospholipid syndrome.*
- Anti-SS-A/La *is associated with primary Sjögren syndrome.*
- Anti-SS-A/Ro *is a predictor of congenital heart block in neonates born to mothers with SLE.*
- Anti-SS-A/Ro–positive patients *have photosensitivity.*

Decreased in: N/A

NURSING IMPLICATIONS

POTENTIAL NURSING PROBLEMS: ASSESSMENT & NURSING DIAGNOSIS

Problems	Signs and Symptoms
Nonadherence risk *(related to failure to adhere to recommended therapeutic interventions, failure to accept diagnosis)*	Acute episode of lupus triggered by excessive sun exposure during peak periods
Protection *(related to open sores, decreased immune response, steroid use)*	Fever, tenderness, redness, warmth, drainage, and swelling of open sores
Skin *(related to rash and lesions associated with the disease process)*	Butterfly rash across bridge of nose, lesions on exposed areas of the skin, nose and mouth ulcers

BEFORE THE STUDY: PLANNING AND IMPLEMENTATION

Teaching the Patient What to Expect

▶ Inform the patient this test can assist in evaluating immune system function.
▶ Explain that a blood sample is needed for the test.

AFTER THE STUDY: POTENTIAL NURSING ACTIONS

Avoiding Complications

▶ Provide education on good hand hygiene skills and caring for open sores to prevent infection.

Treatment Considerations

▶ Nonadherence: Ensure the patient understands the diagnosis and disease process; discuss the risks of nonadherence on overall health.
▶ Protection: Stress the importance of vigilant hand hygiene to protect from infection, which is a significant cause of death in immunosuppressed individuals. Monitor temperature and report any fever, monitor open sores for signs of infection, and white blood count. Initiate protective isolation if immune system is compromised.
▶ Skin: Explain the relationship between sun exposure and triggering an acute lupus episode. Explain that wearing loose, long-legged, and long-sleeved clothing can enhance sun protection. Encourage patient to avoid sun exposure during high-UV times, teach correct application of sunscreen with a UV protection greater than SPF 15 prior to sun exposure, to reapply sunscreen frequently as needed, and to apply therapeutic creams or ointments to skin as prescribed by the health-care provider.

Safety Considerations

▶ Progressive changes in body function, joint pain, fatigue, and fibrosis can lead to increased fall risk and injury. Institute steps to keep the patient safe.

Nutritional Considerations

▶ Discuss the importance of adequate nutrients in supporting the immune system, preventing infection, and promotion of healing.

Follow-Up, Evaluation, and Desired Outcomes

▶ Acknowledges contact information provided for the American College of Rheumatology (www.rheumatology .org), the Lupus Foundation of America (www.lupus.org), or the Arthritis Foundation (www.arthritis.org).
▶ Understands the implications of abnormal test results on lifestyle choices and changes that need to be made to decrease infection risk and development of cardiovascular disease. Recognizes that collagen and connective tissue diseases are chronic, and as such, they must be addressed on a continuous basis.
▶ Accepts the importance of adherence to the treatment regimen. Understands to contact the health-care provider (HCP) immediately if new SLE symptoms present, including vague or common symptoms such as fever.
▶ Acknowledges the importance of avoiding direct exposure to sunlight or other sources of UV light, such as tanning beds *(related to hypersensitivity of skin cells in people with lupus to UV light. The exact mechanism for this is not clearly understood, but it is believed that in people with lupus, damaged or dead skin cells are not sloughed as efficiently as occurs in individuals without lupus. It is also believed that cell contents released from damaged or dead skin cells may instigate an immune response leading to development of a skin rash. Sun exposure is known to damage skin; therefore, avoiding direct exposure reduces the amount of damage incurred).*
▶ Acknowledges that pregnancy should be discussed with the HCP as the medication regimen may present significant risks to both mother and child; pregnancies should be carefully planned.
▶ Agrees to keep immunizations updated as recommended by their HCP, typically given during periods of remission.

A

Antisperm Antibody

SYNONYM/ACRONYM: Antispermatozoal antibody, infertility screen.

RATIONALE: To evaluate testicular fertility and identify causes of infertility such as congenital defects, cancer, and torsion.

PATIENT PREPARATION: There are no food, fluid, activity, or medication restrictions unless by medical direction. Advise the patient that additional specimens may be needed.

NORMAL FINDINGS: Method: Immunoassay.

Result	Sperm Bound by Immunobead (%)
Negative	0–15
Weak positive	16–30
Moderate positive	31–50
Strong positive	51–100

CRITICAL FINDINGS AND POTENTIAL INTERVENTIONS: N/A

OVERVIEW: (**Study type:** Blood collected in a red-top tube; **related body system:** Immune and Reproductive systems.) Normally, sperm develop in the seminiferous tubules of the testes separated from circulating blood by the blood-testes barrier. Any situation that disrupts this barrier can expose sperm to detection by immune response cells in the blood and subsequent antibody formation against the sperm. Antisperm antibodies attach to the head, midpiece, or tail of the sperm, impairing motility and ability to penetrate the cervical mucosa. The antibodies can also cause clumping of sperm, which may be noted on a semen analysis. A major cause of infertility in men is blocked efferent testicular ducts. Reabsorption of sperm from the blocked ducts may also result in development of sperm antibodies. Another more specific and sophisticated method than measurement of circulating antibodies is the immunobead sperm antibody test used to identify antibodies directly attached to the sperm. Semen and cervical mucus can also be tested for antisperm antibodies.

INDICATIONS
• Evaluation of infertility.

INTERFERING FACTORS
Factors that may alter the results of the study
• The patient should not ejaculate for 3 to 4 days before specimen collection if semen will be evaluated; results may be affected if specimens are collected within 48 hr of ejaculating or after no ejaculation for longer than 5 days.

Other considerations
• Sperm antibodies have been detected in pregnant women and in women with primary infertility.

POTENTIAL MEDICAL DIAGNOSIS: CLINICAL SIGNIFICANCE OF RESULTS

Increased in

Conditions that affect the integrity of the blood-testes barrier can result in antibody formation.

- Blocked testicular efferent duct *(related to absorption of sperm by blocked vas deferens)*
- Congenital absence of the vas deferens *(related to absorption of sperm by blocked vas deferens)*
- Cryptorchidism *(related to disruption in the integrity of the blood-testes barrier)*
- Infection (orchitis, prostatitis) *(related to disruption in the integrity of the blood-testes barrier)*
- Inguinal hernia repair prior to puberty *(related to disruption in the integrity of the blood-testes barrier)*
- Testicular biopsy *(related to disruption in the integrity of the blood-testes barrier)*
- Testicular cancer *(related to disruption in the integrity of the blood-testes barrier)*
- Testicular torsion *(related to disruption in the integrity of the blood-testes barrier)*

- Varicocele *(related to disruption in the integrity of the blood-testes barrier)*
- Vasectomy *(related to absorption of sperm by blocked vas deferens)*
- Vasectomy reversal *(related to interaction between sperm and autoantibodies developed after vasectomy)*

Decreased in: N/A

NURSING IMPLICATIONS

BEFORE THE STUDY: PLANNING AND IMPLEMENTATION

Teaching the Patient What to Expect
- Inform the patient this test can assist in the evaluation of infertility and provide guidance through assistive reproductive techniques.
- Explain that a blood sample is needed for the test.

AFTER THE STUDY: POTENTIAL NURSING ACTIONS

Follow-Up, Evaluation, and Desired Outcomes
- Adheres to therapeutic management recommendations tailored to specific needs based on prognosis and response to treatment.

Antistreptococcal Deoxyribonuclease-B Antibody

SYNONYM/ACRONYM: ADNase-B, AntiDNase-B titer, antistreptococcal DNase-B titer, streptodornase.

RATIONALE: To assist in assessing the cause of recent infection, such as streptococcal exposure, by identification of antibodies.

PATIENT PREPARATION: There are no food, fluid, activity, or medication restrictions unless by medical direction.

NORMAL FINDINGS: Method: Nephelometry.

A

Age	Normal Results
1–6 yr	Less than 250 units
7–17 yr	Less than 375 units
18 yr and older	Less than 300 units

CRITICAL FINDINGS AND POTENTIAL INTERVENTIONS: N/A

OVERVIEW: (**Study type:** Blood collected in a red-top tube; related body system: Immune system.) The presence of streptococcal deoxyribonuclease (DNase)-B antibodies is an indicator of recent group A, beta hemolytic streptococcal infection, especially if a rise in antibody titer can be shown. This test is more sensitive than the antistreptolysin O (ASO) test. Anti-DNase B titers rise more slowly than ASO titers, peaking 4 to 8 wk after infection. They also decline much more slowly, remaining elevated for several months. A rise in titer of two or more dilution increments between acute and convalescent specimens is clinically significant.

INDICATIONS

• Investigate the presence of streptococcal antibodies as a source of recent infection.

INTERFERING FACTORS: N/A

POTENTIAL MEDICAL DIAGNOSIS: CLINICAL SIGNIFICANCE OF RESULTS

Increased in
Presence of antibodies, especially a rise in titer, is indicative of exposure.

• Post streptococcal glomerulonephritis
• Rheumatic fever
• Streptococcal infections (systemic)

Decreased in: N/A

NURSING IMPLICATIONS

BEFORE THE STUDY: PLANNING AND IMPLEMENTATION

Teaching the Patient What to Expect
◗ Inform the patient this test can assist in documenting recent streptococcal infection.
◗ Explain that a blood sample is needed for the test.

Potential Nursing Actions
◗ Confirm that ordered cultures have been completed prior to initiating antibiotic therapy if possible.

AFTER THE STUDY: POTENTIAL NURSING ACTIONS

Treatment Considerations
◗ Promote good hygiene and assist with hygiene as needed. Administer prescribed antibiotics and antipyretics. Institute cooling measures and administer ordered IV fluids. Monitor vital signs and trend temperatures. Encourage oral fluids. Adhere to standard or universal precautions. Implement isolation as appropriate and ensure ordered cultures are submitted.

Follow-Up, Evaluation, and Desired Outcomes
◗ Understands that a convalescent specimen may be requested in 7 to 10 days to assess disease progress and treatment effectiveness.
◗ Acknowledges the importance of completing the entire course of antibiotic therapy, even if signs and symptoms disappear before completion of therapy.

Antistreptolysin *O* Antibody

A

SYNONYM/ACRONYM: Streptozyme, ASO.

RATIONALE: To assist in the diagnosis of streptococcal infection.

PATIENT PREPARATION: There are no food, fluid, activity, or medication restrictions unless by medical direction.

NORMAL FINDINGS: (Method: Immunoturbidimetric) Adult/older adult: Less than 200 international units/mL; 17 yr and younger: Less than 150 international units/mL.

CRITICAL FINDINGS AND POTENTIAL INTERVENTIONS: N/A

OVERVIEW: (Study type: Blood collected in a red-top tube; related body system: Immune system.) Group A β-hemolytic streptococci secrete streptolysin *O*, a toxin that can hemolyze red blood cells. Circulating toxin stimulates the immune system to develop streptolysin *O* antibodies. These antistreptolysin *O* (ASO) antibodies form within 1 wk after the onset of a streptococcal infection and peak 2 to 3 wk later. The ASO titer usually returns to preinfection levels within 6 to 12 mo, assuming reinfection has not occurred. Up to 95% of patients with acute glomerulonephritis and up to 85% of patients with rheumatic fever demonstrate a rise in titer. ASO titer may not become elevated in some patients who experience sequelae involving the skin or kidneys, and the antideoxyribonuclease-B streptococcal test may a better test for these patients.

INDICATIONS

• Assist in establishing a diagnosis of streptococcal infection.

• Evaluate patients with streptococcal infections for the development of acute rheumatic fever or nephritis.
• Monitor response to therapy in streptococcal illnesses.

INTERFERING FACTORS

Factors that may alter the results of the study

• Drugs and other substances that may decrease ASO titers include antibiotics and corticosteroids because therapy suppresses antibody response.
• False-positive ASO titers can be caused by elevated levels of serum β-lipoprotein (observed in liver disease).

POTENTIAL MEDICAL DIAGNOSIS: CLINICAL SIGNIFICANCE OF RESULTS

Increased in

Presence of antibodies, especially a rise in titer, is indicative of exposure.

• Endocarditis
• Glomerulonephritis
• Rheumatic fever
• Scarlet fever

Decreased in: N/A

NURSING IMPLICATIONS

BEFORE THE STUDY: PLANNING AND IMPLEMENTATION

Teaching the Patient What to Expect

▶ Inform the patient this test can assist in documenting exposure to streptococcal bacteria.
▶ Explain that a blood sample is needed for the test. Advise the patient that repeat blood draws may be necessary to identify the highest point of increase in results.

AFTER THE STUDY: POTENTIAL NURSING ACTIONS

Avoiding Complications
▶ Advise the patient to strictly adhere to the therapeutic regime developed by the health-care provider for the best chance of a positive outcome.

Treatment Considerations
▶ Promote good hygiene and assist with hygiene as needed. Administer prescribed antibiotics, antipyretics, and IV fluids. Institute cooling measures, monitor and trend vital signs, and encourage oral fluids. Adhere to standard or universal precautions, isolate as appropriate, and submit ordered cultures.
▶ Remind the patient of the importance of completing the entire course of antibiotic therapy even if signs and symptoms disappear or diminish before completion of therapy.

Antithrombin III

SYNONYM/ACRONYM: Heparin cofactor assay, AT-III.

RATIONALE: To assist in diagnosing heparin resistance or disorders resulting from a hypercoagulable state such as thrombus.

PATIENT PREPARATION: There are no food, fluid, activity, or medication restrictions unless by medical direction.

NORMAL FINDINGS: Method: Chromogenic immunoturbidimetric.

Age	AT-III Activity Conventional Units (% of Normal)
Newborn	39–87
Child	82–139
Adult–older adult	80–120
Age	**AT-III antigen**
Newborn	40–60
6 mo–adult	82–136

CRITICAL FINDINGS AND POTENTIAL INTERVENTIONS: N/A

OVERVIEW: (Study type: Blood collected in a completely filled blue-top [3.2% sodium citrate] tube; related body system: Circulatory/Hematopoietic system.) If the patient's Hct exceeds 55%, the volume of citrate in the collection tube must be adjusted. *Important note:* The collection tube should be completely filled. When multiple specimens are drawn, the blue-top tube should be collected after sterile (i.e., blood culture) tubes. Otherwise, when using a standard vacutainer system, the blue top is the first tube collected. When a butterfly is used, due to the added tubing, an extra red-top tube should be collected before the blue-top tube to ensure complete filling of the blue-top tube. Antithrombin III (AT-III) is a non-vitamin K–dependent protein that can inhibit thrombin (factor IIa) and factors IX, X, XI, and XII. It is a heparin cofactor, produced by the liver, interacting with heparin and thrombin. AT-III acts to increase the rate at which thrombin is neutralized or inhibited, and it decreases the total quantity of thrombin inhibited. Patients with low levels of AT-III show some level of resistance to heparin therapy and are at risk for venous thrombosis. AT-III deficiency can be acquired (most common) or can be an inherited autosomal dominant condition. Acquired AT-III deficiency is the result of overconsumption of AT-III related to conditions that include, among others, disseminated intravascular coagulation (DIC) and venous thrombosis. Tests that measure the level of AT-III activity are used to identify individuals with AT-III deficiency. If a deficiency is identified, AT antigen testing is used to provide information regarding subtyping. Decreased AT-III activity and decreased antigen levels correspond to type I or classic deficiency in which there is a quantitative deficiency of AT-III. Decreased AT-III activity and normal antigen levels correspond to type II or a functional deficiency; the antigen level is normal in the presence of decreased activity levels, which reflects an abnormality in the protein structure of AT-III.

INDICATIONS
- Investigate tendency for thrombosis.

INTERFERING FACTORS
Factors that may alter the results of the study
- Drugs and other substances that may increase AT-III levels include anabolic steroids, gemfibrozil, and warfarin.
- Drugs and other substances that may decrease AT-III levels include asparaginase, estrogens, heparin, and oral contraceptives.
- Hct greater than 55% may cause falsely prolonged results because of anticoagulant excess relative to plasma volume.
- Incompletely filled collection tubes, specimens contaminated with heparin, clotted specimens, or unprocessed specimens not delivered to the laboratory within 1 to 2 hr of collection should be rejected.
- Placement of the tourniquet for longer than 1 min can result in venous stasis and changes in the concentration of the plasma proteins to be measured. Platelet activation may also occur under these conditions, resulting in erroneous measurements.

POTENTIAL MEDICAL DIAGNOSIS: CLINICAL SIGNIFICANCE OF RESULTS

Increased in

- **Acute hepatitis**
- **Kidney transplantation** *(Some studies have demonstrated high levels of AT-III in proximal tubule epithelial cells at the time of kidney transplant. The exact relationship between the kidneys and AT-III levels is unknown. It is believed the kidneys may play a role in maintaining plasma levels of AT-III, as evidenced by the correlation between kidney disease and low AT-III levels.)*
- **Vitamin K deficiency** *(decreased consumption related to impaired coagulation factor function)*

Decreased in

- **Cancer** *(related to decreased synthesis)*
- **Chronic liver failure** *(related to decreased synthesis)*
- **Cirrhosis** *(related to decreased synthesis)*
- **Congenital deficiency**
- **DIC** *(related to increased consumption)*
- **Liver transplantation or partial hepatectomy** *(related to decreased synthesis)*
- **Nephrotic syndrome** *(related to increased protein loss)*
- **Pulmonary embolism** *(related to increased consumption)*
- **Septic shock** *(related to increased consumption and decreased synthesis due to hepatic impairment)*
- **Venous thrombosis** *(related to increased consumption)*

NURSING IMPLICATIONS

BEFORE THE STUDY: PLANNING AND IMPLEMENTATION

Teaching the Patient What to Expect
- Inform the patient this test can assist in diagnosing clotting disorders.
- Explain that a blood sample is needed for the test.

AFTER THE STUDY: POTENTIAL NURSING ACTIONS

Avoiding Complications
- Consider activity limitations for those patients who are diagnosed with pulmonary or venous thrombus.

Treatment Considerations
- Increase frequency of vital sign assessment and note variances in results. Administer blood or blood products as ordered. Administer stool softeners as needed. Encourage intake of foods rich in vitamin K, such as kale, spinach, and other leafy green vegetables.
- Assess for physical cause of fatigue and pace activities to preserve energy stores. Rate fatigue on a numeric scale to trend degree of fatigue over time. Identify what aggravates and decreases fatigue. Assess for physiologic factors such as anemia.
- Monitor blood pressure; assess for dizziness, skin temperature, color, and warmth. Assess capillary refill, pedal pulses, numbness, tingling, and hyperesthesia or hypoesthesia. Monitor for deep vein thrombosis (DVT). Exercise careful use of heat and cold on affected areas and use a foot cradle to keep pressure off of effected body parts.

Safety Considerations
- Consider implementation of bleeding precautions for patients with coagulation disorders.

Follow-Up, Evaluation, and Desired Outcomes
- States necessary bleeding precautions that should be instituted to decrease injury risk.
- Understands that ongoing fatigue can impact the ability to meet personal role performance expectations.
- Agrees to alter personal lifestyle choices and limit risky behavior that could result in injury due to altered coagulation status.

Antithyroglobulin Antibody and Antithyroid Peroxidase Antibody

A

SYNONYM/ACRONYM: Thyroid antibodies, antithyroid peroxidase antibodies (thyroid peroxidase [TPO] antibodies were previously called thyroid antimicrosomal antibodies).

RATIONALE: To assist in diagnosing hypothyroid and hyperthyroid disease.

PATIENT PREPARATION: There are no food, fluid, activity, or medication restrictions unless by medical direction.

NORMAL FINDINGS: Method: Immunoassay.

Antibody	Conventional Units
Antithyroglobulin antibody	Less than 20 international units/mL
Antiperoxidase antibody	
Newborn–3 days	0–9 international units/mL
4–30 days	0–26 international units/mL
1–12 mo	0–13 international units/mL
13 mo–19 yr	0–20 international units/mL
20 yr–older adult	0–34 international units/mL

CRITICAL FINDINGS AND POTENTIAL INTERVENTIONS: N/A

OVERVIEW: (**Study type:** Blood collected in a red-top tube; **related body system:** Endocrine and Immune systems.) Thyroid peroxidase (TPO) is a key enzyme in the formation of thyroid hormones, and thyroglobulin is the stored precursor to the active, iodinated thyroid hormones. Antibodies to both may form and affect normal thyroid function. Both tests are normally requested together. Thyroid antibodies are mainly immunoglobulin G–type antibodies. Antithyroid peroxidase antibodies (anti-TPO antibodies) bind with microsomal antigens on cells lining the microsomal membrane of thyroid tissue. They are thought to destroy thyroid tissue as a result of stimulation by lymphocytic killer cells.

These antibodies are present in hypothyroid and hyperthyroid conditions. Anti-TPO antibodies are present in Hashimoto autoimmune thyroiditis, a major cause of hypothyroidism. Hypothyroidism in women of childbearing age is a significant concern because of the deleterious effects of insufficient thyroxine levels on fetal brain development. Anti-TPO antibodies are also demonstrable in Graves disease, a major cause of hyperthyroidism. Graves disease is the most common type of thyrotoxicosis in women of childbearing age, impairing fertility and increasing risk of miscarriage to 26%. Transplacental passage of anti-TPO antibodies in pregnant patients may affect the developing fetus or lead to thyroid disease in the

A

neonate. Mild depression is more common in postpartum women with anti-TPO antibodies.

INDICATIONS
- Assist in confirming suspected inflammation of thyroid gland.
- Assist in the diagnosis of suspected hypothyroidism caused by thyroid tissue destruction.
- Assist in the diagnosis of suspected thyroid autoimmunity in patients with other autoimmune disorders.

INTERFERING FACTORS
Factors that may alter the results of the study
- Lithium may increase thyroid antibody levels.

POTENTIAL MEDICAL DIAGNOSIS: CLINICAL SIGNIFICANCE OF RESULTS
Increased in
The presence of these antibodies differentiates the autoimmune origin of these disorders from nonautoimmune causes, which may influence treatment decisions.

- Autoimmune disorders
- Graves disease
- Goiter
- Hashimoto thyroiditis
- Idiopathic myxedema
- Pernicious anemia
- Thyroid cancer

Decreased in: N/A

NURSING IMPLICATIONS

BEFORE THE STUDY: PLANNING AND IMPLEMENTATION
Teaching the Patient What to Expect
- Inform the patient this test can assist in evaluating thyroid gland function.
- Explain that a blood sample is needed for the test.

AFTER THE STUDY: POTENTIAL NURSING ACTIONS
Follow-Up, Evaluation, and Desired Outcomes
- Acknowledges the importance of following the appropriate therapeutic plan when diagnosed with autoimmune thyroid disease.

Apolipoproteins: A, B, and E

SYNONYM/ACRONYM: Apo A (Apo A1), Apo B (Apo B100), and Apo E.

RATIONALE: To identify levels of circulating lipoprotein to evaluate the risk of coronary artery disease (CAD).

PATIENT PREPARATION: There are no food, fluid, activity, or medication restrictions unless by medical direction. However, if the test is ordered in conjunction with a lipid profile or triglyceride level, instruct the patient to abstain from food for 6 to 12 hr before specimen collection.

NORMAL FINDINGS: Method: Immunonephelometry for Apo A and Apo B; polymerase chain reaction (PCR) with restriction length enzyme digestion and polyacrylamide gel electrophoresis for Apo E.

A

Apolipoprotein A-1

Age	Conventional Units	SI Units (Conventional Units × 0.01)
Newborn	38–106 mg/dL	0.38–1.06 g/L
Child	60–150 mg/dL	0.6–1.5 g/L
Adult		
Male	81–166 mg/dL	0.81–1.66 g/L
Female	80–214 mg/dL	0.8–2.14 g/L

Apolipoprotein B

Age	Conventional Units	SI Units (Conventional Units × 0.01)
Newborn–5 yr	11–31 mg/dL	0.11–0.31 g/L
Child		
Male	47–139 mg/dL	0.47–1.39 g/L
Female	41–96 mg/dL	0.41–0.96 g/L
Adult		
Male	46–174 mg/dL	0.46–1.74 g/L
Female	46–142 mg/dL	0.46–1.42 g/L

Normal Apo E: Homozygous phenotype for e3/e3.

CRITICAL FINDINGS AND POTENTIAL INTERVENTIONS: N/A

OVERVIEW: (Study type: Blood collected in a gold-, red-, red/gray-, green- [heparin], or lavender-top [EDTA] tube; related body system: Circulatory system.) Apolipoproteins assist in the regulation of lipid metabolism by activating and inhibiting enzymes required for this process. The apolipoproteins also help keep lipids in solution as they circulate in the blood and direct the lipids toward the correct target organs and tissues in the body. A number of types of apolipoproteins have been identified (A, B, C, D, E, H, J), each of which contains subgroups. Apolipoprotein A (Apo A), the major component of high-density lipoprotein (HDL), is synthesized in the liver and intestines. Apo A-I activates the enzyme lecithin-cholesterol acyltransferase (LCAT),

whereas Apo A-II inhibits LCAT. It is believed that Apo A measurements may be more important than HDL cholesterol measurements as a predictor of coronary artery disease (CAD). For additional information regarding screening guidelines for *atherosclerotic cardiovascular disease (ASCVD)*, refer to the study titled "Cholesterol, Total and Fractions." There is an inverse relationship between Apo A levels and risk for developing CAD. Because of difficulties with method standardization, the above-listed reference ranges should be used as a rough guide in assessing abnormal conditions. Values for people of African descent are 5 to 10 mg/dL (0.05–0.1 g/L) higher than values for individuals of European descent. Apolipoprotein B

(Apo B), the major component of the low-density lipoproteins (chylomicrons, low-density lipoprotein [LDL], and very-low-density lipoprotein [VLDL]), is synthesized in the liver and intestines. Apolipoprotein E is found in most lipoproteins, except LDL, and is synthesized in a variety of cell types, including liver, brain astrocytes, spleen, lungs, adrenals, ovaries, kidneys, muscle cells, and in macrophages. The largest amount is produced by the liver; the next significant amount is produced by the brain. There are three forms of Apo E: Apo-E2, Apo-E3, and Apo-E4, and six possible combinations; of these, Apo-E3 (e3/3e) is the fully functioning form. The varied roles of Apo E include removal of chylomicrons and VLDL from the circulation by binding to LDL. The Apo E2 isoform demonstrates significantly less LDL receptor binding, which results in impaired clearance of chylomicrons, VLDL, and triglyceride remnants. The presence of Apo E isoforms E2 and E4 is associated with high cholesterol levels, high triglyceride levels, and the premature development of atherosclerosis. The presence of the E2 isoform is associated with type III hyperlipidemia, a familial dyslipidemia, which is important to distinguish from other causes of hyperlipidemia to determine the correct treatment regimen. Apo E4 is being used in association with studies of predisposing factors in the development of Alzheimer disease. Additional information is found in the study titled "Alzheimer Disease Markers."

INDICATIONS
• Evaluation for risk of CAD.

INTERFERING FACTORS
Factors that may alter the results of the study
• Drugs and other substances that may increase Apo A levels include anticonvulsants, beclobrate, bezafibrate, ciprofibrate, estrogens, ethanol (misuse), furosemide, lovastatin, pravastatin, prednisolone, and simvastatin.
• Drugs and other substances that may decrease Apo A levels include androgens, beta blockers, diuretics, and probucol.
• Drugs and other substances that may increase Apo B levels include amiodarone, androgens, beta blockers, catecholamines, cyclosporine, diuretics, ethanol (misuse), etretinate, glucogenic corticosteroids, oral contraceptives, and phenobarbital.
• Drugs and other substances that may decrease Apo B levels include beclobrate, captopril, cholestyramine, fibrates, ketanserin, lovastatin, niacin, nifedipine, pravastatin, prazosin, probucol, and simvastatin.
• Drugs and other substances that may decrease Apo E levels include bezafibrate, fluvastatin, gemfibrozil, ketanserin, lovastatin, niacin, nifedipine, oral contraceptives, pravastatin, probucol, and simvastatin.
• Lipemic specimens will be rejected for analysis as lipemia interferes with the immunonephelometry test method.

POTENTIAL MEDICAL DIAGNOSIS: CLINICAL SIGNIFICANCE OF RESULTS
Apolipoproteins are the protein portion of lipoproteins. Their function is to transport and to assist in cell surface receptor recognition and cellular absorption of lipoproteins to be used as energy. While studies of the exact role of apolipoproteins in health and

disease continue, there is a very strong association between Apo A and HDL "good" cholesterol and Apo B and LDL "bad" cholesterol.

Apolipoprotein A
Increased in
- Familial hyper-α-lipoproteinemia
- Pregnancy
- Weight reduction

Decreased in
- Abetalipoproteinemia
- Cholestasis
- Chronic kidney disease
- CAD
- Diabetes (uncontrolled)
- Diet high in carbohydrates or polyunsaturated fats
- Familial deficiencies of related enzymes and lipoproteins (e.g., Tangier disease)
- Hemodialysis
- Hepatocellular disorders
- Hypertriglyceridemia
- Nephrotic syndrome
- Premature CAD
- Smoking

Apolipoprotein B
Increased in
- Anorexia nervosa
- Biliary obstruction
- Chronic kidney disease
- CAD
- Cushing syndrome
- Diabetes
- Dysglobulinemia
- Emotional stress
- Hemodialysis
- Hepatic disease
- Hepatic obstruction
- Hyperlipoproteinemias
- Hypothyroidism
- Infantile hypercalcemia
- Nephrotic syndrome
- Porphyria
- Pregnancy
- Premature CAD
- Werner syndrome

Decreased in
- Acute stress (burns, illness)
- Chronic anemias
- Chronic pulmonary disease
- Familial deficiencies of related enzymes and lipoproteins (e.g., Tangier disease)
- Hyperthyroidism
- Inflammatory joint disease
- Intestinal malabsorption
- α-Lipoprotein deficiency (Tangier disease)
- Malnutrition
- Myeloma
- Reye syndrome
- Weight reduction

NURSING IMPLICATIONS

BEFORE THE STUDY: PLANNING AND IMPLEMENTATION

Teaching the Patient What to Expect
▸ Inform the patient this test can assist in assessing and monitoring risk for CAD.
▸ Explain that a blood sample is needed for the test.

Potential Nursing Actions
▸ Investigate the presence of other risk factors, such as family history of heart disease, smoking, obesity, diet, lack of physical activity, hypertension, diabetes, previous myocardial infarction, and previous vascular disease. Knowledge of genetics assists in identifying those who may benefit from additional education, risk assessment, and counseling. The combined activity or combined expression of groups of genes allows assumptions or predictions to be made. As an example, genomic studies measure the levels of activity in multiple genes to predict how they, along with environmental and lifestyle decisions, influence the development of type 2 diabetes, CAD, myocardial infarction, or ischemic stroke. Further information regarding inheritance of genes can be found in the study titled "Genetic Testing."

A

AFTER THE STUDY: POTENTIAL NURSING ACTIONS

Treatment Considerations

♦ Asses peripheral pulses and capillary refill. Monitor blood pressure and check for orthostatic changes. Assess respiratory rate, breath sounds, skin color, temperature, and level of consciousness. Monitor urinary output. Use pulse oximetry to monitor oxygenation, and administer ordered oxygen. Monitor sodium, potassium, and B-type natriuretic peptide levels. Administer ordered angiotensin-converting enzyme inhibitors, beta-blockers, diuretics, aldosterone antagonists, and vasodilators.

♦ Assess diet, smoking, and alcohol use. Teach the importance of adequate calcium intake with diet and supplements. Refer to smoking cessation and alcohol treatment programs. Collaborate with health-care provider for bone density evaluation and discuss the value of regular participation in weight bearing exercise.

Nutritional Considerations

♦ Discuss ideal body weight and the purpose of and relationship between ideal weight and caloric intake to support cardiac health. Review ways to decrease intake of saturated fats and increase intake of polyunsaturated fats. Discuss limiting intake of refined processed sugar and sodium; discuss limiting cholesterol intake to less than 300 mg per day. Encourage the intake of fresh fruits and vegetables, unprocessed carbohydrates, poultry, and grains.

♦ Nutritional therapy is recommended for those with identified CAD risk, especially for those with elevated LDL cholesterol levels, other lipid disorders, diabetes, insulin resistance, or metabolic syndrome. Always consider cultural influences with dietary choices to ensure better adherence to a change in lifestyle. A variety of dietary patterns are beneficial for people with ASCVD. For additional information regarding nutritional guidelines, refer to the study titled "Cholesterol, Total and Fractions."

♦ Other changeable risk factors warranting education include strategies to encourage regular participation of moderate aerobic physical activity three to four times per week, eliminate tobacco use, and adhere to a heart-healthy diet.

♦ Those with elevated triglycerides should be advised to eliminate or reduce alcohol.

Follow-Up, Evaluation, and Desired Outcomes

♦ Acknowledges contact information provided for the American Heart Association (www.heart.org/HEARTORG), National Heart, Lung, and Blood Institute (www.nhlbi.nih.gov), or the U.S. Department of Agriculture's resource for nutrition (www.choosemyplate.gov).

♦ Understands the relationship between personal health choices (diet, smoking, alcohol use) and cardiac disease.

Arthrogram

SYNONYM/ACRONYM: Joint study.

RATIONALE: To assess and identify the cause of persistent joint pain and monitor the progression of joint disease. Commonly performed on shoulder, elbow, wrist, hip, knee, ankle, temporomandibular joint.

PATIENT PREPARATION: There are no food, fluid, activity or medication restrictions unless by medical direction.

Note: If iodinated contrast medium is scheduled to be used in patients receiving metformin or drugs containing metformin for type 2 diabetes, the drug may be discontinued on the day of the test and continue to be withheld for 48 hr after the test. Regarding the patient's risk for bleeding, the patient should be instructed to avoid taking natural products and medications with known anticoagulant, antiplatelet, or thrombolytic properties or to reduce dosage, as ordered, prior to the procedure. Number of days to withhold medication is dependent on the type of anticoagulant. Note the last time and dose of medication taken. Protocols may vary among facilities.

Pediatric Considerations: Young children may need to be sedated in order to remain still during the procedure. Parents should be encouraged to ask about preparation for sedation prior to the procedure, including any ordered medications or restrictions regarding medications, diet, and activity.

NORMAL FINDINGS

• Normal bursae, menisci, ligaments, and articular cartilage of the joint. (*Note:* The cartilaginous surfaces and menisci should be smooth, without evidence of erosion, tears, or disintegration.)

CRITICAL FINDINGS AND POTENTIAL INTERVENTIONS: N/A

OVERVIEW: (**Study type:** X-ray, special/contrast; **related body system:** Musculoskeletal system.) An arthrogram evaluates the cartilage, ligaments, and bony structures that compose a joint. After a local anesthetic is administered to the area of interest, a fluoroscopically guided small-gauge needle is inserted into the joint space. Fluid in the joint space is aspirated and sent to the laboratory for analysis. A water-based or air-contrast medium is injected into the joint space to outline the soft tissue structures and the contour of the joint. After a brief exercise of the joint, radiographs, computed tomography (CT), or magnetic resonance images (MRIs) are obtained.

Arthrography is instrumental in evaluating ongoing joint pain or dysfunction, damage from recurrent dislocations of a joint, visualizing synovial cysts, and identifying acute or chronic tears in the soft tissue of the joint. Arthrography can also be used therapeutically to remove fluid in the joint space or to inject medications for pain relief.

Pediatrics: Arthrography is usually performed on young athletes with a suspected chronic joint injury or acute joint trauma. Hip arthrography is performed most often in children to evaluate congenital hip dislocation, hip dysplasia, or Perthes disease, before and after treatment.

INDICATIONS
• Evaluate pain, swelling, or dysfunction of a joint.
• Monitor disease progression.

INTERFERING FACTORS
Contraindications

Patients who are pregnant or suspected of being pregnant, unless the potential benefits of a procedure using radiation far outweigh the risk of radiation exposure to the fetus.

◈ Conditions associated with adverse reactions to contrast medium (e.g., asthma, food allergies, or allergy to contrast medium). Although patients are asked specifically if they have a known allergy to iodine or shellfish (shellfish contain high levels of iodine), it has been well established that the reaction is not to iodine; an actual iodine allergy would be problematic because iodine is required for the production of thyroid hormones. In the case of shellfish, the reaction is to a muscle protein called *tropomyosin*; in the case of iodinated contrast medium, the reaction is to the noniodinated part of the contrast molecule. Patients with a known hypersensitivity to the contrast medium may benefit from premedication with corticosteroids and diphenhydramine; the use of nonionic contrast or an alternative noncontrast imaging study, if available, may be considered for patients who have severe asthma or who have experienced moderate to severe reactions to ionic contrast medium.

◈ Patients with infection in the joint of interest.

◈ Patients with active arthritis.

◈ Patients with bleeding disorders receiving an arthrogram, *because the injection site may not stop bleeding.*

◈ Patients with metal in their body, such as shrapnel or ferrous metal in the eye, and who will be having associated MRI studies.

◈ Patients with cardiac pacemakers and who will be having associated MRI studies, *because the pacemaker can be deactivated by MRI.*

◈ Conditions associated with preexisting renal insufficiency (e.g., chronic kidney disease, single kidney transplant, nephrectomy, diabetes, multiple myeloma, treatment with aminoglycosides and NSAIDs), *because iodinated contrast is nephrotoxic.*

◈ Use of gadolinium-based contrast medium (GBCA) is contraindicated in patients with acute or chronic severe kidney disease (glomerular filtration rate less than 30 mL/min/1.73 m²). Patients should be screened for renal dysfunction prior to administration. The use of GBCAs should be avoided in these patients unless the benefits of the studies outweigh the risks and essential diagnostic information is not available using non-contrast-enhanced diagnostic studies.

◈ Patients who are chronically dehydrated before the test, especially older adults and patients whose health is already compromised, *because of their risk of contrast-induced acute kidney injury.*

Factors that may alter the results of the study
• Metallic objects (e.g., jewelry, body rings) within the examination field, which may inhibit organ visualization and cause unclear images.
• Inability of the patient to cooperate or remain still during the procedure, because movement can produce blurred or otherwise unclear images.

POTENTIAL MEDICAL DIAGNOSIS: CLINICAL SIGNIFICANCE OF RESULTS
Abnormal findings related to
• Arthritis
• Cysts
• Diseases of the cartilage (chondromalacia)
• Injury to the ligaments
• Joint derangement
• Meniscal tears or laceration
• Muscle tears
• Osteochondral fractures
• Osteochondritis dissecans
• Synovial tumor
• Synovitis

A

NURSING IMPLICATIONS

BEFORE THE STUDY: PLANNING AND IMPLEMENTATION

Teaching the Patient What to Expect

▶ Inform the patient this procedure can assist in assessing the joint being examined.

▶ Explain that prior to the procedure, laboratory testing may be required to determine the possibility of bleeding risk (coagulation testing) or to assess for impaired kidney function (Cr level and estimated glomerular filtration rate) if use of iodinated contrast medium is anticipated.

▶ Pregnancy is a general contraindication to procedures involving radiation. Explain to the female patient that she will be asked the date of her last menstrual period. Pregnancy testing may be performed to determine the possibility of pregnancy before exposure to radiation.

▶ Review the procedure with the patient. Address concerns about pain and explain that there may be moments of discomfort or pain experienced when the IV line or catheter is inserted to allow infusion of fluids such as saline, anesthetics, sedatives, contrast medium, medications used in the procedure, or emergency medications.

▶ Inform the patient that the procedure is usually performed in the radiology department by a health-care provider (HCP) and takes approximately 30 to 60 min.

▶ Instruct the patient to remove jewelry and other metallic objects from the area of examination.

▶ Baseline vital signs will be recorded and monitored throughout the procedure. Protocols may vary among facilities.

▶ Positioning for this procedure is determined in accordance with procedures ideally suited for the joint being examined after the patient is assisted to an examination table.

▶ Earplugs will be given to the patient having an MRI to block out the loud, banging sounds that occur during the MRI. Assure the patient that communication with the technologist is available at all times during the examination via a microphone within the scanner.

▶ Advise the patient that immediately prior to the procedure, the skin surrounding the joint is aseptically cleaned and anesthetized. A small-gauge needle is inserted into the joint space. During the procedure, any fluid in the space is aspirated and sent to the laboratory for analysis. Contrast medium is inserted into the joint space with fluoroscopic guidance. The needle is removed, and the joint is exercised to help distribute the contrast medium. X-rays or MRIs are then taken of the joint.

▶ Advise taking slow, deep breaths if nausea occurs during the procedure. An ordered antiemetic drug can be administered as needed. An emesis basin can be ready for use.

▶ Explain to the patient that he or she will be monitored for complications related to the procedure (e.g., allergic reaction, anaphylaxis, bronchospasm).

▶ Explain that once the study is completed, the needle or catheter is removed, and a pressure dressing is applied over the puncture site.

Potential Nursing Actions

✹ *Make sure a written and informed consent has been signed prior to the procedure and before administering any medications.*

▶ If iodinated contrast medium is scheduled to be used in patients receiving metformin or drugs containing metformin for type 2 diabetes, the drug may be discontinued on the day of the test and continue to be withheld for 48 hr after the test. Protocols may vary among facilities.

Safety Considerations

▶ Anticoagulants, aspirin, and other salicylates should be discontinued by medical direction for the appropriate number of days prior to a procedure in which bleeding is a potential complication.

A

AFTER THE STUDY: POTENTIAL NURSING ACTIONS

Avoiding Complications

▶ Establishing an IV site and injection of contrast medium are invasive procedures. Complications are rare but include risk for allergic reaction *(related to contrast reaction)*, bleeding from the puncture site *(related to a bleeding disorder or the effects of natural products and medications with known anticoagulant, antiplatelet, or thrombolytic properties)*, cardiac dysrhythmias, hematoma *(related to blood leakage into the tissue following needle insertion)*, infection *(which might occur if bacteria from the skin surface is introduced at the puncture site)*, tissue damage *(related to extravasation or leaking of contrast into the tissues during injection)*, nerve injury *(which might occur if the needle strikes a nerve)*, or nephrotoxicity *(a deterioration of renal function associated with contrast administration)*. Monitor the patient for complications related to the procedure (e.g., allergic reaction, anaphylaxis, bronchospasm, infection, injury). Immediately report symptoms such as difficulty breathing, chest pain, fever, hyperpnea, hypertension, nausea, palpitations, pruritus, rash, tachycardia, urticaria, or vomiting to the appropriate HCP. Observe/assess the needle/catheter insertion site for bleeding, inflammation, or hematoma formation. Administer ordered antihistamines or prophylactic steroids if the patient has an allergic reaction.

▶ Instruct the patient to notify the HCP if fever, increased pain, drainage, warmth, edema, or swelling of the joint occurs. Inform the patient that noises from the joint after the procedure are common and should disappear 24 to 48 hr after the procedure. Advise the patient to avoid strenuous activity, showering, and use of a hot tub or heating pad until approved by the HCP.

Treatment Considerations

▶ Observe and assess the joint for swelling after the test. Assess pain characteristics, location, duration, and intensity. Institute pain management modalities that fit with the patient's view of appropriate pain management. Instruct the patient to use a mild analgesic (aspirin, acetaminophen), as ordered, if there is discomfort. Narcotics may be ordered for severe pain. Rest periods are used to decrease joint aggravation. Teach the patient that appropriate use of ice application can relieve pain and reduce swelling. Suggest using an ice bag wrapped in a small towel and filled with crushed ice. Crushed ice easily conforms to the body site, and a towel helps protect the skin from the ice cold temperature.

▶ Assist patient in meeting activities of daily living. Assess the severity of mobility limitations; implement the use of assistive devices as needed and range of motion exercises for the affected side. Review and adapt environment to physical limitations to prevent injury. Teach the patient to perform circulation exercises and to elevate the affected limb, as ordered and appropriate, to prevent swelling and formation of blood clots *related to pooling of blood during lengthy periods of inactivity.*

▶ Discuss with the patient self-care activities that may require assistance, and collaboratively develop a plan to meet those needs. Encourage the patient to do as much as possible for himself or herself. Medication for pain 30 minutes prior to activity can maximize self-care opportunities and decrease pain.

Safety Considerations

▶ Advise diabetic patients to avoid all medications containing metformin for 48 hr following a procedure with iodinated contrast. Iodinated contrast can temporarily impair kidney function, and failure to withhold metformin may indirectly result in drug-induced lactic acidosis, a dangerous and sometimes fatal adverse effect of metformin (related to renal impairment that does not support sufficient excretion of metformin).

Nutritional Considerations
▶ Consider diet modification if excess body weight places stress on affected joints.

Follow-Up, Evaluation, and Desired Outcomes
▶ Acknowledges contact information provided for the American College of Rheumatology (www.rheumatology .org) or the Arthritis Foundation (www.arthritis.org).
▶ Understands the importance of rehabilitation in accomplishing a full recovery.

▶ Agrees to participate in a home-based exercise program or physical therapy to assist in recovering strength and range of motion.
▶ Acknowledges that a balanced exercise regime during recovery that avoids both excessive and insufficient use of the affected muscles will provide the best outcome. Excessive use can cause inflammation, pain, and swelling, and insufficient use can cause stiffness and atrophy. Agrees to avoid strenuous activity until approved by the HCP.

Arthroscopy

SYNONYM/ACRONYM: N/A

RATIONALE: To obtain direct visualization of a specific joint to assist in diagnosis of joint injury or disease and assessment of response to treatment.

PATIENT PREPARATION: There are no activity restrictions unless by medical direction. Food and fluids will be restricted to reduce aspiration risk from nausea and vomiting related to anesthesia during the procedure. Some institutions may allow clear liquids up to 2 hr prior to receiving regional anesthesia, or sedation/ analgesia (monitored anesthesia). Those having general anesthesia are usually required to be NPO (nothing by mouth) at midnight the night before the procedure. The American Society of Anesthesiologists has fasting guidelines for risk levels according to patient status. More information can be located at www.asahq.org.

Patients on beta blockers before the surgical procedure should be instructed to take their medication, as ordered, during the perioperative period. Regarding the patient's risk for bleeding, the patient should be instructed to avoid taking natural products and medications with known anticoagulant, antiplatelet, or thrombolytic properties or to reduce dosage, as ordered, prior to the procedure. Number of days to withhold medication is dependent on the type of anticoagulant. Note the last time and dose of medication taken. Protocols may vary among facilities.

Advice and education regarding pre- and postprocedural skin care is recommended; increased patient engagement levels are linked to decreased risk for a health-care-associated infection.

NORMAL FINDINGS
• Normal muscle, ligament, cartilage, synovial, and tendon structures of the joint, which is lined with a smooth, finely vascularized synovial

A

membrane. The normal appearance of the cable-like ligaments and tendons visible in joints is smooth and silvery; the cartilage appears smooth and white.

CRITICAL FINDINGS AND POTENTIAL INTERVENTIONS: N/A

OVERVIEW: (Study type: Endoscopy; related body system: Musculoskeletal system.) Arthroscopy provides direct visualization of a joint, usually a major joint such as the ankle, knee, hip, or shoulder, through the use of a fiberoptic endoscope. The arthroscope has a light, fiberoptics, and lenses; it connects to a monitor, and the images are recorded for future study and comparison. This procedure is used for inspection of joint structures, performance of a biopsy, and surgical repairs to the joint. Meniscus removal, spur removal, and ligamentous repair are some of the surgical procedures that may be performed. This procedure can also be used to monitor disease progression.

INDICATIONS
• Detect torn ligament or tendon.
• Evaluate joint pain and damaged cartilage.
• Evaluate meniscal, patellar, condylar, extrasynovial, and synovial injuries or diseases of the knee.
• Evaluate the extent of arthritis.
• Evaluate the presence of gout.
• Monitor effectiveness of therapy.
• Remove loose objects.

INTERFERING FACTORS
Contraindications
✳ Patients with bleeding disorders undergoing arthroscopy, *because the insertion site may not stop bleeding.*

✳ Patients with infection in the joint of interest or on the skin surrounding the area of the insertion site, *because the infection can be introduced into the joint by the contaminated arthroscope.*

✳ Patients who have had an arthrogram within the last 14 days *related to residual inflammation.*

Factors that may alter the results of the study
• Fibrous ankylosis of the joint preventing effective use of the arthroscope.
• Joints with flexion of less than 50 degrees.

POTENTIAL MEDICAL DIAGNOSIS: CLINICAL SIGNIFICANCE OF RESULTS
Abnormal findings related to
• Arthritis (rheumatoid)
• Chondromalacia
• Cysts
• Degenerative joint changes (osteoarthritis)
• Fractures
• Ganglion or Baker cyst
• Gout or pseudogout
• Hemarthrosis
• Infection
• Joint tumors
• Loose bodies
• Meniscal disease
• Osteochondritis
• Rheumatoid arthritis
• Subluxation, fracture, or dislocation
• Synovial rupture
• Synovitis
• Torn cartilage
• Torn ligament
• Torn rotator cuff
• Trapped synovium

A

NURSING IMPLICATIONS

POTENTIAL NURSING PROBLEMS: ASSESSMENT & NURSING DIAGNOSIS

Problems	Signs and Symptoms
Mobility *(related to joint pain, stiffness, the presence of muscle weakness, fear of pain)*	Hesitant or refuses to move for fear of pain, limited muscle strength on the affected side, anxiety
Pain (acute, chronic) *(related to degradation of the joint, damaged cartilage, altered bone growth)*	Self-report of pain that is acute or chronic; presence of facial grimace, crying, irritability; difficulty concentrating; social withdrawal; refusal or reluctance to participate in activities
Self-care, insufficient *(related to the presence of pain, fear, limited range of motion, anxiety)*	Observed physical limitations in the completion of activities of daily living, self-report of need of assistance for self-care activities

BEFORE THE STUDY: PLANNING AND IMPLEMENTATION

Teaching the Patient What to Expect

◗ Inform the patient this procedure can assist in assessing the joint being examined.

◗ Review the procedure with the patient. Address concerns about pain and explain that there may be moments of discomfort or pain experienced when the IV line or catheter is inserted to allow infusion of fluids such as saline, anesthetics, sedatives, medications used in the procedure, or emergency medications.

◗ Explain that reducing health-care-associated infections is an important patient safety goal, and a number of different safety practices will be implemented during the procedure. Advise the patient that hair around the joint area and areas 5 to 6 in. above and below the joint may be clipped or shaved and the area cleaned with an antiseptic solution to remove bacteria from the skin in order to reduce the risk for infection. *Note:* The World Health Organization, Centers for Disease Control and Prevention, and Association of periOperative Registered Nurses recommend that hair not be removed at all unless it interferes with the incision site or other aspects of the procedure because hair removal by any means is associated with increased infection rates. Clipping immediately before the procedure and in a location outside the procedure area is preferred to shaving with a razor. Shaving can create a break in skin integrity and provide a way for bacteria on the skin to enter the incision site.

◗ Inform the patient that the procedure is performed by a health-care provider (HCP), usually in the surgery department, and takes approximately 30 to 120 min, depending on the joint studied.

◗ The extremity is scrubbed, elevated, and wrapped with an elastic bandage from the distal portion of the extremity to the proximal portion to drain as much blood as possible from the limb. A pneumatic tourniquet placed around the proximal portion of the limb is inflated, and the elastic bandage is removed. As an alternative to a tourniquet, a mixture of lidocaine with epinephrine and sterile normal saline may be instilled into the joint to help reduce bleeding.

◗ Explain that at the start of the procedure, the joint is placed in a 45-degree angle, a local anesthetic is injected at the site, and a small incision is made in the skin in the lateral or medial aspect of the joint. The arthroscope is inserted into the joint spaces, and the joint is manipulated as it is visualized. Added puncture sites may be needed to provide a full view of the joint. Biopsy or treatment can be performed at this time, and images may be taken for future reference. After inspection, specimens may be obtained for cultures, cytology, or synovial fluid analysis.

▶ At the conclusion of the procedure, the joint is irrigated, and the arthroscope is removed. Steroids may be injected to reduce inflammation. Manual pressure is applied to the joint to remove remaining irrigation solution. The incision sites are sutured, and a pressure dressing is applied.

Potential Nursing Actions

❉ *Make sure a written and informed consent has been signed prior to the procedure and before administering any medications.*

▶ Explain that crutch walking might be taught before the procedure if it is anticipated postoperatively.

Safety Considerations

▶ Anticoagulants, aspirin, and other salicylates should be discontinued by medical direction for the appropriate number of days prior to a procedure in which bleeding is a potential complication.

AFTER THE STUDY: POTENTIAL NURSING ACTIONS

Avoiding Complications

▶ Possible complications include infection, phlebitis, hemarthrosis, hematoma, swelling, formation of blood clots, and synovial sac rupture. Monitor the patient's circulation and sensations in the joint area. Instruct the patient to immediately report symptoms such as fever, excessive bleeding, difficulty breathing, incision site redness, swelling, coldness, numbness, tingling, change in skin color (blue or dusky), and tenderness. Instruct the patient to elevate the joint when sitting and to avoid flexion of the joint to reduce swelling and formation of blood clots. Advise the patient to shower after 48 hr but to avoid strenuous activity and use of a hot

tub or heating pad until approved by the HCP. The patient may be asked to limit joint use for a specific period of time.

Treatment Considerations

▶ Mobility: Assist patient in meeting activities of daily living. Assess the severity of mobility limitations and implement the use of assistive devices as needed, including range-of-motion exercises for the affected side. Review and adapt environment to physical limitations to prevent injury.

▶ Pain: Assess pain characteristics (location, duration, intensity); institute pain management modalities that fit with the patient's view of appropriate pain management. Administer ordered analgesics and narcotics. Promote rest periods to decrease joint aggravation with the application of ordered hot or cold packs.

▶ Self-Care: Discuss with the patient self-care activities that may require assistance, and collaborate to develop a plan to meet those needs. Encourage the patient to do as much as possible for himself or herself. Medicate for pain 30 minutes prior to activity, and pace activities to maximize self-care opportunities and decrease pain.

Safety Considerations

▶ Ensure correct use of assistive devices such as crutches to decrease the risk of joint re-injury.

▶ Mobility limitations may make driving risky; confirm with the HCP when it is safe to resume driving.

Follow-Up, Evaluation, and Desired Outcomes

▶ Acknowledges contact information provided for the American College of Rheumatology (www.rheumatology.org) or for the Arthritis Foundation (www.arthritis.org).

▶ Patient/family understands the necessity of accurately reporting pain characteristics so that an appropriate pain management plan can be developed, and patient agrees to take ordered medication (NSAIDs, corticosteroids, muscle relaxants) for joint discomfort after the procedure.

▶ Recognizes the importance of decreasing joint stress and pain in order to promote healing. Acknowledges the importance of refraining from activities that will impair healing and understands the importance of ordered heat and cold therapy for decreasing joint pain and improving mobility.

▶ Accepts the importance of continuing physical or occupational therapy services and correctly demonstrates range-of-motion exercises.

A

Aspartate Aminotransferase

SYNONYM/ACRONYM: AST.

RATIONALE: Considered an indicator of cellular damage in liver disease, such as hepatitis or cirrhosis.

PATIENT PREPARATION: There are no food, fluid, activity, or medication restrictions unless by medical direction.

NORMAL FINDINGS: Method: Spectrophotometry, enzymatic at 37°C.

Age	Conventional and SI Units	SI Units Expressed as microkat/L = (Units/L × 0.017)
Newborn	25–75 units/L	0.43–1.28 microkat/L
10 days–3 yr	15–60 units/L	0.26–1.02 microkat/L
Child	20–39 units/L	0.34–0.66 microkat/L
Adult–older adult		
Male	20–40 units/L	0.34–0.68 microkat/L
Female	15–30 units/L	0.26–0.51 microkat/L

Values may be slightly elevated in older adults due to the effects of medications and the presence of multiple chronic or acute diseases with or without muted symptoms.

CRITICAL FINDINGS AND POTENTIAL INTERVENTIONS: N/A

OVERVIEW: (**Study type:** Blood collected in a gold-, red-, or red/gray-top tube; **related body system:** Digestive system.) Aspartate aminotransferase (AST) is an enzyme that catalyzes the reversible transfer of an amino group between aspartate and α-ketoglutaric acid in the citric acid or Krebs cycle, a powerful and essential biochemical pathway for releasing stored energy. AST exists in large amounts in liver and myocardial cells and in smaller but significant amounts in skeletal muscle, kidneys, pancreas, red blood cells, and the brain. Serum AST rises when there is damage to the tissues and cells where the enzyme is found, and levels directly reflect the extent of damage. AST values greater than 500 units/L (SI = 8.5 microkat/L) are usually associated with hepatitis and other hepatocellular diseases in an acute phase. AST levels are very elevated at birth, decrease with age to adulthood, and increase slightly in older adults.

A

INDICATIONS

- Compare serially with alanine aminotransferase levels to track the course of hepatitis.
- Monitor response to therapy with potentially hepatotoxic or nephrotoxic drugs.
- Monitor response to treatment for various disorders of hepatic function in which AST may be elevated, with tissue repair indicated by declining levels.

INTERFERING FACTORS

Factors that may alter the results of the study

- Drugs and other substances that may increase AST levels by causing cholestasis include amitriptyline, anabolic steroids, androgens, benzodiazepines, chlorothiazide, chlorpropamide, dapsone, erythromycin, estrogens, ethionamide, gold salts, imipramine, mercaptopurine, nitrofurans, oral contraceptives, penicillins, phenothiazines, progesterone, sulfonamides, tamoxifen, and tolbutamide.
- Drugs and other substances that may increase AST levels by causing hepatocellular damage include acetaminophen, acetylsalicylic acid, allopurinol, amiodarone, anabolic steroids, anticonvulsants, asparaginase, azithromycin, bromocriptine, captopril, cephalosporins, chloramphenicol, clindamycin, clofibrate, danazol, enflurane, ethambutol, ethionamide, fenofibrate, fluconazole, fluoroquinolones, foscarnet, gentamicin, indomethacin, interferon, interleukin-2, levamisole, levodopa, lincomycin, low-molecular-weight heparin, methyldopa, monoamine oxidase inhibitors, naproxen, nifedipine, nitrofurans, oral contraceptives, probenecid, procainamide, quinine, ranitidine, retinol, ritodrine, sulfonylureas, tetracyclines, tobramycin, and verapamil.
- Drugs and other substances that may decrease AST levels include allopurinol, cyclosporine, interferon alpha, naltrexone, progesterone, trifluoperazine, and ursodiol.
- Hemolysis falsely increases AST values.
- Hemodialysis falsely decreases AST values.

POTENTIAL MEDICAL DIAGNOSIS: CLINICAL SIGNIFICANCE OF RESULTS

Increased in

AST is released from any damaged cell in which it is stored, so conditions that affect the liver, kidneys, heart, pancreas, red blood cells, or skeletal muscle and cause cellular destruction demonstrate elevated AST levels.

Significantly increased (greater than five times normal levels) in:

- Acute hepatitis *(AST is very elevated in acute viral hepatitis)*
- Acute hepatocellular disease *(especially related to chemical toxicity or drug overdose; moderate doses of acetaminophen have initiated severe hepatocellular disease in patients who are alcoholics)*
- Acute pancreatitis
- Shock

Moderately increased (three to five times normal levels) in:

- Alcohol misuse (chronic)
- Biliary tract obstruction
- Cardiac dysrhythmias
- Cardiac catheterization, angioplasty, or surgery
- Cirrhosis
- Chronic hepatitis
- Heart failure
- HELLP (hemolysis, elevated liver enzymes, low platelet count) syndrome of pregnancy
- Infectious mononucleosis
- Liver tumors
- Muscle diseases (e.g., dermatomyositis, dystrophy, gangrene, polymyositis, trichinosis)
- Myocardial infarction
- Reye syndrome
- Trauma *(related to injury or surgery of liver, head, and other sites where AST is found)*

Slightly increased (two to three times normal) in:

- Cerebrovascular accident
- Cirrhosis, fatty liver *(related to obesity, diabetes, jejunoileal bypass, administration of total parenteral nutrition)*
- Delirium tremens
- Hemolytic anemia
- Pericarditis
- Pulmonary infarction

Decreased in

- Hemodialysis *(presumed to be related to a corresponding deficiency of vitamin B₆ observed in hemodialysis patients)*
- Uremia *(related to a buildup of toxins that modify the activity of coenzymes required for transaminase activity)*
- Vitamin B₆ deficiency *(related to the lack of vitamin B₆, a required cofactor for the transaminases)*

NURSING IMPLICATIONS

BEFORE THE STUDY: PLANNING AND IMPLEMENTATION

Teaching the Patient What to Expect

⏵ Inform the patient this test can assist in assessing liver function.

⏵ Explain that a blood sample is needed for the test.

Potential Nursing Actions

⏵ Measuring and trending abdominal girth can assist in monitoring the progression of ascites with liver disease.

AFTER THE STUDY: POTENTIAL NURSING ACTIONS

Avoiding Complications

⏵ The patient with cirrhosis should be observed carefully for the development of ascites, in which case fluid and electrolyte balance requires strict attention.

Nutritional Considerations

⏵ Increased AST levels may be associated with liver disease. In general, patients should be encouraged to eat a well-balanced diet that includes foods high in fiber. Dietary recommendations will vary depending on the condition and its severity. For example, recommend a diet of soft foods if esophageal varices develop, fat substitutes for bile duct disease, or limitations on salt intake if ascites develop.

⏵ Other options include enteral and parenteral nutrition as replacement strategies. Correlate laboratory values with IV fluid infusion and collaborate with the health-care provider and pharmacist to adjust to patient needs. Adequate pain and nausea control can improve caloric intake.

Audiometry, Hearing Loss

SYNONYM/ACRONYM: N/A

RATIONALE: To evaluate hearing loss in newborns and school-age children but can be used for all ages.

PATIENT PREPARATION: There are no food, fluid, activity, or medication restrictions unless by medical direction.

NORMAL FINDINGS

- Normal pure tone average of –10 to 15 dB for infants, children, or adults.

CRITICAL FINDINGS AND POTENTIAL INTERVENTIONS: N/A

OVERVIEW: (**Study type:** Sensory (auditory); **related body system:** Nervous system.) Tests to estimate hearing ability can be performed on patients of any age (e.g., at birth before discharge from a hospital or birthing center, as part of a school screening program, or as adults if indicated). Hearing loss audiometry includes quantitative testing for a hearing deficit. An audiometer is used to measure and record thresholds of hearing by air-conduction and bone-conduction tests. The test results determine if hearing loss is conductive, sensorineural, or a combination of both. An elevated air-conduction threshold with a normal bone-conduction threshold indicates a conductive hearing loss. An equally elevated threshold for both air and bone conduction indicates a sensorineural hearing loss. An elevated threshold of air conduction that is greater than an elevated threshold of bone conduction indicates a composite of both types of hearing loss. A conductive hearing loss is caused by an abnormality in the external auditory canal or middle ear, and a sensorineural hearing loss by an abnormality in the inner ear or of the VIII (auditory) nerve. Sensorineural hearing loss can be further differentiated clinically by sensory (cochlear) or neural (VIII nerve) lesions. Sensorineural hearing loss is permanent. Additional information for comparing and differentiating between conductive and sensorineural hearing loss can be obtained from hearing loss tuning fork tests. Every state and territory in the United States has a newborn screening program that includes early hearing loss detection and intervention (EHDI). The goal of EHDI is to assure that permanent hearing loss is identified before 3 mo of age, appropriate and timely intervention services are provided before 6 mo of age, families of infants with hearing loss receive culturally competent support, and tracking and data management systems for newborn hearing screens are linked with other relevant public health information systems.

INDICATIONS

- Determine the need for a type of hearing aid and evaluate its effectiveness.
- Determine the type and extent of hearing loss and whether further radiological, audiological, or vestibular procedures are needed to identify the cause.
- Evaluate communication disabilities and plan for rehabilitation interventions.
- Evaluate degree and extent of preoperative and postoperative hearing loss following stapedectomy in patients with otosclerosis.
- Screen for hearing loss in infants and children and determine the need for a referral to an audiologist.

INTERFERING FACTORS

Factors that may alter the results of the study

- Effects of ototoxic medications can cause temporary, intermittent, or permanent hearing loss.
- Improper earphone fit or audiometer calibration can affect results.
- Tinnitus or other sensations can cause abnormal responses.

POTENTIAL MEDICAL DIAGNOSIS: CLINICAL SIGNIFICANCE OF RESULTS

If findings are normal, the patient should have normal hearing. The test is conducted using earphones and/or a device placed behind the ear to deliver sounds of varying intensities. Results are categorized using ranges of pure tone recorded in decibels.

ASHA Category	Pure Tone Averages
Normal range or no impairment	−10–15 dB
Slight loss	16–25 dB
Mild loss	26–40 dB
Moderate loss	41–55 dB
Moderately severe loss	56–70 dB
Severe loss	71–90 dB
Profound loss	Greater than 91 dB

dB = decibel.

Abnormal findings related to
• Causes of conductive hearing loss
  Impacted cerumen
  Hole in eardrum
  Malformed outer ear, ear canal, or middle ear
  Obstruction of external ear canal *(related to presence of a foreign body)*
  Otitis externa *(related to infection in ear canal)*
  Otitis media *(related to poor eustachian tube function or infection)*
  Otitis media serous *(related to fluid in middle ear due to allergies or a cold)*
  Otosclerosis
• Causes of sensorineural hearing loss
  Congenital damage or malformations of the inner ear
  Ménière disease
  Ototoxic drugs administered orally, topically, as otic drops, by IV, or passed to the fetus in utero *(aminoglycoside antibiotics, e.g., gentamicin or tobramycin, and chemotherapeutic drugs, e.g., cisplatin and carboplatin, are known to cause permanent hearing loss; quinine, loop diuretics, and salicylates, e.g., aspirin, are known to cause temporary hearing loss; other categories of drugs known to be ototoxic include anesthetics, cardiac medications, mood altering medications, and glucocorticosteroids, e.g., cortisone, steroids)*
  Presbycusis *(gradual hearing loss experienced in advancing age related to degeneration of the cochlea)*
  Serious infections *(meningitis, measles, mumps, other viral, syphilis)*
  Trauma to the inner ear *(related to exposure to noise in excess of 90 dB or as a result of physical trauma)*

Tumor *(e.g., acoustic neuroma, cerebellopontine angle tumor, meningioma)*
Vascular disorders

NURSING IMPLICATIONS

BEFORE THE STUDY: PLANNING AND IMPLEMENTATION

Teaching the Patient What to Expect
▸ Inform the patient/caregiver this procedure can assist in detecting hearing loss.
▸ Review the procedure with the patient. Address concerns about pain and explain that no discomfort will be experienced during the test.
▸ Inform the patient that an audiologist or health-care provider specializing in this procedure performs the test in a quiet, soundproof room and that the test can take up to 20 min to evaluate both ears.
▸ Explain that each ear will be tested separately by using earphones and/or a device placed behind the ear to deliver sounds of varying intensities. The ear not being tested is masked to prevent crossover of test tones, and the earphones are positioned on the head and over the ear canals. Infants and children may be tested using earphones that are inserted into the ear, unless contraindicated. An oscillating probe may be placed over the mastoid process behind the ear or on the forehead if bone-conduction testing is to be performed as part of the hearing assessment.

A

• Explain that the test results are plotted on a graph called an *audiogram*. Symbols are used to indicate the ear tested and whether responses were obtained using earphones (air conduction) or an oscillator (bone conduction). Explain that the patient will be asked to press a button each time a tone is heard, no matter how loudly or faintly it is perceived. The study is conducted using individualized determinations appropriate for the patient. In children between 6 mo and 2 yr of age, minimal response levels can be determined by behavioral responses to test tone. In the child 2 yr and older, play audiometry that requires the child to perform a task or raise a hand in response to a specific tone is performed. In children 12 yr and older, the child is asked to follow directions in identifying objects; response to speech of specific intensities can be used to evaluate hearing loss that is affected by speech frequencies.

Potential Nursing Actions

✺ *Make sure a written and informed consent has been signed prior to the procedure and before administering any medications.*

• Obtain a history of the patient's health concerns (especially the patient's known or suspected hearing loss, including type and cause; ear conditions with treatment regimens), symptoms, surgical procedures (especially related to the ears), and results of previously performed laboratory and diagnostic studies.

• Otoscopy examination may be necessary to ensure that the external ear canal is free from any obstruction and is clear of impacted cerumen. Test for closure of the canal from the pressure of the earphones by compressing the tragus. Tendency for the canal to close (often the case in children and older adult patients) can be corrected by the careful insertion of a small, stiff plastic tube into the anterior canal.

Safety Considerations

• Address concerns about claustrophobia, as appropriate. Describe and demonstrate to the patient how to communicate with the audiologist and how to exit from the room.

AFTER THE STUDY: POTENTIAL NURSING ACTIONS

Avoiding Complications

• Ensure the culture for ear drainage is completed prior to beginning antibiotic therapy, if possible, for accurate organism identification.

Safety Considerations

• Communication with a patient with hearing deficits will require that the nurse take special effort to ensure messages are clearly sent and received. Make sure you are facing the patient when speaking with him or her. Use agreed-upon alternative communication methods that are easily understood and age/culture appropriate.

Follow-Up, Evaluation, and Desired Outcomes

• Acknowledges contact information provided for the National Center for Hearing Assessment and Management (http://infanthearing.org) or the American Speech-Language-Hearing Association (www.asha.org).

• Understands that profound hearing loss can have a long-range impact personally, socially, and professionally. The patient and family will consider support groups that may help provide guidance toward a realistic transition into life management with an auditory deficit.

• Demonstrates how to use, clean, and store a hearing aid.

• Acknowledges that a follow-up appointment to examine the ear is necessary to ensure complete healing and prevent complications that may lead to significant hearing loss.

• Describes the correct use of over-the-counter medications for pain management (acetaminophen and ibuprofen).

β₂-Microglobulin, Blood and Urine

SYNONYM/ACRONYM: β_2-M, BMG.

RATIONALE: To assist in diagnosing malignancy such as lymphoma, leukemia, or multiple myeloma. Also valuable in assessing for chronic severe inflammatory and kidney diseases.

PATIENT PREPARATION: There are no food, fluid, activity, or medication restrictions unless by medical direction. Usually, a 24-hr urine collection is ordered. As appropriate, provide the required urine collection container and specimen collection instructions.

NORMAL FINDINGS: Method: Immunochemiluminometric assay.

Sample	Conventional and SI Units
Serum	Less than 2.5 mg/L
Urine	0–300 mcg/L

CRITICAL FINDINGS AND POTENTIAL INTERVENTIONS: N/A

OVERVIEW: (**Study type:** Blood collected in a red- or red/gray-top tube or urine from a timed collection in a clean plastic container with 1 N NaOH as a preservative; **related body system:** Immune and Urinary systems.) Urine from an unpreserved random collection may also be requested. β_2-Microglobulin (BMG) is a protein component of human leukocyte antigen (HLA) complexes. BMG is on the surface of most cells and is therefore a useful indicator of cell death or unusually high levels of cell production. BMG is a small protein and is readily reabsorbed by kidneys with normal function. Cerebrospinal fluid (CSF) levels parallel serum levels. BMG increases in inflammatory conditions and when lymphocyte turnover increases, such as in lymphocytic leukemia or when T-lymphocyte helper (OKT4) cells are attacked by HIV. Serum BMG becomes elevated with malfunctioning glomeruli but decreases with malfunctioning tubules because it is metabolized by the renal tubules. Conversely, urine BMG decreases with malfunctioning glomeruli but becomes elevated with malfunctioning tubules.

INDICATIONS
- Detect aminoglycoside toxicity.
- Detect chronic lymphocytic leukemia, multiple myeloma, lung cancer, hepatoma, or breast cancer.
- Detect HIV infection. (*Note:* Levels do not correlate with stages of infection.)
- Evaluate kidney disease to differentiate glomerular from tubular dysfunction.
- Evaluate kidney transplant viability and predict rejection.
- Monitor antiretroviral therapy.

INTERFERING FACTORS
Factors that may alter the results of the study
- Drugs and other substances that may increase serum BMG levels include cyclosporin A, gentamicin, interferon alfa, and lithium.
- Drugs and other substances that may decrease serum BMG levels include zidovudine.

B

- Drugs and other substances that may increase urine BMG levels include azathioprine, cisplatin, cyclosporin A, furosemide, gentamicin, iodixanol, iopentol, mannitol, nifedipine, sisomicin, and tobramycin.
- Urinary BMG is unstable at pH less than 5.5.
- All urine voided for the timed collection period must be included in the collection, or else falsely decreased values may be obtained. Compare output records with volume collected to verify that all voids were included in the collection.

POTENTIAL MEDICAL DIAGNOSIS: CLINICAL SIGNIFICANCE OF RESULTS
Increased in
- AIDS *(related to increased lymphocyte turnover)*
- Aminoglycoside toxicity *(related to acute kidney injury; urine BMG becomes elevated before creatinine)*
- Amyloidosis *(related to chronic inflammatory conditions associated with increased BMG and other acute-phase reactant proteins; also related to deposition of amyloid in joints and tissues of patients receiving long-term hemodialysis)*
- Autoimmune disorders *(related to increased lymphocyte turnover)*
- Breast cancer *(related to increased lymphocyte turnover; serum BMG indicates tumor growth rate, size, and response to treatment)*
- Crohn disease *(related to chronic inflammatory conditions associated with increased BMG and other acute-phase reactant proteins)*
- Felty syndrome *(related to chronic inflammatory conditions associated with increased BMG and other acute-phase reactant proteins)*
- Heavy metal poisoning
- Hepatitis *(related to increased lymphocyte turnover in response to viral infection)*
- Hepatoma *(related to increased lymphocyte turnover; serum BMG indicates tumor growth rate, size, and response to treatment)*
- Hyperthyroidism *(related to increased lymphocyte turnover in immune thyroid disease)*
- Kidney dialysis *(related to ability of kidney tubule to reabsorb BMG)*
- Kidney disease (glomerular): serum only *(related to ability of kidney tubule to reabsorb BMG)*
- Kidney disease (tubular): urine only *(related to ability of kidney tubule to reabsorb BMG)*
- Leukemia (chronic lymphocytic) *(related to increased lymphocyte turnover; serum BMG indicates tumor growth rate, size, and response to treatment)*
- Lung cancer *(related to increased lymphocyte turnover; serum BMG indicates tumor growth rate, size, and response to treatment)*
- Lymphoma *(related to increased lymphocyte turnover; serum BMG indicates tumor growth rate, size, and response to treatment)*
- Multiple myeloma *(related to increased lymphocyte turnover)*
- Poisoning with heavy metals, such as mercury or cadmium *(related to kidney damage that decreases BMG absorption)*
- Sarcoidosis
- Sjögren disease
- Systemic lupus erythematosus *(related to chronic inflammatory conditions associated with increased BMG and other acute-phase reactant proteins)*
- Vasculitis *(related to chronic inflammatory conditions associated with increased BMG and other acute-phase reactant proteins)*
- Viral infections (e.g., cytomegalovirus) *(related to increased lymphocyte turnover)*

Decreased in
- Kidney disease (glomerular): urine only
- Kidney disease (tubular): serum only

- Response to zidovudine (ZVD), also known as *azidothymidine* (AZT) *(related to decreased viral replication and lymphocyte destruction)*

B

NURSING IMPLICATIONS

POTENTIAL NURSING PROBLEMS: ASSESSMENT & NURSING DIAGNOSIS

Problems	Signs and Symptoms
Bleeding *(related to altered bone marrow function secondary to radiation therapy and chemotherapy)*	Decreased platelet count, altered level of consciousness, hypotension, increased heart rate, decreased hemoglobin (Hgb) and hematocrit (Hct), capillary refill greater than 3 sec, cool extremities
Fatigue *(related to metastatic disease, tumor, pain, radiation therapy, chemotherapy, anemia, insufficient nutrition, anxiety)*	Report of tiredness, inability to maintain activities of daily living at current level, inability to restore energy after rest or sleep
Infection *(related to altered immune response associated with chemotherapy and radiation therapy, opportunistic hosts)*	Fever; evidence of local or systemic infection, blood cultures positive for infection, sputum culture positive for infection, increased heart rate and respiratory rate, chills, change in mental status, fatigue, malaise, weakness, anorexia, headache, nausea, elevated blood glucose, hypotension, diminished oxygen saturation, elevated white blood cell (WBC) count, elevated C-reactive protein
Spirituality *(related to diagnosis of terminal illness, active dying, ongoing chronic illness, anxiety, fear, hopelessness)*	Disharmony between personal beliefs, value system, and threat to life; anger; lack of courage; no purpose or meaning to life; lack of acceptance of diagnosis, disease process; separation from support system; disinterest in connecting with others

BEFORE THE STUDY: PLANNING AND IMPLEMENTATION

Teaching the Patient What to Expect
- Inform the patient that the test is used to evaluate kidney disease, AIDS, and certain malignancies.
- Explain that a blood or urine sample is needed for the test. Information regarding specimen collection is presented with other general guidelines in Appendix A: Patient Preparation and Specimen Collection.

Potential Nursing Actions
- Include on the collection container's label urine total volume, test start and stop times/dates, and any medications that may interfere with test results.

AFTER THE STUDY: POTENTIAL NURSING ACTIONS

Treatment Considerations
- Bleeding: Administer prescribed platelets or blood as ordered, monitor and trend platelet count. Increase

frequency of vital sign assessment with variances and trends in results. Administer stool softeners as needed and monitor stool for blood. Encourage intake of foods rich in vitamin K, monitor and trend Hgb/Hct. Assess skin for petechiae, purpura, hematoma; monitor for blood in emesis or sputum. Institute bleeding precautions (prevent unnecessary venipuncture; avoid intramuscular [IM] injections; prevent trauma; be gentle with oral care, suctioning; avoid use of a sharp razor). Coordinate laboratory draws to decrease number of venipunctures, and review transfusion reaction symptoms.

- Fatigue: Discuss the implementation of energy conservation activities (even pace when working, frequent rest periods, frequent items in easy reach, push items instead of pulling) and set priorities for energy expenditures. Limit naps to increase nighttime sleeping. Administer ordered transfusion of blood or blood products to treat anemia. Administer ordered psychostimulants as appropriate and encourage participation in ordered psychotherapy.
- Infection: Use standard precautions in the provision of care. Correlate symptoms with laboratory values and disease process, and trend vital signs and laboratory values to monitor for improvement or decline. Administer prescribed antibiotics and medications for fever reduction with appropriate cooling measures. Encourage vigilant hand hygiene and educate patient and family regarding good hand hygiene with rationale. Infuse ordered IV fluids to support adequate hydration. Ensure implementation of infection prevention measures with consideration of age and culture, such as adequate nutrition; perform aseptic wound care. Ensure skin care, oral care, and adequate rest. Avoid exposure to opportunistic hosts, send cultures to the laboratory as ordered, and correlate culture findings with selected antibiotics.

Avoid mouthwashes with high alcohol content. Notify health-care provider (HCP) of temperature spikes or flu-like symptoms; discuss implementation of protective isolation for neutrophil count less than 0.5 to 1 × 10³/microL.

- Spirituality: Assess for the presence of religious affiliation and cultural factors that influence spirituality. Encourage verbalization of feelings. Work proactively to develop a positive relationship with the patient, assist decision making working within patient's value system. Facilitate interaction with spiritual leaders and support faith-based rituals.

Nutritional Considerations
- Stress the importance of good nutrition, and suggest that the patient meet with a registered dietitian. Also, stress the importance of following the care plan for medications and follow-up visits.

Follow-Up, Evaluation, and Desired Outcomes
- Acknowledges contact information provided for the American Cancer Society (www.cancer.org). Provide contact information, if desired, for AIDS information provided by the National Institutes of Health (https://aidsinfo.nih.gov), American College of Obstetricians and Gynecologists (www.acog.org), or Centers for Disease Control and Prevention (www.cdc.gov).
- Victims of sexual assault accept offered emotional support.
- Agrees to discuss risks of sexually transmitted infections in a non-judgmental, nonthreatening atmosphere. Acknowledges the risk of transmission and proper prophylaxis and accepts the importance of strict adherence to the treatment regimen.
- Acknowledges that retesting may be necessary.
- Understands the risk of infection related to immunosuppressed inflammatory response and fatigue related to decreased energy production.

Barium Enema

SYNONYM/ACRONYM: Air-contrast barium enema, double-contrast barium enema, lower GI series, BE.

RATIONALE: To assist in diagnosing bowel disease in the colon such as tumors and polyps.

PATIENT PREPARATION: Instruct the patient to eat a low-residue diet for several days before the procedure and consume only clear liquids during the 24 hr before the procedure, including the evening before the test. There are no activity restrictions unless by medical direction. Instruct the patient to fast and restrict fluids for 8 hr, or as ordered, prior to the procedure. Fasting may be ordered as a precaution against aspiration related to possible nausea and vomiting. The American Society of Anesthesiologists has fasting guidelines for risk levels according to patient status. More information can be located at www.asahq.org.

Note: If iodinated contrast medium is scheduled to be used in patients receiving metformin or drugs containing metformin for type 2 diabetes, the drug may be discontinued on the day of the test and continue to be withheld for 48 hr after the test.

Regarding the patient's risk for bleeding, the patient should be instructed to avoid taking natural products and medications with known anticoagulant, anti-platelet, or thrombolytic properties or to reduce dosage, as ordered, prior to the procedure. Number of days to withhold medication is dependent on the type of anticoagulant. Note the last time and dose of medication taken. Protocols may vary among facilities.

Inform the patient that a laxative and cleansing enema may be needed the day before the procedure, with cleansing enemas on the morning of the procedure, depending on the institution's policy. Patients with a colostomy will be ordered special preparations and colostomy irrigation.

If studies involving the entire digestive tract are required (e.g., upper GI or barium swallow), verify that the barium enema is performed first to avoid retention in the abdomen of residual barium from the swallow study, which may obscure details of interest.

Pediatric Preps

2 years or younger	Clear liquid diet 24 hr prior to the procedure; a pediatric Fleet enema (a half or whole suppository [glycerin or bisacodyl (Dulcolax)] may be ordered instead of the enema) on the evening before and morning of the procedure up to 3 hr prior to the procedure; NPO for 4 hr before procedure

(table continues on page 132)

3–16 years	• Low-residue diet for 48 hr prior to procedure
	• Clear liquid diet for 24 hr prior to procedure; castor oil or Neoloid, a flavored castor oil, may be ordered the night before the procedure; dose is based on either weight or age—for castor oil, 26–80 lb, give 1 oz, 81 lb or greater, give 2 oz; for Neoloid, 2–5 yr give 2 teaspoons (9.9 mL), 6–8 yr give 1 tablespoon (14.8 mL), 8–18 yr give 2 tablespoons (29.6 mL)—or bisacodyl oral tablet may be substituted based on age (3–8 yr give 1 tablet, 9 yr and older give 2 tablets)
	• Fleet enemas, until fecal return is clear, up to 3 hr prior to procedure
	• NPO for 4 hr prior to procedure

NORMAL FINDINGS
• Normal size, filling, shape, position, and motility of the colon
• Normal filling of the appendix and terminal ileum.

CRITICAL FINDINGS AND POTENTIAL INTERVENTIONS: N/A

OVERVIEW: (Study type: X-ray Contrast/Special; related body system: Digestive system.) This radiological examination of the colon, distal small bowel, and occasionally the appendix follows instillation of barium (single-contrast study) using a rectal tube inserted into the rectum or an existing ostomy; the patient retains the contrast while a series of images are obtained. Visualization can be improved by draining the barium and using air contrast (double-contrast study). Some of the barium remains on the surface of the colon wall, allowing for greater detail in the images. A combination of x-ray and fluoroscopic techniques are used to complete the study. This test is especially useful in the evaluation of patients experiencing lower abdominal pain, changes in bowel habits, or the passage of stools containing blood or mucus, and for visualizing polyps, diverticula, and tumors. A barium enema may be therapeutic by reducing an obstruction caused by intussusception, or telescoping of the small intestine into the large intestine; this is a condition that most commonly affects children.

INDICATIONS
• Determine the cause of rectal bleeding, blood, pus, or mucus in feces.
• Evaluate suspected inflammatory process, congenital anomaly, motility disorder, or structural change.
• Evaluate unexplained weight loss, anemia, or a change in bowel pattern.
• Identify and locate benign or malignant polyps or tumors.

INTERFERING FACTORS
Contraindications
Patients who are pregnant or suspected of being pregnant, unless

the potential benefits of a procedure using radiation far outweigh the risk of radiation exposure to the fetus and mother.

✦ Patients with suspected perforation of the colon should receive a water-soluble iodinated contrast medium, such as Gastrografin, *to prevent barium from spilling into the retroperitoneum and causing an inflammatory reaction in the surrounding tissue.*

✦ Conditions associated with adverse reactions to contrast medium (e.g., asthma, food allergies, or allergy to contrast medium). Although patients are asked specifically if they have a known allergy to iodine or shellfish (shellfish contain high levels of iodine), it has been well established that the reaction is not to iodine; an actual iodine allergy would be problematic because iodine is required for the production of thyroid hormones. In the case of shellfish, the reaction is to a muscle protein called *tropomyosin*; in the case of iodinated contrast medium, the reaction is to the noniodinated part of the contrast molecule. Patients with a known hypersensitivity to the medium may benefit from premedication with corticosteroids and diphenhydramine; the use of nonionic contrast or an alternative noncontrast imaging study, if available, may be considered for patients who have severe asthma or who have experienced moderate to severe reactions to ionic contrast medium.

✦ Patients with conditions such as rapid heart rate, intestinal obstruction, megacolon, acute ulcerative colitis, acute diverticulitis, or suspected rupture of the colon; *barium or water from the enema may make the condition worse.*

Factors that may alter the results of the study
- Gas or feces in the gastrointestinal (GI) tract resulting from inadequate cleansing or failure to restrict food intake before the study can interfere with visualization. Residual stool can mimic a polyp.
- Retained barium from a previous radiological procedure.
- Spasm of the colon, which can mimic the radiographic signs of cancer. (*Note:* The use of IV glucagon minimizes spasm.)
- Inability of the patient to tolerate introduction of or retention of barium, air, or both, in the bowel.
- Metallic objects (e.g., jewelry, body rings) within the examination field, which may inhibit organ visualization and cause unclear images.
- Inability of the patient to cooperate or remain still during the procedure because movement can produce blurred or otherwise unclear images.

POTENTIAL MEDICAL DIAGNOSIS: CLINICAL SIGNIFICANCE OF RESULTS
Abnormal findings related to
- Appendicitis
- Colorectal cancer
- Congenital anomalies
- Crohn disease
- Diverticular disease
- Fistulas
- Gastroenteritis
- Granulomatous colitis
- Hirschsprung disease
- Intussusception
- Perforation of the colon
- Polyps
- Sarcoma
- Sigmoid torsion
- Sigmoid volvulus
- Stenosis
- Tumors
- Ulcerative colitis

B

NURSING IMPLICATIONS

POTENTIAL NURSING PROBLEMS: ASSESSMENT & NURSING DIAGNOSIS

Problems	Signs and Symptoms
Altered gastrointestinal elimination *(related to bowel disease, inflammation, infection, tumor)*	Altered bowel sounds, compromised GI motility, diarrhea, constipation
Pain *(related to abdominal distention, GI inflammation, postoperative incision)*	Crying, holding abdomen with guarding, verbalization of pain and pain characteristics, facial grimace

BEFORE THE STUDY: PLANNING AND IMPLEMENTATION

Teaching the Patient What to Expect

▶ Inform the patient this procedure can assist in assessing the colon.

▶ Pregnancy is a general contraindication to procedures involving radiation. Explain to the female patient that she will be asked the date of her last menstrual period. Pregnancy testing may be performed to determine the possibility of pregnancy before exposure to radiation.

▶ Review the procedure with the patient. Address concerns about pain and explain that there may be moments of discomfort or pain experienced when the rectal tube is inserted.

▶ **Pediatric Considerations:** Preparing children for a barium enema depends on the age of the child. Encourage parents to be truthful about unpleasant sensations (cramping, pressure, fullness) the child may experience during the procedure and to use words that they know their child will understand. Toddlers and preschool-age children have a short attention span, so the best time to talk about the test is right before the procedure. The child should be assured that he or she will be allowed to bring a favorite comfort item into the examination room and, if appropriate, that a parent will be with him or her during the procedure. Explain that there will be monitors in the room, and the child and parent will

be able to watch the procedure along with the health-care team.

▶ Inform the patient that the procedure is performed in a radiology department, by a health-care provider (HCP) specializing in this procedure, with support staff, and takes approximately 30 min.

▶ Instruct the patient to remove jewelry and other metallic objects from the area of examination.

▶ Baseline vital signs will be recorded and monitored throughout the procedure. Protocols may vary among facilities.

▶ Explain that during the procedure the initial image will be taken in the supine position. Afterwards, the position will change to lying in the Sim position on the left side. A rectal tube is then inserted into the anus and an attached balloon is inflated once situated against the anal sphincter.

▶ **Older Adult and Pediatric Considerations:** Reduced muscle tone occurs with advanced age, and fully developed muscle tone may not be present in children. Therefore, older adult patients and children may have difficulty holding the barium in the colon while the images are taken. A balloon tip may be used to assist with retention of the barium; the buttocks may be gently held together with tape if necessary.

▶ Explain that barium is instilled into the colon by gravity, and its movement through the colon is observed by fluoroscopy. For patients with a colostomy, an indwelling urinary catheter is inserted into the stoma and barium is administered.

‣ Images are taken with the patient in different positions to aid in the diagnosis. If a double-contrast barium enema has been ordered, air is then instilled in the intestine and additional images are taken.

‣ After the procedure, most of the barium is removed using the rectal tube. The patient is helped to the bathroom to expel residual barium or placed on a bedpan if unable to ambulate.

‣ A postevacuation image is taken of the colon to verify expulsion of the barium.

Potential Nursing Actions

✦ *Make sure a written and informed consent has been signed prior to the procedure and before administering any medications.*

‣ Ask the patient about known allergens, especially allergies or sensitivities to latex (if a latex balloon tip is to be used) and administer ordered premedication with corticosteroids and diphenhydramine before the procedure.

‣ If iodinated contrast medium is scheduled to be used in patients receiving metformin or drugs containing metformin for type 2 diabetes, the drug may be discontinued on the day of the test and continue to be withheld for 48 hr after the test. Protocols may vary among facilities.

Safety Considerations

‣ **Older Adult Considerations:** Older adult patients present with a variety of concerns when undergoing diagnostic procedures. Level of cooperation and fall risk may be complicated by underlying problems such as visual and hearing impairment, joint and muscle stiffness, physical weakness, mental confusion, and the effects of medications. A fall injury can be avoided by clear communication to the radiation team ensuring assistance is provided in getting on and off the x-ray table and on and off the toilet at the end of the examination. Older adult patients are often chronically dehydrated; anticipating the effects of hypovolemia and orthostasis can also help prevent falls.

AFTER THE STUDY: POTENTIAL NURSING ACTIONS

Avoiding Complications

‣ Complications are rare but include risk for abdominal discomfort and cramping *(related to retention of barium),* allergic reaction *(related to contrast reaction),* constipation, fecal impaction, or bowel obstruction *(related to dehydration and/or retained barium),* or peritonitis *(related to leakage of barium into the peritoneal cavity, perforation of the colon or hemorrhage, resulting from changes in hydrostatic pressure during administration of the enema or manipulations of the tip of the enema tubing during barium administration to patients with a weak colon; a rare complication that may occur in children, immunocompromised patients, or patients whose colon is already weakened by disease).* Monitor the patient for complications related to the procedure.

Treatment Considerations

‣ Altered GI elimination: Assess and trend bowel sounds, abdominal distention, and abdominal girth. Ensure adherence to nothing by mouth (NPO) to rest the GI tract. Once taking an oral diet, encourage selections that will decrease gastric irritation; a dietary consult may assist. Monitor diarrhea and check stool for occult blood. Administer ordered medication to treat constipation or diarrhea.

‣ After the barium enema instruct the patient to resume usual diet, fluids, medications, or activity, as directed by the HCP. Kidney function should be assessed before metformin is resumed.

‣ Instruct the patient to take an ordered mild laxative and increase fluid intake (four 8-oz glasses) to aid in elimination of barium, unless contraindicated.

‣ Carefully monitor the patient for fatigue and fluid and electrolyte imbalance.

‣ **Pediatric Considerations:** Advise the parents of pediatric patients to hydrate the child with electrolyte fluid post barium enema.

‣ **Older Adult Considerations:** Chronic dehydration can also result in frequent bouts of constipation. Therefore, after the procedure, older adult patients should be encouraged to hydrate with fluids containing electrolytes (e.g., Gatorade, Gatorade low calorie for individuals with diabetes, or Pedialyte) and to use a mild laxative daily until the stool is back to normal color.

▶ Pain: Administer prescribed analgesics or opioids. Encourage movement to relieve gas, assist the patient to move to a more comfortable position, and discuss and identify alternative methods of pain relief that work for the patient.

▶ Educate the patient that stools will be white or light in color for 2 to 3 days. If the patient is unable to eliminate the barium, or if stools do not return to normal color, the patient should notify the HCP. Advise patients with a colostomy that tap water colostomy irrigation may aid in barium removal.

Safety Considerations
▶ Advise diabetic patients to avoid all medications containing metformin for 48 hr following a procedure with iodinated contrast. Iodinated contrast can temporarily impair kidney function, and failure to withhold metformin may indirectly result in drug-induced lactic acidosis, a dangerous and sometimes fatal adverse effect of metformin (related to renal impairment that does not support sufficient excretion of metformin).

Nutritional Considerations
▶ Teach the patient and family dietary changes that are necessary to decrease pain and GI irritation.

Follow-Up, Evaluation, and Desired Outcomes
▶ Recognizes colon cancer screening options and understands that decisions regarding the need for and frequency of occult blood testing, colonoscopy, or other cancer screening procedures may be made after consultation between the patient and HCP. Colonoscopy should be used to follow up abnormal findings obtained by any of the screening tests. The most current guidelines for colon cancer screening of the general population as well as of individuals with increased risk are available from the American Cancer Society (www.cancer.org), U.S. Preventive Services Task Force (www.uspreventiveservicestaskforce.org), and American College of Gastroenterology (http://gi.org). For additional information regarding screening guidelines, refer to the study titled "Colonoscopy."

▶ Surgical patients successfully demonstrate how to splint the abdomen when moving to decrease incisional pain postoperatively.

▶ Acknowledges the necessity of close collaboration with the HCP to develop a treatment plan that fits with personal health-care goals.

▶ Recognizes the value of contact information to attend a support group for grief counseling and end-of-life care.

Barium Swallow

SYNONYM/ACRONYM: Esophagram, video swallow, esophagus x-ray, swallowing function, esophagography.

RATIONALE: To assist in diagnosing disease of the esophagus such as stricture or tumor.

PATIENT PREPARATION: There are no activity restrictions unless by medical direction. Instruct the patient to fast and restrict fluids for 8 hr, or as ordered, prior to the procedure. Fasting may be ordered as a precaution against aspiration related to possible nausea and vomiting. The American Society of Anesthesiologists has fasting guidelines for risk levels according to patient status. More information can be located at www.asahq.org.

Note: If iodinated contrast medium is substituted for barium contrast in patients receiving metformin or drugs containing metformin for type 2 diabetes, the drug may be discontinued on the day of the test and continue to be withheld for 48 hr after the test.

Regarding the patient's risk for bleeding, the patient should be instructed to avoid taking natural products and medications with known anticoagulant, antiplatelet, or thrombolytic properties or to reduce dosage, as ordered, prior to the procedure. Number of days to withhold medication is dependent on the type of anticoagulant. Note the last time and dose of medication taken. Protocols may vary among facilities.

Pediatric Considerations: The fasting period prior to the time of the examination depends on the child's age. General guidelines are as follows: birth to 6 mo, 3 hr; 7 months to 2 yr, 4 hr; 3 yr and older, 6 hr.

Ensure that this procedure is performed before an upper gastrointestinal (GI) study or modified (video) swallow and after cholangiography and barium enema, if these tests are ordered, to avoid retention of residual barium in the abdomen, which may obscure details of interest in the upper GI or modified swallow study.

NORMAL FINDINGS

• Normal peristalsis through the esophagus into the stomach with normal size, filling, patency, and shape of the esophagus.

CRITICAL FINDINGS AND POTENTIAL INTERVENTIONS: N/A

OVERVIEW: (**Study type:** X-ray Contrast/Special; **related body system:** Digestive system.) This radiological examination of the esophagus evaluates motion and anatomic structures of the esophageal lumen by recording images of the lumen while the patient swallows a barium solution of milkshake consistency and a chalky taste. The procedure is a dynamic study and uses fluoroscopic and cineradiographic techniques. A dynamic study is one in which there is continuous monitoring of the motion being studied as opposed to a static study in which the patient and equipment are held in one position until the image has been taken. The barium swallow is often performed as part of an upper GI series or cardiac series and is indicated for patients with a history of dysphagia and gastric reflux. The standard barium swallow study focuses on the esophageal structures of the GI tract and may identify reflux of the barium from the stomach back into the esophagus. Muscular abnormalities such as achalasia, as well as diffuse esophageal spasm, can be easily detected with this procedure. Gastroesophageal reflux disease (GERD) is a disorder of the GI system commonly seen in older adults. Because of the physiological changes associated with the aging process, numerous factors may negatively impact quality of life and contribute to the development of significant complications in older adult patients as a result of GERD.

The *modified (video) barium swallow* focuses on the oropharyngeal structures and is also used to evaluate dysphagia, or difficulty swallowing. The test may be performed and observed in the presence of a radiologist and radiology technician with or without a feeding specialist or speech pathologist, depending on the reason for the examination. Nurses will encounter patients who struggle with swallowing disorders in different settings, such as intensive care units, nurseries, rehabilitative units, and skilled nursing care units. Situations that might indicate a modified barium swallow include the evaluation of a patient's ability to swallow food after a stroke or the inability of a child to swallow food of varying consistencies without gagging and choking during feeding.

INDICATIONS

- Confirm the integrity of esophageal anastomoses in the postoperative patient.
- Detect esophageal reflux, tracheoesophageal fistulas, and esophageal varices.
- Determine the cause of dysphagia or heartburn.
- Determine the type and location of foreign bodies within the pharynx and esophagus.
- Evaluate suspected esophageal motility disorders.
- Evaluate suspected polyps, strictures, Zenker diverticula, tumor, or inflammation.

INTERFERING FACTORS

Contraindications

✷ Patients who are pregnant or suspected of being pregnant, unless the potential benefits of a procedure using radiation far outweigh the risk of radiation exposure to the fetus and mother.

✷ Patients with an obstruction, ulcer, or suspected esophageal rupture, unless water-soluble iodinated contrast medium is used; *barium is not used because leakage of the dye could worsen any existing infection.*

✷ Conditions associated with adverse reactions to contrast medium (e.g., asthma, food allergies, or allergy to contrast medium). Although patients are asked specifically if they have a known allergy to iodine or shellfish (shellfish contain high levels of iodine), it has been well established that the reaction is not to iodine; an actual iodine allergy would be problematic because iodine is required for the production of thyroid hormones. In the case of shellfish, the reaction is to a muscle protein called *tropomyosin*; in the case of iodinated contrast medium, the reaction is to the noniodinated part of the contrast molecule. Patients with a known hypersensitivity to the medium may benefit from premedication with corticosteroids and diphenhydramine; the use of nonionic contrast or an alternative noncontrast imaging study, if available, may be considered for patients who have severe asthma or who have experienced moderate to severe reactions to ionic contrast medium.

✷ Patients with severe constipation or bowel obstruction, as barium may make the condition worse.

✷ Patients with a severe swallowing disorder *to the extent that aspiration might occur.*

Factors that may alter the results of the study

- Metallic objects (e.g., jewelry, body rings) within the examination field, which may inhibit organ visualization and cause unclear images.

- Inability of the patient to cooperate or remain still during the procedure, because movement can produce blurred or otherwise unclear images.

POTENTIAL MEDICAL DIAGNOSIS: CLINICAL SIGNIFICANCE OF RESULTS
Abnormal findings related to
- Achalasia
- Acute or chronic esophagitis
- Benign or malignant tumors
- Chalasia
- Congenital diaphragmatic hernia
- Diverticula
- Dysphagia with or without pain *(related to constrictions, arteria lusoria, paralysis, muscle spasms, etc.)*
- Esophageal motility issues *(related to other conditions, such as scleroderma or advancing age)*
- Esophageal ulcers
- Esophageal varices
- Gastroesophageal reflux disease
- Hiatal hernia
- Perforation of the esophagus
- Strictures or polyps

NURSING IMPLICATIONS

POTENTIAL NURSING PROBLEMS: ASSESSMENT & NURSING DIAGNOSIS

Problems	Signs and Symptoms
Bleeding *(related to inflammation, infection, ulceration, trauma, alcohol misuse, cancer)*	Dark stools, tarry stools; foul-smelling stools; fatigue; dizziness; pallor; shortness of breath; bloody or coffee ground emesis; tachycardia; hypotension
Insufficient fluid volume *(related to gastrointestinal bleeding secondary to ulceration, inflammation, infection, trauma, cancer, alcohol misuse)*	Bloody or coffee ground emesis. tachycardia, orthostatic hypotension, altered level of consciousness, weakness, poor skin turgor, dry mucous membranes

BEFORE THE STUDY: PLANNING AND IMPLEMENTATION

Teaching the Patient What to Expect
- Inform the patient this procedure can assist in assessing the esophagus.
- Pregnancy is a general contraindication to procedures involving radiation. Explain to the female patient that she will be asked the date of her last menstrual period. Pregnancy testing may be performed to determine the possibility of pregnancy before exposure to radiation.
- Review the procedure with the patient. Address concerns about pain and explain that no pain should be experienced during the test.
- Explain that barium contrast medium will need to be swallowed.

- Inform the patient that the procedure is performed in a radiology department by a health-care provider (HCP) and takes approximately 15 to 30 min.
- Instruct the patient to remove jewelry and other metallic objects from the area of examination.
- Baseline vital signs will be recorded and monitored throughout the procedure. Protocols may vary among facilities.
- Positioning for this procedure is to stand in front of the x-ray fluoroscopy screen. Those who are unable to stand will be placed supine on the radiographic table.
- As the procedure begins, an initial image is taken, and the patient is asked to swallow a barium solution with or without a straw.

- Multiple images at different angles may be taken.
- Explain that it may be necessary to drink additional barium to complete the study. Swallowing the additional barium evaluates the passage of barium from the esophagus into the stomach.

Potential Nursing Actions

◈ *Make sure a written and informed consent has been signed prior to the procedure and before administering any medications.*

- If iodinated contrast medium is scheduled to be used in patients receiving metformin or drugs containing metformin for type 2 diabetes, the drug may be discontinued on the day of the test and continue to be withheld for 48 hr after the test. Protocols may vary among facilities.

AFTER THE STUDY: POTENTIAL NURSING ACTIONS

Avoiding Complications

- Although complications are rare, they may include allergic reaction *(related to contrast reaction);* constipation, impaction, or bowel obstruction *(related to retained barium);* and aspiration of barium *(related to extreme swallowing disorders).* Monitor the patient for complications related to the procedure.

Treatment Considerations

- After completion of the barium swallow, instruct the patient to resume usual diet, fluids, medications, and activity, as directed by the HCP. Kidney function should be assessed before metformin is resumed.
- Bleeding: Trend and increase frequency of vital signs assessment. Administer ordered blood or blood products. Administer ordered stool softeners. Encourage intake of foods rich in vitamin K, and avoid foods that may irritate the esophagus. Monitor stools for color consistency, odor, and amount.
- Carefully monitor the patient for fatigue and fluid and electrolyte imbalance.

- Insufficient fluid volume: Monitor and trend hemoglobin (Hgb), hematocrit (Hct), prothrombin time (PT), and international normalized ratio (INR). Assess sensorium frequently. Monitor heart rate and blood pressure, including orthostatic. Administer ordered fluid replacement therapy (crystalloids, blood, platelets) and facilitate procedures to identify causes of bleeding. Administer vitamin K to assist coagulation. Provide information for an alcohol support group.
- Instruct the patient to take a mild laxative and increase fluid intake (four 8-oz glasses) to aid in elimination of barium, unless contraindicated.
- **Pediatric Considerations:** Instruct the parents of pediatric patients to hydrate children with electrolyte fluids post barium swallow.
- **Considerations for Older Adults:** Chronic dehydration can also result in frequent bouts of constipation. Therefore, after the procedure, older adult patients should be encouraged to use a mild laxative daily until the stool is back to normal color.

Safety Considerations

- Advise diabetic patients to avoid all medications containing metformin for 48 hr following a procedure with iodinated contrast. Iodinated contrast can temporarily impair kidney function, and failure to withhold metformin may indirectly result in drug-induced lactic acidosis, a dangerous and sometimes fatal adverse effect of metformin (related to renal impairment that does not support sufficient excretion of metformin).

Follow-Up, Evaluation, and Desired Outcomes

- Understands to monitor stool color and that variances will be white or light in color for 2 to 3 days. If the patient is unable to eliminate the barium, or if stools do not return to normal color, the patient should notify the requesting HCP.
- Acknowledges the importance of monitoring stools and the necessity to record and report color,

consistency, amount, and odor. Emphasize the importance of tracking and reporting bloody or coffee ground emesis.

▶ Correctly states the common signs and symptoms of GI bleeding and actions that can be taken to decrease bleeding risk, and can explain why it is important to avoid taking substances (NSAIDs, aspirin, steroids, alcohol) that can cause gastric irritation and result in bleeding.

▶ Acknowledges the importance of calling for assistance in the presence of hypotension and dizziness to decrease bleeding, fall, and injury risk.

Bilirubin and Bilirubin Fractions

SYNONYM/ACRONYM: Conjugated/direct bilirubin, unconjugated/indirect bilirubin, delta bilirubin, TBil.

RATIONALE: A multipurpose laboratory test that acts as an indicator for various diseases of the liver, for disease that affects the liver, or for conditions associated with red blood cell (RBC) hemolysis.

PATIENT PREPARATION: There are no food, fluid, activity, or medication restrictions unless by medical direction.

NORMAL FINDINGS: (Method: Spectrophotometry) Total bilirubin levels in infants should decrease to adult levels by day 10 as the development of the hepatic circulatory system matures. Values in breastfed infants may take longer to reach normal adult levels. Values in premature infants may initially be higher than in full-term infants and also take longer to decrease to normal levels.

Age	Conventional Units	SI Units (Conventional Units × 17.1)
Total bilirubin		
Newborn–1 d	Less than 5.8 mg/dL	Less than 99 micromol/L
1–2 d	Less than 8.2 mg/dL	Less than 140 micromol/L
3–5 d	Less than 11.7 mg/dL	Less than 200 micromol/L
6–7 d	Less than 8.4 mg/dL	Less than 144 micromol/L
8–9 d	Less than 6.5 mg/dL	Less than 111 micromol/L
10–11 d	Less than 4.6 mg/dL	Less than 79 micromol/L
12–13 d	Less than 2.7 mg/dL	Less than 46 micromol/L
14–30 d	Less than 0.8 mg/dL	Less than 14 micromol/L
1 mo–older adult	Less than 1.2 mg/dL	Less than 21 micromol/L
Unconjugated bilirubin	Less than 1.1 mg/dL	Less than 19 micromol/L
Conjugated bilirubin		
Neonate	Less than 0.6 mg/dL	Less than 10 micromol/L
29 d–older adult	Less than 0.3 mg/dL	Less than 5 micromol/L
Delta bilirubin	Less than 0.2 mg/dL	Less than 3 micromol/L

B

CRITICAL FINDINGS AND POTENTIAL INTERVENTIONS

Adults and Children
- Greater than 15 mg/dL (SI: Greater than 257 micromol/L)

Newborns
- Greater than 13 mg/dL (SI: Greater than 222 micromol/L)

Timely notification to the requesting health-care provider (HCP) of any critical findings and related symptoms is a role expectation of the professional nurse. A listing of these findings varies among facilities.

Consideration may be given to verification of critical findings before action is taken. Policies vary among facilities and may include requesting recollection and retesting by the laboratory.

Sustained hyperbilirubinemia can result in brain damage. *Kernicterus* refers to the deposition of bilirubin in the basal ganglia and brainstem nuclei. There is no exact level of bilirubin that puts infants at risk for developing kernicterus. Symptoms of kernicterus in infants include lethargy, poor feeding, upward deviation of the eyes, and seizures. Intervention for infants may include early frequent feedings to stimulate gastrointestinal (GI) motility, phototherapy, and exchange transfusion.

OVERVIEW: (Study type: Blood collected in gold-, red-, red/gray-, or green-top [heparin] tube; related body system: Digestive system.) A heparinized Microtainer is also acceptable. Protect sample from direct light. The spleen removes old or damaged RBCs from circulation. When RBCs are destroyed, the cellular contents are recycled (e.g., iron from hemoglobin) or excreted (e.g., heme from hemoglobin). Bilirubin is a by-product of heme catabolism from aged RBCs and is primarily produced in the liver and spleen. Unconjugated bilirubin is carried to the liver by albumin, where it is conjugated with glucuronic acid. Conjugated bilirubin is water soluble and more easily excreted. Most of the conjugated bilirubin enters the bile and is transported directly into the small intestine; a small portion of the conjugated bilirubin remains in the bile and is stored in the gallbladder. Bacteria in the small intestine convert the conjugated bilirubin to urobilinogen, which is then converted to stercobilin and urobilin. Stercobilin, a pigmented waste product of bilirubin, is excreted in feces; stercobilin gives feces its normal brown color. Small amounts of urobilin, another pigmented waste product of bilirubin, are excreted in urine; urobilin gives urine its characteristic yellow color. Defects in bilirubin excretion can be identified by the presence of urobilinogen in a routine urinalysis. Increases in levels of bilirubin or its metabolites can result from prehepatic, hepatic, and/or posthepatic conditions, making fractionation useful in determining the cause of the increase in total bilirubin levels. Total bilirubin is the sum of unconjugated or indirect bilirubin, monoglucuronide and diglucuronide (conjugated or direct bilirubin), and albumin-bound delta bilirubin. Delta bilirubin has a longer half-life than the other bilirubin fractions and therefore remains elevated during convalescence after the other fractions have decreased to normal levels. Delta bilirubin can be calculated using this formula:

Delta bilirubin = Total bilirubin
– (Indirect bilirubin
+ Direct bilirubin)

When bilirubin concentration increases, the yellowish pigment deposits in skin and sclera. This increase in yellow pigmentation is termed *jaundice* or *icterus*. Bilirubin levels can also be checked using noninvasive methods. Hyperbilirubinemia in neonates can be reliably evaluated using transcutaneous measurement devices.

INDICATIONS

- Assist in the differential diagnosis of obstructive jaundice.
- Assist in the evaluation of liver and biliary disease.
- Monitor the effects of drug reactions on liver function.
- Monitor the effects of phototherapy on jaundiced newborns.
- Monitor physiological jaundice in newborn patients.

INTERFERING FACTORS

Factors that may alter the results of the study

- Drugs and other substances that may increase bilirubin levels by causing cholestasis include anabolic steroids, androgens, butaperazine, chlorothiazide, chlorpromazine, chlorpropamide, dapsone, dienoestrol, erythromycin, estrogens, ethionamide, gold salts, imipramine, iproniazid, isocarboxazid, isoniazid, meprobamate, mercaptopurine, meropenem, nitrofurans, nortriptyline, oleandomycin, oral contraceptives, penicillins, phenothiazines, prochlorperazine, progesterone, promethazine, protriptyline, sulfonamides, tacrolimus, thiouracil, tolazamide, tolbutamide, thiacetazone, trifluoperazine, and trimeprazine.
- Drugs and other substances that may increase bilirubin levels by causing hepatocellular damage include acetaminophen (toxic), acetylsalicylic acid, allopurinol, aminothiazole, anabolic steroids, asparaginase, azathioprine, azithromycin, carbamazepine, chloramphenicol, clindamycin, clofibrate, chlorambucil, chloramphenicol, chlordane, chloroform, chlorzoxazone, clonidine, colchicine, coumarin, cyclophosphamide, cyclopropane, cycloserine, cyclosporine, dactinomycin, danazol, desipramine, diazepam, diethylstilbestrol, enflurane, ethambutol, ethionamide, ethoxazene, factor IX complex, felbamate, flavaspidic acid, flucytosine, fusidic acid, gentamicin, glycopyrrolate, guanoxan, haloperidol, halothane, hycanthone, hydroxyacetamide, ibuprofen, interferon, interleukin-2, isoniazid, kanamycin, labetalol, levamisole, lincomycin, melphalan, mesoridazine, metahexamide, metaxalone, methotrexate, methoxsalen, methyldopa, nitrofurans, oral contraceptives, oxamniquine, pemoline, penicillin, perphenazine, phenazopyridine, phenelzine, pheniprazine, phenothiazines, piroxicam, probenecid, procainamide, pyrazinamide, quinine, sulfonylureas, thiothixene, timolol, tobramycin, tolcapone, tretinoin, trimethadione, urethan, and verapamil.
- Drugs and other substances that may increase bilirubin levels by causing hemolysis include amphotericin B, carbamazepine, cephaloridine, cephalothin, chloroquine,

B

dimercaprol, dipyrone, furazolidone, mefenamic acid, melphalan, methylene blue, nitrofurans, nitrofurazone, pamaquine, penicillins, pentaquine, phenylhydrazine, piperazine, pipobroman, primaquine, procainamide, quinacrine, quinidine, quinine, stibophen, streptomycin, sulfonamides, triethylenemelamine, tyrothricin, and vitamin K.

- Drugs and other substances that may decrease bilirubin levels include anticonvulsants, barbiturates (newborns), chlorophenothane, cyclosporine, flumecinolone (newborns), and salicylates.
- Bilirubin is light sensitive. Failure to suitably protect the collection container from light between the time of collection and time of analysis may decrease bilirubin levels.

POTENTIAL MEDICAL DIAGNOSIS: CLINICAL SIGNIFICANCE OF RESULTS
Increased in

- Prehepatic (hemolytic) jaundice *(related to excessive amounts of heme released from RBC destruction. Heme is catabolized to bilirubin in concentrations that exceed the liver's conjugation capacity, and indirect bilirubin accumulates)*
  Erythroblastosis fetalis (Hemolytic Disease of the Newborn/HDN)
  Hematoma
  Hemolytic anemia
  Pernicious anemia
  Physiological jaundice of the newborn
  The post–blood transfusion period, when a number of units are rapidly infused or in the case of a delayed transfusion reaction
  RBC enzyme abnormalities (i.e., glucose-6-phosphate dehydrogenase, pyruvate kinase, spherocytosis)
- Hepatic jaundice *(related to bilirubin conjugation failure)*
  Crigler-Najjar syndrome

- Hepatic jaundice *(related to disturbance in bilirubin transport)*
  Dubin-Johnson syndrome (related to preconjugation transport failure)
  Gilbert syndrome (related to postconjugation transport failure)
- Hepatic jaundice *(evidenced by liver damage or necrosis that interferes with excretion into bile ducts either by physical obstruction or drug inhibition and bilirubin accumulates)*
  Alcohol misuse
  Cholangitis
  Cholecystitis
  Cholestatic drug reactions
  Cirrhosis
  Hepatitis
  Hepatocellular damage
  Infectious mononucleosis
- Posthepatic jaundice *(evidenced by blockage that interferes with excretion into bile ducts, resulting in accumulated bilirubin)*
  Advanced tumors of the liver
  Biliary obstruction
- Other conditions
  Anorexia or starvation (related to liver damage)
  HELLP syndrome of pregnancy (hemolysis, elevated liver enzymes, low platelet count) (related to RBC hemolysis)
  Hypothyroidism (related to effect on the liver whereby hepatic enzyme activity for formation of conjugated or direct bilirubin is enhanced in combination with decreased flow of bile and secretion of bile acids; results in accumulation of direct bilirubin)
  Premature or breastfed infants (evidenced by diminished hepatic function of the liver in premature infants; related to inability of neonate to feed in sufficient quantity. Insufficient breast milk intake results in weight loss, decreased stool formation, and decreased elimination of bilirubin)

Decreased in: N/A

NURSING IMPLICATIONS

POTENTIAL NURSING PROBLEMS: ASSESSMENT & NURSING DIAGNOSIS

Problems	Signs and Symptoms
Body image *(related to jaundice; ascites; dry, flaky, itchy skin)*	Yellowing of sclera and skin, open sores due to aggressive itching, repeated self-criticism, refusal to discuss altered physical appearance, withdrawal from social situations, conceals physical self with clothing
Confusion, altered sensory perception *(related to hepatic encephalopathy, acute alcohol consumption, hepatic metabolic insufficiency)*	Altered attention span; unable to follow directions; disoriented to person, place, time, and purpose; inappropriate affect
Gas exchange *(related to accumulation of pleural fluid, atelectasis, ventilation perfusion mismatch, altered oxygen supply)*	Irregular breathing pattern, use of accessory muscles, altered chest excursion, adventitious breath sounds (crackles, rhonchi, wheezes, diminished breath sounds), copious secretions, signs of hypoxia
Nutrition *(related to poor eating habits, excessive alcohol use, altered liver function, nausea, vomiting)*	Known inadequate caloric intake, weight loss, muscle wasting in arms and legs, stool that is pale or gray-colored, skin that is flaky with loss of elasticity

BEFORE THE STUDY: PLANNING AND IMPLEMENTATION

Teaching the Patient What to Expect

▶ Inform the patient this test can assist in assessing liver function and conditions that cause jaundice.
▶ Explain that a blood sample is needed for the test.

AFTER THE STUDY: POTENTIAL NURSING ACTIONS

Avoiding Complications

▶ There are several types of jaundice that may occur in the neonate, and it is important to quickly determine the cause so effective treatment can be initiated.
▶ Physiologic jaundice occurs as a normal response to the neonate's limited ability to excrete bilirubin in the first days of life. Intervention may include early frequent feeding to stimulate GI motility and phototherapy. This type of jaundice usually lasts 10 to 14 days (premature neonates may take up to a month) and resolves in reverse to the pattern of development with the legs looking normal first and the face remaining yellowish longer.
▶ Breastfeeding jaundice is seen in breastfed neonates during the first week of life, peaking during the second or third week. It occurs due to dehydration in neonates who do not nurse well or if the mother's milk is slow to come in; the bilirubin levels are elevated relative to the decreased total fluid volume. The goal is to provide adequate fluid and nutrition to the breastfeeding neonate by providing water or formula between feedings

B

and until the mother's milk supply is adequate. Phototherapy may also be ordered to accelerate the breakdown of bilirubin and prevent accumulation to dangerous levels. Skin turgor, input and output, vital signs, and number/quality of stools should be frequently monitored. Total bilirubin and fractions should be monitored regularly until levels decrease to normal neonatal values.

♦ Breast milk jaundice is different from breastfeeding jaundice, occurs in about 2% of breastfed neonates after the first week of life, takes up to 12 wk to resolve, and is believed to have a familial relationship; assessment for family history is helpful. Hyperbilirubinemia occurs due to substances in the mother's milk that interfere with development of enzymes required to break down bilirubin. The main goals are to increase fluids by more frequent feeding or additional fluids given orally or by IV and through the use of phototherapy. Fiberoptic blankets and special beds that shine light up from the mattresses are available.

♦ Severe jaundice may occur as the result of an ABO or Rh incompatibility between the mother and baby. An ABO incompatibility can occur if a mother with blood type O blood is carrying a baby with blood type A, type B, or type AB. An Rh incompatibility can occur if a mother with Rh negative blood is carrying a baby with Rh positive blood. The jaundice occurs as the result of hemolysis or RBC breakdown due to the incompatibility.

Treatment Considerations

♦ Body Image: Assess for yellowing of the sclera and skin. Assess skin for patches of itching, and provide mitts to decrease scratching and skin damage. Monitor liver function tests and bilirubin levels. Assess patient's perception of self related to current medical status, monitor for self-criticism, and acknowledge normal response to changed appearance.

♦ Confusion: Monitor blood ammonia level, determine last alcohol use, and assess for symptoms of hepatic encephalopathy such as confusion, sleep disturbances, and incoherence. Protect confused patients from physical harm. Administer ordered lactulose.

♦ Gas Exchange: Monitor respiratory rate and effort based on assessment of patient condition. Frequently assess lung sounds, and monitor for secretions and suction as necessary. Perform pulse oximetry to monitor oxygen saturation, collaborate with the HCP to administer oxygen as needed, and elevate the head of the bed 30 degrees. Monitor IV fluids, and avoid aggressive fluid resuscitation. Monitor and document degree of abdominal ascites and abdominal girth.

Nutritional Considerations

♦ Increased bilirubin levels may be associated with liver disease. Dietary recommendations may be indicated depending on the condition and its severity.

♦ Assess barriers to eating and consider using a food diary.

♦ It may be necessary to document food intake with a calorie count.

♦ Consider a consult with a registered dietitian and assessment of cultural food selections.

♦ Administer ordered multivitamin and parenteral or enteral nutrition. Monitor glucose levels and check daily weight.

♦ Assess and trend liver function tests (alanine aminotransferase [ALT], aspartate aminotransferase [AST], alkaline phosphatase [ALKP], total protein, albumin, bilirubin), folic acid, glucose, thiamine, and electrolytes.

♦ Currently, specific drugs are being used to treat different types of viral hepatitis. For example, there are a number of drugs used to treat hepatitis B such as pegylated interferon (adults only), interferon alfa (adults and children), and lamivudine (adults and children); Harvoni (a combination of ledipasvir and sofosbuvir) and Solvaldi (sofosbuvir) are examples of drugs used to treat hepatitis C. There are also drugs that can be given to treat and reverse the symptoms of nonviral hepatitis once the primary cause of hepatic inflammation is identified.

▶ Monitor continued alcohol use, as it is a barrier to adequate nutrition. Elimination of alcohol consumption and a diet optimized for convalescence are commonly included in the treatment plan. Patients who misuse alcohol should be encouraged to avoid alcohol and also to seek appropriate counseling.

▶ Increased bilirubin levels may be associated with liver disease. In general, patients should be encouraged to eat a well-balanced diet that includes foods high in fiber. Dietary recommendations will vary depending on the condition and its severity. For example, recommend a diet of soft foods if esophageal varices develop, fat substitutes for bile duct disease, or limitations on salt intake if ascites develop.

▶ Administer ordered enteral or parenteral nutrition; monitor laboratory values (albumin, protein, potassium) and collaborate with the HCP on replacement strategies; correlate laboratory values with IV fluid infusion and collaborate with the HCP and pharmacist to adjust to patient needs; ensure adequate pain control; monitor vital signs for alterations associated metabolic imbalances.

Follow-Up, Evaluation, and Desired Outcomes

▶ Understands the cause of the hyperbilirubinemia and that jaundice may resolve with treatment of the liver disease.

▶ Acknowledges the importance of adhering to scheduled laboratory appointments to monitor liver function and disease progress.

▶ Agrees with the importance of adequate fluid intake and demonstrates how to perform skin care for the neonate.

▶ Accepts therapeutic management plan and strictly adheres to HCP care strategy.

▶ Agrees to alcohol cessation and attends support group to prevent relapse.

Bioelectric Impedance Analysis

SYNONYM/ACRONYM: BIA.

RATIONALE: To estimate and assess body composition.

PATIENT PREPARATION: There are no food, fluid, activity, or medication restrictions unless by medical direction.

NORMAL FINDINGS
• Healthy adults.

CRITICAL FINDINGS AND POTENTIAL INTERVENTIONS: N/A

OVERVIEW: (Study type: Electrophysiologic; related body system: Multisystem.) Electrical impulses run continuously through the cells, tissues, and organs involved in any type of metabolic process. A few examples include the musculoskeletal, cardiovascular, and nervous systems. The impulses are conducted and sustained through complex chain reactions involving electrolytes such as sodium, potassium, calcium, and magnesium.

B

The ability of tissues to conduct or prevent the passage of electrical energy varies with changes in the concentration of electrolytes in intra- and extracellular fluids, changes in cell membrane permeability, cellular composition, and water content. When an electric current is passed through the body, it is conducted through the intra- and extracellular fluids containing water and electrolytes. Lean tissue contains more water than fatty tissue; therefore, the flow of current occurs easily through muscle but is impeded by fat, which is the basis for bioelectric impedance analysis (BIA). Bioelectric impedance measurements are a reflection of the structure, composition, and function of specific tissues. Measurements of the electrical properties of normal tissue have been expanded to explore tissue profiles along a continuum of cellular change from damaged to expired. These advances may make it possible to diagnose diseases earlier, predict survival, and guide the progress of therapeutic interventions. The technology has appeal because it is simple, portable, noninvasive, relatively inexpensive, and has rapid turnaround to results. In practice, it is usually conducted by contact with electrodes at the site of interest, such as wrist to ankle, hand to hand, or foot to foot. Estimates of body fat percentage are derived from the measurements set against validated formulas that consider factors to include a person's age, height, weight, gender, and ethnicity. The development of medical applications based on BIA include impedance plethysmography; electroencephalography; hydration management

for patients with hemodynamic disturbances; nutritional interventions for malnourished, critically ill patients; and assessment of body composition as a risk factor for developing diseases such as heart disease, diabetes, hypertension, and some types of cancer. Nutritionists, athletic club trainers, and members of sports organizations are using BIA to assess health and assist patients in successful weight management. Health assessment has become part of some employee wellness programs. Participation in health assessment is also tied to some employer-sponsored health insurance plans that offer discounts to employees who participate and penalties for those who do not participate. Drawbacks to some of the simpler equipment used to measure body composition in healthy individuals are inconsistent readings due to variations in hydration level, skin temperature, and testing environment, as well as the skill level of the person administering the measurements.

INDICATIONS
- Assessment of nutritional therapy for the treatment of a chronic disease.
- Assist in evaluating prognosis for patients with chronic conditions such as cancer or liver disease or who are critically ill with an infectious disease.
- Estimation of body composition as part of a biophysical health assessment.

INTERFERING FACTORS
Contraindications

Patients who are pregnant may be excluded from participating in the study; protocols vary among facilities. Fluid volumes change significantly throughout the course of a pregnancy, and interpretation of results may not be accurate or useful.

◈ Patients with a pacemaker·

◈ Patients with extremely abnormal body weight (obese or emaciated) or physical deformities that present an irregular distribution in body composition may be excluded from participating in the study; protocols vary among facilities. Interpretation of results may not be accurate or useful.

◈ Patients with a skin condition that would interfere with placement of electrodes.

◈ Patients with sudden and significant changes in hydration status (hyper- or hypovolemia).

◈ Young patients (neonate to adolescent) and older adult patients may be excluded from participating in the study; protocols vary among facilities. Validated formulas for younger and older adult patients may not be available, and interpretation of results may not be accurate or useful.

Factors that may alter the results of the study
- The quality of the BIA study is dependent on the skill of the person performing the study.
- Poor electrode conduction.

POTENTIAL MEDICAL DIAGNOSIS: CLINICAL SIGNIFICANCE OF RESULTS
Abnormal findings related to
- Chronic conditions (e.g., cancer, HIV, liver disease) *(related to diminished electrical conductivity as a result of cachexia)*
- Patients receiving nutritional therapy related to weight issues or chronic conditions *(in order to assess and monitor the efficacy of therapy)*

NURSING IMPLICATIONS

BEFORE THE STUDY: PLANNING AND IMPLEMENTATION

B

Teaching the Patient What to Expect
▸ Inform the patient that this procedure is performed to measure the amount of fat and lean muscle mass in the body.
▸ Review the procedure with the patient.
▸ Advise the patient that the application of an electrical current is brief, will not be felt, and is not harmful.
▸ Inform the patient that the procedure is performed by a health-care provider (HCP) or other person trained to perform the BIA, and it takes approximately 3 to 5 min to complete.
▸ Instruct the patient to remove jewelry and other metallic objects from the area to be examined.
▸ In some types of studies, the patient may stand and hold a device containing hand-to-hand electrodes to record body composition, and in other types of studies, the patient may stand on a device used to record body composition using foot-to-foot measurements. A third type of measurement is taken with the patient lying down (hand-to-foot study).

Hand-to-Foot Study
▸ Explain to the patient they will be placed in a supine position for 5 to 10 min prior to the study in order to achieve a relatively even distribution of body fluids. Specific positioning includes lying on the examination table facing up with the arms abducted 30 degrees from the sides of the body and legs positioned such that the thighs do not touch. The person performing the study may place a thin piece of acrylic fabric between the arms and trunk or between the thighs if necessary. Skin will be thoroughly cleansed where the electrodes will be placed with alcohol pads to remove any fatty substances such as lotion or other types of residue that may interfere with the study measurements.

B

▶ Two sets of electrodes will be placed: one to the patient's right hand and one to the patient's right foot. Each set of electrodes has one electrode that provides the source of the current and another that serves as a voltage detector. When the procedure is complete, the electrodes will be removed.

AFTER THE STUDY: POTENTIAL NURSING ACTIONS

Avoiding Complications
▶ Monitor electrode sites for inflammation.

Nutritional Considerations
▶ Chronic illness can often require significant diet changes to maximize health. Dietary changes will be made based on a specific diagnosis, and individual study results.

Follow-Up, Evaluation, and Desired Outcomes
▶ Acknowledges that depending on the results of this procedure, additional testing may be performed to evaluate or monitor progression of the disease process and determine the need for a change in therapy.

Biopsy, Bone Marrow

SYNONYM/ACRONYM: N/A

RATIONALE: To assist in diagnosing hematological diseases and in identifying and staging myeloproliferative tumors and leukemias.

PATIENT PREPARATION: There are no food, fluid, activity, or medication restrictions unless by medical direction. However, to reduce the risk of aspiration related to nausea or vomiting, the patient may be requested to abstain from solid food and milk or milk products for at least 6 hr, and clear liquids are restricted for at least 2 hr prior to general anesthesia, regional anesthesia, or sedation/analgesia (monitored anesthesia). The patient may be required to be NPO at midnight. The American Society of Anesthesiologists has fasting guidelines for risk levels according to patient status. More information can be located at www.asahq.org.

Regarding the patient's risk for bleeding, the patient should be instructed to avoid taking natural products and medications with known anticoagulant, antiplatelet, or thrombolytic properties or to reduce dosage, as ordered, prior to the procedure. Number of days to withhold medication is dependent on the type of anticoagulant. Note the last time and dose of medication taken. Protocols may vary among facilities.

NORMAL FINDINGS: (Method: Microscopic study of bone and bone marrow samples, flow cytometry) Reference ranges are subject to many variables, and therefore the laboratory should be consulted for their specific interpretation. Some generalities may be commented on regarding findings as follows:

• Ratio of marrow fat to cellular elements is related to age, with the amount of fat increasing with increasing age.
• Normal cellularity, cellular distribution, presence of megakaryocytes, and absence of fibrosis or tumor cells.

- The myeloid-to-erythrocyte ratio (M:E) is 2:1 to 4:1 in adults. It may be slightly higher in children.

Differential Parameter	Conventional Units
Erythrocyte precursors	18%–32%
Myeloblasts	0%–2%
Promyelocytes	2%–6%
Myelocytes	9%–17%
Metamyelocytes	7%–25%
Bands	10%–16%
Neutrophils	18%–28%
Eosinophils and precursors	1%–5%
Basophils and precursors	0%–1%
Monocytes and precursors	1%–5%
Lymphocytes	9%–19%
Plasma cells	0%–1%

CRITICAL FINDINGS AND POTENTIAL INTERVENTIONS
- Classification or grading of tumor
- Identification of malignancy

Timely notification to the requesting health-care provider (HCP) of any critical findings and related symptoms is a role expectation of the professional nurse. A listing of these findings varies among facilities.

OVERVIEW: (**Study type:** Tissue and cell microscopy, bone marrow aspirate, bone core biopsy, marrow and peripheral smears; **related body system:** Circulatory/Hematopoietic and Immune systems.) Tissue samples placed in properly labelled specimen containers containing formalin solution are promptly transported to the laboratory for processing and analysis. This test involves the removal of a small sample of bone marrow by aspiration, needle biopsy, or open surgical biopsy for a complete hematological analysis. The marrow is a suspension of blood, fat, and developing blood cells, which is evaluated for morphology and examined for all stages of maturation, iron stores, and M:E. Sudan black B and periodic acid–Schiff (PAS) stains

can be performed for microscopic examination to differentiate the types of leukemia, although flow cytometry and cytogenetics have become more commonly used techniques for this purpose. Immunophenotyping by flow cytometry uses markers directed at specific antigens on white blood cell (WBC) membranes to provide rapid enumeration and identification of WBC types as well as detection of abnormal increases or decreases in specific cell lines.

Cytogenetics is a specialization within the area of genetics that includes chromosome analysis or karyotyping. Bone marrow cells are incubated in culture media to increase the number of cells available for study and to allow for hybridization of the cellular DNA with fluorescent DNA probes in a technique called *fluorescence in situ hybridization* (FISH). The probes are designed to target areas of the chromosome known to correlate with genetic risk for a particular disease. When a suitable volume of hybridized sample is achieved, cell growth is chemically inhibited during the prophase and metaphase stages of mitosis (cell division), and cellular DNA is examined to detect fluorescence, which represents chromosomal abnormalities, in the targeted areas. Real-time polymerase chain reaction (RT-PCR) and cell-based polymerase chain reaction (PCR) are newer, more sensitive methods for quantitation of genetic material. There are a number of chromosome markers used to diagnose, develop potential treatment regimens, and monitor treatment outcomes. Some chromosome markers commonly evaluated on whole blood and bone marrow include BCR-ABL1 and/or Philadelphia chromosome to diagnose chronic myelogenous leukemia (CML); JAK2 V617F mutation, which is associated with polycythemia vera (PV), essential thrombocytosis (ET), and primary myelofibrosis (PMF); and promyelocytic leukemia/retinoic acid receptor alpha (PML-RARA), which is used to help diagnose acute promyelocytic leukemia.

INDICATIONS

- Determine marrow differential (proportion of the various types of cells present in the marrow) and M:E.
- Evaluate abnormal results of complete blood count or WBC count with differential showing increased numbers of leukocyte precursors.
- Evaluate hepatomegaly or splenomegaly.
- Identify bone marrow hyperplasia or hypoplasia.
- Identify infectious organisms present in the bone marrow (histoplasmosis, mycobacteria, cytomegalovirus, parvovirus inclusions).
- Monitor effects of exposure to bone marrow depressants.
- Monitor bone marrow response to chemotherapy or radiation therapy.

INTERFERING FACTORS

Contraindications

✦ Patients with bleeding disorders *(related to the potential for prolonged bleeding from the biopsy site).*

Factors that may alter the results of the study

- Recent blood transfusions, iron therapy, or administration of cytotoxic drugs may alter test results.

POTENTIAL MEDICAL DIAGNOSIS: CLINICAL SIGNIFICANCE OF RESULTS

Increased Reticulocytes

- Compensated red blood cell (RBC) loss
- Response to vitamin B_{12} therapy

Decreased Reticulocytes

- Aplastic crisis of sickle cell anemia or hereditary spherocytosis

Increased Leukocytes

- *General associations include compensation for infectious process, leukemias, or leukemoid drug reactions*

Decreased Leukocytes

- *General associations include reduction in the marrow space as seen in myelofibrosis, lack of production of cells, lower production of cells as seen in older adults, or following suppressive therapy such as chemo-therapy or radiation*

Increased Neutrophils (Total)
- Acute myeloid leukemia
- Chronic myeloid leukemia
- Compensation for bone marrow aplasia
- Myelofibrosis
- Polycythemia vera

Decreased Neutrophils (Total)
- Aplastic anemia
- Leukemias (monocytic and lymphoblastic)
- Myelodysplastic syndrome

Increased Lymphocytes
- Compensation for bone marrow aplasia
- Infections (chronic infection, viral infections, e.g., Epstein-Barr, hepatitis, HTLV-1, parvovirus B19)
- Lymphoblastic leukemia
- Lymphomas: Hodgkin disease and all other non-Hodgkin lymphomas; Waldenström macroglobulinemia is a type of non-Hodgkin lymphoma, also called lymphoplasmacytic lymphoma

Decreased Lymphocytes
- Aplastic anemia

Increased Plasma Cells
- Cirrhosis of the liver
- Connective tissue disorders
- Hypersensitivity reactions
- Infections and conditions of chronic inflammation
- Multiple myeloma
- Ulcerative colitis

Increased Monocytes
- Acute monocytic leukemia
- Acute myelomonocytic leukemia
- Chronic myelomonocytic leukemia
- Compensation for bone marrow aplasia
- Hodgkin and non-Hodgkin lymphomas

Decreased Monocytes
- Compensation for bone marrow aplasia
- Hairy cell leukemia

Increased Eosinophils
- Lymphadenoma
- Myeloid leukemia
- Polycythemia vera

Decreased Eosinophils
- Aplastic anemia

Increased Basophils
- Acute basophilic leukemia
- Myelodysplastic syndrome
- Myeloid leukemia
- Polycythemia vera

Decreased Basophils
- Aplastic anemia

Increased Megakaryocytes
- Hemorrhage *(related to bone marrow response for compensatory replacement)*
- Increasing age
- Infections
- Myeloid leukemia
- Polycythemia vera
- Thrombocytopenia *(related to bone marrow response for compensatory replacement)*

Decreased Megakaryocytes
- Aplastic anemia
- Cirrhosis of the liver
- Myelodysplastic syndrome
- Radiation or chemotherapy
- Thrombocytopenic purpura

Increased M:E
- Bone marrow failure
- Infections
- Leukemoid reactions
- Myeloid leukemia

Decreased M:E
- Anemias
- Hepatic disease
- Polycythemia vera
- Posthemorrhagic hematopoiesis

B

Increased Normoblasts
- Anemias
- Chronic blood loss
- Polycythemia vera

Decreased Normoblasts
- Aplastic anemia
- Folic acid or vitamin B$_{12}$ deficiency
- Hemolytic anemia

NURSING IMPLICATIONS

BEFORE THE STUDY: PLANNING AND IMPLEMENTATION

Teaching the Patient What to Expect

▶ Inform the patient this procedure can assist in establishing a diagnosis of bone marrow and immune system disease.

▶ Pregnancy may be a contraindication to procedures involving some types of anesthesia. Explain to the female patient that she will be asked the date of her last menstrual period. Pregnancy testing may be performed to determine the possibility of pregnancy before the biopsy is performed.

▶ Explain that reducing health-care-associated infections is an important patient safety goal and a number of different safety practices will be implemented during their procedure. Advise the patient that hair in the area near the incision site may be clipped or shaved and the area cleaned with an antiseptic solution to cleanse bacteria from the skin in order to reduce the risk for infection. *Note:* The World Health Organization, Centers for Disease Control and Prevention, and Association of periOperative Registered Nurses recommend that hair not be removed at all unless it interferes with the incision site or other aspects of the procedure because hair removal by any means is associated with increased infection rates. When hair removal is necessary, facilities must use a protocol that is based on scientific literature or the endorsement of a professional organization. Clipping immediately before the procedure and in a location outside the procedure area is preferred to shaving with a razor. Shaving creates a break in skin integrity and provides a way for bacteria on the skin to enter the incision site.

▶ Review the procedure with the patient, address concerns about pain, and explain that there may be moments of discomfort or pain experienced when the IV line is inserted to allow infusion of fluids such as saline, anesthetics, antibiotics, sedatives, medications used in the procedure, or emergency medications. Instruct the patient that prophylactic antibiotics may be administered before the procedure. Explain that the patient may feel some pain when the lidocaine is injected and some discomfort at the stage in the procedure when the specimen is aspirated.

▶ Inform the patient that the biopsy is performed under sterile conditions by an HCP specializing in this procedure. A needle biopsy usually takes about 20 min to complete.

▶ Baseline vital signs will be recorded and monitored throughout the procedure. Protocols may vary among facilities.

▶ Assist the patient to the desired position depending on the test site to be used. In young children, the most frequently chosen site is the proximal tibia. Vertebral bodies T10 through L4 are preferred in older children. In adults, the sternum or iliac crests are the preferred sites. Place the patient in the prone, sitting, or side-lying position for the vertebral bodies; the side-lying position for iliac crest or tibial sites; or the supine position for the sternum. The HCP administers a local anesthetic (usually lidocaine), the site is cleaned with an antiseptic solution, and the area is draped with sterile towels.

▶ Explain to the patient that he or she will be monitored for complications related to the procedure (e.g., allergic reaction, etc.).

▶ Explain that once the study is completed, a pressure dressing is applied over the puncture site.

▶ Tissue samples will be placed in a properly labelled specimen container containing formalin solution and promptly transport the specimen to the laboratory for processing and analysis.

Needle Aspiration

▶ The HCP will insert a needle with stylet into the marrow. The stylet is removed, a syringe attached, and a 0.5-mL aliquot of marrow withdrawn. The needle is removed, and pressure is applied to the site. The aspirate is applied to slides, and when dry, a fixative is applied.

Needle Biopsy

▶ Local anesthetic is introduced deeply enough to include periosteum. A cutting biopsy needle is introduced through a small skin incision and bored into the marrow cavity. A core needle is introduced through the cutting needle, and a plug of marrow is removed. Pressure is applied to the site for 3 to 5 min, and then a pressure dressing is applied.

Potential Nursing Actions

Make sure a written and informed consent has been signed prior to the procedure and before administering any medications.

Safety Considerations

▶ Anticoagulants, aspirin, and other salicylates should be discontinued by medical direction for the appropriate number of days prior to a procedure in which bleeding is a potential complication.

AFTER THE STUDY: POTENTIAL NURSING ACTIONS

Avoiding Complications

▶ Bleeding *(related to a bleeding disorder, or the effects of natural products and medications with known anticoagulant, antiplatelet, or thrombolytic properties).* Observe/assess the biopsy site for bleeding, inflammation, or hematoma formation. Instruct the patient in the care and assessment of the site and to report any fever, chills, redness, edema, bleeding, or pain at the biopsy site.

Treatment Considerations

General Information

▶ Always follow the protocols provided by each individual facility.

▶ Monitor vital signs and neurological status every 15 min for 1 hr, then every 2 hr for 4 hr, and then as ordered by the HCP. Monitor temperature every 4 hr for 24 hr and intake and output at least every 8 hr. Notify the HCP if temperature is elevated. Compare and trend with baseline values.

▶ Assess for nausea and pain. Administer antiemetic and analgesic medications as ordered by the HCP. Administer antibiotic therapy if ordered. Remind the patient of the importance of completing the entire course of antibiotic therapy, even if signs and symptoms disappear before completion of therapy.

▶ Instruct the patient in the adverse effects associated with prescribed medications. Encourage him or her to review corresponding literature provided by a pharmacist.

Follow-Up, Evaluation, and Desired Outcomes

▶ Acknowledges contact information provided for the National Marrow Donor Program (https://bethematch.org).

▶ Acknowledges the medical versus surgical options for disease management.

▶ Successfully demonstrates care of surgical and/or biopsy site.

▶ Understands the pathophysiology associated with cancer, disease, and ongoing treatment and screenings. Accepts that a health-care specialist may need to be consulted to manage the disease and therapeutic interventions.

▶ Understands the use of any ordered medications, including the importance of adhering to the therapeutic regimen.

▶ Acknowledges end-of-life treatment options for those with terminal diagnosis.

▶ Agrees to seek psychological counseling to adjust to lifestyle changes associated with positive therapeutic management strategies and attend disease-specific support group meetings.

B

Biopsy, Breast

B

SYNONYM/ACRONYM: N/A

RATIONALE: To assist in establishing a diagnosis of breast disease; in the presence of breast cancer, this test is also used to assist in evaluating prognosis and management of response to therapy.

PATIENT PREPARATION: There are no activity restrictions unless by medical direction. Instruct the patient that to reduce the risk of aspiration related to nausea and vomiting, solid food and milk or milk products are restricted for at least 6 hr, and clear liquids are restricted for at least 2 hr prior to general anesthesia, regional anesthesia, or sedation/analgesia (monitored anesthesia). The patient may be required to be NPO after midnight. The American Society of Anesthesiologists has fasting guidelines for risk levels according to patient status. More information can be located at www .asahq.org.

Regarding the patient's risk for bleeding, the patient should be instructed to avoid taking natural products and medications with known anticoagulant, antiplatelet, or thrombolytic properties or to reduce dosage, as ordered, prior to the procedure. Number of days to withhold medication is dependent on the type of anticoagulant. Note the last time and dose of medication taken. Patients on beta blockers before the surgical procedure should be instructed to take their medication as ordered during the perioperative period. Protocols may vary among facilities.

NORMAL FINDINGS: (Method: Macroscopic and microscopic examination of tissue for biopsy; cytochemical or immunohistochemical for estrogen and progesterone receptors Ki67, PCNA, P53; flow cytometry for DNA ploidy and S-phase fraction; immunohistochemical or FISH for Her-2/neu) Fluorescence in situ hybridization (FISH) is a cytogenic technique that uses fluorescent-labelled DNA probes to detect specific chromosome abnormalities. Favorable findings:

- Biopsy: No abnormal cells or tissue.
- DNA ploidy: Majority diploid cell population.
- SPF: Low fraction of replicating cells in total cell population.
- Her-2/neu, Ki67, PCNA, and P53: Negative to low percentage of stained cells.
- Estrogen and progesterone receptors: High percentage of stained cells.

CRITICAL FINDINGS AND POTENTIAL INTERVENTIONS
- Assessment of clear margins after tissue excision
- Classification or grading of tumor
- Identification of malignancy

Timely notification to the requesting health-care provider (HCP) of any critical findings and related symptoms is a role expectation of the professional nurse. A listing of these findings varies among facilities.

OVERVIEW: (Study type: Tissue and cell microscopy, breast tissue or cells; **related body system:** Immune and Reproductive systems.) Label the appropriate specimen containers with the corresponding patient demographics, initials of the person collecting the specimen, date and time of collection, and site location, especially right or left breast. Breast cancer is the most common newly diagnosed cancer in American women. It is the second leading cause of cancer-related death. Biopsy is the excision of a sample of tissue that can be analyzed microscopically to determine cell morphology and the presence of tissue abnormalities. Fine-needle and open biopsies of the breast have become more commonly ordered in recent years as increasing emphasis on early detection of breast cancer has become stronger. Breast biopsies are used to assist in the identification and prognosis of breast cancer. A number of tests can be performed on breast tissue to assist in identification and management of breast cancer. *Estrogen and progesterone receptor assays (ER and PR)* are used to identify patients with a type of breast cancer that may be more responsive than other types of tumors to estrogen-deprivation (antiestrogen) therapy or removal of the ovaries. Patients with these types of tumors generally have a better prognosis. *DNA ploidy* testing by flow cytometry may also be performed on suspicious tissue. Cancer is the unchecked proliferation of tumor cells that contain abnormal amounts of DNA. The higher the grade of tumor cells, the more

likely abnormal DNA will be detected. The *ploidy* (number of chromosome sets in the nucleus) is an indication of the speed of cell replication and tumor growth. Cells synthesize DNA in the S phase of mitosis. *S-phase fraction* (SPF) is an indicator of the number of cells undergoing replication. Normal tissue has a higher percentage of resting diploid cells, or cells containing two chromosomes. Aneuploid cells contain multiple chromosomes. Genes on the chromosomes are coded to produce specific proteins. *Ki67 and proliferating cell nuclear antigen* (PCNA) are examples of proteins that can be measured to indicate the degree of cell proliferation in biopsied tissue. Overexpression of a protein called *human epidermal growth factor receptor 2* (HER-2/neu oncoprotein) is helpful in establishing histological evidence of metastatic breast cancer. Metastatic breast cancer patients with high levels of HER-2/neu oncoprotein have a poor prognosis. They have rapid tumor progression, increased rate of recurrence, poor response to standard therapies, and a lower survival rate. Herceptin (trastuzumab) is indicated for treatment of HER-2/neu overexpression. *P53* is a suppressor protein that normally prevents cells with abnormal DNA from multiplying. Mutations in the P53 gene cause the loss of P53 functionality; the checkpoint is lost, and cancerous cells are allowed to proliferate.

Knowledge of genetics assists in identifying those who may benefit from additional education, risk assessment, and counseling. Genetics is the study and

B

identification of genes, genetic mutations, and inheritance. For example, genetics provides some insight into the likelihood of inheriting a condition associated with a type of cancer such as breast cancer. Genomic studies evaluate the interaction of groups of genes. The combined activity or combined expression of groups of genes allows assumptions or predictions to be made. As an example, genomic studies measure the levels of activity in multiple genes to predict how they influence the development and growth of a tumor. Further information regarding inheritance of genes can be found in the study titled "Genetic Testing." Presently, there are four genomic tests for breast cancer: Oncotype DX, MammaPrint, Mammostrat, and Prosigna Breast Cancer Prognostic Gene Signature Assay.

- Oncotype DX measures the activity of 21 genes that influence the likelihood that breast cancer will develop and, if so, how well it will respond to chemotherapy (early-stage invasive) or radiation treatments (ductal cancer in situ [DCIS]). Candidates include patients who have been diagnosed with early-stage breast cancer, recently diagnosed with estrogen receptor–positive breast cancer, recently diagnosed with DCIS, or scheduled to have a lumpectomy to remove the ductal cancer in situ. Test results from this assay have been robustly validated in research studies. The assay is included in the National Comprehensive Cancer Network (NCCN) and the American Society of Clinical Oncology (ASCO) treatment guidelines for early-stage breast cancer. Use of the test

for DCIS is growing, but it has not yet been included in the NCCN or ASCO treatment guidelines.
- MammaPrint measures the activity of 70 genes. Candidates include patients who have been diagnosed with state I or state II cancer—whether estrogen receptor positive or negative—that is invasive, smaller than 5 cm, or present in three or fewer lymph nodes.
- Mammostrat measures the activity of five genes. Candidates include patients who have been diagnosed with stage I or stage II cancer. It is not widely used to make treatment decisions.
- Prosigna measures the activity of 58 genes. Candidates are limited to postmenopausal patients who have been diagnosed with
  a. Stage I or stage II breast cancer that is lymph node negative
  b. Stage II breast cancer with one to three positive nodes
  c. Breast cancer and are hormone receptor positive
  d. Breast cancer that is invasive
  e. Breast cancer and have been treated with surgery and hormone therapy
     It is not widely used to make treatment decisions.

Fluid from breast cysts or nipple discharge may be collected by aspiration and examined microscopically for benign or cancerous findings. Mammography should be performed before aspiration of cyst fluid because of the potential interference to the mammogram from bleeding. Potential complications of fluid aspiration include infection, pneumothorax, and hematoma.

Sentinel lymph node biopsy (SLNB) may be considered to assist in the diagnosis of breast cancer. A sentinel lymph node (SLN) is the first lymph node to be infiltrated by cancer cells from the primary tumor, usually in the axilla or armpit area. To identify an SLN, the surgeon injects one or more tracers (such as technetium-99m and isosulfan blue dye) near the tumor, then uses a handheld gamma detector to locate the nodes emitting radioactivity or visually inspects the nearby nodes for any that are stained blue from the dye. Once the SLN is located, a small incision is made and the node is removed. The suspicious tissue is checked microscopically for the presence of cancer cells by a pathologist. Positive SLN samples may warrant immediate removal of additional lymph nodes or removal during a follow-up procedure. SLNB is used to assist in staging cancers, to estimate the risk of metastasis to other parts of the body, and in the case of negative SLN testing to avoid the unnecessary removal of nearby lymph nodes. Adverse effects of lymph node surgery include lymphedema, pain, and increased risk of infection in the affected area.

There are a number of risk factor tools that can be used to estimate an individuals's risk of breast cancer. The tools cannot determine whether a person will get breast cancer. The tools are based on the average risk for a group of women with similar risk factors; the original tools were based on data from women of European ethnicity. Generally, an HCP will consider the number of risk factors a person has and how much each factor contributes to increasing the risk for breast cancer (e.g., a BRCA1 gene mutation contributes a significant amount

of risk). The Gail model, commonly used by HCPs, calculates a woman's short-term risk (within the next 5 years) and long-term risk (within her lifetime, up to age 90) of developing breast cancer. It is based on seven key risk factors.

1. Current age
2. Age at first menstrual period
3. Age at the first birth of a child (or a woman who has not given birth)
4. Family history of breast cancer (mother, sister, daughter)
5. Number of past breast biopsies
6. Number of breast biopsies showing atypical hyperplasia
7. Ethnicity

Women with a 5-year risk of 1.67% or greater are classified as high risk, which is the U.S. Food and Drug Administration's guideline for taking a drug such as tamoxifen or raloxifene to reduce the risk of developing breast cancer. Other commonly used tools include the Claus model and the Tyrer-Cuzick model.

INDICATIONS
- Evidence of breast lesion by palpation, mammography, or ultrasound.
- Identify patients with breast or other types of cancer that may respond to hormone or antihormone therapy.
- Monitor responsiveness to hormone or antihormone therapy.
- Observable breast changes such as peau d'orange skin, scaly skin of the areola, drainage from the nipple, or ulceration of the skin.

INTERFERING FACTORS
Contraindications
Patients with bleeding disorders *(related to the potential for prolonged bleeding from the biopsy site).*

Factors that may alter the results of the study

- Massive tumor necrosis or tumors with low cellular composition falsely decrease results.
- Antiestrogen preparations (e.g., tamoxifen) ingested 2 mo before tissue sampling will affect test results [ER and PR]).
- Pretesting preservation of the tissue is method and test dependent. The testing laboratory should be consulted for proper instructions prior to the biopsy procedure. Failure to transport specimen to the laboratory immediately can result in degradation of tissue. Prompt and proper specimen processing, storage, and analysis are important to achieve accurate results.

POTENTIAL MEDICAL DIAGNOSIS: CLINICAL SIGNIFICANCE OF RESULTS
Positive findings in
- Cancer
- Hormonal therapy (ER and PR)
- Receptor-positive tumors (ER and PR)

NURSING IMPLICATIONS

BEFORE THE STUDY: PLANNING AND IMPLEMENTATION

Teaching the Patient What to Expect
- Inform the patient this procedure can assist in evaluating breast health.
- Explain that prior to the procedure, laboratory testing may be required to determine the possibility of bleeding risk (coagulation testing) or to assess for impaired kidney function (creatinine level and estimated glomerular filtration rate) if use of iodinated contrast medium is anticipated.
- Pregnancy may be a contraindication to procedures involving some types of anesthesia. Explain to the female patient that she will be asked the date

of her last menstrual period. Pregnancy testing may be performed to determine the possibility of pregnancy before the biopsy is performed.
- Explain that reducing health-care-associated infections is an important patient safety goal and a number of different safety practices will be implemented during their procedure. Advise the patient that hair in the area near the incision site may be clipped or shaved and the area cleaned with an antiseptic solution to cleanse bacteria from the skin in order to reduce the risk for infection. *Note:* The World Health Organization, Centers for Disease Control and Prevention, and Association of periOperative Registered Nurses recommend that hair not be removed at all unless it interferes with the incision site or other aspects of the procedure because hair removal by any means is associated with increased infection rates. When hair removal is necessary, facilities must use a protocol that is based on scientific literature or the endorsement of a professional organization. Clipping immediately before the procedure and in a location outside the procedure area is preferred to shaving with a razor. Shaving creates a break in skin integrity and provides a way for bacteria on the skin to enter the incision site.
- Review the procedure with the patient, address concerns about pain, and explain that there may be moments of discomfort or pain experienced when the IV line is inserted to allow infusion of fluids such as saline, anesthetics, sedatives, medications used in the procedure, or emergency medications. Instruct the patient that prophylactic antibiotics may be administered before the procedure.
- Inform the patient that the biopsy is performed under sterile conditions by an HCP specializing in this procedure. The surgical procedure usually takes about 20 to 30 min to complete, and sutures may be necessary to close the site. A needle biopsy usually takes about 15 min to complete.

▶ Baseline vital signs will be recorded and monitored throughout the procedure. Protocols may vary among facilities.

▶ Explain that the patient will be monitored for complications related to the procedure (e.g., allergic reaction, etc.).

▶ Explain that once the study is completed, a pressure dressing is applied over the puncture site.

Open Biopsy

▶ Adhere to organizational policies and the Centers for Medicare and Medicaid Services (CMS) quality measures regarding administration of prophylactic antibiotics. Administer ordered prophylactic antibiotics 1 hr before incision and use antibiotics that are consistent with current guidelines specific to the procedure.

▶ After administration of general anesthetic and surgical preparation are completed, an incision is made, suspicious area(s) are located, and tissue samples are collected.

Needle Biopsy

▶ Direct the patient to take slow, deep breaths when the local anesthetic is injected. Protect the site with sterile drapes. Instruct the patient to take a deep breath, exhale forcefully, and hold the breath while the biopsy needle is inserted and rotated to obtain a core of breast tissue. Once the needle is removed, the patient may breathe. Pressure is applied to the site for 3 to 5 min, then a sterile pressure dressing is applied.

General

▶ Place tissue samples in formalin solution. Label the specimen, indicating site location, and promptly transport the specimen to the laboratory for processing and analysis.

Potential Nursing Actions

✸ *Make sure a written and informed consent has been signed prior to the procedure and before administering any medications.*

Safety Considerations

▶ Anticoagulants, aspirin, and other salicylates should be discontinued by medical direction for the appropriate number of days prior to a procedure in which bleeding is a potential complication.

Avoiding Complications

▶ Bleeding *(related to a bleeding disorder or the effects of natural products and medications with known anticoagulant, antiplatelet, or thrombolytic properties)* or seeding of the biopsy tract with tumor cells. Observe/assess the biopsy site for bleeding, inflammation, or hematoma formation. Instruct the patient in the care and assessment of the biopsy site and to report any fever, chills, redness, edema, bleeding, or pain at the biopsy site.

Treatment Considerations

▶ Do not allow the patient to eat or drink until the gag reflex returns due to aspiration risk.

▶ Monitor vital signs and neurological status every 15 min for 1 hr, then every 2 hr for 4 hr, and then as ordered by the HCP. Monitor temperature every 4 hr for 24 hr. Monitor intake and output at least every 8 hr. Compare with baseline values. Notify the HCP if temperature is elevated. Discontinue prophylactic antibiotics within 24 hr after the conclusion of the procedure.

▶ Assess for nausea and pain. Administer antiemetic and analgesic medications as needed and as directed by the HCP. Administer antibiotic therapy if ordered and emphasize the importance of completing the entire course of antibiotic therapy, even if signs and symptoms disappear before completion of therapy.

Safety Considerations

▶ Assess the patient's ability to swallow before allowing the patient to attempt liquids or solid foods. Instruct the patient to resume preoperative diet, as directed by the HCP.

Follow-Up, Evaluation, and Desired Outcomes

▶ Understands that decisions regarding the need for and frequency of breast self-examination, mammography, magnetic resonance imaging or ultrasound of the breast, or other cancer screening procedures should be made after consultation between the patient and HCP. Acknowledges that the most current guidelines for breast cancer screening of the general population as well as of individuals with increased risk are available from the American Cancer Society (www.cancer.org), the American College of Obstetricians and Gynecologists (www.acog.org), and the American College of Radiology (www.acr.org). Screening guidelines vary depending on the age and health history of those at average risk and those at high risk for breast cancer. Guidelines may not always agree among organizations; therefore, it is important for patients to participate in their health care, be informed, ask questions, and follow their HCP's recommendations regarding frequency and type of screening.

For additional information regarding screening guidelines refer to the study titled "Mammography."
▶ Understands the pathophysiology associated with breast cancer as well as ongoing treatment, screenings, and medical versus surgical options.
▶ Acknowledges that a health-care specialist may need to be consulted to manage the disease and therapeutic interventions.
▶ Agrees to a follow-up appointment for removal of sutures, if indicated. Demonstrates correct care of the surgical site.
▶ Agrees to adhere to the therapeutic regimen, including self-administration of medication. Understands information about adverse effects and the option to review corresponding literature provided by a pharmacist.
▶ Agrees to attend cancer support group meetings and to seek psychological counseling to adjust to body changes and intimacy concerns.

Biopsy, Cervical

SYNONYM/ACRONYM: Cone biopsy, LEEP.

RATIONALE: To assist in diagnosing and staging cervical cancer.

PATIENT PREPARATION: There are no activity restrictions unless by medical direction. Instruct the patient that to reduce the risk of aspiration related to nausea and vomiting, solid food and milk or milk products are restricted for at least 6 hr, and clear liquids are restricted for at least 2 hr prior to general anesthesia, regional anesthesia, or sedation/analgesia (monitored anesthesia). The patient may be required to be NPO after midnight. The American Society of Anesthesiologists has fasting guidelines for risk levels according to patient status. More information can be located at www.asahq.org.

Regarding the patient's risk for bleeding, the patient should be instructed to avoid taking natural products and medications with known anticoagulant, antiplatelet, or thrombolytic properties or to reduce dosage, as ordered, prior to the procedure. Note the last time and dose of medication taken. Number of days to withhold medication is dependent on the type of anticoagulant. Protocols may vary among facilities.

NORMAL FINDINGS: (Method: Microscopic examination of tissue cells) No abnormal cells or tissue.

CRITICAL FINDINGS AND POTENTIAL INTERVENTIONS
- Assessment of clear margins after tissue excision
- Classification or grading of tumor
- Identification of malignancy

Timely notification to the requesting health-care provider (HCP) of any critical findings and related symptoms is a role expectation of the professional nurse. A listing of these findings varies among facilities.

OVERVIEW: (Study type: Tissue and cell microscopy; related body system: Immune and Reproductive systems.) Tissue samples are placed in properly labelled specimen containers containing formalin solution and promptly transport the specimen to the laboratory for processing and analysis. Biopsy is the excision of a sample of tissue that can be analyzed microscopically to determine cell morphology and the presence of tissue abnormalities. The cervical biopsy is used to assist in confirmation of cancer when screening tests are positive. Cervical biopsy is obtained using an instrument that punches into the tissue and retrieves a tissue sample. The Schiller test entails applying an iodine solution to the cervix. Normal cells pick up the iodine and stain brown. Abnormal cells do not pick up any color. Punch biopsy results may indicate the need for a cone biopsy of the cervix. Cone biopsy involves removing a wedge of tissue from the cervix by using a surgical knife, a carbon dioxide laser, or a loop electrosurgical excision procedure (LEEP). LEEP can be performed by placing the patient under a general anesthetic; by a regional anesthesia, such as a spinal or epidural; or by a cervical block whereby a local anesthetic is injected into the cervix. The patient is given oral or IV pain medicine in conjunction with the local anesthetic when this method is used. Following colposcopy or cervical biopsy, LEEP can be used to treat abnormal tissue identified on biopsy.

INDICATIONS
- Follow-up to abnormal Papanicolaou (Pap) smear, Schiller test, or colposcopy.
- Suspected cervical malignancy.

INTERFERING FACTORS
Contraindications

Patients with bleeding disorders *(related to the potential for prolonged bleeding from the biopsy site)* or acute pelvic inflammatory disease.

Factors that may alter the results of the study
- This test should not be performed while the patient is menstruating.

POTENTIAL MEDICAL DIAGNOSIS: CLINICAL SIGNIFICANCE OF RESULTS
Positive findings in
- Cancer in situ
- Cervical dysplasia
- Cervical polyps

NURSING IMPLICATIONS

BEFORE THE STUDY: PLANNING AND IMPLEMENTATION

Teaching the Patient What to Expect
- Inform the patient this procedure can assist in establishing a diagnosis of cervical disease.

B

Pregnancy may be a contraindication to procedures involving some types of anesthesia. Explain to the female patient that she will be asked the date of her last menstrual period. Pregnancy testing may be performed to determine the possibility of pregnancy before the biopsy is performed.

Explain that reducing health-care-associated infections is an important patient safety goal and a number of different safety practices will be implemented during their procedure. Advise the patient that hair in the area near the incision site may be clipped or shaved and the area cleaned with an antiseptic solution to cleanse bacteria from the skin in order to reduce the risk for infection. *Note:* The World Health Organization, Centers for Disease Control and Prevention, and Association of periOperative Registered Nurses recommend that hair not be removed at all unless it interferes with the incision site or other aspects of the procedure because hair removal by any means is associated with increased infection rates. When hair removal is necessary, facilities must use a protocol that is based on scientific literature or the endorsement of a professional organization. Clipping immediately before the procedure and in a location outside the procedure area is preferred to shaving with a razor. Shaving creates a break in skin integrity and provides a way for bacteria on the skin to enter the incision site.

Review the procedure with the patient, address concerns about pain, and explain that there may be moments of discomfort or pain experienced when the IV line is inserted to allow infusion of fluids such as saline, anesthetics, sedatives, medications used in the procedure, or emergency medications. Instruct the patient that prophylactic antibiotics may be administered before the procedure.

Inform the patient the biopsy is performed under sterile conditions by an HCP specializing in this procedure. The biopsy can be performed in the HCP's office and takes approximately 5 to 10 min to complete. The open biopsy is performed in a surgical suite, usually takes about 20 to 30 min to complete, and sutures may be necessary to close the site.

Explain that the patient must remove clothes below the waist after which she will be assisted into a lithotomy position on a gynecological examination table (with feet in stirrups). The patient's legs will be draped.

Punch Biopsy

Iodine solution is used to cleanse the cervix and distinguish normal from abnormal tissue. Local anesthetics, analgesics, or both, are administered to minimize discomfort. A small, round punch is rotated into the skin to the desired depth. The cylinder of skin is pulled upward with forceps and separated at its base with a scalpel or scissors.

LEEP in the HCP's Office

A speculum is inserted into the vagina and is opened to gently spread apart the vagina for inspection of the cervix. Iodine solution is used to cleanse the cervix and distinguish normal from abnormal tissue. Local anesthetics, analgesics, or both, are administered to minimize discomfort. The diseased tissue is removed along with a small amount of healthy tissue along the margins of the biopsy to ensure that no diseased tissue is left in the cervix after the procedure.

Open Biopsy

Adhere to organizational policies and the Centers for Medicare and Medicaid Services (CMS) quality measures regarding administration of prophylactic antibiotics. Administer ordered prophylactic antibiotics 1 hr before incision and use antibiotics that are consistent with current guidelines specific to the procedure.

After administration of general anesthetics and surgical preparation are completed, the procedure is carried out as noted above.

Explain to the patient she will be monitored for complications related to the procedure (e.g., allergic reaction, etc.).

Potential Nursing Actions

✦ *Make sure a written and informed consent has been signed prior to the procedure and before administering any medications.*

▶ Record the date of the last menstrual period and determine the possibility of pregnancy in perimenopausal women.

Safety Considerations

▶ Anticoagulants, aspirin, and other salicylates should be discontinued by medical direction for the appropriate number of days prior to a procedure in which bleeding is a potential complication.

AFTER THE STUDY: POTENTIAL NURSING ACTIONS

Avoiding Complications

▶ Bleeding *(related to a bleeding disorder or the effects of natural products and medications with known anticoagulant, antiplatelet, or thrombolytic properties)* Observe/assess biopsy site for bleeding, inflammation, or hematoma formation.

Treatment Considerations

▶ Instruct the patient to resume usual diet, fluids, and medications, as directed by the HCP.

▶ Monitor vital signs and neurological status every 15 min for 1 hr, then every 2 hr for 4 hr, and then as ordered by the HCP. Monitor temperature every 4 hr for 24 hr. Compare with baseline values.

▶ Discontinue prophylactic antibiotics within 24 hr after the conclusion of the procedure.

▶ Assess for nausea and pain. Administer antiemetic, analgesic medications as needed and antibiotic therapy if ordered. Remind the patient of the importance of completing the entire course of antibiotic therapy, even if signs and symptoms disappear before completion of therapy.

▶ Advise the patient to expect a gray-green vaginal discharge for several days, that some vaginal bleeding may occur for up to 1 wk but should not be heavier than a normal menses, and that some pelvic pain may occur.

Instruct the patient to wear a sanitary pad, and advise the patient that tampons should not be used for 1 to 3 wk. Patients who have undergone a simple cervical punch biopsy can usually resume normal activities immediately following the procedure. Instruct patients who have undergone LEEP or open biopsy to avoid strenuous activity for 8 to 24 hr; to avoid douching or intercourse for 2 to 4 wk or as instructed; and to report excessive bleeding, chills, fever, or any other unusual findings to the HCP.

▶ Instruct the patient in the care and assessment of the biopsy site and to report any fever, chills, redness, edema, bleeding, or pain at the biopsy site.

Safety Considerations

▶ Assess the patient's ability to swallow before allowing the patient to attempt liquids or solid foods. Instruct the patient to resume preoperative diet, as directed by the HCP.

Follow-Up, Evaluation, and Desired Outcomes

▶ Understands that decisions regarding the need for and frequency of conventional or liquid-based Pap tests or other cancer screening procedures should be made after consultation between the patient and HCP. The most current guidelines for cervical cancer screening of the general population as well as of individuals with increased risk are available from the ACS (www.cancer.org) and the American College of Obstetricians and Gynecologists (www.acog.org). For additional information regarding screening guidelines refer to the study titled "Papanicolaou Smear."

▶ Acknowledges the importance of adhering to the therapeutic regimen and prescribed medications. Understands the adverse effects associated with the prescribed medications and the recommendation to review corresponding literature provided by a pharmacist.

▶ Understands the pathophysiology associated with cervical cancer as well as ongoing treatment,

B

screenings, and medical versus surgical options. Consultation with a health-care specialist may need to manage the disease and therapeutic interventions.
▶ Successfully demonstrates care of the surgical site.

▶ Agrees to attend cancer support group meetings and to seek psychological counseling to adjust to body changes and intimacy and fertility concerns.
▶ Acknowledges end-of-life treatment options for those with a terminal diagnosis.

Biopsy, Chorionic Villus

SYNONYM/ACRONYM: N/A

RATIONALE: To assist in diagnosing genetic fetal abnormalities such as Down syndrome.

PATIENT PREPARATION: There are no food, fluid, activity, or medication restrictions unless by medical direction. Instruct the patient to drink 1 to 2 glasses of water about 30 min prior to testing so that the bladder is full. This elevates the uterus higher in the pelvis. The patient should not void before the procedure.

NORMAL FINDINGS: (Method: Tissue culture) Normal karyotype.

CRITICAL FINDINGS AND POTENTIAL INTERVENTIONS
• Identification of abnormalities in chorionic villus tissue

Timely notification to the requesting health-care provider (HCP) of any critical findings and related symptoms is a role expectation of the professional nurse. A listing of these findings varies among facilities.

OVERVIEW: (Study type: Tissue and cell microscopy; related body system: Reproductive system. Tissue samples are placed in formalin solution, labelled indicating site location, and promptly transported to the laboratory for processing and analysis.) This test is used to detect fetal abnormalities caused by numerous genetic disorders. Examples of genetic defects that are commonly tested for and can be identified from a chorionic villus sampling include sickle cell anemia and cystic fibrosis. The advantage over amniocentesis is that it can be performed as early as the eighth week of pregnancy, permitting earlier decisions regarding termination of pregnancy. However, unlike amniocentesis, this test will not detect neural tube defects.

Knowledge of genetics assists in identifying those who may benefit from additional education, risk assessment, and counseling. Genetics is the study and identification of genes, genetic mutations, and inheritance. For example, genetics provides some insight into the likelihood of inheriting a medical condition such as cystic fibrosis, Duchenne muscular dystrophy, hemophilia, sickle cell anemia, Tay-Sachs disease, thalassemia, trisomy 21, or trisomy 18. Some conditions are the result of mutations involving a single gene, and other conditions may involve multiple genes and/or multiple chromosomes. Sickle cell anemia and cystic fibrosis are examples of autosomal recessive, single-gene disorders. Down syndrome is an example of a chromosome disorder in which the cells have three copies of chromosome 21 (trisomy) instead of the normal two copies. Hemophilia is an example of a recessive, sex-linked genetic disorder passed on from a mother to male children. Further information regarding inheritance of genes can be found in the study titled "Genetic Testing."

INDICATIONS

- Assist in the diagnosis of in utero metabolic disorders such as cystic fibrosis or other errors of lipid, carbohydrate, or amino acid metabolism.
- Detect abnormalities in the fetus of women of advanced maternal age.
- Determine fetal gender when the mother is a known carrier of a sex-linked abnormal gene that could be transmitted to male offspring, such as hemophilia or Duchenne muscular dystrophy.
- Evaluate fetus in families with a history of genetic disorders, such as Down syndrome, Tay-Sachs disease, chromosome or enzyme anomalies, or inherited hemoglobinopathies.

INTERFERING FACTORS

Contraindications

✺ Patients with a history of or in the presence of incompetent cervix, vaginal infection, or Rh sensitization.

POTENTIAL MEDICAL DIAGNOSIS: CLINICAL SIGNIFICANCE OF RESULTS

Abnormal karyotype: *Numerous genetic disorders. Generally, the laboratory provides detailed interpretive information regarding the specific chromosome abnormality detected.*

NURSING IMPLICATIONS

BEFORE THE STUDY: PLANNING AND IMPLEMENTATION

Teaching the Patient What to Expect

▶ Inform the patient this procedure can assist in establishing a diagnosis of in utero genetic disorders. Warn the patient that normal results do not guarantee a healthy fetus.

▶ Review the procedure with the patient. Assure the patient that precautions to avoid injury to the fetus will be taken by locating the fetus with ultrasound.

▶ Address concerns about pain related to the procedure. Explain that during the transabdominal procedure, any discomfort with a needle biopsy will be minimized with local anesthetics. Explain that during the transvaginal procedure, some cramping may be experienced as the catheter is guided through the cervix.

▶ Encourage relaxation and controlled breathing during the procedure to aid in reducing any mild discomfort. Inform the patient that specimen collection is performed by an HCP specializing in this procedure and usually takes approximately 10 to 15 min to complete.

▶ The procedure will require the patient to remove clothes below the waist. *Transabdominal:* Positioning for this procedure will require assistance into a supine position on the examination table with abdomen exposed and legs draped. *Transvaginal:* Positioning for this procedure requires assisting the patient into a lithotomy position on a gynecologic examination table (lying on the back with feet in stirrups)

B

with legs draped. Direct the patient to breathe normally and to avoid unnecessary movement during the local anesthetic and the procedure. After the administration of the local anesthetic, use clippers to remove hair from the surgical site if appropriate, cleanse the site with an antiseptic solution, and drape the area with sterile towels.

Transabdominal Biopsy

▶ Positions of the amniotic fluid, fetus, and placenta will be identified using ultrasound.
▶ A needle is inserted through the abdomen into the uterus, avoiding contact with the fetus. A syringe is connected to the needle, and the specimen of chorionic villus cells is withdrawn from the uteroplacental area. Pressure is applied to the site for 3 to 5 min, and then a sterile pressure dressing is applied.

Transvaginal Biopsy

▶ Positions of the fetus and placenta are identified using ultrasound. A speculum is inserted into the vagina and is opened to gently spread apart the vagina for inspection of the cervix. The cervix is cleansed with a swab of antiseptic solution. A catheter is inserted through the cervix into the uterus, avoiding contact with the fetus. A syringe is connected to the catheter, and the specimen of chorionic villus cells is withdrawn from the uteroplacental area.

General

▶ Record maternal and fetal baseline vital signs, and continue to monitor throughout the procedure. Monitor for uterine contractions. Monitor fetal vital signs using ultrasound. Protocols may vary among facilities.
▶ Monitor the patient for complications related to the procedure (e.g., premature labor, allergic reaction, anaphylaxis).

Potential Nursing Actions

✦ *Make sure a written and informed consent has been signed prior to the procedure and before administering any medications.*

▶ Obtain a family history of genetic disorders.
▶ Obtain maternal Rh type. If Rh-negative, check for prior sensitization.
▶ Record the date of the last menstrual period and determine that the pregnancy is in the first trimester between the 10th and 12th weeks.

AFTER THE STUDY: POTENTIAL NURSING ACTIONS

Avoiding Complications

▶ Women at risk for or with known cervical abnormalities should be aware of the risks of miscarriage due to incompetent (loose) cervix *(related to passing a catheter or other instrument through the cervix, weakening the cervix).* Rh-negative women risk mixing of the maternal and fetal blood supply *(related to the invasive nature of the procedure and potentially resulting in development of maternal antibodies directed against fetal blood cells, a situation that can develop into hemolytic disease of the newborn). Administer Rh(D) immune globulin RhoGAM IM or Rhophylac IM or IV to maternal Rh-negative patients to prevent maternal Rh sensitization should the fetus be Rh-positive.* Monitor the patient for bleeding or signs of inflammation. Moderate to severe abdominal pain or cramps, increased or prolonged leaking of amniotic fluid from vagina or abdominal needle site, vaginal bleeding that is heavier than spotting, and chills or fever should be reported to the HCP.

Treatment Considerations

▶ After the procedure, the patient is placed in the left side-lying (Sims) position, and both maternal and fetal vital signs are monitored for at least 30 min. Protocols may vary among facilities.
▶ Instruct the patient in the care and assessment of the site. Instruct the patient to report any redness, edema, bleeding, or pain at the biopsy site.
▶ Administer mild analgesic and antibiotic therapy as ordered. Remind the patient of the importance of completing the entire course of antibiotic therapy, even if signs and symptoms disappear before completion of therapy.

- Advise the patient to expect mild cramping, leakage of small amount of amniotic fluid, and vaginal spotting for up to 2 days following the procedure.

Follow-Up, Evaluation, and Desired Outcomes

- Acknowledges the importance of adhering to the therapeutic regime, including prescribed medications. States the significant adverse effects associated with the prescribed medication, and agrees to review the corresponding literature provided by a pharmacist.
- Understands the implications of abnormal test results on lifestyle choices, including the clinical implications of the test results.
- Acknowledges the risks of delivering a developmentally challenged infant, including options such as termination of pregnancy or adoption. Understands there may be some guilt, depression, or anger if fetal abnormalities are detected.
- Agrees to seek counseling if concerned with pregnancy termination or to seek genetic counseling if chromosomal abnormality is determined. Decisions regarding elective abortion should take place in the presence of both parents.

Biopsy, Various Sites
(Bladder, Bone, Intestinal, Kidney, Liver, Lung, Lymph Node, Muscle, Prostate, Skin, Thyroid)

SYNONYM/ACRONYM: N/A

RATIONALE: To assist in diagnosing cancer or other tissue abnormality.

PATIENT PREPARATION: There are no activity restrictions unless by medical direction. Explain that diet is restricted to clear liquids from the day prior to the day of an intestinal biopsy. Instruct all patients that to reduce the risk of aspiration related to nausea and vomiting, solid food and milk or milk products are restricted for at least 6 hr, and clear liquids are restricted for at least 2 hr prior to general anesthesia, regional anesthesia, or sedation/analgesia (monitored anesthesia). Patients may be asked to be NPO after midnight. The American Society of Anesthesiologists has fasting guidelines for risk levels according to patient status. More information can be located at www.asahq.org.

Regarding the patient's risk for bleeding, the patient should be instructed to avoid taking natural products and medications with known anticoagulant, antiplatelet, or thrombolytic properties or to reduce dosage, as ordered, prior to the procedure. Number of days to withhold medication is dependent on the type of anticoagulant. Note the last time and dose of medication taken. Patients on beta blockers before the surgical procedure should be instructed to take their medication as ordered during the perioperative period. Protocols may vary among facilities.

Ensure that a barium swallow is not scheduled within 48 hr prior to the small intestine biopsy.

NORMAL FINDINGS: (Method: Macroscopic and microscopic examination of tissue) No abnormal tissue or cells.

B

CRITICAL FINDINGS AND POTENTIAL INTERVENTIONS

General
- Assessment of clear margins after tissue excision
- Classification or grading of tumor
- Identification of malignancy

Lung
- Shortness of breath, cyanosis, or rapid pulse during the procedure must be reported immediately. Any postprocedural decrease in breath sounds noted at the biopsy site should be reported immediately

Timely notification to the requesting health-care provider (HCP) of any critical findings and related symptoms is a role expectation of the professional nurse. A listing of these findings varies among facilities.

OVERVIEW: (Study type: Tissue and cell microscopy, from the selected site; **related body system:** Digestive, Endocrine, Immune, Integumentary, Lymphatic, Musculoskeletal, Reproductive, Respiratory, Urinary systems.) Instructions regarding the appropriate transport container for molecular diagnostic studies should be obtained from the laboratory prior to the procedure. Specimens are placed in a labelled container, including site and laterality, with formalin solution, and promptly transport the specimen to the laboratory for processing and analysis. Biopsy is the excision of a sample of tissue that can be analyzed microscopically to determine cell morphology and the presence of tissue abnormalities. This test is used to assist in confirming the diagnosis of cancer or other disease when clinical symptoms or diagnostic findings (e.g., ultrasound or x-ray) are suspicious. Samples can be obtained by aspiration of fluid and tumor cells from the tumor site. Needle biopsies are often performed using guidance by CT scan or ultrasound. There are two types of needle biopsy:

fine-needle biopsy in which fluid and tumor cells are aspirated from the tumor site and core-needle biopsy in which a plug of tissue is removed using a special serrated needle. The choice of biopsy method is based on the type of tumor expected, whether the tumor is benign or malignant, and the surgeon's anticipated plan regarding removal of the tumor. If the diagnostic imaging examinations indicate the cancer has spread outside the suspicious area, confirmatory samples can be obtained by surgical biopsy. A sample of suspicious tissue is then excised and examined macroscopically and microscopically to determine the presence of cell morphology and tissue abnormalities.

Endoscopic Biopsy
Biopsy specimens may be obtained during endoscopic examinations. Bladder biopsy is performed by a urologist with visualization of the urethra and bladder during cystoscopic examination. A biopsy of the bladder is taken after the bladder is filled with saline for irrigation. The cystoscopy and biopsy are

performed either in the urologist's office with local anesthetics or in the operating room under general anesthesia. Prostate biopsy using a transurethral approach is accomplished when the endoscope is inserted into the urethra and tissue is excised with a cutting loop. An intestinal biopsy specimen is also usually obtained during endoscopic examination.

Many other biopsy specimens are obtained either percutaneously or after surgical incision:

Lung

The lung biopsy specimen can be obtained transbronchially or by open lung biopsy. In a transbronchial biopsy, forceps pass through the bronchoscope to obtain the specimen. In a transbronchial needle aspiration biopsy, a needle passes through a bronchoscope to obtain the specimen. In a transcatheter bronchial brushing, a brush is inserted through the bronchoscope. In an open lung biopsy, the chest is opened and a small thoracic incision is made to remove tissue from the chest wall. Lung biopsies are used to differentiate between infection and other sources of disease indicated by initial radiology studies, computed tomography scans, or sputum analysis. Specimens are also cultured to detect pathogenic organisms or directly examined for the presence of malignant cells.

Lymph Node

Biopsies most commonly performed on types of lymph nodes include cervical nodes, which drain the face and scalp; axillary nodes, which drain the arms, breasts, and upper chest; and inguinal nodes, which drain the legs, external genitalia, and lower abdominal wall.

Muscle

A muscle biopsy specimen is usually obtained from the deltoid or gastrocnemius muscle after a surgical incision.

Prostate

Biopsy of the prostate gland is performed to identify cancerous cells, especially if serum prostate-specific antigen (PSA) is increased. Serial measurements of PSA in the blood are often performed before and after surgery. Approximately 15% to 40% of patients who have had their prostate removed will encounter an increase in PSA. Patients treated for prostate cancer and who have had a PSA recurrence can still develop a metastasis as much as 8 yr after the postsurgical PSA level increased. The majority of tumors develop slowly and require minimal intervention, but patients with an increase in PSA greater than 2 ng/mL in a year are more likely to have an aggressive form of prostate cancer with a greater risk of death. The Prostate Health Index (PHI) is another multimarker strategy used to improve the positive prediction rate of prostate cancer, especially when PSA levels are considered to be moderately increased (4–10 ng mL). The PHI applies information provided by the results of prostate marker blood tests to a mathematical formula and offers additional information for clinical decision making. The three tests used in the formula are the total PSA, free PSA, and p2PSA (an isoform of PSA, where PHI = p2PSA/[free PSA] × square root of free PSA). Precision medicine provides a technology to predict the progression of prostate cancer, likelihood of recurrence, or development of related metastatic disease. New technology makes it possible to combine data such as analysis of molecular biomarkers and cellular structure specific to the individual's biopsy tissue, standard tissue biopsy results, Gleason score, number of positive tumor cores, tumor stage, presurgical and postsurgical PSA levels, and postsurgical margin status with computerized mathematical programs to create a personalized report that predicts the likelihood of post-prostatectomy disease progression.

Skin

A skin biopsy can be obtained by any of four methods:

- Curettage biopsy in which the skin is scraped with a curette to obtain specimen.
- Shaving biopsy in which a scalpel is used to remove a portion of the lesion that protrudes above the epidermis.
- Excision biopsy in which a scalpel is used to remove the entire lesion.
- Punch biopsy in which a small, round punch about 4 to 6 mm in diameter is rotated into the skin to the desired depth. The cylinder of skin is pulled upward with forceps and separated at its base with a scalpel or scissors.

A Tzanck smear may be prepared from vesicles (blisters) present on the skin. Skin cells in the vesicles can be evaluated microscopically to indicate the presence of certain viruses, especially herpes, that cause cells to become enlarged and otherwise abnormal in appearance. Sentinel lymph node biopsy (SLNB) may be considered to assist in the diagnosis of melanoma. A sentinel lymph node (SLN) is the first lymph node to be infiltrated by cancer cells from the primary tumor. To identify an SLN, the surgeon injects one or more tracers (such as technetium-99m and isosulfan blue dye) near the tumor, then uses a handheld gamma detector to locate the nodes emitting radioactivity or visually inspects the nearby nodes for any that are stained blue from the dye. Once the SNL is located, a small incision is made and the node is removed. The suspicious tissue is checked microscopically for the presence of cancer cells by a pathologist. Lymph node positive samples may warrant immediate removal of additional lymph nodes or removal during a follow-up procedure.

Thyroid

A thyroid biopsy specimen can be obtained by needle aspiration or by surgical excision.

INDICATIONS

General

- Assist in the diagnosis of the cause of organ-/site-specific disease.
- Confirm suspected malignancy based on evidence provided by diagnostic study results.
- Confirm suspicious findings during endoscopic visualization.

- Monitor existing recurrent benign lesions for malignant changes.
- Monitor therapeutic response.

Bladder

- Assist in the evaluation of cases in which symptoms such as hematuria persist after previous treatment (e.g., removal of polyps or kidney stones).

Bone

- Differentiation of a benign from a malignant bone lesion.

Intestinal

- Assist in the diagnosis of various intestinal disorders, such as lactose and other enzyme deficiencies, celiac disease, and parasitic infections.

Kidney

- Determine extent of involvement in systemic lupus erythematosus or other immunological disorders.
- Monitor progression of nephrotic syndrome.
- Monitor kidney function after transplantation.

Liver

- Assist in confirming suspected hepatic parenchymal disease.
- Assist in diagnosing the cause of persistently elevated liver enzymes, hepatomegaly, or jaundice.

Lung

- Assist in the diagnosis of fibrosis and degenerative or inflammatory diseases of the lung.
- Assist in the diagnosis of sarcoidosis.

Lymph Node

- Assist in confirming suspected fungal or parasitic infections of the lymphatics.
- Determine the stage of metastatic cancer.
- Differentiate between benign and malignant disorders that may cause lymph node enlargement.

- Evaluate persistent enlargement of one or more lymph nodes for unknown reasons.

Muscle

- Assist in confirming suspected fungal infection or parasitic infestation of the muscle.
- Assist in diagnosing the cause of neuropathy or myopathy.
- Assist in the diagnosis of Duchenne muscular dystrophy.

Skin

- Assist in the diagnosis of keratoses, warts, moles, keloids, fibromas, cysts, or inflamed lesions.
- Assist in the diagnosis of inflammatory process of the skin, especially herpes infection.
- Evaluate suspicious skin lesions.

Prostate

- Evaluate prostatic hyperplasia of unknown etiology.
- Investigate suspected cancer of the prostate.

Thyroid

- Determine the cause of inflammatory thyroid disease.
- Determine the cause of hyperthyroidism.
- Evaluate enlargement of the thyroid gland.

INTERFERING FACTORS

Contraindications

◆ Patients with bleeding disorders *(related to the potential for prolonged bleeding from the biopsy site)* or an acute infection of the biopsy site of interest.

Factors that may alter the results of the study

Intestinal Biopsy

- Barium swallow within 48 hr of small intestine biopsy *(related to retained barium, which may obscure clear visualization and guidance of the biopsy needle).*

B

Kidney Biopsy

- Obesity and severe spinal deformity can make percutaneous biopsy impossible.

Liver Biopsy

◈ Patients with suspected vascular tumor of the liver that may increase the risk of bleeding, ascites that may obscure proper insertion site for needle biopsy, subdiaphragmatic or right hemothoracic infection, or biliary tract infection.

Lung Biopsy

◈ Conditions such as vascular anomalies of the lung, bleeding abnormalities, or pulmonary hypertension may increase the risk of bleeding.

◈ Conditions such as bullae or cysts and respiratory insufficiency increase the risk of pneumothorax.

Muscle Biopsy

- If electromyography is performed before muscle biopsy, residual inflammation may lead to false-positive biopsy results.

Prostate Biopsy

- The various sampling approaches have individual drawbacks that should be considered: Transurethral sampling does not always ensure that malignant cells will be included in the specimen, whereas transrectal sampling carries the risk of perforating the rectum and creating a channel through which malignant cells can seed normal tissue.

POTENTIAL MEDICAL DIAGNOSIS: CLINICAL SIGNIFICANCE OF RESULTS
Abnormal findings related to

Bladder

- Positive findings in tumor of the bladder or ureter

Bone

- Ewing sarcoma
- Multiple myeloma
- Osteoma
- Osteosarcoma

Intestinal

- Cancer
- Celiac disease
- Lactose deficiency
- Parasitic infestation
- Tropical sprue

Kidney

- Acute and chronic poststreptococcal glomerulonephritis
- Amyloidosis infiltration
- Cancer
- Disseminated lupus erythematosus
- Goodpasture syndrome
- Immunological rejection of transplanted kidney
- Nephrotic syndrome
- Pyelonephritis
- Renal venous thrombosis

Liver

- Benign tumor
- Cancer
- Cholesterol ester storage disease
- Cirrhosis
- Galactosemia
- Hemochromatosis
- Hepatic involvement with systemic lupus erythematosus, sarcoidosis, or amyloidosis
- Hepatitis
- Parasitic infestations (e.g., amebiasis, malaria, visceral larva migrans)
- Reye syndrome
- Wilson disease

Lung

- Amyloidosis
- Cancer
- Granulomas
- Infections caused by *Blastomyces*, *Histoplasma*, *Legionella* spp., and *Pneumocystis jiroveci*

- Sarcoidosis
- Systemic lupus erythematosus
- Tuberculosis

Lymph Node
- Chancroid
- Fungal infection (e.g., cat scratch disease)
- Immunodeficiency
- Infectious mononucleosis
- Lymph involvement of systemic diseases (e.g., systemic lupus erythematosus, sarcoidosis)
- Lymphangitis
- Lymphogranuloma venereum
- Malignancy (e.g., lymphomas, leukemias)
- Metastatic disease
- Parasitic infestation (e.g., pneumoconiosis)

Muscle
- Amyotrophic lateral sclerosis
- Duchenne muscular dystrophy
- Fungal infection
- Myasthenia gravis
- Myopathy (chronic alcohol misuse)
- Myotonia congenita
- Parasitic infestation

- Polymyalgia rheumatica
- Polymyositis

Skin
- Basal cell cancer
- Cysts
- Dermatitis
- Dermatofibroma
- Keloids
- Malignant melanoma
- Neurofibroma
- Pemphigus
- Pigmented nevi
- Seborrheic keratosis
- Skin involvement in systemic lupus erythematosus, discoid lupus erythematosus, and scleroderma
- Squamous cell cancer
- Viral infection (herpes, varicella)
- Warts

Prostate
- Prostate cancer

Thyroid
- Benign thyroid cyst
- Granulomatous thyroiditis
- Hashimoto thyroiditis
- Nontoxic nodular goiter
- Thyroid cancer

NURSING IMPLICATIONS

POTENTIAL NURSING PROBLEMS: ASSESSMENT & NURSING DIAGNOSIS

Problems	Signs and Symptoms
Bladder, prostate: Altered urination *(related to disease, obstruction, inflammation, tumor, infection)*	Decreased urinary output less than 30 mL/hr, distended bladder, high residual urine, urinary retention, urinary dribbling, complaints of full bladder with inability to void
Bone: Mobility *(related to inflammation, trauma, pain, infection, tumor)*	Inability to meet physical demands associated with activities of daily living, ineffective range of motion, pain
Intestinal: Altered fecal elimination *(related to blockage, inflammation, infection, tumor)*	Abdominal distention, high-pitched or absent bowel sounds, nausea and vomiting, fecal odor of emesis

(table continues on page 176)

B

Problems	Signs and Symptoms
Kidney: Infection *(related to obstruction, infection, cyst, abscess, inflammation, tumor, trauma, injury)*	Positive culture, fever, chills, elevated temperature, elevated white blood cell count, flank pain, hematuria, urinary frequency
Liver: Nutrition *(related to pain, nausea, vomiting, anorexia)*	Weight loss, emaciation, malabsorption, poor intake
Lung: Gas exchange *(related to obstruction, infection, inflammation, tumor, malignancy)*	Difficulty breathing, dyspnea, hypoxia, cyanosis, increased heart and respiratory rates, restlessness, anxiety, sense of impending death and doom, hemoptysis, abnormal arterial blood gas
Lymph node: Grief *(related to diagnosis, fear, poor prognosis, surgery, disease staging)*	Verbalization of fear and distress, crying, expressions of anxiety, restlessness
Muscle: Self-care deficit *(related to loss of mobility and function, malignancy, tumor)*	Unable to complete the activities of daily living (eating, bathing, dressing, toileting) without assistance
Skin: Body image *(related to physical changes associated with the disease process)*	Expressions of feelings or concerns about visual physical changes, fear of rejection by others due to appearance
Thyroid: Altered thought processes *(related to decreased cardiac output and impaired cerebral perfusion secondary to a deficit of thyroid hormone)*	Altered memory, mental impairment, decreased concentration, depression, inaccurate environmental perception, inappropriate thinking, memory deficits

BEFORE THE STUDY: PLANNING AND IMPLEMENTATION

Teaching the Patient What to Expect

▶ Inform the patient this procedure can assist in establishing a diagnosis of cancer or other disease (in the tissue of interest).

▶ Advise the patient that small procedures may be performed in a clinic or HCP's office, and larger procedures will be performed in the operating room. Explain that prior to the procedure, laboratory testing may be required to determine the possibility of bleeding risk (coagulation testing).

▶ Pregnancy may be a contraindication to procedures involving some types of anesthesia. Explain to the female patient that she will be asked the date of her last menstrual period. Pregnancy testing may be performed to determine the possibility of pregnancy before the biopsy is performed.

▶ Explain that reducing health-care-associated infections is an important patient safety goal and a number of different safety practices will be implemented during their procedure. Advise the patient that hair in the area near the incision site may be clipped or shaved and the area cleaned with an antiseptic solution to cleanse bacteria from the skin in order to reduce the risk for infection. *Note:* The World Health Organization, Centers for Disease Control and Prevention, and Association of periOperative Registered Nurses recommend that hair not be removed at all unless it interferes with the incision site or other aspects of the procedure because hair removal by any means is associated with increased infection rates. When hair removal is necessary, facilities must use a protocol that is based on scientific literature or the endorsement of a professional organization. Clipping immediately before the procedure and in a location outside the procedure area is preferred to shaving with a razor. Shaving creates a break in skin integrity and provides a way for bacteria on the skin to enter the incision site.

▶ Review the procedure with the patient, address concerns about pain, and explain that there may be moments of discomfort or pain experienced when the IV line is inserted to allow infusion of fluids such as saline, anesthetics, antibiotics, sedatives, medications used in the procedure, or emergency medications. Instruct the patient that prophylactic antibiotics may be administered before the procedure.

▶ Inform the patient that the biopsy is performed under sterile conditions by an HCP specializing in this procedure. The estimated time of completion for the procedure can be provided to the patient and family as described in the table below.

▶ Baseline vital signs will be recorded and monitored throughout the procedure. Protocols may vary among facilities.

▶ The patient will be assisted to the position that gives the safest and most effective access: for example, supine position for deltoid biopsy; prone position for gastrocnemius biopsy; on a urological examination table with the feet in stirrups for transurethral prostate biopsy; or left, lateral Sims position for transrectal prostate biopsy. A sandbag or roll may be used to properly position the patient. For example, a sandbag may be placed under the abdomen to aid in moving the kidneys to the desired position

▶ After the administration of general or local anesthesia, the site will be cleansed with an antiseptic solution and the area draped with sterile towels.

▶ Explain to the patient he or she will be monitored for complications related to the procedure (e.g., allergic reaction, etc.).

▶ Explain that once the study is completed, a pressure dressing is applied over the puncture site.

Open Biopsy

▶ Adhere to organizational policies and the Centers for Medicare and Medicaid Services (CMS) quality measures regarding administration of prophylactic antibiotics. Administer ordered prophylactic antibiotics 1 hr before incision, and use antibiotics that are consistent with current guidelines specific to the procedure. After administration of general anesthesia and surgical preparation are completed, an incision is made, suspicious area(s) are located, and tissue samples are collected.

▶ *Lung:* The patient is prepared for thoracotomy under general anesthesia in the operating room. Tissue specimens are collected from suspicious sites. The specimen from needle aspiration or brushing is placed on clean glass microscope slides. Tissue or aspirate specimens will be placed in the appropriate sterile container for culture or appropriate fixative container for histological studies. Patients will be carefully observed and assessed for any signs of respiratory distress during the procedure. A chest tube is inserted after the procedure. Chest tube insertion, or thoracostomy, is a common procedure indicated for prevention of pleural effusions associated with hemothorax in the postsurgical setting. In these situations, preventing the accumulation of blood or other drainage is imperative to allow for lung reexpansion. Thoracostomy (a small incision or opening [ostomy]), made in the chest wall to facilitate the insertion of a tube through which fluids can be removed from the chest) can be confused with thoracotomy (a large, surgical incision used to access the internal organs in the chest [-otomy, or "to cut"]).

▶ *Prostate perineal approach:* The patient is assisted to the lithotomy position. The perineum is cleansed with an antiseptic solution, and the biopsy site is protected with sterile drapes. A small

B

incision is made, and the sample is removed by needle biopsy or biopsy punch and placed in formalin solution.

Needle Biopsy
▸ After the local anesthetic is administered, a small incision is made and the biopsy needle is inserted to remove the specimen. The patient is directed to take slow, deep breaths when the local anesthetic is injected, and the site is protected with sterile drapes. The patient is instructed to take a deep breath, exhale forcefully, and hold the breath while the biopsy needle is inserted and rotated to obtain a core of tissue. Once the needle is removed, the patient may breathe. Pressure is applied to the site for 3 to 20 min, depending on the site, and then a sterile pressure dressing is applied.
▸ *Lung:* The patient will be instructed to avoid coughing during the procedure. The needle is inserted through the posterior chest wall and into the intercostal space. The needle is rotated to obtain the sample and then withdrawn. Pressure is applied to the site with a petroleum jelly gauze, and a pressure dressing is applied over the petroleum jelly gauze.
▸ *Prostate transrectal approach:* A rectal examination is performed to locate suspicious nodules. A biopsy needle guide is placed at the biopsy site, and the biopsy needle is inserted through the needle guide for aspiration of cells.

Endoscopy Biopsy
▸ *Intestinal:* A local anesthetic is sprayed into the throat. A protective tooth guard and a bite block may be placed in the mouth. The flexible endoscope is passed into and through the mouth, and the patient is asked to swallow. Once the endoscope passes into the

esophagus, the patient is assisted into the left lateral (Sims) position. A suction device is used to drain saliva. The esophagus, stomach, and duodenum are visually examined as the endoscope passes through each section. A biopsy specimen can be taken from any suspicious sites. Tissue samples are obtained by inserting a cytology brush or biopsy forceps through the endoscope.
▸ *Lung:* After administration of general anesthetics, the patient is placed in a supine position with the neck hyperextended. If a local anesthetic is used, the patient is seated while the tongue and oropharynx are sprayed and swabbed with anesthetic. An emesis basin is provided for the increased saliva, and the patient is encouraged to spit out the saliva because the gag reflex may be impaired. When loss of sensation is adequate, the patient is placed in a supine or side-lying position. The fiberoptic scope can be introduced through the nose, the mouth, an endotracheal tube, a tracheostomy tube, or a rigid bronchoscope. Most common insertion is through the nose. Patients with copious secretions or massive hemoptysis, or in whom airway complications are more likely, may be intubated before the bronchoscopy. Additional local anesthetic is applied through the scope as it approaches the vocal cords and the carina, eliminating reflexes in these sensitive areas. The fiberoptic approach allows visualization of airway segments without having to move the patient's head through various positions. After visual inspection of the lungs, tissue samples are collected from suspicious sites by bronchial brush or biopsy forceps to be used for cytological and microbiological studies.

Procedure	Approximate Time to Complete
Cystoscopy and bladder biopsy	30–45 min
Bone biopsy	Surgical procedure: 30 min, and sutures may be necessary to close the site Needle biopsy: 20 min

Procedure	Approximate Time to Complete
Intestinal biopsy	60 min
Kidney biopsy	Surgical procedure: 60 min, and sutures may be necessary to close the site Needle biopsy: 40 min
Liver biopsy	Surgical procedure: 90 min, and sutures may be necessary to close the site Needle biopsy: 15 min
Lung biopsy	Surgical procedure: 30 min, and sutures may be necessary to close the site Needle biopsy: 15 to 30 min
Lymph node biopsy	Surgical procedure: 30 min, and sutures may be necessary to close the site Needle biopsy: 15 min
Prostate biopsy	Needle biopsy: 20 min
Skin biopsy	Surgical procedure: 20 min, and sutures may be necessary to close the site
Thyroid biopsy	Surgical procedure: 30 min, and sutures may be necessary to close the site Needle biopsy: 15 min

Potential Nursing Actions

❖ *Make sure a written and informed consent has been signed prior to the procedure and before administering any medications.*

▶ Intestinal biopsy or lung biopsy by endoscopy: As appropriate, provide mouth care to reduce oral bacterial flora. Instruct the patient to remove dentures. Inform the HCP if the patient has any crowns, caps on the teeth, or loose teeth.

Safety Considerations

▶ Anticoagulants, aspirin, and other salicylates should be discontinued by medical direction for the appropriate number of days prior to a procedure in which bleeding is a potential complication.

AFTER THE STUDY: POTENTIAL NURSING ACTIONS

Avoiding Complications

▶ *Bladder: Related to perforation of the bladder; a bleeding disorder; or the effects of natural products and medications with known anticoagulant, antiplatelet, or thrombolytic properties* or seeding of the biopsy tract with tumor

cells. The patient should be instructed to avoid taking natural products and medications with known anticoagulant, antiplatelet, or thrombolytic properties or to reduce dosage, as ordered, prior to the procedure. Number of days to withhold medication is dependent on the type of anticoagulant.

▶ *Liver:* After the procedure the patient may be placed in the right decubitus position for the first hour, followed by placement in the supine position for an additional 2 to 3 hr in order to avoid post procedural bleeding.

▶ *Lung: Related to a bleeding disorder or the effects of natural products and medications with known anticoagulant, antiplatelet, or thrombolytic properties,* pneumothorax *(related to the presence of bullae or cysts and respiratory insufficiency),* hemoptysis, air embolism, or seeding of the biopsy tract with tumor cells.

▶ *Lung:* Avoid using morphine sulfate in those with asthma or other pulmonary disease. This drug can further exacerbate bronchospasms and respiratory impairment.

▶ *Lymph node: Related to a bleeding disorder, or the effects of natural products*

B

and medications with known anticoagulant, antiplatelet, or thrombolytic properties or seeding of the biopsy tract with tumor cells.

♦ Observe/assess the biopsy site for bleeding, inflammation, or hematoma formation. Instruct the patient in the care and assessment of the site. Immediately report to the appropriate HCP any redness, edema, bleeding, pain at the biopsy site, or any chills or fever.

Treatment Considerations

General

♦ Do not allow the patient to eat or drink until the gag reflex returns due to aspiration risk; then instruct the patient to resume usual diet, fluids, and medications, as directed by the HCP.

♦ Monitor vital signs and neurological status every 15 min for 1 hr, then every 2 hr for 4 hr, and then as ordered by the HCP. Monitor temperature every 4 hr for 24 hr. Compare with baseline values.

♦ Monitor intake and output at least every 8 hr.

♦ Administer ordered antibiotic therapy. Remind the patient of the importance of completing the entire course of antibiotic therapy, even if signs and symptoms disappear before completion of therapy. Discontinue prophylactic antibiotics within 24 hr after the conclusion of the procedure. Protocols may vary among facilities.

♦ Assess for nausea, pain, and bladder spasms. Administer antiemetic, analgesic, and antispasmodic medications as needed and as directed by the HCP.

Site Specific

♦ *Bladder/Prostate:* Altered urination— Assess for bladder distention every 4 hr or as needed. Observe urinary pattern and palpate the bladder for retention. Measure residual urine directly after voiding or urine retention with a bladder scan. Administer ordered medication to facilitate urination, send ordered urine culture, and administer prescribed antibiotics. Instruct the patient on intake and output recording and provide appropriate measuring containers. After the bladder biopsy, assess

for bladder spasms, hemorrhage, or perforation of the urethra or rectum. Inform the patient that blood may be seen in the urine after the first or second postprocedural voiding. Instruct the patient to report any further changes in urinary pattern, volume, or appearance. Encourage fluid intake of 3,000 mL in 24 hr unless contraindicated.

♦ *Bone:* Mobility—Facilitate the use of assistive devices and physical therapy. Administer ordered medications (analgesics, steroids, antibiotics). Institute fall risk protocols.

♦ *Intestinal:* Altered fecal elimination— Assess for active bowel sounds in all four quadrants, keep NPO until bowel sounds are active. Administer parenteral fluids until taking oral adequately. Implement ostomy care as appropriate and provide education related to new dietary restrictions.

♦ *Kidney:* Advise the patient that blood may be seen in the urine after the first or second postprocedural void with strict intake and output for 24 hr. Ask the patient to report any changes in urinary pattern, volume, or appearance. If urinary volume is less than 200 mL in the first 8 hr, oral liquids may need to be increased unless contraindicated by another medical condition. Monitor and trend laboratory studies for signs of infection (BUN, Cr, WBC count, Hgb, Hct, electrolytes; urine cultures), and evaluate results of complementary diagnostic studies (KUB, CT, MRI, IVP). Administer ordered antibiotics and monitor and trend temperature.

♦ *Liver:* Nutrition—Monitor daily weight. Complete a nutrition history, evaluate intake with a calorie count, and consider a dietary consult. Monitor and trend albumin.

♦ *Lung:* Gas exchange—Assess respiratory status to establish a baseline (rate, rhythm, depth). Use pulse oximetry to monitor the effectiveness of administered oxygen. Monitor and trend arterial blood gas results and administer ordered medications (anticoagulants, antibiotics, bronchodilators, steroids, diuretics). Elevating the head of the bed may be helpful. Instruct the patient to remain in a semi-Fowler position after bronchoscopy or fine-needle aspiration to maximize ventilation and to stay in bed lying on the affected side for at least 2 hr with a pillow or rolled towel under the site to prevent bleeding. The patient will also need to remain on bedrest for 24 hr. Provide ordered lozenges or gargle for throat discomfort. Monitor the patient's sputum for blood when a biopsy is taken, since a large amount of blood may indicate the development of a problem; a small amount of streaking is expected. Signs of bleeding include tachycardia, hypotension, or restlessness.

▶ *Lymph node:* Grief—Assess coping mechanisms to mitigate anxiety and concerns related to possible death and poor prognosis. Facilitate spiritual support and integrate cultural aspects of grieving in planning care. Discuss treatment options.

▶ *Muscle:* Self-care deficit—Identify areas where the patient can provide own care and encourage them. Evaluate the family's ability to assist with self-care needs. Complete a home health evaluation and provide assistive devices to assist with self-care.

▶ *Skin:* Body image—Assure the patient that his or her feelings of distress over an altered appearance is normal. Consider the cultural aspects of body image and incorporate them into the plan of care. Ensure privacy to explore personal grief, listen to the patient, and support positive coping strategies.

▶ *Thyroid:* Altered thought process—Collaborate with the HCP to manage medical problem associated with decreased cerebral perfusion. Promote comprehension and understanding of current events. Create a safe environment. Monitor injury risk (violence, fall risk, self-harm risk). Administer prescribed thyroid hormone replacement medication.

Safety Considerations

▶ *Lung:* Emergency resuscitation equipment should be readily available if the vocal cords become spastic after intubation. Monitor the patient for hemoptysis, dyspnea, tachypnea, air hunger, excessive coughing, pain, hemothorax, or pneumothorax. Monitor chest tube (thoracostomy) patency and drainage after a thoracotomy. A chest x-ray may be ordered to check for the presence of complications.

Nutritional Considerations

▶ *Bladder:* Recommend a consult with a registered dietitian, if necessary, as many adverse effects of treatment for bladder cancer, such as fatigue, bowel disturbances, and weight loss, can result in malnutrition and increased risk for infection.

▶ *Lung:* Malnutrition is commonly seen in patients with severe respiratory disease for numerous reasons, including fatigue, lack of appetite, and gastrointestinal distress. Adequate intake of vitamins A and C are also important to prevent pulmonary infection and to decrease the extent of lung tissue damage. The importance of following the prescribed diet should be stressed to the patient and caregiver.

▶ *Prostate:* There is growing evidence that inflammation and oxidation play key roles in the development of numerous diseases, including prostate cancer. Research also shows that diets containing dried beans, fresh fruits and vegetables, nuts, spices, whole grains, and smaller amounts of red meats can increase the amount of protective antioxidants. Regular exercise, especially in combination with a healthy diet, can bring about changes in the body's metabolism that decrease inflammation and oxidation.

Follow-Up, Evaluation, and Desired Outcomes

General

▶ Acknowledges the time and date for suture removal, if indicated.

▶ Agrees to attend a smoking cessation program, as appropriate. Cigarette smokers have a higher risk than nonsmokers of developing bladder cancer.

▶ Acknowledges the importance of taking prescribed medications and adhering to the therapeutic regimen. States significant adverse effects associated with the prescribed medication. Understands that a pharmacist is available to review corresponding literature upon request.

▶ Correctly states the medical versus surgical options for disease management.
▶ Those with terminal diagnosis understand end-of-life treatment options.
▶ Surgical patients correctly demonstrate care of surgical site, biopsy site.
▶ Acknowledges contact information provided for the American Cancer Society (ACS) (www.cancer.org). Educate the patient regarding access to counseling services.

Lung
▶ Agrees to report symptoms of empyema, such as fever, tachycardia, malaise, or elevated WBC count.

Prostate
▶ Understands that decisions regarding the need for and frequency of routine PSA testing or other prostate cancer screening procedures should be made after consultation between the patient and HCP. Recommendations made by various medical associations and national health organizations regarding prostate cancer screening are moving away from routine PSA screening and toward informed decision making. The most current guidelines for prostate cancer screening of the general population as well as of individuals with increased risk are available from the ACS (www.cancer.org) and the American Urological Association (www.auanet.org). Counsel the patient, as appropriate, that sexual dysfunction related to altered body function, drugs, or radiation may occur. For additional information regarding screening guidelines, refer to the study titled "Prostate-Specific Antigen."

Skin
▶ Acknowledges that DNA testing for mutations in the CDKN2A, CDK4, or BRAF V600 genes may be requested to identify those at high risk for developing cutaneous melanoma. The test for TA90 (melanoma-associated antigen) is used to evaluate the status of postoperative patients who have had localized areas of melanoma removed. Methods for these genetic markers include microarray, reverse transcriptase polymerase chain reaction (RT-PCR), and enzyme-linked immunosorbent assay (ELISA). Evaluate test results in relation to the patient's symptoms and other tests performed.

Thyroid
▶ Understands that genetic testing may be conducted to search for mutations in various genes associated with types of thyroid cancer. Markers associated with a significant incidence of thyroid cancers include BRAF (associated with papillary thyroid cancer), RAS (associated with follicular and papillary thyroid cancers), RET/PTC (associated with an increased risk of developing inherited medullary thyroid cancer, also known as *multiple endocrine neoplasia*, or MEN), and PAX8/PPAR (associated with congenital hypothyroidism and thyroid dysgenesis).

Bioterrorism and Public Health Safety Concerns: Testing for Toxins and Infectious Agents

SYNONYM/ACRONYM: N/A

RATIONALE: To assist in confirming the diagnosis of infection or poisoning in cases of accidental or intentional exposure to agents of high risk to public health safety.

PATIENT PREPARATION: There are no food or fluid restrictions unless by medical direction; as a general rule, specimens should be collected prior to administration of antibiotics whenever possible.

NORMAL FINDINGS: (Method: Disease specific) Negative findings for the organism or toxin of interest; negative serology; negative PCR.

B

CRITICAL FINDINGS AND POTENTIAL INTERVENTIONS
- Positive findings for a disease listed in the Overview section leads to a high likelihood of being required for reporting to the appropriate agencies.

Timely notification to the requesting health-care provider (HCP) of any critical findings and related symptoms is a role expectation of the professional nurse. A listing of these findings varies among facilities.

OVERVIEW: (Study type: Collect the appropriate specimen as described in the related blood, stool, body fluid analysis, tissue biopsy, or culture study. The facility or testing laboratory should be contacted for guidelines regarding chain of custody, specimen collection requirements, and specimen packaging and shipping instructions; related body system: Multisystem.) All local and state health departments and the Centers for Disease Control and Prevention (CDC) require HCPs to report specific diseases/pathogens when they are identified by the requesting HCP or the testing laboratory. Information regarding bioterrorism and emergency response plans can be accessed at (https://emergency.cdc.gov/bioterrorism). Information regarding reportable diseases can be accessed at the CDC Web site (www.bt.cdc.bov/agent/agentlist-category.asp).

This study addresses some of the pathogens and toxins of biological origin that pose a national security risk through unintended exposure or transmission, use in a military action, or to perpetrate terrorist attacks against civilians. The biological agents of most significant concern are grouped into three categories based on the types of impact to public health that include ease of transmission, high mortality or morbidity rates, and level of action required for intervention by public health services. Category A includes infectious organisms and toxins that pose the highest risk, Category B includes the next highest risk group, and Category C includes emerging infectious diseases.

The subspecialty of microbiology has been revolutionized by molecular diagnostics. Molecular diagnostics involves the identification of specific sequences of DNA. The application of molecular diagnostics techniques, such as polymerase chain reaction (PCR), has led to the development of automated instruments that can identify a single infectious agent or multiple pathogens from a small amount of specimen in less than 2 hr.

(text continues on page 193)

B

Infectious Organism/ Toxin	Disease	Mode of Transmission and Site of Entry	Incubation Period, Signs, Symptoms, and Treatment	Specimen Required and Test Method
Category A				
Bacillus anthracis is a gram-positive, aerobic, rod-shaped, spore-forming bacteria; spores are a dormant form of the bacteria. The composition of the spore confers resistance to unfavorable conditions for growth until a suitable environment is attained.	Anthrax	*Bacillus anthracis* is found naturally in soil and causes disease in humans when spores from the bacteria are ingested into the gastrointestinal (GI) system in contaminated water or undercooked meat or cutaneously by handling meat, wool, or hides from infected animals (usually hoofed animals in close contact with humans); by inhalation of spores or introduction of spores through breaks in the skin from contaminated animal products; or by an intentional and targeted release of spores in a bioterrorist attack. Infected individuals are not contagious; the disease is not transmitted directly from person to person.	The incubation period for anthrax infection is between 1 and 7 d and may vary according to the site of entry with inhalation anthrax having the most rapid progression of symptoms. Symptoms may also vary according to the site of entry. General symptoms include fever, malaise, and vomiting. Papules escalating to skin ulceration and eschar formation are associated with cutaneous anthrax; bloody diarrhea is associated with GI anthrax; severe respiratory distress, pulmonary edema, and development of pleural effusions are associated with inhalation anthrax, advancing to shock, coma, and possible death within 1–3 d after inhalation. Treatment for all forms of anthrax with antibiotics (penicillin, doxycycline, and ciprofloxacin) is usually successful, especially if administered early in the course of the disease. Untreated anthrax of any type or late-stage inhaled anthrax may be fatal. Prevention can be enhanced through a veterinary vaccine	Specimens considered for testing include blood, stool, skin lesions, sputum, throat culture, body fluids (sputum, ascites, cerebrospinal fluid [CSF], pleural fluid), tissue biopsy, and contaminated food (in the original container if possible). Test methods include culture and gram stain, PCR, immunochemical techniques (tissue samples), serology, enzyme-linked immunosorbent assays (ELISA). Specimen handling, testing, and culture handling should be performed in a Biosafety Level (BSL) 2 environment.

used for periodic immunization of livestock, where appropriate. A cell-free culture filtrate vaccine prepared from a non-encapsulated strain of *Bacillus anthracis* is available to individuals in high-risk groups (military personnel and other individuals with high exposure risk due to the nature of their jobs). The vaccine is given in a series of five doses (initial dose and then at 1, 6, 12, and 18 mo after the first dose) followed by a yearly booster dose. The effectiveness is not well established, and there is a possibility of significant adverse effects.

The most common type of botulism is food borne, and the incubation period is a few hours to 3 d. Incubation periods for other types of botulism may vary according to the site of entry and can extend up to 1 wk for exposure by wound. Neuromuscular symptoms are the hallmark of how the toxin achieves its effect on the body and include blurred vision, difficulty swallowing, and muscle weakness that progresses to paralysis. Irreversible binding of the toxin to sites where neuromuscular activity is normally initiated prevent the release of the

Specimens considered for testing include blood, stool, vomitus, and contaminated food (in the original container if possible). Test methods include mouse neutralization test (to detect the toxin), culture. Specimen handling, testing, and culture handling should be performed in a BSL2 environment.

(table continues on page 186)

Botulism

Clostridium botulinum is found naturally in soil and other types of environments, including the human intestine. There are four forms of botulism. The foodborne disease occurs when the bacteria, toxin, or spores are ingested into the GI system in undercooked, contaminated meat, fish, vegetables, sauces, and home-canned foods, especially when kept at

Clostridium botulinum is a gram-positive, anaerobic, rod-shaped, spore-forming bacteria that produces a potent neurotoxin; spores are a dormant

B

B

Infectious Organism/ Toxin	Disease	Mode of Transmission and Site of Entry	Incubation Period, Signs, Symptoms, and Treatment	Specimen Required and Test Method
form of the bacteria. The composition of the spore confers resistance to unfavorable conditions for growth until a suitable environment is attained.		room temperature after cooking. Infants under 1 yr of age are susceptible to a type of botulism linked to ingestion of spores in honey. Wound botulism occurs when the bacteria, toxin, or spores are introduced through breaks in the skin. Botulism can also occur by inhalation of spores from a contaminated source or by an intentional and targeted release of spores in a bioterrorist attack. Infected individuals are not contagious; the disease is not transmitted directly from person to person. Seven distinct botulism neurotoxin types are known to affect humans, identified as A, B, C, D, E, F, and G.	neurotransmitter acetylcholine. Normal neuromuscular function halts as the body's muscles are irreversibly paralyzed. Respiratory symptoms may also occur with inhalation botulism. Additional symptoms of infant botulism include other indications of altered neuromuscular function, such as poor feeding (due to loss of muscle function related to sucking), constipation (due to loss of muscle function related to elimination), pooled oral secretions (due to loss of muscle function related to swallowing), and loss of head control related to loss of neck muscle strength and function. There is no prescribed treatment for botulism other than palliative care. As the paralysis advances and organ function diminishes, mechanical support is required for breathing and nutrition. A heptavalent vaccine is available for individuals identified as high risk and is effective for clostridial toxin strains A through G. An intravenous botulism immune globulin is available for infant botulism and is	

Francisella tularensis is a gram-negative, aerobic coccobacillus.	Tularemia	Tularemia can be contracted in a number of different ways: ingestion of the bacteria into the GI system from contaminated water or plants; cutaneously through a break in the skin when handling infected animal products or from the bite of an infected insect, such as a tick or deerfly; or breathing the bacteria into the lungs. Infected individuals are not contagious; the disease is not transmitted directly from person to person.	approved for the treatment of botulism types A and B. More information can be obtained from www.infantbotulism.org.
			The incubation period for tularemia averages 3–5 d but can take as long as 2 wk, depending on the site of entry. Symptoms may also vary according to the site of entry. The general symptoms include fever, chills, headache, diarrhea, weakness, muscle aches, and joint pain. Ingestion of the bacteria can cause symptoms that affect the entire alimentary canal, including mouth ulcers, sore throat, swollen and painful lymph glands, intestinal pain, vomiting, and diarrhea. Inhalation of the bacteria can cause symptoms that resemble influenza or pneumonia, such as chest pain from difficulty breathing or bloody sputum. When the infection is introduced cutaneously, skin ulcers and swelling of the associated lymph nodes are evident. The disease can be fatal if it is not treated in a timely manner. Treatment for infection is a 2-wk course of the antibiotic doxycycline or ciprofloxacin. Currently, no vaccine is available in the United States; there is ongoing research to identify an effective vaccine.	Specimens considered for testing include serum, blood, sputum/throat swab, bronchial/tracheal wash, and stool. Test methods include serology, gram stain, and culture. Specimen handling and testing should be performed in a BSL2 environment; culture handling should be performed in a BSL3 environment.

(table continues on page 188)

B

B

Infectious Organism/ Toxin	Disease	Mode of Transmission and Site of Entry	Incubation Period, Signs, Symptoms, and Treatment	Specimen Required and Test Method
Variola major is a severe and potentially lethal strain of the variola DNA virus.	Smallpox	The smallpox virus is transmitted by an infected human through the respiratory system in droplets that become aerosolized and are inhaled by another person in very close proximity. The smallpox virus can also be transmitted by direct contact with contaminated fomites or direct contact with body fluids from an infected person (secretions from rashes, pustules, or scabs), or by an intentional and targeted bioterrorist attack. The disease can be directly transmitted from person to person.	The incubation period for smallpox averages 12–14 d after which general symptoms develop to include fever, headache, and body aches followed by the development of a rash in the mouth and on the skin; the most infectious period is during the first 7–10 d following development of the rash. In the next stage of the infection, the rash becomes pustular. Eventually, the pustules dry up and scab formation occurs. Viable viral particles are present in the scabs; therefore, a person is considered contagious until after the last scab has fallen off. There is no specified treatment for smallpox, and the only prevention is by vaccination. Routine vaccination in the United States ended in 1972 after the disease was eradicated.	Specimens considered for testing include culture, vesicular fluid, skin scraping, and biopsy specimens. Test methods include viral culture or identification from a sample using electron microscopy. Specimen handling, testing, and culture handling should be performed in a BSL4 environment.
Filoviruses (e.g., Ebola, Marburg), *arenaviruses* (e.g., Lassa, Machupo),	VHF	VHFs are a group of severe infections caused by different RNA viruses. The viruses are transmitted to humans cutaneously by way of a bite from an	The incubation period for VHFs varies from 3–21 d. Beginning symptoms include fever, headache, body aches, fatigue, jaundice, and vomiting; some cases progress with bleeding, shock, and multiorgan failure. There is no	Specimens considered for testing include serum, blood, sputum, and tissue. Test methods include viral isolation, PCR, ELISA,

flaviviruses (including the virus that causes yellow fever), and *Bunyaviridae* (e.g., Haantan). The viruses responsible for viral hemorrhagic fevers (VHFs) are RNA viruses.

infected reservoir host (e.g., rodent) or infected arthropod vector (e.g., mosquito or tick that has bitten an infected host). Some viruses (e.g., Ebola, Marburg, Lassa) can be directly transmitted from person to person by way of contact with contaminated blood or body fluids. The infection is significant; it can result in multisystem failure and death. Because some viruses have the potential to cause massive numbers of deaths through contagious infection, they are considered possible weapons for use in an intentional and targeted bioterrorist attack.

prescribed treatment for VHFs, and patients are given supportive treatment for their symptoms. Care should be taken in the selection of medications to reduce fever and pain, avoiding those medications known to increase the risk of bleeding (e.g., salicylates and NSAIDs). Yellow fever is the only VHF for which an effective vaccine is available. Additional preventive measures for yellow fever include avoidance of further exposure to mosquitoes by staying indoors during hours when they are most active and using repellents and mosquito netting. Preventive measures decrease the opportunity for uninfected mosquitoes to feed on infected blood, which in turn decreases the spread of the disease.

immunohistochemistry of tissue, and serology. Specimen handling, testing, and culture handling for yellow fever should be performed in a BSL3 environment; for dengue, they should be performed in a BSL2 environment; for others, they should be performed in a BSL4 environment.

Plague

Yersinia pestis is a gram-negative, facultatively anaerobic, obligate intracellular coccobacillus.

There are three forms of plague. The first and probably best known is bubonic plague. The reservoir host (usually a rodent) carries infected fleas; the fleas spread the disease cutaneously to

The average incubation period for plague is 1–6 d depending on the site of entry; generally, pneumonic plague has a shorter incubation period. General symptoms include fever, chills, enlarged lymph nodes, malaise, septicemia, hemorrhagic skin changes, pneumonia (pneumonic plague), shock,

Specimens considered for testing include serum, blood, sputum/throat swab, bronchial/tracheal wash, and lymph node aspirate. Test methods include serology, gram

(table continues on page 190)

B

B

Infectious Organism/ Toxin	Disease	Mode of Transmission and Site of Entry	Incubation Period, Signs, Symptoms, and Treatment	Specimen Required and Test Method
		humans through a bite. The bacteria multiply in the lymph node closest to the site of the flea bite. Septicemic plague occurs when the bacteria is inoculated into the bloodstream by flea bite or by the bite of an infected animal. Pneumonic plague is the most lethal form of plague. It occurs when the infection from either untreated bubonic or septicemic plague spreads to the lungs. Pneumonic is the only form of plague that can be transmitted person to person from inhalation of aerosolized droplets of contaminated fluid, direct contact with contaminated fomites (for short periods of time), or by an intentional and targeted bioterrorist attack.	and death. Early identification and administration of antibiotics (tetracycline or fluoroquinolone) for 7 d, with supportive care, is the most effective treatment for plague.	stain, and culture. Specimen and culture handling should be performed in a BSL2 environment.

Category B

Brucella abortus, *B. suis*, *B. melitensis*, or *B. canis*; the species are gramnegative, aerobic, coccobacilli.	Brucellosis	Infection occurs after ingestion into the GI system from infected meats and contaminated milk products (especially goat's milk), direct puncture of the skin (by butchers and farmers), or by inhalation. It is not a contagious disease that is transmitted from person to person.	The average incubation period for brucellosis infection is 1–2 mo. General symptoms include fever, chills, headache, night sweats, back pain, joint pain, and malaise. The disease is systemic, affecting multiple organs and body systems. Brucellosis can be effectively treated with antibiotics (e.g., doxycycline, tetracycline, streptomycin, sulfamethoxazole and trimethoprim, rifampin, ciprofloxacin, or gentamicin). Currently, no vaccine is available for use in humans.	Specimens considered for testing include serum, blood, bone marrow, spleen or liver tissue, sputum, and food. Test methods include serology, gram stain, culture, and immunofluorescence. Specimen handling should be performed in a BSL2 environment; culture handling should be performed in a BSL3 environment.
Ricinus communis is the name for the castor oil plant. The plant's seeds contain an oil composed mostly of the lipid ricinolein and smaller	Ricin poisoning.	Ricin poisoning occurs by ingestion into the GI system or by inhalation into the respiratory system. The toxin is released after ingestion of castor beans. It is not a contagious disease that is transmitted from person to person, and the likelihood of accidental poisoning is very low. It can	Symptoms of ricin poisoning vary according to the site of entry and concentration of the dose. If the toxin is ingested, GI symptoms such as nausea, pain, and vomiting appear in 6–12 hr; if the toxin is inhaled, respiratory symptoms such as difficulty breathing, coughing, and chest pain appear in 4–6 hr. Over the next 12–24 hr, the symptoms rapidly escalate toward organ failure. Ricin affects the body at the	Environmental samples can be tested for the presence of ricin by time-resolved fluorescence immunoassay and PCR. Specimen handling should be performed in a BSL2 or BSL3 environment depending on the

(table continues on page 192)

B

Infectious Organism/ Toxin	Disease	Mode of Transmission and Site of Entry	Incubation Period, Signs, Symptoms, and Treatment	Specimen Required and Test Method
amounts of ricin, a powerful toxin.		also be purposely made from a waste product generated in the normal production of castor oil. The manufactured toxin can be released as a powder into the air or dissolved in water supplies. Very small amounts could sicken and kill large numbers of people, and for this reason it is considered as a potential weapon for use in an intentional and targeted bioterrorist attack.	cellular level by preventing the production of proteins, an essential process for every living cell, tissue, and organ. Presently there are no methods available for the detection of ricin in biological fluids. Diagnosis of ricin poisoning is made using general laboratory tests for evidence of the effects of the toxin on the body and is arrived at within the context of high suspicion of exposure. Laboratory results of interest might include elevated liver function results, elevated renal function results, abnormal urinalysis findings such as blood in the urine, and moderate to increased WBC count (two to five times normal levels).	possibility of aerosolization and concentration of toxin submitted for testing.

INDICATIONS

- Suspected infection by high-risk pathogen *(demonstrated by associated signs and symptoms or known exposure).*

INTERFERING FACTORS

Other considerations

- Failure to follow the appropriate specimen collection and transport procedures may affect the validity of the results.

POTENTIAL MEDICAL DIAGNOSIS: CLINICAL SIGNIFICANCE OF RESULTS

Positive findings in

- Positive findings for the organism or toxin of interest; positive serology. Refer to the table in the Overview section for details.

NURSING IMPLICATIONS

BEFORE THE STUDY: PLANNING AND IMPLEMENTATION

Teaching the Patient What to Expect

- Inform the patient this test can assist in assessing for infection or poisoning.
- Explain that a blood, stool, body fluid, or tissue sample may be needed for the test. Inform the patient that several tests may be necessary to confirm the diagnosis. Any individual positive serology result may be repeated in 3 wk to monitor a change in detectable level of antibody, as appropriate.

Potential Nursing Actions

- Contact the testing laboratory prior to specimen collection in order to obtain accurate information regarding specimen collection containers, sample volumes, and specific transport instructions. Chain of custody policies may be required in cases of intentional exposure.

AFTER THE STUDY: POTENTIAL NURSING ACTIONS

Avoiding Complications

- Instruct the patient in isolation precautions during time of communicability or contagion, as appropriate. Instruct the patient in the proper way to decontaminate solid surfaces with a 1:10 dilution of household bleach:water to decontaminate clothing; to "cover a cough"; and to perform good hand hygiene.

Safety Considerations

- Follow all provided safety instructions to prevent disease reexposure.

Nutritional Considerations

- Perform a daily weight at the same time each day with the same scale. Closely monitor intake and output with a potential calorie count. Administer prescribed medication to facilitate caloric intake. Evaluate the attitude toward eating and facilitate a dietary consult to evaluate current eating habits and best method of nutritional supplementation. Collaborate with the registered dietitian to develop short-term and long-term eating strategies. Monitor nutritional laboratory values such as albumin, transferrin, RBC, WBC, and serum electrolytes; and encourage cultural home foods. Parenteral or enteral nutrition should be considered if necessary.

Follow-Up, Evaluation, and Desired Outcomes

- Understands the need to return to have a convalescent blood sample taken in 3 wk, if ordered.
- Acknowledges the importance of an advance directive in the overall healthcare plan.
- Agrees to complete the therapeutic regime tailored to the specific disease process.
- Collaborates with the HCP to select end-of-life strategies for terminal conditions.

B

Bladder Cancer Markers, Urine

SYNONYM/ACRONYM: Nuclear matrix protein (NMP) 22, bladder tumor antigen (BTA), cytogenic marker for bladder cancer.

RATIONALE: To assist in diagnosing bladder cancer.

PATIENT PREPARATION: There are no food, fluid, activity, or medication restrictions unless by medical direction. As appropriate, provide the required urine collection container and specimen collection instructions.

NORMAL FINDINGS: Method: Enzyme immunoassay for NMP22 and BTA, fluorescence in situ hybridization (FISH) for cytogenic marker.

NMP22: Negative: Less than 6 units/mL, borderline: 6 to 10 units/mL, positive: greater than 10 units/mL.

BTA: Negative.

Cytogenic Marker: Negative.

CRITICAL FINDINGS AND POTENTIAL INTERVENTIONS

• Bladder cancer

Timely notification to the requesting health-care provider (HCP) of any critical findings and related symptoms is a role expectation of the professional nurse. A listing of these findings varies among facilities.

OVERVIEW: (Study type: Urine, unpreserved random specimen collected in a clean plastic collection container for NMP22 and Bard BTA; urine, first void specimen collected in fixative specific for FISH testing; **related body system:** Urinary system.) Cystoscopy is still considered the gold standard for detection of bladder cancer, but other noninvasive tests have been developed. Compared to cytological studies, these assays are believed to be more sensitive but less specific for detecting transitional cell cancer. FISH is a cytogenic technique that uses fluorescent-labelled DNA probes to detect specific chromosome abnormalities. The FISH bladder cancer assay specifically detects the presence of aneuploidy for chromosomes 3, 7,

and 17 and absence of the 9p21 loci, findings associated with transitional cell cancer of the bladder.

NMP22: Nuclear matrix proteins (NMPs) are involved in the regulation and expression of various genes. The NMP identified as NuMA is abundant in bladder tumor cells. The dying tumor cells release the soluble NMP into the urine. This assay is quantitative.

Bladder tumor antigen (BTA): A human complement factor H–related protein (hCF-Hrp) is thought to be produced by bladder tumor cells as protection from the body's natural immune response. BTA is released from tumor cells into the urine. This assay is qualitative.

INDICATIONS

* Detection of bladder cancer.
* Management of recurrent bladder cancer.

INTERFERING FACTORS

Factors that may alter the results of the study

* *NMP22:* Any condition that results in inflammation of the bladder or urinary tract may cause falsely elevated values.
* *BTA:* Recent surgery, biopsy, or other trauma to the bladder or urinary tract may cause falsely elevated values. Bacterial overgrowth from active urinary tract infection, renal or bladder calculi, gross contamination from blood, and positive leukocyte dipstick may also cause false-positive results.
* *Cytogenic marker:* Incorrect fixative, gross contamination from blood, bacterial overgrowth from active urinary tract infection, or inadequate number of bladder cells in specimen may produce invalid results.

POTENTIAL MEDICAL DIAGNOSIS: CLINICAL SIGNIFICANCE OF RESULTS

Increased in bladder cancer

NURSING IMPLICATIONS

BEFORE THE STUDY: PLANNING AND IMPLEMENTATION

Teaching the Patient What to Expect

* Inform the patient this procedure can assist in establishing a diagnosis of bladder disease.
* Explain that a urine sample is needed for the test. Information regarding specimen collection is presented with other general guidelines in Appendix A:

Patient Preparation and Specimen Collection.

Potential Nursing Actions

* Include on the collection container's label the specimen collection type (e.g., clean catch, catheter), date and time of collection, and any medications that may interfere with test results.

AFTER THE STUDY: POTENTIAL NURSING ACTIONS

Treatment Considerations

* Assess for bladder distention every 4 hr or as appropriate with strict monitoring of intake and output. Assess for a urinary pattern and palpate the lower abdomen for urine retention. Measure residual urine directly after voiding by inserting an ordered urinary catheter or by the use of a bladder scan. Administer ordered medication to facilitate urination. Send ordered urine culture, administer ordered antibiotics, and monitor laboratory studies (BUN, Cr, PSA). Consider limiting evening fluids after 1800.
* Obtain an ordered urine culture and sensitivity; monitor urine characteristics (blood, color, odor, amount). Monitor and trend WBC count. Assess and monitor vital signs (blood pressure, pulse, temperature, heart rate) and administer ordered antibiotics, antipyretics. Facilitate cooling measures as needed and ensure aseptic technique in the presence of an indwelling catheter with good hand hygiene and perineal care.

Follow-Up, Evaluation, and Desired Outcomes

* Acknowledges contact information provided for the American Cancer Society (www.cancer.org) or the National Cancer Institute (www.cancer.gov).
* Understands that the disease progression may require lifestyle choice changes.
* Agrees to smoking cessation counseling. The greatest risk factor for bladder cancer is smoking.

Bleeding Time

SYNONYM/ACRONYM: Mielke bleeding time, Simplate bleeding time, template bleeding time, Surgicutt bleeding time, Ivy bleeding time.

RATIONALE: To evaluate platelet function.

PATIENT PREPARATION: There are no food, fluid, activity, or medication restrictions unless by medical direction. The patient may be instructed to withhold aspirin or related products for at least 1 wk prior to testing, as ordered. Note the last time and dose of medication taken that are known to prolong bleeding to include dietary supplements, anticoagulants, aspirin, and other salicylates.

NORMAL FINDINGS: Method: Timed observation of incision.
Template: 2.5 to 10 min.
Ivy: 2 to 7 min.
Slight differences exist in the disposable devices used to make the incision. Although the Mielke or template bleeding time is believed to offer greater standardization to a fairly subjective procedure, both methods are thought to be of equal sensitivity and reproducibility.

CRITICAL FINDINGS AND POTENTIAL INTERVENTIONS
• Greater than 14 min.

Timely notification to the requesting health-care provider (HCP) of any critical findings and related symptoms is a role expectation of the professional nurse. A listing of these findings varies among facilities.

Potential nursing interventions for bleeding include applying pressure to the incision until the bleeding stops and covering the incision site with a bandage. Some people are more prone than others to develop scars or keloids. Generally, they are pink to reddish in color, raised, and shinier than the surrounding skin. They can be itchy, tender, or even painful to the touch. There is no immediate intervention to prevent the formation of scars or keloids. Treatment options for developed scars and keloids range from cortisone injections to a variety of strategies for removal, each of which can vary widely in degree of success. The site should be observed for subsequent bleeding, bruising, or redness. Fever, localized redness, or warmth of the area to the touch may be indications of infection. Potential nursing interventions include monitoring temperature as well as administering antipyretic and antibiotic medications, as ordered.

OVERVIEW: (Study type: Blood; **related body system:** Circulatory/Hematopoietic system.) There are three main stages of hemostasis. Primary hemostasis includes constriction of injured blood vessels, exposure of subendothelial collagen, platelet aggregation and adhesion, and formation of a plug. Secondary hemostasis involves the coagulation cascade with subsequent formation of a fibrin clot. The third stage of hemostasis is clot retraction and healing. Bleeding time assesses platelet and capillary function.

B

INDICATIONS

Many laboratories have discontinued the use of bleeding time testing in favor of prothrombin time and international normalized ratio (PT/INR), activated partial thromboplastin time (aPTT), platelet count, and platelet function testing as appropriate. This change in laboratory practice is based on the results of studies that do not support the clinical value of bleeding time in either surgical or nonsurgical applications.

INTERFERING FACTORS

Contraindications

❋ The test should not be performed on patients who have excessively cold or edematous arms, have a platelet count less than $50 \times 10^3/\text{microL}$, have an infectious skin disease, or cannot have a blood pressure cuff placed on the arm.

Factors that may alter the results of the study

- Drugs and other substances that may prolong bleeding time include acetylsalicylic acid, aminocaproic acid, ampicillin, asparaginase, aspirin, canola oil, carbenicillin, cilostazol, clopidogrel, dextran, diltiazem, flurbiprofen, ketorolac, moxalactam, nafcillin, naproxen, nifedipine, NSAIDs, penicillin, piroxicam, plicamycin, propranolol, streptokinase, sulindac, ticarcillin, ticlopidine, tolmetin, valproic acid, and warfarin.
- Aspirin or related products should not be taken for at least 1 wk prior to the test.
- Drugs and other substances that may decrease bleeding time include desmopressin and erythropoietin.

POTENTIAL MEDICAL DIAGNOSIS: CLINICAL SIGNIFICANCE OF RESULTS

This test does not predict excessive bleeding during a surgical procedure.

Prolonged In

- Bernard-Soulier syndrome *(evidenced by a rare hereditary condition in which platelet glycoprotein GP1b is deficient and platelet aggregation is decreased)*
- Fibrinogen disorders *(related to the role of fibrinogen to help platelets link together)*
- Glanzmann thrombasthenia *(evidenced by a rare hereditary condition in which platelet glycoprotein IIb/IIIa is deficient and platelet aggregation is decreased)*
- Hereditary telangiectasia *(evidenced by fragile blood vessels that do not permit adequate constriction to stop bleeding)*
- Kidney disease *(related to abnormal platelet function)*
- Liver disease *(related to decreased production of coagulation proteins that affect bleeding time)*
- Some myeloproliferative disorders *(evidenced by disorders of decreased platelet production)*
- Thrombocytopenia *(evidenced by insufficient platelets to stop bleeding)*
- von Willebrand disease *(evidenced by deficiency of von Willebrand factor, necessary for normal platelet adhesion)*

Decreased in: N/A

NURSING IMPLICATIONS

BEFORE THE STUDY: PLANNING AND IMPLEMENTATION

Teaching the Patient What to Expect

▸ Inform the patient this test can assist in evaluating the amount of time it takes for blood to clot.

▸ Explain that blood is needed for the test. Inform the patient that specimen collection takes approximately 2 to 15 min. Address concerns about pain and explain that there may be some discomfort during the procedure. Inform the patient that scarring, keloid formation, or infection may occur.

▶ Explain that prior to the test, a blood pressure cuff will be placed on the arm above the elbow and inflated to 40 mm Hg. The puncture site is cleansed with alcohol and allowed to air-dry. A bleeding time device is used to make a parallel incision about 3 mm deep into the muscular outside area of the forearm distal to the antecubital fossa (in the direction of wrist to elbow). As soon as the incision is made, a stopwatch is used to keep time; at 30-sec intervals, the incision site is blotted in a clockwise fashion, on the edge of a piece of filter paper. The test concludes when the bleeding stops or if bleeding continues longer than 15 min. Bleeding time is determined by adding the total number of blots on the filter paper (30 sec or 0.5 min).

Potential Nursing Actions
▶ Obtain a list of the patient's current medications, including over-the-counter medications, dietary supplements, anticoagulants, aspirin, and other salicylates

---

AFTER THE STUDY: POTENTIAL NURSING ACTIONS

Avoiding Complications
▶ When blood or blood products are ordered, follow specific guidelines for blood type, crossmatch, and transfusion and monitor for transfusion reaction.

Treatment Considerations
▶ Observe/assess the incision site for bleeding. It may be necessary to place a dressing or butterfly bandage on the site after the test.

▶ Assess for the underlying cause of bleeding, monitor and trend coagulation studies (PT/INR) and hemoglobin and hematocrit levels. Observe the skin for bruising, hematoma, oozing bloody drainage from open sores or IV sites; watch for blood in urine and stools as well as for bleeding gums. Avoid at-risk behaviors that could result in injury, unnecessary venipuncture, or invasive procedures. Administer ordered blood or blood products and vitamin K.

▶ Inform the patient with a bleeding disorder of the importance of taking precautions against bruising and bleeding. These precautions may include the use of soft-bristle toothbrush, use of an electric razor, avoidance of constipation, avoidance of acetylsalicylic acid and similar products, and avoidance of intramuscular injections.

Safety Considerations
▶ Institute fall precautions to decrease injury risk.

Nutritional Considerations
▶ May want to include vitamin K–rich foods in the diet. Foods that contain vitamin K include asparagus, beans, cabbage, cauliflower, chickpeas, egg yolks, green tea, pork, liver, milk, soybean products, tomatoes, mayonnaise, vegetable oils, and green leafy vegetables such as leaf lettuce, watercress, parsley, broccoli, brussels sprouts, kale, spinach, swiss chard, and collard, mustard, and turnip greens.

Follow-Up, Evaluation, and Desired Outcomes
▶ Acknowledges the importance of avoiding high-risk activities that could result in personal injury.

Blood Gases

SYNONYM/ACRONYM: Arterial blood gases (ABGs), venous blood gases, capillary blood gases, cord blood gases.

RATIONALE: To assess oxygenation and acid-base balance.

PATIENT PREPARATION: There are no food, fluid, activity, or medication restrictions unless by medical direction.

NORMAL FINDINGS: Method: Selective electrodes for pH, Pco_2, and Po_2.

Blood Gas Value (pH)	Arterial	Venous	Capillary
Scalp	—	—	7.25–7.35
Birth, cord, full term	7.11–7.36	7.25–7.45	7.32–7.49
Adult/child	7.35–7.45	7.32–7.43	7.35–7.45

Note: SI units (conversion factor × 1).

Pco$_2$	Arterial	SI Units (Conventional Units x 0.133)	Venous	SI Units (Conventional Units x 0.133)	Capillary	SI Units (Conventional Units x 0.133)
Scalp	—	—	—	—	40–50 mm Hg	5.3–6.6 kPa
Birth, cord, full term	32–66 mm Hg	4.3–8.8 kPa	27–49 mm Hg	3.6–6.5 kPa	—	—
Newborn–adult	35–45 mm Hg	4.7–6 kPa	41–51 mm Hg	5.4–6.8 kPa	26–41 mm Hg	3.5–5.4 kPa

Po$_2$	Arterial	SI Units (Conventional Units x 0.133)	Venous	SI Units (Conventional Units x 0.133)	Capillary	SI Units (Conventional Units x 0.133)
Scalp	—	—	—	—	20–30 mm Hg	2.7–4 kPa
Birth, cord, full term	8–24 mm Hg	1.1–3.2 kPa	17–41 mm Hg	2.3–5.4 kPa	—	—
0–1 hr	33–85 mm Hg	4.4–11.3 kPa	—	—	—	—
Greater than 1 hr–adult	80–95 mm Hg	10.6–12.6 kPa	20–49 mm Hg	2.7–6.5 kPa	80–95 mm Hg	10.6–12.6 kPa

HCO₃⁻	Arterial Conventional and SI Units	Venous Conventional and SI Units	Capillary Conventional and SI Units
Birth, cord, full term	17–24 mmol/L	17–24 mmol/L	—
2 mo–2 yr	16–23 mmol/L	24–28 mmol/L	18–23 mmol/L
Adult	22–26 mmol/L	24–28 mmol/L	18–23 mmol/L

O₂ Sat	Arterial	Venous	Capillary
Birth, cord, full term	40%–90%	40%–70%	—
Adult/child	95%–99%	70%–75%	95%–98%

Values may be at the lower end of the normal range in older adults.

Oxygen Content: Arterial 6.6–9.7 mmol/L	Oxygen Content: Venous 4.9–7.1 mmol/L

Tco₂	Arterial Conventional and SI Units mmol/L	Venous Conventional and SI Units mmol/L
Birth, cord, full term	13–22 mmol/L	14–22 mmol/L
Adult/child	22–29 mmol/L	25–30 mmol/L

Base Excess Arterial	Conventional and SI Units
Birth, cord, full term	(−10) − (−2) mmol/L
Adult/child	(−2) − (+3) mmol/L

CRITICAL FINDINGS AND POTENTIAL INTERVENTIONS

Timely notification to the requesting health-care provider (HCP) of any critical findings and related symptoms is a role expectation of the professional nurse. A listing of these findings varies among facilities.

Consideration may be given to verification of critical findings before action is taken. Policies vary among facilities and may include requesting recollection and retesting by the laboratory.

	Arterial Blood Gas Parameter	Less Than	Greater Than
Adult/child	pH	7.2	7.6
Adult/child	HCO₃⁻	10 mmol/L	40 mmol/L
Adult/child	Pco₂	20 mm Hg (SI: 2.7 kPa)	67 mm Hg (SI: 8.9 kPa)
Adult/child	Po₂	45 mm Hg (SI: 6 kPa)	
Newborns	Po₂	37 mm Hg (SI: 4.9 kPa)	92 mm Hg (SI: 12.2 kPa)

B

OVERVIEW: (Study type: Whole blood; related body system: Circulatory, Respiratory, and Urinary systems. Specimen volume and collection container may vary with collection method. See section titled "Teaching the patient what to expect" for specific collection instructions. Specimen should be tightly capped and transported in an ice slurry.) Blood gas analysis is used to evaluate respiratory function and provide a measure for determining acid-base balance. Respiratory, renal, and cardiovascular system functions are integrated in order to maintain normal acid-base balance. Therefore, respiratory or metabolic disorders may cause abnormal blood gas findings. The blood gas measurements commonly reported are pH, partial pressure of carbon dioxide (Pco_2), partial pressure of oxygen (Po_2), bicarbonate (HCO_3^-), O_2 saturation, and base excess (BE) or base deficit (BD). pH reflects the number of free hydrogen ions (H^+) in the body. A pH less than 7.35 indicates acidosis. A pH greater than 7.45 indicates alkalosis. Changes in the ratio of free H^+ to HCO_3 will result in a compensatory response from the lungs or kidneys to restore proper acid-base balance.

Pco_2 is an important indicator of ventilation. The level of Pco_2 is controlled primarily by the lungs and is referred to as the *respiratory component* of acid-base balance. The main buffer system in the body is the bicarbonate–carbonic acid system. Bicarbonate is an important alkaline ion that participates along with other anions, such as hemoglobin, proteins, and phosphates, to neutralize acids. For the body to maintain proper balance, there must be a ratio of 20 parts bicarbonate to one part carbonic acid (20:1). Carbonic acid level is indirectly measured by Pco_2. Bicarbonate level is indirectly measured by the total carbon dioxide content (Tco_2). The carbonic acid level is not measured directly but can be estimated because it is 3% of the Pco_2. Bicarbonate can also be calculated from these numbers once the carbonic acid value has been obtained because of the 20:1 ratio. For example, if the Pco_2 were 40, the carbonic acid would be calculated as ($3\% \times 40$), or 1.2, and the HCO_3^- would be calculated as (20×1.2), or 24. The main acid in the acid-base system is carbonic acid. It is the metabolic or nonrespiratory component of the acid-base system and is controlled by the kidney. Bicarbonate levels can either be measured directly or estimated from the Tco_2 in the blood. BE/BD reflects the number of anions available in the blood to help buffer changes in pH. A BD (negative BE) indicates metabolic acidosis, whereas a positive BE indicates metabolic alkalosis.

Extremes in acidosis are generally more life threatening than alkalosis. Acidosis can develop either very quickly (e.g., cardiac arrest) or over a longer period of time (e.g., kidney failure). Infants can develop acidosis very quickly if they are not kept warm and given enough calories. Children with diabetes tend to go into acidosis more quickly than do adults who have been dealing with the disease over a longer period of time. In many cases, a venous or capillary specimen is satisfactory to obtain the necessary information regarding acid-base balance without subjecting the patient to an arterial puncture with its associated risks.

As seen in the table of reference ranges, P_{O_2} is lower in infants than in children and adults owing to the respective level of maturation of the lungs at birth. P_{O_2} tends to trail off after age 30, decreasing by approximately 3 to 5 mm Hg per decade as the organs age and begin to lose elasticity. The formula used to approximate the relationship between age and P_{O_2} is $P_{O_2} = 104 - (age \times 0.27)$.

The oxygen-carrying capacity of the blood indicates how much oxygen could be carried if all the hemoglobin were saturated with oxygen. Percentage of oxygen saturation is [oxyhemoglobin concentration ÷ (oxyhemoglobin concentration + deoxyhemoglobin concentration)] × 100.

Like carbon dioxide, oxygen is carried in the body in a dissolved and combined (oxyhemoglobin) form. Most of the oxygen circulating in the body (98%) is bound to hemoglobin; the rest is dissolved. One gram of hemoglobin can bind 1.34 mL of oxygen, whereas plasma is capable of carrying much less—0.3 mL of dissolved oxygen. Oxygen content is the sum of the dissolved and combined oxygen. Because circulating blood may contain less oxygen than it is capable of carrying, it is useful to know the actual oxygen content. Oxygen content can be calculated on the basis of measured parameters (oxygen saturation, hemoglobin, and P_{O_2}) and a solubility factor (0.003 is the Bunsen solubility factor for dissolved oxygen in blood). The oxygen content in arterial blood is calculated as $C_{AO_2} = 1.34 (S_{AO_2} \times Hgb) + 0.003 (P_{AO_2})$. The oxygen content of venous blood is calculated as $C_{VO_2} = 1.34 (S_{VO_2} \times Hgb) + 0.003 (P_{VO_2})$.

Testing on specimens other than arterial blood is often ordered when oxygen measurements are not needed or when the information regarding oxygen can be obtained by noninvasive techniques such as pulse oximetry. Capillary blood is satisfactory for most purposes for pH and P_{CO_2}; the use of capillary P_{O_2} is limited to the exclusion of hypoxia. Measurements involving oxygen are usually not useful when performed on venous samples; arterial blood is required to accurately measure P_{O_2} and oxygen saturation. Considerable evidence indicates that prolonged exposure to high levels of oxygen can result in injury, such as retinopathy of prematurity in infants or the drying of airways in any patient. Monitoring P_{O_2} from blood gases is especially appropriate under such circumstances.

INDICATIONS

This group of tests is used to assess conditions such as asthma, chronic obstructive pulmonary disease (COPD), embolism (e.g., fatty or other embolism) during coronary arterial bypass surgery, and hypoxia. It is also used to assist in the diagnosis of respiratory failure, which is defined as a P_{O_2} less than 50 mm Hg and P_{CO_2} greater than 50 mm Hg. Blood gases can be valuable in the management of patients on ventilators or being weaned from ventilators. Blood gas values are used to determine acid-base status, the type

B

of imbalance, and the degree of compensation as summarized in the following section.

Acid-base status: Decreased pH indicates acidosis, increased pH indicates alkalosis, and restoration of pH to near-normal values is referred to as *fully compensated balance*. When pH values are moving in the same direction (i.e., increasing or decreasing) as the Pco_2 or HCO_3^-, the imbalance is metabolic. When the pH values are moving in the opposite direction from the Pco_2 or HCO_3^-, the imbalance is caused by respiratory disturbances.

Type of imbalance: To remember this concept, the following mnemonic can be useful: **MetRO = Metabolic Together** (pH, Pco_2 and HCO_3^- all moving in the same direction, i.e., increasing or decreasing); **Respiratory Opposite** (pH is moving in the opposite direction of Pco_2 and HCO_3^-, i.e., pH increases and the other two decrease or pH decreases and the other two increase).

Acid-Base Imbalance	pH	Pco_2 (Respiratory or Compensatory Response to Metabolic Imbalance)	HCO_3^- (Metabolic or Compensatory Response to Respiratory Imbalance)
Respiratory Acidosis			
Uncompensated	Decreased	Increased	Normal
Partially compensated	Decreased	Increased	Increased
Fully compensated	Normal	Increased	Increased
Respiratory Alkalosis			
Uncompensated	Increased	Decreased	Normal
Partially compensated	Increased	Decreased	Decreased
Compensated	Normal	Decreased	Decreased
Metabolic (Nonrespiratory) Acidosis			
Uncompensated	Decreased	Normal	Decreased
Partially compensated	Decreased	Decreased	Decreased
Compensated	Normal	Decreased	Decreased
Metabolic (Nonrespiratory) Alkalosis			
Uncompensated	Increased	Normal	Increased
Partially compensated	Increased	Increased	Increased
Compensated	Normal	Increased	Increased

Romanski method of evaluating (most) blood gas scenarios

1. Determine whether the pH imbalance indicates acidosis or alkalosis.
   a. Decreased pH indicates acidosis.
   b. Increased pH indicates alkalosis.

2. Determine whether the Pco_2 component indicates probability of respiratory cause or rules out respiratory cause.
   a. Increased Pco_2 with decreased pH and normal HCO_3^- indicates

respiratory acidosis because *the blood becomes more acidotic when carbon dioxide is retained and production of carbonic acid increases.*

b. Decreased P_{CO_2} with increased pH and normal HCO_3^- indicates respiratory alkalosis because *the blood becomes alkalotic when more carbon dioxide is being "blown off" by the lungs than is staying in the blood.*

c. If respiratory cause is ruled out (i.e., HCO_3^- is abnormal), assume metabolic cause.

3. Determine which component, respiratory (P_{CO_2}) or metabolic (HCO_3^-), is consistent (increases or decreases) with pH.

4. Determine degree of compensation.

a. Uncompensated: The component that is not consistent with pH is normal, *which indicates that the companion compensatory mechanism, respiratory or metabolic, was unable to compensate.*

b. Partially compensated: The component not consistent with pH and the pH are either increased or decreased, *which indicates that the companion compensatory mechanism, respiratory or metabolic, was able to partially compensate, but not enough to resolve the acid-base imbalance.*

c. Compensated: The component not consistent with pH is increased or decreased and the pH is normal, *which indicates that the companion compensatory mechanism, respiratory or metabolic, was able to compensate and resolved the acid-base imbalance.*

INTERFERING FACTORS
Contraindications
Arterial puncture in any of the following circumstances:

Inadequate circulation, *as evidenced by an abnormal (negative) Allen test or the absence of a radial artery pulse.*

Significant or uncontrolled bleeding disorder, *as the procedure may cause excessive bleeding;* caution should be used when performing an arterial puncture on patients receiving anticoagulant therapy or thrombolytic medications.

Infection at the puncture site *carries the potential for introducing bacteria from the skin surface into the blood stream.*

Congenital or acquired abnormalities of the skin or blood vessels in the area of the anticipated puncture site, such as arteriovenous fistulas, burns, tumors, vascular grafts.

Factors that may alter the results of the study
• Drugs and other substances that may cause an increase in HCO_3^- include acetylsalicylic acid (initially), antacids, carbenicillin, ethacrynic acid, glycyrrhiza (licorice), laxatives, mafenide, and sodium bicarbonate.
• Drugs that may cause a decrease in HCO_3^- include acetazolamide, acetylsalicylic acid (long term or high doses), citrates, dimethadione, ether, ethylene glycol, fluorides, mercury compounds (laxatives), methylenedioxyamphetamine, paraldehyde, and xylitol.
• Drugs and other substances that may cause an increase in P_{CO_2} include acetylsalicylic acid, aldosterone, bicarbonate, carbenicillin, corticosteroids, dexamethasone, ethacrynic acid, laxatives (chronic misuse), and x-ray contrast medium.
• Drugs and other substances that may cause a decrease in P_{CO_2} include acetazolamide, acetylsalicylic acid, ethamivan,

B

B

neuromuscular relaxants (secondary to postoperative hyperventilation), theophylline, tromethamine, and xylitol.

- Drugs and other substances that may cause an increase in Po_2 include theophylline and urokinase.
- Drugs and other substances that may cause a decrease in Po_2 include barbiturates, granulocyte-macrophage colony-stimulating factor, isoproterenol, and meperidine.
- Specimens with extremely elevated white blood cell counts will undergo misleading decreases in pH, resulting from cellular metabolism, if transport to the laboratory is delayed.
- Excessive amounts of heparin in the sample may falsely decrease pH, Pco_2, and Po_2.
- A falsely increased O_2 saturation may occur because of elevated levels of carbon monoxide in the blood.
- Recent blood transfusion may produce misleading values.
- Specimens collected soon after a change in inspired oxygen has occurred will not accurately reflect the patient's oxygenation status.
- Specimens collected within 20 to 30 min of respiratory passage suctioning or other respiratory therapy will not be accurate.
- Excessive differences in actual body temperature relative to normal body temperature will not be reflected in the results. Temperature affects the amount of gas in solution. Blood gas analyzers measure samples at 37°C (98.6°F); therefore, if the patient is hyperthermic or hypothermic, it is important to notify the laboratory of the patient's actual body temperature at the time the specimen was collected. Fever will increase actual Po_2 and Pco_2 values; therefore, the uncorrected

values measured at 37°C will be falsely decreased. Hypothermia decreases actual Po_2 and Pco_2 values; therefore, the uncorrected values measured at 37°C will be falsely increased.

- O_2 saturation is a calculated parameter based on an assumption of 100% hemoglobin A. Values may be misleading when hemoglobin variants with different oxygen dissociation curves are present. Hemoglobin S will cause a shift to the right, indicating decreased oxygen binding. Fetal hemoglobin and methemoglobin will cause a shift to the left, indicating increased oxygen binding.
- Citrates should never be used as an anticoagulant in evacuated collection tubes for venous blood gas determinations because citrates will cause a marked analytic decrease in pH.
- Air bubbles or blood clots in the specimen are cause for rejection. Air bubbles in the specimen can falsely elevate or decrease the results depending on the patient's blood gas status. If an evacuated tube is used for venous blood gas specimen collection, the tube must be removed from the needle before the needle is withdrawn from the arm or else the sample will be contaminated with room air.
- Specimens should be placed in an ice slurry immediately after collection because blood cells continue to carry out metabolic processes in the specimen after it has been removed from the patient. These natural life processes can affect pH, Po_2, Pco_2, and the other calculated values in a short period of time. The cold temperature provided by the ice slurry will slow down, but not completely stop, metabolic changes occurring in the sample over time. Iced specimens not

analyzed within 60 min of collection should be rejected for analysis. Electrolyte analysis from iced specimens should be carried out within 30 min of collection to avoid falsely elevated potassium values.

POTENTIAL MEDICAL DIAGNOSIS: CLINICAL SIGNIFICANCE OF RESULTS

Acid-base imbalance is determined by evaluating pH, PCO_2, and HCO_3^- values. pH less than 7.35 reflects an acidic state, whereas pH greater than 7.45 reflects alkalosis. PCO_2 and HCO_3^- determine whether the imbalance is respiratory or nonrespiratory (metabolic). Because a patient may have more than one imbalance and may also be in the process of compensating, the interpretation of blood gas values may not always seem straightforward.

Respiratory conditions that interfere with normal breathing cause CO_2 to be retained in the blood. This results in an increase of circulating carbonic acid and a corresponding decrease in pH (respiratory acidosis). Acute respiratory acidosis can occur in acute pulmonary edema, severe respiratory infections, bronchial obstruction, pneumothorax, hemothorax, open chest wounds, opiate poisoning, respiratory depressant drug therapy, and inhalation of air with a high CO_2 content. Chronic respiratory acidosis can be seen in patients with asthma, pulmonary fibrosis, COPD, bronchiectasis, and respiratory depressant drug therapy. Respiratory conditions that increase the breathing rate cause CO_2 to be removed from the alveoli more rapidly than it is being produced. This results in an alkaline pH. Acute respiratory alkalosis may be seen in anxiety, hysteria, hyperventilation, and pulmonary embolus and with an increase in artificial ventilation. Chronic respiratory alkalosis may be seen in high fever, administration of drugs (e.g., salicylate and sulfa) that stimulate the respiratory system, hepatic coma, hypoxia of high altitude, and central nervous system (CNS) lesions or injury that result in stimulation of the respiratory center

Metabolic (nonrespiratory) conditions that cause the excessive formation or decreased excretion of organic or inorganic acids result in metabolic acidosis. Some of these conditions include ingestion of salicylates, ethylene glycol, and methanol, as well as uncontrolled diabetes, starvation, shock, kidney disease, and biliary or pancreatic fistula. Metabolic alkalosis results from conditions that increase pH, as can be seen in excessive intake of antacids to treat gastritis or peptic ulcer, excessive administration of HCO_3^-, loss of stomach acid caused by protracted vomiting, cystic fibrosis, or potassium and chloride deficiencies.

Respiratory Acidosis

- Decreased pH
- Decreased O_2 saturation
- Increased PCO_2:

  Acute intermittent porphyria
  Acute respiratory distress syndrome (adult and neonatal)
  Anemia (severe)
  Anorexia
  Anoxia
  Asthma
  Atelectasis
  Bronchitis (chronic)
  Bronchoconstriction
  Carbon monoxide poisoning
  Cardiac disorders
  Congenital heart defects
  COPD
  Cystic fibrosis
  Depression of respiratory center
  Drugs depressing the respiratory system
  Electrolyte disturbances (severe)
  Fever
  Head injury
  Heart failure
  Hypercapnia
  Hypothyroidism (severe)
  Near drowning
  Pleural effusion

Pneumonia
Pneumothorax
Poisoning
Poliomyelitis
Pulmonary edema
Pulmonary embolism
Pulmonary tuberculosis
Respiratory failure
Sarcoidosis
Smoking
Tumor (lung, brain)
- A decreased Po_2 that increases Pco_2:
   Decreased alveolar gas exchange:
      Acute respiratory distress syndrome
      (newborns), cancer, compression or
      resection of lung, sarcoidosis
   Decreased ventilation or perfusion:
      Asthma, bronchiectasis, bronchitis
      (chronic), cancer, croup, cystic fibrosis
      (mucoviscidosis), COPD, granulomata,
      pneumonia, pulmonary infarction, shock
   Hypoxemia: Anesthesia, carbon monox-
      ide exposure, cardiac disorders, high
      altitudes, near drowning, presence of
      abnormal hemoglobins
   Hypoventilation: Cerebrovascular inci-
      dent, drugs depressing the respiratory
      system, head injury
   Right-to-left shunt: Congenital heart
      disease, intrapulmonary venoarterial
      shunting

Compensation
- Increased Po_2:
   Hyperbaric oxygenation
   Hyperventilation
- Increased base excess:
   Increased HCO_3^- to bring pH to (near)
   normal

Respiratory Alkalosis
- Increased pH
- Decreased Pco_2:
   Anxiety
   CNS lesions or injuries that cause stimu-
      lation of the respiratory center
   Excessive artificial ventilation
   Fever
   Head injury
   Hyperthermia
   Hyperventilation
   Hysteria
   Salicylate intoxication

Compensation
- Decreased Po_2:
   Rebreather mask
- Decreased base excess:
   Decreased HCO_3^- to bring pH to (near)
   normal

Metabolic Acidosis
- Decreased pH
- Decreased HCO_3^-
- Decreased base excess
- Decreased Tco_2:
   Decreased excretion of H^+: Acute kidney
      injury, acquired (e.g., drugs, hyper-
      calcemia), Addison disease, chronic
      kidney disease, diabetic ketoacidosis,
      Fanconi syndrome, inherited (e.g., cys-
      tinosis, Wilson disease), renal tubular
      acidosis
   Increased acid intake
   Increased formation of acids: Diabetic
      ketoacidosis, high-fat/low-carbohydrate
      diets
   Increased loss of alkaline body fluids:
      Diarrhea, excess potassium, fistula

Compensation
- Decreased Pco_2:
   Hyperventilation

Metabolic Alkalosis
- Increased pH
- Increased HCO_3^-
- Increased base excess
- Increased Tco_2:
   Alkali ingestion (excessive)
   Anoxia
   Gastric suctioning
   Hypochloremic states
   Hypokalemic states
   Potassium depletion: Cushing dis-
      ease, diarrhea, diuresis, excessive
      vomiting, excessive ingestion of
      licorice, inadequate potassium intake,
      potassium-losing nephropathy, steroid
      administration
   Salicylate intoxication
   Shock
   Vomiting

Compensation
- Increased Tco_2:
   Hypoventilation

NURSING IMPLICATIONS

POTENTIAL NURSING PROBLEMS: ASSESSMENT & NURSING DIAGNOSIS

Problems	Signs and Symptoms
Breathing *(related to inflammation, viral or bacterial infection, muscular impairment, tracheal or bronchial obstruction, compromised neuromuscular function, spinal cord injury)*	Shortness of breath, rapid or slow breathing, nasal flare, use of accessory muscles, changes in respiratory effort and depth, cyanosis, pursed-lip breathing, bending forward to breathe easier
Cardiac output *(related to altered ventricular filling, impaired contractility, increased afterload, altered conductivity, deceased oxygenation, cardiac disease)*	Hypotension; increased heart rate; decreased cardiac output; decreased oxygen saturation, peripheral pulses, urinary output; cool, clammy skin; tachypnea; dyspnea; edema; altered level of consciousness; abnormal heart sounds; crackles in lungs; decreased activity tolerance; weight gain; fatigue; hypoxia; deceased ejection fraction (less than 55%)
Gas exchange *(related to altered alveolar and capillary exchange, ventilation-perfusion mismatch, compromised oxygen supply, inadequate oxygen-carrying capacity of the blood)*	Confusion; restlessness; hypoxia; irritability; shortness of breath; altered blood gases; orthopnea; cyanosis; increased heart rate, respiratory rate; use of respiratory accessory muscles; elevated blood pressure
Tissue perfusion *(related to compromised cardiac contractility, interrupted blood flow, inadequate oxygen transportation, decreased hemoglobin, hypoventilation, hypovolemia)*	Hypotension; dizziness; cool extremities; capillary refill greater than 3 sec; weak pedal pulses; weak or absent peripheral pulses; altered level of consciousness; compromised sensation; poor healing; cool, clammy skin

BEFORE THE STUDY: PLANNING AND IMPLEMENTATION

Teaching the Patient What to Expect

- Inform the patient this test can assist in assessing blood oxygen balance and oxygenation level.
- Explain that a blood sample is needed for the test. Address concerns about pain, and explain there may be some discomfort or pain during the arterial or venous puncture.
- Review the procedure with the patient and advise rest for 30 min before specimen collection. Explain to the patient that an arterial puncture may be painful. The site may be anesthetized with 1% to 2% lidocaine before puncture. Inform the patient that specimen collection and postprocedure care of the puncture site usually take 10 to 15 min. The person collecting the specimen should be notified beforehand if the patient is receiving anticoagulant therapy or taking aspirin or other natural products that may prolong bleeding from the puncture site.

If the sample is to be collected by radial artery puncture, perform an Allen test before puncture to ensure that the patient has adequate collateral circulation to the hand if thrombosis of the radial artery occurs after arterial puncture. The modified Allen test is performed as follows: Extend the patient's wrist over a rolled towel. Ask the patient to make a fist with the hand extended over the towel. Use the second and third fingers to locate the pulses of the ulnar and radial arteries on the palmar surface of the wrist. (The thumb should not be used to locate these arteries because it has a pulse.) Compress both arteries and ask the patient to open and close the fist several times until the palm turns pale. Release pressure on the ulnar artery only. Color should return to the palm within 5 sec if the ulnar artery is functioning. This is a positive Allen test, and blood gases may be drawn from the radial artery site. The Allen test should then be performed on the opposite hand. The hand to which color is restored fastest has better circulation and should be selected for specimen collection.

Arterial

▶ Perform an arterial puncture and collect the specimen in an air-free heparinized syringe. There is no demonstrable difference in results between samples collected in plastic syringes and samples collected in glass syringes. It is very important that no room air be introduced into the collection container because the gases in the room and in the sample will begin equilibrating immediately. The end of the syringe must be stoppered immediately after the needle is withdrawn and removed. Apply a pressure dressing over the puncture site. Samples should be mixed by gently rolling the syringe to ensure proper mixing of the heparin with the sample, which prevents the formation of small clots leading to rejection of the sample. The tightly capped sample should be placed in an ice slurry immediately after collection. Information on the specimen label should be protected from water in the ice slurry by first placing the specimen in a protective plastic bag. Promptly transport the specimen to the laboratory for processing and analysis.

Venous

▶ Central venous blood is collected in a heparinized syringe.
▶ Venous blood is collected percutaneously by venipuncture in a 5-mL green-top (heparin) tube (for adult patients) or a heparinized Microtainer (for pediatric patients). The vacuum collection tube must be removed from the needle before the needle is removed from the patient's arm. Apply a pressure dressing over the puncture site. Samples should be mixed by gently rolling the syringe to ensure proper mixing of the heparin with the sample, which prevents the formation of small clots leading to rejection of the sample. The tightly capped sample should be placed in an ice slurry immediately after collection. Information on the specimen label should be protected from water in the ice slurry by first placing the specimen in a protective plastic bag. Promptly transport the specimen to the laboratory for processing and analysis.

Capillary

▶ Perform a capillary puncture and collect the specimen in two 250-μL heparinized capillaries (scalp or heel for neonatal patients) or a heparinized Microtainer (for pediatric patients). The capillary tubes should be filled as much as possible and capped on both ends. Some hospitals recommend that metal "fleas" be added to the capillary tube before the ends are capped. During transport, a magnet can be moved up and down the outside of the capillary tube to facilitate mixing and prevent the formation of clots, which would cause rejection of the sample. It is important to inform the laboratory or respiratory therapy staff of the number of fleas used so the fleas can be accounted for and removed before the sample is introduced into the blood gas analyzers. Fleas left in the sample may damage the blood gas equipment if allowed to enter the analyzer. Microtainer samples should be mixed by gently rolling the capillary tube to ensure proper mixing of the heparin with the sample, which prevents the formation of small clots leading to rejection of the sample. Promptly transport the specimen to the laboratory for processing and analysis.

Cord Blood

▶ The sample may be collected immediately after delivery from the clamped cord, using a heparinized syringe. The tightly capped sample should be placed in an ice slurry immediately after collection. Information on the specimen label should be protected from water in the ice slurry by first placing the specimen in a protective plastic bag. Promptly transport the specimen to the laboratory for processing and analysis.

Scalp Sample

▶ Samples for scalp pH may be collected anaerobically before delivery in special scalp-sample collection capillaries and transported immediately to the laboratory for analysis. The procedure takes approximately 5 min. Place the patient on her back with her feet in stirrups. The cervix must be dilated at least 3 to 4 cm. A plastic cone is placed in the vagina and fit snugly against the scalp of the fetus. The cone provides access for visualization using an endoscope and to cleanse the site. The site is pierced with a sharp blade. Containment of the blood droplet can be aided by smearing a small amount of silicone cream on the fetal skin site. The blood sample is collected in a thin, heparinized tube. Some hospitals recommend that small metal fleas be added to the scalp tube before the ends are capped. See preceding section on capillary collection for discussion of fleas.

Potential Nursing Actions

▶ Validate the type of oxygen, mode of oxygen delivery, and delivery rate as part of the test requisition process and ensure there is a wait time of 30 min after a change in type or mode of oxygen delivery or rate for specimen collection.

▶ Ensure an ice slurry in a cup or plastic bag is readily available for immediate transport of the specimen to the laboratory.

AFTER THE STUDY: POTENTIAL NURSING ACTIONS

Avoiding Complications

▶ Bleeding, pain, hematoma. Apply pressure to the puncture site for at least 5 min in the unanticoagulated patient and for at least 15 min in the case of a patient taking natural products or medications with known anticoagulant, antiplatelet, or thrombolytic properties. Observe/assess puncture site for bleeding or hematoma formation. Apply pressure bandage.

Treatment Considerations

▶ Breathing: Assess respiratory rate, rhythm, and depth. Assess use of accessory muscles, nasal flare, and adventitious breath sounds. Monitor and trend blood gas results, oxygenation with pulse oximetry, and administration of prescribed oxygen. Discuss positions that will improve ventilation and oxygenation. Administer ordered antibiotics or antivirals. Pace activities to match energy stores. Consider future need for mechanical ventilation. Teach breathing exercises to assist with the appropriate exchange of oxygen and carbon dioxide, including breathing deeply and slowly. Breathing into a paper bag can decrease hyperventilation and quickly help the patient's breathing return to normal. Teach the patient how to properly use the incentive spirometer device or mininebulizer if ordered.

▶ Cardiac Output: Assess peripheral pulses and capillary refill. Monitor blood pressure and check for orthostatic changes. Assess respiratory rate, breath sounds, orthopnea, skin color and temperature, and level of consciousness. Monitor urinary output, oxygenation with pulse oximetry, sodium and potassium levels, and B-type natriuretic peptide (BNP) levels. Administer ordered ACE inhibitors, antidysrhythmics, diuretics, vasodilators, oxygen, and inotropics.

◗ Gas Exchange: Auscultate and trend breath sounds (adventitious breath sound). Assess respiratory rate, rhythm, depth, accessory muscle use, symptoms of infection, atelectasis, consolidation, and pleural effusion. Monitor for restlessness, dizziness, lethargy, disorientation, confusion, and trend Hgb and Hct. Monitor chest x-ray reports and oxygenation with pulse oximetry with administration of ordered oxygen. Consider preparation for intubation and/or mechanical ventilation. Place the head of the bed in high Fowler position (head elevated to 90–degree angle) to improve breathing. Administer ordered diuretics, vasodilators, and ABG results. Observe/assess the patient for signs or symptoms of respiratory and metabolic disturbances. Symptoms of respiratory acidosis are dyspnea, headache, tachycardia, pallor, diaphoresis, apprehension, drowsiness, coma, hypertension, or disorientation. Respiratory alkalosis presents with tachypnea, restlessness, agitation, tetany, numbness, seizures, muscle cramps, dizziness, or tingling fingertips. Symptoms of metabolic acidosis are rapid breathing, flushed skin, nausea, vomiting, dysrhythmias, coma, hypotension, hyperventilation, and restlessness. Metabolic alkalosis presents with shallow breathing, weakness, dysrhythmias, tetany, hypokalemia, hyperactive reflexes, and excessive vomiting.

◗ Tissue Perfusion: Monitor blood pressure (orthostatic). Assess dizziness, capillary refill, and pedal pulses. Monitor level of consciousness and check skin temperature for warmth.

Administer prescribed intravenous fluids, vasodilator, antiplatelet, anticoagulant, inotropic drugs, and oxygen.

◗ Water balance needs to be closely monitored in COPD patients. Fluid retention can lead to pulmonary edema.

◗ Teach the patient the appropriate use of oxygen therapy.

Nutritional Considerations

◗ Abnormal blood gas values may be associated with diseases of the respiratory system. Malnutrition is commonly seen in patients with severe respiratory disease for reasons including fatigue, lack of appetite, and gastrointestinal distress. Research has estimated that the daily caloric intake required for respiration of patients with COPD is 10 times higher than that of healthy individuals. Inadequate nutrition can result in hypophosphatemia, especially in the respirator-dependent patient. During periods of starvation, phosphorus leaves the intracellular space and moves outside the tissue, resulting in dangerously decreased phosphorus levels. Adequate intake of vitamins A and C is also important to prevent pulmonary infection and to decrease the extent of lung tissue damage. The importance of following the prescribed diet should be stressed to the patient and/or caregiver.

Follow-Up, Evaluation, and Desired Outcomes

◗ Demonstrates the ability to position himself or herself in an upright position to improve oxygenation.

◗ Understands the importance of adhering to the request to change position every 2 hr to decrease the risk of atelectasis.

◗ Demonstrates proficiency in the self-administration of medication to treat the underlying cause of the altered blood gas results.

◗ Acknowledges that oxygen therapy can improve blood oxygen levels.

◗ Uses oxygen, as prescribed, to support and improve oxygenation.

Blood Pool Imaging: First Pass and MUGA Scan

B

SYNONYM/ACRONYM: Cardiac blood pool scan, cardiac flow studies, ejection fraction study, gated cardiac scan, multigated acquisition (MUGA) scan, radionuclide ventriculogram, wall motion study.

RATIONALE: To evaluate blood flow through the ventricles of the heart and determine cardiac ejection fraction.

PATIENT PREPARATION: Instruct the patient to fast, restrict fluids (especially those containing caffeine), and abstain from the use of tobacco products for 4 hr prior to the procedure. No other radionuclide scans should be scheduled within 24 to 48 hr before this procedure. Protocols may vary among facilities.

NORMAL FINDINGS

- Normal wall motion, ejection fraction (55%–70%), coronary blood flow, ventricular size and function, and symmetry in contractions of the left ventricle.

CRITICAL FINDINGS AND POTENTIAL INTERVENTIONS: N/A

OVERVIEW: (Study type: Nuclear Scan; related body system: Circulatory system.) Two main types of cardiac blood pool scans are performed on adults and children. They are used to evaluate the direction of blood flow in the major blood vessels, to provide information regarding patency of vessels after vascular surgery, and to evaluate the ejection fraction of the right and left ventricles. First-pass or shunt imaging scans are commonly performed on pediatric patients to measure left-to-right shunts and assess for congenital heart defects. MUGA blood pool imaging, also known as *radionuclide ventriculogram* (RVG), provides information about cardiac function such as ejection fraction, ventricular wall motion, ventricular dilation, stroke volume, and cardiac output. Heart shunt imaging is sometimes done in conjunction with a resting MUGA scan to obtain ejection fraction and assess regional wall motion.

The radionuclide is prepared by one of several in vitro or in vivo methods. One commonly used in vitro method of preparation is performed by adding a radioactive tracer, technetium-99m (Tc-99m) (pertechnetate), to a sample of the patient's blood and reinjecting the labelled blood. The in vivo method involves two steps: first an injection of stannous pyrophosphate (PyP), a "sticky" substance that adheres to the circulating RBCs, followed 20 min later by an injection of Tc-99m (pertechnetate) that adheres to the PyP. The radionuclide is injected into a jugular or antecubital vein. The ventricular blood pool can be imaged during the initial transit of a peripherally injected, IV bolus of radionuclide (first-pass technique) or when the radionuclide has reached equilibrium concentration. For multigated studies, the patient's heartbeat, as measured with an electrocardiogram (ECG), is synchronized to the gamma camera imager and computer and therefore termed *gated*.

MUGA scans can be performed with the heart at rest or additionally as part of a stress test. The MUGA procedure, performed with the heart in motion, is used to obtain multiple images of the heart in contraction and relaxation during an R-to-R cardiac cycle. The resulting images can be displayed in a cinematic mode to visualize cardiac function. They can also be compared to MUGA scans performed at rest. Repetitive data acquisitions are possible during graded levels of exercise, usually a bicycle ergometer or handgrip, to assess ventricular functional response to exercise. The MUGA scan can also be used to evaluate the effectiveness of sublingual nitroglycerin on ventricular function; nitroglycerin is a strong vasodilator used to treat angina.

A related cardiac nuclear study is the myocardial perfusion scan (MPS). The MPS evaluates myocardial tissue perfusion, as demonstrated by presence of the Tc-99m (sestamibi) or Tc-99m (tetrofosmin), which localizes near mitochondria in the myocardial tissue cells, whereas the MUGA scan evaluates blood flow and the pumping action of the heart by following the movement of a radionuclide in the circulating blood. Combined technologies are now being used to offer higher quality, three-dimensional imaging in color. The single-photon emission computed tomography (SPECT) scan is an example of combining conventional nuclear medicine imaging provided by a gamma camera with CT. Stress testing is frequently performed following the MPS. Stress on the heart is induced, either by exercise or with drugs. Scanning may then be performed with a conventional gamma camera or with SPECT/CT.

Comparison of Cardiac Nuclear Scans

	Common Use	Radionuclide/ Radiopharmaceutical/ Action	Alternate Names
Blood pool (MUGA): Gated equilibrium studies	Collect images of heart function and blood flow over numerous cardiac cycles to evaluate the direction of blood flow, wall motion, and most frequently to determine cardiac ejection fraction	Tc-99m (pertechnetate) for in vitro procedure; PyP injection followed by a second injection of Tc-99m (pertechnetate) for in vivo procedure	Blood pool imaging, cardiac flow studies, cardiac equilibrium studies, cardiac nuclear scan, multigated acquisition scan, radionuclide ventriculogram, wall motion study

B

| Blood pool scan: First-pass studies | Determination of direction of blood flow, wall movement, and ejection fraction based on the data collected from the initial movement of the radiopharmaceutical as it passes through the heart | Tc-99m (pertechnetate), Tc-99m (pentetate) | Blood pool imaging, cardiac flow studies, cardiac nuclear scan, radionuclide ventriculogram, wall motion study |

Related studies	Common Use	Radionuclide/ Radiopharmaceutical/ Action	Alternate Names
Myocardial perfusion scan with or without SPECT	Visualizes areas of reversible ischemia and irreversibly infarcted cardiac tissue; heart movement visualized in 3D images with SPECT; used to evaluate the pharmacological stress test	Tc-99m (sestamibi) or Cardiolite, Tc-99m (tetrofosmin) or Myoview, Thallium-201 chloride	Sestamibi scan, cardiac stress scan (because it is often performed with the pharmacological cardiac stress test)
Myocardial infarct scan	Evaluate extent of myocardial damage after acute myocardial infarction; the PyP adheres to calcium deposits in irreversibly damaged myocardium	Tc-99m (PyP)	PyP cardiac scan, infarct scan, pyrophosphate cardiac scan, acute myocardial infarction scan

INDICATIONS

Adult

- Aid in the diagnosis of true or false ventricular aneurysms.
- Aid in the diagnosis of valvular heart disease and determining the optimal time for valve replacement surgery.
- Detect left-to-right shunts and determine pulmonary-to-systemic blood flow ratios.
- Determine cardiomyopathy.
- Determine drug cardiotoxicity to stop therapy before development of heart failure *(related to chemotherapy drugs or other medications known to cause cardiac damage).*
- Determine ischemic coronary artery disease.
- Differentiate between chronic obstructive pulmonary disease and left ventricular failure.
- Evaluate ventricular size, function, and wall motion after an acute episode or in chronic heart disease.
- Quantitate cardiac output by calculating global or regional ejection fraction.

Pediatric
- Detect left-to-right and right-to-left shunts; determine pulmonary-to-systemic blood flow ratios.
- Evaluate for cardiac dysfunction related to diagnosed or undiagnosed congenital heart defects (chambers, valves, or vessels).
- Quantitatively assess valvular regurgitation.

INTERFERING FACTORS

Contraindications

❋ Patients who are pregnant or suspected of being pregnant, unless the potential benefits of a procedure using radiation far outweigh the risk of radiation exposure to the fetus and mother.

❋ Patients with anginal pain at rest or in patients with severe atherosclerotic coronary vessels; dipyridamole testing is not performed in these circumstances.

❋ Chemical stress with vasodilators in patients having asthma *(because bronchospasm can occur).*

Factors that may alter the results of the study
- Conditions such as chest wall trauma, cardiac trauma, angina that is difficult to control, significant cardiac dysrhythmias, or a recent cardioversion procedure may affect test results.
- Atrial fibrillation and extrasystoles invalidate the procedure.
- Suboptimal cardiac stress or patient exhaustion, preventing maximum heart rate testing, will affect results when the procedure is done in conjunction with exercise testing.
- Metallic objects (e.g., jewelry, body rings) within the examination field, other nuclear scans done within the previous 24 to 48 hr, or retained barium from a previous radiological procedure, which may inhibit organ visualization and cause unclear images.
- Improper injection of the radionuclide that allows the tracer to seep deep into the muscle tissue can produce erroneous hot spots.
- Inability of the patient to cooperate or remain still during the procedure, because movement can produce blurred or otherwise unclear images.

POTENTIAL MEDICAL DIAGNOSIS: CLINICAL SIGNIFICANCE OF RESULTS

Abnormal findings related to
Measurements of blood volume and flow are recorded as the concentration of radionuclide is detected by the imaging equipment. The measurements are used to indicate abnormalities identified in the ventricles during different periods of the cardiac cycle. The scan also provides moving images of the heart to assess abnormalities in the size and function of the heart.

- Abnormal wall motion (akinesia or dyskinesia)
- Cardiac hypertrophy
- Cardiac ischemia
- Heart failure
- Enlarged left ventricle
- Infarcted areas are akinetic
- Ischemic areas are hypokinetic

NURSING IMPLICATIONS

BEFORE THE STUDY: PLANNING AND IMPLEMENTATION

Teaching the Patient What to Expect
▶ Inform the patient this procedure can assist in assessing the pumping action of the heart.
▶ Pregnancy is a general contraindication to procedures involving radiation. Explain to the female patient that she will be asked the date of her last menstrual period and pregnancy testing

may be performed to determine the possibility of pregnancy before she is exposed to radiation.

▶ Review the procedure with the patient. Address concerns about pain and explain that there may be moments of discomfort or pain experienced when the IV line is inserted to allow infusion of fluids such as saline, anesthetics, sedatives, radionuclides, medications used in the procedure, or emergency medications.

▶ Inform the patient that the procedure is performed in a nuclear medicine department by a health-care provider (HCP), and staff, specializing in this procedure and takes approximately 60 min.

▶ Reassure the patient that the radionuclide poses no radioactive hazard and rarely produces adverse effects.

▶ Positioning for this procedure is in a supine position on a flat table with foam wedges, which help maintain position and immobilization.

▶ Next, the chest will be exposed and the ECG leads will be attached. Baseline readings will be recorded immediately prior to administration of the IV radionuclide, and the heart is scanned with images taken in various positions over the entire cardiac cycle. Explain that vital signs to monitor oxygen level (pulse oximetry) and blood pressure (sphygmomanometer) will be measured before, during (peak), and after the study.

▶ Reassure the patient that he or she will be closely monitored for any complications related to the procedure (e.g., allergic reaction, anaphylaxis, bronchospasm).

▶ At the conclusion of the study, the needle or catheter is removed and a pressure dressing is applied over the puncture site.

▶ Refer to the study titled "Stress Testing" for further details regarding the exercise and pharmacological stress tests.

Potential Nursing Actions

◈ *Make sure a written and informed consent has been signed prior to*

the procedure and before administering any medications.

▶ Patients who cannot exercise are given dipyridamole before the radionuclide is injected.

Safety Considerations

▶ If nitroglycerin is given, an HCP assessing the baseline MUGA scan injects the medication. Additional scans are repeated until blood pressure reaches the desired level.

AFTER THE STUDY: POTENTIAL NURSING ACTIONS

Avoiding Complications

▶ Establishing an IV site and injection of radionuclides are invasive procedures. Complications are rare but include risk for allergic reaction *(related to contrast reaction)*, hematoma *(related to blood leakage into the tissue following needle insertion)*, bleeding from the puncture site *(related to a bleeding disorder or the effects of natural products and medications with known anticoagulant, antiplatelet, or thrombolytic properties)*, or infection *(which might occur if bacteria from the skin surface is introduced at the puncture site)*. Monitor the patient for complications related to the procedure (e.g., allergic reaction, anaphylaxis, bronchospasm). Immediately report symptoms such as fast heart rate, difficulty breathing, skin rash, itching, or chest pain to the appropriate HCP. Observe/assess the needle/catheter insertion site for bleeding, inflammation, or hematoma formation.

Treatment Considerations

▶ Explain that the radionuclide is eliminated from the body within 6 to 24 hr. Advise the patient to drink increased amounts of fluids for 24 to 48 hr to eliminate the radionuclide from the body, unless contraindicated.

▶ Instruct the patient to resume usual dietary, medication, and activity, as directed by the HCP.

▶ Activity: Identify the patient's normal activity patterns. Maintain bedrest as required to rest the heart and conserve oxygen. Administer ordered oxygen. If the patient is active, he or she should wear oxygen with activity and pace actions to what can be tolerated. Monitor and trend vital signs. Discuss the effects of altered cardiac health on sexual activity.

▶ Inadequate Cardiac Tissue Perfusion: Assess for characteristics of pain, quality, intensity, duration, and location. Monitor and trend vital signs, heart rate, respiratory rate, and blood pressure. Administer ordered oxygen and monitor saturation with continuous pulse oximetry. Continuous cardiac monitoring may be required. Assess skin color and temperature. Evaluate for cyanosis, breath sounds (rate, rhythm), capillary refill, and peripheral pulses. Monitor laboratory studies; arterial blood gases, creatine phosphokinase, creatine kinase-myocardial band (CKMB), C-reactive protein, and troponin. Monitor for confusion and restlessness. Administer ordered medications (thrombolytics, morphine, amiodarone, nitroglycerin, beta blockers). Elevate the head of the bed.

▶ Evaluate the patient's vital signs. Monitor vital signs, and neurological status every 15 min for 1 hr, then every 2 hr for 4 hr, and then as ordered by HCP. Monitor intake and output at least every 8 hr. Monitor ECG tracings until stable. Compare with baseline values. Protocols may vary among facilities.

▶ Pain: Administer ordered oxygen. Assess pain character, location, duration, and intensity. Use an easily understood pain rating scale, place in a position of comfort, and administer ordered medications (morphine, nitroglycerin, calcium channel blockers, beta blockers). Consider alternative measures for pain management (imagery, relaxation, music, etc.). Assess and trend vital signs and facilitate a calm, quiet environment

▶ Instruct the patient in the care and assessment of the injection site.

▶ Explain that application of cold compresses to the puncture site may reduce discomfort or edema.

Safety Considerations

▶ The patient who is breastfeeding should consult with the requesting HCP regarding alternative testing that does not involve radiation. In general, if a woman who is breastfeeding must have a nuclear scan, she should not breastfeed the infant for 72 hr after the scan, until the radionuclide has been eliminated. She should be instructed to express the milk in order to prevent cessation of milk production; the milk can be stored and used after the 3-day period.

▶ Refer to organizational policy for additional precautions that may include instructions on handwashing, toilet flushing, limited contact with others, and other aspects of nuclear medicine safety.

Nutritional Considerations

▶ Nutritional therapy is recommended for the patient identified to be at risk for developing coronary artery disease (CAD) or for individuals who have specific risk factors and/or existing medical conditions (e.g., elevated low-density lipoprotein cholesterol levels, other lipid disorders, diabetes, insulin resistance, or metabolic syndrome).

▶ If triglycerides are elevated, the patient should be advised to eliminate or reduce alcohol.

▶ Always consider cultural influences with dietary choices to ensure better adherence to a change in lifestyle.

▶ A variety of dietary patterns are beneficial for people with CAD.

Follow-Up, Evaluation, and Desired Outcomes

▶ Acknowledges contact information provided for the American Heart Association (www.heart.org/HEARTORG), National Heart, Lung, and Blood Association (www.nhlbi.nih.gov), and U.S. Department of Agriculture's resource for nutrition (www.choosemyplate.gov).

▶ Understands recommended treatment options and expected outcomes in relation to their cardiac status.

▶ Accepts the necessity of lifestyle changes that will need to be made to support positive cardiac health, including participation in cardiac rehabilitation. Changeable risk factors warranting education include strategies to encourage patients, especially those who are overweight and with high blood pressure, to safely decrease sodium intake, achieve a normal weight, ensure regular participation in moderate aerobic physical activity three to four times per week, eliminate tobacco use, and adhere to a heart-healthy diet.

▶ Meets with a registered dietitian to make heart-healthy changes that are culturally congruent.
▶ Agrees to meet with a support group to decrease risk of depression.
▶ Understands education given about basic pathophysiology of the pumping action of the heart and the purpose of the medications that are being administered related to cardiac status.

B

Blood Typing, Antibody Screen, and Crossmatch

SYNONYM/ACRONYM: ABO group and Rh typing, blood group antibodies, type and screen, type and crossmatch.

RATIONALE: To identify ABO blood group and Rh type, typically for prenatal screen and transfusion purposes. These tests are also used to help establish compatibility for cellular therapy and solid organ transplantation (in addition to human leukocyte antigen [HLA] and HLA antibody typing).

PATIENT PREPARATION: There are no food, fluid, activity, or medication restrictions unless by medical direction.

NORMAL FINDINGS: (Method: FDA-approved reagents with glass slides, glass tubes, gel, or automated systems) Compatibility (no clumping or hemolysis).

CRITICAL FINDINGS AND POTENTIAL INTERVENTIONS
Timely notification to the requesting health-care provider (HCP) of any critical findings and related symptoms is a role expectation of the professional nurse. A listing of these findings varies among facilities.

Signs and symptoms of blood transfusion reaction range from mildly febrile to anaphylactic and may include chills, dyspnea, fever, headache, nausea, vomiting, palpitations and tachycardia, chest or back pain, apprehension, flushing, hives, angioedema, diarrhea, hypotension, oliguria, hemoglobinuria, acute kidney injury, sepsis, shock, and jaundice. Complications from disseminated intravascular coagulation (DIC) may also occur.

Possible interventions in mildly febrile reactions include slowing the rate of infusion, then verifying and comparing patient identification, transfusion requisition, and blood bag label. The patient should be monitored closely for further development of signs and symptoms. Administration of epinephrine may be ordered.

Possible interventions in a more severe transfusion reaction may include immediate cessation of infusion, notification of the HCP, keeping the IV line open with saline or lactated Ringer solution, collection of red- and lavender-top tubes for posttransfusion work-up, collection of urine, monitoring vital signs every 5 min, ordering additional testing if DIC is suspected, maintaining patent airway and blood pressure, and administering mannitol.

B

OVERVIEW: (Study type: Blood collected in a red-top or lavender-top [EDTA] tube; related body system: Circulatory/Hematopoietic and Immune systems.) Blood typing is a series of tests that include the ABO and Rh blood-group system performed to detect surface antigens on red blood cells (RBCs) by an agglutination test and compatibility tests to determine antibodies against these antigens. The major antigens in the ABO system are A and B, although AB and O are also common phenotypes. Individuals with A antigens have group A blood; those with B antigens have group B blood. Individuals with both A and B antigens have group AB blood (universal recipient); those with neither A nor B antigens have group O blood (universal donor). Blood group and type is genetically determined. After 6 mo of age, individuals develop serum antibodies that react with A or B antigen absent from their own RBCs. These are called *anti-A* and *anti-B* antibodies.

In ABO blood typing, the patient's RBCs mix with anti-A and anti-B sera, a process known as *forward grouping*. The process then reverses, and the patient's serum mixes with type A and B cells in *reverse grouping*.

Generally, only blood with the same ABO group and Rh type as the recipient is transfused because the anti-A and anti-B antibodies are strong agglutinins that cause a rapid, complement-mediated destruction of incompatible cells. However, blood donations have decreased nationwide, creating shortages in the available supply. Safe substitutions with blood of a different group and/or Rh type

may occur depending on the inventory of available units. Many laboratories require consultation with the requesting HCP prior to issuing Rh-positive units to an Rh-negative individual.

ABO and Rh testing is also performed as a prenatal screen in pregnant women to identify the risk of hemolytic disease of the newborn. Although most of the anti-A and anti-B activity resides in the immunoglobulin M (IgM) class of immunoglobulins, some activity rests with immunoglobulin G (IgG). Anti-A and anti-B antibodies of the IgG class coat the RBCs without immediately affecting their viability and can readily cross the placenta, resulting in hemolytic disease of the newborn. Individuals with type O blood frequently have more IgG anti-A and anti-B than other people; thus, ABO hemolytic disease of the newborn will affect infants of type O mothers almost exclusively (unless the newborn is also type O).

Major antigens of the Rh system are D (or Rh_o), C, E, c, and e. Individuals whose RBCs possess D antigen are called Rh-positive; those who lack D antigen are called Rh-negative, no matter what other Rh antigens are present. Individuals who are Rh-negative produce anti-D antibodies when exposed to Rh-positive cells by either transfusions or pregnancy. These anti-D antibodies cross the placenta to the fetus and can cause hemolytic disease of the newborn or transfusion reactions if Rh-positive blood is administered.

The type and screen (T&S) procedure is performed to determine the ABO/Rh and identify any antibodies that may react with transfused blood products. The T&S may take from 30 to 45 min or longer to complete depending on whether unexpected or unusual antibodies are detected. Every unit of product must be crossmatched against the intended recipient's serum and RBCs for compatibility before transfusion. Knowing the ABO/Rh and antibody status saves time when the patient's sample is crossmatched against units of donated blood products. There are three crossmatch procedures. If no antibodies are identified in the T&S, it is permissible to use either an immediate spin crossmatch or an electronic crossmatch, either of which may take 5 to 10 min to complete. If antibodies are detected, the antiglobulin crossmatch procedure is performed, along with antibody identification testing, or the process is repeated, beginning with the selection of other units for compatibility testing. Typically, specimens for T&S can be held for 72 hr from the time of collection for use in future crossmatch procedures. This timeframe may be extended for up to 14 days for patients with a reliably known history of no prior transfusions or pregnancy within the previous 3 mo. Donated blood products are tested for ABO group, Rh type, unexpected RBC antibodies, and transmissible infectious diseases that include the presence of hepatitis B core antibody (antibodies directed against the hepatitis B core antigen), hepatitis B surface antigen, hepatitis B virus (viral DNA by nucleic acid testing [NAT]), hepatitis C antibody (viral RNA by NAT), HTLV I and II antibody, HIV 1 (viral RNA by NAT) and 2 antibody, syphilis, West Nile virus antibody (viral RNA by NAT), *Trypanosoma cruzi* antibody (negative results on either current or at least one previous test), and most recently Zika virus (RNA using an approved investigational donor NAT or a licensed NAT, once it is available). Additional testing may be performed in cases of specific need and include cytomegalovirus antibody and IgA deficiency. All donated units receiving additional testing will be labelled with the results (positive or negative). Licensed testing for emerging transmissible pathogens (e.g., Zika, a flavivirus transmitted most commonly by the *Aedes aegypti* mosquito) is not always available when the pathogens are identified. Therefore, blood component collection facilities implement a variety of strategies to help ensure the safety of the blood supply. Recommendations may include the addition of specific questions to the donor history questionnaire to evaluate risk of infection, implementation of a waiting period prior to donation, or deferral of donation. Decisions regarding donor eligibility are based on criteria and recommendations developed by national (e.g., AABB, FDA, Centers for Disease Control and Prevention) and international scientific communities (e.g., World Health Organization). Educational material is also available at collection facilities for potential donors to review and determine whether they should self-defer from donation.

Febrile nonhemolytic reaction and urticarial/allergic reaction are the two most common types of reactions that occur in blood product transfusions. Many institutions have a policy that provides for premedication with acetaminophen and diphenhydramine to avoid initiation of mild transfusion reactions, where appropriate.

Many of the same tests used to determine the compatibility and safety of blood products (ABO, Rh, antibody screen, and infectious disease markers) are also used to establish a safe, compatible transplantation between donors and recipients of cellular therapy and solid organs. Cellular therapy uses human cells, such as bone marrow or stem cells, from a donated source to replace or repair damaged cells in a human recipient; solid organ transplantation serves a similar purpose, most commonly with heart, kidney, liver, lungs, pancreas, and skin. Tissue typing, also called *HLA typing,* is additional testing performed to match a compatible donor and recipient for cellular therapy or solid organ transplantation. Blood cell antigens and tissue type are inherited, half from each of the biological parents. The individual antigens and tissue surface antigen patterns are specific for each person and are unique except in the case of identical twins. HLA typing is also performed to identify antibodies the recipient may develop against the donor's foreign tissue cells in order to prevent graft versus host rejection. Although it is possible to find a compatible, nonrelated, donor-recipient pair in the general population, donor compatibility is best matched to a recipient who shares some of the same genetic markers—in other words, a person who is a blood relative.

INDICATIONS

- Determine ABO and Rh compatibility of donor and recipient before transfusion (type and screen or crossmatch).
- Determine anti-D antibody titer of Rh-negative mothers after sensitization by pregnancy with an Rh-positive fetus.
- Determine the need for a microdose of immunosuppressive therapy (e.g., with Rh(D) immune globulin RhoGAM intramuscular (IM) or Rhophylac IM or IV) during the first 12 wk of gestation or a standard dose after 12 wk of gestation for complications such as abortion, miscarriage, vaginal hemorrhage, ectopic pregnancy, or abdominal trauma.
- Determine Rh blood type and perform antibody screen of prenatal patients on initial visit to determine maternal Rh type and to indicate whether maternal RBCs have been sensitized by any antibodies known to cause hemolytic disease of the newborn, especially anti-D antibody. Rh blood type, antibody screen, and antibody titration (if an antibody has been identified) will be rechecked at 28 wk of gestation and prior to injection of a prophylactic standard dose of RhoGAM for Rh-negative mothers. These tests will also be repeated after delivery of an Rh-positive fetus to an Rh-negative mother and prior to injection of prophylactic standard dose of RhoGAM (if maternal Rh-negative blood has not been previously sensitized with Rh-positive cells resulting in a positive anti-D antibody titer). A postpartum blood sample must be evaluated for fetal-maternal bleed on all Rh-negative mothers to determine the need for additional doses of Rh immune

globulin. One in 300 cases will demonstrate hemorrhage greater than 15 mL of blood and require additional RhoGAM.

- Identify donor ABO and Rh blood type for stored blood.
- Identify maternal and infant ABO and Rh blood types to predict risk of hemolytic disease of the newborn.
- Identify the patient's ABO and Rh blood type, especially before a procedure in which blood loss is a threat or blood replacement may be needed.
- Identify any unusual transfusion-related antibodies in the patient's blood, especially before a procedure in which blood replacement may be needed.

INTERFERING FACTORS

Factors that may alter the results of the study

- Drugs and other substances, including cephalexin, levodopa, methyldopa, and methyldopate hydrochloride, may cause a false-positive result in Rh typing and in antibody screens.
- Recent administration of blood, blood products, dextran, or IV contrast medium causes cellular aggregation resembling agglutination in ABO typing.

- Contrast material such as iodine, barium, and gadolinium may interfere with testing.
- Abnormal proteins, cold agglutinins, and bacteremia may interfere with testing.
- History of bone marrow transplant, cancer, or leukemia may cause discrepancy in ABO typing.

Other considerations

- Testing does not detect every antibody and may miss the presence of a weak antibody.

POTENTIAL MEDICAL DIAGNOSIS: CLINICAL SIGNIFICANCE OF RESULTS

- *Agglutination is graded from 1+ to 4+ in manual testing systems; with 4+ being the strongest degree of agglutination. Automated testing systems are capable of reporting 1+ to 4+ graded results, providing images of the tested material so laboratory professionals can interpret the results, or providing computer-assisted interpretation of the test results as positive or negative findings.*
- ABO system: A, B, AB, or O specific to person
- Rh system: Positive or negative specific to person
- Crossmatching: Compatibility between donor and recipient
- Incompatibility indicated by clumping (agglutination) of RBCs

RBC Group and Type	Incidence (%)	Alternative Transfusion Group and Type of Packed Cell Units in Order of Preference If Patient's Own Group and Type Not Available
O positive	37.4	O negative
O negative	6.6	O positive*
A positive	35.7	A negative, O positive, O negative
A negative	6.3	O negative, A positive,* O positive*
B positive	8.5	B negative, O positive, O negative
B negative	1.5	O negative, B positive,* O positive*

(table continues on page 224)

B

RBC Group and Type	Incidence (%)	Alternative Transfusion Group and Type of Packed Cell Units in Order of Preference If Patient's Own Group and Type Not Available
AB positive	3.4	AB negative, A positive, B positive, A negative, B negative, O positive, O negative
AB negative	0.6	A negative, B negative, O negative, AB positive,* A positive,* B positive,* O positive*
Rh Type		
Rh positive	85–90	
Rh negative	10–15	

*If blood units of exact match to the patient's group and type are not available, a switch in ABO blood group is preferable to a change in Rh type. However, in extreme circumstances, Rh-positive blood can be issued to an Rh-negative recipient. It is very likely that the recipient will develop antibodies as the result of receiving Rh-positive red blood cells. Rh antibodies are highly immunogenic, and once the antibodies are developed, the recipient can receive only Rh-negative blood for subsequent red blood cell transfusion.

NURSING IMPLICATIONS

POTENTIAL NURSING PROBLEMS: ASSESSMENT & NURSING DIAGNOSIS

Problems	Signs and Symptoms
Cardiac output *(related to inadequate circulating blood supply secondary to blood loss)*	Decreased peripheral pulses; decreased urinary output; cool, clammy skin; tachypnea; dyspnea; edema; altered level of consciousness; abnormal heart sounds; crackles in lungs; decreased activity tolerance; weight gain; fatigue; hypoxia
Excess fluid volume *(related to increased circulatory volume secondary to blood transfusion and normal saline IV fluids)*	Edema, shortness of breath, increased weight, ascites, rales, rhonchi, and diluted laboratory values
Gas exchange *(related to insufficient oxygen supply secondary to blood loss)*	Decreased activity tolerance, increased shortness of breath with activity, weakness, orthopnea, cyanosis, cough, increased heart rate, weight gain, edema in the lower extremities, weakness, increased respiratory rate, use of respiratory accessory muscles
Injury risk *(related to possible transfusion reaction secondary to protein hypersensitivity, WBC febrile reaction, hemolytic incompatibility)*	Fever, chills, rash, itching, decreased blood flow to organs, acute kidney injury

BEFORE THE STUDY: PLANNING AND IMPLEMENTATION

Teaching the Patient What to Expect

▶ Inform the patient this test can assist in identification of blood type.

▶ Explain that a blood sample is needed for the test.

Potential Nursing Actions

◆ *Make sure a written and informed consent has been signed prior to any transfusion blood products.*

▶ *Sensitivity to Social and Cultural Issues:* as well as concern for modesty, is important in providing psychological support before, during, and after the procedure. Answer questions from the patient and family regarding the risks and benefits of blood transfusion. Provide the opportunity for the patient and family to voice any religious or cultural objections to the ordered transfusion. Provide the opportunity for discussion regarding possible transfusion alternatives other than donor blood.

▶ Provide required blood transfusion education.

▶ Note any recent or past procedures, especially blood or blood product transfusion or bone marrow transplantation, that could complicate or interfere with test results.

Safety Considerations

▶ Strict adherence to protocols regarding type and crossmatch is necessary to prevent inadvertent errors in determining ABO type for the purposes of transfusion of blood and blood products. Mistakes can lead to injury or death.

AFTER THE STUDY: POTENTIAL NURSING ACTIONS

Avoiding Complications

▶ A transfusion reaction may occur in some patients. A transfusion reaction is also a critical finding. Signs, symptoms, and possible interventions are described in the Critical Findings section.

Treatment Considerations

▶ Cardiac Output: Assess peripheral pulses and capillary refill. Monitor blood pressure and check for orthostatic changes. Assess respiratory rate, breath sounds, orthopnea, and skin color and temperature. Assess level of consciousness. Monitor urinary output, oxygenation with pulse oximetry, sodium and potassium levels, and hemoglobin (Hgb) and hematocrit (Hct).

▶ Excess Fluid Volume: Monitor transfusion rate. Transfuse according to standards of care. Monitor respiratory status with establishment of baseline assessment data and administer ordered diuretic.

▶ Gas Exchange: Auscultate and trend breath sounds. Perform pulse oximetry to monitor oxygenation and administer oxygen to meet specific oxygen saturation. Collaborate with the HCP to consider intubation and/or mechanical ventilation for respiratory support. Place the head of the bed in high Fowler position for ease of breathing. Administer ordered diuretics, vasodilators, blood or blood products. Monitor and trend Hgb and Hct.

▶ Injury Risk: Administer ordered premedication to prevent fever and itching during transfusion. Use of a leukocyte filter may be ordered by the requesting HCP for immunosuppressed or other sensitive patient populations; leukocyte-reduced blood products may also be ordered. Follow standard hospital procedure to ensure informed consent and a correct match prior to transfusion. Take vital signs prior to transfusion and within 15 min after the transfusion has started to assess for transfusion reaction (fever and chills). Facilitate ongoing monitoring for fever, chills, itching, and rash during transfusion. Immediately stop transfusion if reaction is noted and follow institutional process for assessing transfusion reaction such as urine and blood sample collection for analysis per institutional policy.

Safety Considerations

▶ Although correct patient identification is important for all test specimens, it is crucial when blood is collected for

B

type and crossmatch because clerical error is the most frequent cause of life-threatening ABO incompatibility. Therefore, additional requirements are necessary, including the verification of two unique identifiers that could include any two unique patient demographics, such as name, date of birth, Social Security number, hospital number, date, or blood bank number on requisition and specimen labels; completing and applying a wristband on the arm with the same information; and placing labels with the same information and blood bank number on blood sample tubes.

Follow-Up, Evaluation, and Desired Outcomes
◗ Acknowledges the importance of transfusion to overall health and recognizes that repeat transfusions may be necessary.
◗ Correctly states symptoms of transfusion reaction and agrees to report any symptoms as they occur.
◗ Records blood and Rh type on a card or other document routinely carried for easy reference.
◗ Women who are Rh-negative understand the importance of communicating that information to their HCP if they become pregnant or need a transfusion.

Bone Mineral Densitometry

SYNONYM/ACRONYM: BMD, DEXA, DXA, SXA, QCT, RA, ultrasound densitometry.

Dual-energy x-ray absorptiometry (DEXA, DXA): Two x-rays of different energy levels measure bone mineral density and predict risk of fracture.

Single-energy x-ray absorptiometry (SXA): A single-energy x-ray measures bone density at peripheral sites.

Quantitative computed tomography (QCT): QCT is used to examine the lumbar vertebrae. It measures trabecular and cortical bone density. Results are compared to a known standard. This test is the most expensive and involves the highest radiation dose of all techniques.

Radiographic absorptiometry (RA): A standard x-ray of the hand. Results are compared to a known standard.

Ultrasound densitometry: Studies bone mineral content in peripheral densitometry sites such as the heel or wrist. It is not as precise as x-ray techniques but is less expensive than other techniques.

RATIONALE: To evaluate bone density related to osteoporosis.

PATIENT PREPARATION: There are no food, fluid, activity, or medication restrictions unless by medical direction. Bone mineral density (BMD) should not be performed until 7 to 10 days after other radiological studies depending on the tracer and dose used.

NORMAL FINDINGS
• Normal bone mass with T-score value not less than –1.

CRITICAL FINDINGS AND POTENTIAL INTERVENTIONS: N/A

B

OVERVIEW: (Study type: X-ray, plain; related body system: Musculoskeletal system.) BMD can be measured at any of several body sites, including the spine, hip, wrist, and heel. Equipment used to measure BMD include computed tomography (CT), radiographic absorptiometry, ultrasound, SXA, and most commonly, DEXA. The radiation exposure from SXA and DEXA machines is approximately one-tenth that of a standard chest x-ray.

Osteoporosis is a condition characterized by low BMD, which results in increased risk of fracture. The National Osteoporosis Foundation estimates that 4 to 6 million postmenopausal women in the United States have osteoporosis, and an additional 13 to 17 million (30%–50%) have low bone density at the hip. It is estimated that one of every two women will experience a fracture as a result of low bone mineral content in her lifetime. The measurement of BMD gives the best indication of risk for a fracture. The lower the BMD, the greater is the risk of fracture. The most common fractures are those of the hip, vertebrae, and distal forearm. Bone mineral loss is a disease of the entire skeleton and is not restricted to the areas listed. The effect of the fractures has a wide range, from complete recovery to chronic pain, disability, and possible death.

The BMD values measured by the various techniques cannot be directly compared. Therefore, they are stated in terms of standard deviation (SD) units. The patient's T-score is the number of SD units above or below the average BMD in young adults. A Z-score is the number of SD units above or below the average value for a person of the same age as the measured patient. Since bone loss occurs naturally as part of the aging process, using a patient's Z-score in comparison to a person of the same age could be misleading, especially in the early development of osteoporosis. The World Health Organization has defined normal bone density as being within (above or below) 1 SD of the mean for young adults. Low bone density is defined as density 1 SD to 2.5 SD below the mean for young adults; bone density 2.5 SD or more below the mean for young adults is indicative of osteoporosis (osteopenia), and bone density more than 2.5 SD below the mean for young adults is defined as severe (established) osteoporosis. The baseline age for young adults is approximately 30 years of age. For most BMD readings, 1 SD is equivalent to 10% to 12% of the average young-normal BMD value. A T-score of –2.5 is therefore equivalent to a bone mineral loss of 30% when compared to a young adult.

INDICATIONS
- Determine the mineral content of bone.
- Determine a possible cause of amenorrhea.
- Establish a diagnosis of osteoporosis.
- Estimate the actual fracture risk compared to young adults.
- Evaluate bone demineralization associated with chronic conditions (e.g., chronic kidney disease) or long-term use of corticosteroids.
- Evaluate bone demineralization associated with immobilization.

B

- Evaluate secondary causes of bone demineralization associated with endocrine disorders (e.g., Cushing syndrome, diabetes, eating disorders, hyperparathyroidism, hyperprolactinemia).
- Monitor changes in BMD due to medical problems (e.g., malabsorption, multiple myeloma) or therapeutic intervention.
- Predict future fracture risk.

INTERFERING FACTORS
Contraindications

✦ Patients who are pregnant or suspected of being pregnant, unless the potential benefits of a procedure using radiation far outweigh the risk of radiation exposure to the fetus and mother.

Factors that may alter the results of the study
- BMD test results may be lower in individuals receiving corticosteroid therapy; ideally BMD testing should be performed before a patient is placed on a regimen of chronic steroid therapy to obtain a valid baseline.
- Residual radionuclide activity from a previous nuclear scan or retained contrast medium (e.g., barium or iodine-based) may affect the image. BMD should not be performed until 7 to 10 days after other radiological studies depending on the tracer and dose used.
- The use of anticonvulsant drugs, cytotoxic drugs, tamoxifen, glucocorticoids, lithium, or heparin, as well as increased alcohol intake, increased aluminum levels, excessive thyroxin, hemodialysis, or smoking, may affect the test results by either increasing or decreasing the bone mineral content.
- Metallic objects (e.g., jewelry, body rings, joint replacement hardware, pins, screws, metallic rods, spinal

fusion hardware, and/or dental amalgams) within the examination field, which may inhibit organ visualization and cause unclear images. A forearm scan can be used in cases where spine or bilateral hip sites are unavailable.
- Inability of the patient to cooperate or remain still during the procedure, because movement can produce blurred or otherwise unclear images.

Other considerations
- BMD scans can be safely performed on patients with a pacemaker or implanted defibrillator.

Other Considerations as a Result of Altered BMD, Not the BMD Testing Process
- Vertebral fractures may cause complications including back pain, height loss, and kyphosis.
- Limited activity, including difficulty bending and reaching, may result.
- Patient may have poor self-esteem resulting from the cosmetic effects of kyphosis.
- Potential restricted lung function may result from fractures.
- Fractures may alter abdominal anatomy, resulting in constipation, pain, distention, and diminished appetite.
- Potential for a restricted lifestyle may result in depression and other psychological symptoms.
- Possible increased dependency on family for basic care may occur.

POTENTIAL MEDICAL DIAGNOSIS: CLINICAL SIGNIFICANCE OF RESULTS
Abnormal findings related to
- Osteoporosis is defined as T-score value less than −2.5.
- Low bone mass or osteopenia has T-scores from −1 to −2.5.
- Fracture risk increases as BMD declines from young-normal levels (low T-scores).

- Low Z-scores in older adults can be misleading because low BMD is very common.

- Z-scores estimate fracture risk compared to others of the same age (versus young-normal adults).

NURSING IMPLICATIONS

POTENTIAL NURSING PROBLEMS: ASSESSMENT & NURSING DIAGNOSIS

Problems	Signs and Symptoms
Pain (acute, chronic) *(related to degradation of the joint, damaged cartilage, fracture, bone mass loss)*	Self-report of pain that is acute or chronic; presence of facial grimace, crying, irritability; difficulty concentrating; social withdrawal; refusal or reluctance to participate in activities
Mobility *(related to joint pain, stiffness, the presence of muscle weakness, fear of pain)*	Hesitant or refuses to move for fear of pain, limited muscle strength on the affected side, anxiety
Self-care *(related to the presence of pain, fear, limited range of motion, anxiety)*	Observed physical limitations, self-report of need of assistance for self-care activities

BEFORE THE STUDY: PLANNING AND IMPLEMENTATION

Teaching the Patient What to Expect

▶ Inform the patient this procedure can assist in assessing bone density.

▶ Pregnancy is a general contraindication to procedures involving radiation. Explain to the female patient that she will be asked the date of her last menstrual period. Pregnancy testing may be performed to determine the possibility of pregnancy before exposure to radiation.

▶ Review the procedure with the patient. Address concerns about pain and explain that no pain should be experienced during the test.

▶ Inform the patient that the procedure is usually performed in a radiology department by a health-care provider (HCP), and staff, specializing in this procedure and takes approximately 60 min.

▶ Explain that prior to the procedure the patient will be placed in a supine position on a flat table with foam wedges, which help maintain position and immobilization.

▶ Images are taken of the spine, femur, and forearm.

AFTER THE STUDY: POTENTIAL NURSING ACTIONS

Treatment Considerations

▶ Pain: Assess pain characteristics, location, duration, and intensity. Institute pain management modalities that fit with the patient's view of appropriate pain management. Administer ordered analgesics or narcotics, institute rest periods to decrease joint aggravation, and apply either hot or cold packs as appropriate.

▶ Mobility: Assist with activity to meet daily living needs. Assess the severity of mobility limitations and implement the use of assistive devices as needed. Review and adapt environment to physical limitations to prevent injury.

▶ Self-Care: Discuss with patients their perception of self-care activities that may require assistance and collaboratively develop a plan to meet those needs. Encourage patients to do as much as possible for themselves. Administer medication for pain

30 min prior to activity. Pace activities to maximize self-care opportunities and decrease pain.

Nutritional Considerations

♦ Educate the patient with vitamin D deficiency, as appropriate, that foods high in calcium and vitamin D should be included in the diet. Examples of foods rich in calcium and vitamin D are yogurt, cheese, cottage cheese, canned sardines with bones, flounder, salmon, dried figs, and dark-green leafy vegetables such as spinach and broccoli. Processed foods with added calcium, such as breads and cereals, can also be included. Avoiding red meat and high-fat foods that bind calcium in the intestine can reduce loss. The excess use of alcohol, salt, or caffeine can also decrease absorption.

Explain to the patient that vitamin D is also synthesized by the body, in the skin, and is activated by sunlight. Daily recommendations for calcium and vitamin D intake are based on age. Calcium and vitamin D supplements may be used if dietary intake is insufficient.

Follow-Up, Evaluation, and Desired Outcomes

♦ Acknowledges contact information provided for the U.S. Department of Agriculture's resource for nutrition (www.choosemyplate.gov).
♦ Acknowledges the importance of using assistive devices to facilitate mobility, self-care, and decrease injury fall risk.
♦ Agrees to diet changes that will include more calcium and vitamin D.

Bone Scan

SYNONYM/ACRONYM: Bone imaging, radionuclide bone scan, bone scintigraphy, whole-body bone scan.

RATIONALE: To assist in diagnosing bone disease such as cancer or other degenerative bone disorders.

PATIENT PREPARATION: There are no food, fluid, activity, or medication restrictions unless by medical direction. No other radionuclide scans should be scheduled within 24 to 48 hr before this procedure. Protocols may vary among facilities.

NORMAL FINDINGS
• No abnormalities, as indicated by homogeneous and symmetric distribution of the radionuclide throughout all skeletal structures.

CRITICAL FINDINGS AND POTENTIAL INTERVENTIONS: N/A

OVERVIEW: (Study type: Nuclear scan; related body system: Musculoskeletal system.) This nuclear medicine scan assists in diagnosing and determining the extent of primary and metastatic bone disease and bone trauma and monitors the progression of degenerative disorders. Abnormalities are identified by scanning 1 to 3 hr after the IV injection of a radionuclide such as technetium-99m attached to methylene diphosphonate (Tc-99m, MDP) which has a specific affinity for areas of altered bone formation.

The radionuclide targets sites of increased bone mineralization and adheres to the surface of crystals in the bone matrix. Areas of increased uptake and activity on the bone scan represent abnormalities unless they occur in normal areas of increased activity, such as the sternum, sacroiliac, clavicle, and scapular joints in adults, and growth centers and cranial sutures in children. A number of types of cancer, such as breast, lung, lymphomas, and prostate, are known to metastasize to bone. The radionuclide mimics calcium physiologically and therefore localizes in bone with an intensity proportional to the degree of metabolic activity. Bone scan is very sensitive; abnormalities can be identified weeks or months before they might be detected by x-ray. Gallium, magnetic resonance imaging (MRI), or white blood cell (WBC) scanning may be performed after a bone scan to obtain a more sensitive study if acute inflammatory conditions such as osteomyelitis or septic arthritis are suspected. In addition, bone scan can detect fractures in patients who continue to have pain even though x-rays have proved negative. A gamma camera detects the radiation emitted from the injected radioactive material. Whole-body or representative images of the skeletal system can be obtained. Single-photon emission computed tomography (SPECT) has significantly improved the resolution and accuracy of bone scanning and may or may not be included as part of the examination. SPECT enables images to be recorded from multiple angles around the body and reconstructed by a computer to produce images or "slices" representing the area of interest at different levels.

INDICATIONS

- Aid in the diagnosis of benign tumors or cysts.
- Aid in the diagnosis of metabolic bone diseases.
- Aid in the diagnosis of osteomyelitis.
- Aid in the diagnosis of primary malignant bone tumors (e.g., osteogenic sarcoma, chondrosarcoma, Ewing sarcoma, metastatic malignant tumors).
- Aid in the detection of traumatic or stress fractures.
- Assess degenerative joint changes or acute septic arthritis.
- Assess suspected child abuse.
- Confirm temporomandibular joint derangement.
- Detect Legg-Calvé-Perthes disease.
- Determine the cause of unexplained bone or joint pain.
- Evaluate the healing process following fracture, especially if an underlying bone disease is present.
- Evaluate prosthetic joints for infection, loosening, dislocation, or breakage.
- Evaluate tumor response to radiation or chemotherapy.
- Identify appropriate site for bone biopsy, lesion excision, or débridement.

INTERFERING FACTORS
Contraindications
Patients who are pregnant or suspected of being pregnant, unless the potential benefits of a procedure using radiation far outweigh the risk of radiation exposure to the fetus and mother.

B

Factors that may alter the results of the study

- A distended bladder may obscure pelvic detail; the patient should be asked to void and empty the bladder immediately before the delayed images are taken.
- The existence of multiple myeloma or cancers that have metastasized to the bones (e.g., thyroid cancer) can result in a false-negative scan for bone abnormalities until a significant amount of bone and bone marrow destruction has occurred; these conditions are better detected using other imaging techniques (radiography for multiple myeloma and radioactive iodine uptake for thyroid cancer).
- Metallic objects (e.g., jewelry, body rings) within the examination field, other nuclear scans done within the previous 24 to 48 hr, or retained barium from a previous radiological procedure, which may inhibit organ visualization and cause unclear images.
- Improper injection of the radionuclide that allows the tracer to seep deep into the muscle tissue can produce erroneous hot spots.
- Inability of the patient to cooperate or remain still during the procedure because movement can produce blurred or otherwise unclear images.

POTENTIAL MEDICAL DIAGNOSIS: CLINICAL SIGNIFICANCE OF RESULTS

Abnormal findings related to

Uneven distribution of the radionuclide, deposited in concentrated "hot spots," indicate areas where lesions, trauma, or degeneration in bone tissue are located.

- Bone necrosis
- Degenerative arthritis
- Fracture
- Legg-Calvé-Perthes disease

- Metastatic bone tumor
- Osteomyelitis
- Paget disease
- Primary metastatic bone tumors
- Renal osteodystrophy
- Rheumatoid arthritis

NURSING IMPLICATIONS

BEFORE THE STUDY: PLANNING AND IMPLEMENTATION

Teaching the Patient What to Expect

◗ Inform the patient this procedure can assist in identification of bone disease before it can be detected with plain x-ray images.

◗ Pregnancy is a general contraindication to procedures involving radiation. Explain to the female patient that she will be asked the date of her last menstrual period and pregnancy testing may be performed to determine the possibility of pregnancy before she is exposed to radiation.

◗ Review the procedure with the patient. Address concerns about pain and explain that there may be moments of discomfort or pain experienced when the IV line is inserted to allow infusion of fluids such as saline, anesthetics, sedatives, radionuclides, medications used in the procedure, or emergency medications.

◗ Inform the patient that the procedure is performed in a nuclear medicine department by a health-care provider (HCP), and staff, specializing in this procedure and takes approximately 30 to 60 min.

◗ **Pediatric Considerations:** Preparing children for a bone scan depends on the age of the child. Encourage parents to be truthful about what the child may experience during the procedure (e.g., there may be a pinch or minor discomfort when the IV needle is inserted) and to use words that they know their child will understand. Toddlers and preschool-age children have a very short attention span, so the best time

B

to talk about the test is right before the procedure. The child should be assured that he or she will be allowed to bring a favorite comfort item into the examination room and, if appropriate, that a parent will be with the child during the procedure.

- Reassure the patient that the radionuclide poses no radioactive hazard and rarely produces adverse effects.
- Instruct the patient to remove jewelry and other metallic objects from the area to be examined prior to the procedure.
- Baseline vital signs and neurological status will be recorded. Protocols may vary among facilities.
- Positioning for this procedure is at rest in the supine position; foam wedges may be used to help maintain position and immobilization.
- After a delay of 2 to 3 hr to allow the radionuclide to be taken up by the bones, multiple images are obtained over the complete skeleton. Delayed views may be taken up to 24 hr after the injection. At the conclusion of the study, the needle or catheter is removed and a pressure dressing is applied over the puncture site.

Potential Nursing Actions

- *Make sure a written and informed consent has been signed prior to the procedure and before administering any medications.*

AFTER THE STUDY: POTENTIAL NURSING ACTIONS

Avoiding Complications

- Establishing an IV site and injection of radionuclides are invasive procedures. Complications are rare but include risk for allergic reaction *(related to contrast reaction),* hematoma *(related to blood leakage into the tissue following needle insertion),* bleeding from the puncture site *(related to a bleeding disorder or the effects of natural products and medications with known anticoagulant, antiplatelet, or thrombolytic properties),* or infection *(which might occur if bacteria from the skin surface is introduced at the puncture site).* Monitor

the patient for complications related to the procedure (e.g., allergic reaction, anaphylaxis, bronchospasm). Immediately report symptoms such as fast heart rate, difficulty breathing, skin rash, itching, or chest pain to the appropriate HCP. Observe/assess the needle/catheter insertion site for bleeding, inflammation, or hematoma formation.

Treatment Considerations

- Explain that the radionuclide is eliminated from the body within 6 to 24 hr. Advise the patient to drink increased amounts of fluids for 24 to 48 hr to eliminate the radionuclide from the body, unless contraindicated.
- Evaluate the patient's vital signs. Monitor vital signs, and neurological status every 15 min for 1 hr, then every 2 hr for 4 hr, and then as ordered by the HCP. Monitor intake and output at least every 8 hr. Monitor ECG tracings until stable. Compare with baseline values. Protocols may vary among facilities.
- Administer ordered antiemetics. Collaborate with the patient to identify the pattern of nausea in relation to chemotherapy to better treat nausea. Monitor hydration with Intake and output. Evaluate skin turgor related to poor intake and administer ordered IV fluids. Consider small frequent meals to decrease nausea risk.
- Decrease exposure to the environment by placing the patient in a private room. Monitor and trend vital signs (temperature, blood pressure, heart and respiratory rates) and laboratory values that would indicate an infection (WBC count, C-reactive protein). Promote good hygiene and assist with hygiene as needed. Administer prescribed antibiotics, antipyretics, and IV fluids. Institute cooling measures, encourage oral fluids where appropriate, and facilitate the use of lightweight clothing and bedding to manage fever. Adhere to standard precautions, use isolation as appropriate, and ensure ordered cultures are completed.

B

◆ Collaborate with the patient to prioritize activities and conserve energy. Discuss limiting daytime napping to facilitate nighttime sleeping. Correct anemia if present with ordered interventions (blood transfusion, etc.). Address emotional distress with the use of social services and inclusion of psychotherapy if appropriate.

◆ Instruct the patient in the care and assessment of the injection site.

◆ Explain that application of cold compresses to the puncture site may reduce discomfort or edema.

Safety Considerations

◆ The patient who is breastfeeding should consult with the requesting HCP regarding alternative testing that does not involve radiation. In general, if a woman who is breastfeeding must have a nuclear scan, she should not breastfeed the infant for 72 hr after the scan, until the radionuclide has been eliminated. She should be instructed to express the milk in order to prevent cessation of milk production; the milk can be stored and used after the 3-day period.

◆ Refer to organizational policy for additional precautions that may include instructions on handwashing, toilet flushing, limited contact with others, and other aspects of nuclear medicine safety.

Nutritional Considerations

◆ Consider a consult with a registered dietitian to maximize caloric intake.

Follow-Up, Evaluation, and Desired Outcomes

◆ Acknowledges contact information provided for the American Cancer Society (www.cancer.org), American College of Rheumatology (www.rheumatology.org), or Arthritis Foundation (www.arthritis.org).

◆ Accepts that some fatigue associated with chemotherapy and radiation therapy is normal. Agrees to bundle activity to conserve energy and decrease fatigue.

◆ Acknowledges that eating in small amounts can decrease nausea. Agrees that spicy, greasy, fried, strong-odor foods that can precipitate nausea should be avoided.

◆ Understands that nausea may be better controlled by taking antiemetics around the clock rather than with each individual episode of nausea.

Bone Turnover Markers

SYNONYM/ACRONYM: NT_x, collagen cross-linked N-telopeptide.

RATIONALE: To evaluate the effectiveness of treatment for osteoporosis.

PATIENT PREPARATION: There are no food, fluid, activity, or medication restrictions unless by medical direction. As appropriate, provide the required urine collection container and specimen collection instructions.

NORMAL FINDINGS: Method: Immunoassay.

Adult male 18–29 yr	Less than 100 mmol bone collagen equivalents (BCE)/mmol creatinine
Adult male 30–59 yr	Less than 65 mmol BCE/mmol creatinine
Adult female (premenopausal)	Less than 65 mmol BCE/mmol creatinine

CRITICAL FINDINGS AND POTENTIAL INTERVENTIONS: N/A

OVERVIEW: (Study type: Urine from a random specimen collected in a clean plastic container; related body system: Musculoskeletal system.) Osteoporosis is often called the "silent disease" because bone loss occurs without symptoms. The formation and maintenance of bone mass is dependent on a combination of factors that include genetics, nutrition, exercise, and hormone function. Normally, the rate of bone formation is equal to the rate of bone resorption. After midlife, the rate of bone loss begins to increase. Osteoporosis is more commonly identified in women than in men. Other risk factors include thin, small-framed body structure; family history of osteoporosis; diet low in calcium; white or Asian ancestry; excessive use of alcohol; cigarette smoking; sedentary lifestyle; long-term use of corticosteroids, thyroid replacement medications, or antiepileptics; history of bulimia, anorexia nervosa, chronic liver disease, or malabsorption disorders; and postmenopausal state. Knowledge of genetics assists in identifying those who may benefit from additional education, risk assessment, and counseling. Genetics is the study and identification of genes, genetic mutations, and inheritance. Genomic studies evaluate the interaction of groups of genes. The combined activity or combined expression of groups of genes allows assumptions or predictions to be made. As an example, genomic studies measure the levels of activity in multiple genes to predict how they, along with environmental and lifestyle decisions, influence the development of reduction in bone mass, type 2 diabetes, coronary artery disease,

or ischemic stroke. Further information regarding inheritance of genes can be found in the study titled "Genetic Testing."

Osteoporosis is a major consequence of menopause in women owing to the decline of estrogen production. Osteoporosis is rare in premenopausal women. Estrogen replacement therapy (after menopause) is one strategy that has been commonly employed to prevent osteoporosis, although its exact protective mechanism is unknown. Results of some recently published studies indicate that there may be significant adverse effects to estrogen replacement therapy; more research is needed to understand the long-term effects (positive and negative) of this therapy. Other treatments include raloxifene (selectively modulates estrogen receptors), calcitonin (interacts directly with osteoclasts), and bisphosphates (inhibit osteoclast-mediated bone resorption).

A noninvasive test to detect the presence of collagen cross-linked N-telopeptide (NT_x) is used to follow the progress of patients who have begun treatment for osteoporosis. NT_x is formed when collagenase acts on bone. Small NT_x fragments are excreted in the urine after bone resorption. A desirable response, 2 to 3 mo after therapy is initiated, is a 30% reduction in NT_x and a reduction of 50% below baseline by 12 mo.

INDICATIONS
- Assist in the evaluation of osteoporosis.
- Assist in the management and treatment of osteoporosis.
- Monitor effects of estrogen replacement therapy.

B

INTERFERING FACTORS
- NT_x levels are affected by urinary excretion, and values may be influenced by the presence of kidney disease.

POTENTIAL MEDICAL DIAGNOSIS: CLINICAL SIGNIFICANCE OF RESULTS
Increased in
Conditions that reflect increased bone resorption are associated with increased levels of N-telopeptide in the urine.

- Alcohol misuse *(related to inadequate nutrition)*
- Chronic immobilization
- Chronic treatment with anticonvulsants, corticosteroids, gonadotropin releasing hormone agonists, heparin, or thyroid hormone
- Conditions that include hypercortisolism, hyperparathyroidism, hyperthyroidism, and hypogonadism
- Gastrointestinal disease *(related to inadequate dietary intake or absorption of minerals required for bone formation and maintenance)*

- Growth disorders (acromegaly, growth hormone deficiency, osteogenesis imperfecta)
- Hyperparathyroidism *(related to imbalance in calcium and phosphorus that affects the rate of bone resorption)*
- Multiple myeloma and metastatic tumors
- Osteomalacia *(related to defective bone mineralization)*
- Osteoporosis
- Paget disease
- Postmenopausal women *(related to estrogen deficiency)*
- Recent fracture
- Renal insufficiency *(related to excessive loss through renal dysfunction)*
- Rheumatoid arthritis and other connective tissue diseases *(related to inadequate diet due to loss of appetite)*

Decreased in
- Effective therapy for osteoporosis

NURSING IMPLICATIONS

POTENTIAL NURSING PROBLEMS: ASSESSMENT & NURSING DIAGNOSIS

Problems	Signs and Symptoms
Fall risk *(related to altered mobility associated with loss of bone mass)*	Postural instability; jerky movement; uncoordinated movement; slow, unsteady movement
Self-care *(related to loss of bone mass and physical deformity, pain, and limited range of motion)*	Difficulty fastening clothing, difficulty performing personal hygiene, inability to maintain appropriate appearance, difficulty with independent mobility

BEFORE THE STUDY: PLANNING AND IMPLEMENTATION

Teaching the Patient What to Expect
- Inform the patient this test can assist in diagnosing osteoporosis and evaluating the effectiveness of therapy.

- Explain that a urine sample is needed for the test. Instruct the patient to collect a second-void morning specimen as follows: (1) void and then drink a glass of water; (2) wait 30 min and then try to void again.

Information regarding specimen collection is presented with other general guidelines in Appendix A: Patient Preparation and Specimen Collection.

Potential Nursing Actions
Include on the collection container's label the specimen collection type (e.g., clean catch, catheter), date and time of collection, and any medications that may interfere with test results.

AFTER THE STUDY: POTENTIAL NURSING ACTIONS

Treatment Considerations
Self-Care: Reinforce self-care techniques as taught by occupational therapy. Ensure the patient has adequate time to perform self-care, and encourage use of assistive devices to maintain independence. Ask if there is any interference with lifestyle activities.

Safety Considerations
Fall Risk: Teach about fall precautions and assess home environment for fall risk. Evaluate medications for contributory cause related to recent falls. Encourage physical therapy to facilitate moderate exercise. Teach that low, comfortable walking shoes can promote safe ambulation and decrease fall risk.

Nutritional Considerations
Increased NT$_x$ levels may be associated with osteoporosis. Nutritional therapy may be indicated for patients identified as being at high risk for developing osteoporosis. Educate the patient about the National Osteoporosis Foundation's guidelines regarding a regular regimen of weight-bearing exercises, limited alcohol intake, avoidance of tobacco products, and adequate dietary intake of vitamin D and calcium. Dietary calcium can be obtained from animal or plant sources. Almonds (milk, nuts), beet greens, broccoli, cheese, clams, kale, legumes, milk and milk products, oysters, rhubarb, salmon (canned), sardines (canned), spinach, tofu, yogurt, and calcium fortified foods such as orange juice are high in calcium. Milk and milk products also contain vitamin D and lactose, which assist calcium absorption.

Follow-Up, Evaluation, and Desired Outcomes
Acknowledges contact information provided for the National Osteoporosis Foundation (www.nof.org) or American College of Rheumatology (www.rheumatology.org).

Bone X-ray

SYNONYM/ACRONYM: Arm x-rays, bone x-rays, leg x-rays, orthopedic x-rays, radiography bone, rib x-rays, skeletal x-rays, spine x-rays.

RATIONALE: To assist in evaluating bone pain, trauma, and abnormalities related to disorders or events such as dislocation, fracture, physical abuse, and degenerative disease.

PATIENT PREPARATION: There are no food, fluid, activity, or medication restrictions unless by medical direction.

NORMAL FINDINGS
• *Infants and children:* Thin plate of cartilage, known as *growth plate* or *epiphyseal plate,* between the shaft and both ends

- *Adolescents and adults:* By age 17, calcification of cartilage plate; no evidence of fracture, congenital abnormalities, tumors, or infection.

CRITICAL FINDINGS AND POTENTIAL INTERVENTIONS: N/A

OVERVIEW: (Study type: Radiography, plain; related body system: Musculoskeletal system.) Skeletal x-rays are noninvasive studies used to evaluate extremity pain or discomfort due to trauma, bone and spine abnormalities, or fluid within a joint. Serial skeletal x-rays are used to evaluate growth pattern. Radiation emitted from the x-ray machine passes through the patient onto an image receptor. X-rays pass through air freely and are absorbed by the anatomical structures of the body in varying degrees based on density. Bones are very dense and therefore absorb or attenuate most of the x-rays passing into the body and appear white; organs and muscles are denser than air but not as dense as bone, so they appear in various shades of gray. Metals absorb x-rays and appear white, which facilitates the search for foreign bodies in the patient.

INDICATIONS

- Assist in detecting bone fracture, dislocation, deformity, and degeneration.
- Evaluate for child or elder abuse.
- Evaluate growth pattern.
- Identify abnormalities of bones, joints, and surrounding tissues.
- Monitor fracture healing process.

INTERFERING FACTORS

Contraindications

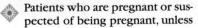 Patients who are pregnant or suspected of being pregnant, unless the potential benefits of a procedure using radiation far outweigh the risk of radiation exposure to the fetus and mother.

Factors that may alter the results of the study

- Retained barium from a previous radiological procedure.
- Metallic objects (e.g., jewelry, body rings) within the examination field, which may inhibit organ visualization and can produce unclear images.
- Inability of the patient to cooperate or remain still during the procedure, because movement can produce blurred or otherwise unclear images.

POTENTIAL MEDICAL DIAGNOSIS: CLINICAL SIGNIFICANCE OF RESULTS

Abnormal findings related to

- Arthritis
- Bone degeneration
- Bone spurs
- Foreign bodies
- Fracture
- Genetic disturbance (achondroplasia, dysplasia, dyostosis)
- Hormonal disturbance
- Infection, including osteomyelitis
- Injury
- Joint dislocation or effusion
- Nutritional or metabolic disturbances
- Osteoporosis or osteopenia
- Soft tissue abnormalities
- Tumor or neoplastic disease (osteogenic sarcoma, Paget disease, myeloma)

B

NURSING IMPLICATIONS

POTENTIAL NURSING PROBLEMS: ASSESSMENT & NURSING DIAGNOSIS

Problems	Signs and Symptoms
Inadequate tissue perfusion *(related to edema, inappropriate cast or appliance application, fracture instability)*	Loss of sensation in effected limb, capillary refill greater than 3 seconds, cool extremity, cyanosis, pain
Mobility *(related to inflammation, trauma, pain, infection, dislocation, genetic disturbance [deformity])*	Inability to meet physical demands associated with activities of daily living, ineffective range of motion, pain
Pain *(related to inflammation, trauma, pain, infection, dislocation, genetic disturbance [deformity], muscle spasms, application of supportive orthopedic equipment)*	Self-report of pain, moaning, crying, restlessness, anxiety, increased heart rate, increased blood pressure

BEFORE THE STUDY: PLANNING AND IMPLEMENTATION

Teaching the Patient What to Expect

▶ Inform the patient this procedure can assist in examining bone structure.
▶ Pregnancy is a general contraindication to procedures involving radiation. Explain to the female patient that she will be asked the date of her last menstrual period. Pregnancy testing may be performed to determine the possibility of pregnancy before exposure to radiation.
▶ Review the procedure with the patient. Address concerns about pain and explain that some pain may be experienced during the test, or there may be moments of discomfort; the extremity's position during the procedure may be uncomfortable, but ask the patient to hold still during the procedure because movement will produce unclear images.
▶ Inform the patient that the procedure is performed in the radiology department by a health-care provider (HCP), with support staff, and takes approximately 10 to 30 min.

▶ Explain that jewelry and other metallic objects must be removed from the area to be examined prior to the procedure.
▶ **Pediatric Considerations:** Preparation of children for a bone radiography depends on the age of the child. Encourage parents to be truthful about what the child may experience during the procedure and to use words that they know their child will understand. Toddlers and preschool-age children have short attention spans, so the best time to talk about the test is right before the procedure. The child should be assured that he or she will be allowed to bring a favorite comfort item into the examination room, and if appropriate, that a parent will be with the child during the procedure. Provide older children with information about the test and allow them to participate in as many decisions as possible (e.g., choice of clothes to wear to the appointment) in order to reduce anxiety and encourage cooperation. If the child will be asked to maintain a certain position for the test, encourage the child to practice

the required position, provide a CD that demonstrates the procedure, and teach strategies to remain calm, such as deep breathing, humming, or counting to himself or herself.

▶ Positioning for this procedure depends on the location of the area of interest; the patient will be positioned in a standing, sitting, or recumbent position in front of the image receptor or in the supine position on an examination table. The selected area will be cleansed and covered with a sterile drape.

AFTER THE STUDY: POTENTIAL NURSING ACTIONS

Avoiding Complications

▶ Teach the patient the signs and symptoms of impinged circulation due to cast or appliance application.

Treatment Considerations

▶ Inadequate Tissue Perfusion: Assess and monitor peripheral pulses, skin warmth, color, capillary refill, and sensation. Monitor for compartment syndrome, which is pain unrelieved by medication or other interventions. Monitor for increasing edema to effected limb, check the cast for pressure points, and monitor and trend vital signs (watch for hypotension that could contribute to poor tissue perfusion).

▶ Mobility: Immobilize the injured extremity. Facilitate the use of assistive devices, assist in maintaining body

alignment, and administer ordered medications (analgesics, steroids, antibiotics). Monitor and trend x-ray results and circulation and sensation with cast application. Facilitate physical therapy, encourage ambulation, and institute applicable fall risk protocols.

▶ Pain: Assess pain character, location, duration, intensity and use an easily understood pain rating scale. Place in a position of comfort and administer ordered medications: analgesics, narcotics, antipyretics, NSAIDs, antibiotics. Consider alternative measures for pain management: imagery, relaxation, music. Assess and trend vital signs and facilitate a calm quiet environment. Use caution when moving extremities; ensure orthopedic appliances are adjusted for best fit. Apply ice packs to affected areas as appropriate and assess and monitor the cast for pressure points.

Safety Considerations

▶ Teach the patient how to decrease fall risk by adhering to fall risk protocols.

Follow-Up, Evaluation, and Desired Outcomes

▶ Acknowledges contact information provided for the American College of Rheumatology (www.rheumatology .org) or the Arthritis Foundation (www .arthritis.org).

▶ Agrees to participate in recommended physical therapy to improve mobility.

▶ Demonstrates how to use assistive devices to support mobility.

Bronchoscopy

SYNONYM/ACRONYM: Flexible bronchoscopy.

RATIONALE: To visualize and assess bronchial structure for disease such as cancer and infection. The procedure has both diagnostic and therapeutic implications.

PATIENT PREPARATION: There are no activity restrictions unless by medical direction. Instruct the patient that to reduce the risk of aspiration related to nausea and vomiting, solid food and milk or milk products are restricted for at least

6 hr, and clear liquids are restricted for at least 2 hr prior to general anesthesia, regional anesthesia, or sedation/analgesia (monitored anesthesia). The patient may be required to be NPO at midnight. The American Society of Anesthesiologists has fasting guidelines for risk levels according to patient status. More information can be located at www.asahq.org.

Patients on beta blockers before the surgical procedure should be instructed to take their medication as ordered during the perioperative period. Regarding the patient's risk for bleeding, the patient should be instructed to avoid taking natural products and medications with known anticoagulant, antiplatelet, or thrombolytic properties or to reduce dosage, as ordered, prior to the procedure. Number of days to withhold medication is dependent on the type of anticoagulant. Note the last time and dose of medication taken. Protocols may vary among facilities.

NORMAL FINDINGS
• Normal larynx, trachea, bronchi, bronchioles, and alveoli.

CRITICAL FINDINGS AND POTENTIAL INTERVENTIONS: N/A

OVERVIEW: (Study type: Endoscopy; related body system: Respiratory system.) This procedure provides direct visualization of the larynx, trachea, and bronchial tree by means of either a rigid or more commonly, a flexible bronchoscope. A bronchoscope with a light incorporated is guided into the tracheobronchial tree. A local anesthetic may be used to allow the scope to be inserted through the mouth or nose into the trachea and into the bronchi. The patient must breathe during insertion and with the scope in place.

The rigid bronchoscope is used under general anesthesia and allows visualization of the larger airways, including the lobar, segmental, and subsegmental bronchi, while maintaining effective gas exchange. Rigid bronchoscopy is preferred when large volumes of blood or secretions need to be aspirated, large foreign bodies are to be removed, or large-sized biopsy specimens are to be obtained. The flexible bronchoscope has a smaller lumen that is designed to allow for visualization of all segments of the bronchial tree. The accessory lumen of the bronchoscope is used for tissue biopsy, bronchial washings, instillation of anesthetic drugs and medications, and to obtain specimens with brushes for cytological examination. In general, flexible bronchoscopy is less traumatic to the surrounding tissues than the larger rigid bronchoscopes. Flexible bronchoscopy is performed under local anesthesia; patient tolerance is better for flexible bronchoscopy than for rigid bronchoscopy.

INDICATIONS
• Detect end-stage bronchogenic cancer.
• Detect lung infections and inflammation.
• Determine etiology of persistent cough, hemoptysis, hoarseness, unexplained chest x-ray abnormalities, and/or abnormal cytological findings in sputum.
• Determine extent of smoke-inhalation or other traumatic injury.
• Evaluate airway patency; aspirate deep or retained secretions.

B

- Evaluate endotracheal tube placement or possible adverse sequelae to tube placement.
- Evaluate possible airway obstruction in patients with known or suspected sleep apnea.
- Evaluate respiratory distress and tachypnea in an infant to rule out tracheoesophageal fistula or other congenital anomaly.
- Identify and, as appropriate, cauterize bleeding sites, and remove clots within the tracheobronchial tree.
- Identify hemorrhagic and inflammatory changes in Kaposi sarcoma.
- Intubate patients with cervical spine injuries or massive upper airway edema.
- Remove foreign body.
- Treat lung cancer through instillation of chemotherapeutic drugs, implantation of radioisotopes, or laser palliative therapy.

INTERFERING FACTORS
Contraindications

Patients with bleeding disorders, especially those associated with uremia and cytotoxic chemotherapy.

Patients with pulmonary hypertension.

Patients with cardiac conditions or dysrhythmias.

Patients with disorders that limit extension of the neck.

Patients with severe obstructive tracheal conditions.

Patients with or having the potential for respiratory failure; *(introduction of the bronchoscope alone may cause a 10–20 mm Hg drop in Pao₂).*

Factors that may alter the results of the study
- Metallic objects within the examination field (e.g., jewelry, earrings, and/or dental amalgams), which may inhibit organ visualization and can produce unclear images.

Other considerations
- Hypoxemic or hypercapnic states require continuous oxygen administration.

POTENTIAL MEDICAL DIAGNOSIS: CLINICAL SIGNIFICANCE OF RESULTS
Abnormal findings related to
- Abscess
- Bronchial diverticulum
- Bronchial stenosis
- Bronchogenic cancer
- *Coccidioidomycosis, histoplasmosis, blastomycosis, phycomycosis*
- Foreign bodies
- Inflammation
- Interstitial pulmonary disease
- Opportunistic lung infections (e.g., *pneumocystitis, nocardia, cytomegalovirus*)
- Strictures
- Tuberculosis
- Tumors

NURSING IMPLICATIONS

POTENTIAL NURSING PROBLEMS: ASSESSMENT & NURSING DIAGNOSIS

Problems	Signs and Symptoms
Activity *(related to ineffective oxygenation secondary to obstruction, infection, inflammation, tumor, trauma, fistula, edema, hemorrhage, foreign body)*	Weakness, fatigue, chest pain with exertion, anxiety, shortness of breath, cyanosis, increased work of breathing, decreasing oxygen saturation, increased heart rate

Problems	Signs and Symptoms
Breathing *(related to obstruction, infection, inflammation, tumor, trauma, fistula, edema, hemorrhage, foreign body)*	Shortness of breath; cool, clammy skin; cyanosis; anxiety; pleuritic chest pain; decreased oxygenation; abnormal blood gas; increased work of breathing (use of accessory muscles); increased respiratory rate
Gas exchange *(related to obstruction, infection, inflammation, tumor, trauma, fistula, edema, hemorrhage, foreign body)*	Dyspnea; chest pain (pleuritic); diminished oxygenation, cyanosis; increased heart rate, respiratory rate, work of breathing; restlessness, anxiety, fear; adventitious breath sounds (rales, crackles); sense of impending death and doom; hemoptysis; abnormal arterial blood gas

BEFORE THE STUDY: PLANNING AND IMPLEMENTATION

Teaching the Patient What to Expect

▶ Inform the patient this procedure can assess the lungs and respiratory system.

▶ Review the procedure with the patient. Address concerns about pain and explain that there may be moments of discomfort or pain experienced when the IV line or catheter is inserted to allow infusion of fluids such as saline, anesthetics, sedatives, medications used in the procedure, or emergency medications.

▶ Baseline vital signs will be recorded and monitored throughout the procedure. Protocols may vary among facilities.

▶ Explain that a sedative and/or analgesia may be administered to promote relaxation and reduce discomfort prior to the bronchoscopy. Atropine is usually given before bronchoscopy examinations to reduce bronchial secretions and prevent vagally induced bradycardia. A local anesthetic such as lidocaine is sprayed in the patient's throat to reduce discomfort caused by the presence of the tube.

▶ Inform the patient that the procedure is performed in a respiratory or gastrointestinal laboratory or radiology department, under sterile conditions, by a health-care provider (HCP) specializing in this procedure. The procedure usually takes about 30 to 60 min to complete. Tissue samples are placed in properly labelled specimen containers containing formalin solution and promptly transported to the laboratory for processing and analysis.

Rigid Bronchoscopy

▶ Inform the patient that he or she will be placed in the supine position using a pillow underneath the head and a shoulder roll to align the pharynx, larynx, and trachea, after which a general anesthetic is administered. The patient's neck is hyperextended, and the lightly lubricated bronchoscope is inserted orally and passed through the glottis. The patient's head is turned or repositioned to aid visualization of various segments. After inspection, the bronchial brush, suction catheter, biopsy forceps, laser, and electrocautery devices are introduced to obtain specimens for cytological or microbiological study or for therapeutic procedures. If a bronchial washing is performed, small amounts of solution are instilled into the airways and removed.

Flexible Bronchoscopy

▶ Explain to the patient that he or she will be placed in a sitting or supine position while the tongue and

B

oropharynx are sprayed or swabbed with local anesthetic. An emesis basin will be provided for the increased saliva. Encourage the patient to spit out the saliva because the gag reflex may be impaired. When loss of sensation is adequate, the patient is placed in a supine or side-lying position. The flexible scope can be introduced through the nose, the mouth, an endotracheal tube, a tracheostomy tube, or a rigid bronchoscope. Most common insertion is through the nose. Patients with copious secretions or massive hemoptysis, or in whom airway complications are more likely, may be intubated before the bronchoscopy. Additional local anesthetic is applied through the scope as it approaches the vocal cords and the carina, eliminating reflexes (e.g., cough) in these sensitive areas. The flexible bronchoscopy approach allows visualization of airway segments without having to move the patient's head through various positions. After visual inspection of the lungs, tissue samples are collected from suspicious sites by bronchial brush or biopsy forceps to be used for cytological and microbiological studies.

Potential Nursing Actions

✺ *Make sure a written and informed consent has been signed prior to the procedure and before administering any medications.*

▶ Provide mouth care to reduce oral bacterial flora.

Safety Considerations

▶ The use of morphine for sedation in patients with asthma or other pulmonary disease should be avoided. This drug can further exacerbate bronchospasms and respiratory impairment.

▶ Anticoagulants, aspirin, and other salicylates should be discontinued by medical direction for the appropriate number of days prior to a procedure where bleeding is a potential complication.

AFTER THE STUDY: POTENTIAL NURSING ACTIONS

Avoiding Complications

▶ Bleeding *(related to a bleeding disorder or the effects of natural products and medications with known anticoagulant, antiplatelet, or thrombolytic properties),* bronchospasm, hemoptysis, hypoxemia, infection *(related to the use of an endoscope),* or pneumothorax. Monitor the patient for complications related to the procedure (e.g., bleeding, bronchospasm, infection, pneumothorax). Immediately report to the appropriate HCP symptoms such as absent breathing sounds, air hunger, excessive coughing, or dyspnea (indications of hemoptysis); elevated white blood cell count, fever, malaise, or tachycardia (indications of infection); dyspnea, tachypnea, anxiety, decreased breathing sounds, or restlessness (symptoms of developing pneumothorax). A chest x-ray may be ordered to check for the presence of pneumothorax. Observe/assess the needle/catheter insertion site for bleeding, inflammation, or hematoma formation. Administer ordered antihistamines or prophylactic steroids if the patient has an allergic reaction. The use of morphine sulfate in those with asthma or other pulmonary disease should be avoided. This drug can further exacerbate bronchospasms and respiratory impairment. Emergency resuscitation equipment should be readily available in the case of respiratory impairment or laryngospasm after intubation or after the procedure.

Establishing an IV site is an invasive procedure. Complications are rare but include risk for bleeding from the puncture site *(related to a bleeding disorder or the effects of natural products and medications with known anticoagulant, antiplatelet, or thrombolytic properties),* hematoma *(related to blood leakage into the tissue following needle insertion),* infection *(that might occur if bacteria from the skin surface is introduced at the puncture site),* or nerve injury *(that might occur if the needle strikes a nerve).*

Treatment Considerations

▶ After the bronchoscopy procedure and the bronchoscope is removed, the patient is placed in a semi-Fowler position (lying on the back, knees slightly bent, with head elevated to 45 degrees) to maximize ventilation during recovery.

▶ Monitor vital signs and neurological status every 15 min for 1 hr, then every 2 hr for 4 hr, and then as ordered by the HCP. Monitor temperature every 4 hr for 24 hr. Monitor intake and output at least every 8 hr. Compare with baseline values. Protocols very among facilities.

▶ Assess for nausea and pain. Administer antiemetic and analgesic medications as needed and as directed by the HCP.

▶ Administer antibiotic therapy if ordered. Remind the patient of the importance of completing the entire course of antibiotic therapy even if signs and symptoms disappear before completion of therapy.

▶ Inform the patient that some throat soreness and hoarseness may be experienced. Instruct the patient to treat throat discomfort with lozenges and warm gargles when the gag reflex returns. Inform the patient of smoking cessation programs as appropriate.

▶ Activity: Identify the patient's normal activity patterns. He or she may need to remain on bedrest to rest the heart and conserve oxygen. Administer ordered oxygen and have the patient wear oxygen with activity. Prioritize, pace, and bundle activities and increase as tolerated. Monitor and trend vital signs.

▶ Breathing: Assess and trend breath sounds, work of breathing, respiratory rate, and arterial blood gases. Use coping mechanisms to decrease anxiety. Position patient to facilitate breathing, elevate the head of the bed or bedrest as appropriate. Administer ordered analgesics. Encourage the patient to cough and deep breathe,

prepare for intubation, and administer ordered oxygen.

▶ Gas Exchange: Assess respiratory status to establish a baseline (rate, rhythm, depth). Administer ordered oxygen and assess saturation with pulse oximetry. Elevate the head of the bed to facilitate breathing and encourage drainage. Monitor and trend arterial blood gas results. Assess for cyanosis and work of breathing. Administer ordered medications, anticoagulants, antibiotics, bronchodilators, steroids, and diuretics.

Safety Considerations

▶ Assess the patient's ability to swallow before allowing the patient to attempt liquids or solid foods.

Nutritional Considerations

▶ Malnutrition is commonly seen in patients with severe respiratory disease for numerous reasons, including fatigue, lack of appetite, and gastrointestinal distress. Adequate intake of vitamins A and C is also important to prevent pulmonary infection and to decrease the extent of lung tissue damage. The importance of following the prescribed diet should be stressed to the patient/caregiver.

Follow-Up, Evaluation, and Desired Outcomes

▶ Correctly describes the pathophysiology behind diminished oxygenation and disease process. Understands that a health-care specialist may need to be consulted to assist managing the disease.

▶ Demonstrates techniques for controlled breathing to improve breathing patterns. Recognizes the value in identifying strategies to bundle and pace activities to improve activity tolerance.

▶ Correctly describes reportable signs and symptoms of poor oxygenation and recognizes the importance of keeping oxygen on at all times.

▶ Agrees to make required lifestyle changes to support positive health.

B-Type Natriuretic Peptide and Pro-B-Type Natriuretic Peptide

SYNONYM/ACRONYM: BNP and proBNP.

RATIONALE: To assist in diagnosing heart failure (HF).

PATIENT PREPARATION: There are no food, fluid, activity, or medication restrictions unless by medical direction.

NORMAL FINDINGS: Method: Chemiluminescent immunoassay for BNP; electrochemiluminescent immunoassay for proBNP.

BNP	Conventional Units	SI Units (Conventional Units × 1)
Male and Female **proBNP (N-terminal)**	Less than 100 pg/mL	Less than 100 ng/L
0–74 yr	Less than 125 pg/mL	Less than 125 ng/L
Greater than 75 yr	Less than 449 pg/mL	Less than 449 ng/L

BNP levels are increased in older adults.

CRITICAL FINDINGS AND POTENTIAL INTERVENTIONS: N/A

OVERVIEW: (Study type: Blood collected in a lavender-top [EDTA] tube; **related body system:** Circulatory system.) The peptides B-type natriuretic peptide (BNP) and atrial natriuretic peptide (ANP) are antagonists of the renin-angiotensin-aldosterone system; they assist in the regulation of electrolytes, fluid balance, and blood pressure. BNP, proBNP, and ANP are useful markers in the diagnosis of heart failure (HF). BNP, first isolated in the brain of pigs, is a neurohormone synthesized primarily in the ventricles of the human heart in response to increases in ventricular pressure and volume. Circulating levels of BNP and proBNP increase in proportion to the severity of heart failure. A rapid BNP point-of-care immunoassay may be performed, in which a venous blood sample is collected, placed on a strip, and inserted into a device that measures BNP. Results are completed in 10 to 15 min. Conditions that can contribute to the development or acceleration of HF include anemia, congenital heart defect, diabetes, hypertension, kidney disease, and thyroid disease.

INDICATIONS

- Assist in determining the prognosis and therapy of patients with heart failure.
- Assist in the diagnosis of heart failure.

- Assist in differentiating heart failure from pulmonary disease.
- Cost-effective screen for left ventricular dysfunction; positive findings would point to the need for echocardiography and further assessment.

INTERFERING FACTORS
Contraindications
Patients receiving nesiritide. Nesiritide (Natrecor) is a recombinant form of BNP that may be given therapeutically by IV to patients in acutely decompensated heart failure; with some assays, BNP levels may be transiently and significantly elevated at the time of administration and must be interpreted with caution. The testing laboratory should be consulted to verify whether test measurements are affected by nesiritide.

Factors that may alter the results of the study
- Age: BNP levels are increased in older adults

POTENTIAL MEDICAL DIAGNOSIS: CLINICAL SIGNIFICANCE OF RESULTS
Increased in
BNP is secreted in response to increased hemodynamic load caused by physiological stimuli, as with ventricular stretch or endocrine stimuli from the aldosterone/renin system. Increasing BNP levels would indicate a worsening condition.

- Acute kidney injury
- Cardiac inflammation (myocarditis, cardiac allograft rejection)
- Chronic kidney disease
- Cirrhosis
- Cushing syndrome
- Heart failure
- Kawasaki disease
- Left ventricular hypertrophy
- Myocardial infarction
- Primary hyperaldosteronism
- Primary pulmonary hypertension
- Ventricular dysfunction

Decreased in
Decreasing BNP levels would indicate improvement.

NURSING IMPLICATIONS

POTENTIAL NURSING PROBLEMS: ASSESSMENT & NURSING DIAGNOSIS

Problems	Signs and Symptoms
Cardiac output *(related to increased preload, increased afterload, impaired cardiac contractility, cardiac muscle disease, altered cardiac conduction)*	Decreased peripheral pulses; decreased urinary output; cool, clammy skin; tachypnea; dyspnea; edema; altered level of consciousness; abnormal heart sounds; crackles in lungs; decreased activity tolerance; weight gain; fatigue; hypoxia
Excess fluid volume *(related to altered cardiac output)*	Edema; shortness of breath; increased weight; ascites, rales, and rhonchi; diluted laboratory values; increased blood pressure; positive jugular venous distention (JVD); orthopnea; cough; restlessness; tachycardia; pulmonary congestion with x-ray

(table continues on page 248)

Problems	Signs and Symptoms
Gas exchange *(related to altered alveolar and capillary exchange secondary to fluid in the alveoli)*	Decreased activity tolerance, increased shortness of breath with activity, weakness, orthopnea, cyanosis, cough, increased heart rate, weight gain, edema in the lower extremities, increased respiratory rate, use of respiratory accessory muscles
Tissue perfusion *(related to compromised cardiac contractility, interrupted blood flow)*	Hypotension, dizziness, cool extremities, capillary refill greater than 3 sec, weak pedal pulses, altered level of consciousness

BEFORE THE STUDY: PLANNING AND IMPLEMENTATION

Teaching the Patient What to Expect

▶ Inform the patient this test can assist in diagnosing heart failure.

▶ Explain that a blood sample is needed for the test.

AFTER THE STUDY: POTENTIAL NURSING ACTIONS

Treatment Considerations

▶ Cardiac Output: Assess peripheral pulses and capillary refill. Monitor blood pressure and check for orthostatic changes (dizziness) related to fluid loss. Assess respiratory rate, breath sounds, orthopnea, skin color and temperature, and level of consciousness. Monitor urinary output, sodium and potassium levels, and BNP levels. Administer ordered oxygen and use pulse oximetry to monitor oxygenation. Administer ordered medications aldosterone antagonists, angiotensin-converting enzyme (ACE) inhibitors, beta blockers, diuretics, inotropic drugs, and vasodilators. Explain the importance of taking prescribed medications to support cardiac health.

▶ Excess Fluid Volume: Daily weight with monitoring of trends. Limit fluid as appropriate. Assess for peripheral edema, JVD, adventitious lung sounds such as crackles. Monitor blood pressure, heart rate, and intake versus output. Administer prescribed diuretics, restrict sodium intake, and order a low-sodium diet. Monitor laboratory values that reflect alterations in fluid status and manage underlying cause of fluid alteration.

▶ Gas Exchange: Auscultate and trend breath sounds. Assess respiratory rate and administer ordered oxygen with pulse oximetry to monitor oxygenation. Collaborate with the health-care provider (HCP) to consider intubation and/or mechanical ventilation as appropriate. Place the head of the bed in high Fowler position. Administer ordered diuretics and vasodilators. Monitor potassium levels.

▶ Tissue Perfusion: Monitor blood pressure. Assess for dizziness, pedal pulses, capillary refill, and skin temperature for warmth.

Nutritional Considerations

▶ Instruct patients to consume a variety of foods within the basic food groups, eat foods high in potassium when taking diuretics, eat a diet high in fiber (25–35 g/day), maintain a healthy weight, be physically active, limit salt intake to 2,000 mg/day, limit alcohol intake, and be a nonsmoker.

▶ Recommend consultation with a registered dietitian. High-potassium foods (bananas, strawberries, oranges; cantaloupes; green leafy vegetables such as spinach and broccoli; dried fruits such as dates, prunes, and raisins; legumes such as peas and pinto beans; nuts and whole grains) can offset the loss of potassium from taking diuretics. Emphasize limiting dietary salt to recommended daily amount.

Follow-Up, Evaluation, and Desired Outcomes

▶ Details the purpose of taking pre-scribed medications: diuretic, ACE inhibitor, and/or beta blocker.

▶ Acknowledges the importance of limiting fluids to decrease cardiac stress, including strategies to limit fluid intake.

▶ Safely self-administers ordered oxygen.

▶ Demonstrates how to keep an accurate intake and output and acknowledges the importance of a daily weight to monitor fluid fluctuations.

▶ Understands the importance of reporting life-threatening changes such as cool extremities, pallor, and diaphoresis to HCP immediately.

Calcitonin

SYNONYM/ACRONYM: Thyrocalcitonin.

RATIONALE: To diagnose and monitor the effectiveness of treatment for medullary thyroid cancer.

PATIENT PREPARATION: There are no fluid, activity, or medication restrictions unless by medical direction. Instruct the patient to fast for 10 to 12 hr before specimen collection. Protocols may vary among facilities. Specimen stability is best maintained if the collection tube is prechilled and then immediately transported to the laboratory in an ice slurry.

NORMAL FINDINGS: Method: Chemiluminescent immunoassay.

	Conventional Units	SI Units (Conventional Units × 1)
Calcitonin *Baseline*		
Male	Less than 10 pg/mL	Less than 10 ng/L
Female	Less than 5 pg/mL	Less than 5 ng/L

CRITICAL FINDINGS AND POTENTIAL INTERVENTIONS: N/A

OVERVIEW: (**Study type:** Blood collected in a gold-, red-, or red/gray-top tube; **related body system:** Endocrine.) Calcitonin, also called *thyrocalcitonin*, is a hormone secreted mainly by the parafollicular or C cells of the thyroid gland in response to elevated serum calcium levels. The lungs and intestinal tract are other tissues that synthesize calcitonin to a lesser degree. Calcitonin is also secreted by tumors of the C cells and is therefore a useful marker for medullary thyroid cancer. Calcitonin participates in the regulation of calcium and phosphorus levels by antagonizing the effects of parathyroid hormone and vitamin D. It inhibits the activity of osteoclasts so that calcium continues to be laid down in bone rather than be reabsorbed with phosphorus into the blood. Calcitonin also inhibits tubular reabsorption of calcium and phosphorus, which increases their renal excretion.

The net result is that calcitonin decreases the serum calcium level. Calcitonin is used therapeutically, by injection or nasal spray, in the case of osteoporosis to help slow down bone loss. The pentagastrin (Peptavlon) provocation test and the calcium pentagastrin provocation test are useful for diagnosing medullary thyroid cancer.

INDICATIONS

- Assist in the diagnosis of hyperparathyroidism.
- Assist in the diagnosis of medullary thyroid cancer.
- Evaluate altered serum calcium levels.
- Monitor response to therapy for medullary thyroid cancer.
- Predict recurrence of medullary thyroid cancer.
- Screen family members of patients with medullary thyroid cancer (20% have a familial pattern).

C

INTERFERING FACTORS
Factors that may alter the results of the study
- Drugs and other substances that may increase calcitonin levels include calcium, epinephrine, estrogens, glucagon, oral contraceptives, pentagastrin, and sincalide.

POTENTIAL MEDICAL DIAGNOSIS: CLINICAL SIGNIFICANCE OF RESULTS
Increased in
- Cancer of the breast, lung, and pancreas *(related to metastasis of calcitonin-producing cells to other organs)*
- Carcinoid syndrome *(related to calcitonin-producing tumor cells)*
- C-cell hyperplasia *(related to increased production due to hyperplasia)*
- Chronic kidney disease *(related to increased excretion of calcium and retention of phosphorus resulting in release of calcium from body stores; C cells respond to an increase in serum calcium levels)*
- Cirrhosis *(related to chronic alcohol misuse)*
- Ectopic secretion *(especially neuroendocrine origins)*
- Hypercalcemia (any cause) *(related to increased production by C cells in response to increased calcium levels)*
- Medullary thyroid cancer *(related to overproduction by cancerous cells)*
- MEN type II *(related to calcitonin-producing tumor cells)*
- Pancreatitis *(related to alcohol misuse or hypercalcemia)*
- Pernicious anemia *(related to hypergastrinemia)*
- Pheochromocytoma *(related to calcitonin-producing tumor cells)*
- Pregnancy (late) *(related to increased maternal loss of circulating calcium to developing fetus; release of calcium from maternal stores stimulates increased release of calcitonin)*
- Pseudohypoparathyroidism *(related to release of calcium from body stores initiates feedback response from C cells)*
- Thyroiditis *(related to calcitonin-producing tumor cells)*
- Zollinger-Ellison syndrome *(related to hypergastrinemia)*

Decreased in: N/A

NURSING IMPLICATIONS

BEFORE THE STUDY: PLANNING AND IMPLEMENTATION
Teaching the Patient What to Expect
- Inform the patient this test can assist in assessing the thyroid gland for disease or can monitor effectiveness of therapy.
- Explain that a blood sample is needed for the test.

AFTER THE STUDY: POTENTIAL NURSING ACTIONS
Follow-Up, Evaluation, and Desired Outcomes
- Acknowledges the importance of strict adherence to the individualized treatment plan to improve overall health.
- Considers instituting advance directive to identify health-care wishes if faced with a terminal prognosis.

Calcium, Blood, Total and Ionized

SYNONYM/ACRONYM: Total and free calcium, Ca (total), unbound calcium (ionized), Ca^{++} (ionized), Ca^{2+} (ionized).

RATIONALE: To investigate various conditions, such as hypercalcemia and hypocalcemia, related to abnormally increased or decreased calcium levels.

PATIENT PREPARATION: There are no food, fluid, activity, or medication restrictions unless by medical direction.

NORMAL FINDINGS: Method: Spectrophotometry for total calcium; ion-selective electrode for ionized calcium.

Calcium, Total

Age	Conventional Units	SI Units (Conventional Units × 0.25)
Cord	8.2–11.2 mg/dL	2.1–2.8 mmol/L
0–10 days	7.6–10.4 mg/dL	1.9–2.6 mmol/L
11 d–2 yr	9–11 mg/dL	2.2–2.8 mmol/L
3–12 yr	8.8–10.8 mg/dL	2.2–2.7 mmol/L
13 yr–adult	8.4–10.2 mg/dL	2.1–2.6 mmol/L
Adult older than 90 yr	8.2–9.6 mg/dL	2.1–2.4 mmol/L

Calcium, Ionized

Age	Conventional Units	SI Units (Conventional Units × 0.25)
Whole blood		
0–11 mo	4.2–5.84 mg/dL	1.05–1.46 mmol/L
1 yr–adult	4.6–5.08 mg/dL	1.15–1.27 mmol/L
Plasma		
Adult	4.12–4.92 mg/dL	1.03–1.23 mmol/L
Serum		
1–18 yr	4.8–5.52 mg/dL	1.2–1.38 mmol/L
Adult and older adult	4.64–5.28 mg/dL	1.16–1.32 mmol/L

CRITICAL FINDINGS AND POTENTIAL INTERVENTIONS

Calcium, Total
- Less than 7 mg/dL (SI: Less than 1.8 mmol/L)
- Greater than 12 mg/dL (SI: Greater than 3 mmol/L) (some patients can tolerate higher concentrations)

Calcium, Ionized
- Less than 3.2 mg/dL (SI: Less than 0.8 mmol/L)
- Greater than 6.2 mg/dL (SI: Greater than 1.6 mmol/L)

C

Timely notification to the requesting health-care provider (HCP) of any critical findings and related symptoms is a role expectation of the professional nurse. A listing of these findings varies among facilities.

Consideration may be given to verification of critical findings before action is taken. Policies vary among facilities and may include requesting immediate recollection and retesting by the laboratory or retesting using a rapid point-of-care testing instrument at the bedside, if available.

Observe the patient for symptoms of critically decreased or elevated calcium levels. Hypocalcemia is evidenced by convulsions, nervousness, dysrhythmias, changes in electrocardiogram (ECG) in the form of prolonged ST segment and Q-T interval, facial spasms (positive Chvostek sign), tetany, lethargy, muscle cramps, tetany, numbness in extremities, tingling, and muscle twitching (positive Trousseau sign). Possible interventions include seizure precautions, increased frequency of ECG monitoring, and administration of calcium or magnesium.

Severe hypercalcemia is manifested by excessive thirst, polyuria, constipation, changes in ECG (shortened QT interval due to shortening of the ST segment and prolonged PR interval), lethargy, confusion, muscle weakness, joint aches, apathy, anorexia, headache, nausea, and vomiting; ultimately, severe hypercalcemia may result in coma. Possible interventions include the administration of normal saline and diuretics to speed up dilution and excretion or administration of calcitonin or steroids to force the circulating calcium into the cells.

OVERVIEW: (Study type: Blood collected in a gold-, red-, red/gray-top tube, or green-top [heparin] tube; **related body system:** Circulatory, Circulatory/Hematopoietic, Digestive, Endocrine, Musculoskeletal, Nervous, and Urinary systems.) Calcium, the most abundant cation in the body, participates in almost all of the body's vital processes. Calcium concentration is largely regulated by the parathyroid glands and by the action of vitamin D. Of the body's calcium reserves, 98% to 99% is stored in the teeth and skeleton. Calcium values are higher in children because of growth and active bone formation. About 45% of the total amount of blood calcium circulates as free ions that participate in numerous regulatory functions, including bone development and maintenance, blood coagulation, transmission of nerve impulses, activation of enzymes, stimulation of the glandular secretion of hormones, and control of skeletal and cardiac muscle contractility. The remaining calcium is bound to circulating proteins (40% bound mostly to albumin) and anions (15% bound to anions such as bicarbonate, citrate, phosphate, and lactate) and plays no physiological role. Calcium values can be adjusted up or down by 0.8 mg/dL (0.2 mmol/L) for every 1 g/dL (10 g/L) that albumin is greater than or less than 4 g/dL (40 g/L). Calcium levels are regulated largely by the parathyroid glands and by vitamin D; calcium levels are inversely proportional to parathyroid hormone (PTH) levels. Vitamin D enhances gastrointestinal (GI) absorption of calcium. Calcium and phosphorus levels are inversely proportional.

Fluid and electrolyte imbalances are often seen in patients with serious illness or injury; in these clinical situations, the normal homeostatic balance of the body is altered. During surgery or in the case of a critical illness, bicarbonate, phosphate, and lactate concentrations can change dramatically. Therapeutic treatments may also cause or contribute to electrolyte imbalance. This is why total calcium values can sometimes be misleading. Abnormal calcium levels are used to indicate general malfunctions in various body systems. Compared to total calcium level, ionized calcium is a better measurement of calcium metabolism. Ionized calcium levels are not influenced by protein concentrations, as seen in patients with hypoalbuminemia, chronic kidney disease, nephrotic syndrome, malabsorption, and multiple myeloma. Levels are also not affected in patients with metabolic acid-base balance disturbances. Elevations in ionized calcium may be seen when the total calcium is normal. Measurement of ionized calcium is useful to monitor patients undergoing cardiothoracic surgery or organ transplantation. It is also useful in the evaluation of patients in cardiac arrest.

Calcium values should be interpreted in conjunction with results of other tests. Normal calcium with an abnormal phosphorus value indicates impaired calcium absorption (possibly because of altered parathyroid hormone level or activity). Normal calcium with an elevated urea nitrogen value indicates possible hyperparathyroidism (primary or secondary). Normal calcium with decreased albumin value is an indication of hypercalcemia. The most common cause of hypocalcemia is hypoalbuminemia. The most common causes of hypercalcemia are hyperparathyroidism and cancer (with or without bone metastases).

INDICATIONS
- Detect ectopic PTH-producing tumors.
- Detect parathyroid gland loss after thyroid or other neck surgery, as indicated by decreased levels.
- Evaluate cardiac dysrhythmias and coagulation disorders to determine if altered serum calcium level is contributing to the problem.
- Evaluate the effect of protein on calcium levels.
- Evaluate the effects of various disorders on calcium metabolism, especially diseases involving bone.
- Identify individuals with hypo- or hypercalcemia.
- Identify individuals with toxic levels of vitamin D.
- Investigate suspected hyperparathyroidism.
- Monitor the effectiveness of therapy being administered to correct abnormal calcium levels, especially calcium deficiencies.
- Monitor patients with chronic kidney disease or organ transplantation in whom secondary hyperparathyroidism may be a complication.
- Monitor patients with sepsis or magnesium deficiency.

INTERFERING FACTORS
Factors that may alter the results of the study
- Drugs and other substances that may increase calcium levels include anabolic steroids, some antacids, calcitriol, calcium salts, danazol, diuretics (long-term), ergocalciferol, hydralazine, isotretinoin, lithium, oral contraceptives, parathyroid extract, parathyroid hormone, prednisone, progesterone, tamoxifen, vitamin A, and vitamin D.

- Hemolysis may cause falsely increased results.
- Patients who ingest large amounts of milk, calcium or vitamin D supplements, or antacid tablets shortly before specimen collection will have increased calcium values.
- Venous hemostasis caused by pro-longed use of a tourniquet during venipuncture can falsely elevate calcium levels.
- Drugs and other substances that may decrease calcium levels include acetazolamide, albuterol, alprostadil, aminoglycosides, anti-convulsants, asparaginase, aspirin, calcitonin, cisplatin, citrates, diuret-ics (initially), estrogens, foscarnet, gastrin, glucagon, glucocorticoids, glucose, heparin, insulin, laxatives (excessive use), magnesium salts, methicillin, phosphates, plicamycin, sodium sulfate (given IV), tetracy-cline (in pregnancy), trazodone, and viomycin.
- Patients on ethylenediaminetctra-acetic acid (EDTA) therapy (chela-tion) may show falsely decreased calcium values.
- Patients receiving massive blood transfusions may experience decreased ionized calcium values related to chelation of the free calcium by the anticoagulant in the blood products.
- Patients with chronic kidney dis-ease, especially those on hemodial-ysis, may have low calcium levels. The inability of the kidneys to filter excess phosphorus from the blood into urine stimulates abnor-mal excretion of calcium, resulting in lower circulating calcium levels. If the calcium concentration in the dialysate fluid is not adjusted to correct the blood levels, the parathyroid glands secrete PTH, which causes calcium to be lost from the bones. Over time, bone

loss results in deformities and loss of function.
- Patients with low albumin levels (e.g., in cases of malnutrition or dilutional effect of IV fluid excess) will have low total calcium levels.

Other considerations
- Calcium exhibits diurnal variation; serial samples should be col-lected at the same time of day for comparison.
- Specimens should never be col-lected above an IV line because of the potential for dilution when the specimen and the IV solution com-bine in the collection container, falsely decreasing the result. There is also the potential of contaminat-ing the sample with the substance of interest if it is present in the IV solution, falsely increasing the result.

POTENTIAL MEDICAL DIAGNOSIS: CLINICAL SIGNIFICANCE OF RESULTS
Increased in
- Acidosis *(related to imbalance in electrolytes; longstanding acido-sis can result in osteoporosis and release of calcium into circulation)*
- Acromegaly *(related to alteration in vitamin D metabolism, resulting in increased calcium)*
- Addison disease *(related to adrenal gland dysfunction; decreased blood volume and dehydration occur in the absence of aldosterone)*
- Cancers (bone, Burkitt lymphoma, Hodgkin lymphoma, leukemia, myeloma, and metastases from other organs)
- Dehydration *(related to a decrease in the fluid portion of blood, causing an overall increase in the concentration of most plasma constituents)*
- Hyperparathyroidism *(related to increased PTH and vitamin D levels,*

which increase circulating calcium levels)
- Idiopathic hypercalcemia of infancy
- Kidney transplant *(related to imbalances in electrolytes; a common post-transplant issue)*
- Lung disease (tuberculosis, histoplasmosis, coccidioidomycosis, berylliosis) *(related to activity by macrophages in the epithelium that interfere with vitamin D regulation by converting it to its active form; vitamin D increases circulating calcium levels)*
- Malignant disease without bone involvement *(some cancers [e.g., squamous cell cancer of the lung and kidney cancer] produce PTH-related peptide that increases calcium levels)*
- Milk-alkali syndrome (Burnett syndrome) *(related to excessive intake of calcium-containing milk or antacids, which can increase calcium levels)*
- PTH-producing tumors *(PTH increases calcium levels)*
- Paget disease *(related to calcium released from bone)*
- Pheochromocytoma *(hyperparathyroidism related to multiple endocrine neoplasia type 2A [MEN2A] syndrome associated with some pheochromocytomas; PTH increases calcium levels)*
- Polycythemia vera *(related to dehydration; decreased blood volume due to excessive production of red blood cells)*
- Sarcoidosis *(related to activity by macrophages in the granulomas that interfere with vitamin D regulation by converting it to its active form; vitamin D increases circulating calcium levels)*
- Thyrotoxicosis *(related to increased bone turnover and release of calcium into the blood)*

- Vitamin D toxicity *(vitamin D increases circulating calcium levels)*

Decreased in
- Acute pancreatitis *(complication of pancreatitis related to hypoalbuminemia and calcium binding by excessive fats)*
- Alcohol misuse *(related to insufficient nutrition)*
- Alkalosis *(increased blood pH causes intracellular uptake of calcium to increase)*
- Burns, severe *(related to increased amino acid release)*
- Chronic kidney disease *(related to decreased synthesis of vitamin D)*
- Cystinosis *(hereditary disorder of the renal tubules that results in excessive calcium loss)*
- Hepatic cirrhosis *(related to impaired metabolism of vitamin D and calcium)*
- Hyperphosphatemia *(phosphorus and calcium have an inverse relationship)*
- Hypoalbuminemia *(related to insufficient levels of albumin, an important carrier protein)*
- Hypomagnesemia *(lack of magnesium inhibits PTH and thereby decreases calcium levels)*
- Hypoparathyroidism (congenital, idiopathic, surgical) *(related to lack of PTH)*
- Inadequate nutrition
- Leprosy *(related to increased bone resorption)*
- Long-term anticonvulsant therapy *(these medications block calcium channels and interfere with calcium transport)*
- Magnesium deficiency *(inhibits release of PTH)*
- Malabsorption (celiac disease, tropical sprue, pancreatic insufficiency) *(related to insufficient absorption)*

- Massive blood transfusion *(related to the presence of citrate preservative in blood product that chelates or binds calcium and removes it from circulation)*
- Multiple organ failure
- Osteomalacia (advanced) *(bone loss is so advanced there is little calcium remaining to be released into circulation)*
- Premature infants with hypoproteinemia and acidosis *(related to alterations in transport protein levels)*
- Pseudohypoparathyroidism *(related to decreased PTH)*
- Sepsis *(related to decreased PTH)*
- The postdialysis period *(result of low-calcium dialysate administration)*
- Trauma (i.e., major surgeries) *(related to decreased PTH)*
- Renal tubular disease *(related to decreased synthesis of vitamin D)*
- Vitamin D deficiency (rickets) *(related to insufficient amounts of vitamin D, resulting in decreased calcium metabolism)*

NURSING IMPLICATIONS

POTENTIAL NURSING PROBLEMS: ASSESSMENT & NURSING DIAGNOSIS

Problems	Signs and Symptoms
Health management *(related to failure to regulate diet, lack of exercise, alcohol use, smoking)*	Inability or failure to recognize or process information toward improving health and preventing illness with associated mental and physical effects
Injury risk *(related to phosphorous retention, bone resorption, inadequate calcium resorption, acute kidney injury or chronic kidney disease, lack of dietary vitamin D, decreased sun exposure, eating disorders)*	Tingling sensation in the fingertips and around the mouth, muscle cramps, tetany, seizures, bone pain, weakness, unsteady gait, laryngospasm, cardiac dysrhythmias, hyperactive tendon reflexes
Nutrition *(related to inability to digest, metabolize, ingest foods; refusal to eat; increased metabolic needs associated with disease process; lack of understanding; inability to obtain healthy foods)*	Unintended weight loss; current weight 20% below ideal weight; pale, dry skin; dry mucous membranes; documented inadequate caloric intake; subcutaneous tissue loss; hair pulls out easily; paresthesia
Pain *(related to organ inflammation and surrounding tissues, infection, bone deformity)*	Emotional symptoms of distress, crying, agitation, facial grimace, moaning, verbalization of pain, rocking motions, irritability, disturbed sleep, diaphoresis, altered blood pressure and heart rate, nausea, vomiting, self-report of pain

BEFORE THE STUDY: PLANNING AND IMPLEMENTATION

Teaching the Patient What to Expect

▶ Inform the patient this test can assist as a general indicator in diagnosing health concerns.
▶ Explain that a blood sample is needed for the test.

AFTER THE STUDY: POTENTIAL NURSING ACTIONS

Treatment Considerations

▶ Health Management: Encourage regular participation in weight-bearing exercises. Assess diet, smoking, and alcohol use. Teach the importance of adequate calcium intake with diet and supplements. Refer to smoking cessation and alcohol treatment programs. Collaborate with HCP for bone density evaluation.
▶ Injury Risk: Assess for signs and symptoms of hypocalcemia. Monitor and trend calcium and phosphorus levels. Administer ordered replacement therapy. Assess for bone pain and alterations in mobility. Increase dietary calcium and encourage the minimum recommended sun exposure.
▶ Pain: Collaborate with the patient and HCP to identify the best pain management modality to provide relief. Refrain from activities that may aggravate pain. Use the application of heat or cold to the best effect in managing the pain. Monitor pain severity.

Nutritional Considerations

▶ Complete an accurate daily weight at the same time each day with the same scale. Obtain an accurate nutritional history and assess attitude toward eating. Promote a dietary consult to evaluate current eating habits and best method of nutritional supplementation. Develop short-term and long-term eating strategies. Monitor nutritional laboratory values such as albumin, hemoglobin (Hgb), iron, red blood cells (RBCs), white blood cells (WBCs), and serum electrolytes. Discourage caffeinated and carbonated beverages. Assess swallowing ability, encourage cultural home foods, and provide a pleasant environment for eating. Alter food seasoning to enhance flavor. Provide parenteral or enteral nutrition as prescribed.
▶ Patients with abnormal calcium values should be informed that daily intake of calcium is important even though body stores in the bones can be called on to supplement circulating levels. Dietary calcium can be obtained from animal or plant sources. Almonds (milk, nuts), beet greens, broccoli, cheese, clams, kale, legumes, milk and milk products, oysters, rhubarb, salmon (canned), sardines (canned), spinach, tofu, yogurt, and calcium-fortified foods such as orange juice are high in calcium. Milk and milk products also contain vitamin D and lactose, which assist calcium absorption.
▶ Teach the patient that good oral hygiene prior to eating can improve the food's flavor. Discuss the importance of adequate dietary calcium intake to maintain health.

Follow-Up, Evaluation, and Desired Outcomes

▶ Acknowledges the value of contact information provided for the U.S. Department of Agriculture's resource for nutrition (www.choosemyplate.gov)
▶ Understands the signs and symptoms associated with a calcium imbalance.
▶ Recognizes the importance of associated studies such as ECG, phosphorus, and albumin so the correct therapeutic measures can be taken. Hypoalbuminemia may initiate symptoms of hypocalcemia in the presence of near-normal calcium levels.
▶ Agrees to meet with a speech therapist to evaluate swallowing ability, as appropriate.
▶ Accurately demonstrates how to perform a daily self-weight and to record the results correctly.
▶ Understands that parenteral or enteral nutrition may be used if oral intake is insufficient to support caloric needs.
▶ Adheres to the request to take prescribed calcium replacement therapy and can accurately self-administer prescribed dietary supplements.

Calcium, Urine

SYNONYM/ACRONYM: N/A

RATIONALE: To indicate sufficiency of dietary calcium intake and rate of absorption. Urine calcium levels are also used to assess bone resorption, kidney stones, and renal loss of calcium.

PATIENT PREPARATION: There are no fluid, activity, or medication restrictions unless by medical direction. Usually, a 24-hr urine collection is ordered. Instruct the patient to follow a normal calcium diet for at least 4 days before test. Protocols may vary among facilities. As appropriate, provide the required urine collection container and specimen collection instructions.

NORMAL FINDINGS: Method: Spectrophotometry.

Age	Conventional Units*	SI Units (Conventional Units × 0.025)*
Infant and child	Up to 6 mg/kg per 24 hr	Up to 0.15 mmol/kg per 24 hr
Adult on average diet	100–300 mg/24 hr	2.5–7.5 mmol/24 hr

*Values depend on diet.

CRITICAL FINDINGS AND POTENTIAL INTERVENTIONS: N/A

OVERVIEW: (Study type: Urine from an unpreserved random or timed specimen collected in a clean plastic collection container; related body system: Endocrine, Musculoskeletal, and Urinary systems.) Regulating electrolyte balance is a major function of the kidneys. In normally functioning kidneys, urine levels increase when serum levels are high and decrease when serum levels are low to maintain homeostasis. Analyzing urinary electrolyte levels can provide important clues to the functioning of the kidneys and other major organs. Tests for calcium in urine usually involve timed urine collections during a 12- or 24-hr period. Measurement of random specimens may also be requested. Urinary calcium excretion may also be expressed as calcium-to-creatinine ratio:

In a healthy individual with constant muscle mass, the ratio is less than 0.14.

INDICATIONS

- Assist in establishing the presence of kidney stones.
- Evaluate bone disease.
- Evaluate dietary intake and absorption.
- Evaluate renal loss.
- Monitor patients on calcium replacement.

INTERFERING FACTORS

Factors that may alter the results of the study

- Drugs and other substances that can increase urine calcium levels include acetazolamide, ammonium chloride, asparaginase, calcitonin, corticosteroids, corticotropin, dexamethasone, dihydroxycholecalciferol, diuretics (initially),

C

ergocalciferol, ethacrynic acid, glucocorticoids, mannitol (initially), meralluride, mercaptomerin, metolazone, parathyroid extract, parathyroid hormone, plicamycin, prednisolone, sodium sulfate, sulfates, torsemide, triamcinolone, triamterene, viomycin, and vitamin D.

- Drugs and other substances that can decrease urine calcium levels include angiotensin, bicarbonate, calcitonin, cellulose phosphate, citrates, diuretics (chronic), lithium, mestranol, methyclothiazide, neomycin, oral contraceptives, parathyroid extract, polythiazide, sodium phytate, spironolactone, thiazides, trichlormethiazide, and vitamin K.
- All urine voided for the timed collection period must be included in the collection or else falsely decreased values may be obtained. Compare output records with volume collected to verify that all voids were included in the collection.

POTENTIAL MEDICAL DIAGNOSIS: CLINICAL SIGNIFICANCE OF RESULTS
Increased in
- Acromegaly *(related to imbalance in vitamin D metabolism)*
- Diabetes *(related to increased loss from damaged kidneys)*
- Fanconi syndrome *(evidenced by hereditary or acquired disorder of the renal tubules that results in excessive calcium loss)*
- Glucocorticoid excess *(related to action of glucocorticoids, which is to decrease the gastrointestinal absorption of calcium and increase urinary excretion)*
- Hepatolenticular degeneration (Wilson disease) *(related to excessive electrolyte loss due to renal damage)*
- Hyperparathyroidism *(related to increased levels of parathyroid hormone [PTH], which result in increased calcium levels)*

- Hyperthyroidism *(related to increased bone turnover; excess circulating calcium is excreted by the kidneys)*
- Idiopathic hypercalciuria
- Immobilization *(related to disruption in calcium homeostasis and bone loss)*
- Kidney stones *(evidenced by excessive urinary calcium; contributes to the formation of kidney stones)*
- Leukemia and lymphoma (some instances)
- Myeloma *(calcium is released from damaged bone; excess circulating calcium is excreted by the kidneys)*
- Tumor of the breast or bladder *(some cancers secrete PTH or PTH-related peptide that increases calcium levels)*
- Osteitis deformans *(calcium is released from damaged bone; excess circulating calcium is excreted by the kidneys)*
- Osteolytic bone metastases (cancer, sarcoma) *(calcium is released from damaged bone; excess circulating calcium is excreted by the kidneys)*
- Osteoporosis *(calcium is released from damaged bone; excess circulating calcium is excreted by the kidneys)*
- Paget disease *(calcium is released from damaged bone; excess circulating calcium is excreted by the kidneys)*
- Renal tubular acidosis *(metabolic acidosis resulting in loss of calcium by the kidneys)*
- Sarcoidosis *(macrophages in the granulomas interfere with vitamin D regulation by converting it to its active form; vitamin D increases circulating calcium levels, and excess is excreted by the kidneys)*
- Schistosomiasis
- Thyrotoxicosis *(increased bone turnover; excess circulating calcium is excreted by the kidneys)*

- Vitamin D intoxication *(increases calcium metabolism; excess is excreted by the kidneys)*

Decreased in

- Hypocalcemia (other than renal disease)
- Hypocalciuric hypercalcemia (familial, nonfamilial)
- Hypoparathyroidism *(PTH instigates release of calcium; if PTH levels are low, calcium levels will be decreased)*
- Hypothyroidism
- Malabsorption (celiac disease, tropical sprue) *(related to insufficient levels of calcium)*
- Malignant bone tumor
- Nephrosis and acute nephritis *(related to decreased synthesis of vitamin D)*
- Osteoblastic metastases
- Osteomalacia *(related to vitamin D deficiency)*
- Pre-eclampsia
- Pseudohypoparathyroidism
- Renal osteodystrophy
- Rickets *(related to deficiency in vitamin D)*
- Vitamin D deficiency *(deficiency in vitamin D results in decreased calcium levels)*

NURSING IMPLICATIONS

BEFORE THE STUDY: PLANNING AND IMPLEMENTATION

Teaching the Patient What to Expect

- Inform the patient this test can assist in evaluating the effectiveness of the body's absorption of calcium.
- Explain that a urine sample is needed for the test. Information regarding specimen collection is presented with other general guidelines in Appendix A: Patient Preparation and Specimen Collection.

Potential Nursing Actions

- Include on the collection container's label urine total volume, test start and stop times/dates, and any medications that may interfere with test results.

AFTER THE STUDY: POTENTIAL NURSING ACTIONS

Treatment Considerations

- Assess pain character, location, duration, and intensity. Use an easily understood pain rating scale. Place the patient in a position of comfort, administer ordered medications, and consider alternative measures for pain management (imagery, relaxation, music, etc.). Assess and trend vital signs, facilitate a calm quiet environment, and encourage oral fluids if not contraindicated. Administer ordered parenteral fluids, monitor voiding patterns (urgency, frequency, incontinence), observe voided urine for the presence of hematuria, and strain urine if kidney stones are suspected.
- Monitor and trend laboratory and diagnostic studies (BUN, CT, Cr, electrolytes, Hgb, Hct, IVP, KUB, MRI, WBC count, and urine cultures). Administer ordered antibiotics, increase oral fluid intake as appropriate, administer ordered parenteral fluids, and monitor and trend temperature.

Nutritional Considerations

- Complete an accurate daily weight at the same time each day with the same scale. Obtain an accurate nutritional history and assess attitude toward eating. Promote a dietary consult to evaluate current eating habits and best method of nutritional supplementation. Develop short-term and long-term eating strategies. Monitor nutritional laboratory values such as albumin, Hgb, iron, RBC count, WBC count, and serum electrolytes. For additional information regarding nutritional recommendations for calcium refer to the study titled, "**Calcium, Blood, Total and Ionized.**"

Follow-Up, Evaluation, and Desired Outcomes

- Increased urine calcium levels may be associated with kidney stones. Educate the patient, if appropriate, about the importance of drinking a sufficient amount of water when kidney stones are suspected. Educate the patient at risk of developing calcium oxalate stones that avoiding calcium in the diet may increase the chances of stone formation. For additional information refer to the study titled, "Kidney Stone Evaluation."

Cancer Markers

SYNONYM/ACRONYM: α_1-*Fetoprotein*, anaplastic lymphoma receptor tyrosine kinase gene (ALK), BRAC-1, BRAC-2, BRAF, carcinoembryonic antigen (CEA), cancer antigen 125 (CA 125), cancer antigen 15-3 (CA 15-3), cancer antigen 19-9 (CA 19-9), cancer antigen 27.29 (CA 27.29), epidermal growth factor receptor gene (EGFR), HCG, HE4, HER-2–Neu, KRAS, methylated Septin 9 DNA.

RATIONALE: To identify the presence of various cancers, such as breast and ovarian, as well as to evaluate the effectiveness of cancer treatment.

PATIENT PREPARATION: There are no food, fluid, activity, or medication restrictions unless by medical direction.

NORMAL FINDINGS: Method: Electrochemiluminometric immunoassay.

α_1-Fetoprotein	Males (Conventional Units)	SI Units (Conventional Units × 1)	Females (Conventional Units)	SI Units (Conventional Units × 1)
Less than 1 mo	0.5–16,387 ng/mL	0.5–16,387 mcg/L	0.5–18,964 ng/mL	0.5–18,964 mcg/L
1–11 mo	0.5–28.3 ng/mL	0.5–28.3 mcg/L	0.5–77 ng/mL	0.5–77 mcg/L
1–3 yr	0.5–7.9 ng/mL	0.5–7.9 mcg/L	0.5–11.1 ng/mL	0.5–11.1 mcg/L
4 yr and older	Less than 6.1 ng/mL	Less than 6.1 mcg/L	Less than 6.1 ng/mL	Less than 6.1 mcg/L

Values may be higher for premature newborns.

Smoking Status	Conventional Units	SI Units (Conventional Units × 1)
CEA		
Smoker	Less than 5 ng/mL	Less than 5 mcg/L
Nonsmoker	Less than 2.5 ng/mL	Less than 2.5 mcg/L

Conventional Units	SI Units (Conventional Units × 1)
CA 125	
Less than 35 units/mL	Less than 35 kilo units/L
CA 15-3	
Less than 25 units/mL	Less than 25 kilo units/L
CA 19-9	
Less than 35 units/mL	Less than 35 kilo units/L
CA 27.29	
Less than 38.6 units/mL	Less than 38.6 kilo units/L
HCG	
Greater than 5 milli-international units/mL in males or nonpregnant females	Greater than 5 international units/L in males or nonpregnant females

CRITICAL FINDINGS AND POTENTIAL INTERVENTIONS: N/A

OVERVIEW: (Study type: Blood collected in a red-top tube; related body system: circulatory/hematopoietic, digestive, endocrine, immune, integumentary, reproductive, respiratory, and urinary systems.) Care must be taken to use the same assay method if serial measurements are to be taken. Today's approach to identifying and treating cancer has changed dramatically from the previous century's approach. Numerous genetic mutations have associations with various types of cancer and are used to identify the potential for that cancer to be expressed in a given individual. Research has shown that cancer is not a distinctive disease with a specific cause and a single cure. In fact, the new wave of precision medicine is being driven by the discovery that cancer cells emerge as the product of a complex interplay between genetic, environmental, and individual lifestyle influences. Traditional therapies such as surgery, chemotherapy, and radiation are still relevant, but molecular approaches are slowly gaining ground as more is learned about targeted therapy. The successful application of targeted therapy involves identifying the unique proteins produced by a growing tumor and developing a therapy that blocks further growth of the tumor. Targeted therapies attack only the malignant cells as opposed to the traditional methods that destroy both diseased and healthy tissue. The challenge for this new, individualized approach to treating cancer is that research also shows that the response to using the same therapy on the same type of cancer but in different individuals does not provide the same response. But many years ago, before the terms *personalized medicine* and *targeted therapy* were coined, scientists in that time were aware that the cure given for one patient could be disastrous if administered to another patient with the same condition. This phenomena is exemplified by the famous immunologist Karl Landsteiner who discovered the major blood groups. As our understanding expands of how the body works at the cellular level, progress continues. Another emerging area of cancer treatment is immunotherapy. Drugs are being developed to target proteins associated with immune function that have been modified in the process of a cancer's development, such that the immune system's ability to recognize and destroy the malignant cells has been turned off.

Non-small-cell lung cancer (NSCLC) is the most common type of lung cancer and the worldwide cause of death from cancer. A small percentage of NSCLC demonstrate changes in the ALK gene that make them more responsive to drug treatments than are NSCLC associated with other risk factors or genetic mutations.

CA 125 or Muc16 is a glycoprotein member of the mucin family and is present in normal endometrial tissue. It appears in the blood when natural endometrial protective barriers are destroyed, as occurs in cancer or endometriosis. CA 125 is most useful in monitoring the progression or recurrence of known ovarian cancer. It is not useful as a screening test because elevations can occur with numerous other conditions, such as endometriosis, other diseases of the ovary, menstruation, pregnancy, and uterine fibroids. Persistently rising levels indicate a poor prognosis. Levels may also rise in pancreatic, liver, colon, breast, and lung cancers. Absence of detectable levels of CA 125 does not rule out the presence of tumor. Human epididymis protein 4 (HE4) is a newer protein marker associated with various types of cancer, including ovarian cancer. Significant or persistent elevations of HE4 may indicate the appearance, recurrence, or progression of epithelial ovarian cancer. A significant elevation would be an increase of greater than 25% over normal findings. Normal findings for HE4 are less than 70 pmol/L in females who are premenopausal and less than 140 pmol/L in females who are postmenopausal.

CA 15-3 monitors patients for recurrence or metastasis of breast cancer.

CA 19-9 is a carbohydrate antigen used for post-therapeutic monitoring of patients with gastrointestinal (GI), pancreatic, liver, and colorectal cancer.

CA 27.29 is a glycoprotein product of the muc-1 gene. It is most useful as a serial monitor for response to therapy or recurrence of breast cancer.

Carcinoembryonic antigen (CEA) is a family of 36 different glycoproteins whose function is believed to be involved in cell adhesion. These structurally related proteins are part of the immunoglobulin superfamily. CEA is normally produced during fetal development and rapid multiplication of epithelial cells, especially those of the digestive system. A small amount of circulating

CEA is detectable in the blood of healthy adults; normal half-life is 7 days. The liver is the main site for metabolism of CEA. Because of the variability in CEA molecules, the test is not diagnostic for any specific disease and is not useful as a screening test for cancer. However, it is very useful for monitoring response to therapy in breast, liver, colon, and GI cancer. Serial monitoring is also a useful indicator of recurrence or metastasis in colon or liver cancer. CEA levels are higher in the blood of individuals who smoke than in those who do not smoke, so most laboratories will have a normal range for each group.

Human chorionic gonadotropin (HCG) is a hormone secreted in large quantity by the placenta after conception; however, the test has also been established for use as a tumor marker. In the absence of a pregnancy, an elevated HCG level in blood or some body fluids (e.g., peritoneal fluid) may indicate the presence of a germ cell tumor such as testicular cancer in males and ovarian or molar (hydatidiform) cancer in females. Gestational trophoblastic disease (GTD) is a group of rare tumors, affecting females, that develop from cells that would normally become placental tissue during pregnancy. The most common types of GTD include hydatidiform mole (complete or partial), choriocarcinoma, placental-site trophoblastic tumor, and epithelioid trophoblastic tumor.

A growing number of studies are used to identify cancer occurring at various sites in the body. Further detail for some of these tumor markers can be reviewed in the individual studies indicated in the table below.

INDICATIONS

- Assist in the diagnosis of various cancers.
- Determine stage of cancer and test for recurrence or metastasis.
- Monitor response to treatment of cancers.
- Predict recurrence of some cancers.

Cancer Marker	Cancer Site Commonly Associated with Marker	Additional Associated Studies for Further Information That Can Be Found in This Book
AFP (α_1-fetoprotein)	Liver, germ cell lines (reproductive organs)	
ALK gene	Lung (NSCLC)	
Antithyroglobulin antibody	Thyroid	Antithyroglobulin Antibody and Antithyroid Peroxidase Antibody
β_2 microglobulin	Blood (CLL, multiple myeloma), liver, lung	β_2 Microglobulin, Blood and Urine
Bladder cancer markers: Nuclear matrix protein (NMP) 22, bladder tumor antigen (BTA)	Bladder	Bladder Cancer Markers, Urine
BRAF	Skin (melanoma)	Biopsy, Various Sites (Bladder, Bone, Intestinal, Kidney, Liver, Lung, Lymph Node, Muscle, Prostate, Skin, Thyroid); Genetic Testing
BRCA1 and BRCA2	Breast, ovarian	Biopsy, Breast; Genetic Testing
Calcitonin	Thyroid (medullary)	Calcitonin
CEA	Colon, liver	
CA 125	Ovary	
CA 15–3	Breast	
CA 19–9	Colon, GI, liver, pancreas	
CA 27.29	Breast	
EGFR	Breast, colon, lung	Genetic Testing
Fecal occult blood test	Colon	Fecal Analysis
HE4	Breast	
HER-2–NEU	Breast	Biopsy, Breast; Genetic Testing
HCG	Choriocarcinoma, ectopic locations (breast, colon, GI, liver, lung, pancreas), germ cell lines (reproductive organs)	Human Chorionic Gonadotropin

(table continues on page 266)

Cancer Marker	Cancer Site Commonly Associated with Marker	Additional Associated Studies for Further Information That Can Be Found in This Book
Quantitative immunoglobulins	Blood (multiple myeloma, Waldenström macroglobulinemia)	Immunoglobulins A, D, G, E, and M
KRAS	Breast, colon, lung	Genetic Testing
Methylated Septin 9 DNA	Colon	
PSA	Prostate	Prostate-Specific Antigen

INTERFERING FACTORS

Other considerations

• CA 19-9 is absent in individuals with the Lewis blood group, Le(a-b-).

POTENTIAL MEDICAL DIAGNOSIS: CLINICAL SIGNIFICANCE OF RESULTS

Increased in

• Conditions such as an inflammatory process (abscess, endometriosis, inflammatory bowel disease, pancreatitis, pelvic inflammatory disease), benign tumors, or cancer affecting the target organ.

Decreased in

• Effective therapy or removal of the tumor

NURSING IMPLICATIONS

BEFORE THE STUDY: PLANNING AND IMPLEMENTATION

Teaching the Patient What to Expect

◗ Inform the patient this test can assist in identifying cancer, monitoring the progress of various types of disease, and evaluating response to therapy.
◗ Explain that a blood sample is needed for the test.

Potential Nursing Actions

◗ Determine if the patient smokes because people who smoke may have false elevations of CEA.

AFTER THE STUDY: POTENTIAL NURSING ACTIONS

Treatment Considerations

◗ Assure the patient that his or her feelings of distress are normal. Consider the cultural aspects of body image and incorporate them into the plan of care. Ensure privacy to explore personal grief, listen, and support positive coping strategies. Encourage viewing surgical site because the imagined is sometimes worse than the real.
◗ Assess pain intensity and characteristics using an appropriate rating scale. Administer ordered analgesics and evaluate the effectiveness of the plan making appropriate changes. Consider alternative pain management (imagery, relaxation, music).

Follow-Up, Evaluation, and Desired Outcomes

◗ Recognizes the importance of contact information provided for the American Cancer Association (ACS) (www.cancer.org) and U.S. Preventive Services Task Force (www.uspreventiveservicestaskforce.org) for various types of cancer.

Breast Cancer

◗ Understands that decisions regarding the need for and frequency of breast self-examination, mammography, magnetic resonance imaging (MRI) or ultrasound of the breast, or other cancer screening procedures should be made after consultation between the patient and health-care provider (HCP). Acknowledges that the most current guidelines for breast cancer screening of the general population as well as of individuals with increased risk are available from the ACS (www.cancer.org), the American College of Obstetricians and Gynecologists (www.acog.org), and the American College of Radiology (www.acr.org). Screening guidelines vary depending on the age and health history of those at average risk and those at high risk for breast cancer. Guidelines may not always agree between organizations; therefore, it is important for patients to participate in their health care, be informed, ask questions, and follow their HCP's recommendations regarding frequency and type of screening. For additional information regarding screening guidelines, refer to the study titled "Mammography."

Colon Cancer

▶ Recognizes colon cancer screening options and understands that decisions regarding the need for and frequency of occult blood testing, colonoscopy, or other cancer screening procedures may be made after consultation between the patient and HCP. Colonoscopy should be used to follow up abnormal findings obtained by any of the screening tests. The most current guidelines for colon cancer screening of the general population as well as of individuals with increased risk are available from the ACS (www.cancer.org), U.S. Preventive Services Task Force (www.uspreventiveservicestaskforce.org), and American College of Gastroenterology (www.gi.org). For additional information regarding screening guidelines, refer to the study titled "Colonoscopy."

Prostate Cancer

▶ Understands that decisions regarding the need for and frequency of routine PSA testing or other prostate cancer screening procedures should be made after consultation between the patient and HCP. Recommendations made by various medical associations and national health organizations regarding prostate cancer screening are moving away from routine PSA screening and toward informed decision making. The most current guidelines for prostate cancer screening of the general population as well as of individuals with increased risk are available from the ACS (www.cancer.org) and the American Urological Association (www.auanet.org). Counsel the patient, as appropriate, that sexual dysfunction related to altered body function, drugs, or radiation may occur. For additional information regarding screening guidelines, refer to the study titled "Prostate Specific Antigen."

▶ Agrees to strict adherence to specified therapeutic interventions.

▶ Further information regarding genetic markers for cancer can be found in the study titled "Genetic Testing."

Capsule Endoscopy

SYNONYM/ACRONYM: Pill GI endoscopy.

RATIONALE: To assist in visualization of the gastrointestinal (GI) tract to identify disease such as tumor and inflammation.

PATIENT PREPARATION: The patient with an implanted cardiac device should contact his or her health-care provider (HCP) for evaluation regarding compatibility with the capsule device prior to the procedure. There are no activity restrictions unless by medical direction. Inform the patient to stop taking medications that have a coating effect, such as sucralfate and Pepto-Bismol,

3 days before the procedure; they may prevent the camera from providing clear images. Instruct the patient to abstain from the use of tobacco products for 24 hr prior to the procedure and not to take any medication for 2 hr prior to the procedure, by medical direction. Instruct the patient to start a liquid diet on the day before the procedure, then from 2200 the evening before the procedure, the patient should not eat or drink except for necessary medication with a sip of water. As appropriate, provide information for the patient to take a standard bowel prep the night before the procedure. Protocols may vary among facilities. Ensure that this procedure is performed before an upper GI series or barium swallow. Ask the patient to wear loose, two-piece clothing on the day of the procedure because this assists with the placement of the sensors on the patient's abdomen.

NORMAL FINDINGS

- Esophageal mucosa is normally yellow-pink. At about 9 in. from the incisor teeth, a pulsation indicates the location of the aortic arch. The gastric mucosa is orange-red and contains rugae. The proximal duodenum is reddish and contains a few longitudinal folds, whereas the distal duodenum has circular folds lined with villi. No abnormal structures or functions are observed in the esophagus, stomach, or duodenum.

CRITICAL FINDINGS AND POTENTIAL INTERVENTIONS: N/A

OVERVIEW: (Study type: Endoscopy; related body system: Digestive system.) This outpatient procedure involves ingesting a small (size of a large vitamin pill) capsule that is wireless and contains a small video camera that will pass naturally through the digestive system while taking pictures of the intestine. The capsule is 11 mm by 30 mm and contains a camera, light source, radio transmitter, and battery. The patient swallows the capsule, and the camera takes and transmits two images per second. The images are transmitted to a recording device, which saves all images for later review by an HCP. The recording device is approximately the size of a personal compact disk player. It is worn on a belt around the patient's waist, and the video images are transmitted to aerials taped to the body and are stored on the device. After 8 hr, the device is removed and returned to the HCP for processing. Thousands of images are downloaded onto a computer for viewing by an HCP specialist. The capsule is disposable and will be excreted naturally in the patient's bowel movements. In the rare case that it is not excreted naturally, it will need to be removed endoscopically or surgically.

INDICATIONS

- Assist in differentiating between benign and neoplastic tumors
- Detect gastric or duodenal ulcers.
- Detect GI inflammatory disease.
- Determine the presence and location of GI bleeding and vascular abnormalities.
- Evaluate the extent of esophageal injury after ingestion of chemicals.
- Evaluate stomach or duodenum after surgical procedures.
- Evaluate suspected gastric obstruction.

- Identify Crohn disease, infectious enteritis, and celiac sprue.
- Identify source of chronic diarrhea.
- Investigate the cause of abdominal pain, celiac syndrome, and other malabsorption syndromes.

INTERFERING FACTORS
Contraindications

Patients who have had surgery involving the stomach or duodenum, *which can make locating the duodenal papilla difficult.*

Patients with unstable cardiopulmonary status, a bleeding disorder, blood coagulation defects, known aortic arch aneurysm, large esophageal Zenker diverticulum, recent GI surgery, esophageal varices, known esophageal perforation, or cholangitis (unless the patient received prophylactic antibiotic therapy before the test; otherwise, the examination must be rescheduled).

Patients with swallowing disorders or intestinal blockages or obstructions that may prevent passage of the capsule through the GI tract.

Patients who are unable to have surgery in the case of recovering a retained capsule.

Patients with implanted electronic devices such as pacemakers or cardiac defibrillators *because normal function of the implanted device may be affected by the capsule device's electromagnetic field.*

Factors that may alter the results of the study

- Gas or feces in the GI tract resulting from inadequate cleansing or failure to restrict food intake before the study.
- Retained barium from a previous radiological procedure may obscure images.
- Rapid capsule transit times may produced blurred images.

Other considerations
- Delayed capsule transit times may be a result of narcotic use, somatostatin use, gastroparesis, or drugs used to treat psychiatric illness.

POTENTIAL MEDICAL DIAGNOSIS: CLINICAL SIGNIFICANCE OF RESULTS
Abnormal findings related to
- Achalasia
- Acute and chronic gastric and duodenal ulcers
- Crohn disease, infectious enteritis, and celiac sprue
- Diverticular disease
- Duodenal cancer, diverticula, and ulcers
- Duodenitis
- Esophageal or pyloric stenosis
- Esophageal varices
- Esophagitis or strictures
- Gastric cancer, tumors, and ulcers
- Gastritis
- Hiatal hernia
- Mallory-Weiss syndrome
- Perforation of the esophagus, stomach, or small bowel
- Polyps
- Small bowel tumors
- Strictures

NURSING IMPLICATIONS

BEFORE THE STUDY: PLANNING AND IMPLEMENTATION

Teaching the Patient What to Expect

▶ Inform the patient this procedure can assist in assessing the esophagus, stomach, and upper intestines for disease.

▶ Review the procedure with the patient. Address concerns about pain and explain that no pain will be experienced during the procedure.

▶ Inform the patient that the capsule is a single-use device that does not harbor any environmental hazards.

▶ Explain that the procedure is started in a GI laboratory or office, usually by an HCP or support staff, and that it takes approximately 30 to 60 min to begin the procedure.

▶ Advise the patient that prior to the procedure an accurate weight and abdominal girth measurement will be taken. Once the capsule is ingested, the patient should not eat or drink for at least the next 2 hr. After 4 hr, the patient may have a light snack. The procedure lasts approximately 8 hr.

▶ Instruct the patient not to disconnect the equipment or remove the belt at any time during the test. If the data recorder stops functioning, instruct the patient to record the time and the nature of any event such as eating or drinking. Instruct the patient to keep a timed diary for the day detailing the food and liquids ingested and symptoms during the recording period. The patient should be instructed to avoid any strenuous physical activity, bending, or stooping during the test.

▶ Explain that the patient will also be asked to ingest the capsule with a full glass of water. The water may have simethicone in it to reduce gastric and bile bubbles that may produce unclear images.

Potential Nursing Actions

※ *Make sure a written and informed consent has been signed prior to the procedure and before administering any medications.*

▶ Verify the patient is able to swallow without aspiration risk.

▶ Ensure that the patient with an implanted cardiac device has been cleared to have the procedure.

Safety Considerations

▶ The patient should be instructed to avoid close proximity to any strong electromagnetic source, such as magnetic resonance imaging (MRI) or amateur (ham) radio equipment until the capsule has been eliminated from the body; magnetic fields can disrupt the function of the capsule device and serious damage could be caused to the patient's GI tract if he or she is exposed to the strong magnetic force of MRI equipment.

AFTER THE STUDY: POTENTIAL NURSING ACTIONS

Avoiding Complications

▶ Possibility of intestinal obstruction is associated with the procedure. Obtain post-test weight and abdominal girth; comparison of pre- and post-test measurements may assist in early identification and resolution of obstruction or retained capsule. Emphasize that any abdominal pain, fever, nausea, vomiting, or difficulty breathing must be immediately reported to the HCP.

Treatment Considerations

▶ Instruct the patient to resume normal activity, medication, and diet after the test is ended or as tolerated after the examination, as directed by the HCP.

▶ Assess skin turgor, perform a daily weight, monitor and trend laboratory studies (blood urea nitrogen, creatinine, hemoglobin, hematocrit, electrolytes). Complete frequent vital signs; monitor and trend blood pressure, heart rate, temperature; and assess capillary refill. Administer ordered parenteral fluids and replacement electrolytes. Ensure strict intake and output; monitor for fluid overload; and administer ordered antiemetics, analgesics, or antibiotics.

▶ Initiate ordered nasogastric intubation (NGT), and monitor for patency and amount of drainage. Assess hydration status, assess bowel sounds, and measure abdominal girth to monitor degree of abdominal distention. Keep NPO as required with implementation of fluid replacement strategies.

▶ Instruct the patient to remove the recorder and return it to the HCP. Patients are asked to verify the elimination of the capsule but not to retrieve the capsule.

Safety Considerations

▶ Patients with an NGT should have placement verified according to best practice guidelines and organizational policy.

Nutritional Considerations

▶ Dietary changes may be necessary based on prognosis to meet therapeutic goals. Dietary consult with a registered dietitian can assist the patient to structure diet changes to meet therapeutic and cultural needs.

Follow-Up, Evaluation, and Desired Outcomes

▸ Recognizes colon cancer screening options and understands that decisions regarding the need for and frequency of occult blood testing, colonoscopy, or other cancer screening procedures may be made after consultation between the patient and HCP. Colonoscopy should be used to follow up abnormal findings obtained by any of the screening tests. The most current guidelines for colon cancer screening of the general population as well as of individuals with increased risk are available from the American Cancer Society (www.cancer.org), U.S. Preventive Services Task Force (www.uspreventiveservicestaskforce.org), and American College of Gastroenterology (www.gi.org) For additional information regarding screening guidelines, refer to the study titled "Colonoscopy."

Carbon Dioxide

SYNONYM/ACRONYM: CO_2 combining power, CO_2, TCO_2.

RATIONALE: To assess the effect of total carbon dioxide levels on respiratory and metabolic acid-base balance.

PATIENT PREPARATION: There are no food, fluid, activity, or medication restrictions unless by medical direction.

NORMAL FINDINGS: Method: Colorimetry, enzyme assay, or PCO_2 electrode.

Carbon Dioxide	Conventional and SI Units
Plasma or serum (venous)	
Infant–2 yr	13–29 mEq/L or mmol/L
2 yr–older adult	23–29 mEq/L or mmol/L
Whole blood (venous)	
Infant–2 yr	18–28 mEq/L or mmol/L
2 yr–older adult	22–26 mEq/L or mmol/L

CRITICAL FINDINGS AND POTENTIAL INTERVENTIONS

• Less than 15 mEq/L or mmol/L (SI: Less than 15 mmol/L).
• Greater than 40 mEq/L or mmol/L (SI: Greater than 40 mmol/L).

Timely notification to the requesting health-care provider (HCP) of any critical findings and related symptoms is a role expectation of the professional nurse. A listing of these findings varies among facilities.

Consideration may be given to verification of critical findings before action is taken. Policies vary among facilities and may include requesting immediate recollection and retesting by the laboratory or retesting using a rapid point-of-care testing instrument at the bedside, if available.

Observe the patient for signs and symptoms of excessive or insufficient CO_2 levels, and report these findings to the HCP. If the patient has been vomiting for several days and is breathing shallowly, or if the patient has had gastric suctioning and is breathing shallowly, this may indicate elevated CO_2 levels. Decreased CO_2 levels are evidenced by deep, vigorous breathing and flushed skin.

OVERVIEW: (**Study type:** Blood collected in a gold-, red-, red/gray-, green-top [lithium or sodium heparin] tube or heparinized syringe; **related body system:** Respiratory and Urinary systems.) Serum or plasma carbon dioxide (CO_2) measurement is usually done as part of an electrolyte panel. Total CO_2 (T_{CO_2}) is an important component of the body's buffering capability, and measurements are used mainly in the evaluation of acid-base balance. It is important to understand the differences between T_{CO_2} (CO_2 content) and CO_2 gas (P_{CO_2}). Total CO_2 reflects the majority of CO_2 in the body, mainly in the form of bicarbonate (HCO_3^-); is present as a base; and is regulated by the kidneys. CO_2 gas contributes little to the T_{CO_2} level, is acidic, and is regulated by the lungs (see study titled "Blood Gases").

CO_2 provides the basis for the principal buffering system of the extracellular fluid system, which is the bicarbonate–carbonic acid buffer system. CO_2 circulates in the body either bound to protein or physically dissolved. Constituents in the blood that contribute to T_{CO_2} levels are bicarbonate, carbamino compounds, and carbonic acid (carbonic acid includes undissociated carbonic acid and dissolved CO_2). Bicarbonate is the second-largest group of anions in the extracellular fluid (chloride is the largest). T_{CO_2} levels closely reflect bicarbonate levels in the blood, because 90% to 95% of CO_2 circulates as HCO_3^-.

INDICATIONS

- Evaluate decreased venous CO_2 in the case of compensated metabolic acidosis.
- Evaluate increased venous CO_2 in the case of compensated metabolic alkalosis.
- Monitor decreased venous CO_2 as a result of compensated respiratory alkalosis.
- Monitor increased venous CO_2 as a result of compensation for respiratory acidosis secondary to significant respiratory system infection or cancer, decreased respiratory rate.

INTERFERING FACTORS

Factors that may alter the results of the study

- Drugs and other substances that may cause an increase in T_{CO_2} levels include acetylsalicylic acid, aldosterone, bicarbonate, carbenicillin, corticosteroids, dexamethasone, ethacrynic acid, laxatives (chronic misuse), and x-ray contrast.
- Drugs and other substances that may cause a decrease in T_{CO_2} levels include acetazolamide, acetylsalicylic acid (initially), amiloride, ammonium chloride, fluorides, metformin, methicillin, nitrofurantoin, paraldehyde, tetracycline, triamterene, and xylitol.
- Prompt and proper specimen processing, storage, and analysis are important to achieve accurate results. The specimen should be stored under anaerobic conditions after collection to prevent the diffusion of CO_2 gas from the specimen. Falsely decreased values result from uncovered specimens. It is estimated that CO_2 diffuses from the sample at the rate of 6 mmol/hr.

POTENTIAL MEDICAL DIAGNOSIS: CLINICAL SIGNIFICANCE OF RESULTS

Increased in

- *Interpretation requires clinical information and evaluation of other electrolytes*
- Acute intermittent porphyria *(related to severe vomiting associated with acute attacks)*
- Airway obstruction *(related to impaired elimination from weak breathing responses)*
- Asthmatic shock *(related to impaired elimination from abnormal breathing responses)*
- Brain tumor *(related to abnormal blood circulation)*
- Bronchitis (chronic) *(related to impaired elimination from weak breathing responses)*
- Cardiac disorders *(related to lack of blood circulation)*
- Chronic obstructive pulmonary disease (COPD) *(related to impaired elimination from weak breathing responses)*
- Depression of respiratory center *(related to impaired elimination from weak breathing responses)*
- Electrolyte disturbance (severe) *(response to maintain acid-base balance)*
- Hypothyroidism *(related to impaired elimination from weak breathing responses)*
- Hypoventilation *(related to impaired elimination from weak breathing responses)*
- Metabolic alkalosis *(various causes; excessive vomiting)*
- Myopathy *(related to impaired ventilation)*
- Pneumonia *(related to impaired elimination from weak breathing responses)*
- Poliomyelitis *(related to impaired elimination from weak breathing responses)*
- Respiratory acidosis *(related to impaired elimination)*
- Tuberculosis (pulmonary) *(related to impaired elimination from weak breathing responses)*

Decreased in

- *Interpretation requires clinical information and evaluation of other electrolytes*
- Acute kidney injury *(response to buildup of ketoacids)*
- Anxiety *(related to hyperventilation; too much CO_2 is exhaled)*
- Dehydration *(response to metabolic acidosis that develops)*
- Diabetic ketoacidosis *(response to buildup of ketoacids)*
- Diarrhea (severe) *(acidosis related to loss of base ions such as HCO_3; most of CO_2 content is in this form)*
- High fever *(response to neutralize acidosis present during fever)*
- Metabolic acidosis *(response to neutralize acidosis)*
- Respiratory alkalosis *(hyperventilation; too much CO_2 is exhaled)*
- Salicylate intoxication *(response to neutralize related metabolic acidosis)*
- Starvation *(CO_2 buffer system used to neutralize buildup of ketoacids)*

NURSING IMPLICATIONS

BEFORE THE STUDY: PLANNING AND IMPLEMENTATION

Teaching the Patient What to Expect

- Inform the patient this test can assist in measuring the amount of carbon dioxide in the body.
- Explain that a blood sample is needed for the test.

Safety Considerations

- Confusion caused by acid-base imbalances and increased fall and injury risk. Fall safety interventions may be necessary.

AFTER THE STUDY: POTENTIAL NURSING ACTIONS

Avoiding Complications
▸ Timely and appropriate interventions are necessary to reverse the effects of acid-base imbalances.

Treatment Considerations
▸ Identify the underlying cause of the metabolic disturbance. Monitor and trend vital signs: heart rate, blood pressure, pulse rate, and respirations. Assess, monitor, and trend both cardiac and peripheral vascular status. Administer ordered sodium bicarbonate and evaluate effectiveness. Monitor and trend arterial blood gas.
▸ Encourage slow deep breathing to slow respiratory rate. Obtain a history related to respiratory disease. Provide emotional support to reduce anxiety and enhance coping skills.
▸ Treat the medical condition and correlate confusion with the need to reverse altered electrolytes. Evaluate medications; prevent falls and injury through appropriate use of postural support, bed alarm, or the appropriate use of restraints; consider pharmacological interventions, initiate accurate intake and output to assess fluid status.

Nutritional Considerations
▸ Abnormal CO_2 values may be associated with diseases of the respiratory system. Malnutrition is commonly seen in patients with severe respiratory disease for reasons including fatigue, lack of appetite, and gastrointestinal distress. Research has estimated that the daily caloric intake required for respiration of patients with chronic obstructive pulmonary disease is 10 times higher than that of healthy individuals. Adequate intake of vitamins A and C is also important to prevent pulmonary infection and to decrease the extent of lung tissue damage. The importance of following the prescribed diet should be stressed to the patient and/or caregiver.

Carbon Monoxide

SYNONYM/ACRONYM: Carboxyhemoglobin, CO, COHb, COH.

RATIONALE: To identify the amount of carbon monoxide in the blood related to poisoning, toxicity from smoke inhalation, or exhaust from cars.

PATIENT PREPARATION: There are no food, fluid, activity, or medication restrictions unless by medical direction.

NORMAL FINDINGS: Method: Spectrophotometry, co-oximetry.

	% Saturation of Hemoglobin
Newborns	10%–12%
Nonsmokers	Up to 2%
Smokers	Up to 10%

CRITICAL FINDINGS AND POTENTIAL INTERVENTIONS

% Total Hemoglobin	Symptoms
10%–20%	Asymptomatic
10%–30%	Disturbance of judgment, headache, dizziness
30%–40%	Dizziness, muscle weakness, vision problems, confusion, increased heart rate, increased breathing rate
50%–60%	Loss of consciousness, coma
Greater than 60%	Death

Timely notification to the requesting health-care provider (HCP) of any critical findings and related symptoms is a role expectation of the professional nurse. A listing of these findings varies among facilities.

Consideration may be given to verification of critical findings before action is taken. Policies vary among facilities and may include requesting immediate recollection and retesting by the laboratory or retesting using a rapid point-of-care testing instrument at the bedside, if available.

Women and children may suffer more severe symptoms of carbon monoxide poisoning at lower levels of carbon monoxide than do men because women and children usually have lower red blood cell (RBC) counts.

A possible intervention in moderate CO poisoning is the administration of supplemental oxygen given at atmospheric pressure. In severe CO poisoning, hyperbaric oxygen treatments may be used.

OVERVIEW: (Study type: Blood collected in a green-top [heparin] or lavender-top [EDTA] tube; related body system: Respiratory system.) Carboxyhemoglobin is stable at room temperature; however, the specimen should be transported tightly capped (anaerobic) and in an ice slurry if blood gases are to be performed simultaneously. Exogenous carbon monoxide (CO) is a colorless, odorless, tasteless by-product of incomplete combustion derived from the exhaust of automobiles, coal and gas burning, and tobacco smoke. Endogenous CO is produced as a result of RBC catabolism. CO levels are elevated in newborns as a result of the combined effects of high hemoglobin turnover and the inefficiency of the infant's respiratory system. CO binds tightly to hemoglobin with an affinity 250 times greater than oxygen, competitively and dramatically reducing the oxygen-carrying capacity of hemoglobin. The increased percentage of bound CO reflects the extent to which normal transport of oxygen has been negatively affected. Overexposure causes hypoxia, which results in headache, nausea, vomiting, vertigo, collapse, or convulsions. Toxic exposure causes anoxia, increased levels of lactic acid, and irreversible tissue damage, which can result in coma or death. Acute exposure may be evidenced by a cherry red color to the lips, skin, and nailbeds; this observation may not be apparent in cases of chronic exposure. A direct correlation has been implicated between carboxyhemoglobin levels and symptoms of atherosclerotic disease, angina, and myocardial infarction.

INDICATIONS

- Assist in the diagnosis of suspected CO poisoning.
- Evaluate the effect of smoking on the patient.
- Evaluate exposure to fires and smoke inhalation.

INTERFERING FACTORS

Factors that may alter the results of the study

Specimen should be collected before administration of oxygen therapy.

POTENTIAL MEDICAL DIAGNOSIS: CLINICAL SIGNIFICANCE OF RESULTS

Increased in

- CO poisoning
- Hemolytic disease *(CO released during RBC catabolism)*
- Tobacco smoking

Decreased in: N/A

NURSING IMPLICATIONS

BEFORE THE STUDY: PLANNING AND IMPLEMENTATION

Teaching the Patient What to Expect

- Inform the patient this test can assist in evaluating the extent of carbon monoxide poisoning or toxicity.
- Explain that a blood sample is needed for the test. Explain to the patient or family members that the cause of the headache, vomiting, dizziness, convulsions, or coma could be related to CO exposure.

AFTER THE STUDY: POTENTIAL NURSING ACTIONS

Follow-Up, Evaluation, and Desired Outcomes

- Recognizes the importance of avoiding gas heaters and indoor cooking fires without adequate ventilation and the need to have gas furnaces checked yearly for CO leakage.

Cardiac Catheterization

SYNONYM/ACRONYM: Angiography of heart, angiocardiography, cardiac angiography, cardiac catheterization, cineangiocardiography, coronary angiography, coronary arteriography.

RATIONALE: To visualize and assess the heart and surrounding structure for abnormalities, defects, aneurysm, atherosclerosis, and tumors

PATIENT PREPARATION: There are no activity restrictions unless by medical direction. Instruct the patient to fast and restrict fluids for 2 to 4 hr, or as ordered, prior to the procedure. Fasting may be ordered as a precaution against aspiration related to possible nausea and vomiting. The American Society of Anesthesiologists has fasting guidelines for risk levels according to patient status. More information can be located at www.asahq.org.

Note: If iodinated contrast medium is scheduled to be used in patients receiving metformin or drugs containing metformin for type 2 diabetes, the drug may be discontinued on the day of the test and continue to be withheld for 48 hr after the test.

Regarding the patient's risk for bleeding, the patient should be instructed to avoid taking natural products and medications with known anticoagulant, antiplatelet, or thrombolytic properties or to reduce dosage, as ordered, prior to the procedure. Number of days to withhold medication is dependent on the type of anticoagulant. Note the last time and dose of medication taken.

Patients on beta blockers before the surgical procedure should be instructed to take their medication as ordered during the perioperative period. Protocols may vary among facilities.

NORMAL FINDINGS

• Normal great vessels and coronary arteries.

Normal Adult Hemodynamic Pressures and Volumes Monitored During Coronary Angiography (Cardiac Catheterization)

Pressures	Description of What Measured Parameter Represents	Normal Value
Arterial blood pressure (also known as *routine blood pressure*)	The pressure in the brachial artery; one of the significant vital signs, it reflects the pressure the heart exerts to pump blood through the circulatory system	Systolic (90–140) mm Hg/diastolic (60–90) mm Hg
Mean arterial pressure (MAP)	The average arterial pressure of one cardiac cycle; considered a better indicator of perfusion than routine blood pressure but obtainable only by direct measurement during cardiac catheterization	70–100 mm Hg
Left ventricular pressures	Peak pressure in the left ventricle during systole/peak pressure in the left ventricle at the end of diastole; indication of contractility of the heart muscle	Systolic (90–140) mm Hg/diastolic (4–12) mm Hg
Central venous pressure (CVP); also right atrial pressure (RAP)	The right-sided ventricular pressures exerted by the central veins closest to the heart (jugular, subclavian, or femoral); used to estimate blood volume and venous return	2–6 mm Hg
Pulmonary artery pressure (PAP)	The pressures in the pulmonary artery	Systolic (15–30) mm Hg/diastolic (4–12) mm Hg
Pulmonary capillary wedge pressure (PCWP); also pulmonary artery occlusion pressure (PAOP)	The pressure in the pulmonary vessels; used to provide an estimate of left atrial filling pressure, to provide an estimate of left ventricle pressure during end diastole, and as a way to measure ventricular preload	4–12 mm Hg

(table continues on page 278)

Volumes	Description of What Measured Parameter Represents	Normal Value
Cardiac output	The amount of blood pumped out by the ventricle of the heart in 1 min	4–8 L/min
Cardiac index	The cardiac output adjusted for body surface to provide the index, which is a more precise measurement; used to assess the function of the ventricle	2.5–4 L/min/m²
Arterial oxygen saturation	The concentration of oxygen in the blood	95%–100%
Stroke volume (SV)	The amount of blood pumped by each ventricle with each contraction in a heartbeat	60–100 mL/beat
Stroke volume index (SVI)	The stroke volume adjusted for body surface to provide the index, which is a more precise measurement	25–45 mL/m²
Ejection fraction (EF)	Stroke volume expressed as a percentage of end diastolic volume	55%–70%

CRITICAL FINDINGS AND POTENTIAL INTERVENTIONS
- Aneurysm
- Aortic dissection

Timely notification to the requesting health-care provider (HCP) of any critical findings and related symptoms is a role expectation of the professional nurse. A listing of these findings varies among facilities.

OVERVIEW: (Study type: X-ray, special/contrast; related body system: Circulatory system.) Angiography allows x-ray visualization of the heart, aorta, inferior vena cava, pulmonary artery and vein, and coronary arteries after injection of contrast medium through a catheter; cardiac pressures and volumes are recorded through the same catheter. The insertion site for a right heart catheterization is into a peripheral vein, usually the femoral, brachial, or subclavian vein. The insertion site for a left heart catheterization is into an artery, usually the femoral, radial, or brachial artery. Fluoroscopy is used to guide catheter placement, and angiograms (high-speed x-ray images) provide images of the heart and associated vessels, which are displayed on a monitor and are recorded for future viewing and evaluation. Digital subtraction angiography (DSA) is a computerized method of removing undesired structures, such as bone, from the surrounding area of interest. A digital image is taken prior to injection of the contrast and then again after the contrast has been injected. By subtracting the preinjection image from the postinjection image, a higher-quality, unobstructed image can be created. Patterns of circulation, cardiac output, cardiac functions, and changes in vessel wall appearance can be viewed to help diagnose the presence of vascular abnormalities or lesions. Pulmonary artery abnormalities are seen with right heart views, and coronary artery and thoracic aorta abnormalities are seen with left heart views. Coronary angiography is useful for evaluating cardiovascular disease and various types of cardiac abnormalities.

Coronary angiography, more commonly called *cardiac catheterization*, is a definitive test for coronary artery disease (CAD). CAD is a condition in which the blood vessels to the heart lose their elasticity and become narrowed by atherosclerotic deposits of plaque. Significant blockage is treatable using coronary artery bypass grafting (CABG) surgery. Cardiac catheterization can also be used in conjunction with less invasive interventional alternatives to CABG surgery, such as percutaneous transluminal coronary angioplasty (PTCA), with or without placement of stents. PTCA is also known as *balloon angioplasty* because once the blockage is identified and determined to be treatable, a balloon catheter is used to help correct the problem. The balloon in the catheter is inflated to compress the plaque against the sides of the affected vessel. The balloon may be inflated multiple times and with increasing size to increase the diameter of the vessel's lumen, which restores more normal blood flow. A stent, which is a small mesh tube, may be placed in the affected vessel to keep it open after the angioplasty is completed. For additional information regarding screening guidelines for *atherosclerotic cardiovascular disease* (ASCVD), which includes

coronary artery disease (CAD) refer to the study titled "Cholesterol, Total and Fractions."

Applications of Cardiac Catheterization for Infants and Pediatric Patients: Cardiac catheterization is very useful in identification of the type of heart defect, determination of the exact location of the defect, and indications regarding the severity of the defect. Some of the common operable heart defects in infants and children include repairs for ventricular septal defects, atrial septal defects, tetralogy of Fallot, valve defects, and arterial switches. Cardiac catheterization can also be used as a palliative procedure prior to arterial switch repair. The catheterization, called a *balloon atrial septostomy,* is used to create a small hole in the inner wall of the heart between the atria that allows a greater volume of oxygenated blood to enter the circulatory system. The improved quality of circulating blood provides some time for very young patients to gain strength prior to the surgical repair. The hole is closed when the corrective surgery is completed.

INDICATIONS

- Allow infusion of thrombolytic drugs into an occluded coronary.
- Detect narrowing of coronary vessels or abnormalities of the great vessels in patients with angina, syncope, abnormal electrocardiogram, hypercholesteremia with chest pain, and persistent chest pain after revascularization.
- Evaluate cardiac muscle function.
- Evaluate cardiac valvular and septal defects.
- Evaluate disease associated with the aortic arch.

- Evaluate previous cardiac surgery or other interventional procedures.
- Evaluate peripheral arterial disease (PAD).
- Evaluate peripheral vascular disease (PVD).
- Evaluate ventricular aneurysms.
- Monitor pulmonary pressures and cardiac output.
- Perform angioplasty, perform atherectomy, or place a stent.
- Quantify the severity of atherosclerotic, occlusive CAD.

INTERFERING FACTORS

Contraindications

✳ Patients who are pregnant or suspected of being pregnant, unless the potential benefits of a procedure using radiation far outweigh the risk of radiation exposure to the fetus and mother.

✳ Conditions associated with adverse reactions to contrast medium (e.g., asthma, food allergies, or allergy to contrast medium). Although patients are asked specifically if they have a known allergy to iodine or shellfish (shellfish contain high levels of iodine), it has been well established that the reaction is not to iodine; an actual iodine allergy would be problematic because iodine is required for the production of thyroid hormones. In the case of shellfish, the reaction is to a muscle protein called *tropomyosin*; in the case of iodinated contrast medium, the reaction is to the noniodinated part of the contrast molecule. Patients with a known hypersensitivity to the medium may benefit from premedication with corticosteroids and diphenhydramine; the use of nonionic contrast or an alternative noncontrast imaging study, if available, may be considered for patients who have severe asthma or who have experienced moderate to severe reactions to ionic contrast medium.

✳ Conditions associated with pre-existing renal insufficiency (e.g., chronic kidney disease, single kidney transplant, nephrectomy, diabetes, multiple myeloma, treatment with aminoglycosides and NSAIDs), *because iodinated contrast is nephrotoxic.*

✳ Patients who are chronically dehydrated before the test, especially older adults and patients whose health is already compromised, *because of their risk of contrast-induced acute kidney injury.*

✳ Patients with pheochromocytoma, *because iodinated contrast may cause a hypertensive crisis.*

✳ Patients with bleeding disorders or receiving anticoagulant therapy, *because the puncture site may not stop bleeding.*

Factors that may alter the results of the study

- Gas or feces in the gastrointestinal tract resulting from inadequate cleansing or failure to restrict food intake before the study.
- Retained barium from a previous radiological procedure; barium studies should be performed more than 4 days before angiography.
- Metallic objects (e.g., jewelry, body rings) within the examination field, which may inhibit organ visualization and cause unclear images.
- Inability of the patient to cooperate or remain still during the procedure, because movement can produce blurred or otherwise unclear images.

POTENTIAL MEDICAL DIAGNOSIS: CLINICAL SIGNIFICANCE OF RESULTS

Abnormal findings related to

Areas where the contrast medium was not able to circulate will appear dark against the normally white blood vessels and vascular areas of cardiac tissue.

- Aortic atherosclerosis
- Aortic dissection

- Aortitis
- Aneurysms
- Cardiomyopathy
- Congenital anomalies
- Coronary artery atherosclerosis and degree of obstruction
- Graft occlusion
- Heart failure

- PAD
- PVD
- Pulmonary artery abnormalities
- Septal defects
- Trauma causing tears or other disruption
- Tumors
- Valvular disease

C

NURSING IMPLICATIONS

POTENTIAL NURSING PROBLEMS: ASSESSMENT & NURSING DIAGNOSIS

Problems	Signs and Symptoms
Inadequate cardiac output *(related to anomalies, dissection, occlusion, plaque, rupture, tumors)*	Altered level of consciousness, anxiety, cool skin, delayed capillary refill, diaphoresis, diminished peripheral pulses, hypotension, increased pulse that may be thready, restlessness
Pain *(related to aneurysm, dissection, inflammation, injury, obstruction, trauma, tumor)*	Self-report of pain, moaning, crying, restlessness, anxiety, increased heart rate, increased blood pressure, guarding

BEFORE THE STUDY: PLANNING AND IMPLEMENTATION

Teaching the Patient What to Expect

▶ Inform the patient this procedure can assist with assessment of cardiac function and check for heart disease.

▶ Explain that prior to the procedure, laboratory testing may be required to determine the possibility of bleeding risk (coagulation testing) or to assess for impaired kidney function (creatinine level and estimated glomerular filtration rate) if use of iodinated contrast medium is anticipated.

▶ Pregnancy is a general contraindication to procedures involving radiation. Explain to the female patient that she will be asked the date of her last menstrual period. Pregnancy testing may be performed to determine the possibility of pregnancy before exposure to radiation.

▶ Review the procedure with the patient. Address concerns about pain and explain that there may be moments of discomfort or pain experienced

when the IV line or catheter is inserted to allow infusion of fluids such as saline, anesthetics, sedatives, contrast medium, medications used in the procedure, or emergency medications.

▶ Explain that contrast medium will be injected, by catheter, at a separate site from the IV line.

▶ Advise that a burning and flushing sensation may be felt throughout the body during injection of the contrast medium, and the patient may experience an urge to cough, flushing, nausea, or a salty or metallic taste.

▶ Explain that reducing health-care-associated infections is an important patient safety goal, and a number of different safety practices will be implemented during their procedure. Advise the patient that hair in the area near the catheter insertion site may be clipped or shaved and the area cleaned with an antiseptic solution to cleanse bacteria from the skin in order to reduce the risk for infection. *Note:* The World Health Organization, Centers for Disease Control and Prevention, and

Association of periOperative Registered Nurses recommend that hair not be removed at all unless it interferes with the incision site or other aspects of the procedure because hair removal by any means is associated with increased infection rates. When hair removal is necessary, facilities must use a protocol that is based on scientific literature or the endorsement of a professional organization. Clipping immediately before the procedure and in a location outside the procedure area is preferred to shaving with a razor. Shaving creates a break in skin integrity and provides a way for bacteria on the skin to enter the incision site.

▶ Inform the patient that the procedure is usually performed in a radiology or vascular suite by an HCP and takes approximately 30 to 60 min. Address concerns about pain and explain that there may be moments of discomfort and some pain experienced during the procedure.

▶ Instruct the patient to remove jewelry and other metallic objects from the area of examination.

▶ Baseline vital signs will be recorded and monitored throughout the procedure. Protocols may vary among facilities.

▶ Explain that electrocardiographic electrodes will be placed for cardiac monitoring to establish a baseline rhythm and identify any ventricular dysrhythmias.

▶ Explain that peripheral pulses will be marked with a pen before the venography, allowing for a quicker and more consistent assessment of the pulses after the procedure.

▶ Positioning for this procedure is in the supine position on an examination table. The selected area will be cleansed and covered with a sterile drape.

▶ A local anesthetic will be injected at the site, and a small incision is made or a needle inserted under fluoroscopy.

▶ Once contrast medium is injected, a rapid series of images is taken during and after the filling of the vessels to be examined. Delayed images may be taken to examine the vessels after a time and to monitor the venous phase of the procedure.

▶ Advise patients that they will be instructed to inhale deeply and hold their breath while the x-ray images are taken, and then to exhale.

▶ Advise taking slow, deep breaths if nausea occurs during the procedure. An ordered antiemetic drug can be administered as needed. An emesis basin can be ready for use.

▶ Explain to patients that they will be monitored for complications related to the procedure (e.g., allergic reaction, anaphylaxis, bronchospasm).

▶ Explain that once the study is completed, the needle or catheter is removed, and a pressure dressing is applied over the puncture site.

Potential Nursing Actions

Make sure a written and informed consent has been signed prior to the procedure and before administering any medications.

▶ Glucagon or an anticholinergic drug may be given to stabilize movement of the stomach muscles; peristaltic contractions (motion) may alter study findings.

▶ If iodinated contrast medium is scheduled to be used in patients receiving metformin or drugs containing metformin for type 2 diabetes, the drug may be discontinued on the day of the test and continue to be withheld for 48 hr after the test. Protocols may vary among facilities.

▶ Investigate the presence of other risk factors, such as family history of heart disease, smoking, obesity, diet, lack of physical activity, hypertension, diabetes, previous myocardial infarction (MI), and previous vascular disease. Knowledge of genetics assists in identifying those who may benefit from additional education, risk assessment, and counseling. Genetics is the study and identification of genes, genetic mutations, and inheritance. For example, genetics provides some insight into the likelihood of inheriting a medical condition such as CAD. Genomic studies evaluate the interaction of groups of genes. The combined activity or combined expression of groups of genes allows assumptions or predictions to be made. As an example, genomic studies measure the levels of activity in multiple genes to predict how they, along with environmental and lifestyle decisions, influence the development of type 2 diabetes, CAD, MI, or ischemic stroke. Further information regarding inheritance of genes can be found in the study titled "Genetic Testing."

Safety Considerations

▶ Anticoagulants, aspirin, and other salicylates should be discontinued by medical direction for the appropriate number of days prior to a procedure where bleeding is a potential complication. Note the last time and dose of medication taken.

AFTER THE STUDY: POTENTIAL NURSING ACTIONS

Avoiding Complications

▶ Establishing an IV site and injection of contrast medium are invasive procedures. Complications are rare but include risk for allergic reaction *(related to contrast reaction)*, bleeding from the puncture site *(related to a bleeding disorder or the effects of natural products and medications with known anticoagulant, antiplatelet, or thrombolytic properties; postprocedural bleeding from the site is rare because at the conclusion of the procedure, a resorbable device, composed of non-latex-containing arterial anchor, collagen plug, and suture, is deployed to seal the puncture site)*, blood clot formation *(related to thrombus formation on the tip of the catheter sheath surface or in the lumen of the catheter; the use of a heparinized saline flush during the procedure decreases the risk of emboli)*, dysrhythmia/extrasystole *(related to contact between the catheter tip and the myocardium)*, hematoma *(related to blood leakage into the tissue following needle insertion)*, infection *(which might occur if bacteria from the skin surface is introduced at the puncture site)*, ischemic

stroke *(caused by debris [plaque, thrombus] dislodged from the vessel wall or air embolism introduced during catheter advancement or injection of contrast)*, tissue damage *(related to extravasation or leaking of contrast into the tissues during injection)*, nerve injury or damage to a nearby organ *(which might occur if the catheter strikes a nerve or perforates an organ)*, nephrotoxicity *(a deterioration of renal function associated with contrast administration)*, or perforation of blood vessel or heart wall. Monitor the patient for complications related to the procedure (e.g., allergic reaction, anaphylaxis, bronchospasm, infection, injury). Immediately report symptoms such as difficulty breathing, chest pain, fever, hyperpnea, hypertension, nausea, palpitations, pruritus, rash, tachycardia, urticaria, or vomiting to the appropriate HCP. Observe/assess the needle/catheter insertion site for bleeding, inflammation, or hematoma formation. Administer ordered antihistamines or prophylactic steroids if the patient has an allergic reaction. Assess extremities for signs of ischemia or absence of distal pulse caused by a catheter-induced thrombus.

Treatment Considerations

▶ Instruct the patient to resume usual diet, fluids, medications, or activity, as directed by the HCP. Kidney function should be assessed before metformin is resumed.
▶ Monitor vital signs and neurological status every 15 min for 1 hr, then every 2 hr for 4 hr, and then as ordered by the HCP. Take temperature every 4 hr for 24 hr.
▶ Monitor peripheral pulses as well as changes in the color or temperature of the skin around the insertion site that may be indicative of bleeding.
▶ Maintain bedrest in supine position *to prevent stress on the puncture site* for 2 to 6 hr, depending on the location of insertion site.
▶ Monitor intake and output and renal status at least every 8 hr. Compare with baseline values. Protocols may vary among facilities.

C

C

▶ Cardiac Output: Provide IV fluid to support blood pressure (rapid rate as appropriate) or blood transfusion as ordered. Monitor and trend vital signs; heart rate, blood pressure, and respiratory rate. Continuous ECG monitoring. Monitor for decreased urinary output, changes in level of consciousness, shortness of breath, cyanosis, pallor, and cool skin.

▶ Pain: Assess pain character, location, duration, and intensity. Use an easily understood pain rating scale and place in a position of comfort. Administer ordered medications and consider alternative measures for pain management (imagery, relaxation, music, etc.). Assess and trend vital signs. Facilitate a calm, quiet environment.

Safety Considerations

▶ Advise diabetic patients to avoid all medications containing metformin for 48 hr following a procedure with iodinated contrast. Iodinated contrast can temporarily impair kidney function, and failure to withhold metformin may indirectly result in drug-induced lactic acidosis, a dangerous and sometimes fatal adverse effect of metformin (related to renal impairment that does not support sufficient excretion of metformin).

Nutritional Considerations

▶ Discuss ideal body weight and the purpose of and relationship between ideal weight and caloric intake to support cardiac health. Review ways to decrease intake of saturated fats and increase intake of polyunsaturated fats. Discuss limiting intake of refined processed sugar and sodium; discuss limiting cholesterol intake to less than 300 mg per day. Encourage the intake of fresh fruits and vegetables, unprocessed carbohydrates, poultry, and grains.

▶ Nutritional therapy is recommended for those with identified CAD risk, especially for those with elevated low-density lipoprotein (LDL) cholesterol levels, other lipid disorders, diabetes, insulin resistance, or metabolic syndrome. Always consider cultural influences with dietary choices to ensure better adherence to a change in lifestyle. A variety of dietary patterns are beneficial for people with CAD; for additional information regarding nutritional guidelines refer to the study titled "Cholesterol, Total and Fractions."

▶ Other changeable risk factors warranting education include strategies to encourage regular participation of moderate aerobic physical activity three to four times per week, eliminate tobacco use, and adhere to a heart-healthy diet.

▶ Those with elevated triglycerides should be advised to eliminate or reduce alcohol.

Follow-Up, Evaluation, and Desired Outcomes

▶ Acknowledges contact information provided for the American Heart Association (www.heart.org/HEARTORG), National Heart, Lung, and Blood Institute (www.nhlbi.nih.gov), the U.S. Department of Agriculture's resource for nutrition (www.choosemyplate.gov), and Legs for Life (www.legsforlife.org)

▶ Understands that bedrest should be maintained at home for 4 to 6 hr after the procedure or as ordered and to apply cold compresses to the puncture site as needed to reduce discomfort or edema. Verbalizes the correct process for the care and assessment of the site and the need to observe for bleeding, hematoma formation, and inflammation.

▶ Demonstrates correct self-administration of ordered medications. Understands the importance of adhering to the therapy regimen and understands any significant adverse effects associated with the prescribed medication. Agrees to review corresponding literature provided by a pharmacist.

Catecholamines, Blood and Urine

SYNONYM/ACRONYM: Epinephrine, norepinephrine, dopamine.

RATIONALE: To assist in diagnosing catecholamine-secreting tumors, such as those found in the adrenal medulla, and in the investigation of hypertension. The urine test is used to assist in diagnosing pheochromocytoma and as a work-up of neuroblastoma.

PATIENT PREPARATION: Instruct the patient to follow a normal-sodium diet for 3 days before testing, to avoid consumption of foods high in amines for 48 hr before testing, and to withhold food and fluids for 10 to 12 hr before the test. Instruct the patient to avoid self-prescribed medications for 2 wk before testing (especially appetite suppressants and cold and allergy medications, such as nose drops, cough suppressants, and bronchodilators). Instruct the patient to withhold prescribed medication (especially methyldopa, epinephrine, levodopa, and methenamine mandelate) by medical direction. Protocols may vary among facilities. The patient should also abstain from smoking tobacco for 24 hr before testing. Usually, a 24-hr urine collection is ordered. Instruct the patient to avoid excessive exercise and stress during the 24-hr collection of urine. As appropriate, provide the required urine collection container and specimen collection instructions.

NORMAL FINDINGS: Method: High-performance liquid chromatography.

Blood	Conventional Units	SI Units
(Conventional Units × 5.46)		
Epinephrine (supine)		
Child	Less than 450 pg/mL	Less than 2,457 pmol/L
Adult	Less than 50 pg/mL	Less than 273 pmol/L
(Conventional Units × 5.91)		
Norepinephrine (supine)		
Child	Less than 1,200 pg/mL	Less than 7,100 pmol/L
Adult	Less than 410 pg/mL	Less than 2,420 pmol/L
(Conventional Units × 6.53)		
Dopamine (supine or upright)		
Child	Less than 40 pg/mL	Less than 260 pmol/L
Adult	Less than 20 pg/mL	Less than 130 pmol/L

Generally, higher values are expected in specimens collected when the patient has been standing; dopamine values are unaffected by position.

Urine	Conventional Units	SI Units
(Conventional Units × 5.46)		
Epinephrine		
Child	Less than 11 mcg/24 hr	Less than 60 nmol/24 hr
Adult	Less than 20 mcg/24 hr	Less than 100 nmol/24 hr
(Conventional Units × 5.91)		
Norepinephrine		
Child	Less than 50 mcg/24 hr	Less than 300 nmol/24 hr
Adult	Less than 90 mcg/24 hr	Less than 500 nmol/24 hr
(Conventional Units × 6.53)		
Dopamine		
Child	Less than 414 mcg/24 hr	Less than 2,703 nmol/24 hr
Adult	Less than 300 mcg/24 hr	Less than 1,960 nmol/24 hr

Due to the numerous factors that can elevate catecholamines, urine specimens are thought to provide more reliable results in the pediatric population.

CRITICAL FINDINGS AND POTENTIAL INTERVENTIONS: N/A

OVERVIEW: (**Study type:** Blood collected in green-top [heparin] tube and urine from a timed specimen collected in a clean, plastic, amber collection container with 6N hydrochloric acid as a preservative; **related body system:** Endocrine system.) Prior to blood specimen collection, prepare an ice slurry in a cup or plastic bag to have ready for immediate transport of the specimen to the laboratory. The collection tube should be prechilled in the ice slurry. Catecholamines are produced by the chromaffin tissue of the adrenal medulla. They also are found in sympathetic nerve endings and in the brain. The major catecholamines are epinephrine, norepinephrine, and dopamine. They prepare the body for the fight-or-flight stress response, help to regulate metabolism, and are excreted from the body by the kidneys. Levels are affected by diurnal variations,

fluctuating in response to stress, postural changes, diet, smoking, drugs, and temperature changes. As a result, blood measurement is not as reliable as a 24-hr timed urine test. For test results to be valid, all of the previously mentioned environmental variables must be controlled when the test is performed. Results of blood specimens are most reliable when the specimen is collected during a hypertensive episode. Catecholamines are measured when there is high suspicion of pheochromocytoma but urine results are normal or borderline. Use of a clonidine suppression test with measurement of plasma catecholamines may be requested. Failure to suppress production of catecholamines after administration of clonidine supports the diagnosis of pheochromocytoma. Elevated homovanillic acid levels rule out pheochromocytoma because this tumor primarily secretes epinephrine. Elevated catecholamines without hypertension suggest neuroblastoma or ganglioneuroma. Findings should be compared with metanephrines and vanillylmandelic acid, which are the metabolites of epinephrine and norepinephrine. Findings should also be compared with homovanillic acid, which is the product of dopamine metabolism.

INDICATIONS

- Assist in the diagnosis of neuroblastoma, ganglioneuroma, or dysautonomia.
- Assist in the diagnosis of pheochromocytoma.
- Evaluate acute hypertensive episode.
- Evaluate hypertension of unknown origin.
- Screen for pheochromocytoma among family members with an autosomal dominant inheritance pattern for von Hippel-Lindau disease or multiple endocrine neoplasia.

INTERFERING FACTORS

Factors that may alter the results of the study

- Drugs and other substances that may increase plasma catecholamine levels include ajmaline, chlorpromazine, cyclopropane, diazoxide, ether, monoamine oxidase inhibitors, nitroglycerin, pentazocine, perphenazine, phenothiazines, promethazine, and theophylline.
- Drugs and other substances that may decrease plasma catecholamine levels include captopril and reserpine.
- Drugs and other substances that may increase urine catecholamine levels include atenolol, isoproterenol, methyldopa,

niacin, nitroglycerin, prochlorperazine, rauwolfia, reserpine, and theophylline.

- Drugs and other substances that may decrease urine catecholamine levels include bretylium tosylate, clonidine, decaborane, guanethidine, guanfacine, methyldopa, ouabain, radiographic substances, and reserpine.
- Stress, hypoglycemia, smoking, and drugs can produce elevated catecholamines.
- Diets high in amines (e.g., bananas, avocados, beer, aged cheese, chocolate, cocoa, coffee, fava beans, grains, tea, vanilla, walnuts, Chianti wine) can produce elevated catecholamine levels.

Other considerations

- Secretion of catecholamines exhibits diurnal variation, with the lowest levels occurring at night.
- Secretion of catecholamines varies during the menstrual cycle, with higher levels excreted during the luteal phase and lowest levels during ovulation.
- All urine voided for the timed collection period must be included in the collection or else falsely decreased values may be obtained. Compare output records with volume collected to verify that all voids were included in the collection.

POTENTIAL MEDICAL DIAGNOSIS: CLINICAL SIGNIFICANCE OF RESULTS

Increased in

- Diabetic acidosis (epinephrine and norepinephrine) *(related to metabolic stress; are released to initiate glycogenolysis, gluconeogenesis, and lipolysis)*
- Ganglioblastoma (epinephrine, slight increase; norepinephrine, large increase) *(related to production by the tumor)*

C

- Ganglioneuroma (all are increased; norepinephrine, largest increase) *(related to production by the tumor)*
- Hypothyroidism (epinephrine and norepinephrine) *(possibly related to interactions among the immune, endocrine, and nervous systems)*
- Long-term bipolar disorder (epinephrine and norepinephrine) *(some studies indicate a relationship between decreased catecholamine levels and bipolar disorder; the pathophysiology is not well understood)*
- Myocardial infarction (epinephrine and norepinephrine) *(related to physical stress)*
- Neuroblastoma (all are increased; norepinephrine and dopamine, largest increase) *(related to production by the tumor)*
- Pheochromocytoma (epinephrine, continuous or intermittent increase; norepinephrine, slight increase) *(related to production by the tumor)*
- Shock (epinephrine and norepinephrine) *(related to physical stress)*
- Strenuous exercise (epinephrine and norepinephrine) *(related to physical stress)*

Decreased in
- Autonomic nervous system dysfunction (norepinephrine)
- Orthostatic hypotension caused by central nervous system disease (norepinephrine) *(related to inability of sympathetic nervous system to activate postganglionic neuron)*
- Parkinson disease (dopamine) *(some studies indicate a relationship between decreased catecholamine levels and Parkinson disease; the pathophysiology is not well understood)*

NURSING IMPLICATIONS

BEFORE THE STUDY: PLANNING AND IMPLEMENTATION

Teaching the Patient What to Expect
- Inform the patient this test can assist in the diagnosis of a type of tumor that produces excessive amounts of hormones related to physical and emotional stress.
- Explain that a blood or urine sample is needed for the test. Inform the patient that multiple blood specimens may be required and that he or she may be asked to keep warm and to rest for 45 to 60 min before the blood sample is collected. Inform the patient that a saline lock for blood sample collection may be inserted before the test, at the direction of the requesting health-care provider (HCP), because the stress of repeated venipunctures may increase catecholamine levels. Typically, the blood is collected between 0600 and 0800; the patient is asked to stand, and a second sample is collected.
- Information regarding specimen collection is presented with other general guidelines in Appendix A: Patient Preparation and Specimen Collection.

Potential Nursing Actions
- Include on the collection container's label urine total volume, test start and stop times/dates, and any medications that may interfere with test results.

AFTER THE STUDY: POTENTIAL NURSING ACTIONS

Treatment Considerations
- Instruct the patient to resume usual diet, fluids, medications, and activity, as directed by the HCP.

Follow-Up, Evaluation, and Desired Outcomes
- Considers recommendation for screening for pheochromocytoma among family members with an autosomal dominant inheritance pattern for von Hippel-Lindau disease or multiple endocrine neoplasia.

CD4/CD8 Enumeration and Viral Load Testing

SYNONYM/ACRONYM: T-cell profile, cell surface immunotyping.

RATIONALE: To monitor myeloproliferative diseases, immunodeficiency conditions, and HIV disease progression including the effectiveness of retroviral therapy.

PATIENT PREPARATION: There are no food, fluid, activity, or medication restrictions unless by medical direction.

NORMAL FINDINGS: (Method: Flow cytometry) Results are not interchangeable from method to method. Therefore, it is important to use the same method for serial testing.

	Mature T Cells (CD3)		Helper T Cells (CD4)		Suppressor T Cells (CD8)		CD4/ CD8
	Absolute (cells/ microL)	%	Absolute (cells/ microL)	%	Absolute (cells/ microL)	%	
Adult	527–2,846	49–81	332–1,642	28–51	170–811	12–38	1–2

CRITICAL FINDINGS AND POTENTIAL INTERVENTIONS: N/A

OVERVIEW: (**Study type:** Blood collected in a green-top [heparin] tube; **related body system:** Circulatory/Hematopoietic and Immune systems.) Enumeration of lymphocytes, identification of cell lineage, and identification of cellular stage of development are used to diagnose and classify malignant myeloproliferative diseases and to plan treatment. T-cell enumeration is also useful in the evaluation and management of immunodeficiency and autoimmune disease. The CD4 count is a reflection of immune status. It is used to make decisions regarding initiation of antiretroviral therapy (ART) and is also an excellent predictor of imminent opportunistic infection. CD4 counts greater than 500 cells/microL are associated with asymptomatic HIV infection; CD4 counts less than 200 cells/microL are associated with a high risk of developing HIV infection. A sufficient response for patients receiving ART is defined as an increase of CD4 of 50 to 150 (cells/microL) per year with rapid response during the first 3 mo of treatment followed by an annual increase of 50 to 100 (cells/microL) until stabilization is achieved. HIV viral load is another important test used to establish a baseline for viral activity when a person is first diagnosed with HIV and then afterward to monitor response to ART. Viral load testing, also called *plasma HIV RNA*, is performed on plasma from a whole blood sample. The viral load demonstrates how actively the virus is reproducing and helps determine whether treatment is necessary. Optimal viral load is considered to be less than 20 to 75 copies/mL or below the level of detection, but the actual level of detection varies somewhat by test method. Methods commonly used to perform viral load testing include nucleic acid amplification (NAAT) and polymerase chain reaction (PCR). Public health guidelines recommend CD4 counts and viral load testing upon initiation of care for HIV; 3 to 4 mo before commencement of ART; every 3 to 4 mo, but no later than 6 mo, thereafter; and if treatment failure is suspected or otherwise when clinically indicated. Additionally, viral load testing should be requested 2 to 4 wk, but no later than 8 wk, after initiation of ART to verify success of therapy. In clinically stable patients, CD4 testing may be recommended every 6 to 12 mo rather than every 3 to 6 mo. Guidelines also state that treatment of asymptomatic patients should begin when CD4 count is less than 350 cells/microL; treatment is recommended when the patient is symptomatic regardless of test results or when the patient is asymptomatic and CD4 count is between 350 and 500 cells/microL. Failure to respond to therapy is defined as a viral load greater than 200 copies/mL. Increased viral load may be indicative of viral mutations, drug resistance, or nonadherence to the therapeutic regimen. Testing

for drug resistance is recommended if viral load is greater than 1,000 copies/mL.

INDICATIONS
- Assist in the diagnosis of AIDS and plan treatment.
- Evaluate malignant myeloproliferative diseases and plan treatment.
- Evaluate thymus-dependent or cellular immunocompetence.

INTERFERING FACTORS
Factors that may alter the results of the study
- Drugs and other substances that may increase T-cell count include interferon.
- Drugs and other substances that may decrease T-cell count include chlorpromazine and prednisone.
- Recent radioactive scans or radiation can decrease T-cell counts.

Other considerations
- Values may be abnormal in patients with severe recurrent illness or after recent surgery requiring general anesthesia.
- Specimens should be stored at room temperature.

POTENTIAL MEDICAL DIAGNOSIS: CLINICAL SIGNIFICANCE OF RESULTS
Increased in
- Malignant myeloproliferative diseases (e.g., acute and chronic lymphocytic leukemia, lymphoma)

Decreased in
- AIDS
- Aplastic anemia
- Hodgkin disease

NURSING IMPLICATIONS

POTENTIAL NURSING PROBLEMS: ASSESSMENT & NURSING DIAGNOSIS

Problems	Signs and Symptoms
Gas exchange *(related to insufficient oxygen supply secondary to pulmonary infiltrates, sepsis, hyperventilation)*	Decreased activity tolerance, increased shortness of breath with activity, weakness, orthopnea, cyanosis, cough, increased heart rate, weight gain, edema in the lower extremities, weakness, increased respiratory rate, use of respiratory accessory muscles
Infection *(related to altered immune system, malnutrition, chemotherapy)*	Symptoms of infection (increased temperature, increased heart rate, increased blood pressure, shaking, chills, mottled skin, lethargy, fatigue, swelling, edema, pain, localized pressure, diaphoresis, night sweats, confusion, vomiting, nausea, headache), night sweats, persistent cough, adventitious breath sounds (crackles, course, diminished)
Nutrition *(related to fatigue; malabsorption, nausea [adverse effects of medication], effects of chemotherapy)*	Unintended weight loss; current weight 20% below ideal weight; skin tone loss and pale dry skin; dry mucous membranes; documented inadequate caloric intake; subcutaneous tissue loss; hair pulls out easily; paresthesia; muscle wasting
Tissue integrity *(related to insufficient nutrition; vomiting and diarrhea secondary to adverse effects of medications, chemotherapy; altered mobility)*	Area on the skin that is warm or tender to touch; skin that turns red, purple, or black; localized pain; swelling of affected area

BEFORE THE STUDY: PLANNING AND IMPLEMENTATION

Teaching the Patient What to Expect

▶ Inform the patient this test can assist in diagnosing disease and monitoring the effectiveness of disease therapy.

▶ Explain that a blood sample is needed for the test.

AFTER THE STUDY: POTENTIAL NURSING ACTIONS

Treatment Considerations

▶ Gas Exchange: Auscultate and trend breath sounds. Use pulse oximetry to monitor oxygenation and administer oxygen as ordered. Collaborate with health-care provider (HCP) to consider intubation and/or mechanical ventilation if required.

C

Place the head of the bed in high Fowler position to improve ventilatory effort. Administer ordered diuretics, vasodilators, prescribed medications for *Pneumocystis jiroveci*, and steroids. Monitor and trend arterial blood gas (ABG) results. Monitor color and character of sputum. Encourage periods of rest.

▶ Infection: Decrease exposure to environment by placing the patient in a private room. Monitor and trend vital signs and laboratory values that would indicate an infection (white blood cells [WBC], C-reactive protein [CRP]). Promote good hygiene and assist with hygiene as needed. Administer prescribed antibiotics, IV fluids, and antipyretics. Provide cooling measures and encourage oral fluids. Adhere to standard precautions with appropriate use of isolation. Obtain ordered cultures. Provide lightweight clothing and bedding, assess for night sweats. Evaluate cough and sputum color (if cough is productive, check for blood in sputum); use isolation as appropriate (e.g., in the case of tuberculosis); encourage use of incentive spirometer.

▶ Nutrition: Obtain accurate daily weight at the same time each day with the same scale. Obtain an accurate nutritional history and assess attitude toward eating. Promote a dietary consult to evaluate current eating habits and the best method of nutritional supplementation. Develop short-term and long-term eating strategies, monitor nutritional laboratory values such as albumin, transferrin, RBCs, WBCs, and serum electrolytes. Discourage caffeinated and carbonated beverages. Assess swallowing ability and encourage cultural home foods as appropriate. Provide a pleasant environment for eating and alter food seasoning to enhance flavor. Administer ordered parenteral or enteral nutrition. If used, check gastric residual every 4 hr or per facility policy. Encouraging good oral hygiene. Small, frequent meals with prescribed antiemetics can improve appetite.

▶ Tissue Integrity: Conduct baseline skin assessment and frequent reassessment using a standardized organizational evidenced-based approved scale. Monitor and note the presence of herpes lesions. Encourage the use of hypoallergenic soap and lanolin products and to pat rather than rub skin dry. Avoid bed wrinkles and ensure sheets are soft and gentle on the skin. Encourage adequate nutrition and administer prescribed vitamin supplements. Encourage and assist range of motion. Assess the characteristics of a wound (color, size, length, width, depth, drainage, and odor). Monitor for fever and identify the cause of the tissue damage.

Nutritional Considerations

▶ As appropriate, stress the importance of good nutrition and suggest that the patient meet with a registered dietitian.

Follow-Up, Evaluation, and Desired Outcomes

▶ Acknowledges contact information provided for the National Institutes of Health (https://aidsinfo.nih.gov), American College of Obstetricians and Gynecologists (www.acog.org), or Centers for Disease Control and Prevention (www.cdc.gov).

▶ Understands that there will be requests for follow-up blood work at regular intervals.

▶ Acknowledges the risk of transmission and proper prophylaxis, and the importance of strict adherence to the treatment regimen, including consultation with a pharmacist. Understands the importance of following the care plan for medications and follow-up visits.

▶ Accepts there may be anxiety related to test results, perceived loss of independence, and fear of shortened life expectancy. Understands the potential for infection risk related to immunosuppressed inflammatory response and fatigue related to decreased energy production. Counseling services may assist with coping with health and lifestyle changes.

Cerebrospinal Fluid Analysis

SYNONYM/ACRONYM: CSF analysis, lumbar puncture with analysis of CSF, spinal tap.

RATIONALE: To assist in the differential diagnosis of infection or hemorrhage of the brain. Also used in the evaluation of other conditions with significant neuromuscular effects, such as multiple sclerosis.

PATIENT PREPARATION: There are no food, fluid, activity, or medication restrictions unless by medical direction.

NORMAL FINDINGS: Method: Macroscopic evaluation of appearance; spectrophotometry for glucose, lactic acid, and protein; immunoassay for myelin basic protein; nephelometry for immunoglobulin G (IgG); electrophoresis for oligoclonal banding; Gram stain, India ink preparation, and culture or polymerase chain reaction (PCR) for microbiology; microscopic examination of fluid for cell count; flocculation for Venereal Disease Research Laboratory (VDRL).

Lumbar Puncture	Conventional Units	SI Units
Color and appearance	Crystal clear	
Protein		*(Conventional Units × 10)*
0–1 mo	Less than 150 mg/dL	Less than 1,500 mg/L
1–6 mo	30–100 mg/dL	300–1,000 mg/L
7 mo–adult	15–45 mg/dL	150–450 mg/L
Older adult	15–60 mg/dL	150–600 mg/L
Glucose		*(Conventional Units × 0.0555)*
Infant or child	60–80 mg/dL	3.3–4.4 mmol/L
Adult/older adult	40–70 mg/dL	2.2–3.9 mmol/L
Lactic acid		*(Conventional Units × 0.111)*
Neonate	10–60 mg/dL	1.1–6.7 mmol/L
3–10 d	10–40 mg/dL	1.1–4.4 mmol/L
Adult	Less than 25.2 mg/dL	Less than 2.8 mmol/L
IgG		*(Conventional Units × 10)*
	Less than 3.4 mg/dL	Less than 34 mg/L
Myelin basic protein		*(Conventional Units × 1)*
	Less than 4 ng/mL	Less than 4 mcg/L
Oligoclonal bands	Absent	
Gram stain	Negative	
India ink	Negative	
Culture	No growth	
RBC count	0	0

(table continues on page 294)

Lumbar Puncture	Conventional Units	SI Units
WBC count		*(Conventional Units × 1)*
Neonate–1 mo	0–30/microL	0–30/mm³
1 mo–1 yr	0–10/microL	0–10/mm³
1–5 yr	0–8/microL	0–8/mm³
5 yr–adult	0–5/microL	0–5/mm³
VDRL	Nonreactive	
Cytology	No abnormal cells seen	

RBC = red blood cell; VDRL = Venereal Disease Research Laboratory; WBC = white blood cell.
CSF glucose should be 60%–70% of plasma glucose level.
Color should be assessed after sample is centrifuged.

WBC Differential	Adult	Children
Lymphocytes	40%–80%	5%–13%
Monocytes	15%–45%	50%–90%
Neutrophils	0%–6%	0%–8%

CRITICAL FINDINGS AND POTENTIAL INTERVENTIONS

- Positive Gram stain, India ink preparation, or culture
- Presence of malignant cells or blasts
- Elevated WBC count
- Adults: Glucose less than 37 mg/dL (SI: Less than 2.1 mmol/L); greater than 440 mg/dL (SI: Greater than 24.4 mmol/L)
- Children: Glucose less than 31 mg/dL (SI: Less than 1.7 mmol/L); greater than 440 mg/dL (SI: Greater than 24.4 mmol/L)

Timely notification to the requesting health-care provider (HCP) of any critical findings and related symptoms is a role expectation of the professional nurse. A listing of these findings varies among facilities.

Important signs to note include allergic or other reaction to the anesthesia, bleeding or CSF drainage at the puncture sight, changes in level of consciousness, changes to or inequality of pupil size, or respiratory failure.

OVERVIEW: (**Study type:** Body fluid, CSF collected in three or four separate plastic conical tubes; **related body system:** Immune and Nervous systems.) Tube 1 is used for chemistry and serology testing, tube 2 is used for microbiology, tube 3 is used for cell count, and tube 4 is used for miscellaneous testing. CSF circulates in the subarachnoid space and has a twofold function: to protect the brain and spinal cord from injury and to transport products of cellular metabolism and neurosecretion. The total volume of CSF is 90 to 150 mL in adults and 60 mL in infants. CSF analysis helps determine the presence and cause of bleeding and assists in diagnosing cancer, infections, and degenerative and autoimmune diseases of the brain and spinal cord. Specimens for analysis are most frequently obtained by lumbar puncture and sometimes by ventricular or cisternal puncture. Lumbar puncture can also have therapeutic uses, including injection of drugs and anesthesia. Lumbar puncture is performed as a sterile procedure with the use of a spinal needle to capture a spinal fluid specimen for analysis. Needle size is important, as the smaller the bevel, the more time it will take to collect a sufficient volume of fluid; usually a 22-gauge needle is used. Once the needle has been properly placed, the stylet is removed, allowing CSF to drip from the needle. A stopcock and manometer are attached to the hub of the needle to measure initial CSF pressure. Normal pressure for an adult in the lateral recumbent position is 90 to 180 mm H_2O. Four or five vials of fluid, according to the HCP's request, may be collected in separate tubes (1–3 mL in each) and labelled numerically (1–4 or 5) in the order they were filled. A final pressure reading is taken, and the needle is removed. After the CSF has been removed, the puncture site is cleansed with an antiseptic solution and direct pressure is applied with dry gauze to stop bleeding or CSF leakage. The subspeciality of microbiology has been revolutionized by molecular diagnostics. Molecular diagnostics involves the identification of specific sequences of DNA. The application of molecular diagnostics techniques, such as PCR, has led to the development of automated instruments that can identify a single infectious organism or multiple pathogens from a CSF sample in less than 2 hr. The instruments can detect the presence of bacteria, viruses, and yeast commonly associated with meningitis and encephalitis.

INDICATIONS

- Assist in the diagnosis and differentiation of subarachnoid or intracranial hemorrhage.
- Assist in the diagnosis and differentiation of viral or bacterial meningitis or encephalitis.
- Assist in the diagnosis of diseases such as multiple sclerosis, autoimmune disorders, or degenerative brain disease.
- Assist in the diagnosis of neurosyphilis and chronic central nervous system (CNS) infections.
- Detect obstruction of CSF circulation due to hemorrhage, tumor, or edema.
- Establish the presence of any condition decreasing the flow of oxygen to the brain.
- Monitor for metastases of cancer into the CNS.
- Monitor severe brain injuries.

INTERFERING FACTORS

Contraindications

Patients with infection present at the needle insertion site.

Patients with degenerative joint disease or coagulation defects.

Patients with increased intracranial pressure; extreme caution should be used *because overly rapid removal of CSF can result in herniation.*

Factors that may alter the results of the study

- Drugs and other substances that may decrease CSF protein levels include cefotaxime and dexamethasone.
- Interferon-β may increase myelin basic protein levels.
- Drugs and other substances that may increase CSF glucose levels include cefotaxime and dexamethasone.
- RBC count may be falsely elevated with a traumatic spinal tap.

- Delays in analysis may present a false-positive appearance of xanthochromia due to RBC lysis that begins within 4 hr of a bloody tap.

Other considerations
- CSF pressure may be elevated if the patient is anxious, holding his or her breath, tensing muscles, or if the patient's knees are flexed too firmly against the abdomen. If the initial pressure is elevated, the HCP may perform Queckenstedt test. This would be performed by the application of pressure to the jugular vein for about 10 sec. CSF pressure usually rises in response to the occlusion, then rapidly returns to normal within 10 sec after the pressure is released. A sluggish response may indicate CSF obstruction.

POTENTIAL MEDICAL DIAGNOSIS: CLINICAL SIGNIFICANCE OF RESULTS
Increased in
- Color and appearance *(xanthochromia is any pink, yellow, or orange color; bloody—hemorrhage; xanthochromic—old hemorrhage, RBC breakdown, methemoglobin, bilirubin [greater than 6 mg/dL (SI: 102.6 micromol/L)], increased protein [greater than 150 mg/dL (SI: 1,500 mg/L)], melanin [meningeal melanosarcoma], carotene [systemic carotenemia]; hazy—meningitis; pink to dark yellow—aspiration of epidural fat; turbid—cells, microorganisms, protein, fat, or contrast medium; turbidity related to increased cell count is called pleocytosis)*
- Protein *(related to alterations in blood-brain barrier that allow permeability to proteins):* Type 2 diabetes *(related to relative increase in plasma glucose)*, encephalitis, Guillain-Barré syndrome (elevated protein with normal WBC count—also called *albuminocytological dissociation*), meningitis, trauma, tumors
- Lactic acid *(related to cerebral hypoxia and correlating anaerobic metabolism):* Bacterial, tubercular, fungal meningitis
- Myelin basic protein *(related to accumulation as a result of nerve sheath demyelination):* Trauma, stroke, tumor, multiple sclerosis, subacute sclerosing panencephalitis
- IgG and oligoclonal banding *(related to autoimmune or inflammatory response):* Multiple sclerosis, CNS syphilis, and subacute sclerosing panencephalitis
- Gram stain: *Meningitis due to Escherichia coli, Streptococcus agalactiae, S. pneumoniae, Haemophilus influenzae, Mycobacterium avium-intracellulare, M. leprae, M. tuberculosis, Neisseria meningitidis, Cryptococcus neoformans*
- India ink preparation: *Meningitis due to C. neoformans*
- Culture: *Encephalitis or meningitis due to herpes simplex virus,* S. pneumoniae, H. influenzae, N. meningitidis, C. neoformans
- RBC count: *Hemorrhage*
- WBC count:

  General increase—injection of contrast media or anticancer drugs in subarachnoid space, CSF infarct, metastatic tumor in contact with CSF, reaction to repeated lumbar puncture

  Elevated WBC count with a predominance of neutrophils indicative of abscess, bacterial meningitis, tubercular meningitis

  Elevated WBC count with a predominance of lymphocytes indicative of viral, tubercular, parasitic, or fungal meningitis; multiple sclerosis

  Elevated WBC count with a predominance of monocytes indicative of chronic bacterial meningitis, amebic meningitis, multiple sclerosis, toxoplasmosis

Increased plasma cells indicative of acute
viral infections, demyelinating diseases,
multiple sclerosis, neurosyphilis, sarcoidosis, syphilitic meningoencephalitis,
subacute sclerosing panencephalitis,
tubercular meningitis, parasitic infections,
Guillain-Barré syndrome
Presence of eosinophils indicative of parasitic
and fungal infections, acute polyneuritis,

idiopathic hypereosinophilic syndrome,
reaction to drugs or a shunt in CSF
- VDRL: *Syphilis*

Positive findings in
- Cytology: *Malignant cells*

Decreased in
- Glucose: *Bacterial and tubercular
  meningitis*

C

NURSING IMPLICATIONS

POTENTIAL NURSING PROBLEMS: ASSESSMENT & NURSING DIAGNOSIS

Problems	Signs and Symptoms
Mobility *(related to nerve demyelination, spastic muscle movement, weakness, muscle tremors)*	Weak or unsteady gait, uncoordinated movement, difficult purposeful movement, limited range of motion
Skin *(related to limited mobility, sensory changes)*	Development of pressure ulcers, open sores that are unattended due to lack of sensation and recognition, skin injury from burn
Visual disturbance *(related to optic nerve demyelination)*	Blurred vision, some visual loss or blind spots, nystagmus, double vision, altered color perception

BEFORE THE STUDY: PLANNING AND IMPLEMENTATION

Teaching the Patient What to Expect

- Inform the patient this procedure can assist in evaluating health by providing a sample of fluid from around the spinal cord to be tested for disease and infection.
- Explain that a spinal fluid sample is needed for the test. Address concerns about pain, and explain there may be some discomfort during the lumbar puncture.
- Inform the patient/caregiver that the CSF specimen collection will be performed by an HCP trained to perform the procedure and takes approximately 20 min.
- Explain that the lumbar puncture is performed using sterile technique to avoid infection; the site (usually between L3 and L4 or L4 and L5) is prepped with

an antiseptic cleanser and covered with a sterile drape prior to injection of the local anesthetic and CSF needle/stylet. Warn the patient that the antiseptic will feel cold when it is applied to the skin.
- Baseline vital signs and assessment of neurological status will be recorded prior to the lumbar puncture for post-procedure comparison.
- Positioning is typically the knee-chest lateral recumbent (lateral decubitus, Sims, or side-lying) position for maximum spinal flexion and widening of intervertebral spaces. Pillows may need to be placed between the legs to support the spine.
- Local anesthetic is injected with a spinal needle through the spinous processes of the vertebrae into the subarachnoid space to decrease discomfort.
- Observe/assess the puncture site for bleeding, CSF leakage, or hematoma

formation, cover the site with a gauze, and secure the gauze with an adhesive bandage.

▶ Specimens should be promptly transported to the laboratory for processing and analysis. It is possible that there may be a postprocedure headache.

Potential Nursing Actions

◈ *Make sure a written and informed consent has been signed prior to the procedure and before administering any medications.*

▶ Assess the patient's ability to maintain required position and provide assistance as needed.

AFTER THE STUDY: POTENTIAL NURSING ACTIONS

Avoiding Complications

▶ Headache is a common minor complication experienced after lumbar puncture and is caused by leakage of the spinal fluid from around the puncture site, *most probably related to the tear in the dura after the needle has been withdrawn.* On a rare occasion, the headache may require treatment with an epidural blood patch in which an anesthesiologist or pain management specialist injects a small amount of the patient's blood in the epidural space of the puncture site. The blood patch forms a clot and seals the puncture site to prevent further leakage of CSF and provides relief within 30 min. Other complications include lower back pain after the procedure, infection that might occur if bacteria from the skin surface is introduced at the puncture site, bleeding near the puncture site, or brainstem herniation due to increased intracranial pressure.

Treatment Considerations

▶ After the procedure, position the patient flat, either on the back or abdomen, although some HCPs allow 30 degrees of elevation. Maintain this position for 8 hr. Changing position is acceptable as long as the body remains horizontal.

▶ Observe/assess the puncture site for leakage, and frequently monitor body signs, such as temperature and blood pressure.

▶ Observe/assess the patient for neurological changes, such as altered level of consciousness, change in pupils, reports of tingling or numbness, and irritability.

▶ Monitor vital signs and neurologic status every 15 min for 1 hr, then every 2 hr for 4 hr, and as ordered after lumbar puncture. Take the temperature every 4 hr for 24 hr. Compare with baseline values. Protocols may vary among facilities.

▶ To prevent or relieve headache due to lumbar puncture, administer ordered or permitted caffeinated fluids to replace lost CSF. The use of a flexible straw facilitates intake of fluids while the patient is lying flat. Advise the patient that headache may begin within a few hours up to 2 days after the procedure and may be associated with dizziness, nausea, and vomiting. The length of time for the headache to resolve varies considerably.

▶ Mobility: Assess the patient's muscle strength and coordination and use assistive devices if necessary. Encourage self-care and appropriate and safe activity.

▶ Skin: Careful use of heat and cold to prevent skin damage and unintended burns. Ensure water used for personal hygiene is tested for temperature prior to use. Change position a minimum of every 2 hr.

Safety Considerations

▶ Visual Disturbance: Check the immediate environment for items that could cause fall and injury. Encourage the patient to wear assistive devices such as glasses or contacts to improve vision. Provide information for support group related to vision loss. Encourage the use of an eye patch as appropriate.

Follow-Up, Evaluation, and Desired Outcomes

▶ Agrees to keep frequently used items within easy reach, and states the importance of creating a safe home environment to prevent injury due to vision loss.

- Understands the importance of changing position frequently to prevent pressure ulcers.
- Recognizes that the disease process may be accompanied by periods of exacerbation.

- Demonstrates the ability to use assistive devices safely and to complete activities of daily living.
- Agrees to use assistive devices to decrease fall risk and associated injury.

C

Ceruloplasmin

SYNONYM/ACRONYM: Copper oxidase, Cp.

RATIONALE: To assist in the evaluation of copper intoxication and liver disease, especially Wilson disease.

PATIENT PREPARATION: There are no food, fluid, activity, or medication restrictions unless by medical direction.

NORMAL FINDINGS: Method: Nephelometry.

Age	Conventional Units	SI Units (Conventional Units × 10)
Newborn–3 mo	5–18 mg/dL	50–180 mg/L
6–12 mo	33–43 mg/dL	330–430 mg/L
1–5 yr	26–55 mg/dL	260–550 mg/L
6 yr–older adult	20–40 mg/dL	200–400 mg/L

CRITICAL FINDINGS AND POTENTIAL INTERVENTIONS: N/A

OVERVIEW: (Study type: Blood collected in a gold-, red-, or red/gray-top tube; related body system: Circulatory/Hematopoietic and Digestive systems.) Ceruloplasmin is an α_2-globulin produced by the liver that binds copper for transport in the blood after it is absorbed from the gastrointestinal system. Decreased production of this transport protein results in the deposition of unbound copper in body tissues such as the brain, liver, corneas, and kidneys. Ceruloplasmin, a ferroxidase, also plays a role in regulating iron homeostasis.

Knowledge of genetics assists in identifying those who may benefit from additional education, risk assessment, and counseling. Genetics is the study and identification of genes, genetic mutations, and inheritance. For example, genetics provides some insight into the likelihood of inheriting a medical condition such as Menkes disease (syndrome) or Wilson disease. Some conditions are the result of mutations involving a single gene, whereas other conditions may involve multiple genes and/or multiple chromosomes. Menkes disease is an example of a recessive sex-linked genetic disorder passed from a mother to a male child; approximately 30% of cases result from "new" mutations in the affected gene, which means those patients will not have a family history of the disease. Wilson disease is an example of an autosomal recessive disorder in which the offspring inherits a copy of the defective gene from each parent. Molecular genetic testing for the respective gene mutations can confirm a diagnosis of Menkes and Wilson disease. Further information regarding inheritance of genes can be found in the study titled "Genetic Testing."

INDICATIONS

- Assist in the diagnosis of Menkes (kinky hair) disease.
- Assist in the diagnosis of Wilson disease.
- Determine genetic predisposition to Wilson disease.
- Monitor patient response to total parenteral nutrition (hyperalimentation).

INTERFERING FACTORS

Factors that may alter the results of the study

- Drugs and other substances that may increase ceruloplasmin levels include anticonvulsants, norethindrone, oral contraceptives, and tamoxifen.
- Drugs and other substances that may decrease ceruloplasmin levels include asparaginase and levonorgestrel.

Other considerations

- Excessive therapeutic intake of zinc may interfere with intestinal absorption of copper.

POTENTIAL MEDICAL DIAGNOSIS: CLINICAL SIGNIFICANCE OF RESULTS

Increased in

Ceruloplasmin is an acute-phase reactant protein and will be increased in many inflammatory conditions, including cancer

- Acute infections
- Biliary cholangitis
- Cancer of the bone, lung, stomach
- Copper intoxication
- Hodgkin disease
- Leukemia
- Pregnancy (last trimester) *(estrogen increases copper levels)*
- Rheumatoid arthritis
- Tissue necrosis

Decreased in

- Menkes disease *(severe X-linked defect causing failed transport to the liver and tissues)*
- Nutritional deficiency of copper
- Wilson disease *(genetic defect causing failed transport to the liver and tissues)*

NURSING IMPLICATIONS

BEFORE THE STUDY: PLANNING AND IMPLEMENTATION

Teaching the Patient What to Expect

- Inform the patient this test can determine copper levels in the blood.
- Explain that a blood sample is needed for the test.

AFTER THE STUDY: POTENTIAL NURSING ACTIONS

Treatment Considerations

- Recommend a consult with a registered dietitian to assist the patient to identify culturally appropriate copper rich foods.

Nutritional Considerations

- Instruct the patient with copper deficiency to increase intake of foods rich in copper, as appropriate. Organ meats, shellfish, nuts, and legumes are good sources of dietary copper. High intake of zinc, iron, calcium, and manganese interferes with copper absorption. Copper deficiency does not normally occur in adults; however, patients receiving long-term total parenteral nutrition should be evaluated if signs and symptoms of copper deficiency appear, such as jaundice or eye color changes.

Follow-Up, Evaluation, and Desired Outcomes
▶ Understands that Kayser-Fleischer rings (green-gold rings) in the cornea and a liver biopsy specimen showing elevated copper levels are findings indicative of Wilson disease. Acknowledges that depending on the results of this procedure additional testing may be performed to evaluate or monitor progression of the disease process and determine the need for a change in therapy.

C

Chest X-Ray

SYNONYM/ACRONYM: Chest radiography, CXR, lung radiography.

RATIONALE: To assist in the evaluation of cardiac, respiratory, and skeletal structure within the lung cavity and diagnose multiple diseases such as pneumonia and heart failure.

PATIENT PREPARATION: There are no food, fluid, activity, or medication restrictions unless by medical direction.

NORMAL FINDINGS
- Normal lung fields, cardiac size and shape, mediastinal structures, thoracic spine, ribs, and diaphragm.

CRITICAL FINDINGS AND POTENTIAL INTERVENTIONS
- Foreign body
- Malposition of tube, line, or postoperative device (pacemaker)
- Pneumonia
- Pneumoperitoneum
- Pneumothorax
- Spine fracture

Timely notification to the requesting health-care provider (HCP) of any critical findings and related symptoms is a role expectation of the professional nurse. A listing of these findings varies among facilities.

OVERVIEW: (Study type: X-ray, plain; **related body system:** Circulatory, Musculoskeletal, and Respiratory systems.) Chest radiography, commonly called chest x-ray, is one of the most frequently performed diagnostic imaging studies. This study yields information about the pulmonary, cardiac, and skeletal systems. The lungs, filled with air, are easily penetrated by x-rays and appear black on chest images. A routine chest x-ray includes

C

a posteroanterior projection, in which x-rays pass from the posterior to the anterior, and a left lateral projection. Additional projections that may be requested are obliques, lateral decubitus, or lordotic views. Portable x-rays, done in acute or critical situations, can be done at the bedside and usually include only the anteroposterior projection with additional images taken in a lateral decubitus position if the presence of free pleural fluid or air is in question. Chest images should be taken on full inspiration and erect when possible to minimize heart magnification and demonstrate fluid levels. Expiration images may be added to detect a pneumothorax or locate foreign bodies. Rib detail images may be taken to delineate bone pathology, useful when chest radiographs suggest fractures or metastatic lesions. Fluoroscopic studies of the chest can also be done to evaluate lung and diaphragm movement. In the beginning of the disease process of tuberculosis, asthma, and chronic obstructive pulmonary disease, the results of a chest x-ray may not correlate with the clinical status of the patient and may even be normal.

INDICATIONS

- Aid in the diagnosis of diaphragmatic hernia, lung tumors, and metastasis.
- Evaluate known or suspected pulmonary disorders, chest trauma, cardiovascular disorders, and skeletal disorders.
- Evaluate placement and position of an endotracheal tube, tracheostomy tube, nasogastric feeding tube, pacemaker wires, central venous catheters, Swan-Ganz catheters, chest tubes, and intra-aortic balloon pump.
- Evaluate positive purified protein derivative (PPD) or Mantoux tests.
- Monitor resolution, progression, or maintenance of disease.
- Monitor effectiveness of the treatment regimen.

INTERFERING FACTORS
Contraindications

✧ Patients who are pregnant or suspected of being pregnant, unless the potential benefits of a procedure using radiation far outweigh the risk of radiation exposure to the fetus and mother.

Factors that may alter the results of the study
- Metallic objects (e.g., jewelry, body rings) within the examination field, which may inhibit organ visualization and cause unclear images.
- Inability of the patient to cooperate or remain still during the procedure, because movement can produce blurred or otherwise unclear images.

POTENTIAL MEDICAL DIAGNOSIS: CLINICAL SIGNIFICANCE OF RESULTS
Abnormal findings related to
- Atelectasis
- Bronchitis
- Curvature of the spinal column (scoliosis)
- Enlarged heart
- Enlarged lymph nodes
- Flattened diaphragm
- Foreign bodies lodged in the pulmonary system *as seen by a radiopaque object*
- Fractures of the sternum, ribs, and spine
- Lung pathology, including tumors
- Malposition of tubes or wires
- Mediastinal tumor and pathology
- Pericardial effusion
- Pericarditis

- Pleural effusion
- Pneumonia
- Pneumothorax

- Pulmonary bases, fibrosis, infiltrates
- Tuberculosis
- Vascular abnormalities

C

NURSING IMPLICATIONS

POTENTIAL NURSING PROBLEMS: ASSESSMENT & NURSING DIAGNOSIS

Problems	Signs and Symptoms
Gas exchange *(related to inflammation of lung tissues, impaired alveolar membrane with decreased oxygen supply, consolidation)*	Restlessness; altered level of consciousness; tachypnea; shortness of breath; cyanosis; activity intolerance; nasal flare; use of accessory muscles; adventitious, diminished breath sounds
Infection *(related to inflammation, trauma)*	Fever, chills, elevated white blood cell (WBC) count, cough, purulent sputum, tachycardia, increased respiratory rate
Insufficient fluid volume (water) *(related to fluid loss from fever, diaphoresis)*	Decreased urinary output, weight loss, dry oral mucous membranes, dehydration, poor skin turgor

BEFORE THE STUDY: PLANNING AND IMPLEMENTATION

Teaching the Patient What to Expect

▶ Inform the patient this procedure can assist in assessing the heart and lungs for disease.

▶ Pregnancy is a general contraindication to procedures involving radiation. Explain to the female patient that she will be asked the date of her last menstrual period. Pregnancy testing may be performed to determine the possibility of pregnancy before exposure to radiation.

▶ Review the procedure with the patient. Address concerns about pain and explain that no pain should be experienced during the test.

▶ Inform the patient that the procedure is performed in the radiology department or at the bedside, by a registered radiological technologist, and takes approximately 5 to 15 min. Instruct the patient to remove all metallic objects from the area to be examined.

▶ **Pediatric Considerations:** Preparing children for a chest x-ray depends on the age of the child. Encourage parents to be truthful about what the child may experience during the procedure and to use words that they know their child will understand. Toddlers and preschool-age children have a very short attention span, so the best time to talk about the test is right before the procedure. The child should be assured that he or she will be allowed to bring a favorite comfort item into the examination room, and if appropriate, that a parent will be with the child during the procedure. Provide older children with information about the test, and allow them to participate in as many decisions as possible (e.g., choice of clothes to wear to the appointment) in order to reduce anxiety and encourage cooperation. If the child will be asked to maintain a certain position for the test, encourage the child to practice the required position, provide a CD that demonstrates the procedure, and teach strategies to remain calm, such as deep breathing, humming, or counting to himself or herself.

▶ Instruct the patient to remove jewelry and other metallic objects from the area of examination.

> ▸ Routine chest view is taken by placing the patient in the standing position, facing the cassette or image detector, with hands on hips, neck extended, and shoulders rolled forward. The chest is positioned with the left side against the image holder for a lateral view. For portable examinations, the head of the bed is elevated to the high Fowler position (90 degrees). The patient will be asked to inhale deeply and hold his or her breath while the x-ray images are taken, and then to exhale after the images are taken.

Potential Nursing Actions

> ▸ Verify the patient will be able to cooperate fully and to follow directions. The patient will be asked to assume specific positions and remain still throughout the procedure because movement produces unreliable results.

AFTER THE STUDY: POTENTIAL NURSING ACTIONS

Treatment Considerations

> ▸ Gas Exchange: Use continuous pulse oximetry to monitor oxygen saturation, and administer ordered oxygen. Monitor and trend arterial blood gases results and chest x-ray results. Position the patient with the head elevated to improve ventilation. Pace activities and assess respiratory effort, rate, and work of breathing.
> ▸ Infection: Evaluate current immunizations. Monitor and trend WBC count and vital signs (blood pressure, pulse, temperature, heart rate). Administer ordered antibiotics and antipyretics. Monitor breath sounds and ensure any ordered sputum culture and sensitivity has been submitted to the laboratory. Evaluate hydration and consider the use of cooling measures for elevated temperature.
> ▸ Insufficient Fluid Volume (Water): Monitor intake and output and trend results. Perform a daily weight. Fluid intake can be increased by oral or parenteral means or a combination of both. Keep mucous membranes (oral) moist with good oral care.

Safety Considerations

> ▸ Avoid overly aggressive fluid replacement. Observe for symptoms of fluid overload; shortness of breath, tachycardia, hypertension, positive jugular vein distention, edema, and sodium/potassium electrolyte imbalance.

Follow-Up, Evaluation, and Desired Outcomes

> ▸ Demonstrates how to accurately perform and document daily weight and intake and output.
> ▸ Acknowledges the importance of good hand hygiene to decrease infection risk.
> ▸ Choose activities that decrease the risk of fatigue leading to a compromised respiratory status.
> ▸ Demonstrates effective cough and deep-breathing techniques to improve oxygenation and understands the importance of keeping oxygen on to support respiratory status.

Chlamydia Testing

SYNONYM/ACRONYM: N/A

RATIONALE: To diagnose some of the more common chlamydia infections such as community-acquired pneumonia transmitted by *Chlamydophila pneumoniae* and chlamydia disease that is sexually transmitted by *Chlamydia trachomatis*.

PATIENT PREPARATION: There are no food, fluid, activity, or medication restrictions unless by medical direction.

NORMAL FINDINGS: (Method: Transcription-mediated amplification [TMA], viral culture with monoclonal antibody detection) Negative for TMA, not isolated for viral culture.

Method: Enzyme Immunofluorescent (EIF) Assay	
Chlamydia trachomatis, C. pneumoniae, C. psittaci antibody IgG	*Chlamydia trachomatis,* C. pneumoniae, C. psittaci antibody IgM
Less than 1:64	Less than 1:20

CRITICAL FINDINGS AND POTENTIAL INTERVENTIONS: N/A

OVERVIEW: (**Study type:** Blood collected in a red-top tube [EIF]; endocervical, vaginal, or male urethral swab, urine, cervical brush [TMA—positive findings must be confirmed by alternative nucleic acid target]; swabs or tissue from various body sites or fluids in special viral culture transport media that supports *Chlamydia* species; **related body system:** Immune, Reproductive, and Respiratory systems.) *Chlamydia trachomatis* is the cause of one of the most common sexually transmitted infections. These gram-negative bacteria are called *obligate cell parasites* because they require living cells for growth. There are three serotypes of *C. trachomatis*. One group causes lymphogranuloma venereum, with symptoms of the first phase of the disease appearing 2 to 6 wk after infection; another causes a genital tract infection different from lymphogranuloma venereum, in which symptoms in men appear 7 to 28 days after intercourse (women are generally asymptomatic); and the third causes the ocular disease trachoma (incubation period 7–10 days). *C. psittaci* is the cause of psittacosis in birds and humans. It is increasing in prevalence as a pathogen responsible for other significant diseases of the respiratory system. The incubation period for *C. psittaci* infections in humans is 7 to 15 days and is followed by chills, fever, and a persistent nonproductive cough. Another chlamydia, *C. pneumoniae*, is a common cause of community-acquired pneumonia.

Chlamydia is difficult to culture and grow, so antibody testing has become the technology of choice to identify antibodies to *C. psittaci* and *C. pneumoniae*. A limitation of antibody screening is that positive results may not distinguish past from current infection. Antibody testing may also be used to identify sexually transmitted chlamydial disease; however, nucleic acid amplification and DNA probes are more commonly used to identify the *Chlamydia* species. Assays can specifically identify *C. trachomatis* and require special collection and transport kits. They also have specific collection instructions, and the specimens are collected on swabs. The laboratory performing this testing should be consulted before specimen collection. Culture- or liquid-based Pap test may also be requested for identification of oculogenital chlamydia infections.

INDICATIONS

- Establish *Chlamydia* as the cause of atypical pneumonia.
- Establish *Chlamydia* as the cause of sexually transmitted chlamydial disease.
- Establish the presence of other types of chlamydial infection.

INTERFERING FACTORS

Factors that may alter the results of the study

- Positive antibody test results may demonstrate evidence of past infection and not necessarily indicate current infection.
- Specimen rejection criteria for culture samples is determined by the laboratory performing the procedure.

Other considerations

- Hemolysis or lipemia may interfere with antibody testing analysis.

POTENTIAL MEDICAL DIAGNOSIS: CLINICAL SIGNIFICANCE OF RESULTS

Positive findings in

- Chlamydial infection
- Community-acquired pneumonia
- Infantile pneumonia *(related to transmission at birth from an infected mother)*
- Infertility *(related to scarring of ovaries or fallopian tubes from untreated chlamydial infection)*
- Lymphogranuloma venereum
- Ophthalmia neonatorum *(related to transmission at birth from an infected mother)*
- Pelvic inflammatory disease
- Urethritis

NURSING IMPLICATIONS

POTENTIAL NURSING PROBLEMS: ASSESSMENT & NURSING DIAGNOSIS

Problems	Signs and Symptoms
Infection *(related to exposure to* C. pneumoniae*); (related to sexual exposure to* C. trachomatis*)*	*C. pneumoniae* exposure: Temperature, increased heart rate, increased blood pressure, shaking, chills, mottled skin, lethargy, fatigue, swelling, elevated white blood cell (WBC) count, sputum culture positive for infecting organism, tachypnea, dyspnea, productive cough, tachycardia *C. trachomatis* sexual exposure: Purulent penile or vaginal drainage; dysuria; lower abdominal pain in women (pelvic inflammatory disease); testicular pain and swelling (epididymitis); pain, bleeding, and discharge from the rectum (proctitis); sometimes there are no symptoms
Airway *(related to congestion, sputum production as a result of exposure to* C. pneumoniae*)*	Ineffective cough, purulent sputum, dyspnea, tachypnea, documented infiltrates, decreased or diminished breath sounds

C

Problems	Signs and Symptoms
Gas exchange *(related to congestion [fluid in alveoli or mucus in airways], mucous secretions, ventilation and perfusion mismatch, lung consolidation as a result of exposure to* C. pneumoniae*)*	Decreased activity tolerance, increased shortness of breath with activity, weakness, orthopnea, cyanosis (pale, dusky), cough, increased heart rate, increased respiratory rate, use of respiratory accessory muscles, tachypnea, tachycardia, hypotension, restlessness, irritability, confusion, lethargy, disorientation, hypercapnia

BEFORE THE STUDY: PLANNING AND IMPLEMENTATION

Teaching the Patient What to Expect

▶ Inform the patient this test can assist in diagnosing chlamydial infection.

▶ Explain that a blood, urine, or genital swab sample is needed for the test depending on the infection site.

▶ Explain that several tests may be necessary to confirm diagnosis.

▶ Advise the patient that any individual positive antibody result should be repeated in 7 to 10 days to monitor a change in titer

Chlamydia Vaginal Swab Collection Followed by Nucleic Acid Amplification

▶ *Care provider specimen:* Explain that a vaginal fluid sample will be collected using the vaginal swab kit by contacting the swab to the lower third of the vaginal wall, and rotating the swab for 10 to 30 sec to absorb the fluid. The swab will be immediately placed into a transport tube, the swab shaft carefully broken against the side of the tube, and the cap tightly screwed on.

▶ *Patient self-collection instructions:* If the patient is doing a self-collection, provide these instructions and verify understanding for accurate results.

▶ First, partially open the package and do not touch the soft tip or lay the swab down.

▶ Explain that if the soft tip is touched, the swab is laid down, or the swab is dropped, a new vaginal swab

specimen collection kit will need to be used.

▶ Next, remove the swab and carefully insert the swab into the vagina about 2 in. past the introitus. Gently rotate the swab for 10 to 30 sec, making sure the swab touches the walls of the vagina so that moisture is absorbed by the swab.

▶ Finally, withdraw the swab without touching the skin. Immediately place the swab into the transport tube, and carefully break the swab shaft against the side of the tube. Tightly screw on the cap.

Chlamydia Endocervical Swab

▶ Explain that excess mucus will be removed from the cervical os and surrounding mucosa using a cleaning swab (white shaft swab in the package with red printing). This swab will be discarded.

▶ Explain that a collection swab (blue shaft swab in the package with green printing) will be inserted into the endocervical canal and gently rotated clockwise for 10 to 30 sec in the endocervical canal to ensure adequate sampling.

▶ The collection swab will be carefully withdrawn to avoid contact with the vaginal mucosa and immediately placed in a transport tube. The swab shaft will be carefully broken at the scoreline, using care to avoid splashing of the contents, then tightly recapped.

Chlamydia Male Urethral Swab

▶ Explain to the male patient that it is important not to urinate at least 1 hr prior to specimen collection. Withdraw the swab carefully. Remove the cap from the swab specimen transport tube, and immediately place the specimen collection swab into the specimen transport tube. Carefully break the swab shaft at the scoreline, using care to avoid splashing of contents. Recap the swab specimen transport tube tightly.

▶ Explain that a specimen collection swab (blue shaft swab in the package with the green printing) will be inserted 2 to 4 cm into the urethra and gently rotated clockwise for 2 to 3 sec to ensure adequate sampling.

Urine Specimen

▶ Explain to the patient that it is important not to urinate at least 1 hr prior to specimen collection.

▶ Instruct the patient to provide a first-catch urine (approximately 20 to 30 mL of the initial urine stream) into a urine collection cup free of any preservatives.

▶ Collection of larger volumes of urine may result in specimen dilution that may reduce test sensitivity; lesser volumes may not adequately rinse organisms into the specimen.

▶ Advise female patients not to cleanse the labial area prior to providing the specimen.

▶ Explain that the final volume must be between the two black lines on the device (about 2 mL). Add urine to the urine collection device.

General

▶ Place samples in properly labelled specimen container and promptly transport the specimen to the laboratory for processing and analysis.

AFTER THE STUDY: POTENTIAL NURSING ACTIONS

Treatment Considerations

▶ Offer support resources to victims of sexual assault and access to counseling services.

▶ Infection *(related to exposure to C. pneumoniae):* Promote good hygiene and assist with hygiene as needed. Administer prescribed antibiotics, antipyretics, and IV fluids. Institute cooling measures, monitor vital signs, and trend temperatures. Encourage oral fluids, adhere to standard precautions, and provide isolation as appropriate. Obtain ordered cultures. Lightweight clothing and bedding can assist to keep the fevered patient cool. Monitor and trend WBC count and chest x-ray results.

▶ Infection *(related to sexual exposure to C. trachomatis):* Provide written information about sexually transmitted infections. Complete a thorough history and physical assessment. Administer prescribed antibiotics and teach the patient to refrain from sexual activity until the course of antibiotics is completed. Explain that it may be necessary to have repeat testing 3 mo after initial treatment to assess for reinfection from sexual partner.

▶ Airway *(related to exposure to C. pneumoniae):* Assess respiratory characteristics, rate, rhythm, depth, and accessory muscle use. Assess effectiveness of cough and amount of productivity including sputum characteristics (color, viscosity). Assess hydration status and encourage increased fluid intake. Emphasize the importance of increasing fluid intake to thin and mobilize secretions. Auscultate lungs for adventitious breath sounds (crackles), use pulse oximetry to monitor the effectiveness of prescribed oxygen. Suction as needed, consider oxygen humidification, encourage use of incentive spirometer, facilitate chest physiotherapy and nebulized treatments with mucolytic and bronchodilator medications. Facilitate ordered bronchoscopy or thoracentesis.

▶ Gas exchange *(related to exposure to C. pneumoniae):* Auscultate and trend breath sounds, assess for hypoxia (nailbeds, mucous membranes), administer ordered oxygen, and use pulse oximetry to monitor oxygenation. Collaborate with the HCP to consider intubation and/or mechanical ventilation. Place the head of the bed in high Fowler position to improve ventilation. Administer ordered diuretics and vasodilators. Monitor and trend blood pressure and heart rate and for changes in level of consciousness.

Safety Considerations
⬧ Counsel the patient with chlamydial infection, as appropriate, to the risk of sexual transmission and educate the patient regarding proper prophylaxis.
⬧ Provide a nonjudgmental, nonthreatening atmosphere to victims of sexual assault for a discussion during which you explain the risks of sexually transmitted infections. It is also important to discuss emotions the patient may experience: guilt, depression, and anger.

Follow-Up, Evaluation, and Desired Outcomes
⬧ Understands that a chlamydial infection during pregnancy places the newborn at risk for pneumonia and conjunctivitis.
⬧ Recognizes the importance of completing course of antibiotics for chlamydial infection prior to engaging in sexual activity and adherence to the request to collect a convalescent blood sample taken in 7 to 14 days, or 3 mo retesting for persistent chlamydial infection, as requested.
⬧ Understands that positive results of *C. trachomatis* must be reported to a local public health department official, who will question the patient regarding his or her sexual partners.

Chloride, Blood

SYNONYM/ACRONYM: Cl⁻.

RATIONALE: To evaluate electrolytes, acid-base balance, and hydration level.

PATIENT PREPARATION: There are no food, fluid, activity, or medication restrictions unless by medical direction.

NORMAL FINDINGS: Method: Ion-selective electrode.

Age	Conventional and SI Units
Newborn	98–113 mEq/L or mmol/L
2 mo–older adult	97–107 mEq/L or mmol/L

CRITICAL FINDINGS AND POTENTIAL INTERVENTIONS
• Less than 80 mEq/L or mmol/L (SI: Less than 80 mmol/L)
• Greater than 115 mEq/L or mmol/L (SI: Greater than 115 mmol/L)

Timely notification to the requesting health-care provider (HCP) of any critical findings and related symptoms is a role expectation of the professional nurse. A listing of these findings varies among facilities.

Consideration may be given to verification of critical findings before action is taken. Policies vary among facilities and may include requesting immediate recollection and retesting by the laboratory or retesting using a rapid point-of-care testing instrument at the bedside, if available.

The following may be seen in hypochloremia: twitching or tremors, which may indicate excitability of the nervous system; slow and shallow breathing;

and decreased blood pressure as a result of fluid loss. Possible interventions relate to treatment of the underlying cause.

Signs and symptoms associated with hyperchloremia are weakness; lethargy; and deep, rapid breathing. Proper interventions include treatments that correct the underlying cause.

OVERVIEW: (Study type: Blood collected in a gold-, red-, red/gray-, or green-top [heparin] tube; related body system: Circulatory, Endocrine, Respiratory, and Urinary systems.) Chloride is the most abundant anion in the extracellular fluid. Its most important function is in the maintenance of acid-base balance, in which it competes with bicarbonate for sodium. Chloride levels generally increase and decrease proportionally to sodium levels and inversely proportional to bicarbonate levels. Chloride also participates with sodium in the maintenance of water balance and aids in the regulation of osmotic pressure. Chloride contributes to gastric acid (hydrochloric acid) for digestion and activation of enzymes. The chloride content of venous blood is slightly higher than that of arterial blood because chloride ions enter red blood cells (RBCs) in response to absorption of carbon dioxide into the cell. As carbon dioxide enters the blood cell, bicarbonate leaves and chloride is absorbed in exchange to maintain electrical neutrality within the cell.

Chloride is provided by dietary intake, mostly in the form of sodium chloride. It is absorbed by the gastrointestinal system, filtered out by the glomeruli, and reabsorbed by the renal tubules. Excess chloride is excreted in the urine. Serum values normally remain fairly stable. A slight decrease may be detectable after meals because chloride is used to produce hydrochloric acid as part of the digestive process. Measurement of chloride levels is not as essential as measurement of other electrolytes such as sodium or potassium. Chloride is usually included in standard electrolyte panels to detect the presence of unmeasured anions via calculation of the anion gap. Chloride levels are usually not interpreted apart from sodium, potassium, carbon dioxide, and anion gap.

The patient's clinical picture needs to be considered in the evaluation of electrolytes. Fluid and electrolyte imbalances are often seen in patients with serious illness or injury because in these cases the clinical situation has affected the normal homeostatic balance of the body. It is also possible that therapeutic treatments being administered are causing or contributing to the electrolyte imbalance. Children and older adults are at high risk for fluid and electrolyte imbalances when chloride levels are depleted. Children are considered to be at high risk during chloride imbalance because a positive serum chloride balance is important for expansion of the extracellular fluid compartment. Anemia, the result of decreased hemoglobin levels, is a frequent issue for older adult patients. Because hemoglobin participates in a major buffer system in the body, depleted hemoglobin levels affect the efficiency of chloride ion exchange for bicarbonate in RBCs, which in turn affects acid-base balance. Older adult patients are also at high risk because their renal response to change in pH is slower, resulting in a more rapid development of electrolyte imbalance.

INDICATIONS

- Assist in confirming a diagnosis of disorders associated with abnormal chloride values, as seen in acid-base and fluid imbalances.
- Differentiate between types of acidosis (hyperchloremic versus anion gap).
- Monitor effectiveness of drug therapy to increase or decrease serum chloride levels.

INTERFERING FACTORS

Factors that may alter the results of the study

- Drugs or other substances that may cause an increase in chloride levels include acetazolamide, acetylsalicylic acid, ammonium chloride, androgens, bromide, cholestyramine, cyclosporine, hydrochlorothiazide, estrogens, guanethidine, lithium, methyldopa, NSAIDs, phenylbutazone, and triamterene.
- Drugs or other substances that may cause a decrease in chloride levels include aldosterone, bicarbonate, corticosteroids, corticotropin, cortisone, diuretics, ethacrynic acid, furosemide, hydroflumethiazide, laxatives (chronic misuse), mannitol, meralluride, mersalyl, methyclothiazide, metolazone, and triamterene. Many of these drugs can cause a diuretic action that inhibits the tubular reabsorption of chloride. *Note:* Triamterene has nephrotoxic and azotemic effects, and when organ damage has occurred, increased serum chloride levels result. Potassium

chloride (found in salt substitutes) can lower blood chloride levels and raise urine chloride levels.

- Specimens should never be collected above an IV line because of the potential for dilution when the specimen and the IV solution combine in the collection container, falsely decreasing the result. There is also the potential of contaminating the sample with the normal saline contained in the IV solution, falsely increasing the result.
- Elevated triglyceride or protein levels may cause a volume-displacement error in the specimen, reflecting falsely decreased chloride values when chloride measurement methods employing predilution specimens are used (e.g., indirect ion-selective electrode, flame photometry).

Other considerations

- Specimens should not be collected during hemodialysis *(the replacement fluid infused during hemofiltration is composed of constituents that simulate normal plasma and may not represent the patient's actual chloride level).*

POTENTIAL MEDICAL DIAGNOSIS: CLINICAL SIGNIFICANCE OF RESULTS

Increased in

- Acute kidney injury *(related to decreased renal excretion)*
- Cushing disease *(related to sodium retention as a result of increased levels of aldosterone; typically, chloride levels follow sodium levels)*
- Dehydration *(related to hemoconcentration)*
- Diabetes insipidus *(hemoconcentration related to excessive urine production)*
- Excessive infusion of normal saline *(related to excessive intake)*
- Head trauma with hypothalamic stimulation or damage

C

- Hyperparathyroidism (primary) *(high chloride-to-phosphate ratio is used to assist in diagnosis)*
- Metabolic acidosis *(associated with prolonged diarrhea)*
- Renal tubular acidosis *(acidosis related to net retention of chloride ions)*
- Respiratory alkalosis (e.g., hyperventilation) *(related to metabolic exchange of intracellular chloride replaced by bicarbonate; chloride levels increase)*
- Salicylate intoxication *(related to acid-base imbalance resulting in a hyperchloremic acidosis)*

Decreased in

- Addison disease *(related to insufficient production of aldosterone; potassium is retained while sodium and chloride are lost)*
- Burns *(dilutional effect related to sequestration of extracellular fluid)*
- Heart failure *(related to dilutional effect of fluid buildup)*
- Diabetic ketoacidosis *(related to acid-base imbalance with accumulation of ketone bodies and increased chloride)*
- Excessive sweating *(related to excessive loss of chloride without replacement)*
- Gastrointestinal loss from vomiting (severe), diarrhea, nasogastric suction, or fistula
- Metabolic alkalosis *(related to homeostatic response in which intracellular chloride increases to reduce alkalinity of extracellular fluid)*
- Overhydration *(related to dilutional effect)*
- Respiratory acidosis (chronic)
- Salt-losing nephritis *(related to excessive loss)*
- Syndrome of inappropriate antidiuretic hormone secretion *(related to dilutional effect)*
- Water intoxication *(related to dilutional effect)*

NURSING IMPLICATIONS

BEFORE THE STUDY: PLANNING AND IMPLEMENTATION

Teaching the Patient What to Expect

- Inform the patient this test can assist in evaluating the amount of chloride in the blood.
- Explain that a blood sample is needed for the test.

AFTER THE STUDY: POTENTIAL NURSING ACTIONS

Treatment Considerations

- Observe the patient on saline IV fluid replacement therapy for signs of overhydration, especially in cases in which there is a history of heart or kidney disease. Signs of overhydration include constant, irritable cough; chest rales; dyspnea; and engorgement of neck and hand veins.
- Evaluate the patient for signs and symptoms of dehydration. Check the patient's skin turgor, mucous membrane moisture, and ability to produce tears. Dehydration is a significant and common finding in older adult and other patients in whom kidney function has deteriorated.
- Monitor daily weights as well as intake and output to determine whether fluid retention is occurring because of sodium and chloride excess. Patients at risk for or with a history of fluid imbalance are also at risk for electrolyte imbalance.

Nutritional Considerations

- Careful observation of the patient on IV fluid replacement therapy is important. A patient receiving a continuous 5% dextrose solution (D_5W) may not be taking in an adequate amount of chloride to meet the body's needs. The patient, if allowed, should be encouraged to drink fluids such as broths, tomato juice, and colas and to eat foods such as meats, seafood, and eggs, which contain sodium and chloride. The use of table salt may also be appropriate.

Instruct patients with elevated chloride levels to avoid eating or drinking anything containing sodium chloride salt. The patient or caregiver should also be encouraged to read food labels to determine which products are suitable for a low-sodium diet.

Instruct patients with low chloride levels that a decrease in iron absorption may occur as a result of less chloride available to form gastric acid, which is essential for iron absorption. In prolonged periods of chloride deficit, iron-deficiency anemia could develop.

Follow-Up, Evaluation, and Desired Outcomes

Acknowledges contact information provided for the U.S. Department of Agriculture's resource for nutrition (www.choosemyplate.gov).

Demonstrates how to accurately perform daily weight, intake and output, and document results.

Chloride, Sweat

SYNONYM/ACRONYM: Sweat test, pilocarpine iontophoresis sweat test, sweat chloride.

RATIONALE: To assist in diagnosing cystic fibrosis (CF).

PATIENT PREPARATION: There are no food, fluid, activity, or medication restrictions unless by medical direction.

NORMAL FINDINGS: Method: Ion-specific electrode or titration.

	Conventional and SI Units	Interpretation
Birth–6 mo		
	0–29 mEq/L or mmol/L	Normal
	30–59 mEq/L or mmol/L	Borderline
	Greater than 60 mEq/L or mmol/L	Consistent with the diagnosis of CF
6 mo–adult		
	0–39 mEq/L or mmol/L	Normal
	40–59 mEq/L or mmol/L	Borderline
	Greater than 60 mEq/L or mmol/L	Consistent with the diagnosis of CF

CRITICAL FINDINGS AND POTENTIAL INTERVENTIONS

• Greater than 60 mEq/L or mmol/L (SI greater than 60 mEq/L) is considered diagnostic of CF.

Timely notification to the requesting health-care provider (HCP) of any critical findings and related symptoms is a role expectation of the professional nurse. A listing of these findings varies among facilities

Consideration may be given to verification of critical findings before action is taken. Policies vary among facilities and may include requesting recollection and retesting by the laboratory.

The validity of the test result is affected tremendously by proper specimen collection and handling. Before proceeding with appropriate patient education and counseling, it is important to perform duplicate testing on patients whose results are in the diagnostic or intermediate ranges. A negative test should be repeated if test results do not support the clinical picture.

OVERVIEW: (Study type: Body fluid, sweat collected by pilocarpine iontophoresis; **related body system:** Endocrine and Respiratory systems.) The preweighed specimen container or filter paper must not be directly touched by hand, either before or after specimen collection. Powder-free gloves should be used in order to avoid transferring contaminants of any kind that would erroneously affect the sweat concentration or final weight of the sample. The specimen should be promptly transported to the laboratory for processing and analysis. CF is a genetic disease that affects normal functioning of the exocrine glands, causing them to excrete large amounts of electrolytes. Patients with CF have sweat electrolyte levels two to five times normal. Sweat test values, with family history and signs and symptoms, are required to establish a diagnosis of CF. CF is transmitted as an autosomal recessive trait in which the offspring inherits a copy of the defective cystic fibrosis transmembrane conductance regulator (CFTR) gene from each parent. Mutations of this gene disrupt the regulation of chloride and sodium transport between cells within the lungs, pancreas, small intestine, bile ducts, and skin, and the disease is characterized by abnormal exocrine secretions. Clinical presentation may include chronic problems of the gastrointestinal and/or respiratory system. CF is more common in Caucasians. Sweat conductivity is a screening method that estimates chloride levels. Sweat conductivity values greater than or equal to 50 mmol/L should be referred for quantitative analysis of sweat chloride. Testing of stool samples for decreased trypsin activity has been used as a screen for CF in infants and children, but this is a much less reliable method than the sweat test.

Knowledge of genetics assists in identifying those who may benefit from additional education, risk assessment, and counseling. Genetics is the study and identification of genes, genetic mutations, and inheritance. For example, genetics provides some insight into the likelihood of inheriting a medical condition such as CF. Every person receives a copy of the CFTR gene from each parent. If each parent provides an abnormal or mutated CFTR gene, the baby will likely develop CF. Babies who inherit a normal and abnormal copy of the CFTR gene are considered "carriers" because they provide the potential for transmitting the condition to the next generation. More than 2,000 mutations of the CFTR gene have been documented. Some conditions are the result of mutations involving a single gene, whereas other conditions may involve multiple genes and/or multiple chromosomes. Further information regarding inheritance of genes can be found in the study titled "Genetic Testing." The American College of Obstetricians and Gynecologists (ACOG) suggests that carrier screening be discussed as an option to patients (and couples) who are pregnant or are considering pregnancy. Laboratories generally offer a panel of the current and most common CF mutations recommended by ACOG and the American College of Medical Genetics. All 50 states include CF in the neonatal screening performed at birth. Genetic testing can also be reliably performed on DNA material harvested from whole blood, amniotic fluid (submitted with maternal blood sample), chorionic villus samples (submitted with maternal blood sample), or buccal swabs to screen for genetic mutations associated with CF and can assist in confirming a diagnosis of CF, but the sweat electrolyte test is still considered the gold standard diagnostic for CF. Genetic testing for confirmation by polymerase chain reaction (PCR) may be indicated when the sweat chloride test results are indeterminate and the patient demonstrates symptoms, especially in the presence of family history for CF.

The sweat test is a noninvasive study done to assist in the diagnosis of CF when considered with other test results and physical assessments. This test is usually performed on children, although adults may also be tested; it is not usually ordered on adults or infants in the first few weeks of life because results can be highly variable and should be interpreted with caution. Sweat for specimen collection is induced by a small electrical current carrying the drug pilocarpine. The test measures the concentration of chloride produced by the sweat glands of the skin. A high concentration of chloride in the specimen indicates the presence of CF. The sweat test is used less commonly to measure the concentration of sodium ions for the same purpose.

INDICATIONS
- Assist in the diagnosis of CF.
- Screen for CF in individuals with a family history of the disease.
- Screen for suspected CF in children with recurring respiratory infections.
- Screen for suspected CF in infants with failure to thrive and infants who pass meconium late.
- Screen for suspected CF in individuals with malabsorption syndrome.

INTERFERING FACTORS
Contraindications

Patients with skin disorders (e.g., rash, erythema, eczema).

Factors that may alter the results of the study
- An inadequate amount of sweat may produce inaccurate results.
- Improper cleaning of the skin or improper application of gauze pad or filter paper for collection affects test results.
- Hot environmental temperatures may reduce the sodium chloride concentration in sweat; cool environmental temperatures may reduce the amount of sweat collected.
- If the specimen container that stores the gauze or filter paper is handled without gloves, the test results may show a false increase in the final weight of the collection container.

POTENTIAL MEDICAL DIAGNOSIS: CLINICAL SIGNIFICANCE OF RESULTS

Increased in

Conditions that affect electrolyte distribution and excretion may produce false-positive sweat test results.

- Addison disease
- Alcohol related pancreatitis *(dysfunction of CF gene is linked to pancreatic disease susceptibility)*
- CF
- Chronic kidney disease
- Chronic pulmonary infections *(related to undiagnosed CF)*
- Congenital adrenal hyperplasia
- Diabetes insipidus
- Familial cholestasis
- Familial hypoparathyroidism
- Fucosidosis
- Glucose-6-phosphate dehydrogenase deficiency
- Hypothyroidism
- Mucopolysaccharidosis
- Nephrogenic diabetes insipidus

Decreased in

Conditions that affect electrolyte distribution and retention may produce false-negative sweat test results.

- Edema
- Hypoaldosteronism
- Hypoproteinemia
- Sodium depletion

NURSING IMPLICATIONS

BEFORE THE STUDY: PLANNING AND IMPLEMENTATION

Teaching the Patient What to Expect

- Inform the patient this test can assist in diagnosing an inherited disease that affects the lungs. Explain that a positive sweat test alone is not diagnostic of CF; confirmation of borderline and positive tests is generally recommended.
- Explain that a sweat sample is required. The caregiver will be encouraged to stay with and support the child during the test. The iontophoresis and specimen collection are performed in a setting approved for sweat chloride testing and usually takes approximately 75 to 90 min. Address concerns about pain and explain that there is no pain or needle associated with the test, but a stinging sensation may be experienced when the low electrical current is applied at the site.
- Explain that prior to specimen collection, the site is washed with distilled water (which contains no electrolytes) and dried. Then, one electrode is covered with a pad saturated with pilocarpine and attached to the collection site on the right forearm or right thigh. The second electrode is attached, and a low electrical current is applied for 12 to 15 min. The combination of pilocarpine and low current stimulates the skin to produce sweat. At the end of the iontophoresis period, the electrodes are removed, and the site is washed with distilled water and then dried to remove any possible contaminants on the skin. Preweighed disks made of filter paper are placed on the site with a forceps; to prevent evaporation of sweat collected at the site, the disks are covered with paraffin or plastic and sealed at the edges. The child can be distracted with books or games while the disks are left in place for about 1 hr. After 1 hr, the paraffin covering is removed, and disks are placed in a preweighed container with a forceps. The container is sealed and sent immediately to the laboratory for weighing and analysis of chloride content. The sample is weighed prior to analysis because at least 100 mg of sweat is required for accurate results.

Potential Nursing Actions

- Inquire about the patient's health concerns and history (especially failure to thrive or CF in other family members).

Safety Considerations

- The test should be terminated if the patient complains of burning at the electrode site. The electrodes can be repositioned before the test is resumed.

❋ The test should not be performed if the patient is receiving oxygen by means of an open system related to the remote possibility of explosion from an electrical spark. If the patient can temporarily receive oxygen via a facemask or nasal cannula, then sweat testing can be done.

❋ The patient is placed in a position that will allow exposure of the site on the forearm or thigh. To ensure collection of an adequate amount of sweat in a small infant, two sites (right forearm and right thigh) can be used. The patient should be covered to prevent cool environmental temperatures from affecting sweat production. The site selected for iontophoresis should never be the chest or left side because of the risk of cardiac arrest from the electrical current.

▶ Battery-powered equipment is preferred over an electrical outlet to supply the current.

AFTER THE STUDY: POTENTIAL NURSING ACTIONS

Treatment Considerations

▶ Observe/assess the site for unusual color, sensation, or discomfort. Inform the patient and caregiver that redness at the site fades in 2 to 3 hr.

▶ Monitor for disturbed gas exchange with compromised airway clearance. Symptoms include restlessness, altered level of consciousness, tachypnea, cyanosis, nasal flare, and use of accessory muscles.

Nutritional Considerations

▶ If appropriate, instruct the patient and caregiver that nutrition may be altered because of impaired digestive processes associated with CF.

Increased viscosity of exocrine gland secretion may lead to poor absorption of digestive enzymes and fat-soluble vitamins, necessitating oral intake of digestive enzymes with each meal and calcium and vitamin (A, D, E, and K) supplementation. Malnutrition also is seen commonly in patients with chronic, severe respiratory disease for many reasons, including fatigue, lack of appetite, and gastrointestinal distress. Research has estimated that the daily caloric intake needed for children with CF between 4 and 7 yr may be 2,000 to 2,800 and for teens 3,000 to 5,000. Tube feeding may be necessary to supplement regular high-calorie meals. To prevent pulmonary infection and decrease the extent of lung tissue damage, adequate intake of vitamins A and C is also important. Excessive loss of sodium chloride through the sweat glands of a patient with CF may necessitate increased salt intake, especially in environments where increased sweating is induced. The importance of following the prescribed diet should be stressed to the patient and caregiver.

Follow-Up, Evaluation, and Desired Outcomes

▶ Acknowledges contact information provided for the Cystic Fibrosis Foundation (www.cff.org) or ACOG (www.acog.org).

▶ Understands that ineffective airway clearance related to excessive production of mucus and decreased ciliary action may occur. Demonstrates how to perform chest physical therapy and use aerosolized antibiotics and mucus-thinning drugs as part of the daily treatment regimen.

Cholangiography, Percutaneous Transhepatic

SYNONYM/ACRONYM: Percutaneous cholecystogram, PTC, PTHC.

RATIONALE: To visualize and assess biliary ducts for causes of obstruction and jaundice, such as cancer or stones.

C

PATIENT PREPARATION: There are no activity restrictions unless by medical direction. Instruct the patient to fast and restrict fluids for 4 to 8 hr, or as ordered, prior to the procedure. Fasting is ordered because an empty stomach provides better visualization and as a precaution against aspiration related to possible nausea and vomiting. The American Society of Anesthesiologists has fasting guidelines for risk levels according to patient status. More information can be located at www.asahq. org. The patient may be instructed to prepare the bowel with a laxative the night before and a cleansing enema the morning of the procedure, by medical direction.

Note: If iodinated contrast medium is scheduled to be used in patients receiving metformin or drugs containing metformin for type 2 diabetes, the drug may be discontinued on the day of the test and continue to be withheld for 48 hr after the test.

Patients with heart valve disease may be premedicated with antibiotics.

Regarding the patient's risk for bleeding, the patient should be instructed to avoid taking natural products and medications with known anticoagulant, antiplatelet, or thrombolytic properties or to reduce dosage, as ordered, prior to the procedure. Number of days to withhold medication is dependent on the type of anticoagulant. Note the last time and dose of medication taken.

Patients on beta blockers before the surgical procedure should be instructed to take their medication as ordered during the perioperative period. Protocols may vary among facilities.

Ensure that this procedure is performed before an upper gastrointestinal (GI) study or barium swallow.

NORMAL FINDINGS

- Biliary ducts are normal in diameter, with no evidence of dilation, filling defects, duct narrowing, or extravasation
- Contrast medium fills the ducts and flows freely
- Gallbladder appears normal in size and shape.

CRITICAL FINDINGS AND POTENTIAL INTERVENTIONS: N/A

OVERVIEW: (Study type: X-ray, special/contrast; **related body system:** Digestive system.) Percutaneous transhepatic cholangiography (PTC) is a test used to visualize the biliary system in order to evaluate persistent upper abdominal pain after cholecystectomy and to determine the presence and cause of obstructive jaundice. The liver capsule is punctured with a thin needle under fluoroscopic guidance, and contrast medium is injected as the needle is slowly withdrawn. This study visualizes the biliary ducts without depending on the gallbladder's concentrating ability. The intrahepatic and extrahepatic biliary ducts, and occasionally the gallbladder, can be visualized to determine possible obstruction. In obstruction of the extrahepatic ducts, a catheter can be placed in the duct to allow external drainage of bile. Endoscopic retrograde cholangiopancreatography (ERCP) and PTC are the only methods available to view the biliary tree in the presence of jaundice. PTC is more invasive and painful to undergo than ERCP.

INDICATIONS

- Aid in the diagnosis of obstruction caused by gallstones, benign strictures, malignant tumors, congenital cysts, and anatomic variations.
- Determine the cause, extent, and location of mechanical obstruction.
- Determine the cause of upper abdominal pain after cholecystectomy.
- Distinguish between obstructive and nonobstructive jaundice.

INTERFERING FACTORS

Contraindications

⟐ Patients who are pregnant or suspected of being pregnant, unless the potential benefits of a procedure using radiation far outweigh the risk of radiation exposure to the fetus and mother.

⟐ Patients with conditions associated with adverse reactions to contrast medium (e.g., asthma, food allergies, or allergy to contrast medium). Although patients are asked specifically if they have a known allergy to iodine or shellfish (shellfish contain high levels of iodine), it has been well established that the reaction is not to iodine; an actual iodine allergy would be problematic because iodine is required for the production of thyroid hormones. In the case of shellfish, the reaction is to a muscle protein called *tropomyosin*; in the case of iodinated contrast medium, the reaction is to the noniodinated part of the contrast molecule. Patients with a known hypersensitivity to the medium may benefit from premedication with corticosteroids and diphenhydramine; the use of nonionic contrast or an alternative noncontrast imaging study, if available, may be considered for patients who have severe asthma or who have experienced moderate to severe reactions to ionic contrast medium.

⟐ Patients with conditions associated with preexisting renal insufficiency (e.g., chronic kidney disease, single kidney transplant, nephrectomy, diabetes, multiple myeloma, treatment with aminoglycosides and NSAIDs), *because iodinated contrast is nephrotoxic.*

⟐ Patients who are chronically dehydrated before the test, especially older adults and patients whose health is already compromised, *because of their risk of contrast-induced acute kidney injury.*

⟐ Patients with bleeding disorders or receiving anticoagulant therapy, *because the puncture site may not stop bleeding.*

⟐ Patients with cholangitis; *the injection of the contrast medium can increase biliary pressure, leading to bacteremia, septicemia, and shock.*

Factors that may alter the results of the study

- Gas or feces in the GI tract resulting from inadequate cleansing or failure to restrict food intake before the study.
- Retained barium from a previous radiological procedure.
- Metallic objects (e.g., jewelry, body rings) within the examination field, which may inhibit organ visualization and cause unclear images.
- Inability of the patient to cooperate or remain still during the procedure, because movement can produce blurred or otherwise unclear images.

POTENTIAL MEDICAL DIAGNOSIS: CLINICAL SIGNIFICANCE OF RESULTS

Abnormal findings related to

- Anatomic biliary or pancreatic duct variations
- Biliary cholangitis
- Cholangiocarcinoma
- Cirrhosis
- Common bile duct cysts
- Gallbladder cancer
- Gallstones
- Hepatitis

- Nonobstructive jaundice
- Pancreatitis
- Tumors, strictures, inflammation, or gallstones of the common bile duct

NURSING IMPLICATIONS

BEFORE THE STUDY: PLANNING AND IMPLEMENTATION

Teaching the Patient What to Expect

▶ Inform the patient this procedure can assist in assessing the bile ducts of the gallbladder and pancreas.

▶ Explain that prior to the procedure, laboratory testing may be required to determine the possibility of bleeding risk (coagulation testing) or to assess for impaired kidney function (creatinine level and estimated glomerular filtration rate) if use of iodinated contrast medium is anticipated. The liver is a vascular organ; therefore, a type and screen of the patient's blood may be ordered for possible transfusion in the event of bleeding. Percutaneous bile drainage may have infected bile, and as such an antibiotic will be administered at least 1 hr before the procedure in order to avoid spreading the infection to other parts of the body.

▶ Pregnancy is a general contraindication to procedures involving radiation. Explain to the female patient that she will be asked the date of her last menstrual period. Pregnancy testing may be performed to determine the possibility of pregnancy before exposure to radiation.

▶ Review the procedure with the patient. Address concerns about pain and explain that there may be moments of discomfort or pain experienced when the IV line or catheter is inserted to allow infusion of fluids such as saline, anesthetics, sedatives, contrast medium, medications used in the procedure, or emergency medications.

▶ Explain that contrast medium will be injected, by catheter, at a separate site from the IV line.

▶ Advise that a burning and flushing sensation may be felt throughout the body during injection of the contrast medium, and the patient may experience an urge to cough, flushing, nausea, or a salty or metallic taste.

▶ Inform the patient that the procedure is usually performed in the radiology department by a health-care provider (HCP), with support staff, and takes approximately 60 min.

▶ Instruct the patient to remove jewelry and other metallic objects from the area of examination.

▶ Baseline vital signs will be recorded and monitored throughout the procedure. Protocols may vary among facilities.

▶ Adhere to organizational policies and the Centers for Medicare and Medicaid Services (CMS) quality measures regarding administration of prophylactic antibiotics. Administer ordered prophylactic antibiotics 1 hr before incision, and use antibiotics that are consistent with current guidelines specific to the procedure.

▶ Positioning for this procedure is in the supine position on a tilting examination table where a kidney, ureter, and bladder (KUB) or plain film is taken to ensure that no stool or barium from a previous study will obscure visualization of the biliary system.

▶ Advise the patient they will be instructed to inhale deeply and hold their breath as the needle is inserted. An area over the upper right quadrant of the abdomen is prepped and draped and local anesthetic is given to the abdominal wall. The needle is inserted and advanced under fluoroscopic guidance. Contrast medium is injected when placement is confirmed by the free flow of bile. A specimen of bile may be sent to the laboratory for culture and cytological analysis. If an obstruction is found during the procedure, a catheter is inserted into the bile duct to allow drainage of bile. At the end of the procedure, the contrast medium is aspirated from the biliary ducts, relieving pressure on the dilated ducts. A closed and sterile drainage system will be established if a catheter is left in place.

▶ Advise taking slow, deep breaths if nausea occurs during the procedure. An ordered antiemetic drug can be administered as needed. An emesis basin can be ready for use.

▶ Explain to the patient they will be monitored for complications related to the procedure (e.g., allergic reaction, anaphylaxis, bronchospasm).

▶ Explain that once the study is completed, the needle or catheter is removed, and a pressure dressing is applied over the puncture site.

Potential Nursing Actions

✧ *Make sure a written and informed consent has been signed prior to the procedure and before administering any medications.*

▶ If iodinated contrast medium is scheduled to be used in patients receiving metformin or drugs containing metformin for type 2 diabetes, the drug may be discontinued on the day of the test and continue to be withheld for 48 hr after the test.

Safety Considerations

▶ Anticoagulants, aspirin, and other salicylates should be discontinued by medical direction for the appropriate number of days prior to a procedure where bleeding is a potential complication.

AFTER THE STUDY: POTENTIAL NURSING ACTIONS

Avoiding Complications

▶ PTC, establishing an IV site, and injection of contrast medium are invasive procedures. Complications are rare but include risk for allergic reaction *(related to contrast reaction),* bile peritonitis, bleeding from the puncture site *(related to a bleeding disorder or the effects of natural products and medications with known anticoagulant, antiplatelet, or thrombolytic properties),* extravasation of bile, hematoma *(related to blood leakage into the tissue following needle insertion),* hemoperitoneum, infection *(which might occur if bacteria from the skin surface is introduced at the puncture site),* tissue damage *(related to extravasation or leaking of contrast into the tissues during injection),* nerve injury or damage to a nearby organ *(which might occur if the needle strikes a nerve or perforates an organ),* nephrotoxicity *(a deterioration of renal function associated with contrast administration),* and septicemia. Monitor

the patient for complications related to the procedure (e.g., allergic reaction, anaphylaxis, bronchospasm, infection, injury). Immediately report symptoms such as difficulty breathing, chest pain, fever, hyperpnea, hypertension, nausea, palpitations, pruritus, rash, tachycardia, urticaria, or vomiting to the appropriate HCP. Observe/assess the needle/catheter insertion site for bleeding, inflammation, or hematoma formation. Administer ordered antihistamines or prophylactic steroids if the patient has an allergic reaction.

Treatment Considerations

▶ Do not allow the patient to eat or drink for several hours after the procedure as a precaution in the event a return to surgery is required *related to postprocedural bleeding.* If no complications present, the patient can resume usual diet, fluids, medications, and activity as directed by the HCP.

▶ Symptoms of bleeding to monitor for are hypotension, tachycardia, confusion with altered level of consciousness, pallor, anxiety and restlessness, shortness of breath.

▶ Pressure should be maintained over the needle insertion site for several hours if bleeding is persistent. The patient may be placed in the right decubitus position for the first hour, followed by placement in the supine position for an additional 2 to 3 hr in order to avoid significant post procedural bleeding. Observe/assess the puncture site for signs of bleeding, hematoma formation, inflammation, ecchymosis, or leakage of bile. Notify the HCP if any of these is present.

▶ Monitor vital signs and neurological status every 15 min for 1 hr, then every 2 hr for 4 hr, and as ordered. Take temperature every 4 hr for 24 hr. Monitor intake and output at least every 8 hr. Compare with baseline values. Notify the HCP if temperature is elevated. Protocols may vary among facilities.

Safety Considerations

▶ Renal function should be assessed before metformin is resumed. Advise diabetic patients to avoid all medications containing metformin for 48 hr following a procedure with iodinated contrast. Iodinated contrast can temporarily impair kidney function, and failure to withhold metformin may indirectly result in drug-induced lactic acidosis, a dangerous and sometimes fatal adverse effect of metformin (related to renal impairment that does not support sufficient excretion of metformin).

Follow-Up, Evaluation, and Desired Outcomes

♦ Generally no specific postprocedural care is required. The complication rate is relatively low and most complications, such as discomfort at the puncture site, are of limited duration.
♦ Demonstrates proficiency in the care of the site and dressing changes.

Cholangiography, Postoperative

SYNONYM/ACRONYM: T-tube cholangiography.

RATIONALE: A postoperative evaluation to provide ongoing assessment of the effectiveness of bile duct or gallbladder surgery.

PATIENT PREPARATION: There are no activity restrictions unless by medical direction. Instruct the patient to fast and restrict fluids for 4 to 8 hr, or as ordered, prior to the procedure. Fasting is ordered because an empty stomach provides better visualization and as a precaution against aspiration related to possible nausea and vomiting. The American Society of Anesthesiologists has fasting guidelines for risk levels according to patient status. More information can be located at www.asahq.org. The patient may be instructed to prepare the bowel with a cleansing enema the morning of the procedure, by medical direction.

Note: If iodinated contrast medium is scheduled to be used in patients receiving metformin or drugs containing metformin for type 2 diabetes, the drug may be discontinued on the day of the test and continue to be withheld for 48 hr after the test.

Regarding the patient's risk for bleeding, the patient should be instructed to avoid taking natural products and medications with known anticoagulant, antiplatelet, or thrombolytic properties or to reduce dosage, as ordered, prior to the procedure. Number of days to withhold medication is dependent on the type of anticoagulant. Note the last time and dose of medication taken.

Patients on beta blockers before the surgical procedure should be instructed to take their medication as ordered during the perioperative period. Protocols may vary among facilities.

This test should be performed before any gastrointestinal (GI) studies using barium and after any studies involving the measurement of iodinated compounds.

NORMAL FINDINGS

• Biliary ducts are normal in size
• Contrast medium fills the ductal system and flows freely.

CRITICAL FINDINGS AND POTENTIAL INTERVENTIONS: N/A

OVERVIEW: (Study type: X-ray, special/contrast; related body system: Digestive system.) After cholecystectomy, a self-retaining, T-shaped tube may be inserted into the common bile duct. Postoperative (T-tube) cholangiography is a fluoroscopic and radiographic examination of the biliary tract that involves the injection of a contrast medium such as sodium diatrizoate (Hypaque) through the T-tube inserted during surgery. This test may be performed during surgery and again 5 to 10 days after cholecystectomy to assess the patency of the common bile duct and to detect any remaining calculi. The procedure will also help identify areas of stenosis or the presence of fistulae (as a result of the surgery). T-tube placement may also be done after a liver transplant because biliary duct obstruction or anastomotic leakage is possible.

INDICATIONS
- Determine biliary duct patency before T-tube removal.
- Identify the cause, extent, and location of obstruction after surgery.

INTERFERING FACTORS
Contraindications

✳ Patients who are pregnant or suspected of being pregnant, unless the potential benefits of a procedure using radiation far outweigh the risk of radiation exposure to the fetus and mother.

✳ Patients with conditions associated with adverse reactions to contrast medium (e.g., asthma, food allergies, or allergy to contrast medium). Although patients are asked specifically if they have a known allergy to iodine or shellfish (shellfish contain high levels of iodine), it has been well established that the reaction is not to iodine; an actual iodine allergy would be problematic because iodine is required for the production of thyroid hormones. In the case of shellfish, the reaction is to a muscle protein called *tropomyosin*; in the case of iodinated contrast medium, the reaction is to the noniodinated part of the contrast molecule. Patients with a known hypersensitivity to the medium may benefit from premedication with corticosteroids and diphenhydramine; the use of nonionic contrast or an alternative noncontrast imaging study, if available, may be considered for patients who have severe asthma or who have experienced moderate to severe reactions to ionic contrast medium.

✳ Patients with conditions associated with preexisting renal insufficiency (e.g., chronic kidney disease, single kidney transplant, nephrectomy, diabetes, multiple myeloma, treatment with aminoglycosides and NSAIDs), *because iodinated contrast is nephrotoxic.*

Patients who are chronically dehydrated before the test, especially older adults and patients whose health is already compromised, *because of their risk of contrast-induced acute kidney injury.*

✳ Patients with bleeding disorders or receiving anticoagulant therapy, *because the puncture site may not stop bleeding.*

✳ Patients with cholangitis; *the injection of the contrast medium can increase biliary pressure, leading to bacteremia, septicemia, and shock.*

✳ Patients with acute cholecystitis or severe liver disease; *the procedure may worsen the condition.*

Factors that may alter the results of the study
- Gas or feces in the GI tract resulting from inadequate cleansing or failure to restrict food intake before the study.

- Retained barium from a previous radiological procedure.
- Air bubbles resembling calculi may be seen if there is inadvertent injection of air.
- Metallic objects (e.g., jewelry, body rings) within the examination field, which may inhibit organ visualization and cause unclear images.
- Inability of the patient to cooperate or remain still during the procedure because movement can produce blurred or otherwise unclear images.

POTENTIAL MEDICAL DIAGNOSIS: CLINICAL SIGNIFICANCE OF RESULTS
Abnormal findings related to
- Appearance of channels of contrast medium outside of the biliary ducts, indicating a fistula.
- Filling defects, dilation, or radiolucent shadows within the biliary ducts, indicating calculi or tumor

NURSING IMPLICATIONS

BEFORE THE STUDY: PLANNING AND IMPLEMENTATION

Teaching the Patient What to Expect
- Inform the patient this procedure can assist in assessing the bile ducts of the gallbladder and pancreas.
- Pregnancy is a general contraindication to procedures involving radiation. Explain to the female patient that she will be asked the date of her last menstrual period. Pregnancy testing may be performed to determine the possibility of pregnancy before exposure to radiation.
- Review the procedure with the patient. Address concerns about pain and explain that there may be moments of discomfort or pain experienced when the IV line or catheter is inserted to allow infusion of fluids such as saline, anesthetics, sedatives, contrast

medium, medications used in the procedure, or emergency medications.
- The T-tube will be clamped 24 hr before and during the procedure, if ordered, to help prevent air bubbles from entering the ducts.
- Explain that contrast medium will be injected through the T-tube that was left in place.
- Inform the patient that the procedure is usually performed in the radiology department by a health-care provider (HCP), with support staff, and takes approximately 60 to 90 min.
- Instruct the patient to remove jewelry and other metallic objects from the area of examination.
- Baseline vital signs will be recorded and monitored throughout the procedure. Protocols may vary among facilities.
- Positioning for this procedure is in the supine position on an examination table. A kidney, ureter, and bladder (KUB) or plain film will be taken to ensure that no stool or barium from a previous study will obscure visualization of the biliary system.
- The area around the T-tube is draped; the end of the T-tube is cleansed with 70% alcohol. If the T-tube site is inflamed and painful, a local anesthetic (e.g., lidocaine) may be injected around the site. A needle is inserted into the open end of the T-tube, and the clamp is removed. Contrast medium is injected, and fluoroscopy is performed to visualize contrast medium moving through the duct system. Explain that there may be a bloating sensation in the upper right quadrant as the contrast medium is injected. The tube is clamped, and images are taken. A delayed image may be taken 15 min later to visualize passage of the contrast medium into the duodenum.
- For procedures done after surgery, the T-tube is removed if findings are normal; a dry, sterile dressing is applied to the site.
- Explain to the patient they will be monitored for complications related to the procedure (e.g., allergic reaction, anaphylaxis, bronchospasm).

C

▶ Explain that once the study is completed, the needle or catheter is removed, and a pressure dressing is applied over the puncture site.

▶ If retained calculi are identified, the T-tube is left in place for 4 to 6 wk until the tract surrounding the T-tube is healed to perform a percutaneous removal.

Potential Nursing Actions

✦ *Make sure a written and informed consent has been signed prior to the procedure and before administering any medications.*

▶ If iodinated contrast medium is scheduled to be used in patients receiving metformin or drugs containing metformin for type 2 diabetes, the drug may be discontinued on the day of the test and continue to be withheld for 48 hr after the test. Protocols may vary among facilities.

AFTER THE STUDY: POTENTIAL NURSING ACTIONS

Avoiding Complications

▶ Cholangiography, establishing an IV site, and injection of contrast medium are invasive procedures. Complications are rare but include risk for allergic reaction *(related to contrast reaction),* bile peritonitis, bleeding from the puncture site *(related to a bleeding disorder or the effects of natural products and medications with known anticoagulant, antiplatelet, or thrombolytic properties),* extravasation of bile, hematoma *(related to blood leakage into the tissue following needle insertion),* infection *(which might occur if bacteria from the skin surface is introduced at the puncture site),* tissue damage *(related to extravasation or leaking of contrast into the tissues during injection),* nerve injury or damage to a nearby organ *(which might occur if the needle strikes a nerve or perforates an organ),* nephrotoxicity *(a deterioration of renal function associated with contrast administration),* and septicemia. Monitor the patient for complications related to the procedure (e.g., allergic reaction,

anaphylaxis, bronchospasm, infection, injury). Immediately report symptoms such as difficulty breathing, chest pain, fever, hyperpnea, hypertension, nausea, palpitations, pruritus, rash, tachycardia, urticaria, or vomiting to the appropriate HCP. Observe/assess the needle/catheter insertion site for bleeding, inflammation, or hematoma formation. Administer ordered antihistamines or prophylactic steroids if the patient has an allergic reaction.

Treatment Considerations

▶ Monitor vital signs and neurological status every 15 min for 1 hr, then every 2 hr for 4 hr, and as ordered. Take temperature every 4 hr for 24 hr. Monitor intake and output at least every 8 hr. Compare with baseline values. Notify the HCP if temperature is elevated. Protocols may vary among facilities.

▶ Carefully monitor the patient for fatigue and fluid and electrolyte imbalance.

Safety Considerations

▶ Renal function should be assessed before metformin is resumed. Advise diabetic patients to avoid all medications containing metformin for 48 hr following a procedure with iodinated contrast. Iodinated contrast can temporarily impair kidney function, and failure to withhold metformin may indirectly result in drug-induced lactic acidosis, a dangerous and sometimes fatal adverse effect of metformin *(related to renal impairment that does not support sufficient excretion of metformin).*

Follow-Up, Evaluation, and Desired Outcomes

▶ Understands there are no food or fluid restrictions for a postsurgical study and that the usual diet, fluids, medications, and activity, may be resumed as directed by the HCP.

▶ Acknowledges the importance of monitoring the T-tube site and changing sterile dressing, as ordered. Demonstrates proficiency in the care of the site and dressing changes.

Cholangiopancreatography, Endoscopic Retrograde

SYNONYM/ACRONYM: ERCP.

RATIONALE: To visualize and assess the pancreas and common bile ducts for occlusion or stricture.

PATIENT PREPARATION: There are no activity restrictions unless by medical direction. Instruct the patient to fast and restrict fluids for 4 to 8 hr, or as ordered, prior to the procedure. Fasting is ordered because an empty stomach provides better visualization and as a precaution against aspiration related to possible nausea and vomiting. The American Society of Anesthesiologists has fasting guidelines for risk levels according to patient status. More information can be located at www .asahq.org. The patient may be instructed to prepare the bowel with a laxative or enema the night before or morning of the procedure, by medical direction.

Note: If iodinated contrast medium is scheduled to be used in patients receiving metformin or drugs containing metformin for type 2 diabetes, the drug may be discontinued on the day of the test and continue to be withheld for 48 hr after the test.

Patients with heart valve disease may be premedicated with antibiotics.

Regarding the patient's risk for bleeding, the patient should be instructed to avoid taking natural products and medications with known anticoagulant, antiplatelet, or thrombolytic properties or to reduce dosage, as ordered, prior to the procedure. Number of days to withhold medication is dependent on the type of anticoagulant. Note the last time and dose of medication taken.

Patients on beta blockers before the surgical procedure should be instructed to take their medication as ordered during the perioperative period. Protocols may vary among facilities.

Ensure that this procedure is performed before an upper gastrointestinal (GI) study or barium swallow.

NORMAL FINDINGS
• Normal appearance of the duodenal papilla
• Patency of the pancreatic and common bile ducts.

CRITICAL FINDINGS AND POTENTIAL INTERVENTIONS: N/A

OVERVIEW: (**Study type:** Endoscopy combined with X-ray, special/contrast; **related body system:** Digestive system.) Tissue specimens collected during the procedure should be placed in appropriate containers, properly labelled, and promptly transported to the laboratory. Endoscopic retrograde cholangiopancreatography (ERCP) allows direct visualization of the pancreatic and biliary ducts with a flexible endoscope and, after injection of contrast material, with x-rays. It allows the health-care provider (HCP) performing the procedure to view the pancreatic, hepatic, and common bile ducts and the ampulla of Vater. ERCP and percutaneous transhepatic cholangiography (PTC) are the only procedures that allow direct visualization of the biliary and pancreatic ducts. ERCP is less invasive and has less morbidity than PTC. It is useful in the evaluation of patients with jaundice, because the ducts can be visualized even when the patient's bilirubin level is high. (In contrast, oral cholecystography and IV cholangiography cannot visualize the biliary system when the patient has high bilirubin levels.) With endoscopy, the distal end of the common bile duct can be widened, and gallstones can be removed and stents placed in narrowed bile ducts to allow bile to be drained in jaundiced patients. During the endoscopic procedure, specimens of suspicious tissue can be taken for pathological review, and manometry pressure readings can be obtained from the bile and pancreatic ducts. ERCP is used in the diagnosis and follow-up of pancreatic disease; it can also be used therapeutically to remove small lesions called *choleliths,* perform sphincterotomy (biliary or pancreatic repair for stenosis), perform stent placement, repair stenosis using dilation balloons, or accomplish the extraction of stones using dilation balloons.

INDICATIONS

- Assess jaundice of unknown cause to differentiate biliary tract obstruction from liver disease.
- Collect specimens for cytology.
- Identify obstruction caused by calculi, cysts, ducts, strictures, stenosis, and anatomic abnormalities.

- Retrieve calculi from the distal common bile duct and release strictures.
- Perform therapeutic procedures, such as sphincterotomy and placement of biliary drains.

INTERFERING FACTORS

Contraindications

Patients who are pregnant or suspected of being pregnant, unless the potential benefits of a procedure using radiation far outweigh the risk of radiation exposure to the fetus and mother.

Patients with conditions associated with adverse reactions to contrast medium (e.g., asthma, food allergies, or allergy to contrast medium). Although patients are asked specifically if they have a known allergy to iodine or shellfish (shellfish contain high levels of iodine), it has been well established that the reaction is not to iodine; an actual iodine allergy would be problematic because iodine is required for the production of thyroid hormones. In the case of shellfish, the reaction is to a muscle protein called *tropomyosin*; in the case of iodinated contrast medium, the reaction is to the noniodinated part of the contrast molecule. Patients with a known hypersensitivity to the medium may benefit from premedication with corticosteroids and diphenhydramine; the use of nonionic contrast or an alternative noncontrast imaging study, if available, may be considered for patients who have severe asthma or who have experienced moderate to severe reactions to ionic contrast medium.

Patients with conditions associated with preexisting renal insufficiency (e.g., chronic kidney disease, single kidney transplant, nephrectomy, diabetes, multiple myeloma, treatment with aminoglycosides and NSAIDs), *because iodinated contrast is nephrotoxic.*

Patients who are chronically dehydrated before the test,

especially older adults and patients whose health is already compromised, *because of their risk of contrast-induced acute kidney injury.*

✦ Patients with bleeding disorders or receiving anticoagulant therapy, *because the puncture site may not stop bleeding.*

✦ Patients with an acute infection of the biliary system (cholangitis, pancreatitis, or possible pseudocyst of the pancreas), pharyngeal or esophageal obstruction (e.g., Zenker's diverticulum).

Factors that may alter the results of the study
• Gas or feces in the GI tract resulting from inadequate cleansing or failure to restrict food intake before the study.
• Retained barium from a previous radiological procedure.
• Previous surgery involving the stomach or duodenum, which can make locating the duodenal papilla difficult.
• Metallic objects (e.g., jewelry, body rings) within the examination field, which may inhibit organ visualization and cause unclear images.
• Inability of the patient to cooperate or remain still during the procedure, because movement can produce blurred or otherwise unclear images.

Other considerations
• Blood specimens for bilirubin, amylase, or lipase, if ordered, should be collected before the procedure; results will be elevated after the procedure.

POTENTIAL MEDICAL DIAGNOSIS: CLINICAL SIGNIFICANCE OF RESULTS
Abnormal findings related to
• Anatomical deviations of biliary or pancreatic ducts
• Biliary cholangitis
• Cancer of the bile ducts
• Duodenal papilla tumors
• Gallstones
• Pancreatic cancer
• Pancreatic cysts or pseudocysts
• Pancreatic fibrosis
• Pancreatitis
• Stenosis of biliary or pancreatic ducts

NURSING IMPLICATIONS

POTENTIAL NURSING PROBLEMS: ASSESSMENT & NURSING DIAGNOSIS

Problems	Signs and Symptoms
Nausea *(related to pain, inflammation, blockage)*	Self-report of nausea, excess salivation, bad taste in the mouth, gagging, avoidance of food, inability to eat
Pain *(related to blockage, tumor, infection, inflammation)*	Self-report of pain; facial grimace; crying; restlessness; diaphoresis; nausea; vomiting; guarding; social withdrawal; elevated blood pressure, heart rate, respiratory rate; pallor

BEFORE THE STUDY: PLANNING AND IMPLEMENTATION

Teaching the Patient What to Expect

▶ Inform the patient this procedure can assist in assessing the bile ducts of the gallbladder and pancreas.

▶ Explain that prior to the procedure, laboratory testing may be required to determine the possibility of bleeding risk (coagulation testing) or to assess for impaired kidney function (creatinine level and estimated glomerular filtration rate) if use of iodinated contrast medium is anticipated.

▶ Pregnancy is a general contraindication to procedures involving radiation. Explain to the female patient that she will be asked the date of her last menstrual period. Pregnancy testing may be performed to determine the possibility of pregnancy before exposure to radiation.

▶ Review the procedure with the patient. Address concerns about pain and explain that there may be moments of discomfort or pain experienced when the IV line or catheter is inserted to allow infusion of fluids such as saline, anesthetics, sedatives, contrast medium, medications used in the procedure, or emergency medications; no pain should be experienced during the procedure because a narcotic will be given prior to the procedure and a sedative will be given to promote relaxation, but there may be moments of discomfort when the endoscope is inserted. IV glucagon or anticholinergics can be administered to minimize duodenal spasm and to facilitate visualization of the ampulla of Vater.

▶ Explain that contrast medium will be injected, by catheter, at a separate site from the IV line.

▶ Inform the patient that the procedure is performed in a GI lab or radiology department, usually by an HCP, with support staff, and takes approximately 30 to 60 min. If the procedure is done in an outpatient setting, the patient must make arrangements for someone to drive him or her home.

▶ An x-ray of the abdomen is obtained to determine if any residual contrast medium is present from previous studies. The oropharynx is sprayed or swabbed with a topical local anesthetic to help prevent gagging as the endoscope is passed down the throat.

▶ Positioning for the study will be in the left lateral position (Sims) or on the stomach. A protective guard is inserted into the mouth to cover the teeth. A bite block can also be inserted to maintain adequate opening of the mouth and to protect the teeth. Record baseline vital signs, and continue to monitor throughout the procedure. Protocols may vary among facilities.

▶ The endoscope is passed through the mouth with a dental suction device in place to drain secretions such as saliva that collects in the mouth during the procedure. A side-viewing flexible fiberoptic endoscope is passed into the duodenum to the biliary tree, and a small cannula is inserted into the duodenal papilla (ampulla of Vater). The duodenal papilla is visualized and cannulated with a catheter. Occasionally, the patient can be turned slightly to the right side to aid in visualization of the papilla.

▶ ERCP manometry can be done at this time to measure the pressure in the bile duct, pancreatic duct, and sphincter of Oddi at the papilla area via the catheter as it is placed in the area before the contrast medium is injected.

▶ When the catheter is in place, contrast medium is injected into the pancreatic and biliary ducts via the catheter, and fluoroscopic images are taken. Biopsy specimens for cytological analysis may be obtained.

▶ Explain that once the study is completed, the needle or catheter is removed, and a pressure dressing is applied over the puncture site.

Potential Nursing Actions

Make sure a written and informed consent has been signed prior to the procedure and before administering any medications.

- If iodinated contrast medium is scheduled to be used in patients receiving metformin or drugs containing metformin for type 2 diabetes, the drug may be discontinued on the day of the test and continue to be withheld for 48 hr after the test. Protocols may vary among facilities.
- Provide mouth care to reduce oral bacterial flora, as appropriate. Ensure that the patient has removed dentures, jewelry, and external metallic objects in the area to be examined prior to being transported for the procedure.

AFTER THE STUDY: POTENTIAL NURSING ACTIONS

Avoiding Complications

- Cholangiography, establishing an IV site, and injection of contrast medium are invasive procedures. Complications are rare but include risk for allergic reaction *(related to contrast reaction)*, bleeding from the puncture site *(related to a bleeding disorder or the effects of natural products and medications with known anticoagulant, antiplatelet, or thrombolytic properties)*, extravasation of bile, hematoma *(related to blood leakage into the tissue following needle insertion)*, infection *(which might occur if bacteria from the skin surface is introduced at the puncture site)*, tissue damage *(related to extravasation or leaking of contrast into the tissues during injection)*, nerve injury or damage to a nearby organ *(which might occur if the needle strikes a nerve or perforates an organ)*, nephrotoxicity *(a deterioration of renal function associated with contrast administration)*, pancreatitis *(the most common post-procedural complication of ERCP; also associated with significant morbidity and mortality)*, perforation, respiratory depression, and septicemia. Monitor the patient for complications related to the procedure (e.g., allergic reaction, anaphylaxis, bronchospasm, infection, injury). Immediately report symptoms such as difficulty breathing, chest pain, fever, hyperpnea, hypertension, nausea, palpitations, pruritus, rash, tachycardia, urticaria, or vomiting to

the appropriate HCP. Observe/assess the needle/catheter insertion site for bleeding, inflammation, or hematoma formation. Administer ordered antihistamines or prophylactic steroids if the patient has an allergic reaction. A rectal suppository containing an NSAID, such as indomethacin or diclofenac, may be administered to help prevent postprocedural pancreatitis in certain high-risk patients.

Treatment Considerations

- Do not allow the patient to eat or drink until the gag reflex returns due to aspiration risk.
- Monitor vital signs and neurological status every 15 min for 1 hr, then every 2 hr for 4 hr, and as ordered. Take temperature every 4 hr for 24 hr. Monitor intake and output at least every 8 hr. Compare with baseline values. Protocols may vary among facilities.
- If nausea is present, administer ordered antiemetics while assessing the frequency and duration of the nausea. Evaluate hydration status, monitor intake and output, and administer ordered parenteral fluids. Provide oral care and identify any factors that precipitate the experience of nausea.
- Manage pain by using a pain rating scale appropriate to the age, mental status, and language barrier. Administer ordered pain medications and identify alternative methods of pain management that work for the patient (imagery, diversion, etc.). Evaluate response to pain management and adjust as appropriate. Tell the patient to expect some throat soreness and possible hoarseness. Advise the patient to use warm gargles, lozenges, ice packs to the neck, or cool fluids to alleviate throat discomfort.
- Inform the patient that any belching, bloating, or flatulence is the result of air insufflation.

Safety Considerations

- Advise diabetic patients to avoid all medications containing metformin for 48 hr following a procedure with iodinated contrast. Iodinated contrast can temporarily impair kidney function, and failure to withhold metformin may indirectly result in drug-induced lactic acidosis, a dangerous and sometimes fatal adverse effect of metformin (related to renal impairment that does not support sufficient excretion of metformin).

Nutritional Considerations
▶ When safe, the patient is permitted to eat lightly for 12 to 24 hr and then to resume usual diet, fluids, medications, and activity as directed by the HCP.

Renal function should be assessed before metformin is resumed.

Follow-Up, Evaluation, and Desired Outcomes
▶ Understands that pain may be better managed by a combination of pharmacological and nonpharmacological treatment choices.
▶ Acknowledges which foods and odors to avoid to prevent nausea.
▶ Describes how antiemetics can assist to relieve nausea and improve oral intake.

Cholesterol, Total and Fractions

SYNONYM/ACRONYM: α_1-Lipoprotein cholesterol, high-density lipoprotein cholesterol (HDLC); and β-lipoprotein cholesterol, low-density lipoprotein cholesterol (LDLC), very-low-density lipoprotein (VLDL); lipid fractionation; lipoprotein phenotyping.

RATIONALE: To assess and monitor risk for coronary artery disease (CAD); to assist in categorizing lipoprotein as an indicator of cardiac health.

PATIENT PREPARATION: There are no medication restrictions unless by medical direction. Instruct the patient to fast 6 to 12 hr before specimen collection if lipoprotein fractionation or triglyceride measurements are ordered and recommend fasting if cholesterol levels alone are measured for screening. Instruct the patient to avoid excessive exercise for at least 12 hr before lipoprotein fractionation testing and to refrain from alcohol consumption for 24 hr before lipoprotein fractionation testing. Protocols may vary among facilities.

NORMAL FINDINGS: Method: Spectrophotometry for total cholesterol, HDLC and LDLC. Lipoprotein fractionation: Electrophoresis and 4°C test for specimen appearance. There is no quantitative interpretation of this test. The specimen appearance and electrophoretic pattern are visually interpreted.

Total Cholesterol		
Risk	Conventional Units	SI Units (Conventional Units × 0.0259)
Children and adolescents (less than 20 yr)		
Desirable	Less than 170 mg/dL	Less than 4.4 mmol/L
Borderline	170–199 mg/dL	4.4–5.2 mmol/L
High	Greater than 200 mg/dL	Greater than 5.2 mmol/L

(table continues on page 332)

C

Total Cholesterol

Risk	Conventional Units	SI Units (Conventional Units × 0.0259)
Adults and older adults		
Desirable	Less than 200 mg/dL	Less than 5.2 mmol/L
Borderline	200–239 mg/dL	5.2–6.2 mmol/L
High	Greater than 240 mg/dL	Greater than 6.2 mmol/L

HDLC	Conventional Units	SI Units (Conventional Units × 0.0259)
Birth	6–56 mg/dL	0.16–1.45 mmol/L
Children, adults, and older adults		
Desirable	Greater than 60 mg/dL	Greater than 1.55 mmol/L
Acceptable	40–60 mg/dL	1–1.55 mmol/L
Low	Less than 40 mg/dL	Less than 1 mmol/L

LDLC	Conventional Units	SI Units (Conventional Units × 0.0259)
Optimal	Less than 100 mg/dL	Less than 2.59 mmol/L
Near optimal	100–129 mg/dL	2.59–3.34 mmol/L
Borderline high	130–159 mg/dL	3.37–4.11 mmol/L
High	160–189 mg/dL	4.14–4.9 mmol/L
Very high	Greater than 190 mg/dL	Greater than 4.92 mmol/L

Hyperlipoproteinemia: Fredrickson Type	Specimen Appearance	Electrophoretic Pattern
Type I	Clear with creamy top layer	Heavy chylomicron band
Type IIa	Clear	Heavy β band
Type IIb	Clear or faintly turbid	Heavy β and pre-β bands
Type III	Slightly to moderately turbid	Heavy β band
Type IV	Slightly to moderately turbid	Heavy pre-β band
Type V	Slightly to moderately turbid with creamy top layer	Intense chylomicron band and heavy β and pre-β bands

CRITICAL FINDINGS AND POTENTIAL INTERVENTIONS: N/A

OVERVIEW: (Study type: Blood collected in a gold-, red-, red/gray, or green-top [Na or Li heparin] tube; related body system: Circulatory system.) Plasma values (Na or Li heparin) may be 10% lower than serum values. Cholesterol is a lipid needed to form cell membranes, bile salts, adrenal corticosteroid hormones, and other hormones such as estrogen and the androgens. Cholesterol is obtained from the diet and also synthesized in the body, mainly by the liver and intestinal mucosa. Very low cholesterol values, as are sometimes seen in critically ill patients, can be as life-threatening as very high levels. Maintaining cholesterol levels less than 200 mg/dL (SI: Less than 5.2 mmol/L) significantly reduces the risk of coronary heart disease. Beyond the total cholesterol and HDLC values, other important risk factors must be considered. Many myocardial infarctions (MI) occur even in patients whose cholesterol levels are considered to be within acceptable limits or who are in a moderate-risk category. Evidence-based risk factors include age, sex, ethnicity, total cholesterol, HDLC, LDLC, blood pressure, blood-pressure treatment status, diabetes, and current use of tobacco products. The combination of risk factors and lipid values helps identify individuals at risk so that appropriate interventions can be taken. If the cholesterol level is greater than 200 mg/dL (SI: greater than 5.2 mmol/L), repeat testing after a 12- to 24-hr fast is recommended.

HDLC and LDLC are the major transport proteins for cholesterol in the body. It is believed that HDLC may have protective properties in that its role includes transporting cholesterol from the arteries to the liver. LDLC is the major transport protein for cholesterol to the arteries from the liver. LDLC can be calculated using total cholesterol, total triglycerides, and HDLC levels.

Studies have shown that CAD is inversely related to LDLC particle number and size. The nuclear magnetic resonance (NMR) lipid profile uses NMR imaging spectroscopy to determine LDLC particle number and size in addition to measurement of the traditional lipid markers.

HDLC levels less than 40 mg/dL or less than 1 mmol/L in men and women represent a coronary risk factor. There is an inverse relationship between HDLC and risk of CAD (i.e., lower HDLC levels represent a higher risk of CAD). Levels of LDLC in terms of risk for CAD are directly proportional to risk and vary by age group. The LDLC can be estimated using the Friedewald formula:

LDLC = (Total Cholesterol) − (HDLC) − (VLDLC)

Very-low-density lipoprotein cholesterol (VLDLC) is estimated by dividing the triglycerides (conventional units) by 5. Triglycerides in SI units would be divided by 2.18 to estimate VLDLC. It is important to note that the formula is valid only if the triglycerides are less than 400 mg/dL or 4.52 mmol/L.

Lipoprotein electrophoresis measures lipoprotein fractions to determine abnormal distribution and concentration of lipoproteins in the serum, an important risk factor in the development of CAD.

C

The lipoprotein fractions, in order of increasing density, are (1) chylomicrons, (2) VLDL, (3) low-density lipoprotein (LDL), and (4) high-density lipoprotein (HDL). Chylomicrons and VLDL contain the highest levels of triglycerides and lower amounts of cholesterol and protein. LDL and HDL contain the lowest amounts of triglycerides and relatively higher amounts of cholesterol and protein. Studies have shown that CAD is directly related to elevated LDLC and inversely related to LDL particle size. An electrophoretic pattern demonstrating the presence of small, dense LDL particles (non-A) carries a threefold risk for developing CAD over the presence of larger, more buoyant LDL particles (pattern A).

Ceramides are a class of naturally occurring lipids. They are synthesized in tissue cells from saturated fats and sphingosine, are involved in cell cycle regulation, and share some of the same cellular functions as other lipids, such as maintenance of cell membrane integrity. Ceramides have long been associated with skin care products. The application of ceramide levels as a predictor of CAD is fairly recent; specifically ceramides Cer 16:0, Cer 18:0, and Cer 24:1. Ceramides are believed to be a strong, independent predictor of MI, stroke, and death. Ceramides are involved in the various processes that result in atherosclerosis, and ceramide levels increase as the degree of atherosclerotic development advances. Dyslipidemias and excessive caloric intake stimulate the transport of ceramides by LDLs into blood vessel tissue cells, which are not normally used for fat storage. The infiltration of LDL and accumulation of ceramides in the blood vessel wall causes an inflammatory response that signals monocytes to come into the endothelium and phagocytize the lipoproteins. The chain reaction intensifies with the release of cytokines and results in increased endothelial cell adhesion and platelet activation (in response to endothelial cell damage). Release of cytokines stimulates further ceramide synthesis.

There are other nonlipid markers used to provide evidence of ASCVD. For example, elevated levels of C-reactive protein are associated with increased risk for ASCVD related to the effects of inflammation on the cardiovascular system. Complex macro-interrelationships of the various body systems are only beginning to be better understood. Environmental and lifestyle factors also significantly influence and interact at the genetic level to regulate bodily functions. The rapid expansion of molecular technologies has led to the development of DNA sequencing techniques now used to identify some of the genetic determinants of kidney and heart disease. Blood pressure is controlled by the renin-angiotensin—aldosterone system, which affects the kidneys, heart, lungs, blood vessels, and central nervous system. Mutations of the angiotensin-converting enzyme gene (AGT) and angiotensin II type 1 receptor (AGTR1) gene in the renin-angiotensin-aldosterone system are strongly associated with an increased risk for hypertension and cerebrovascular disease (CVD), chronic kidney disease, and stroke secondary to hypertension. Identification of these associations is the initial step. Hypertension affects millions of people in the United States and is called a "silent killer" because it does not present with noticeable symptoms, so people are often unaware of their condition. Treatment regimens based on test results are still in development due to the number of genetic variants that have been identified, the variety of genetic expressions within the same mutation, and inconsistent associations between different ethnic populations that have been studied.

Guidelines for the prevention of CAD have been developed by the American College of Cardiology (ACC) and the American Heart Association (AHA) in conjunction with members of the National Heart, Lung, and Blood Institute's (NHLBI) ATP IV Expert Panel. The updated, evidence-based guidelines redefine the condition of concern as ASCVD, which involves atherosclerotic disease in any of the blood vessels in the body and expand ASCVD to include CAD, which specifically involves vessels that supply the heart, cerebrovascular disease (CVD), which involves vessels that supply the brain (e.g. stroke), and peripheral arterial/venous disease (PAD/PVD), which involves vessels that supply the arms and legs. Some of the important highlights include the following:

- Movement away from the use of LDL cholesterol targets in determining treatment with statins. Recommendations that focus on selecting (1) the patients who fall into four groups most likely to benefit from statin therapy and (2) the level of statin intensity most likely to affect or reduce development of ASCVD.

- Development of a new 10-yr risk assessment tool based on findings from a large, diverse population. Evidence-based risk factors include age, gender, ethnicity, total cholesterol, HDLC, blood pressure, blood-pressure treatment status, diagnosis of diabetes, and current use of tobacco products.

- Recommendations for aspects of lifestyle that would encourage prevention of ASCVD to include adherence to a Mediterranean-style or DASH (Dietary Approaches to Stop Hypertension)-style diet; dietary restriction of saturated fats, trans fats, sugar, and sodium; and regular participation in aerobic exercise. The guidelines contain reductions in body mass index (BMI) cutoffs for men and women designed to promote discussions between health-care providers (HCPs) and their patients regarding the benefits of maintaining a healthy weight.

- Recognition that additional biological markers, such as family history, high-sensitivity C-reactive protein, ankle-brachial index (ABI), and coronary artery calcium score, may be selectively used with the assessment tool to assist in predicting and evaluating risk.

- Recognition that other biomarkers, such as apolipoprotein B, estimated glomerular filtration rate (eGFR), creatinine, lipoprotein (a) or Lp(a), and microalbumin, warrant further study and may be considered for inclusion in future guidelines.

INDICATIONS

- Assist in determining risk of CAD.
- Assist in the diagnosis of nephrotic syndrome, hepatic disease, pancreatitis, and thyroid disorders.
- Evaluate known or suspected disorders associated with altered lipoprotein levels.
- Evaluate patients with serum cholesterol levels greater than 250 mg/dL, which indicate a high risk for CAD and need for dietary or drug therapy.
- Evaluate the response to dietary and drug therapy for high cholesterol.
- Investigate hypercholesterolemia in light of family history of CAD.

INTERFERING FACTORS

Factors that may alter the results of the study

- Drugs and other substances that may increase cholesterol levels include amiodarone, androgens, β-blockers, calcitriol, cortisone, cyclosporine, danazol, diclofenac, disulfiram, glucogenic corticosteroids, ibuprofen, isotretinoin, levodopa, methyclothiazide, miconazole (owing to castor oil vehicle, not the drug), nafarelin, some oral contraceptives, phenobarbital, phenothiazines, prochlorperazine, sotalol, thiabendazole, thiouracil, tretinoin, and trifluoperazine.
- Drugs and other substances that may increase HDLC levels include albuterol, anticonvulsants, cholestyramine, cimetidine, clofibrate and other fibric acid derivatives, estrogens, ethanol (moderate use), lovastatin, niacin, oral contraceptives, pindolol, pravastatin, prazosin hydrochloride, and simvastatin.
- Drugs and other substances that may increase LDLC levels include androgens, catecholamines, chenodiol, cyclosporine, danazol, diuretics, etretinate, glucogenic corticosteroids, and progestins.
- Drugs and other substances that may decrease cholesterol levels include acebutolol, amiloride, aminosalicylic acid, androsterone, ascorbic acid, asparaginase, atenolol, atorvastatin, beclobrate, bezafibrate, cerivastatin, cholestyramine, ciprofibrate, clofibrate, colestipol, doxazosin, enalapril, estrogens, fenofibrate, fluvastatin, gemfibrozil, haloperidol, hormone replacement therapy, hydralazine, hydrochlorothiazide, interferon, isoniazid, kanamycin, ketoconazole, lincomycin, lisinopril, lovastatin, metformin, neomycin, niacin, nicotinic acid, nifedipine, paromomycin, pravastatin, probucol, simvastatin, tamoxifen, terazosin, thyroxine, trazodone, triiodothyronine, ursodiol, valproic acid, and verapamil.
- Drugs and other substances that may decrease HDLC levels include acebutolol, atenolol, danazol, diuretics, etretinate, interferon, isotretinoin, linseed oil, metoprolol, neomycin, nonselective β-adrenergic blocking drugs, probucol, progesterone, steroids, and thiazides.
- Drugs and other substances that may decrease LDLC levels include alirocumab, aminosalicylic acid, cholestyramine, colestipol estrogens, evolocumab, fibric acid derivatives, interferon, lovastatin, neomycin, niacin, pravastatin, prazosin, probucol, simvastatin, terazosin, and thyroxine.
- Positioning can affect results; lower cholesterol levels are obtained if the specimen is from a patient who has been supine for 20 min.

Other considerations

- Ingestion of drugs that alter cholesterol levels within 12 hr of the test may give a false impression of cholesterol levels, unless the test is done to evaluate such effects.

- Some of the drugs used to lower total cholesterol and LDLC or increase HDLC may cause liver damage.
- Grossly elevated triglyceride levels invalidate the Friedewald formula for mathematical estimation of LDLC; if the triglyceride level is greater than 400 mg/dL (SI: 4.52 mmol/L), the formula should not be used.
- Fasting before specimen collection is highly recommended. Ideally, the patient should be on a stable diet for 3 wk and fast for 12 hr before specimen collection.

POTENTIAL MEDICAL DIAGNOSIS: CLINICAL SIGNIFICANCE OF RESULTS
Increased in

Total Cholesterol
Although the exact pathophysiology is unknown, cholesterol is required for many functions at the cellular and organ level. Elevations of cholesterol are associated with conditions caused by an inherited defect in lipoprotein metabolism, liver disease, kidney disease, or a disorder of the endocrine system.

- Acute intermittent porphyria
- Alcohol misuse
- Anorexia nervosa
- Cholestasis
- Chronic kidney disease
- Diabetes (with poor control)
- Diets high in cholesterol and fats
- Familial hyperlipoproteinemia
- Glomerulonephritis
- Glycogen storage disease (von Gierke disease)
- Gout
- Hypothyroidism (primary)
- Ischemic heart disease
- Metabolic syndrome
- Nephrotic syndrome

- Obesity
- Pancreatic and prostatic malignancy
- Pregnancy
- Werner syndrome

HDLC Increased In
- Alcohol misuse
- Biliary cholangitis
- Chronic hepatitis
- Exercise
- Familial hyper-α-lipoproteinemia

LDLC Increased In
- Anorexia nervosa
- Chronic kidney disease
- Corneal arcus
- Cushing syndrome
- Diabetes
- Diet high in cholesterol and saturated fat
- Dysglobulinemias
- Hepatic disease
- Hepatic obstruction
- Hyperlipoproteinemia types IIA and IIB
- Hypothyroidism
- Metabolic syndrome
- Nephrotic syndrome
- Porphyria
- Pregnancy
- Premature CAD
- Tendon and tuberous xanthomas

Decreased in
Total Cholesterol
Although the exact pathophysiology is unknown, cholesterol is required for many functions at the cellular and organ level. Decreases in cholesterol levels are associated with conditions caused by malnutrition, malabsorption, liver disease, and sudden increased utilization.

- Burns
- Chronic myelocytic leukemia
- Chronic obstructive pulmonary disease
- Hyperthyroidism
- Liver disease (severe)

- Malabsorption and malnutrition syndromes
- Myeloma
- Pernicious anemia
- Polycythemia vera
- Severe illness
- Sideroblastic anemias
- Tangier disease
- Thalassemia
- Waldenström macroglobulinemia

HDLC Decreased In
- Abetalipoproteinemia
- Cholestasis
- Chronic kidney disease
- Fish-eye disease
- Genetic predisposition or enzyme/cofactor deficiency
- Hepatocellular disorders
- Hypertriglyceridemia
- Metabolic syndrome
- Nephrotic syndrome
- Obesity
- Premature CAD
- Sedentary lifestyle
- Smoking
- Tangier disease
- Uncontrolled diabetes

LDLC Decreased In
- Acute stress (severe burns, illness)
- Chronic anemias
- Chronic pulmonary disease
- Genetic predisposition or enzyme/cofactor deficiency
- Hyperthyroidism
- Hypolipoproteinemia and abetalipoproteinemia
- Inflammatory joint disease
- Myeloma
- Reye syndrome
- Severe hepatocellular destruction or disease
- Tangier disease

Lipoprotein Fractionation
- *Type I:* Hyperlipoproteinemia, or increased chylomicrons, can be primary *resulting from an inherited deficiency of lipoprotein lipase* or secondary *caused by uncontrolled diabetes, systemic lupus erythematosus, and dysgammaglobulinemia.* Total cholesterol is normal to moderately elevated, and triglycerides (mostly exogenous chylomicrons) are grossly elevated. If the condition is inherited, symptoms will appear in childhood.
- *Type IIa:* Hyperlipoproteinemia can be primary *resulting from inherited characteristics* or secondary *caused by uncontrolled hypothyroidism, nephrotic syndrome, and dysgammaglobulinemia.* Total cholesterol is elevated, triglycerides are normal, and LDLC is elevated. If the condition is inherited, symptoms will appear in childhood.
- *Type IIb:* Hyperlipoproteinemia *can occur for the same reasons as in type IIa.* Total cholesterol, triglycerides, and LDLC are all elevated.
- *Type III:* Hyperlipoproteinemia can be primary *resulting from inherited characteristics* or secondary *caused by hypothyroidism, uncontrolled diabetes, alcohol misuse, and dysgammaglobulinemia.* Total cholesterol and triglycerides are elevated, whereas LDLC is normal.
- *Type IV:* Hyperlipoproteinemia can be primary *resulting from inherited characteristics* or secondary *caused by poorly controlled diabetes, alcohol misuse, nephrotic syndrome, chronic kidney disease, and dysgammaglobulinemia.* Total cholesterol is normal to moderately elevated, triglycerides are moderately to grossly elevated, and LDLC is normal.
- *Type V:* Hyperlipoproteinemia can be primary *resulting from inherited characteristics* or secondary *caused by uncontrolled diabetes, alcohol misuse, nephrotic syndrome, and dysgammaglobulinemia.* Total cholesterol is normal to moderately elevated, triglycerides are grossly elevated, and LDLC is normal.

NURSING IMPLICATIONS

POTENTIAL NURSING PROBLEMS: ASSESSMENT & NURSING DIAGNOSIS

Problems	Signs and Symptoms
Cardiac output (related to increased preload, increased afterload, impaired cardiac contractility, cardiac muscle disease, altered cardiac conduction)	Decreased peripheral pulses; decreased urinary output; cool, clammy skin; tachypnea; dyspnea; edema; altered level of consciousness; abnormal heart sounds; crackles in lungs; decreased activity tolerance; weight gain; fatigue; hypoxia
Health management (related to failure to regulate diet, lack of exercise, alcohol use, smoking)	Inability or failure to recognize or process information toward improving health and preventing illness with associated mental and physical effects
Nutrition (related to excess caloric intake with large amounts of dietary sodium and fat; cultural lifestyle; overeating associated with anxiety, depression, compulsive disorder; genetics; inadequate or unhealthy food resources)	Observable obesity, high-fat or sodium food selections, high BMI, high consumption of ethnic foods, sedentary lifestyle, dietary religious beliefs and food selections, binge eating, diet high in refined sugar, repetitive dieting and failure
Pain (related to myocardial ischemia, MI; pericarditis, coronary vasospasm, ventricular hypertrophy, embolism, epicardial artery inflammation)	Reports of chest pain, new onset of angina, shortness of breath, pallor, weakness, diaphoresis, palpitations, nausea, vomiting, epigastric pain or discomfort, increased blood pressure, increased heart rate

BEFORE THE STUDY: PLANNING AND IMPLEMENTATION

Teaching the Patient What to Expect

▶ Inform the patient this test can assist with evaluation of lipid levels.
▶ Explain that a blood sample is needed for the test.

Potential Nursing Actions

▶ Evaluate for the presence of other risk factors, such as family history of heart disease, smoking, obesity, diet, lack of physical activity, hypertension, diabetes, previous MI, and previous vascular disease, which should be investigated.

▶ Understanding genetics assists in identifying those who may benefit from additional education, risk assessment, and counseling.

AFTER THE STUDY: POTENTIAL NURSING ACTIONS

Treatment Considerations

▶ Cardiac Output: Assess peripheral pulses and capillary refill. Monitor orthostatic blood pressure changes, respiratory rate, and breath sounds. Assess skin color and temperature and level of consciousness. Monitor urinary output; provide oxygen and use pulse oximetry to monitor oxygenation; trend sodium, potassium, and B-type natriuretic peptide levels. Administer ordered ACE inhibitors, beta blockers, diuretics, aldosterone antagonists, and vasodilators.

▸ Health Management: Encourage regular participation in weight-bearing exercise. Evaluate diet, smoking, and alcohol use. Refer to smoking cessation and alcohol treatment programs. Teach the importance of adequate calcium intake with diet and supplements. Collaborate with the HCP for bone density evaluation.

▸ Nutrition: Discuss ideal body weight and the purpose of and relationship between ideal weight and caloric intake to support cardiac health. Encourage consultation with a registered dietitian to learn how to plan and prepare healthy meals for the entire family.

▸ Pain: Assess pain characteristics, squeezing pressure, location in substernal back, neck, or jaw; assess pain duration and onset (minimal exertion, sleep, or rest). Identify pain modalities that have relieved pain in the past. Monitor and trend cardiac biomarkers, CK-MB, troponin, and myoglobin. Collaborate with ancillary departments to complete ordered echocardiography, exercise stress testing, and pharmacological stress testing. Administer prescribed pain medication and evaluate effectiveness. Monitor and trend vital signs. Administer prescribed oxygen, prescribed anticoagulants, antiplatelets, beta blockers, calcium channel blockers, ACE inhibitors, angiotensin II receptor blockers, or thrombolytic drugs.

Nutritional Considerations

▸ Nutritional therapy is recommended for the patient identified to be at risk for developing CAD or for individuals who have specific risk factors and/or existing medical conditions (e.g., elevated LDLC levels, other lipid disorders, diabetes, insulin resistance, or metabolic syndrome). Other changeable risk factors warranting patient education include strategies to encourage patients, especially those who are overweight and with high blood pressure, to safely decrease sodium intake, achieve a normal weight, ensure regular participation of moderate aerobic physical activity three to four times per week, eliminate tobacco use, and adhere to a heart-healthy diet. If triglycerides are elevated, the patient should be advised to eliminate or reduce alcohol. Always consider cultural influences with dietary choices to ensure better adherence to a change in lifestyle. A variety of dietary patterns are beneficial for people with CAD, and there are many meal-planning approaches with nutritional goals endorsed by the American Diabetes Association (ADA). The *2013 AHA/ ACC Guideline on Lifestyle Management to Reduce Cardiovascular Risk,* published by the ACC and AHA in conjunction with the NHLBI, recommends a Mediterranean-style diet rather than a low-fat diet. The guideline emphasizes inclusion of vegetables, whole grains, fruits, low-fat dairy, nuts, legumes, and nontropical vegetable oils (e.g., olive, canola, peanut, sunflower, flaxseed) along with fish and lean poultry. The DASH diet makes additional recommendations for the reduction of dietary sodium. Both dietary styles emphasize a reduction in consumption of red meats, which are high in saturated fats and cholesterol, and other foods containing sugar, saturated fats, trans fats, and sodium. The ADA also includes a vegetarian diet as well as other potential weight loss diets such as Weight Watchers. The nutritional needs of each patient need to be determined individually (especially during pregnancy) with the appropriate HCPs, such as registered dietitians.

▸ *Sensitivity to Social and Cultural Issues:* Numerous studies point to the prevalence of excess body weight in American children and adolescents. Findings from the 2015–2016 National Health and Nutrition Examination Survey (NHANES), regarding the prevalence of obesity in younger members of the population, estimate that obesity is present in 13.9% of the population ages 2 to 5 yr, 18.4% ages 6 to 11 yr, and 20.6% ages 12 to 19 yr. The medical, social, and emotional consequences of excess body weight are significant. Special attention should be given to instructing the pediatric patient and caregiver regarding health risks and weight control education.

Follow-Up, Evaluation, and Desired Outcomes

◗ Acknowledges contact information provided for the AHA (www.heart.org/HEARTORG), NHLBI (www.nhlbi.nih.gov), and the U.S. Department of Agriculture's resource for nutrition (www.choosemyplate.gov).

◗ Understands risk factors for CAD, necessary lifestyle changes (diet, smoking, alcohol use), the importance of weight control, and reportable signs and symptoms of heart attack.

Chromosome Analysis, Blood

SYNONYM/ACRONYM: Chromosome karyotyping.

RATIONALE: To test for suspected chromosomal disorders that result in birth defects such as Down syndrome.

PATIENT PREPARATION: There are no food, fluid, activity, or medication restrictions unless by medical direction.

NORMAL FINDINGS: (Method: Tissue culture and microscopic analysis) No chromosomal abnormalities identified.

CRITICAL FINDINGS AND POTENTIAL INTERVENTIONS: N/A

OVERVIEW: (**Study type:** Blood collected in a green-top [sodium heparin] tube; **related body system:** Reproductive system.) Cytogenetics is a specialization within the area of genetics that includes chromosome analysis or karyotyping. Chromosome analysis or karyotyping involves comparison of test samples against normal chromosome patterns of number and structure. A normal karyotype consists of 22 pairs of autosomal chromosomes and one pair of sex chromosomes, XX for female and XY for male. Variations in number or structure can be congenital or acquired. Variations can range from a small, single-gene mutation to abnormalities in an entire chromosome or set of chromosomes due to duplication, deletion, substitution, translocation, or other rearrangement. Molecular probe techniques are used to detect smaller, more subtle changes in chromosomes. Cells are incubated in culture media to increase the number of cells available for study and to allow for hybridization of the cellular DNA with fluorescent DNA probes in a technique called *fluorescence in situ hybridization* (FISH). The probes are designed to target areas of the chromosome known to correlate with genetic risk

C

for a particular disease. When a suitable volume of hybridized sample is achieved, cell growth is chemically inhibited during the prophase and metaphase stages of mitosis (cell division), and cellular DNA is examined to detect fluorescence, which represents chromosomal abnormalities, in the targeted areas. Amniotic fluid, chorionic villus sampling, and cells from fetal tissue or products of conception can also be evaluated for chromosomal abnormalities.

Cell free fetal DNA (cffDNA) analysis is a newer noninvasive cytogenetic screening option for women with an increased risk for fetal aneuploidy (an abnormal number of fetal chromosomes). CffDNA is released by the placenta as early as the 10th week of pregnancy and is detectable in circulating maternal blood. Analysis of a maternal blood sample can be performed to identify trisomy 13 (Patau syndrome), trisomy 18 (Edwards syndrome), trisomy 21 (Down syndrome), and Klinefelter syndrome (XXY). It should be noted that there are a number of limitations with cffDNA testing that would not be encountered with conventional maternal screening and diagnostic testing strategies. Discussion regarding the limitations and benefits should occur between every patient who chooses this testing and the appropriate health-care provider (HCP). The most current screening recommendations for aneuploidy include a requirement that all cffDNA screens be confirmed by a diagnostic test such as amniocentesis or chorionic villus sampling, regardless of whether the screening test results were normal or abnormal.

Knowledge of genetics assists in identifying those who may benefit from additional education, risk assessment, and counseling. Genetics is the study and identification of genes, genetic mutations, and inheritance. For example, genetics provides some insight into the likelihood of inheriting a medical condition such as Down syndrome. Down syndrome is an example of a chromosome disorder in which the cells have three copies of chromosome 21 (trisomy) instead of the normal two copies. Further information regarding inheritance of genes can be found in the study titled "Genetic Testing."

INDICATIONS

- Evaluate conditions related to cryptorchidism, hypogonadism, primary amenorrhea, and infertility.
- Evaluate congenital anomaly, delayed development (physical or mental), intellectual disability, and ambiguous sexual organs.
- Investigate the carrier status of patients or relatives with known genetic abnormalities.
- Investigate the cause of still birth or multiple miscarriages.
- Investigate types of solid tumor or hematological malignancies.
- Provide prenatal care or genetic counseling.

INTERFERING FACTORS
Contraindications

Circumstances in which the parents are not emotionally capable of understanding the test results and managing the ramifications of the test results.

POTENTIAL MEDICAL DIAGNOSIS: CLINICAL SIGNIFICANCE OF RESULTS

The following tables list some common genetic defects.

Syndrome	Autosomal Chromosome Defect	Features
Angelman	Deletion 15q11–q13	Developmental delays (physical growth, communication, and motor skills); hyperactive behavior; overall happy demeanor with frequent laughter and hand-flapping actions; fascination with water
Beckwith-Wiedemann	Duplication 11p15	Macroglossia, omphalocele, earlobe creases
Bloom	Mutations of BLM, 15	Birth weight and length are below normal, and stature remains below normal to adulthood; skin changes in response to sun exposure; increased risk of cancers that develop early in life; high-pitched voice; distinctive facial features (long, narrow face with a small jaw; large nose and ears)
Canavan	Mutations of ASPA, 17p13.3	Developmental delays that become obvious at 3 to 5 months of age; hypotonia that contributes to inability to roll over, sit upright, or swallow; macrocephaly; and intellectual disability
Cat's eye	Trisomy 2q11	Anal atresia, coloboma
Cri du chat	Deletion 5p	Catlike cry, microcephaly, hypertelorism, intellectual disability, retrognathia
Cystic fibrosis	Mutations of CFTR, 7	Impaired transport of chloride affects the movement of water in and out of the cells lining the lungs and pancreas, resulting in production of thick mucus that obstructs airways and prevents normal function of the affected organs; life-threatening, permanent lung damage
DiGeorge	Deletion 22q11.2	The wide variety in type and severity of problems associated with this syndrome of impaired development of body systems most commonly includes cardiac abnormalities or defects, poor immune system function (hypothymic or absent thymus), cleft palate, hypoparathyroidism (low calcium), behavioral disorders, distinctive facial features (long face with downturned mouth, asymmetric face when crying, microcephaly, hooded eye lids, malformed ears)

(table continues on page 344)

C

Syndrome	Autosomal Chromosome Defect	Features
Down	Trisomy 21	Epicanthal folds, simian crease of palm, flat nasal bridge, intellectual disability, congenital heart disease
Edwards	Trisomy 18	Micrognathia, clenched third/fourth fingers with the fifth finger overlapping, rocker-bottom feet, intellectual disability, congenital heart disease
Gaucher	Mutations of GBA, 1	Hepatomegaly and splenomegaly related to accumulation of lipids, anemia, thrombocytopenia, bone disease (bone pain, fractures, and arthritis)
Maple syrup	Mutations of BCKDHA, BCKDHB, DBT, and DLD, 19	Developmental delays, poor feeding, lethargy, distinctive maple syrup odor in urine
Miller-Dieker	Deletion 17	Lissencephaly (incomplete or absent development of the folds of the cerebrum); microcephaly; developmental delays, especially in growth; intellectual disability with seizures; difficulty feeding and failure to thrive; cardiac malformations
Niemann-Pick	Chromosome 14q24.3 (type C2); 18q11.2 (type C1); 11p15.4–p15.1 (types A & B)	All types demonstrate symptoms that reflect abnormalities in liver and lung function; blood tests show hyperlipidemia (cholesterol and other fats) and thrombocytopenia
Pallister-Killian	Trisomy 12p	Psychomotor delay, sparse anterior scalp hair, micrognathia, hypotonia
Patau	Trisomy 13	Microcephaly, cleft palate or lip, polydactyly, intellectual disability, congenital heart disease
Prader-Willi	Deletion 15q11–q13	Delayed development; distinctive facial features (narrow forehead, almond-shaped eyes, triangular-shaped mouth, diminished stature with small hands and feet); hypotonia; childhood development of an insatiable appetite, hyperphagia, and obesity; mild to moderate intellectual disability; behavioral problems (outbursts of anger and compulsive behavior such as picking at the skin)

Syndrome	Autosomal Chromosome Defect	Features
Smith-Magenis	Deletion 17p11.2	Major features include mild to moderate intellectual disability, delayed speech and language skills, distinctive facial features, sleep disturbances, and behavioral problems
Tay-Sachs	Mutations of HEXA, 15q24.1	Normal development until age 3 to 6 mo when development slows and hypotonia affects motor skills such as ability to turn over, sit upright, and crawl; exaggerated startle reaction to loud noises; seizures; eventual loss of vision (cherry red spot upon eye examination is characteristic) and hearing; intellectual disability
Warkam	Mosaic trisomy 8	Malformed ears, bulbous nose, deep palm creases, absent or hypoplastic patellae
Wolf-Hirschhorn	Deletion 4p16.3	Microcephaly, growth retardation, intellectual disability, carp mouth

Syndrome	Sex-Chromosome Defect	Features
Fragile X	Xq27.3	Intellectual disability, autism and autism spectrum disorders
XYY	47,XYY	Tall, increased risk of behavior problems
Klinefelter	47,XXY	Hypogonadism, infertility, underdeveloped secondary sex characteristics, learning disabilities
Rett	Mutations of Xq28	Severe and progressive developmental problems related to brain functions such as speech, motor, and intelligence begin after 6 to 18 mo of normal growth; brain disorder almost exclusively affecting females; slower than normal physical growth; microcephaly; meaningful use of hands is lost in early childhood and replaced by repetitive random hand motions such as clapping or wringing
Triple X	47,XXX	Increased risk of infertility and learning disabilities
Ullrich-Turner	45,X	Short, gonadal dysgenesis, webbed neck, low posterior hairline, renal and cardiovascular abnormalities

C

NURSING IMPLICATIONS

BEFORE THE STUDY: PLANNING AND IMPLEMENTATION

Teaching the Patient What to Expect
▶ Inform the patient this test can assist in identification of potential birth defects.
▶ Explain that a blood sample is needed for the test.

AFTER THE STUDY: POTENTIAL NURSING ACTIONS

Treatment Considerations
▶ *Sensitivity to Social and Cultural Issues:* Encourage the family to seek counseling if they are contemplating pregnancy termination or to seek genetic counseling if a chromosomal abnormality

is determined. Decisions regarding elective abortion should occur in the presence of both parents. Provide a nonjudgmental, nonthreatening atmosphere for discussing the risks and difficulties of delivering and raising a developmentally challenged infant, as well as for exploring other options (termination of pregnancy or adoption). It is also important to discuss feelings the mother and father may experience (e.g., guilt, depression, anger) if fetal abnormalities are detected. Educate the patient and family regarding access to counseling services, as appropriate.

Follow-Up, Evaluation, and Desired Outcomes
▶ Considers all aspects of chromosomal analysis and implied ramifications when deciding how to proceed with pregnancy.

Clot Retraction

SYNONYM/ACRONYM: N/A

RATIONALE: To assist in the diagnosis of bleeding disorders.

PATIENT PREPARATION: There are no food, fluid, activity, or medication restrictions unless by medical direction.

NORMAL FINDINGS: (Method: Macroscopic observation of sample) A normal clot, gently separated from the side of the test tube and incubated at 37°C, shrinks to about half of its original size within 1 hr. The result is a firm, cylindrical fibrin clot that contains red blood cells and is sharply demarcated from the clear serum. Complete clot retraction can take 6 to 24 hr.

CRITICAL FINDINGS AND POTENTIAL INTERVENTIONS: N/A

OVERVIEW: (**Study type:** Blood— Whole blood collected in a full red-top tube; **related body system:** Circulatory/Hematopoietic system.) The clot retraction test helps assess the adequacy of platelet function by measuring the speed and extent of clot retraction away from the side of a collection tube without any additives. Once collected, the specimen must be transported to the laboratory within 1 hr of collection and promptly placed in a 37°C waterbath to simulate the temperature at which hemostasis would occur in the body; the specimen must be observed at 2 and 24 hr. Platelets play a major role in the process of clot formation. When platelets are adequate in number and function is normal, the blood will form a clot in the collection tube and retract away from the sides of the tube within 1 to 2 hr. The blood will appear in a firm, clearly distinguishable clot surrounded by serum, the liquid portion of coagulated blood. When platelets are decreased or their function is impaired, there is little serum surrounding a soft, poorly demarcated clot. In addition to normal platelet count and function, clot retraction depends on the contractile protein thrombosthenin, magnesium, adenosine triphosphate (ATP), and pyruvate kinase. Clot retraction is also influenced by a normal red blood cell (RBC) volume (hematocrit) and by fibrinogen structure and concentration.

INDICATIONS

- Evaluate the adequacy of platelet function.
- Evaluate thrombocytopenia of unknown origin.
- Investigate the possibility of Glanzmann disease.
- Investigate suspected abnormalities of fibrinogen or fibrinolytic activity.

INTERFERING FACTORS

Factors that may alter the results of the study

- Drugs that may produce a decreased result include carbenicillin and plicamycin.

Other considerations

- Platelet count less than 30×10^3/microL (SI: Less than 30×10^9/L),

acetylsalicylic acid therapy, altered fibrinogen/fibrin structure, hypofibrinogenemia, polycythemia or hemoconcentration, and multiple myeloma are conditions in which abnormal clot retraction may occur, limiting the ability to form a valid assessment of platelet function.

- Prompt and proper specimen processing, storage, and analysis are important to achieve accurate results. Specimens received in the laboratory more than 1 hr after collection should be rejected.

POTENTIAL MEDICAL DIAGNOSIS: CLINICAL SIGNIFICANCE OF RESULTS

Increased in

- Anemia (severe) *(related to inadequate numbers of RBCs that quickly produce a clot)*
- Hypofibrinogenemia, dysfibrinogenemia, disseminated intravascular coagulation *(evidenced by rapid formation of a small, loosely formed clot; absence of functional fibrinogen reduces fibrinolysis)*
- Medications such as aspirin *(related to effect of acetylsalicylic acid as a potentiator of platelet aggregation)*

Decreased in

- Glanzmann thrombasthenia *(related to autosomal recessive abnormality of platelet glycoprotein IIb–IIIa required for platelet aggregation)*
- Polycythemia *(related to excessive numbers of RBCs that physically limit the extent to which the clot can retract)*
- Thrombocytopenia *(related to inadequate numbers of platelets to produce a well-formed clot)*
- von Willebrand disease *(related to deficiency of von Willebrand factor required for platelet aggregation)*

- Waldenström macroglobulinemia
  (*related to excessive production of
  paraproteins that physically obstruct
  platelet aggregation*)

NURSING IMPLICATIONS

BEFORE THE STUDY: PLANNING AND IMPLEMENTATION

Teaching the Patient What to Expect
- Inform the patient this test can assist in evaluating the effectiveness of blood clotting.
- Explain that a blood sample is needed for the test.

AFTER THE STUDY: POTENTIAL NURSING ACTIONS

Avoiding Complications
- Inform the patient with abnormal clot retraction of the importance of taking precautions against bruising and bleeding. These precautions may include the use of a soft bristle toothbrush, use of an electric razor, avoidance of constipation, avoidance of acetylsalicylic acid and similar products, and avoidance of intramuscular injections.

Follow-Up, Evaluation, and Desired Outcomes
- Understands the importance of timely reporting of bleeding occurrences to health-care provider.

Coagulation Factors

SYNONYM/ACRONYM: See table on the next page.

RATIONALE: To detect factor deficiencies and related coagulopathies such as found in disseminated intravascular coagulation (DIC).

PATIENT PREPARATION: There are no food, fluid, activity, or medication restrictions unless by medical direction.

NORMAL FINDINGS: (Method: Photo-optical clot detection) Activity from 50% to 150%.

Preferred Name	Synonym	Role in Modern Coagulation Cascade Model	Coagulation Test Responses in the Presence of Factor Deficiency
Fibrinogen	—	Assists in the formation of the fibrin clot	PT prolonged, aPTT prolonged
Prothrombin	Prethrombin	Assists factor Xa in formation of trace thrombin in the initiation phase and assists factors VIIIa, IXa, Xa, and Va to form thrombin in the propagation phase of hemostasis	PT prolonged, aPTT prolonged
Tissue factor (TF) (formerly known as factor III)	Tissue thromboplastin	Assists factor VII and Ca²⁺ in the activation of factors IX and X during the initiation phase of hemostasis	PT prolonged, aPTT prolonged
Calcium (formerly known as factor IV)	Ca²⁺	Essential to the activation of multiple clotting factors	N/A
Proaccelerin	Labile factor, accelerator globulin (AcG)	Assists factors VIIIa, IXa, Xa, and II in the formation of thrombin during the amplification and propagation phases of hemostasis	PT prolonged, aPTT prolonged
Proconvertin	Stable factor, serum prothrombin conversion accelerator, autoprothrombin I	Assists TF and Ca²⁺ in the activation of factors IX and X	PT prolonged, aPTT normal
Antihemophilic factor (AHF)	Antihemophilic globulin (AHG), antihemophilic factor A, platelet cofactor 1	Activated by trace thrombin during the initiation phase of hemostasis to amplify formation of additional thrombin	PT normal, aPTT prolonged

(table continues on page 350)

C

	Preferred Name	Synonym	Role in Modern Coagulation Cascade Model	Coagulation Test Responses in the Presence of Factor Deficiency
Factor IX	Plasma thromboplastin component (PTC)	Christmas factor, antihemophilic factor B, platelet cofactor 2	Assists factors Va and VIIIa in the amplification phase and factors VIIIa, Xa, Va, and II to form thrombin in the propagation phase	PT normal, aPTT prolonged
Factor X	Stuart-Power factor	Autoprothrombin III, thrombokinase	Assists with formation of trace thrombin in the initiation phase and acts with factors VIIIa, IXa, Va, and II to form thrombin in the propagation phase	PT prolonged, aPTT prolonged
Factor XI	Plasma thromboplastin antecedent (PTA)	Antihemophilic factor C	Activated by thrombin produced in the extrinsic pathway to enhance production of additional thrombin inside the fibrin clot via the intrinsic pathway; this factor also participates in slowing down the process of fibrinolysis	PT normal, aPTT prolonged
Factor XII	Hageman factor	Glass factor, contact factor	Contact activator of the kinin system (e.g., prekallikrein, and high-molecular-weight kininogen)	PT normal, aPTT prolonged
Factor XIII	Fibrin-stabilizing factor (FSF)	Laki-Lorand factor (LLF), fibrinase, plasma transglutaminase	Activated by thrombin and assists in formation of bonds between fibrin strands to complete secondary hemostasis	PT normal, aPTT normal
von Willebrand factor	von Willebrand factor	vWF	Assists in platelet adhesion and thrombus formation	Ristocetin cofactor decreased

C

CRITICAL FINDINGS AND POTENTIAL INTERVENTIONS
• Fibrinogen: Less than 80 mg/dL (SI: Less than 2.4 micromol/L)

Timely notification to the requesting health-care provider (HCP) of any critical findings and related symptoms is a role expectation of the professional nurse. A listing of these findings varies among facilities.

Signs and symptoms of microvascular thrombosis include cyanosis, ischemic tissue necrosis, hemorrhagic necrosis, tachypnea, dyspnea, pulmonary emboli, venous distention, abdominal pain, and oliguria. Possible interventions include identification and treatment of the underlying cause, support through administration of required blood products (cryoprecipitate or fresh frozen plasma), and administration of heparin. Cryoprecipitate may be a more effective product than fresh frozen plasma in cases where the fibrinogen level is less than 100 mg/dL (SI: 2.94 micromol/L), the minimum level required for adequate hemostasis, because it delivers a concentrated amount of fibrinogen without as much plasma volume. Further information regarding fibrinogen can be found in the study titled "Fibrinogen."

OVERVIEW: (**Study type:** Blood collected in a completely filled blue-top [3.2% sodium citrate] tube; **related body system:** Circulatory/Hematopoietic system.) If the patient's hematocrit exceeds 55%, the volume of citrate in the collection tube must be adjusted. The collection tube should be completely filled. *Important note:* When multiple specimens are drawn, the blue-top tube should be collected after sterile (i.e., blood culture) tubes. Otherwise, when using a standard vacutainer system, the blue-top tube is the first tube collected. When a butterfly is used, due to the added tubing, an extra red-top tube should be collected before the blue-top tube to ensure complete filling of the blue-top tube. Promptly transport the specimen to the laboratory for processing and analysis. The recommendation for processed and unprocessed samples stored in unopened tubes is that testing should be completed within 1 to 4 hr of collection. Hemostasis involves three components: blood vessel walls, platelets, and plasma coagulation proteins. Primary hemostasis has three major stages involving platelet adhesion, platelet activation, and platelet aggregation. Platelet adhesion is initiated by exposure of the endothelium as a result of damage to blood vessels. Exposed TF-bearing cells trigger the simultaneous binding of von Willebrand factor to exposed collagen and circulating platelets. Activated platelets release a number of procoagulant factors, including thromboxane, a very potent platelet activator, from storage granules. These factors enter the circulation and activate other platelets, and the cycle continues. The activated platelets aggregate at the site of vessel injury, and at this stage of hemostasis, the glycoprotein IIb/IIIa receptors on the activated platelets bind fibrinogen, causing the platelets to stick together and form a plug. There is a balance in health between the prothrombotic or clot formation process and the antithrombotic or clot disintegration process. Simultaneously, the coagulation process or secondary hemostasis occurs. In secondary hemostasis, the coagulation proteins respond to blood vessel injury in an overlapping chain of events. The contact activation and TF pathways (also known respectively as the intrinsic and extrinsic pathways) of secondary hemostasis are a series of reactions involving the substrate protein fibrinogen, the coagulation factors (also known as *enzyme precursors* or *zymogens*), nonenzymatic cofactors (Ca^{2+}), and phospholipids. The factors were assigned Roman numerals in the order of their discovery, not their place in the coagulation sequence. Factor VI was originally thought to be a separate clotting factor. It was subsequently proved to be the same as a modified form of factor Va, and therefore, the number is no longer used.

The antithrombotic process includes tissue factor pathway inhibitor (TFPI), antithrombin, protein C, and fibrinolysis.

The coagulation factors are formed in the liver. They can be divided into three groups based on their common properties:

1. The contact group is activated in vitro by a surface such as glass and is activated in vivo by collagen. The contact group includes factor XI, factor XII, prekallikrein, and high-molecular-weight kininogen.
2. The prothrombin or vitamin K–dependent group includes factors II, VII, IX, and X.
3. The fibrinogen group includes factors I, V, VIII, and XIII. They are the most labile of the factors and are consumed during the coagulation process. The factors listed in the table are the ones most commonly measured.

For many years, our understanding of the process of coagulation has been explained by the traditional model (the *coagulation cascade*), comprised of the intrinsic and extrinsic pathways. While this model is still valid, a more modern and dynamic concept of the coagulation process is presented on page 354. The cellular-based model includes four overlapping phases in the formation of thrombin: initiation, amplification, propagation, and termination. It is now known that the TF pathway is the primary pathway for the initiation of blood coagulation. TF-bearing cells (e.g., endothelial cells, smooth muscle cells, monocytes) can be induced to express TF and are the primary initiators of the coagulation cascade either by contact activation or trauma. The contact activation pathway is more related to inflammation, and although it plays an important role in the body's reaction to damaged endothelial surfaces, a deficiency in factor XII does not result in development of a bleeding disorder, which demonstrates the minor role of the intrinsic pathway in the process of blood coagulation. Substances such as endotoxins, tumor necrosis factor alpha, and lipoproteins can also stimulate expression of TF. TF, in combination with factor VII and calcium, forms a complex that then activates factors IX and X in the initiation phase. Activated factor X in the presence of factor II (prothrombin) leads to the formation of thrombin. TFPI quickly inactivates this stage of the pathway so that limited or trace amounts of thrombin are produced, which results in the activation of factors VIII and V. Activated factor IX, assisted by activated factors V and VIII, initiate amplification and propagation of thrombin in the cascade.

Thrombin activates factor XIII and begins converting fibrinogen into fibrin monomers, which spontaneously polymerize and then become cross-linked into a stable clot by activated factor XIII.

Qualitative and quantitative factor deficiencies can affect the function of the coagulation pathways. Factor V and factor II (prothrombin) mutations are examples of qualitative deficiencies and are the most common inherited predisposing factors for blood clots. Hemophilia A is an inherited deficiency of factor VIII and occurs at a prevalence of about 1 in 5,000 to 10,000 male births. Hemophilia B is an inherited deficiency of factor IX and occurs at a prevalence of about 1 in about 20,000 to 34,000 male births. Genetic testing is available for inherited mutations associated with inherited coagulopathies. The tests are performed on samples of whole blood. Counseling and informed written consent are generally required for genetic testing.

Knowledge of genetics assists in identifying those who may benefit from additional education, risk assessment, and counseling. Genetics is the study and identification of genes, genetic mutations, and inheritance. For example, genetics provides some insight into the likelihood of inheriting a medical condition such as hemophilia. Some conditions are the result of mutations involving a single gene, whereas other conditions may involve multiple genes and/or multiple chromosomes. Hemophilia is an example of a recessive sex-linked genetic disorder passed from a mother to male children. The factor V Leiden mutation in the F5 gene is an inherited autosomal genetic disorder that results in thrombophilia and the development of blood clots. Severity of the disorder depends on whether a single F5 mutation is inherited from one parent or two mutations are inherited, one from each parent. The risk of forming abnormal blood clots is also increased in people who have multiple mutations in the F5 gene or mutations in a different gene that also codes for products involved in the coagulation process, including factor V Leiden. Genomic studies evaluate the interaction of groups of genes. The combined activity or combined expression of groups of genes allows assumptions or predictions to be made. As an example, genomic studies measure the levels of activity in multiple genes to predict how they and other factors influence the prolonged development of abnormal blood clots. Other factors that may contribute to the development of blood clots in people with the factor V Leiden mutation include obesity, tissue injury (e.g., from surgery or trauma), smoking, pregnancy, exposure to hormones (e.g., oral contraceptives or hormone replacement therapy), and advancing age. Further information regarding inheritance of genes can be found in the study titled "Genetic Testing."

The PT/INR measures the function of the tissue factor pathway of coagulation and is used to monitor patients receiving warfarin or coumarin-derivative anticoagulant therapy. The aPTT measures the function of the contact activation pathway of coagulation and is used to monitor patients receiving heparin anticoagulant therapy.

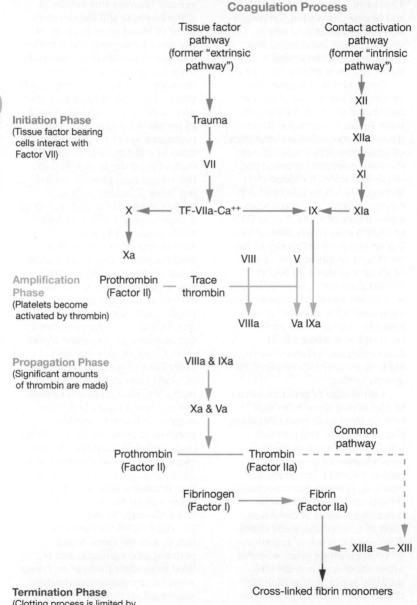

Coagulation Process

Tissue factor pathway (former "extrinsic pathway")

Contact activation pathway (former "intrinsic pathway")

Initiation Phase (Tissue factor bearing cells interact with Factor VII)

XII
↓
Trauma
↓
VII
↓
XIIa
↓
XI
↓
X ← TF-VIIa-Ca⁺⁺ → IX ← XIa
↓
Xa

Amplification Phase (Platelets become activated by thrombin)

VIII   V
Prothrombin (Factor II) — Trace thrombin
VIIIa   Va IXa

Propagation Phase (Significant amounts of thrombin are made)

VIIIa & IXa
↓
Xa & Va
↓

Common pathway

Prothrombin (Factor II) — Thrombin (Factor IIa) - - - ¬

Fibrinogen (Factor I) → Fibrin (Factor IIa)

XIIIa ← XIII

Termination Phase (Clotting process is limited by Antithrombin III, Protein C, Protein S, thrombomodulin, and TF pathway inhibitor in order to prevent occlusion of the vessel)

Cross-linked fibrin monomers

INDICATIONS
- Identify the presence of inherited bleeding disorders.
- Identify the presence of qualitative or quantitative factor deficiency.

INTERFERING FACTORS
Factors that may alter the results of the study
- Drugs and other substances that may decrease factor II levels include warfarin.
- Drugs and other substances that may increase factor V, VII, and X levels include anabolic steroids and oral contraceptives.
- Drugs and other substances that may decrease factor V levels include streptokinase.
- Drugs and other substances that may decrease factor VII levels include acetylsalicylic acid, asparaginase, cefamandole, ceftriaxone, dextran, dicumarol, gemfibrozil, oral contraceptives, and warfarin.
- Drugs and other substances that may increase factor VIII levels include chlormadinone.
- Drugs and other substances that may decrease factor VIII levels include asparaginase.
- Drugs and other substances that may increase factor IX levels include chlormadinone and oral contraceptives.
- Drugs and other substances that may decrease factor IX levels include asparaginase and warfarin.
- Drugs that may decrease factor X levels include chlormadinone, dicumarol, oral contraceptives, and warfarin.

- Drugs that may decrease factor XI levels include asparaginase and captopril.
- Drugs that may decrease factor XII levels include captopril.

Other considerations
- Test results of patients on anticoagulant therapy are unreliable.
- Placement of tourniquet for longer than 1 min can result in venous stasis and changes in the concentration of plasma proteins to be measured. Platelet activation may also occur under these conditions, causing erroneous results.
- Vascular injury during phlebotomy can activate platelets and coagulation factors, causing erroneous results.
- Hemolyzed specimens must be rejected because hemolysis is an indication of platelet and coagulation factor activation.
- Icteric or lipemic specimens interfere with optical testing methods, producing erroneous results.
- Incompletely filled collection tubes, specimens contaminated with heparin, clotted specimens, or unprocessed specimens not delivered to the laboratory within 1 to 2 hr of collection should be rejected.

POTENTIAL MEDICAL DIAGNOSIS: CLINICAL SIGNIFICANCE OF RESULTS
Increased in: N/A

Decreased in
- Congenital deficiency
- DIC *(related to consumption of factors as part of the coagulation cascade)*
- Liver disease *(related to inability of damaged liver to synthesize coagulation factors)*

C

NURSING IMPLICATIONS

POTENTIAL NURSING PROBLEMS: ASSESSMENT & NURSING DIAGNOSIS

Problems	Signs and Symptoms
Bleeding *(related to alerted clotting factors secondary to heparin use or depleted clotting factors)*	Altered level of consciousness, hypotension, increased heart rate, decreased hemoglobin/hematocrit (Hgb/Hct), capillary refill greater than 3 sec, cool extremities
Confusion *(related to an alteration in the oxygen-carrying capacity of the blood, blood loss, compromised clotting factor)*	Disorganized thinking; restlessness; irritability; altered concentration and attention span; changeable mental function over the day; hallucinations; inability to follow directions; disorientation to person, place, time, and purpose; inappropriate affect
Gas exchange *(related to deficient oxygen capacity of the blood)*	Irregular breathing pattern, use of accessory muscles, altered chest excursion, adventitious breath sounds (crackles, rhonchi, wheezes, diminished breath sounds), copious secretions, signs of hypoxia, altered blood gas results, confusion, lethargy, cyanosis
Tissue perfusion *(related to compromised clotting factor, blood loss, deficient oxygen-carrying capacity of the blood)*	Hypotension, dizziness, cool extremities, capillary refill greater than 3 sec, weak pedal pulses, altered level of consciousness

BEFORE THE STUDY: PLANNING AND IMPLEMENTATION

Teaching the Patient What to Expect

▶ Inform the patient this test can assist in evaluating the effectiveness of blood clotting and identify deficiencies in blood factor levels.
▶ Explain that a blood sample is needed for the test.

AFTER THE STUDY: POTENTIAL NURSING ACTIONS

Avoiding Complications

▶ Inform the patient with abnormal clotting of the importance of taking precautions against bruising and bleeding. These precautions may include the use of a soft bristle toothbrush, use of an electric razor, avoidance of constipation, avoidance of acetylsali-cylic acid and similar products, and avoidance of intramuscular injections.

Treatment Considerations

▶ Bleeding: Increase frequency of vital sign assessment with variances in results and monitor for trends. Administer ordered blood or blood products and stool softeners. Monitor stool, emesis, and sputum for blood. Trend Hgb/Hct, and assess skin for petechiae, purpura, or hematoma. Institute bleeding precautions; prevent unnecessary venipuncture, avoid intramuscular injections, prevent trauma, be gentle with oral care and suctioning, and avoid use of a sharp razor. Administer prescribed medications: recombinant human activated protein C or epsilon aminocaproic acid.

● Confusion: Treat the medical condition. Correlate confusion with the need to reverse altered electrolytes. Evaluate medications and consider pharmacological interventions. Prevent falls and injury through appropriate use of postural support, bed alarm, or restraints. Accurate intake and output to assess fluid status, administer ordered blood or blood products, and monitor and trend Hgb/Hct.

● Gas Exchange: Monitor respiratory rate and effort based on assessment of patient condition and frequently assess lung sounds. Evaluate for secretions or bloody sputum with gentle suction as necessary. Use pulse oximetry to monitor oxygen saturation with administered oxygen. Elevate the head of the bed 30 degrees or higher to ease breathing. Monitor IV fluids and avoid aggressive fluid resuscitation. Assess level of consciousness and anticipate the need for possible intubation.

● Tissue Perfusion: Monitor blood pressure, level of consciousness, and dizziness. Check skin temperature for warmth and assess capillary refill and pedal pulses. Administer ordered vasodilators and inotropic drugs, and oxygen.

Safety Considerations
● Inform the patient with decreased factor levels of the importance of taking precautions against bruising and bleeding.
● Explain the importance of monitoring stool, sputum, and urine for blood and reporting any occurrences to the HCP.

Nutritional Considerations
● Vitamin K is a fat-soluble vitamin that plays an important role in blood clotting. The patient with bleeding tendencies may be encouraged to increase intake of foods rich in vitamin K.

Follow-Up, Evaluation, and Desired Outcomes
● Recognizes the importance of immediately reporting any signs of unusual bleeding or bruising.
● Successfully states bleeding precautions that include the use of a soft bristle toothbrush, use of an electric razor, avoidance of constipation, avoidance of acetylsalicylic acid and similar products, and avoidance of intramuscular injections.

Cold Agglutinin Titer

SYNONYM/ACRONYM: Mycoplasma serology.

RATIONALE: To identify and confirm the presence of viral infections such as found in atypical pneumonia.

PATIENT PREPARATION: There are no food, fluid, activity, or medication restrictions unless by medical direction.

NORMAL FINDINGS: (Method: Patient serum containing autoantibodies titered against type O red blood cells [RBCs] at 2°C to 8°C. Type O cells are used because they have no antigens on the cell membrane surface. Agglutination with patient sera would not occur because of reaction between RBC blood type antigens and patient blood type antibodies.) Negative: Single titer less than 1:32 or less than a fourfold increase in titer over serial samples. High titers may appear spontaneously in older adult patients and persist for many years.

CRITICAL FINDINGS AND POTENTIAL INTERVENTIONS: N/A

OVERVIEW: (Study type: Blood collected in a red-top tube; related body system: Immune and Respiratory systems.) Cold agglutinins are antibodies that cause clumping or agglutination of RBCs at cold temperatures in individuals with certain conditions or who are infected by particular organisms. Cold agglutinins are associated with *Mycoplasma pneumoniae* infection. *M. pneumoniae* has i antigen specificity to human RBC membranes. Fetal cells largely contain i antigens, but by 18 mo most cells carry the I antigen. The agglutinins are usually immunoglobulin M (IgM) antibodies and cause agglutination of cells at temperatures in the range of 0°C to 10°C. The temperature of circulating blood in the extremities may be lower than core temperatures. RBCs of affected individuals may agglutinate and obstruct blood vessels in fingers, toes, and ears, or they may initiate the complement cascade. Affected cells may be lysed immediately within the capillaries and blood vessels as a result of the action of complement on the cell wall, or they may return to the circulatory system and be lysed in the spleen by macrophages.

The titer endpoint is the highest dilution of serum that shows a specific antigen-antibody reaction. Single titers greater than 1:64, or a fourfold increase in titer between specimens collected 5 or more days apart, are clinically significant. Patients affected with primary atypical viral pneumonia exhibit a rise in titer 8 to 10 days after the onset of illness. IgM antibodies peak in 12 to 25 days and begin to diminish 30 days after onset. Mycoplasma pneumonia is a self-limiting condition, routinely treated with antibiotics.

INDICATIONS
- Assist in the confirmation of primary atypical pneumonia, influenza, or pulmonary embolus.
- Provide additional diagnostic support for cold agglutinin disease associated with viral infections or lymphoreticular cancers.

INTERFERING FACTORS
Factors that may alter the results of the study
- Antibiotic use may interfere with or decrease antibody production.
- Prompt and proper specimen processing, storage, and analysis are important to achieve accurate results. Specimens should always be transported to the laboratory as quickly as possible after collection. The specimen must clot in a 37°C water bath for 1 hr before separation. Refrigeration of the sample before serum separates from the RBCs may falsely decrease the titer.

Other considerations
- A high antibody titer may interfere with blood typing and crossmatching procedures.
- High titers may appear spontaneously in older adult patients and persist for many years.

POTENTIAL MEDICAL DIAGNOSIS: CLINICAL SIGNIFICANCE OF RESULTS
Increased in
Mycoplasma infection stimulates production of antibodies against specific RBC antigens in affected individuals.

- Cirrhosis
- Gangrene
- Hemolytic anemia
- Infectious diseases (e.g., staphylococcemia, influenza, tuberculosis)
- Infectious mononucleosis
- Malaria

- *M. pneumoniae* (primary atypical pneumonia)
- Multiple myeloma
- Pulmonary embolism
- Raynaud disease (severe)
- Systemic lupus erythematosus
- Trypanosomiasis

Decreased in: N/A

NURSING IMPLICATIONS

BEFORE THE STUDY: PLANNING AND IMPLEMENTATION

Teaching the Patient What to Expect

▶ Inform the patient this test can assist in diagnosing primary atypical pneumonia

versus other infectious diseases or immune-related conditions. Explain that the test detects antibodies developed during an infection that attack RBCs when the patient's body is exposed to cold temperatures.
▶ Explain that a blood sample is needed for the test.

Potential Nursing Actions
▶ Note any recent medications that can interfere with test results.

AFTER THE STUDY: POTENTIAL NURSING ACTIONS

Follow-Up, Evaluation, and Desired Outcomes
▶ Acknowledges the importance of completing the entire course of antibiotic therapy even if no symptoms are present.

Colonoscopy

SYNONYM/ACRONYM: Full colonoscopy, lower endoscopy, lower panendoscopy.

RATIONALE: To visualize and assess the lower colon for tumor, cancer, and infection.

PATIENT PREPARATION: Inform the patient that a laxative and cleansing enema may be needed the day before the procedure, with cleansing enemas on the morning of the procedure, depending on the institution's policy. Instruct the patient that to reduce the risk of aspiration related to nausea and vomiting, solid food and milk or milk products are restricted for at least 6 hr, and clear liquids are restricted for at least 2 hr prior to general anesthesia, regional anesthesia, or sedation/analgesia (monitored anesthesia). The patient may be asked to be NPO after midnight. The American Society of Anesthesiologists has fasting guidelines for risk levels according to patient status. More information can be located at www.asahq.org.

Patients on beta blockers before the surgical procedure should be instructed to take their medication as ordered during the perioperative period.

Regarding the patient's risk for bleeding, the patient should be instructed to avoid taking natural products and medications with known anticoagulant, antiplatelet, or thrombolytic properties or to reduce dosage, as ordered, prior to the procedure. Number of days to withhold medication is dependent on the type of anticoagulant. Note the last time and dose of medication taken.

Patients on beta blockers before the surgical procedure should be instructed to take their medication as ordered during the perioperative period. Protocols may vary among facilities.

Ensure that this procedure is performed before an upper gastrointestinal (GI) study or barium swallow to avoid interference from retained barium. If a computed tomography (CT) scan is requested, ensure that barium studies were performed more than 4 days before the CT scan.

NORMAL FINDINGS
- Normal intestinal mucosa with no abnormalities of structure, function, or mucosal surface in the colon or terminal ileum.

CRITICAL FINDINGS AND POTENTIAL INTERVENTIONS: N/A

OVERVIEW: (**Study type:** Endoscopy; **related body system:** Digestive system.) Colonoscopy, a radiological examination of the colon, follows instillation of barium (single contrast study) using a rectal tube inserted into the rectum. The patient retains the contrast while a series of images are obtained, recorded, and available for viewing. Visualization can be improved by draining the barium and using air contrast (double contrast study); some of the barium remains on the surface of the colon wall, allowing for greater detail in the images. A combination of x-ray and fluoroscopic techniques are used to allow inspection of the mucosa of the entire colon, ileocecal valve, and terminal ileum using a flexible fiberoptic colonoscope inserted through the anus and advanced to the terminal ileum. The colonoscope, a multichannel instrument, allows viewing of the GI tract lining, insufflation of air, aspiration of fluid, collection of tissue biopsy samples, and passage of a laser beam for obliteration of tissue and control of bleeding. Mucosal surfaces of the lower GI tract are examined for ulcerations, polyps, chronic diarrhea, hemorrhagic sites, tumors, and strictures. During the procedure, tissue samples may be obtained for cytology, and some therapeutic procedures may be performed, such as excision of small tumors or polyps, coagulation of bleeding sites, and removal of foreign bodies. CT colonoscopy may be indicated for patients who have diseases rendering them unable to undergo conventional colonoscopy (e.g., bleeding disorders, lung or heart disease) and for patients who are unable to undergo the sedation required for traditional colonoscopy.

INDICATIONS
- Assess GI function in a patient with a personal or family history of colon cancer, polyps, or ulcerative colitis.
- Confirm diagnosis of colon cancer and inflammatory bowel disease.
- Detect Hirschsprung disease and determine the areas affected by the disease.
- Determine cause of lower GI disorders, especially when barium enema and proctosigmoidoscopy are inconclusive.
- Determine source of rectal bleeding and perform hemostasis by coagulation.
- Evaluate postsurgical status of colon resection.
- Evaluate stools that show a positive occult blood test, lower GI bleeding, or change in bowel habits.

- Follow up on previously diagnosed and treated colon cancer.
- Investigate iron-deficiency anemia of unknown origin.
- Reduce volvulus and intussusception in children.
- Remove colon polyps.
- Remove foreign bodies and sclerosing strictures by laser.

INTERFERING FACTORS

Contraindications

Patients with bleeding disorders or cardiac conditions.

Patients with bowel perforation, acute peritonitis, acute colitis, ischemic bowel necrosis, toxic colitis, recent bowel surgery, advanced pregnancy, severe cardiac or pulmonary disease, recent myocardial infarction, known or suspected pulmonary embolus, and large abdominal aortic or iliac aneurysm.

Patients who have had a colon anastomosis within the past 14 to 21 days, *because an anastomosis may break down with gas insufflation.*

Factors that may alter the results of the study

- Gas or feces in the GI tract resulting from inadequate cleansing or failure to restrict food intake before the study.
- Retained barium from a previous radiological procedure.
- Severe lower GI bleeding or the presence of feces, barium, blood, or blood clots, which can interfere with visualization.
- Spasm of the colon, which can mimic the radiographic signs of cancer. (*Note:* The use of IV glucagon minimizes spasm.)
- Inability of the patient to tolerate introduction of or retention of barium, air, or both in the bowel.
- Metallic objects (e.g., jewelry, body rings) within the examination field, which may inhibit organ visualization and cause unclear images.

Other considerations

- Bowel preparations that include laxatives or enemas should be avoided in pregnant patients or patients with inflammatory bowel disease unless specifically directed by a health-care provider (HCP).

POTENTIAL MEDICAL DIAGNOSIS: CLINICAL SIGNIFICANCE OF RESULTS

Abnormal findings related to

- Benign lesions
- Bleeding sites
- Bowel distention
- Bowel infection or inflammation
- Colitis
- Colon cancer
- Crohn disease
- Diverticula
- Foreign bodies
- Hemorrhoids
- Polyps
- Proctitis
- Tumors
- Vascular abnormalities

NURSING IMPLICATIONS

BEFORE THE STUDY: PLANNING AND IMPLEMENTATION

Teaching the Patient What to Expect

- Inform the patient this procedure can assist in assessing the colon for disease.
- Explain that prior to the procedure, laboratory testing may be required to determine the possibility of bleeding risk (coagulation testing) or to assess for impaired kidney function (creatinine level and estimated glomerular filtration rate) if use of iodinated contrast medium is anticipated.
- Review the procedure with the patient. Address concerns about pain and explain that there may be moments of discomfort or pain experienced when the IV line or catheter is inserted to allow infusion of fluids such as saline, anesthetics, sedatives, medications

used in the procedure, or emergency medications; explain that there may be moments of discomfort during the procedure.

▶ Inform the patient that the procedure is performed in a GI laboratory, by an HCP, with support staff, and takes approximately 30 to 60 min.

▶ Baseline vital signs will be recorded and monitored throughout the procedure. Protocols may vary among facilities.

▶ Medications will be administered, as ordered, to reduce discomfort and to promote relaxation and sedation. Positioning for the study is on an examination table in the left lateral decubitus position, draped with the buttocks exposed. Explain that the HCP will initially perform a visual inspection of the perianal area and a digital rectal examination. Tell the patient he or she will be asked to bear down as if having a bowel movement as the fiberoptic tube or colonoscope (scope) is inserted through the rectum.

▶ Explain that the scope is advanced through the sigmoid and the patient's position is changed to supine to facilitate passage into the transverse colon. Advise the patient that he or she will be asked to take deep breaths to aid in movement of the scope downward through the ascending colon to the cecum and into the terminal portion of the ileum. Air is insufflated through the tube during passage to distend the GI tract, as needed, which aids in visualization. Biopsies, cultures, or any endoscopic surgery is performed. Foreign bodies or polyps are removed and placed in appropriate specimen containers, labelled, and sent to the laboratory. Images are obtained for future reference. At the end of the procedure, excess air and secretions are aspirated through the scope, and the colonoscope is removed.

Potential Nursing Actions

✳ *Make sure a written and informed consent has been signed prior to the procedure and before administering any medications.*

▶ Note intake of oral iron preparations within 1 wk before the procedure

because these cause black, sticky feces that are difficult to remove with bowel preparation.

Safety Considerations

▶ Anticoagulants, aspirin, and other salicylates should be discontinued by medical direction for the appropriate number of days prior to a procedure where bleeding is a potential complication.

AFTER THE STUDY: POTENTIAL NURSING ACTIONS

Avoiding Complications

▶ Complications of the procedure may include bleeding and cardiac dysrhythmias. Instruct the patient to immediately report symptoms such as fast heart rate, difficulty breathing, skin rash, itching, chest pain, or abdominal pain.

Treatment Considerations

▶ After the procedure, monitor vital signs and neurological status every 15 min for 1 hr, then every 2 hr for 4 hr, or as ordered. Monitor the patient for signs of respiratory depression. Take temperature every 4 hr for 24 hr. Monitor intake and output at least every 8 hr. Compare with baseline values. Notify the HCP if temperature is elevated. Protocols may vary among facilities.

▶ Observe the patient until the effects of the sedation have worn off. Carefully monitor the patient for fatigue and fluid and electrolyte imbalance. Instruct the patient to resume usual diet, fluids, medications, and activity, as directed by the HCP.

▶ Monitor for any rectal bleeding. Instruct the patient to expect slight rectal bleeding for 2 days after removal of polyps or biopsy specimens but that an increasing amount of bleeding or sustained bleeding should be reported to the HCP immediately.

▶ Advise the patient that belching, bloating, or flatulence is the result of air insufflation.

▶ Encourage the patient to drink several glasses of water to help replace fluids lost during the preparation for the test.

Follow-Up, Evaluation, and Desired Outcomes

▶ Recognizes cancer screening options and understands that decisions regarding the need for and frequency of occult blood testing, colonoscopy, or other cancer screening procedures may be made after consultation between the patient and HCP. The American Cancer Society (ACS) screening recommendations regarding regular screening for colon cancer begins at age 50 yr for individuals with average risk and sooner for those with increased or high risk for developing colon cancer. Its recommendations for frequency of screening are to use one of the following:

Tests That Can Identify Polyps and Cancer

▶ Colonoscopy every 10 yr
▶ CT colonography (virtual colonoscopy) every 5 yr

▶ Flexible sigmoidoscopy every 5 yr
▶ Double contrast barium enema every 5 yr

Tests That Primarily Identify Cancer

▶ Fecal immunochemical test (FIT) annually
▶ Fecal occult blood test (guaiac based) annually
▶ Stool DNA test every 3 yr
▶ Colonoscopy should be used to follow up abnormal findings obtained by any of the other screening tests. The most current guidelines for colon cancer screening of the general population as well as of individuals with increased risk are available from the ACS (www.cancer.org), U.S. Preventive Services Task Force (www.uspreventiveservicestaskforce .org), and American College of Gastroenterology (www.gi.org).

Color Perception Test

SYNONYM/ACRONYM: Color blindness test, Ishihara color perception test, Ishihara pseudoisochromatic plate test.

RATIONALE: To assist in the diagnosis of color blindness.

PATIENT PREPARATION: There are no food, fluid, activity, or medication restrictions unless by medical direction.

NORMAL FINDINGS

• Normal visual color discrimination; no difficulty in identification of color combinations.

CRITICAL FINDINGS AND POTENTIAL INTERVENTIONS: N/A

OVERVIEW: (Study type: Sensory (ocular); related body system: Nervous system.) Defects in color perception can be hereditary or acquired. Color blindness occurs in 8% of males and 0.4% of females. It may be partial or complete. The partial form is the hereditary form, and in the majority of patients, the color deficiency is in the red-green area of the spectrum. Knowledge of genetics assists in identifying those who may benefit from additional education, risk assessment, and counseling. Genetics is the study and identification of genes, genetic mutations, and inheritance. For example, genetics provides some insight into the likelihood of inheriting a condition such as color blindness. Some conditions are the result of mutations involving a single gene, whereas other conditions may involve multiple genes and/or multiple chromosomes. Color blindness is an example of a recessive sex-linked genetic disorder passed from a mother to male children. Further information regarding inheritance of genes can be found in the study titled "Genetic Testing."

Acquired color blindness may occur as a result of diseases of the retina or optic nerve. Color perception tests are performed to determine the acuity of color discrimination. The most common test uses pseudoisochromatic plates with numbers or letters buried in a maze of dots. Misreading the numbers or letters indicates a color perception deficiency and may indicate color blindness, a genetic dysfunction, or retinal pathology.

Color perception is important in some occupations, and testing for color perception may be a requirement for employment, especially for health-care workers whose responsibilities include assessment and monitoring of symptoms or changes in patients' conditions. Some common examples of color -based assessments in a health-care environment include interpreting the results of color pads on blood or urine test strips, identifying changes in body color (e.g., pallor, cyanosis, jaundice), determining the presence of blood or bile in body fluids and feces, and evaluating pH test strips to verify correct placement of a nasopharyngeal tube.

INDICATIONS
- Detect deficiencies in color perception.
- Evaluate because of family history of color visual defects.
- Investigate suspected retinal pathology affecting the cones.

INTERFERING FACTORS
- Inability of the patient to cooperate or remain still during the procedure because of age, significant pain, or mental status.
- Inability of the patient to read.
- Poor visual acuity or poor lighting.
- Failure of the patient to wear corrective lenses (glasses or contact lenses).
- Damaged or discolored test plates.

POTENTIAL MEDICAL DIAGNOSIS: CLINICAL SIGNIFICANCE OF RESULTS
Abnormal findings related to
- Identification of some but not all colors

NURSING IMPLICATIONS

BEFORE THE STUDY: PLANNING AND IMPLEMENTATION

Teaching the Patient What to Expect
- Inform the patient or parent/child this procedure can assist in detection of color vision impairment.
- Review the procedure with the patient. Address concerns about pain and explain that no discomfort will be experienced during the test.
- Inform the patient that a health-care provider (HCP) performs the test in a quiet, darkened room, and that to evaluate both eyes, the test can take 5 to 15 or up to 30 min, depending on the complexity of testing required.

▶ Explain that once the patient is seated comfortably, one eye is occluded while a test booklet is held 12 to 14 in. in front of the exposed eye. Next the patient is asked to identify the numbers or letters buried in the maze of dots or to trace the objects with a handheld pointed object. The test is repeated on the other eye.

Potential Nursing Actions

▶ Ask the patient if he or she wears corrective lenses; also inquire about the importance of color discrimination in his or her work, as applicable.

AFTER THE STUDY: POTENTIAL NURSING ACTIONS

Treatment Considerations
▶ Provide emotional support to those who fail the color perception test.

Follow-Up, Evaluation, and Desired Outcomes
▶ Acknowledges contact information regarding impaired color perception provided for the American Academy of Ophthalmology (www.aao.org/eye-health/diseases/what-is-color-blindness).

C

Colposcopy

SYNONYM/ACRONYM: Cervical biopsy, endometrial biopsy.

RATIONALE: To visualize and assess the cervix and vagina related to suspected cancer or other disease.

PATIENT PREPARATION: There are no food, fluid, activity, or medication restrictions unless by medical direction.

NORMAL FINDINGS
• Normal appearance of the vagina and cervix
• No abnormal cells or tissues.

CRITICAL FINDINGS AND POTENTIAL INTERVENTIONS: N/A

OVERVIEW: (**Study type:** Endoscopy; **related body system:** Reproductive system.) In this procedure, the vagina and cervix are viewed using a colposcope, a special binocular microscope and light system that magnifies the mucosal surfaces. Colposcopy is usually performed after suspicious Papanicolaou (Pap) test results or when suspected lesions cannot be visualized fully by the naked eye. The procedure is useful for identifying areas of cellular dysplasia and diagnosing cervical cancer because it provides the best view of the suspicious lesion, ensuring that the most representative area of the lesion is obtained for cytological analysis to confirm malignant changes. Colposcopy is also valuable for assessing women with a history of exposure to diethylstilbestrol (DES) in utero. The goal is to identify precursor changes in cervical tissue before the changes advance from benign or atypical cells to cervical cancer. Photographs (cervicography) can also be taken of the cervix.

C

INDICATIONS

- Evaluate the cervix after abnormal Pap smear.
- Evaluate vaginal lesions.
- Localize the area from which cervical biopsy samples should be obtained because such areas may not be visible to the naked eye.
- Monitor conservatively treated cervical intraepithelial neoplasia.
- Monitor women whose mothers took DES during pregnancy.

INTERFERING FACTORS

Contraindications

⁎ Patients with bleeding disorders or receiving anticoagulant therapy, especially if cervical biopsy specimens are to be obtained, *because the biopsy site may not stop bleeding.*

⁎ Women who are currently menstruating, *as bleeding may obscure abnormal findings.*

Factors that may alter the results of the study

- Inadequate cleansing of the cervix of secretions and medications.
- Scarring of the cervix.
- Severe bleeding or the presence of feces, blood, or blood clots, which can interfere with visualization.

POTENTIAL MEDICAL DIAGNOSIS: CLINICAL SIGNIFICANCE OF RESULTS

Abnormal findings related to

- Atrophic changes
- Cervical erosion
- Cervical intraepithelial neoplasia
- Infection
- Inflammation
- Invasive cancers
- Leukoplakia
- Papilloma, including condyloma

NURSING IMPLICATIONS

BEFORE THE STUDY: PLANNING AND IMPLEMENTATION

Teaching the Patient What to Expect

- Inform the patient this procedure can assist in assessing the cervix for disease.
- Review the procedure with the patient. Address concerns about pain and explain that there may be moments of discomfort or pain experienced when the IV line or catheter is inserted to allow infusion of fluids such as saline, anesthetics, sedatives, contrast medium, medications used in the procedure, or emergency medications. Medications to reduce discomfort and to promote relaxation and sedation will be administered.
- Advise the patient that if a biopsy is performed, she may feel menstrual-like cramping during the procedure and experience a minimal amount of bleeding.
- Inform the patient that the procedure is performed by a health-care provider (HCP), with support staff, and takes approximately 30 to 60 min
- Baseline vital signs will be recorded and monitored throughout the procedure. Protocols may vary among facilities.
- Explain positioning for the study is on an examination table draped in the lithotomy position, and the external genitalia is cleansed with an antiseptic solution.
- When a Pap smear is performed, the cervix is swabbed and a speculum is inserted into the vagina using water as a lubricant. A lighted magnification scope is used to carefully examine the cervix. Photographs can be taken for future reference.
- Afterwards, the vagina is rinsed with sterile saline or water to remove the acetic acid and prevent burning after the procedure. If bleeding persists, a tampon may be inserted after removal of the speculum.

▶ Biopsy samples are placed in appropriately labelled containers with special preservative solution and promptly transported to the laboratory.

Potential Nursing Actions

◈ *Make sure a written and informed consent has been signed prior to the procedure and before administering any medications.*

AFTER THE STUDY: POTENTIAL NURSING ACTIONS

Avoiding Complications

▶ Complications of the procedure may include bleeding, infection, and cardiac dysrhythmias. Monitor for any bleeding. Bleeding may occur after undergoing biopsy and may be controlled by cautery, suturing, or application of silver nitrate or ferric subsulfate (Monsel solution) to the site.

Treatment Considerations

▶ Perform postprocedure vital signs as ordered, and indicated. Compare with baseline values. Protocols may vary among facilities.

Follow-Up, Evaluation, and Desired Outcomes

▶ Understands to remove the vaginal tampon, if inserted, within 8 to 24 hr and afterwards to wear pads if there is bleeding or drainage.
▶ Acknowledges that there may be slight bleeding and/or a discharge for a few days after removal of biopsy specimens but that persistent vaginal bleeding or abnormal vaginal discharge, an increasing amount of bleeding, abdominal pain, and fever must be reported to the HCP immediately.
▶ Agrees to avoid strenuous exercise 8 to 24 hr after the procedure and to avoid douching and intercourse for about 2 wk or as directed by the HCP.

Complement, Total, C3, and C4

SYNONYM/ACRONYM: Total hemolytic complement, CH_{50}, CH_{100}.

RATIONALE: To detect inborn complement deficiency, evaluate immune diseases related to complement activity, and follow up on a patient's response to therapy such as treatment for rheumatoid arthritis and systemic lupus erythematosus (SLE), in which complement is consumed at an increased rate.

PATIENT PREPARATION: There are no food, fluid, activity, or medication restrictions unless by medical direction.

NORMAL FINDINGS: Method: Quantitative hemolysis for total complement; immunoturbidimetric for C3 and C4.

CH_{50}

100–300 CH_{50} units/mL

C3

Age	Conventional Units	SI Units (Conventional Units × 0.01)
Newborn	57–116 mg/dL	0.57–1.16 g/L
6 mo–adult	74–166 mg/dL	0.74–1.66 g/L
Adult	83–177 mg/dL	0.83–1.77 g/L

C4

Age	Conventional Units	SI Units (Conventional Units × 0.01)
Newborn	10–31 mg/dL	0.1–0.31 g/L
6 mo–6 yr	15–52 mg/dL	0.15–0.52 g/L
7–12 yr	19–40 mg/dL	0.19–0.4 g/L
13–15 yr	19–57 mg/dL	0.19–0.57 g/L
16–18 yr	19–42 mg/dL	0.19–0.42 g/L
Adult	12–36 mg/dL	0.12–0.36 g/L

CRITICAL FINDINGS AND POTENTIAL INTERVENTIONS: N/A

OVERVIEW: (**Study type:** Blood collected in a red-top tube; **related body system:** Immune system.)

Complement is a system of 25 to 30 distinct cell membrane and plasma proteins, numbered C1 through C9. It is an important part of the body's natural defense against allergic and immune reactions. It is activated by plasmin and is interrelated with the coagulation and fibrinolytic systems. Once activated, the proteins interact with each other in a specific sequence called the *complement cascade*. The classical pathway is triggered by antigen-antibody complexes and includes participation of all complement proteins C1 through C9. The alternate pathway occurs when C3, C5, and C9 are activated without participation of C1, C2, and C4 or the presence of antigen-antibody complexes. Activation of the complement system results in cell lysis, release of histamine, chemotaxis of white blood cells, increased vascular permeability, and contraction of smooth muscle. The activation of this system can sometimes occur with uncontrolled self-destructive effects on the body. Other methods for measuring total complement levels have

been developed. They are easier to perform and have demonstrated equal sensitivity to the classical hemolytic method of measuring total complement. The newer methods include the enzyme immunoassay (normal range = 60–140 complement activity enzyme [CAE] units) and liposome immunoassay (normal range = 23–60 units/mL).

Serum complement levels are also used to detect autoimmune diseases. In the total complement assay, a patient's serum is mixed with sheep red blood cells (RBCs) coated with antibodies. If complement is present in sufficient quantities, 50% of the RBCs are lysed. Lower amounts of lysed cells are associated with decreased complement levels. C3 and C4 are the most frequently assayed complement proteins, along with total complement. Circulating C3 is synthesized in the liver and comprises 70% of the complement system, but cells in other tissues can also produce C3. C3 is an essential activating protein in the classic and alternate complement cascades. It is decreased in patients with immunological diseases, in whom it is consumed at an increased rate. C4 is produced primarily in the liver but can also be produced by monocytes, fibroblasts, and macrophages. C4 participates in the classic complement pathway.

INDICATIONS
- Assist in the diagnosis of hereditary angioedema.
- Detect genetic deficiencies.
- Evaluate complement activity in autoimmune disorders.
- Evaluate and monitor therapy for immunological diseases such as SLE.
- Screen for complement deficiency.

INTERFERING FACTORS
Factors that may alter the results of the study
- Drugs that may increase total complement levels include cyclophosphamide and oral contraceptives.
- Drugs and other substances that may increase C3 levels include cimetidine and cyclophosphamide.
- Drugs and other substances that may decrease C3 levels include danazol, methyldopa, and phenytoin.
- Drugs and other substances that may increase C4 levels include cimetidine, cyclophosphamide, and danazol.
- Drugs and other substances that may decrease C4 levels include dextran and penicillamine.

Other considerations
- Specimen should not remain at room temperature longer than 1 hr.

POTENTIAL MEDICAL DIAGNOSIS: CLINICAL SIGNIFICANCE OF RESULTS

Normal C4 and decreased C3	Acute glomerulonephritis, membranous glomerulonephritis, immune complex diseases, SLE, C3 deficiency
Decreased C4 and normal C3	Immune complex diseases, cryoglobulinemia, C4 deficiency, hereditary angioedema
Decreased C4 and decreased C3	Immune complex diseases

Increased in
Total Complement, C3 and C4
- Acute-phase immune response *(related to sudden response to increased demand)*

C3
Amyloidosis
Cancer
Diabetes
Myocardial infarction
Pneumococcal pneumonia
Pregnancy
Rheumatic disease
Thyroiditis
Viral hepatitis

C4
Certain malignancies

Decreased in
Total Complement
- **Autoimmune diseases** *(related to continuous demand)*
- **Autoimmune hemolytic anemia** *(related to consumption during hemolytic process)*
- **Burns** *(related to increased consumption from initiation of complement cascade)*
- **Cryoglobulinemia** *(related to increased consumption)*
- **Hereditary deficiency** *(related to insufficient production)*
- **Infections** *(bacterial, parasitic, viral; related to increased consumption during immune response)*

- **Liver disease** *(related to decreased production by damaged liver cells)*
- **Malignancy** *(related to consumption during cellular immune response)*
- **Membranous glomerulonephritis** *(related to consumption during cellular immune response)*
- **Rheumatoid arthritis** *(related to consumption during immune response)*
- **SLE** *(related to consumption during immune response)*
- **Trauma** *(related to consumption during immune response)*
- **Vasculitis** *(related to consumption during cellular immune response)*

Total Complement, C3 and C4
Related to Overconsumption During Immune Response
Hereditary deficiency *(insufficient production)*
Liver disease *(insufficient production related to damaged liver cells)*
SLE

C3
Chronic infection (bacterial, parasitic, viral)
Post-membranoproliferative glomerulonephritis
Poststreptococcal infection
Rheumatic arthritis

C4
Angioedema *(hereditary and acquired)*
Autoimmune hemolytic anemia
Autoimmune thyroiditis
Cryoglobulinemia
Glomerulonephritis
Juvenile dermatomyositis
Meningitis (bacterial, viral)
Pneumonia
Streptococcal or staphylococcal sepsis

NURSING IMPLICATIONS

BEFORE THE STUDY: PLANNING AND IMPLEMENTATION

Teaching the Patient What to Expect
- Inform the patient this test can assist in diagnosing diseases of the immune system and evaluating response to treatment for infection or disease.
- Explain that a blood sample is needed for the test.

AFTER THE STUDY: POTENTIAL NURSING ACTIONS

Treatment Considerations
- Review test results in relation to the patient's symptoms and other tests performed and potential changes in the plan of care.

Complete Blood Count

SYNONYM/ACRONYM: CBC.

RATIONALE: To evaluate numerous conditions involving red blood cells (RBCs), white blood cells (WBCs), and platelets. This test is also used to indicate inflammation, infection, and response to chemotherapy.

PATIENT PREPARATION: There are no food, fluid, activity, or medication restrictions unless by medical direction.

NORMAL FINDINGS: (Method: Automated, computerized, multichannel analyzers. Many of these analyzers are capable of determining a five- or six-part WBC differential.) This battery of tests includes hemoglobin, hematocrit, RBC count, RBC morphology, RBC indices, RBC distribution width index (RDWCV and RDWSD), platelet count, platelet size, immature platelet fraction (IPF), WBC count, and WBC differential. The six-part automated WBC differential identifies and enumerates neutrophils, lymphocytes, monocytes, eosinophils, basophils, and immature granulocytes (IG), where IG represents the combined enumeration of promyelocytes, metamyelocytes, and myelocytes as both an absolute number and a percentage. The five-part WBC differential includes all but the IG parameters.

Hemoglobin

Age	Conventional Units	SI Units (Conventional Units × 10)
Cord blood	13.5–20.7 g/dL	135–207 g/L
0–1 wk	15.2–23.6 g/dL	152–236 g/L
2–3 wk	13.3–18.7 g/dL	133–187 g/L
1–2 mo	10.7–18 g/dL	107–180 g/L
3–6 mo	11.7–16.3 g/dL	117–163 g/L
7 mo–15 yr	10.3–14.3 g/dL	103–143 g/L
16–18 yr	11–15 g/dL	110–150 g/L
Adult		
Male	14–17.3 g/dL	140–173 g/L
Female	11.7–15.5 g/dL	117–155 g/L
Pregnant Female		
First trimester	11.6–13.9 g/dL	116–139 g/L
Second and third trimesters	9.5–11 g/dL	95–110 g/L

Values are slightly lower in older adults.
Reference range values may vary among laboratories.
Note: See "Hemoglobin and Hematocrit" study for more detailed information.

Hematocrit

Age	Conventional Units (%)	SI Units (Conventional Units × 0.01) (Volume Fraction)
Cord blood	42–62	0.42–0.62
0–1 wk	46–68	0.46–0.68
2–3 wk	41–56	0.41–0.56
1–2 mo	39–59	0.39–0.59
3–6 mo	35–49	0.35–0.49
7 mo–15 yr	31–43	0.31–0.43
16–18 yr	33–45	0.33–0.45
Adult		
Male	42–52	0.42–0.52
Female	36–48	0.36–0.48
Pregnant Female		
First trimester	35–42	0.35–0.42
Second and third trimesters	28–33	0.28–0.33

Values are slightly lower in older adults.
Reference range values may vary among laboratories.
Note: See "Hemoglobin and Hematocrit" study for more detailed information.

WBC Count and Differential

Age	Conventional Units WBC × 10⁹/microL	Neutrophils (Absolute) and %	Lymphocytes (Absolute) and %	Monocytes (Absolute) and %	Eosinophils (Absolute) and %	Basophils (Absolute) and %
Birth	9.1–30.1	(5.5–18.3) 24%–58%	(2.8–9.3) 26%–56%	(0.5–1.7) 7%–13%	(0.02–0.7) 0%–8%	(0.1–0.2) 0%–2.5%
1–23 mo	6.1–17.5	(1.9–5.4) 21%–67%	(3.7–10.7) 20%–64%	(0.3–0.8) 4%–11%	(0.2–0.5) 0%–3.3%	(0–0.1) 0%–1%
2–10 yr	4.5–13.5	(2.4–7.3) 30%–77%	(1.7–5.1) 14%–50%	(0.2–0.6) 4%–9%	(0.1–0.3) 0%–5.8%	(0–0.1) 0%–1%
11 yr–older adult	4.5–11.1	(2.7–6.5) 40%–75%	(1.5–3.7) 12%–44%	(0.2–0.4) 4%–9%	(0.05–0.5) 0%–5.5%	(0–0.1) 0%–1%

Notes: SI Units (Conventional Units × 1 or WBC × 10⁹/L).

See "WBC Count, Blood Smear and Differential" study for more detailed information.

WBC Count and Differential

Age	Immature Granulocytes (Absolute) (10^3/microL)	Immature Granulocyte Fraction (IGF) (%)
Birth–9 yr	0–0.03	0%–0.4%
10 yr–older adult	0–0.09	0%–0.9%

C

RBC Count

Age	Conventional Units (10^6 cells/microL)	SI Units (10^{12} cells/L) (Conventional Units × 1)
Cord blood	3.61–5.81	3.61–5.81
0–1 wk	4.51–6.01	4.51–6.01
2–3 wk	3.99–6.11	3.99–6.11
1–2 mo	3.71–6.11	3.71–6.11
3–6 mo	3.81–5.61	3.81–5.61
7 mo–15 yr	3.81–5.21	3.81–5.21
16–18 yr	4.21–5.41	4.21–5.41
Adult		
Male	4.21–5.81	4.21–5.81
Female	3.61–5.11	3.61–5.11

Values are decreased in pregnancy related to the dilutional effects of increased fluid volume and potential nutritional deficiency related to decreased intake, nausea, and/or vomiting. Values are slightly lower in older adults associated with potential nutritional deficiency. Values are slightly lower in older adults.

Note: See "RBC Count, Indices, Morphology, and Inclusions" study for more detailed information.

RBC Indices

Age	MCV (fl)	MCH (pg/cell)	MCHC (g/dL)	RDWCV	RDWSD
Cord blood	107–119	35–39	31–35	14.9–18.7	51–66
0–1 wk	104–116	29–45	24–36	14.9–18.7	51–66
2–3 wk	95–117	26–38	26–34	14.9–18.7	51–66
1–2 mo	81–125	25–37	26–34	14.9–18.7	44–55
3–11 mo	78–110	22–34	26–34	14.9–18.7	35–46
1–15 yr	74–94	24–32	30–34	11.6–14.8	35–42
16 yr–adult					
Male	77–97	26–34	32–36	11.6–14.8	38–48
Female	78–98	26–34	32–36	11.6–14.8	38–48
Older adult					
Male	79–103	27–35	32–36	11.6–14.8	38–48
Female	78–102	27–35	32–36	11.6–14.8	38–48

MCH = mean corpuscular hemoglobin; MCHC = mean corpuscular hemoglobin concentration; MCV = mean corpuscular volume; RDWCV = coefficient of variation in RBC distribution width index; RDWSD = standard deviation in RBC distribution width index

Note: See "RBC Count, Indices, Morphology, and Inclusions" study for more detailed information.

RBC Morphology

Morphology	Within Normal Limits	1+	2+	3+	4+
Size					
Anisocytosis	0–5	5–10	10–20	20–50	Greater than 50
Macrocytes	0–5	5–10	10–20	20–50	Greater than 50
Microcytes	0–5	5–10	10–20	20–50	Greater than 50
Shape					
Poikilocytes	0–2	3–10	10–20	20–50	Greater than 50
Burr cells	0–2	3–10	10–20	20–50	Greater than 20
Acanthocytes	Less than 1	2–5	5–10	10–20	Greater than 20
Schistocytes	Less than 1	2–5	5–10	10–20	Greater than 20
Dacryocytes (teardrop cells)	0–2	2–5	5–10	10–20	Greater than 20
Codocytes (target cells)	0–2	2–10	10–20	20–50	Greater than 50
Spherocytes	0–2	2–10	10–20	20–50	Greater than 50
Ovalocytes	0–2	2–10	10–20	20–50	Greater than 50
Stomatocytes	0–2	2–10	10–20	20–50	Greater than 50
Drepanocytes (sickle cells)	Absent	Reported as present or absent			
Helmet cells	Absent	Reported as present or absent			
Agglutination	Absent	Reported as present or absent			
Rouleaux	Absent	Reported as present or absent			
Hemoglobin Content					
Hypochromia	0–2	3–10	10–50	50–75	Greater than 75
Polychromasia					
Adult	Less than 1	2–5	5–10	10–20	Greater than 20
Newborn	1–6	7–15	15–20	20–50	Greater than 50

Note: See "RBC Count, Indices, Morphology, and Inclusions" study for more detailed information.

RBC Inclusions

Inclusions	Within Normal Limits	1+	2+	3+	4+
Cabot rings	Absent	Reported as present or absent			
Basophilic stippling	0–1	1–5	5–10	10–20	Greater than 20
Howell-Jolly bodies	Absent	1–2	3–5	5–10	Greater than 10
Heinz bodies	Absent	Reported as present or absent			
Hemoglobin C crystals	Absent	Reported as present or absent			
Pappenheimer bodies	Absent	Reported as present or absent			
Intracellular parasites (e.g., *Plasmodium, Babesia,* trypanosomes)	Absent	Reported as present or absent			

Note: See "RBC Count, Indices, Morphology, and Inclusions" study for more detailed information.

Platelet Count

Age	Conventional Units	SI Units (Conventional Units × 1)	MPV (fl)	IPF (%)
Birth	150–450 × 10³/microL	150–450 × 10⁹/L	7.1–10.2	1.1–7.1
Child/adult/ older adult	140–400 × 10³/microL	140–400 × 10⁹/L	7.1–10.2	1.1–7.1

Platelet counts may decrease slightly with age. *Note:* See "Platelet Count" study for more detailed information.

CRITICAL FINDINGS AND POTENTIAL INTERVENTIONS

Hemoglobin
Adults and Children
• Less than 6.6 g/dL (SI: Less than 66 mmol/L)
• Greater than 20 g/dL (SI: Greater than 200 mmol/L)

Newborns
• Less than 9.5 g/dL (SI: Less than 95 mmol/L)
• Greater than 22.3 g/dL (SI: Greater than 223 mmol/L)

Hematocrit
Adults and Children
- Less than 19.8% (SI: Less than 0.2 volume fraction)
- Greater than 60% (SI: Greater than 0.6 volume fraction)

Newborns
- Less than 28.5% (SI: Less than 0.28 volume fraction)
- Greater than 66.9% (SI: Greater than 0.67 volume fraction)

WBC Count (on Admission)
- Less than 2×10^3/microL (SI: Less than 2×10^9/L)
- Absolute neutrophil count of less than 0.5×10^3/microL (SI: Less than 0.5×10^9/L)
- Greater than 30×10^3/microL (SI: Greater than 30×10^9/L)

Platelet Count
- Less than 30×10^3/microL (SI: Less than 30×10^9/L)
- Greater than $1,000 \times 10^3$/microL (SI: Greater than $1,000 \times 10^9$/L)

Consideration may be given to verifying the critical findings before action is taken. Policies vary among facilities and may include requesting immediate recollection and retesting by the laboratory or retesting using a rapid point-of-care instrument at the bedside, if available.

Timely notification to the requesting health-care provider (HCP) of any critical findings and related symptoms is a role expectation of the professional nurse. A listing of these findings varies among facilities.

The presence of abnormal cells, other morphological characteristics, or cellular inclusions may signify a potentially life-threatening or serious health condition and should be investigated. Examples are the presence of sickle cells, moderate numbers of spherocytes, marked schistocytosis, oval macrocytes, basophilic stippling, eosinophil count greater than 10%, monocytosis greater than 15%, nucleated RBCs (if patient is not an infant), malarial organisms, hypersegmented neutrophils, agranular neutrophils, blasts or other immature cells, Auer rods, Döhle bodies, marked toxic granulation, or plasma cells.

OVERVIEW: (**Study type:** Blood collected in a lavender-top [EDTA] tube or Microtainer; **related body system:** Circulatory/Hematopoietic and Immune systems.) Blood from a green-top (lithium or sodium heparin) tube may be submitted, but the following automated values may not be reported: WBC count, WBC differential, platelet count, IPF, and mean platelet volume. The specimen should be analyzed within 24 hr when stored at room temperature or within 48 hr if stored at refrigerated temperature. If it is anticipated the specimen will not be analyzed within 24 hr, two blood smears should be made immediately after the venipuncture and submitted with the blood sample. Smears made from specimens older than 24 hr may contain an unacceptable number of misleading artifactual abnormalities of the RBCs, such as echinocytes and spherocytes, as well as necrobiotic WBCs. A complete blood count (CBC) is a group of tests used for basic screening purposes. It is probably the most widely ordered laboratory test. Results provide the enumeration of the cellular elements of the blood, measurement of RBC indices, and determination of cell morphology by automation and evaluation of stained smears. The results can provide valuable diagnostic information regarding the overall health of the patient and the patient's response to disease and treatment. Detailed information is found in studies titled "Hemoglobin and Hematocrit," "RBC Count, Indices, Morphology, and Inclusions," "Platelet Count," and "WBC Count, Blood Smear and Differential."

INDICATIONS

- Detect hematological disorder, tumor, leukemia, or immunological abnormality.
- Determine the presence of hereditary hematological abnormality.
- Evaluate known or suspected anemia and related treatment.
- Monitor blood loss and response to blood replacement.
- Monitor the effects of physical or emotional stress.
- Monitor fluid imbalances or treatment for fluid imbalances.
- Monitor hematological status during pregnancy.
- Monitor progression of nonhematological disorders, such as chronic obstructive pulmonary disease, malabsorption syndromes, cancer, and kidney disease.
- Monitor response to chemotherapy and evaluate undesired reactions to drugs that may cause blood dyscrasias.
- Provide screening as part of a general physical examination, especially on admission to a health-care facility or before surgery.

INTERFERING FACTORS

Factors that may alter the results of the study

- Failure to fill the tube sufficiently (less than three-fourths full) may yield inadequate sample volume for automated analyzers and may be a reason for specimen rejection.
- Hemolyzed or clotted specimens should be rejected for analysis.
- Elevated serum glucose or sodium levels may produce elevated mean corpuscular volume values because of swelling of erythrocytes.
- Recent transfusion history should be considered when evaluating the CBC.

POTENTIAL MEDICAL DIAGNOSIS: CLINICAL SIGNIFICANCE OF RESULTS

- See studies titled "Hemoglobin and Hematocrit," "RBC Count, Indices, Morphology, and Inclusions," "Platelet Count," and "WBC Count, Blood Smear and Differential."

Increased in
- See above-listed studies.

Decreased in
- See above-listed studies.

NURSING IMPLICATIONS

BEFORE THE STUDY: PLANNING AND IMPLEMENTATION

Teaching the Patient What to Expect

- Inform the patient this test can assist in evaluating general health and the body's response to illness.
- Explain that a blood sample is needed for the test.

Safety Considerations

Make sure a written and informed consent has been signed prior to administering any blood or blood products.

AFTER THE STUDY: POTENTIAL NURSING ACTIONS

Treatment Considerations

♦ The results of a CBC should be carefully evaluated during transfusion or acute blood loss because the body is not in a state of homeostasis and values may be misleading. Considerations for draw times after transfusion include the type of product, the amount of product transfused, and the patient's clinical situation. Generally, specimens collected an hour after transfusion will provide an acceptable reflection of the effects of the transfused product.

Measurements taken during a massive transfusion are an exception, providing essential guidance for therapeutic decisions during critical care.

Nutritional Considerations

♦ Instruct patient to consume a variety of foods within the basic food groups, maintain a healthy weight, be physically active, limit salt intake, limit alcohol intake, and avoid use of tobacco.

Follow-Up, Evaluation, and Desired Outcomes

♦ Acknowledges the importance of adhering to the recommended diet and medications.

Computed Tomography, Various Sites
(Abdomen, Angiography, Biliary Tract and Liver, Brain and Head, Cardiac Scoring, Chest, Colon, Kidneys, Pancreas, Pelvis, Pituitary, Spine, Spleen)

SYNONYM/ACRONYM: Computed axial tomography (CAT), computed transaxial tomography (CTT), helical/spiral CT.

RATIONALE: To visualize and assess internal organs/structures for abnormal or absent anatomical features, abscess, aneurysm, cancer or other masses, infection, or presence of disease. Used as an evaluation tool for surgical, radiation, and medical therapeutic interventions.

PATIENT PREPARATION: There are no activity restrictions unless by medical direction. Instruct the patient to fast and restrict fluids, as ordered, for 2 to 4 hr prior to the procedure; CT studies performed without contrast usually do not require the patient to fast before the procedure (e.g., CTA). Fasting may be ordered as a precaution against aspiration related to possible nausea and vomiting. The American Society of Anesthesiologists has fasting guidelines for risk levels according to patient status. More information can be located at www.asahq.org.

Note: If iodinated contrast medium is scheduled to be used in patients receiving metformin or drugs containing metformin for type 2 diabetes, the drug may be discontinued on the day of the test and continue to be withheld for 48 hr after the test.

Regarding the patient's risk for bleeding, the patient should be instructed to avoid taking natural products and medications with known anticoagulant, antiplatelet, or thrombolytic properties or to reduce dosage, as ordered, prior to the procedure. Number of days to withhold medication is dependent on the type of anticoagulant. Note the last time and dose of medication taken. Protocols may vary among facilities.

Ensure that barium studies were performed more than 4 days before the CT scan. Protocols may vary among facilities.

NORMAL FINDINGS

General

- Normal structure, function, contour, and patency of organ and related vessels
- Contrast medium normally circulates throughout area of inquiry, symmetrically and without interruption
- No variations in number and size of vessels and organs; no evidence of infection, edema, obstruction, aneurysm, stenosis, malformations, trauma, cysts, polyps, or tumors

Cardiac Scoring

- If the Agatston score is 100 or less, the probability of having significant CAD is minimal or is unlikely to be causing a narrowing at the time of the examination.

CRITICAL FINDINGS AND POTENTIAL INTERVENTIONS

General

- Abscess
- Aneurysm
- Tumor with significant mass effect
- Visceral injury; significant solid organ laceration

Abdomen

- Acute GI bleed
- Leaking aortic aneurysm
- Aortic dissection
- Appendicitis
- Bowel perforation
- Bowel obstruction
- Mesenteric torsion

Angiography

- Brain or spinal cord ischemia
- Emboli
- Hemorrhage
- Occlusion

Brain and Head

- Acute hemorrhage
- Aneurysm
- Infarction
- Infection

Chest

- Pneumothorax
- Pulmonary embolism

Pelvis

- Ectopic pregnancy

Spine

- Cord compression
- Fracture

Spleen
- Hemorrhage
- Laceration

Timely notification to the requesting health-care provider (HCP) of any critical findings and related symptoms is a role expectation of the professional nurse. A listing of these findings varies among facilities.

OVERVIEW: (Study type: X-ray, special/CT with or without contras.) Computed tomography (CT) is a noninvasive procedure used to enhance certain anatomic views of an organ with its surrounding structures and vessels. The table is moved in and out of a circular opening in a doughnut-like device called a *gantry,* which houses the x-ray tube and associated electronics. A beam of x-rays irradiates the patient as the table moves in and out of the scanner in a series of phases. The x-rays penetrate liquids and solids of different densities by varying degrees. Multiple detectors rotate around the patient to collect numeric data associated with the density coefficients assigned to each degree of tissue density. The imaging system's computer converts the numeric data obtained from the scanner into digital images. Air appears black; bone appears white; and body fluids, fat, and soft tissue structures are represented in various shades between black and white.

Cardiac Scoring CT
Cardiac scoring CT is used to enhance certain anatomic views of the heart for quantifying coronary artery calcium content. Coronary artery disease (CAD) occurs when the arteries that carry blood and oxygen to the heart muscle become clogged or built up with plaque. Plaque buildup slows the flow of blood to the heart muscle, causing ischemia and

increasing the risk of heart failure. The cross-sectional views of the arteries demonstrate the location and degree of plaque accumulation (calcium score). The Agatston score is the most frequently used scale to quantitate the amount of calcium in atherosclerotic plaque. The score is graded in levels from 0 to greater than 400, where a score of 0 is associated with a finding of no evidence of CAD, and a score of greater than 400 is associated with a finding of extensive evidence of CAD. Levels of 1 to 10, 11 to 100, and 101 to 400 respectively define minimal, mild, and moderate evidence of CAD. For additional information regarding screening guidelines for *atherosclerotic cardiovascular disease* (ASCVD) refer to the study titled "Cholesterol, Total and Fractions."

A CT scan may be repeated after administration of contrast medium given orally, by IV injection, or rectally. CT becomes invasive when contrast medium is used. The cross-sectional views, or *slices,* of the vascular system that supports major organs (brain, heart, liver and biliary tract, lungs, kidneys and adrenal glands, pancreas, spleen, thyroid gland) and anatomical areas such as the abdomen, chest, head, neck, arms, legs, and spine can be reviewed individually or as a three-dimensional image to allow differentiations of solid, cystic, or vascular obstructions as well as identification of suspected hematomas and aneurysms. Contrast is used to differentiate, enhance, or "light up" areas of interest depending on the type of study to be performed, type of contrast medium to be used, and method of administration. The medium works by creating a contrast between areas of interest based on density; penetration of the x-rays is weaker in areas where the contrast medium is detected by the scanner, showing the blood vessels, organs, and tissue as whitish areas that either outline the area of interest or completely fill it. Oral ingestion of contrast medium can be used for opacification to distinguish the bowel, adjacent abdominal organs, other types of tissue, and blood vessels as the medium moves through the digestive tract. IV injection of contrast medium is used for evaluation of blood flow through vessels and greater enhancement of tissue density and organ visualization. These images are helpful when blood vessels are heavily calcified, and the images give the most precise information regarding the true extent of stenosis. They can also evaluate intracerebral aneurysms. Small ulcerations and plaque irregularity are readily seen with CTA; the degree of stenosis can be closely estimated with CTA because of the increased number of imaging planes. Multislice or multidetector CT scanners continuously collect images in a helical or spiral fashion instead of a series of individual images, as with standard scanners. Helical CT can collect many images over a short period of time (seconds), is sensitive in identifying small abnormalities, and produces high-quality images. Images can be recorded on photographic or

x-ray film or stored in digital format as digitized computer data.

CT Colonoscopy/Colonography (Virtual Colonoscopy)

The procedure is used primarily to detect polyps, which are growths of tissue in the colon or rectum. Some types of polyps increase the risk of colon cancer, especially if they are large or if a patient has several polyps. Compared to conventional colonoscopy, CT colonoscopy is less effective in detecting polyps smaller than 5 mm, more effective when the polyps are between 5 and 9.9 mm, and most effective when the polyps are 10 mm or larger. This test may be valuable for patients who have diseases rendering them unable to undergo conventional colonoscopy (e.g., bleeding disorders, lung or heart disease) and for patients who are unable to undergo the sedation required for traditional colonoscopy. The procedure is less invasive than conventional colonoscopy, with little risk of complications and no recovery time. CT colonoscopy can be done as an outpatient procedure, and the patient may return to work or usual activities the same day. CT colonoscopy and conventional colonoscopy require the bowel to be cleansed before the examination. The screening procedure requires no contrast medium injections, but if a suspicious area or abnormality is detected, a repeat series of images may be completed after IV contrast medium is given. These density measurements are sent to a computer that produces a digital analysis of the anatomy, enabling HCP to look at slices or thin sections of certain anatomic views of the colon and vascular system. A drawback of CT colonoscopy is that polyp removal and biopsies of tissue in the colon must be done using conventional colonoscopy. Therefore, if polyps are discovered during CT colonoscopy and biopsy becomes necessary, the patient must undergo bowel preparation a second time.

Brain and Head CT
In some cases, scans may be repeated after multiple types of contrast are administered. For example, xenon-enhanced CT scanning is an imaging method used to assess cerebral blood flow. Xenon-133 is an odorless, colorless radioactive gas that can be either inhaled or injected. The isotope moves rapidly through the blood into the brain. The diffused gas demonstrates how much blood goes to each area of the brain. Sensitivity of stroke detection in the acute phase is increased by using Xenon. Combinations of diagnostic modalities are also becoming more common. Positron emission tomography (PET) and single-photon emission tomography (SPECT) are types of nuclear medicine studies that offer insights into functionality such as movement of blood flow or uptake and distribution of metabolites into tumors. PET/CT and SPECT/CT are imaging applications that superimpose PET or SPECT and CT findings. The images are collected and produced by a single gantry system. The coregistered or image fusion of PET/CT or SPECT/CT findings can provide a detailed combination of anatomical and functional images. Images can be recorded on photographic or x-ray film or stored in digital format as digitized computer data. The CT scan can be used to guide biopsy needles into areas of suspected tumors to obtain tissue for laboratory analysis and to guide placement of catheters for angioplasty or drainage of cysts or abscesses. Tumor staging and progression, before and after therapy, and effectiveness of medical interventions may be monitored by PET/CT or SPECT/CT scanning. The images can be reevaluated and manipulated for further detailed examination without having to repeat the procedure.

INDICATIONS
- Assist in differentiating between benign and malignant tumors.
- Detect aneurysms and vascular abnormalities.
- Detect tumor extension of masses and metastasis into other areas.
- Differentiate between infectious and inflammatory processes.
- Evaluate bleeding, cysts, hematomas, infarct, stenosis and obstructions, and trauma.
- Monitor and evaluate the effectiveness of medical, radiation, or surgical therapies.

Abdomen
- Differentiate aortic aneurysms from tumors near the aorta.
- Evaluate renal calculi.
- Evaluate retroperitoneal lymph nodes.

Angiography
- Detect fistula.
- Detect peripheral arterial disease (PAD).
- Differentiate aortic aneurysms from tumors near the aorta.
- Evaluate atherosclerosis.
- Evaluate hemorrhage or trauma.

Biliary Tract and Liver

- Detect dilation or obstruction of the biliary ducts with or without calcification or gallstone.
- Detect liver abnormalities, such as cirrhosis with ascites and fatty liver.
- Differentiate aortic aneurysms from tumors near the aorta.
- Differentiate between obstructive and nonobstructive jaundice.

Brain and Head

- Detect ventricular enlargement or displacement by increased cerebrospinal fluid.
- Determine cause of increased intracranial pressure.
- Determine presence and type of hemorrhage in infants and children experiencing signs and symptoms of intracranial trauma or congenital conditions such as hydrocephalus and arteriovenous malformations (AVMs).
- Determine presence of multiple sclerosis, as evidenced by sclerotic plaques.
- Differentiate hematoma location after trauma (e.g., subdural, epidural, cerebral) and determine extent of edema, as evidenced by higher blood densities.
- Differentiate between cerebral infarction and hemorrhage.
- Evaluate abnormalities of the middle ear ossicles, auditory nerve, and optic nerve.
- Evaluate for thyroid cancer.

Cardiac Scoring

- Detect and quantify coronary artery calcium content.

  CAD is the leading cause of death in most industrialized nations.

  Estimation of 10-year cardiovascular risk using a scoring system such as the gender-specific Framingham risk score is a more powerful predictor of CAD than cholesterol screening.

  Of all myocardial infarctions (MIs), 45% occur in people younger than age 65.

  Of women who have had MIs, 44% will die within 1 yr after the attack.

  Women are more likely to die of heart disease than of breast cancer.

- Family history of heart disease.
- Screening for coronary artery calcium in patients with

  Diabetes

  High blood pressure

  High cholesterol

  High-stress lifestyle

  Overweight by 20% or more

  Personal history of smoking

  Sedentary lifestyle

- Screen for coronary artery plaque in patients with chest pain of unknown cause.

Chest

- Detect aortic aneurysms.
- Detect bronchial abnormalities, such as stenosis, dilation, or tumor.
- Detect lymphomas, especially Hodgkin disease.
- Detect mediastinal and hilar lymphadenopathy.
- Determine blood, fluid, or fat accumulation in tissues, pleuritic space, or vessels.
- Differentiate aortic aneurysms from tumors near the aorta.
- Evaluate cardiac chambers and pulmonary vessels.
- Evaluate the presence of plaque in cardiac vessels.
- Identify or rule out thymoma in cases of diagnosed myasthenia gravis.

Colon

- Detect polyps in the colon.
- Evaluate the colon for metachronous lesions.
- Evaluate the colon in patients with obstructing rectosigmoid disease.
- Evaluate polyposis syndromes.
- Evaluate the site of resection for local recurrence of lesions.
- Examine the colon in patients with heart or lung disease, patients unable to be sedated,

and patients unable to undergo colonoscopy.
- Failure to visualize the entire colon during conventional colonoscopy.
- Identify metastases.
- Investigate cause of positive occult blood test.
- Investigate further after an abnormal barium enema.
- Investigate further when flexible sigmoidoscopy is positive for polyps.

Kidneys
- Aid in the diagnosis of congenital anomalies, such as polycystic kidney disease, horseshoe kidney, absence of one kidney, or kidney displacement.
- Assist in localizing perirenal hematomas and abscesses for drainage.
- Detect bleeding or hyperplasia of the adrenal glands.
- Determine kidney size and location in relation to the bladder in post-transplant patients.
- Determine presence and type of adrenal tumor, such as benign adenoma, cancer, or pheochromocytoma.
- Evaluate abnormal fluid accumulation around the kidney.
- Evaluate renal calculi.

Pancreas
- Detect dilation or obstruction of the pancreatic ducts.
- Differentiate between pancreatic disorders and disorders of the retroperitoneum.
- Evaluate unexplained weight loss, jaundice, and epigastric pain.

Pelvis
- Evaluate pelvic lymph nodes.

Pituitary
- Detect congenital anomalies, such as partially empty sella.
- Determine pituitary size and location in relation to surrounding structures.

Spine
- Detect congenital spinal anomalies, such as spina bifida, meningocele, and myelocele.
- Detect herniated intervertebral disks.
- Detect paraspinal cysts.
- Detect vascular malformations.

Spleen
- Evaluate the presence of an accessory spleen, polysplenia, or asplenia.
- Evaluate splenic vein thrombosis.

INTERFERING FACTORS
Contraindications

⁂ Patients who are pregnant or suspected of being pregnant, unless the potential benefits of a procedure using radiation far outweigh the risk of radiation exposure to the fetus and mother.

⁂ Patients who are claustrophobic.

⁂ Patients with conditions associated with adverse reactions to contrast medium (e.g., asthma, food allergies, or allergy to contrast medium). Although patients are asked specifically if they have a known allergy to iodine or shellfish (shellfish contain high levels of iodine), it has been well established that the reaction is not to iodine; an actual iodine allergy would be problematic because iodine is required for the production of thyroid hormones. In the case of shellfish, the reaction is to a muscle protein called *tropomyosin*; in the case of iodinated contrast medium, the reaction is to the noniodinated part of the contrast molecule. Patients with a known hypersensitivity to the medium may benefit from premedication with corticosteroids and diphenhydramine; the use of nonionic contrast or an alternative noncontrast imaging study, if available, may be considered for patients who have severe asthma or who have experienced moderate to severe reactions to ionic contrast medium.

C

❖ Patients with conditions associated with preexisting renal insufficiency (e.g., chronic kidney disease, single kidney transplant, nephrectomy, diabetes, multiple myeloma, treatment with aminoglycosides and NSAIDs), *because iodinated contrast is nephrotoxic.*

❖ Patients who are chronically dehydrated before the test, especially older adults and patients whose health is already compromised, *because of their risk of contrast-induced acute kidney injury.*

❖ Patients with pheochromocytoma, *because iodinated contrast may cause a hypertensive crisis.*

❖ Patients with bleeding disorders or receiving anticoagulant therapy, *because the puncture site may not stop bleeding.*

Factors that may alter the results of the study
- Gas or feces in the GI tract resulting from inadequate cleansing or failure to restrict food intake before the study.
- Retained barium from a previous radiological procedure.
- Metallic objects within the examination field (e.g., jewelry, body rings), which may inhibit organ visualization and cause unclear images.

POTENTIAL MEDICAL DIAGNOSIS: CLINICAL SIGNIFICANCE OF RESULTS
Abnormal findings related to
Identification of abnormal findings is assisted by comparison of parameters such as size, shape, symmetry, density, and location. For example, areas of altered density in either an expected or unexpected location may indicate enlargement of an organ or the presence of blood or other fluids, tumors, or cysts. Comparison by type of abnormal findings may also assist in evaluating areas of altered density.

For example, well-defined round or oval areas, smaller in size and having lower density than a primary tumor, may indicate a cyst; a crescent-shaped area of abnormal density that alters the proximity of the liver to the Glisson capsule may indicate a hematoma; areas of less than normal density may indicate hepatic lesions; and dilation of the associated ducts may indicate an obstruction.

Abdomen
- Abdominal abscess
- Abdominal aortic aneurysm
- Abnormal accumulations of blood, fat, or body fluid
- Adrenal tumor or hyperplasia
- Appendicitis
- Bowel obstruction
- Bowel perforation
- Cirrhosis
- Dilation of the common hepatic duct, common bile duct, or gallbladder
- Diverticulitis or irritable bowel
- Gallstones
- GI bleeding
- Hematomas
- Hemoperitoneum
- Hepatic cysts or abscesses
- Infarction (e.g., intestinal, omental)
- Infection
- Pancreatic pseudocyst
- Primary and metastatic tumors in bone, organs, glands, ducts, or ligaments
- Renal calculi
- Splenic laceration
- Trauma

Angiography
- Aortic aneurysm
- Cysts or abscesses
- Dissected aorta
- Emboli
- Hemorrhage
- Occlusion
- PAD
- Pericarditis
- Shunting

- Stenosis
- Tumor

Biliary Tract and Liver
- Dilation of the common hepatic duct, common bile duct, or gallbladder
- Gallstones
- Hematomas
- Hepatic cysts or abscesses
- Jaundice (obstructive or nonobstructive)
- Primary and metastatic tumors
- Dilation of the common hepatic duct, common bile duct, or gallbladder
- Gallstones
- Hematomas
- Hepatic cysts or abscesses
- Jaundice (obstructive or nonobstructive)
- Primary and metastatic tumors

Brain and Head
- Abscess
- Alzheimer disease
- Aneurysm
- AVMs
- Cerebral atrophy
- Cerebral edema
- Cerebral infarction
- Congenital abnormalities
- Craniopharyngioma
- Cysts
- Foreign body
- Hematomas (e.g., epidural, subdural, intracerebral)
- Hemorrhage
- Hydrocephaly
- Increased intracranial pressure or trauma
- Infarction
- Infection
- Pheochromocytoma
- Sclerotic plaques suggesting multiple sclerosis
- Sinusitis
- Trauma
- Tumor
- Ventricular or tissue displacement or enlargement

Cardiac Scoring
Calcified plaque in the coronary arteries is similar in composition to bone and if present will appear as areas of whiteness depending on the amount of accumulated calcification.

- If the Agatston score is between 100 and 400, a significant amount of calcified plaque was found in the coronary arteries. There is an increased risk of a future MI, and a medical assessment of cardiac risk factors needs to be done. Additional testing may be needed.
- If the Agatston score is greater than 400, the procedure has detected extensive calcified plaque in the coronary arteries, which may have caused a critical narrowing of the vessels. A full medical assessment is needed as soon as possible. Further testing may be needed, and treatment may be needed to reduce the risk of MI.

Chest
- Aortic aneurysm
- Chest, mediastinal, spine, or rib lesions
- Cysts or abscesses
- Enlarged lymph nodes
- Esophageal pathology, including tumors
- Hodgkin disease
- Pleural effusion
- Pneumonitis
- Pneumothorax
- Pulmonary embolism

Colon
- Abnormal endoluminal wall of the colon
- Extraluminal extension of primary cancer
- Mesenteric and retroperitoneal lymphadenopathy
- Metachronous lesions
- Metastases of cancer
- Polyps or growths in colon or rectum
- Tumor recurrence after surgery

Kidneys
- Adrenal tumor or hyperplasia
- Congenital anomalies, such as polycystic kidney disease, horseshoe kidney, absence of one kidney, or kidney displacement
- Dilation of the common hepatic duct, common bile duct, or gallbladder
- Renal artery aneurysm
- Renal calculi and ureteral obstruction
- Renal cell cancer
- Renal cysts or abscesses
- Renal laceration, fracture, tumor, and trauma
- Perirenal abscesses and hematomas
- Primary and metastatic tumors

Pancreas
- Acute or chronic pancreatitis
- Obstruction of the pancreatic ducts
- Pancreatic abscesses
- Pancreatic cancer
- Pancreatic pseudocyst
- Pancreatic tumor

Pelvis
- Bladder calculi
- Ectopic pregnancy
- Fibroid tumors
- Hydrosalpinx

- Ovarian cyst or abscess
- Primary and metastatic tumors

Pituitary
- Abscess
- Adenoma
- Aneurysm
- Chordoma
- Craniopharyngioma
- Cyst
- Meningioma
- Metastasis
- Pituitary hemorrhage

Spine
- Congenital spinal malformations, such as meningocele, myelocele, or spina bifida
- Herniated intervertebral disks
- Paraspinal cysts
- Spinal tumors
- Spondylosis (cervical or lumbar)
- Vascular malformations

Spleen
- Abdominal aortic aneurysm
- Hematomas
- Hemoperitoneum
- Primary and metastatic tumors
- Splenic cysts or abscesses
- Splenic laceration, tumor, infiltration, and trauma

NURSING IMPLICATIONS

POTENTIAL NURSING PROBLEMS: ASSESSMENT & NURSING DIAGNOSIS

Problems	Signs and Symptoms
Abdomen and CT Angiography: Inadequate cardiac output *(related to dissection, rupture)*	Altered level of consciousness, hypotension, increased pulse that may be thready, delayed capillary refill, diminished peripheral pulses, cool skin, restlessness, anxiety
Biliary Tract and Liver: Insufficient fluid volume (water) *(related to vomiting, nausea)*	Dry mucous membranes, low blood pressure, increased heart rate, slow capillary refill, diminished skin turgor, diminished urine output

(table continues on page 388)

C

Problems	Signs and Symptoms
Brain and Head: Inadequate cerebral tissue perfusion *(related to infarct, hemorrhage, mass, edema, infection, plaque, atrophy)*	Diminished or altered level of consciousness, aphasia that can be expressive or receptive, loss of sensory functionality, slurred speech, dysphagia, difficulty in completing a learned activity or in recognizing familiar objects (apraxia, agnosia), motor function deficits, spatial neglect, facial droop and/or varying degrees of flaccid extremities
Cardiac Scoring and Chest: Fluid excess *(related to diminished renal perfusion with release of antidiuretic hormone, inadequate cardiac pumping)*	Weight gain, edema, decreased urinary output, tachycardia, dyspnea, elevated blood pressure, jugular venous distention, restlessness
Colonoscopy: Bowel elimination *(altered related to operative bowel elimination)*	Silent bowel sounds with auscultation, does not pass stool or flatus, bloating, nausea, abdominal distention
Kidneys: Infection *(related to obstruction, aneurysm, infection, cyst, abscess, inflammation, tumor, trauma, injury)*	Positive culture, fever, chills, elevated temperature, elevated white blood cell (WBC) count, flank pain, hematuria, urinary frequency
Pancreas: Inadequate nutrition *(related to decreased oral intake associated with pain, NPO status)*	Self-report of pain with eating, presence of nausea and vomiting, NPO order, inflammation
Pelvis: Pain *(related to tumor, inflammation, abdominal pressure)*	Self-report of pain, facial grimace, crying, restlessness, anxiety, elevated blood pressure and heart rate
Pituitary: Infection risk *(related to a combination of surgical procedure and immunosuppression secondary to chemotherapy)*	Redness, warmth or drainage at the incision site, elevated temperature, elevated WBC and C-reactive protein (CRP)
Spine: Mobility *(related to pain, muscular spasms, nerve compression)*	Slow, guarded movement; pain; difficulty standing upright
Spleen: Bleeding *(related to trauma, injury)*	Decreasing hemoglobin (Hgb) and hematocrit (Hct), hypotension, tachycardia, shortness of breath, weakness, fatigue, pallor

BEFORE THE STUDY: PLANNING AND IMPLEMENTATION

Teaching the Patient What to Expect

◆ Inform the patient this procedure can assist in assessing internal organs and other anatomical areas of interest.

◆ Explain that prior to the procedure, laboratory testing may be required to determine the possibility of bleeding risk (coagulation testing) or to assess for impaired kidney function (creatinine level and estimated glomerular filtration rate) if use of iodinated contrast medium is anticipated.

▶ Pregnancy is a general contraindication to procedures involving radiation. Explain to the female patient that she will be asked the date of her last menstrual period. Pregnancy testing may be performed to determine the possibility of pregnancy before exposure to radiation.

▶ Review the procedure with the patient. Address concerns about pain and explain that there may be moments of discomfort or pain experienced when the IV line or catheter is inserted to allow infusion of fluids such as saline, anesthetics, sedatives, contrast medium, medications used in the procedure, or emergency medications.

▶ Explain that contrast medium will be injected, by catheter, at a separate site from the IV line.

▶ Advise that a burning and flushing sensation may be felt throughout the body during injection of the contrast medium, and the patient may experience an urge to cough, flushing, nausea, or a salty or metallic taste.

▶ Explain that reducing health-care-associated infections is an important patient safety goal and a number of different safety practices will be implemented during their procedure. Advise the patient that hair in the area near the catheter insertion site may be clipped or shaved and the area cleaned with an antiseptic solution to cleanse bacteria from the skin in order to reduce the risk for infection. *Note:* The World Health Organization, Centers for Disease Control and Prevention, and Association of periOperative Registered Nurses recommend that hair not be removed at all unless it interferes with the incision site or other aspects of the procedure because hair removal by any means is associated with increased infection rates. When hair removal is necessary, facilities must use a protocol that is based on scientific literature or the endorsement of a professional organization. Clipping immediately before the procedure and in a location outside the procedure area is preferred to shaving with a razor. Shaving creates a break in skin integrity and provides

a way for bacteria on the skin to enter the incision site.

▶ Advise the patient that the procedure is usually performed in the radiology department by an HCP specializing in this procedure, with support staff, and takes approximately 15 to 30 min depending on factors such as the type of study ordered, whether contrast is used, and the type of contrast used; cardiac scoring takes about 10 to 15 min.

▶ Ask the patient to remove all external metallic objects immediately prior to the procedure.

▶ Baseline vital signs will be recorded and monitored throughout the procedure. Protocols may vary among facilities.

▶ *Cardiac Scoring:* ECG electrodes will be placed to the appropriate locations on the patient's chest. The CT scanner will be synchronized with the patient's heart rate in order to record images when the heart is at rest.

▶ *Abdomen, Angiography, Biliary, Colonoscopy, Kidney, Pancreas, Pelvis, Spleen:* Advise the patient that he or she may be requested to drink approximately 450 mL of a dilute barium solution (approximately 1% barium) or a water-soluble oral contrast; the oral contrast is given within a specified time period prior to the study. Oral contrast is administered to distinguish GI organs from the other abdominal organs and to enhance other areas of interest.

▶ Placement for the patient is in the supine position on an examination table.

▶ For cardiac scoring or if IV contrast media is used, a rapid series of images is taken during and after the filling of the vessels to be examined. Delayed images may be taken to examine the vessels after a time and to monitor the venous phase of the procedure.

▶ The patient will be asked to inhale deeply and hold his or her breath while the images are taken, and then to exhale after the images are taken.

▶ Advise taking slow, deep breaths if nausea occurs during the procedure. An ordered antiemetic drug can be administered as needed. An emesis basin can be ready for use.

◆ Explain to the patient that he or she will be monitored for complications related to the procedure (e.g., allergic reaction, anaphylaxis, bronchospasm).

◆ Explain that once the study is completed, the needle or catheter is removed, and a pressure dressing is applied over the puncture site.

Potential Nursing Actions

✻ *Make sure a written and informed consent has been signed prior to the procedure and before administering any medications.*

◆ *Angiography and Cardiac Scoring:* Investigate the presence of other risk factors, such as family history of heart disease, smoking, obesity, diet, lack of physical activity, hypertension, diabetes, previous MI, and previous vascular disease. Knowledge of genetics assists in identifying those who may benefit from additional education, risk assessment, and counseling. Genetics is the study and identification of genes, genetic mutations, and inheritance. For example, genetics provides some insight into the likelihood of inheriting a medical condition such as CAD. Genomic studies evaluate the interaction of groups of genes. The combined activity or combined expression of groups of genes allows assumptions or predictions to be made. As an example, genomic studies measure the levels of activity in multiple genes to predict how they, along with environmental and lifestyle decisions, influence the development of type 2 diabetes, CAD, MI, or ischemic stroke. Further information regarding inheritance of genes can be found in the study titled "Genetic Testing."

◆ Glucagon or an anticholinergic drug may be given to stabilize movement of the stomach muscles; peristaltic contractions (motion) may alter study findings.

◆ If iodinated contrast medium is scheduled to be used in patients receiving metformin or drugs containing metformin for type 2 diabetes, the drug may be discontinued on the day of the test and continue to be withheld for 48 hr after the test. Protocols may vary among facilities.

Safety Considerations

◆ Anticoagulants, aspirin, and other salicylates should be discontinued by medical direction for the appropriate number of days prior to a procedure where bleeding is a potential complication.

AFTER THE STUDY: POTENTIAL NURSING ACTIONS

Avoiding Complications

◆ Establishing an IV site and injection of contrast medium are invasive procedures. Complications are rare but include risk for allergic reaction *(related to contrast reaction),* bleeding from the puncture site *(related to a bleeding disorder or the effects of natural products and medications with known anticoagulant, antiplatelet, or thrombolytic properties),* hematoma *(related to blood leakage into the tissue following needle insertion),* infection *(which might occur if bacteria from the skin surface is introduced at the puncture site),* tissue damage *(related to extravasation or leaking of contrast into the tissues during injection),* nerve injury or damage to a nearby organ *(which might occur if the catheter strikes a nerve or perforates an organ),* or nephrotoxicity *(a deterioration of renal function associated with contrast administration).* Monitor the patient for complications related to the procedure (e.g., allergic reaction, anaphylaxis, bronchospasm, infection, injury). Immediately report symptoms such as difficulty breathing, chest pain, fever, hyperpnea, hypertension, nausea, palpitations, pruritus, rash, tachycardia, urticaria, or vomiting to the appropriate HCP. Observe/assess the needle/catheter insertion site for bleeding, inflammation, or hematoma formation. Administer ordered antihistamines or prophylactic steroids if the patient has an allergic reaction. Monitor peripheral pulses as well as changes in the color or temperature of the skin around the insertion site that may be indicative of bleeding. Assess extremities for signs of ischemia or absence of distal pulse caused by a catheter-induced thrombus.

Treatment Considerations
General

▶ Instruct the patient to resume pretesting diet, as directed by the HCP. Assess the patient's ability to swallow before allowing the patient to attempt liquids or solid foods. Kidney function should be assessed before metformin is resumed.

▶ Monitor vital signs and neurological status every 15 min for 1 hr, then every 2 hr for 4 hr, and then as ordered by the HCP. Monitor temperature every 4 hr for 24 hr. Monitor intake and output at least every 8 hr. Compare with baseline values.

▶ Maintain bedrest in the supine position for 2 to 6 hr, depending on the location of the insertion site, *to prevent stress on the puncture site.* Protocols may vary among facilities.

▶ Procedures that include oral contrast: Inform the patient that diarrhea may occur after ingestion of oral contrast media.

▶ Provide IV fluid to support blood pressure (rapid rate as appropriate) or blood transfusion as ordered.

▶ Pain: Assess pain character, location, duration, and intensity. Use an easily understood pain rating scale. Place in a position of comfort and administer ordered medications. Consider alternative measures for pain management (imagery, relaxation, music, etc.). Assess and trend vital signs; facilitate a calm, quiet environment.

CT Abdomen and CT Angiography

▶ Inadequate Cardiac Output: IV fluid to support blood pressure (rapid rate as appropriate). Administer ordered blood and blood products. Monitor and trend vital signs, ECG, assess for changes in sensorium, and monitor intake and output and renal status.

CT Biliary Tract and Liver

▶ Insufficient Fluid Volume: Monitor and trend vital signs. Administer ordered parenteral fluids and encourage oral fluids appropriately. Implement strict intake and output, monitor color of urine, and administer ordered antiemetics.

CT Brain and Head

▶ Inadequate Cerebral Tissue Perfusion: Complete a baseline neurological assessment for ongoing comparison to evaluate improvement or deterioration. Monitor and trend vital signs. Prepare the patient for and facilitate complementary diagnostic studies; magnetic resonance imaging (MRI), PET, ultrasound, or subtraction angiography. Elevate the head of the bed. Administer ordered antiplatelet, anticoagulant, or thrombolytic medications. Administer ordered antihypertensive medication, steroids, diuretics, calcium channel blockers, or antiseizure medications. Maintain a quiet, restful environment.

Cardiac Scoring and CT Chest

▶ Fluid Overload: Monitor fluid and electrolytes, monitor heart rate and blood pressure, daily weight, low-sodium diet, and administer prescribed antihypertensive medication and diuretics.

CT Colonoscopy

▶ Patient may need to remain NPO until bowel function returns. If nasogastric tube (NGT) is in use, ensure patency, measure and record output. Provide good oral care.

▶ Encourage the patient to follow colon cancer screening guidelines. The American Cancer Society (ACS) screening recommendations regarding regular screening for colon cancer begins at age 50 yr for individuals with average risk and sooner for those with increased or high risk for developing colon cancer. Its recommendations for frequency of screening are to use one of the following: (1) annual occult blood testing (fecal occult blood testing or fecal immunochemical testing); (2) every 5 yr for flexible sigmoidoscopy, double-contrast barium enema, or CT colonography; (3) every 10 yr for colonoscopy; or (4) every 3 yr for stool DNA testing. Abnormal findings should be followed up by standard colonoscopy. There are both advantages and disadvantages to the screening tests that are available today. The stool DNA test is designed to identify abnormal changes in DNA from the cells in the lining of the colon that are normally shed and excreted in stool. Unlike some of the current screening methods, the DNA tests would be able to detect precancerous polyps.

CT Kidneys

▶ Infection: Monitor and trend laboratory studies; blood urea nitrogen, creatinine, WBC count, Hgb, Hct, electrolytes, urine cultures. Monitor for results of complementary diagnostic studies: KUB; CT; MRI; IVP. Administer ordered antibiotics. Increase oral fluid intake appropriately and administer ordered parenteral fluids. Monitor and trend temperature.

CT Pancreas

▶ Inadequate Nutrition: Complete a culturally appropriate nutritional assessment; daily weight; intake and output; administer ordered IV fluids with supplements such as electrolytes; NPO as ordered with NGT to low suction; monitor and trend specific laboratory studies (lipase, amylase, albumin, total protein, electrolytes, glucose, calcium, iron, folic acid); dietary consultation and collaboration when oral fluids and diet are ordered; administer ordered dietary supplements.

CT Pituitary

▶ Infection Risk: Monitor and trend temperature, WBC count, and CRP. Evaluate the surgical site for redness, warmth, and drainage. Obtain an ordered culture and sensitivity of drainage if present. Administer ordered antibiotics if necessary.

CT Spine

▶ Mobility: Facilitate physical therapy to review proper movement and positioning: push instead of pull, use large muscles to lift objects, avoid twisting, place pillows under the knees or between knees in bed.

CT Spleen

▶ Review and trend Hgb and Hct. Administer ordered blood and blood products. Monitor and trend vital signs. Provide ordered oxygen as necessary.

Safety Considerations

▶ Advise diabetic patients to avoid all medications containing metformin for 48 hr following a procedure with iodinated contrast. Iodinated contrast can temporarily impair kidney function, and failure to withhold metformin may indirectly result in drug-induced lactic acidosis, a dangerous and sometimes fatal adverse effect of metformin (related to renal impairment that does not support sufficient excretion of metformin).

Nutritional Considerations

▶ Discuss ideal body weight and the purpose of and relationship between ideal weight and caloric intake to support cardiac health. Review ways to decrease intake of saturated fats and increase intake of polyunsaturated fats. Discuss limiting intake of refined processed sugar and sodium; discuss limiting cholesterol intake to less than 300 mg per day. Encourage the intake of fresh fruits and vegetables, unprocessed carbohydrates, poultry, and grains.

▶ Nutritional therapy is recommended for those with identified CAD risk, especially for those with elevated low-density lipoprotein cholesterol levels, other lipid disorders, diabetes, insulin resistance, or metabolic syndrome. Always consider cultural influences with dietary choices to ensure better adherence to a change in lifestyle. A variety of dietary patterns are beneficial for people with ASCVD; for additional information regarding nutritional guidelines, refer to the study titled "Cholesterol, Total and Fractions."

▶ Other changeable risk factors warranting education include strategies to encourage regular participation of moderate aerobic physical activity three to four times per week, eliminate tobacco use, and adhere to a heart-healthy diet.

▶ Those with elevated triglycerides should be advised to eliminate or reduce alcohol.

Follow-Up, Evaluation, and Desired Outcomes

▶ After CT colonoscopy, recognizes colon cancer screening options and understands that decisions regarding the need for and frequency of occult blood testing, colonoscopy, or other cancer screening procedures may be made after consultation between the patient and HCP. Colonoscopy should be used to follow up abnormal findings obtained by any of the screening tests. The most current guidelines for colon cancer screening of the general population as well as of individuals with increased risk are available from the ACS (www.cancer .org), U.S. Preventive Services Task Force (www.uspreventiveservices taskforce.org), and American College of Gastroenterology (http://gi.org). For additional information regarding screening guidelines, refer to the study titled "Colonoscopy."

▶ After CT angiography or cardiac scoring, acknowledges contact information provided for the American Heart Association (www.heart.org/HEARTORG), National Heart, Lung, and Blood Institute (www.nhlbi.nih.gov), or the U.S. Department of Agriculture's resource for nutrition (www.choosemyplate.gov).

▶ After all CT studies, recognizes the importance of taking ordered medications and adhering to the therapy regimen.

Coombs Antiglobulin, Direct

SYNONYM/ACRONYM: Direct antiglobulin testing (DAT).

RATIONALE: To detect associated conditions or drug therapies that can result in cell hemolysis, such as found in hemolytic disease of newborns, and hemolytic transfusion reactions.

PATIENT PREPARATION: There are no food, fluid, activity, or medication restrictions unless by medical direction.

NORMAL FINDINGS: (Method: Agglutination) Negative (no agglutination).

CRITICAL FINDINGS AND POTENTIAL INTERVENTIONS: N/A

OVERVIEW: (Study type: Blood collected in a red-top tube and whole blood collected in a lavender-top [EDTA] tube; related body system: Circulatory/Hematopoietic and Immune systems.) DAT detects in vivo antibody sensitization of red blood cells (RBCs). Immunoglobulin G (IgG) produced in certain disease states or in response to certain drugs can coat the surface of RBCs, resulting in cellular damage and hemolysis. When DAT is performed, RBCs are taken from the patient's blood sample, washed with saline to remove residual globulins, and mixed with anti–human globulin reagent. If the anti–human globulin reagent causes agglutination of the patient's RBCs, specific antiglobulin reagents can be used to determine whether the patient's RBCs are coated with IgG, complement, or both. (See study titled "Blood Typing, Antibody Screen, and Crossmatch" for more information regarding transfusion reactions.)

C

INDICATIONS

- Detect autoimmune hemolytic anemia or hemolytic disease of the newborn.
- Evaluate hemolytic anemia (autoimmune or induced by drugs or other substances).
- Evaluate transfusion reaction.

INTERFERING FACTORS

Factors that may alter the results of the study

- Drugs and other substances that may cause a positive DAT include acetaminophen, aminosalicylic acid, ampicillin, antihistamines, aztreonam, cephalosporins, chlorinated hydrocarbon insecticides, chlorpromazine, chlorpropamide, cisplatin, clonidine, dipyrone, ethosuximide, hydralazine, hydrochlorothiazide, ibuprofen, insulin, isoniazid, levodopa, mefenamic acid, melphalan, methadone, methicillin, methyldopa, moxalactam, penicillin, phenytoin, probenecid, procainamide, quinidine, quinine, rifampin, stibophen, streptomycin, sulfonamides, and tetracycline.
- Wharton's jelly may cause a false-positive DAT.
- Cold agglutinins and large amounts of paraproteins in the specimen may cause false-positive results.
- Newborns' cells may give negative results in ABO hemolytic disease.

Other considerations

- Tube methods for DAT are less sensitive than gel methods, and false-negative findings are possible in cases where weak, incompletely developed antigen sites on newborns' RBCs may not allow detectable amounts of anti-A and/or anti-B to bind to the RBC membrane. Neonates who have received multiple intrauterine transfusions of antigen-negative (group O) cells may also have a negative DAT because the results represent circulating donated red blood cells rather than the neonate's native red blood cells.

POTENTIAL MEDICAL DIAGNOSIS: CLINICAL SIGNIFICANCE OF RESULTS

Positive findings in

Antibodies formed during these circumstances or conditions attach to the patient's RBCs, and hemolysis occurs. Agglutination is graded from 1+ to 4+ in manual testing systems, with 4+ being the strongest degree of agglutination. Automated testing systems can report 1+ to 4+ graded results, provide images of the tested material so laboratory professionals can interpret the results, or provide computer-assisted interpretation of the test results as positive or negative findings).

- **Anemia** *(autoimmune hemolytic, drug-induced)*
- Hemolytic disease of the newborn *(related to ABO or Rh incompatibility)*
- Infectious mononucleosis
- Lymphomas
- Mycoplasma pneumonia
- Paroxysmal cold hemoglobinuria *(idiopathic or disease related)*
- Passively acquired antibodies from plasma products
- Post–cardiac vascular surgery *(increased incidence of positive DAT has been reported in patients following cardiac surgery, possibly related to mechanical RBC destruction while the patient is on cardiac bypass)*
- Systemic lupus erythematosus and other connective tissue immune disorders
- Transfusion reactions *(related to blood incompatibility)*

Negative findings in

- Samples in which sensitization of erythrocytes has not occurred

NURSING IMPLICATIONS

POTENTIAL NURSING PROBLEMS: ASSESSMENT & NURSING DIAGNOSIS

Problems	Signs and Symptoms
Gas exchange *(related to destruction of RBCs secondary to maternal-child Rh incompatibility)*	Shortness of breath, orthopnea, cyanosis, increased heart rate, increased respiratory rate, use of respiratory accessory muscles
Injury risk *(related to Rh incompatibility, blood incompatibility)*	Jaundice in newborn, infant cardiac stress (heart failure), infant death

BEFORE THE STUDY: PLANNING AND IMPLEMENTATION

Teaching the Patient What to Expect

▶ Inform the patient/parent this test can assist in assessing for disorders that break down RBCs.

▶ Explain that a blood sample is needed for the test. If a cord sample is to be taken from a newborn, inform parents that the sample will be obtained at the time of delivery and will not result in blood loss to the infant. Cord specimens are obtained by inserting a needle attached to a syringe into the umbilical vein. The specimen is drawn into the syringe and gently expressed into the appropriate collection container.

Potential Nursing Actions

✦ *Verify informed and written consent has been obtained if blood transfusion is likely.*

AFTER THE STUDY: POTENTIAL NURSING ACTIONS

Avoiding Complications

▶ Acute hemolytic reactions can be immediate and life threatening for patients of any age. Chronic hemolytic anemia is also a significant condition that requires timely identification of the problem in order to treat the condition. Assess the newborn's bilirubin and hematocrit (Hct) levels. Increased bilirubin and decreased Hct may be indicative of RBC breakdown. Kernicterus, or deposition of bilirubin in the brain, is a serious and significant development that can lead to permanent brain damage or death.

A transfusion reaction may occur in some patients. A transfusion reaction is also a critical finding. Signs and symptoms of blood transfusion reaction range from mildly febrile to anaphylactic and may include chills, dyspnea, fever, headache, nausea, vomiting, palpitations and tachycardia, chest or back pain, apprehension, flushing, hives, angioedema, diarrhea, hypotension, oliguria, hemoglobinuria, acute kidney injury, sepsis, shock, and jaundice. Complications from disseminated intravascular coagulation (DIC) may also occur.

Possible interventions in mildly febrile reactions include slowing the rate of infusion, then verifying and comparing patient identification, transfusion requisition, and blood bag label. The patient should be monitored closely for further development of signs and symptoms. Administration of epinephrine may be ordered.

Possible interventions in a more severe transfusion reaction may include immediate cessation of infusion, notification of the HCP, keeping the IV line open with saline or lactated Ringer solution, collection of red- and lavender-top tubes for posttransfusion work-up, collection of urine, monitoring vital signs every 5 min, ordering additional testing if DIC is suspected, maintaining patent airway and blood pressure, and administering mannitol.

C

C

Treatment Considerations

▶ Gas Exchange: Auscultate and trend breath sounds. Administer ordered oxygen and use pulse oximetry to monitor effectiveness. Collaborate with the health-care provider (HCP) to consider intubation and/or mechanical ventilation. Elevate the infant's head. Administer ordered blood or blood products and monitor Hgb and Hct.

Safety Considerations

▶ Explain the implications of positive test results in cord blood and newborn's bilirubin and Hct levels. Results may indicate the need for immediate exchange transfusion of fresh whole blood that has been typed and crossmatched with the mother's serum in order to identify the presence of unusual antibodies. Observation of the neonatal patient, especially for the development of jaundice, is an important way to identify a hemolytic process. Facilities not equipped for neonatal exchange transfusion may elect to transfer the neonate to a facility where the appropriate level of care can be provided. Handoff communication is a standardized approach to sharing information in an effort to minimize the risk of error or injury during transition between caregivers. The SBAR-R

(situation, background, assessment, recommendation, and read-back) format may be used as a communication tool to ensure mutual understanding of the clinical situation.

▶ Injury Risk: Administer prescribed Rh(D) immune globulin RhoGAM intramuscular (IM) or Rhophylac IM or IV to the infant's mother. Obtain maternal blood type and crossmatch. Use bilirubin light for newborn. Administer prescribed iron supplements, erythropoietin, and blood transfusion to infant within blood transfusion guidelines. Monitor degree of jaundice and associated laboratory results, bilirubin, hemoglobin, and Hct.

Follow-Up, Evaluation, and Desired Outcomes

▶ Acknowledges the implications of positive test results in the event of a transfusion-associated reaction.

▶ Acknowledges the implications of positive test results in cord blood and reasons for recommendation of blood transfusion.

▶ Mother states the purpose of RhIG (Rh immune globulin) or RhoGam injection in relation to future pregnancies.

▶ Parents demonstrate proficiency in placing the infant under the bilirubin light and adhering to identified precautions.

Coombs Antiglobulin, Indirect

SYNONYM/ACRONYM: Indirect antiglobulin test (IAT), antibody screen.

RATIONALE: To check recipient serum for antibodies prior to blood transfusion.

PATIENT PREPARATION: There are no food, fluid, activity, or medication restrictions unless by medical direction.

NORMAL FINDINGS: (Method: Agglutination) Negative (no agglutination).

CRITICAL FINDINGS AND POTENTIAL INTERVENTIONS: N/A

OVERVIEW: (Study type: Blood collected in a red-top tube; **related body system:** Circulatory/Hematopoietic and Immune systems.) IAT detects and identifies unexpected circulating complement molecules or antibodies in the patient's serum. The first use of this test was for the detection and identification of anti-D using an indirect method. The test is now commonly used to screen a patient's serum for the presence of antibodies that may react against transfused red blood cells (RBCs). During testing, the patient's serum is allowed to incubate with reagent RBCs. The reagent RBCs used are from group O donors and have most of the clinically signifi-cant antigens present (D, C, E, c, e, K, M, N, S, s, Fy^a, Fy^b, Jk^a, and Jk^b). Antibodies present in the patient's serum coat antigenic sites on the RBC membrane. The reagent cells are washed with saline to remove any unbound antibody. Antihuman globulin is added in the final step of the test. If the patient's serum con-tains antibodies, the antihuman globulin will cause the antibody-coated RBCs to stick together or agglutinate. (See study titled "Blood Typing, Antibody Screen, and and Crossmatch" for more information regarding transfusion reactions.)

INDICATIONS

- Detect other antibodies in maternal blood that can be potentially harm-ful to the fetus.
- Determine antibody titers in Rh-negative women sensitized by an Rh-positive fetus.
- Screen for antibodies before blood transfusions.
- Test for the weak Rh-variant antigen D^u. Development of anti-D antibodies occur when Rh-negative women become sensitized by an Rh-positive fetus. Antibody titers should be performed as soon as a subsequent pregnancy becomes

known in order to appropriately anticipate management of hemo-lytic disease of the newborn. Mod-ern technology and more potent reagents provide better sensitivity, and for this reason, women who have the D^u variant will likely be typed as Rh-positive. Consequently, the AABB has determined weak D testing is no longer necessary to be used on obstetric patients. Women who have the weak D variant are tested using less sensitive reagents, and those typed as Rh-negative are candidates for immunization with Rh(D) immune globulin RhoGAM IM or Rhophylac IM or IV. Admin-istration of RhIG (Rh immune globulin) or RhoGam to these can-didates is not harmful. Whether the test is used currently varies among facilities.

INTERFERING FACTORS
Factors that may alter the results of the study

- Drugs and other substances that may cause a positive IAT include meropenem, methyldopa, penicillin, quinidine, and rifampin.
- Recent administration of dextran, whole blood or fractions, or IV contrast media can result in a false-positive reaction.

POTENTIAL MEDICAL DIAGNOSIS: CLINICAL SIGNIFICANCE OF RESULTS
Positive findings in

Circulating antibodies or medications attach to the patient's RBCs, and hemo-lysis occurs. Agglutination is graded from 1+ to 4+ in manual testing sys-tems, with 4+ being the strongest degree of agglutination. Automated testing systems are capable of report-ing 1+ to 4+ graded results, providing images of the tested material so labo-ratory professionals can interpret the results, or providing computer-assisted interpretation of the test results as positive or negative findings.

- Hemolytic anemia *(autoimmune or induced by drugs or other substances)*
- Hemolytic disease of the newborn *(related to ABO or Rh incompatibility)*
- Incompatible crossmatch
- Infections (mycoplasma pneumonia, mononucleosis)

Negative findings in

- Samples in which the patient's antibodies exhibit dosage effects (i.e., stronger reaction with homozygous than with heterozygous expression of an antigen) and reagent erythrocyte antigens contain single-dose expressions of the corresponding antigen (heterozygous)
- Samples in which reagent erythrocyte antigens are unable to detect low-prevalence antibodies
- Samples in which sensitization of erythrocytes has not occurred (true negative, complete absence of antibodies)

NURSING IMPLICATIONS

BEFORE THE STUDY: PLANNING AND IMPLEMENTATION

Teaching the Patient What to Expect
▶ Inform the patient this test can assist in assessing for blood compatibility prior to transfusion.
▶ Explain that a blood sample is needed for the test. Prenatal mothers may be concerned about blood collection from their newborn. Explain that a cord sample of blood taken from the infant at the time of delivery does not result in infant blood loss.

Potential Nursing Actions
▶ Discussion of the patient's transfusion history, especially any problems encountered during blood product transfusion, is important. Note any recent or past blood or blood product transfusion or bone marrow transplantation that could complicate or interfere with test results.

◈ *If transfusion is expected, ensure that informed and written consent is obtained prior to blood administration.*

AFTER THE STUDY: POTENTIAL NURSING ACTIONS

Avoiding Complications
▶ Acute hemolytic reactions, whether immune mediated or developed due to sensitivities to drugs or other substances, can be immediate and life threatening. Chronic hemolytic anemia is also a significant condition that requires timely identification of the problem in order to treat the condition.

Positive findings in the pregnant patient may require further investigation by amniocentesis. Any sampling method that involves penetration of natural tissue barriers carries the risk of infection. Incidental maternal Rh sensitization can result from fetal RBCs mixing with blood of an Rh-negative mother carrying an Rh-positive fetus.

Treatment Considerations
▶ Negative tests during the first 12 wk of gestation should be repeated at 28 wk to rule out the presence of an antibody.
▶ Positive test results in pregnant women after 28 wk of gestation indicate the need for antibody identification testing.

Safety Considerations
▶ It is important for the patient to be made aware of the presence of unusual antibodies. A person may have circulating antibodies, other than ABO/Rh group antibodies, which may respond to transfused blood. The antibodies attach to the person's RBCs, damaging the integrity of the cell wall, and hemolysis occurs. Therefore, it is important to screen for the presence of antibodies

in the recipient's serum prior to transfusion. Unexpected antibodies, other than ABO/Rh, can develop at any time. If present in maternal blood, they can be potentially harmful to the fetus, which makes antibody screening an important test in prenatal care.

Follow-Up, Evaluation, and Desired Outcomes

▶ Acknowledges the importance of knowing transfusion history and the presence of unusual antibodies in order to prevent a potentially fatal transfusion reaction should the need for a blood product transfusion arise.

Copper

SYNONYM/ACRONYM: Cu.

RATIONALE: To evaluate and monitor exposure to copper and to assist in diagnosing Wilson disease.

PATIENT PREPARATION: There are no food, fluid, activity, or medication restrictions unless by medical direction.

NORMAL FINDINGS: Method: Inductively coupled plasma-mass spectrometry.

Age	Conventional Units	SI Units (Conventional Units × 0.157)
Newborn	9–46 mcg/dL	1.4–7.2 micromol/L
Child	80–150 mcg/dL	12.6–23.6 micromol/L
15–19 yr	80–171 mcg/dL	12.6–26.8 micromol/L
Adult		
Male	71–141 mcg/dL	11.1–22.1 micromol/L
Female	80–155 mcg/dL	12.6–24.3 micromol/L
Pregnant female	118–302 mcg/dL	18.5–47.4 micromol/L

Values for people of African descent are 8% to 12% higher. Values increase in older adults.

CRITICAL FINDINGS AND POTENTIAL INTERVENTIONS: N/A

OVERVIEW: (**Study type:** Blood collected in a royal blue-top, trace element–free tube; **related body system:** Circulatory/Hematopoietic and Digestive systems.) Copper is an important cofactor for the enzymes that participate in the formation of hemoglobin and collagen. Copper is also a component of coagulation factor V and assists in the oxidation of glucose. It is required for melanin pigment formation and maintenance of myelin sheaths and is used to synthesize ceruloplasmin. Copper levels vary with intake. Levels vary diurnally and peak during morning hours. This mineral is absorbed in the stomach and duodenum, stored in the liver, and excreted in urine and in feces with bile salts. Copper deficiency results in neutropenia and a hypochromic, microcytic anemia that is not responsive to iron therapy. Other signs and symptoms of copper deficiency include osteoporosis, depigmentation of skin and hair, impaired immune system response, and possible neurological and cardiac abnormalities.

Knowledge of genetics assists in identifying those who may benefit from additional education, risk assessment, and counseling. Genetics is the study and identification of genes, genetic mutations, and inheritance. For example, genetics provides some insight into the likelihood of inheriting a medical condition such as Menkes disease (syndrome) or Wilson disease. Some conditions are the result of mutations involving a single gene, whereas other conditions may involve multiple genes and/or multiple chromosomes. Menkes disease is an example of a recessive sex-linked genetic disorder passed on from a mother to male children; approximately 30% of cases result from "new" mutations in the affected gene, which means those patients will not have a family history of the disease. Wilson disease is an example of an autosomal recessive disorder in which the offspring inherits a copy of the defective gene from each parent. Further information regarding inheritance of genes can be found in the study titled "Genetic Testing."

INDICATIONS

• Assist in establishing a diagnosis of Menkes disease.

• Assist in establishing a diagnosis of Wilson disease.
• Monitor patients receiving long-term parenteral nutrition therapy.

INTERFERING FACTORS

Factors that may alter the results of the study

• Drugs and other substances that may increase copper levels include anticonvulsants and oral contraceptives.
• Drugs and other substances that may decrease copper levels include citrates, penicillamine, and valproic acid.

Other considerations

• Excessive therapeutic intake of zinc may interfere with intestinal absorption of copper.

POTENTIAL MEDICAL DIAGNOSIS: CLINICAL SIGNIFICANCE OF RESULTS

Increased in

Ceruloplasmin is an acute-phase reactant protein and the main protein binder of copper; therefore, copper levels will be increased in many inflammatory conditions, including cancer. Estrogens increase levels of binding protein; therefore, copper is elevated in pregnancy and estrogen therapy.

• Anemias *(related to increased red blood cell [RBC] production)*
• Ankylosing rheumatoid spondylitis
• Biliary cholangitis *(related to release from damaged liver tissue)*
• Collagen diseases
• Complications of hemodialysis *(trace element disturbances related to contamination from dialysate fluid and the disease process itself can be significant and can compound over time)*
• Hodgkin disease
• Infections

- Inflammation
- Leukemia
- Malignant tumors
- Myocardial infarction (MI) *(a correlation exists among copper levels, creatine kinase, and lactate dehydrogenase in MI; the pathophysiology is unclear, but some studies indicate a relationship between trace metal levels and risk of acute MI)*
- Pellagra *(related to niacin deficiency; niacin is an essential cofactor in reactions involving copper)*
- Poisoning from copper-contaminated solutions or insecticides *(related to excessive accumulation due to environmental exposure)*
- Pregnancy
- Pulmonary tuberculosis
- Rheumatic fever
- Rheumatoid arthritis
- Systemic lupus erythematosus
- Thalassemias *(related to zinc deficiency of thalassemia and increased rate of release from hemolyzed RBCs; copper and zinc compete for the same binding sites so that a deficiency in one results in an increase of the other)*
- Thyroid disease (hypothyroid or hyperthyroid) *(related to stimulation of thyroid hormone production by copper)*
- Trauma
- Typhoid fever
- Use of copper intrauterine device *(related to copper leaching from the device)*

Decreased in

- Burns *(related to loss of stores in tissue and possibly to competitive inhibition of zinc-containing medications or vitamins administered as part of burn therapy)*
- Cystic fibrosis *(related to inadequate intake and absorption)*

- Dysproteinemia *(related to decreased transport to and from stores)*
- Infants *(related to inadequate intake of milk or consumption of milk deficient in copper; especially premature infants)*
- Iron-deficiency anemias (some) *(related to decreased absorption of iron from the intestines and transfer from tissues to plasma; iron is essential to hemoglobin formation)*
- Long-term total parenteral nutrition *(related to inadequate intake)*
- Malabsorption disorders (celiac disease, tropical sprue) *(related to inadequate absorption)*
- Malnutrition *(related to inadequate intake)*
- Menkes disease *(evidenced by a severe genetic X-linked defect causing failed transport to the liver and tissues)*
- Nephrotic syndrome *(related to loss of transport proteins)*
- Occipital horn syndrome *(evidenced by an inherited disorder of copper metabolism; similar to Menkes disease)*
- Wilson's disease *(evidenced by a genetic defect causing failed transport to the liver and tissues)*

NURSING IMPLICATIONS

BEFORE THE STUDY: PLANNING AND IMPLEMENTATION

Teaching the Patient What to Expect

▶ Inform the patient this test can assist in monitoring the amount of copper in the body.
▶ Explain that a blood sample is needed for the test.

C

AFTER THE STUDY: POTENTIAL NURSING ACTIONS

Nutritional Considerations
- Instruct the patient with increased copper levels to avoid foods rich in copper and to increase intake of elements (zinc, iron, calcium, and manganese) that interfere with copper absorption.
- Copper deficiency does not normally occur in adults, but patients receiving long-term total parenteral nutrition should be evaluated if signs and symptoms of copper deficiency appear. These patients should be informed that organ meats, shellfish, nuts, and legumes are good sources of dietary copper.

Follow-Up, Evaluation, and Desired Outcomes
- Acknowledges contact information provided for the U.S. Department of Agriculture's resource for nutrition (www.choosemyplate.com).

Cortisol and Challenge Tests

SYNONYM/ACRONYM: Hydrocortisone, compound F.

RATIONALE: To assist in diagnosing adrenocortical insufficiency such as found in Cushing syndrome and Addison disease.

Procedure	Indications	Medication Administered	Recommended Collection Times
ACTH stimulation, rapid test	Suspect adrenal insufficiency (Addison disease) or congenital adrenal hyperplasia	1 mcg (low-dose physiologic protocol) cosyntropin intramuscular (IM) or IV; 250 mcg (standard pharmacologic protocol) cosyntropin IM or IV	3 cortisol levels: Baseline immediately before bolus, 30 min after bolus, and 60 min after bolus Note: Baseline and 30-min levels are adequate for accurate diagnosis using either dosage; low-dose protocol sensitivity is most accurate for 30 min level only

Procedure	Indications	Medication Administered	Recommended Collection Times
CRH stimulation	Differential diagnosis between ACTH-dependent conditions such as Cushing disease (pituitary source) or Cushing syndrome (ectopic source) and ACTH-independent conditions such as Cushing syndrome (adrenal source)	IV dose of 1 mg/kg ovine or human CRH	0800 cortisol and 0800 ACTH levels: Baseline collected 15 min before injection, 0 min before injection, and then 5, 15, 30, 60, 120, and 180 min after injection
Dexamethasone suppression (overnight)	Differential diagnosis between ACTH-dependent conditions such as Cushing disease (pituitary source) or Cushing syndrome (ectopic source) and ACTH-independent conditions such as Cushing syndrome (adrenal source)	Oral dose of 1 mg dexamethasone (Decadron) at 2300	Collect cortisol at 0800 on the morning after the dexamethasone dose
Metyrapone stimulation (overnight)	Suspect hypothalamic/pituitary disease such as adrenal insufficiency, ACTH-dependent conditions such as Cushing disease (pituitary source) or Cushing syndrome (ectopic source), and ACTH-independent conditions such as Cushing syndrome (adrenal source)	Oral dose of 30 mg/kg metyrapone with snack at midnight	Collect cortisol and ACTH at 0800 on the morning after the metyrapone dose

ACTH = adrenocorticotropic hormone; CRH = corticotropin-releasing hormone.

PATIENT PREPARATION: There are no food, fluid, activity, or medication restrictions unless by medical direction. Drugs that enhance steroid metabolism may be withheld by medical direction prior to metyrapone stimulation testing.

NORMAL FINDINGS: Method: Immunochemiluminescent assay.

Cortisol

Time	Conventional Units	SI Units (Conventional Units × 27.6)
0800		
Birth–1 wk	2–11 mcg/dL	55–304 nmol/L
1 wk–adult/older adult	5–25 mcg/dL	138–690 nmol/L
1600		
1 wk–dult/older adult	3–16 mcg/dL	83–442 nmol/L

Long-term use of corticosteroids in patients, especially older adults, may be reflected by elevated cortisol levels. After the first week of life, cortisol levels approach adult levels.

ACTH Challenge Tests

ACTH (Cosyntropin) Stimulated, Rapid Test	Conventional Units	SI Units (Conventional Units × 27.6)
Baseline	Cortisol greater than 5 mcg/dL	Greater than 138 nmol/L
30- or 60-min response	Cortisol 18–20 mcg/dL or incremental increase of 7 mcg/dL over baseline value	497–552 nmol/L or incremental increase of 193 nmol/L over baseline value

Corticotropin-Releasing Hormone Stimulated Test	Conventional Units	
		SI Units (Conventional Units × 27.6)
	Cortisol peaks at greater than 20 mcg/dL within 30–60 min	Greater than 552 nmol/L
		SI Units (Conventional Units × 0.22)
	ACTH increases twofold to fourfold within 30–60 min	Twofold to fourfold increase within 30–60 min

Dexamethasone Suppressed Overnight Test	Conventional Units	SI Units (Conventional Units × 27.6)
	Cortisol less than 1.8 mcg/dL next day	Less than 49.7 nmol/L

Metyrapone Stimulated Overnight Test	Conventional Units	
		SI Units (Conventional Units × 27.6)
	Cortisol less than 3 mcg/dL next day	Less than 83 nmol/L
		SI Units (Conventional Units × 0.22)
	ACTH greater than 75 pg/mL	Greater than 16.5 pmol/L
		SI Units (Conventional Units × 28.9)
	11-Deoxycortisol greater than 7 mcg/dL	Greater than 202 nmol/L

CRITICAL FINDINGS AND POTENTIAL INTERVENTIONS: N/A

OVERVIEW: (**Study type:** Blood collected in a red-, green-, or red/gray-top tube; **related body system:** Endocrine system.) Cortisol (hydrocortisone) is the predominant glucocorticoid secreted by the adrenal glands in response to pituitary ACTH. Cortisol is responsible for a number of regulatory functions, which include stimulation of gluconeogenesis (generation of glucose from amino acids by the liver), breaking down fats to generate energy, acting as an insulin antagonist by increasing glucose levels, responding to stress, and suppressing inflammation. Measuring levels of cortisol in blood is the best indicator of adrenal function.

Cortisol secretion varies diurnally, with highest levels occurring on awakening and lowest levels occurring late in the day, although bursts of cortisol excretion can occur at night. This pattern may be reversed in individuals who sleep during daytime hours and are active during nighttime hours. Cortisol and ACTH test results are evaluated together because they each control the other's concentrations (i.e., any change in one causes a change in the other). ACTH levels exhibit a diurnal variation, peaking between 0600 and 0800 and reaching the lowest point between 1800 and 2300. (See study titled "Adrenocorticotropic Hormone (and Challenge

Tests).") Salivary cortisol levels are known to parallel blood levels and can be used to screen for Cushing disease and Cushing syndrome.

There are three main conditions that can result from an imbalance in cortisol levels. Cushing syndrome is a complex condition that results from excessive levels of cortisol, regardless of the cause. Cushing disease is a condition in which the pituitary gland releases too much ACTH, resulting in overproduction of cortisol. Addison disease is caused by failure of the adrenal glands to produce cortisol.

INDICATIONS
- Detect adrenal hyperfunction (Cushing syndrome).
- Detect adrenal hypofunction (Addison disease).

INTERFERING FACTORS
Contraindications
Patients with suspected adrenal insufficiency should not undergo the metyrapone stimulation test because it may induce an acute adrenal crisis, a life-threatening condition, in patients whose adrenal function is already compromised.

Factors that may alter the results of the study
- Drugs and other substances that may increase cortisol levels include anticonvulsants, clomipramine, corticotropin, cortisone, CRH, ether, gemfibrozil, hydrocortisone, insulin, lithium, methadone, metoclopramide, mifepristone, naloxone, opiates, oral contraceptives, ranitidine, tetracosactrin, and vasopressin.
- Drugs and other substances that may decrease cortisol levels include barbiturates, beclomethasone, betamethasone, clonidine, desoximetasone, dexamethasone, ephedrine, etomidate, fluocinolone, ketoconazole, levodopa, lithium, methylprednisolone, metyrapone, midazolam, morphine, nitrous oxide, oxazepam, phenytoin, ranitidine, and trimipramine.
- Test results are affected by the time this test is done because cortisol levels vary diurnally.
- Stress and excessive physical activity can produce elevated levels.

Other considerations
- Normal values can be obtained in the presence of partial pituitary deficiency.

POTENTIAL MEDICAL DIAGNOSIS: CLINICAL SIGNIFICANCE OF RESULTS
The dexamethasone suppression test is useful in differentiating the causes for increased cortisol levels. Dexamethasone is a synthetic steroid that suppresses secretion of ACTH. With this test, a baseline morning cortisol level is collected, and the patient is given a 1-mg dose of dexamethasone at bedtime. A second specimen is collected the following morning. If cortisol levels have not been suppressed, adrenal adenoma may be suspected. The dexamethasone suppression test also produces abnormal results in patients with mental health disorders.

The CRH stimulation test works as well as the dexamethasone suppression test in distinguishing Cushing disease from conditions in which ACTH is secreted ectopically. In this test, cortisol levels are measured after an injection of CRH. A fourfold increase in cortisol levels above baseline is seen in Cushing disease. No increase in cortisol is seen if ectopic ACTH secretion is the cause.

The ACTH (cosyntropin)-stimulated rapid test is used when adrenal insufficiency is suspected. Cosyntropin is a synthetic form of ACTH. A baseline cortisol level is collected before the injection of cosyntropin. Specimens are subsequently collected at 30- and 60-min intervals. If the adrenal glands are functioning normally, cortisol levels rise significantly after administration of cosyntropin.

The metyrapone stimulation test is used to distinguish corticotropin-dependent (pituitary Cushing disease and ectopic Cushing disease) from corticotropin-independent (cancer of the lung or thyroid) causes of increased cortisol levels. Metyrapone inhibits the conversion of 11-deoxycortisol to cortisol. Cortisol levels should decrease to less than 3 mcg/dL (SI: 83 nmol/L) if normal pituitary stimulation by ACTH occurs after an oral dose of metyrapone. Specimen collection and administration of

the medication are performed as with the overnight dexamethasone test.

Increased in
Conditions that result in excessive production of cortisol.

- Adrenal adenoma
- Cushing syndrome
- Ectopic ACTH production
- Hyperglycemia
- Pregnancy
- Stress

Decreased in
Conditions that result in adrenal hypofunction and corresponding low levels of cortisol.

- Addison disease
- Adrenogenital syndrome
- Hypopituitarism

Summary of the Relationship Between Cortisol and ACTH Levels in Conditions Affecting the Adrenal and Pituitary Glands

Disease	Cortisol Level	ACTH Level
Addison disease (adrenal insufficiency)	Decreased	Increased
Cushing disease (pituitary adenoma)	Increased	Increased
Cushing syndrome related to ectopic source of ACTH	Increased	Increased
Cushing's syndrome (ACTH independent; adrenal cancer or adenoma)	Increased	Decreased
Congenital adrenal hyperplasia	Decreased	Increased

NURSING IMPLICATIONS

POTENTIAL NURSING PROBLEMS: ASSESSMENT & NURSING DIAGNOSIS

Problems	Signs and Symptoms
Body image (related to increased androgen production [virilism, hirsutism], wasting of muscle and bone matrix, capillary fragility, purple striae, slender limbs, abnormal fat distribution [buffalo hump])	Negative verbalization of altered physical appearance, preoccupation with physical body changes, distress and refusal to talk about changed appearance, negative verbalization about changes in appearance, using clothing to conceal body changes

(table continues on page 408)

Problems	Signs and Symptoms
Fluid volume excess (water) *(related to sodium and water retention secondary to elevated cortisol levels)*	Edema, shortness of breath, increased weight, ascites, rales, rhonchi, and diluted laboratory values
Infection risk *(related to impaired immune response secondary to elevated cortisol level)*	Delayed wound healing, inhibited collagen formation, impaired blood flow to edematous tissues, symptoms of infection (temperature, increased heart rate, increased blood pressure, shaking, chills, mottled skin, lethargy, fatigue, swelling, edema, pain, localized pressure, diaphoresis, night sweats, confusion, vomiting, nausea, headache)
Injury risk *(related to poor wound healing, decreased bone density, capillary fragility)*	Easy bruising, blood in stool, skin breakdown, fracture, poor wound healing

C

BEFORE THE STUDY: PLANNING AND IMPLEMENTATION

Teaching the Patient What to Expect
- Inform the patient this test can assist in assessing for the amount of cortisol in the blood.
- Explain that a blood sample is needed for the test.

Potential Nursing Actions
- Weigh patient and report weight to pharmacy for dosing of metyrapone (30 mg/kg body weight to a maximum dose of 3 g).
- Instruct the patient to minimize stress to avoid raising cortisol levels.

AFTER THE STUDY: POTENTIAL NURSING ACTIONS

Avoiding Complications
- Adverse reactions to metyrapone include nausea and vomiting, abdominal pain, headache, dizziness, sedation, allergic rash, decreased white blood cell count, or bone marrow depression. Monitor the patient for hypotension, rapid and weak pulse, rapid respiratory rate, pallor, and extreme weakness that may indicate the patient is in acute adrenocortical insufficiency (addisonian crisis). Other signs and symptoms include cardiac arrhythmias, hypotension, dehydration, anxiety, confusion, impairment of consciousness, epigastric pain, diarrhea, hyponatremia, and hyperkalemia.

Metyrapone may cause gastrointestinal (GI) distress and/or confusion. Administer oral dose of metyrapone with milk and snack.

Treatment Considerations
- Body Image: Assess the patient's perception of ongoing physical changes. Note the frequency of negative comments about changed physical state. Assist in the identification of positive coping strategies to address changed physical appearance. Provide reassurance that changes in physical appearance will improve as hormones return to normal level. Provide a referral to local support groups.
- Fluid Volume Overload: Weigh daily and record trends. Ensure accurate intake and output. Monitor laboratory values that reflect alterations in fluid status: potassium, sodium, blood urea nitrogen, creatinine, calcium, hemoglobin, and hematocrit. Manage underlying cause of fluid overload.

Assess and trend heart rate, respiratory rate, and blood pressure. Assess for symptoms of fluid overload such as jugular venous distention, shortness of breath, dyspnea, crackles. Administer prescribed diuretic, and antihypertensive. Elevate feet when sitting and monitor oxygenation with pulse oximetry.

▶ Infection Risk: Decrease exposure to environment by placing the patient in a private room. Monitor and trend vital signs and laboratory values that would indicate an infection: white blood cells and C-reactive protein (CRP). Promote good hygiene and assist with hygiene as needed. Administer prescribed antibiotics and antipyretics. Ensure careful, judicious use of ordered IV fluids. Monitor vital signs, trend temperatures, and encourage oral fluids. Adhere to standard precautions, isolate as appropriate, obtain cultures as ordered, and encourage use of lightweight clothing and bedding.

▶ Observe/assess the patient who has been administered metyrapone for signs and symptoms of an acute adrenal (addisonian) crisis, which may include abdominal pain, nausea, vomiting, hypotension, tachycardia, tachypnea, dehydration, excessively increased perspiration of the face and hands, sudden and significant fatigue or weakness, confusion, loss of consciousness, shock, coma. Potential interventions include immediate corticosteroid replacement (IV or IM), airway protection and maintenance, administration of dextrose for hypoglycemia, correction of electrolyte imbalance, and rehydration with IV fluids.

Safety Considerations
▶ Injury Risk: Assess for bruising, skin breakdown, and the progress of wound healing. Facilitate ordered bone density screening.
▶ Teach patient to use devices that will decrease injury risk, such as soft toothbrush or electric razor.

Nutritional Considerations
▶ The patient identifies and selects a diet that is high in fiber and drinks plenty of fluids to prevent constipation and potential GI bleed.
▶ Assess the patient with regard to the effects of abnormal cortisol levels, and monitor blood glucose levels to identify hyperglycemia associated with elevated cortisol.

Follow-Up, Evaluation, and Desired Outcomes
▶ Acknowledges contact information provided for the Cushing's Support and Research Foundation (https://csrf.net).
▶ Adheres to health-care provider's recommendation to increase the intake of calcium and vitamin D.
▶ Adheres to the request to maintain good personal hygiene, including frequent hand hygiene.

C-Peptide

SYNONYM/ACRONYM: Connecting peptide insulin, insulin C-peptide, proinsulin C-peptide.

RATIONALE: To evaluate hypoglycemia, assess beta cell function, and monitor insulin production.

PATIENT PREPARATION: There are no fluid, activity, or medication restrictions unless by medical direction. Instruct the patient to fast for at least 10 hr before specimen collection. Protocols may vary among facilities.

NORMAL FINDINGS: Method: Immunochemiluminometric assay (ICMA).

Age	Conventional Units	SI Units (Conventional Units × 0.333)
Child	0–3.3 ng/mL	0–1.1 nmol/L
Adult	0.8–3.5 ng/mL	0.3–1.2 nmol/L
1-hr response to glucose	2.3–11.8 ng/mL	0.8–3.9 nmol/L

CRITICAL FINDINGS AND POTENTIAL INTERVENTIONS: N/A

OVERVIEW: (**Study type:** Blood collected in a red-top tube; **related body system:** Endocrine system.) C-peptide is a biologically inactive peptide formed when beta cells of the pancreas convert proinsulin to insulin; therefore, C-peptide and insulin levels normally correlate. Most of C-peptide is excreted by the kidneys. C-peptide levels provide a reliable indication of how well the pancreatic beta cells secrete insulin. Release of C-peptide is not affected by exogenous insulin administration and levels can assist the healthcare provider (HCP) to determine when to begin treatment with insulin. C-peptide values increase after stimulation with glucose or glucagon, and measurement of C-peptide levels are very useful in the evaluation of hypoglycemia. An insulin/C-peptide ratio of 1 or less indicates endogenous insulin secretion, whereas a ratio greater than 1 indicates an excess of exogenous insulin. For additional information regarding screening guidelines and management of diabetes refer to the study titled "Glucose."

INDICATIONS
- Assist in the diagnosis of insulinoma: Serum levels of insulin and C-peptide are elevated.

- Detect suspected factitious cause of hypoglycemia (excessive insulin administration): An increase in blood insulin from injection does not increase C-peptide levels.
- Determine beta cell function when insulin antibodies preclude accurate measurement of serum insulin production.
- Evaluate hypoglycemia *(related to excessive consumption of alcohol, insulinoma, kidney disease, liver disease, or liver enzyme deficiencies [inherited glycogen storage enzyme deficiencies]).*
- Evaluate viability of beta cell or pancreatic transplant.

INTERFERING FACTORS
Factors that may alter the results of the study
- Drugs and other substances that may increase C-peptide levels include betamethasone, chloroquine, danazol, deferoxamine, ethinyl estradiol, glibenclamide, glimepiride, indapamide, oral contraceptives, piretanide, prednisone, and rifampin.
- Drugs and other substances that may decrease C-peptide levels include atenolol and calcitonin.

Other considerations
- C-peptide and endogenous insulin levels do not always correlate in obese patients.

POTENTIAL MEDICAL DIAGNOSIS: CLINICAL SIGNIFICANCE OF RESULTS

Increased in

- **Chronic kidney disease or end stage renal disease** *(increase in circulating levels of C-peptide related to decreased renal excretion)*
- **Islet cell tumor (e.g., insulinoma)** *(related to excessive endogenous insulin production)*
- **Pancreas or beta cell transplants** *(related to increased insulin production)*
- **Type 2 diabetes** *(related to increased insulin production)*

Decreased in

- **Factitious hypoglycemia** *(related to decrease in blood glucose levels in response to insulin injection)*
- **Pancreatectomy** *(evidenced by absence of the pancreas)*
- **Type 1 diabetes** *(evidenced by insufficient production of insulin by the pancreas)*

NURSING IMPLICATIONS

BEFORE THE STUDY: PLANNING AND IMPLEMENTATION

Teaching the Patient What to Expect

- Inform the patient this test can assist in assessing for low blood sugar.
- Explain that a blood sample is needed for the test.

AFTER THE STUDY: POTENTIAL NURSING ACTIONS

Avoiding Complications

- Emphasize, as appropriate, that good management of glucose levels delays the onset and slows the progression of diabetic retinopathy, nephropathy,

and neuropathy. Teach the patient that diabetes that is unmanaged can cause multiple health issues, including chronic kidney disease, amputation of limbs, and ultimately death. Emphasize the importance of adhering to the HCP-recommended therapeutic regime to manage diabetes. Discuss the advantages of attendance in support group meetings to learn how to manage the disease process from other people with diabetes.

Nutritional Considerations

- Increased levels of C-peptide may be associated with diabetes. There is no "diabetic diet"; however, many meal-planning approaches with nutritional goals are endorsed by the American Diabetes Association. Patients who adhere to dietary recommendations report a better general feeling of health, better weight management, greater management of glucose and lipid values, and improved use of insulin. Instruct the patient, as appropriate, in nutritional management of diabetes. A variety of dietary patterns are beneficial for people with diabetes. Encourage consultation with a registered dietitian who is a certified diabetes educator.

Follow-Up, Evaluation, and Desired Outcomes

- Acknowledges contact information provided for the American Heart Association (www.heart.org/HEARTORG), the National Heart, Lung, and Blood Institute (www.nhlbi.nih.gov), or the U.S. Department of Agriculture's resource for nutrition (www.choosemyplate.gov).
- Demonstrates how to perform a self-check glucose accurately and to correctly self-administer insulin or to take oral antihyperglycemic drugs. Understands the importance of reporting signs and symptoms of hypoglycemia (weakness, confusion, diaphoresis, rapid pulse) or hyperglycemia (thirst, polyuria, hunger, lethargy).

C

C-Reactive Protein

SYNONYM/ACRONYM: CRP.

RATIONALE: Conventional CRP assay indicates a nonspecific inflammatory response; the high-sensitivity test is used to assess risk for cardiovascular and peripheral arterial disease.

PATIENT PREPARATION: There are no food, fluid, activity, or medication restrictions unless by medical direction.

NORMAL FINDINGS: Method: Nephelometry.

High-Sensitivity Immunoassay (Cardiac Applications)	Conventional and SI Units
Low risk	Less than 1 mg/L
Average risk	1–3 mg/L
High risk	Greater than 3 mg/L (after repeat testing)

Conventional Assay	Conventional and SI Units
Adult	Less than 10 mg/L

CRITICAL FINDINGS AND POTENTIAL INTERVENTIONS: N/A

OVERVIEW: (**Study type:** Blood collected in a gold-, red-, or red/gray-top tube; **related body system:** Circulatory and Immune systems.) CRP is a glycoprotein produced by the liver in response to acute inflammation. The CRP assay is a nonspecific test that determines the presence (not the cause) of inflammation; it is often ordered in conjunction with erythrocyte sedimentation rate (ESR). CRP assay is a more sensitive and rapid indicator of the presence of an inflammatory process than ESR. CRP disappears from the serum rapidly when inflammation has subsided. The inflammatory process and its association with atherosclerosis make the presence of CRP, as detected by highly sensitive CRP assays, a potential marker for coronary artery disease (CAD). It is believed that the inflammatory process may instigate the conversion of a stable plaque to a weaker one that can rupture and occlude an artery.

INDICATIONS

Conventional Assay

• Assist in the differential diagnosis of appendicitis and acute pelvic inflammatory disease.

- Assist in the differential diagnosis of Crohn disease and ulcerative colitis.
- Assist in the differential diagnosis of rheumatoid arthritis and uncomplicated systemic lupus erythematosus (SLE).
- Detect the presence or exacerbation of inflammatory processes.
- Monitor response to therapy for autoimmune disorders such as rheumatoid arthritis.

High-Sensitivity Assay
- Assist in the evaluation of CAD.
- Detect the presence or exacerbation of inflammatory processes.

INTERFERING FACTORS

Factors that may alter the results of the study
- Drugs and other substances that may increase CRP levels include chemotherapy, interleukin-2, oral contraceptives, and pamidronate.
- Drugs and other substances that may decrease CRP levels include aurothiomalate, dexamethasone, gemfibrozil, leflunomide, methotrexate, NSAIDs, oral contraceptives (progestogen effect), penicillamine, pentopril, prednisolone, prinomide, and sulfasalazine.
- NSAIDs, salicylates, and steroids may cause false-negative results because of suppression of inflammation.
- Falsely elevated levels may occur with the presence of an intrauterine device.

Other considerations
- Lipemic samples that are turbid in appearance may be rejected for analysis when nephelometry is the test method.

POTENTIAL MEDICAL DIAGNOSIS: CLINICAL SIGNIFICANCE OF RESULTS

Increased in

Conditions associated with an inflammatory response stimulate production of CRP.

- Acute bacterial infections
- Crohn disease
- Inflammatory bowel disease
- Metabolic syndrome *(inflammation of the coronary vessels is associated with increased CRP levels and increased risk for coronary vessel injury, which may result in distal vessel plaque occlusions)*
- Myocardial infarction *(inflammation of the coronary vessels is associated with increased CRP levels and increased risk for coronary vessel injury, which may result in distal vessel plaque occlusions)*
- Pregnancy (second half)
- Rheumatic fever
- Rheumatoid arthritis
- SLE

Decreased in: N/A

NURSING IMPLICATIONS

BEFORE THE STUDY: PLANNING AND IMPLEMENTATION

Teaching the Patient What to Expect
- Inform the patient this test can assist in assessing for inflammation.
- Explain that a blood sample is needed for the test.

AFTER THE STUDY: POTENTIAL NURSING ACTIONS

Follow-Up, Evaluation, and Desired Outcomes
- Acknowledges that additional testing may be performed in order to evaluate or monitor progression of the disease process and determine the need for a change in therapy.

Creatine Kinase and Isoenzymes

SYNONYM/ACRONYM: CK and isoenzymes.

RATIONALE: To monitor MI and some disorders of the musculoskeletal system, such as Duchenne muscular dystrophy.

PATIENT PREPARATION: There are no food, fluid, activity, or medication restrictions unless by medical direction.

NORMAL FINDINGS: Method: Enzymatic for CK, electrophoresis for isoenzymes; enzyme immunoassay techniques are in common use for CK-MB.

	Conventional and SI Units
Total CK	
Newborn–1 yr	Up to 2 × adult values
Male (children and adults)	50–204 units/L
Female (children and adults)	36–160 units/L
CK Isoenzymes by Electrophoresis	
CK-BB	Absent
CK-MB	0–4%
CK-MM	96–100%
CK-MB by Immunoassay	0–5 ng/mL
CK-MB Index	0–2.5

CK = creatine kinase; CK-BB = CK isoenzyme in brain; CK-MB = CK isoenzyme in heart; CK-MM = CK isoenzyme in skeletal muscle.

The CK-MB index is the CK-MB (by immunoassay) divided by the total CK and then multiplied by 100. For example, a CK-MB by immunoassay of 25 ng/mL with a total CK of 250 units/L would have a CK-MB index of 10.

Elevations in total CK occur after exercise. Values in older adults may decline slightly related to loss of muscle mass.

CRITICAL FINDINGS AND POTENTIAL INTERVENTIONS: N/A

OVERVIEW: (**Study type:** Blood collected in a red- or red/gray-top tube; **related body system:** Circulatory and Musculoskeletal systems. Serial specimens are highly recommended. Care must be taken to use the same type of collection container if serial measurements are to be taken.) CK is an enzyme that exists almost exclusively in skeletal muscle, heart muscle, and, in smaller amounts, in the brain and lungs. This enzyme is important for intracellular storage and release of energy. Three isoenzymes, based on primary location, have been identified by electrophoresis: brain and lungs CK-BB, cardiac CK-MB, and skeletal muscle CK-MM. When injury to these tissues occurs, the enzymes are released into the bloodstream. Levels increase and decrease in a predictable timeframe. Measuring the serum levels can help determine the extent and timing of the damage. Noting the presence of the specific isoenzyme helps determine the location of the tissue damage. Atypical forms of CK can be identified. Macro-CK, an immunoglobulin complex of normal CK isoenzymes, has no clinical significance. Mitochondrial-CK is sometimes identified in the sera of seriously ill patients, especially those with metastatic cancers.

Acute MI releases CK into the serum within the first 48 hr; values return to normal in about 3 days. The isoenzyme CK-MB appears in the first 4 to 6 hr, peaks in 24 hr, and usually returns to normal in 72 hr. Recurrent elevation of CK suggests reinfarction or extension of ischemic damage. Significant elevations of CK are expected in early phases of muscular dystrophy, even before the clinical signs and symptoms appear. CK elevation diminishes as the disease progresses and muscle mass decreases. Differences in total CK with age and gender relate to the fact that the predominant isoenzyme is muscular in origin. Body builders have higher values, whereas older individuals have lower values because of deterioration of muscle mass.

Serial use of the mass assay for CK-MB with serial cardiac troponin I, myoglobin, and serial electrocardiograms in the assessment of MI has largely replaced the use of CK isoenzyme assay by electrophoresis. CK-MB mass assays are more sensitive and rapid than electrophoresis. Studies have demonstrated a high positive predictive value for acute MI when the CK-MB (by immunoassay) is greater than 10 ng/mL with a relative CK-MB index greater than 3.

Timing for Appearance and Resolution of Serum/Plasma Cardiac Markers in Acute MI

Cardiac Marker	Appearance (hr)	Peak (hr)	Resolution (d)
CK (total)	4–6	24	2–3
CK-MB	4–6	15–20	2–3
LDH	12	24–48	10–14
Myoglobin	1–3	4–12	1
Troponin I	2–6	15–20	5–7

INDICATIONS

- Assist in the diagnosis of acute MI and evaluate cardiac ischemia (CK-MB). For additional information regarding screening guidelines for *atherosclerotic cardiovascular disease* (ASCVD), refer to the study titled "Cholesterol, Total and Fractions."
- Detect musculoskeletal disorders that do not have a neurological basis, such as dermatomyositis or Duchenne muscular dystrophy (CK-MM).
- Determine the success of coronary artery reperfusion after fibrinolytic therapy or percutaneous transluminal angioplasty, as evidenced by a decrease in CK-MB.

INTERFERING FACTORS

Factors that may alter the results of the study

- Drugs and other substances that may increase total CK levels include aspirin, captopril, clofibrate, ethyl alcohol, propranolol, and statins.

- Drugs and other substances that may decrease total CK levels include dantrolene.

Other considerations
- Any intramuscularly injected preparations will increase CK levels because of tissue trauma caused by the injection.

POTENTIAL MEDICAL DIAGNOSIS: CLINICAL SIGNIFICANCE OF RESULTS
Increased in
CK is released from any damaged cell in which it is stored, so conditions that affect the brain, heart, or skeletal muscle and cause cellular destruction demonstrate elevated CK levels and correlating iso-enzyme source CK-BB, CK-MB, CK-MM.

- Alcohol misuse *(CK-MM)*
- Brain infarction (extensive) *(CK-BB)*
- Delirium tremens *(CK-MM)*
- Dermatomyositis *(CK-MM)*
- Gastrointestinal (GI) tract infarction *(CK-MM)*
- Head injury *(CK-BB)*
- Heart failure *(CK-MB)*
- Hypothyroidism *(CK-MM related to metabolic effect on and damage to skeletal muscle tissue)*

- Hypoxic shock *(CK-MM related to muscle damage from lack of oxygen)*
- Loss of blood supply to any muscle *(CK-MM)*
- Malignant hyperthermia *(CK-MM related to skeletal muscle injury)*
- MI *(CK-MB)*
- Muscular dystrophies *(CK-MM)*
- Myocarditis *(CK-MB)*
- Tumors of the prostate, bladder, and GI tract *(CK-MM)*
- Polymyositis *(CK-MM)*
- Pregnancy, during labor *(CK-MM)*
- Prolonged hypothermia *(CK-MM)*
- Pulmonary edema *(CK-MM)*
- Pulmonary embolism *(CK-MM)*
- Reye syndrome *(CK-BB)*
- Rhabdomyolysis *(CK-MM)*
- Surgery *(CK-MM)*
- Tachycardia *(CK-MB)*
- Tetanus *(CK-MM related to muscle injury from injection)*
- Trauma *(CK-MM)*

Decreased in
- Small stature *(related to lower muscle mass than average stature)*
- Sedentary lifestyle *(related to decreased muscle mass)*

NURSING IMPLICATIONS

POTENTIAL NURSING PROBLEMS: ASSESSMENT & NURSING DIAGNOSIS

Problems	Signs and Symptoms
Cardiac output *(related to prolonged myocardial ischemia, acute MI, reduced cardiac muscle contractility, ruptured papillary muscle, mitral insufficiency)*	Weak peripheral pulses; slow capillary refill; decreased urinary output; cool, clammy skin; tachypnea; dyspnea; altered level of consciousness; abnormal heart sounds; fatigue; hypoxia; loud holosystolic murmur; ECG changes; increased jugular venous distention
Pain *(related to myocardial ischemia, myocardial infarction)*	Reports of chest pain, new onset of angina, shortness of breath, pallor, weakness, diaphoresis, palpitations, nausea, vomiting, epigastric pain or discomfort, increased blood pressure, increased heart rate

C

Teaching the Patient What to Expect

▶ Inform the patient this test can assist in assessing for heart muscle cell damage.
▶ Explain that a blood sample is needed for the test. Inform the patient that a series of samples will be required. (Samples at time of admission and 2 to 4 hr, 6 to 8 hr, and 12 hr after admission are the minimal recommendations. Protocols may vary among facilities. Additional samples may be requested.)

Treatment Considerations

▶ Cardiac Output: Assess peripheral pulses and capillary refill. Monitor blood pressure and check for orthostatic changes. Assess respiratory rate, breath sounds, skin color and temperature, and level of consciousness. Monitor urinary output. Use pulse oximetry to monitor oxygenation and provide oxygen as ordered. Monitor ECG and administer ordered inotropic and peripheral vasodilator medications, nitrates.
▶ Pain: Assess pain characteristics, squeezing pressure, location in substernal back, neck, or jaw. Assess pain duration and onset; minimal exertion, sleep, or rest. Identify pain modalities that have relieved pain in the past. Monitor cardiac biomarkers: CK-MB, troponin, and myoglobin. Collaborate with ancillary departments to complete ordered echocardiography, exercise stress testing, or pharmacological stress testing. Administer prescribed pain medication, oxygen, anticoagulants, antiplatelets, beta blockers, calcium channel blockers, angiotensin-converting enzyme inhibitors, angiotensin II receptor blockers, or thrombolytic drugs.

Nutritional Considerations

▶ Discuss ideal body weight and the purpose of and relationship between ideal weight and caloric intake to support cardiac health. Review ways to decrease intake of saturated fats and increase intake of polyunsaturated fats. Discuss limiting intake of refined processed sugar and sodium; discuss limiting cholesterol intake to less than 300 mg per day. Encourage the intake of fresh fruits and vegetables, unprocessed carbohydrates, poultry, and grains.
▶ Nutritional therapy is recommended for those with identified CAD risk, especially for those with elevated low-density lipoprotein cholesterol levels, other lipid disorders, diabetes, insulin resistance, or metabolic syndrome. Always consider cultural influences with dietary choices to ensure better adherence to a change in lifestyle. A variety of dietary patterns are beneficial for people with ASCVD; for additional information regarding nutritional guidelines refer to the study titled "Cholesterol, Total and Fractions."
▶ Other changeable risk factors warranting education include strategies to encourage regular participation of moderate aerobic physical activity three to four times per week, eliminate tobacco use, and adhere to a heart-healthy diet.
▶ Those with elevated triglycerides should be advised to eliminate or reduce alcohol.

Follow-Up, Evaluation, and Desired Outcomes

▶ Acknowledges contact information provided for the American Heart Association (www.heart.org/HEARTORG), National Heart, Lung, and Blood Institute (www.nhlbi.nih.gov), or U.S. Department of Agriculture's resource for nutrition (www.choosemyplate.gov).
▶ Recognizes the importance of adequate rest, following a heart-healthy diet, and adherence to therapeutic regime to their overall health.

Creatinine, Blood

SYNONYM/ACRONYM: N/A

RATIONALE: To assess kidney function found in acute kidney injury and chronic kidney disease, related to drug reaction and disease such as diabetes.

PATIENT PREPARATION: There are no food, fluid, or medication restrictions unless by medical direction. Instruct the patient to refrain from excessive exercise for 8 hr before the test.

NORMAL FINDINGS: Method: Spectrophotometry.

Creatinine

Age	Conventional Units	SI Units (Conventional Units × 88.4)
Newborn	0.31–1.21 mg/dL	27–107 micromol/L
Infant	0.31–0.71 mg/dL	27–63 micromol/L
1–5 yr	0.31–0.51 mg/dL	27–45 micromol/L
6–10 yr	0.51–0.81 mg/dL	45–72 micromol/L
Adult male	0.61–1.21 mg/dL	54–107 micromol/L
Adult female	0.51–1.11 mg/dL	45–98 micromol/L

Cystatin C

Age	Conventional Units	SI Units (Conventional Units × 74.9)
1–50 yr	0.56–0.9 mg/L	41.9–67.4 mmol/L
Greater than 50 yr	0.58–1.08 mg/L	43.4–80.9 mmol/L

Values in older adults remain relatively stable after a period of decline related to loss of muscle mass during the transition from adult to older adult.

The National Kidney Foundation recommends the use of two decimal places in reporting serum creatinine for use in calculating estimated glomerular filtration rate.

CRITICAL FINDINGS AND POTENTIAL INTERVENTIONS

Adults
Potential critical finding is greater than 7.4 mg/dL (SI: 654.2 micromol/L) (patient not on dialysis).

Children
Potential critical finding is greater than 3.8 mg/dL (SI: 336 micromol/L) (patient not on dialysis).

Timely notification to the requesting health-care provider (HCP) of any critical findings and related symptoms is a role expectation of the professional nurse. A listing of these findings varies among facilities.

Consideration may be given to verification of critical findings before action is taken. Policies vary among facilities and may include requesting immediate recollection and retesting by the laboratory or retesting using a rapid point-of-care testing instrument at the bedside, if available.

Chronic renal insufficiency is identified by creatinine levels between 1.5 and 3 mg/dL (SI: 132.6 and 265.2 micromol/L); CKD is present at levels greater than 3 mg/dL (SI: 265.2 micromol/L).

Possible interventions may include renal or peritoneal dialysis and organ transplant, but early discovery of the cause of elevated creatinine levels might avoid such drastic interventions.

OVERVIEW: (**Study type:** Blood collected in a red-, green-, or red/gray-top tube; **related body system:** Musculoskeletal and Urinary systems.) Creatine resides almost exclusively in skeletal muscle, where it participates in energy-requiring metabolic reactions. A small amount of creatine is irreversibly converted to creatinine by the liver, which then circulates to the kidneys and is excreted. The amount of creatinine generated in an individual is proportional to the mass of skeletal muscle present and remains fairly constant throughout the life span; its consistency in production and clearance is the reason that creatinine is used as an indicator of kidney function. Creatinine values normally decrease with age owing to diminishing muscle mass. Conditions involving degenerative muscle wasting or massive muscle trauma from a crushing injury will also result in decreased creatinine levels. Blood urea nitrogen (BUN) is often ordered with creatinine for comparison. The BUN/creatinine ratio is also a useful indicator of kidney disease. The ratio should be between 10:1 and 20:1. The creatinine clearance test measures a blood sample and a urine sample to determine the rate at which the kidneys are clearing creatinine from the blood; this reflects the glomerular filtration rate, or GFR (see study titled "Creatinine, Urine, and Creatinine Clearance, Urine").

Chronic kidney disease (CKD) is a significant health concern worldwide. International studies have been undertaken to evaluate the risk factors common to cardiovascular disease, diabetes, and hypertension; these three diseases are all associated with CKD. Albuminuria, which can result from increased glomerular permeability to proteins, is considered an independent risk factor predictive of kidney or cardiovascular disease. There has also been an international effort by the National Kidney Disease Education Program (NKDEP), International Confederation of Clinical Chemistry and Laboratory Medicine, and European Communities Confederation of Clinical Chemistry (since renamed *European Federation of Clinical Chemistry and Laboratory Medicine*) to standardize methods to identify and monitor CKD. International efforts have resulted in development of an isotope dilution mass spectrometry (IDMS) reference method for standardized measurement of creatinine and use of equations to estimate glomerular filtration rate (eGFR) for both adults and children under the age of 18 yr. The equation for adults is based on factors identified in either the National Kidney Foundation (NKF)'s Modification of Diet in Renal Disease study or the Chronic Kidney Disease Epidemiology Collaboration equation using creatinine results from a method that has calibration traceable to IDMS. The equation includes four factors: serum or plasma creatinine value, age in years, gender, and race. The equation for adults is valid only for patients between the ages of 18 and 70. A correction factor is incorporated in the equation if the patient is of African descent because CKD is more prevalent in individuals of African descent; results are approximately 20% higher. An IDMS-traceable equation using serum creatinine results from a method that has a calibration traceable to the IDMS, referred to as the *bedside Schwartz equation,* is recommended for estimating GFR for children under 18 yr of age. The formula uses the patient's height in centimeters and the serum creatinine value where the GFR (mL/min/1.73 m2) = (0.41 × height cm)/serum creatinine mg/dL (SI Units: GFR (mL/min/1.73 m2) = (36.2 × height cm)/serum creatinine micromol/L. For consistency in the interpretation of test results, it is important to know whether the creatinine has been measured using IDMS-traceable test methods and equations. The equations have not been validated for pregnant women (GFR is significantly increased in pregnancy); patients older than 70; patients with serious comorbidities; or patients with extremes in body size, muscle mass, or nutritional status. eGFR calculators can be found at the NKDEP Web site (www.niddk.nih.gov/health-information/communication-programs/nkdep); links are provided for various calculators (e.g., adult and pediatric patients), select the appropriate link to access the desired calculator.

Cystatin C, also known as cystatin 3 and CST3, is now recognized as a useful marker for kidney damage and monitor of function in transplanted kidneys. It is a low-molecular-weight molecule belonging in the family of proteinase inhibitors. Cystatin C is produced by all nucleated cells in the body and is freely filtered by the glomerular membrane in the kidney. It is not secreted by the kidney tubules, and although a small amount is reabsorbed by the kidney tubules, it is metabolized in the tubules and does not reenter circulation. Therefore, its serum concentration is directly proportional to kidney function. It is believed to be a better marker of kidney function than creatinine because levels are independent of weight and height, diet, muscle mass, age, and sex.

INDICATIONS
- Assess a known or suspected disorder involving muscles in the absence of kidney disease.
- Evaluate known or suspected impairment of kidney function.

INTERFERING FACTORS
Factors that may alter the results of the study
- Drugs and other substances that may increase creatinine levels include acebutolol, acetaminophen (overdose), acetylsalicylic acid, amikacin, amiodarone, amphotericin B, arginine, arsenicals, ascorbic acid, asparaginase, barbiturates, capreomycin, captopril, carbutamide, carvedilol, cephalothin, chlorthalidone, cimetidine, cisplatin, clofibrate, colistin, corn oil (Lipomul),

cyclosporine, dextran, doxycycline, enalapril, ethylene glycol, gentamicin, indomethacin, ipodate, kanamycin, levodopa, mannitol, methicillin, mitomycin, neomycin, netilmicin, nitrofurantoin, NSAIDs, oxyphenbutazone, paromomycin, penicillin, pentamidine, phosphorus, plicamycin, radiographic medium, semustine, streptokinase, streptozocin, tetracycline, thiazides, tobramycin, triamterene, vancomycin, vasopressin, viomycin, and vitamin D.

- Drugs and other substances that may decrease creatinine levels include citrates, dopamine, ibuprofen, and lisinopril.
- High blood levels of bilirubin and glucose can cause false decreases in creatinine.
- A diet high in meat can cause increased creatinine levels.
- Ketosis can cause a significant increase in creatinine.

Other considerations
- Hemolyzed specimens are unsuitable for analysis.

POTENTIAL MEDICAL DIAGNOSIS: CLINICAL SIGNIFICANCE OF RESULTS
Increased in
- Acromegaly *(related to increased muscle mass)*
- Dehydration *(related to hemoconcentration)*

- Gigantism *(related to increased muscle mass)*
- Heart failure *(related to decreased renal blood flow)*
- Kidney disease, acute kidney injury, and CKD *(related to decreased urinary excretion)*
- Poliomyelitis *(related to increased release from damaged muscle)*
- Pregnancy-induced hypertension *(related to reduced GFR and decreased urinary excretion)*
- Renal calculi *(related to decreased kidney excretion due to obstruction)*
- Rhabdomyolysis *(related to increased release from damaged muscle)*
- Shock *(related to increased release from damaged muscle)*

Decreased in
- Decreased muscle mass *(related to debilitating disease or increasing age)*
- Hyperthyroidism *(related to increased GFR)*
- Inadequate protein intake *(related to decreased muscle mass)*
- Liver disease (severe) *(related to fluid retention)*
- Muscular dystrophy *(related to decreased muscle mass)*
- Pregnancy *(related to increased GFR and renal clearance)*
- Small stature *(related to decreased muscle mass)*

NURSING IMPLICATIONS

POTENTIAL NURSING PROBLEMS: ASSESSMENT & NURSING DIAGNOSIS

Problems	Signs and Symptoms
Cardiac output *(related to excess fluid volume, pericarditis, electrolyte imbalance, toxin accumulation)*	Weak peripheral pulses, slow capillary refill, decreased urinary output, cool clammy skin, tachypnea, dyspnea, altered level of consciousness, abnormal heart sounds, fatigue, hypoxia, loud holosystolic murmur, ECG changes, increased jugular venous distention (JVD)

(table continues on page 422)

Problems	Signs and Symptoms
Fluid volume excess (water)*(related to excess fluid and sodium intake, compromised renal function)*	Edema, shortness of breath, increased weight, ascites, rales, rhonchi, diluted laboratory values, distended neck veins, tachycardia, restlessness

C

BEFORE THE STUDY: PLANNING AND IMPLEMENTATION

Teaching the Patient What to Expect

▶ Inform the patient this test can assist in assessing kidney function.
▶ Explain that a blood sample is needed for the test.

AFTER THE STUDY: POTENTIAL NURSING ACTIONS

Treatment Considerations

▶ Cardiac Output: Assess peripheral pulses and capillary refill. Monitor blood pressure and check for orthostatic changes. Assess respiratory rate, breath sounds, skin color and temperature, and level of consciousness. Monitor urinary output. Use pulse oximetry to monitor oxygenation, administer ordered oxygen, and schedule ECG. Administer ordered inotropic and peripheral vasodilator medications, nitrates, sodium bicarbonate, glucose, and insulin drip.
▶ Fluid Volume Excess: Record daily weight and ensure accurate intake and output. Monitor laboratory values that reflect alterations in fluid status; potassium, BUN, Cr, calcium, Hgb, Hct, and sodium. Manage underlying cause of fluid alteration. Monitor urine characteristics. Establish baseline assessment data; heart rate, blood pressure, JVD, shortness of breath, dyspnea, or crackles. Ensure adherence to a low-sodium diet, administer prescribed diuretic and antihypertensive. Elevate feet when sitting and head of the bed when resting. Monitor oxygenation with pulse oximetry and ordered oxygen.

Nutritional Considerations

▶ Increased creatinine levels may be associated with kidney disease. The nutritional needs of patients with kidney disease vary widely and are in constant flux. Anorexia, nausea, and vomiting commonly occur, prompting the need for continuous monitoring for malnutrition, especially among patients receiving long-term hemodialysis therapy.

Follow-Up, Evaluation, and Desired Outcomes

▶ Acknowledges contact information provided for the American Diabetes Association (www.diabetes.org), NKF (www.kidney.org), or NKDEP (www.nkdep.nih.gov).

Creatinine, Urine, and Creatinine Clearance, Urine

SYNONYM/ACRONYM: N/A

RATIONALE: To assess and monitor kidney function related to acute kidney injury or chronic kidney disease.

PATIENT PREPARATION: There are no fluid or medication restrictions unless by medical direction. Instruct the patient to refrain from eating meat during the test and to refrain from excessive exercise for 8 hr before the test. Protocols may vary among facilities. Usually, a 24-hr urine collection is ordered. As appropriate, provide the required urine collection container and specimen collection instructions.

NORMAL FINDINGS: Method: Spectrophotometry.

Normal Urine Volume per 24 hr

These ranges are very general averages and were not calculated on the basis of normal average body weights. Literature shows that expected urinary output can be estimated by a formula in which the expected output is as follows:

Infants: 1–2 mL/kg/hr
Children and adolescents: 0.5–1 mL/kg/hr
Adults and older adults: 1 mL/kg/hr

Newborns	15–60 mL
Infants	
3–10 days	100–300 mL
11–59 days	250–450 mL
2–12 mo	400–500 mL
Children and adolescents	
13 mo–4 yr	500–700 mL
5–7 yr	650–1,000 mL
8–14 yr	800–1,400 mL
Adults and older adults	800–2,500 mL (average 1,200 mL)

Normally, more urine is produced during the day than at night. With advancing age, the reverse often occurs. The total expected outcome for adults appears to remain the same regardless of age.

Urine Creatinine		
Age	Conventional Units	SI Units
		Urine Creatinine (Conventional Units × 8.84)
2–3 yr	6–22 mg/kg/24 hr	53–194 micromol/kg/24 hr
4–18 yr	12–30 mg/kg/24 hr	106–265 micromol/kg/24 hr
Adult male	14–26 mg/kg/24 hr	124–230 micromol/kg/24 hr
Adult female	11–20 mg/kg/24 hr	97–177 micromol/kg/24 hr
	Creatinine Clearance	
		Creatinine Clearance (Conventional Units × 0.0167)
Children	70–140 mL/min/1.73 m²	1.17–2.33 mL/s/1.73 m²
Adult male	85–125 mL/min/1.73 m²	1.42–2.08 mL/s/1.73 m²
Adult female	75–115 mL/min/1.73 m²	1.25–1.92 mL/s/1.73 m²
For each decade after 40 yr	Decrease of 6–7 mL/ min/1.73 m²	Decrease of 0.06–0.07 mL/s/ 1.73 m²

The 24-hr urine volume is recorded and provided with the results of the creatinine measurement.

CRITICAL FINDINGS AND POTENTIAL INTERVENTIONS
- Degree of impairment:
  Borderline: 62.5–80 mL/min/1.73 m² (SI: 1–1.3 mL/s/1.73 m²)
  Slight: 52–62.5 mL/min/1.73 m² (SI: 0.9–1 mL/s/1.73 m²)
  Mild: 42–52 mL/min/1.73 m² (SI: 0.7–0.9 mL/s/1.73 m²)
  Moderate: 28–42 mL/min/1.73 m² (SI: 0.5–0.7 mL/s/1.73 m²)
  Marked: Less than 28 mL/min/1.73 m² (SI: Less than 0.5 mL/s/1.73 m²)

Timely notification to the requesting health-care provider (HCP) of any critical findings and related symptoms is a role expectation of the professional nurse. A listing of these findings varies among facilities.

OVERVIEW: (**Study type:** Urine from an unpreserved random or timed specimen collected in a clean plastic collection container; **related body system:** Urinary system.) Creatinine is the end product of creatine metabolism. Creatine resides almost exclusively in skeletal muscle, where it participates in energy-requiring metabolic reactions. In these processes, a small amount of creatine is irreversibly converted to creatinine, which then circulates to the kidneys and is excreted. The amount of creatinine generated in an individual is proportional to the mass of skeletal muscle present and remains fairly constant, unless there is massive muscle damage resulting from crushing injury or degenerative muscle disease. Creatinine values decrease with advancing age owing to diminishing muscle mass. Although the measurement of urine creatinine is an effective indicator of kidney function, the creatinine clearance test is more precise. The creatinine clearance test measures a blood sample and a urine sample to determine the rate at which the kidneys are clearing creatinine from the blood; this reflects the glomerular filtration rate (GFR) and is based on an estimate of body surface.

Chronic kidney disease (CKD) is a significant health concern worldwide. International studies have been undertaken to evaluate the risk factors common to cardiovascular disease, diabetes, and hypertension; these three diseases are all associated with CKD. Albuminuria, which can result from increased glomerular permeability to proteins, is considered an independent risk factor predictive of kidney or cardiovascular disease. There has also been an international effort by the National Kidney Disease Education Program (NKDEP), International Confederation of Clinical Chemistry and Laboratory Medicine, and European Communities Confederation of Clinical Chemistry (since renamed *European Federation of Clinical Chemistry and Laboratory Medicine*) to standardize methods to identify and monitor CKD. International efforts have resulted in development of an isotope dilution mass spectrometry (IDMS) reference method for standardized measurement of creatinine and use of equations to estimate glomerular filtration rate (eGFR) for both adults and children under the age of 18 yr. The equation for adults is based on factors identified in either the National Kidney Foundation (NKF)'s Modification of Diet in Renal Disease study or the Chronic Kidney Disease Epidemiology Collaboration (CKD-EPI) equation using creatinine results from a method that has calibration traceable to IDMS. The equation includes four factors: serum or plasma creatinine value, age in years, gender, and race. The equation for adults is valid only for patients between the ages of 18 and 70. A correction factor is incorporated in the equation if the patient is of African descent because CKD is more prevalent in individuals of African descent; results are approximately 20% higher. An IDMS-traceable equation using serum creatinine results from a method that has a calibration traceable to the IDMS, referred to as the *bedside Schwartz equation,* is recommended for estimating GFR for children under 18 yr of age. The formula uses the patient's height in centimeters and the serum creatinine value where the GFR (mL/min/1.73 m2) = (0.41 × height cm)/serum creatinine mg/dL (SI Units: GFR (mL/min/1.73 m2) = (36.2 × height cm)/serum creatinine micromol/L. For consistency in the interpretation of test results, it is important to know whether the creatinine has been measured using IDMS-traceable test methods and equations. The equations have not been validated for pregnant women (GFR is significantly increased in pregnancy); patients older than 70; patients with serious comorbidities; or patients with extremes in body size, muscle mass, or nutritional status. eGFR calculators can be found at the NKDEP Web site (www.niddk .nih.gov/health-information/communication-programs/

nkdep); links are provided for various calculators (e.g. adult and pediatric patients), select the appropriate link to access the desired calculator.

- **Creatinine clearance can be estimated from a blood creatinine level:**

  Creatinine clearance
  = [1.2 × (140 − age in years)
  × (weight in kg)]/blood
  creatinine level.

The result is multiplied by 0.85 if the patient is female; the result is multiplied by 1.18 if the patient is of African descent.

INDICATIONS

- Determine the extent of nephron damage in known kidney disease (at least 50% of functioning nephrons must be lost before values are decreased).
- Determine renal function before administering nephrotoxic drugs.
- Evaluate accuracy of a 24-hr urine collection based on the constant level of creatinine excretion.
- Evaluate glomerular function.
- Monitor effectiveness of treatment in kidney disease.

INTERFERING FACTORS

Factors that may alter the results of the study

- Drugs and other substances that may increase urine creatinine levels include ascorbic acid, cefoxitin, cephalothin, corticosteroids, levodopa, methotrexate, methyldopa, nitrofurans (including nitrofurazone), phenolphthalein, and prednisone.
- Drugs and other substances that may increase urine creatinine clearance include enalapril, oral contraceptives, prednisone, and ramipril.

- Drugs and other substances that may decrease urine creatinine levels include anabolic steroids, androgens, captopril, and thiazides.
- Drugs and other substances that may decrease the urine creatinine clearance include acetylsalicylic acid, amphotericin B, chlorthalidone, cimetidine, cisplatin, cyclosporine, guancidine, ibuprofen, indomethacin, mitomycin, oxyphenbutazone, probenecid (coadministered with digoxin), puromycin, and thiazides.
- Excessive ketones in urine may cause falsely decreased values.
- Failure to refrigerate specimen throughout urine collection period allows decomposition of creatinine, causing falsely decreased values.

Other considerations
- All urine voided for the timed collection period must be included in the collection or else falsely decreased values may be obtained. Compare output records with volume collected to verify that all voids were included in the collection.

POTENTIAL MEDICAL DIAGNOSIS: CLINICAL SIGNIFICANCE OF RESULTS
Increased in
- Acromegaly *(related to increased muscle mass)*
- Carnivorous diets *(related to increased intake of creatine, which is metabolized to creatinine and excreted by the kidneys)*
- Exercise *(related to muscle damage; increased renal blood flow)*
- Gigantism *(related to increased muscle mass)*

Decreased in
Conditions that decrease GFR, impair kidney function, or reduce renal blood flow will decrease renal excretion of creatinine.

- Acute or chronic glomerulonephritis

- Chronic bilateral pyelonephritis
- Kidney disease, acute kidney injury, and CKD *(related to decreased urinary excretion)*
- Leukemia
- Muscle wasting diseases *(related to abnormal creatinine production; decreased production reflected in decreased excretion)*
- Paralysis *(related to abnormal creatinine production; decreased production reflected in decreased excretion)*
- Polycystic kidney disease
- Pregnancy induced hypertension *(related to reduced GFR)*
- Shock
- Urinary tract obstruction (e.g., from calculi)
- Vegetarian diets *(evidenced by diets that exclude intake of animal muscle, the creatine source metabolized to creatinine and excreted by the kidneys)*

NURSING IMPLICATIONS

BEFORE THE STUDY: PLANNING AND IMPLEMENTATION

Teaching the Patient What to Expect
- Inform the patient this test can assist in assessing kidney function.
- Explain that a urine sample is needed for the test. Information regarding specimen collection is presented with other general guidelines in Appendix A: Patient Preparation and Specimen Collection.
- Inform the patient that a blood sample for creatinine will be required on the day urine collection begins or at some point during the 24-hr collection period (see study titled "Creatinine, Blood" for additional information).

Potential Nursing Actions
- Include on the collection container's label urine total volume, test start and stop times/dates, and any medications that may interfere with test results.

AFTER THE STUDY: POTENTIAL NURSING ACTIONS

Follow-Up, Evaluation, and Desired Outcomes

♦ Acknowledges contact information provided for the American Diabetes Association (www.diabetes.org), NKF (www.kidney.org), or NKDEP (www.nkdep.nih.gov).

♦ Recognizes the importance of counseling services to assist in coping with long-term disease implications associated with a chronic disorder.

Cryoglobulin

SYNONYM/ACRONYM: Cryo.

RATIONALE: To assist in identifying the presence of certain immunological disorders such as Reynaud phenomenon.

PATIENT PREPARATION: There are no food, fluid, activity, or medication restrictions unless by medical direction.

NORMAL FINDINGS: (Method: Visual observation for changes in appearance) Negative.

CRITICAL FINDINGS AND POTENTIAL INTERVENTIONS: N/A

OVERVIEW: (**Study type:** Blood collected in a red-top tube; **related body system:** Immune system.) Cryoglobulins are abnormal serum proteins that cannot be detected by protein electrophoresis. Cryoglobulins cause vascular problems because they can precipitate in the blood vessels of the fingers when exposed to cold, causing Raynaud phenomenon. They are usually associated with immunological disease. The laboratory procedure to detect cryoglobulins is a two-step process. The serum sample is observed for cold precipitation after 72 hr of storage at 4°C. True cryoglobulins disappear on warming to room temperature, so in the second step of the procedure, the sample is rewarmed to confirm reversibility of the reaction.

INDICATIONS

• Assist in diagnosis of neoplastic diseases, acute and chronic infections, and collagen diseases.
• Detect cryoglobulinemia in patients with symptoms indicating or mimicking Raynaud disease.
• Monitor course of collagen and rheumatic disorders.

INTERFERING FACTORS

Factors that may alter the results of the study

• Testing the sample prematurely (before total precipitation) may yield incorrect results.
• Failure to maintain sample at normal body temperature before centrifugation can affect results.

Other considerations

• A recent fatty meal can increase turbidity of the blood, decreasing visibility.

POTENTIAL MEDICAL DIAGNOSIS: CLINICAL SIGNIFICANCE OF RESULTS

Increased in

Cryoglobulins are present in varying degrees in associated conditions.

Type I cryoglobulin (monoclonal)
• Chronic lymphocytic leukemia
• Lymphoma
• Multiple myeloma

Type II cryoglobulin (mixtures of monoclonal immunoglobulin [Ig] M and polyclonal IgG)
• Autoimmune hepatitis
• Rheumatoid arthritis
• Sjögren syndrome
• Waldenström macroglobulinemia

Type III cryoglobulin (mixtures of polyclonal IgM and IgG)
• Acute poststreptococcal glomerulonephritis
• Chronic infection (especially hepatitis C)
• Cirrhosis
• Endocarditis
• Infectious mononucleosis
• Polymyalgia rheumatica
• Rheumatoid arthritis
• Sarcoidosis
• Systemic lupus erythematosus

Decreased in: N/A

NURSING IMPLICATIONS

BEFORE THE STUDY: PLANNING AND IMPLEMENTATION

Teaching the Patient What to Expect
▶ Inform the patient this test can assist in assessing for immune system disorders.
▶ Explain that a blood sample is needed for the test.

AFTER THE STUDY: POTENTIAL NURSING ACTIONS

Follow-Up, Evaluation, and Desired Outcomes
▶ Acknowledges that additional testing may be performed in order to evaluate or monitor progression of the disease process and determine the need for a change in therapy.

Culture, Bacterial Various Sites
(Anal/Genital, Ear, Eye, Skin, Wound, Blood, Sputum, Stool, Throat/Nasopharyngeal, Urine)

SYNONYM/ACRONYM: N/A

RATIONALE: To identify pathogenic bacterial organisms as an indicator for appropriate therapeutic interventions for multiple sites of infection, sepsis, and screen for methicillin-resistant *Staphylococcus aureus* (MRSA).

PATIENT PREPARATION: There are no food, fluid, or activity restrictions unless by medical direction. Whenever possible, specimens for culture should be collected before antimicrobial therapy begins as these medications will delay or inhibit growth of pathogens. As appropriate, provide the required urine collection container and specimen collection instructions.

NORMAL FINDINGS

Site	Method	Normal Findings
Anal/genital, ear, eye, skin, and wound	Culture aerobic and/or anaerobic on selected media; cell culture followed by use of direct immunofluorescence, nucleic acid amplification, polymerase chain reaction (PCR), and DNA probe assays (e.g., Gen-Probe) are available for identification of *Neisseria gonorrhoeae, Streptococcus agalactiae* (group B streptococcus [GBS]), and *Chlamydia trachomatis*	Culture, negative: No growth of pathogens Culture-enhanced PCR or other DNA assays, negative: None detected
Blood	Growth of organisms in standard culture media identified by radiometric or infrared automation, by manual reading of subculture, or PCR	Negative: No growth of pathogens
Sputum	Aerobic culture on selective and enriched media; microscopic examination of sputum by Gram stain	The presence of normal upper respiratory tract flora should be expected. Tracheal aspirates and bronchoscopy samples can be contaminated with normal flora, but transtracheal aspiration specimens should show no growth. Normal respiratory flora include *Neisseria catarrhalis, Candida albicans,* diphtheroids, α-hemolytic streptococci, and some staphylococci. The presence of normal flora does not rule out infection. A normal Gram stain of sputum contains polymorphonuclear leukocytes, alveolar macrophages, and a few squamous epithelial cells

(table continues on page 430)

Site	Method	Normal Findings
Stool	Culture on selective media for identification of pathogens usually to include *Salmonella, Shigella, Escherichia coli* 0157:H7, *Yersinia enterocolitica*, and *Campylobacter;* latex agglutination or enzyme immunoassay for *Clostridium* (A and B toxins). PCR may be used to identify bacterial, protozoan, or viral pathogens	Negative: No growth of pathogens. Normal fecal flora is 96% to 99% anaerobes and 1% to 4% aerobes. Normal flora present may include *Bacteroides, Candida albicans, Clostridium, Enterococcus, Escherichia coli, Proteus, Pseudomonas,* and *Staphylococcus aureus*
Throat/ nasopharyngeal	Aerobic culture	No growth
Urine	Culture on selective and enriched media	Negative: No growth

CRITICAL FINDINGS AND POTENTIAL INTERVENTIONS

Anal/Genital, Ear, Eye, Skin, and Wound Culture

- *Listeria* in genital cultures (Listeriosis in pregnant women may result in premature birth, miscarriage, or stillbirth. The earlier in pregnancy the infection occurs, the more likely that it will lead to miscarriage or fetal death. After 20 weeks' gestation, listeriosis is more likely to cause premature labor and birth.)
- Methicillin-resistant *Staphylococcus aureus* in skin or wound cultures
- GBS in urine or anal/genital cultures

Blood Culture

- Positive findings in any sterile body fluid such as blood

Sputum

- *Corynebacterium diphtheriae*
- *Legionella*

Stool

- Bacterial pathogens: *Campylobacter, Clostridium difficile, Escherichia coli* including 0157:H7, *Listeria, Rotavirus* (especially in pediatric patients), *Salmonella, Shigella, Vibrio, Yersinia,* or parasites *Acanthamoeba, Ascaris* (hookworm), *Cyclospora, Cryptosporidium, Entamoeba histolytica, Giardia,* and *Strongyloides* (tapeworm), parasitic ova, proglottid, and larvae.

Throat/Nasopharyngeal

- Culture: Growth of *Corynebacterium* or MRSA

Urine

- Gram-negative extended spectrum beta lactamases *Escherichia coli* or *Klebsiella*

- Gram-negative *Legionella*
- Gram-positive Vancomycin-resistant *Enterococci*

Timely notification to the requesting health-care provider (HCP) of any critical findings and related symptoms is a role expectation of the professional nurse. Lists of specific organisms may vary among facilities; specific organisms are required to be reported to local, state, and national departments of health.

Assess for signs and symptoms of sepsis or development of septic shock to include change in body temperature (greater than 101.3°F or less than 95°F); decreased systolic blood pressure (less than 90 mm Hg); increased heart rate (greater than 90 beats/min); sudden change in mental status (restlessness, agitation, or confusion); significantly decreased urine output (less than 30 mL/hr); increased respirations (greater than 20 breaths/min); change in extremities (pale, mottled, and/or cyanotic in appearance); decreased or absent peripheral pulses.

OVERVIEW: (Study type: Blood collected in bottles containing standard aerobic and anaerobic culture media, sterile body fluid [such as amniotic, cerebrospinal fluid, pericardial fluid, peritoneal fluid, pleural fluid, synovial], sputum, stool, throat/nasopharynx, urine or swab from affected area placed in transport media tube provided by laboratory. Stool sample should be a random, freshly collected specimen submitted in a clean plastic container. Urine should be collected in a sterile plastic collection container; transport tubes containing a preservative are highly recommended if urine testing will not occur within 2 hr of collection; related body system: Circulatory, Digestive, Immune, Integumentary, Nervous, Reproductive, Respiratory, and Urinary systems.)

Optimally, specimens should be obtained before antibiotic use. The method used to culture and grow the organism depends on the suspected infectious organism. There are transport media specifically for bacterial organisms. The laboratory will select the appropriate media for suspect organisms and will initiate antibiotic sensitivity testing if indicated by test results. Sensitivity testing identifies the antibiotics to which organisms are susceptible to ensure an effective treatment plan.

Anal and Genital Cultures
When indicated by patient history, anal and genital cultures may be performed to isolate the organism responsible for sexually transmitted infections (STIs). Chlamydia, gonorrhea, and syphilis are reportable STIs. Anal and genital cultures may also be performed on pregnant women to identify the presence of GBS, a significant and serious neonatal infection transmitted as the newborn passes through the birth canal of colonized mothers. Neonatal GBS is the most common cause of sepsis, pneumonia, and meningitis in newborns. The disease is classified as either early onset (first week of life) or late onset (after the first week of life). The Centers for Disease Control and Prevention (CDC), American Academy of Family Physicians, American Academy of Pediatrics, American College of Nurse-Midwives, and American College of Obstetricians and Gynecologists recommend universal screening for all pregnant women at 35 to 37 weeks' gestation. Pregnant patients with positive results for a GBS urinary tract infection (UTI) at

any time during pregnancy should receive appropriate medical treatment at the time of diagnosis and also receive intrapartum antibiotic prophylaxis to offer continued protection in the absence of complete eradication of the infection at the time of delivery. Rapid GBS test kits can provide results within minutes on vaginal or rectal fluid swab specimens submitted in a sterile red-top tube. Negative rapid test findings should be followed up with culture and Gram stain or culture-enhanced molecular methods.

Blood Cultures

Pathogens can enter the bloodstream from soft-tissue infection sites, contaminated IV lines, or invasive procedures (e.g., surgery, tooth extraction, cystoscopy). Blood cultures are collected whenever bacteremia (bacterial infection of the blood) or septicemia (a condition of systemic infection caused by pathogenic organisms or their toxins) is suspected.

Although mild bacteremia is found in many infectious diseases, a persistent, continuous, or recurrent bacteremia indicates a more serious condition that may require immediate treatment. Early detection of pathogens in the blood may aid in making clinical and etiological diagnoses.

Blood cultures can detect the presence of bacteria and fungi. Organisms can be classified in a number of ways; blood culture findings use oxygen requirements to categorize findings into one of two groups. Blood culture begins with the introduction of a blood specimen into two types of culture medium. The medium is designed to promote the growth of organisms; one group of organisms require oxygen (aerobic) and the other either requires sparing amounts to no oxygen at all (anaerobic).

A blood culture may also be done with an antimicrobial removal device (ARD) if antibiotic therapy is initiated prior to specimen collection. This involves transferring some of the blood sample into a special vial containing absorbent resins that remove antibiotics from the sample before the culture is performed.

Traditional automated culture methods entail incubation of inoculated culture containers for a specific length of time, at a specific temperature, and under other conditions suitable for growth. If organisms are present, they will produce carbon dioxide as they metabolize the nutrients in the culture media. The presence of carbon dioxide in the culture is detected when the culture bottles are "read" by an instrument at specified intervals over a period of time. There are a number of automated blood culture systems with sophisticated computerized algorithms. The complex software allows for frequent monitoring of growth throughout the day and rapid interpretation of culture findings. With these systems, as soon as a positive culture is detected, usually within 24 to 72 hr, the bottle can be removed from the system and a Gram stain performed to provide a preliminary identification of the bacteria present. This preliminary report provides an opportunity for the HCP to initiate therapy. A sample from the positive blood culture bottle is then subcultured on the appropriate plated media for growth, isolation, and positive identification of the organism.

The plated organisms are also used for sensitivity testing, if indicated. Sensitivity testing identifies the antibiotics to which the organisms are susceptible to ensure an effective treatment plan and can take several days. Negative cultures are generally removed from the automated culture system after 5 days and finalized as having "no growth." The subspecialty of microbiology has been revolutionized by molecular diagnostics. Molecular diagnostics involves the identification of specific sequences of DNA. The application of molecular diagnostics techniques, such as PCR, has led to the development of automated instruments that can identify a single infectious organism or multiple pathogens from a small amount of blood in less than 2 hr. The instruments can detect the presence of gram-negative bacteria, gram-positive bacteria, and yeast commonly associated with bloodstream infections. The instruments can also detect mutations in the genetic material of specific pathogens that code for antibiotic resistance.

Ear and Eye Cultures

Ear and eye cultures are performed to isolate the organism responsible for chronic or acute infectious disease of the ear and eye.

Skin and Soft Tissue Cultures

Skin and soft tissue samples from infected sites must be collected carefully to avoid contamination from the surrounding normal skin flora. Skin and tissue infections may be caused by both aerobic and anaerobic organisms. Therefore, a portion of the sample should be placed in aerobic and a portion in anaerobic transport media. Care must be taken to use transport media that are approved by the laboratory performing the testing.

Sputum Cultures

This test involves collecting a sputum specimen so the pathogen can be isolated and identified. The test results will reflect the type and number of organisms present in the specimen as well as the antibiotics to which the identified pathogenic organisms are susceptible. Sputum collected by expectoration or suctioning with catheters and by bronchoscopy cannot be cultured for anaerobic organisms; instead, transtracheal aspiration or lung biopsy must be used.

Sterile Fluid Cultures

Sterile fluids can be collected from the affected site. Refer to related body fluid studies (i.e., amniotic fluid, cerebrospinal fluid, pericardial fluid, peritoneal fluid, pleural fluid, synovial fluid) for specimen collection.

Stool Cultures

Stool culture involves collecting a sample of feces so that organisms present can be isolated and identified. Certain bacteria are normally found in feces. However, when overgrowth of these organisms occurs or pathological organisms are present, diarrhea or other signs and symptoms of systemic infection occur. These symptoms are the result of damage to the intestinal tissue by the pathogenic organisms. Routine stool culture normally screens for a small number of common pathogens associated with food poisoning, such as *Staphylococcus aureus, Salmonella,* and *Shigella.* Identification of other bacteria is initiated by special request or upon consultation

C

with a microbiologist when there is knowledge of special circumstances. An example of this situation is an outbreak of *Clostridium difficile* in a long-term care facility or hospital unit where the infection can spread rapidly from one person to the next. A life-threatening *Clostridium difficile* infection of the bowel may occur in patients who are immunocompromised or are receiving broad-spectrum antibiotic therapy (e.g., clindamycin, ampicillin, cephalosporins). The bacteria release a toxin that causes necrosis of the colon tissue. The toxin can be more rapidly identified from a stool sample using an immunochemical method than from a routine culture. Appropriate interventions can be quickly initiated and might include intravenous replacement of fluid and electrolytes, cessation of broad-spectrum antibiotic administration, and institution of vancomycin or metronidazole antibiotic therapy. The laboratory will initiate antibiotic sensitivity testing if indicated by test results. Sensitivity testing identifies the antibiotics to which organisms are susceptible to ensure an effective treatment plan.

The subspecialty of microbiology has been revolutionized by molecular diagnostics. Molecular diagnostics involves the identification of specific sequences of DNA. The application of molecular diagnostics techniques, such as PCR, has led to the development of automated instruments that can identify a single infectious agent or multiple pathogens from a small amount of stool in less than 2 hr. The instruments can detect the presence of bacteria, viruses, or protozoans commonly associated with gastrointestinal infections. Additional information about identification of pathogens in stool specimens (e.g., *Rotavirus, Clostridium difficile*) can be found in the study titled "Fecal Analysis."

Throat/Nasopharyngeal Cultures
The routine throat culture is a commonly ordered test to screen for the presence of group A β-hemolytic streptococci. *Streptococcus pyogenes* is the gram-positive organism that most commonly causes acute pharyngitis. The more dangerous sequelae of scarlet fever, rheumatic heart disease, and glomerulonephritis are less frequently seen because of the early treatment of infection at the pharyngitis stage. There are a number of other bacterial organisms responsible for pharyngitis. Specific cultures can be set up to detect other pathogens such as *Bordetella* (gram negative), *Corynebacteria* (gram positive), *Haemophilus* (gram negative), or *Neisseria* (gram negative) if they are suspected or by special request from the HCP. *Corynebacterium diphtheriae* is the causative pathogen of diphtheria. *Neisseria gonorrhoeae* is a sexually transmitted pathogen. In children, a positive throat culture for *Neisseria* usually indicates sexual abuse.

Urine Cultures
A urine culture involves collecting a urine specimen so that the organism causing disease can be isolated and identified. Urine can be collected by clean catch, urinary catheterization, or suprapubic aspiration. The severity of the infection or contamination of the specimen can be determined

by knowing the type and number of organisms (colonies) present in the specimen.

Commonly detected organisms are those normally found in the genitourinary tract, including gram-negative *Enterococci, Escherichia coli, Klebsiella, Proteus,* and *Pseudomonas.* A culture showing multiple organisms indicates a contaminated specimen.

Colony counts of 100,000/mL or more indicate UTI.

Colony counts of 1,000/mL or less suggest contamination resulting from poor collection technique.

Colony counts between 1,000 and 10,000/mL may be significant depending on a variety of factors, including patient's age, gender, number of types of organisms present, method of specimen collection, and presence of antibiotics.

Wound Cultures

A wound culture involves collecting a specimen of exudates, drainage, or tissue so that the causative organism can be isolated and pathogens identified. Specimens can be obtained from superficial and deep wounds.

INDICATIONS

General
- Determine effective antimicrobial therapy specific to the identified pathogen.
- Isolate and identify pathogenic microorganisms responsible for infection being investigated.

Anal/Genital
- Assist in the diagnosis of STIs.
- Determine the cause of genital itching or purulent drainage.
- Routine prenatal screening for vaginal and rectal GBS colonization.

Blood
- Determine sepsis in the newborn as a result of prolonged labor, early rupture of membranes, maternal infection, or neonatal aspiration.
- Evaluate chills and fever in patients with infected burns, UTI, rapidly progressing tissue infection, postoperative wound sepsis, and indwelling venous or arterial catheter.
- Evaluate intermittent or continuous temperature elevation of unknown origin.
- Evaluate persistent, intermittent fever associated with a heart murmur.
- Evaluate a sudden change in pulse and temperature with or without chills and diaphoresis.
- Evaluate suspected bacteremia after invasive procedures.
- Identify the cause of shock in the postoperative period.

Ear
- Isolate and identify organisms responsible for outer-, middle-, or inner-ear infection, ear pain, drainage, or changes in hearing.

Skin
- Isolate and identify organisms responsible for skin eruptions, drainage, or other evidence of infection.

Sputum
Additional Indications Regarding the Gram Stain
- Assist in the differentiation of gram-positive from gram-negative bacteria in respiratory infection.
- Assist in the differentiation of sputum from upper respiratory tract secretions, the latter being indicated by excessive squamous cells or absence of polymorphonuclear leukocytes.

Sterile Fluids
- Isolate and identify organisms before surrounding tissue becomes infected.

Stool
- Assist in establishing a diagnosis for diarrhea of unknown etiology.
- Identify pathogenic organisms causing gastrointestinal disease and carrier states.

Throat/Nasopharyngeal
- Assist in the diagnosis of bacterial infections such as tonsillitis, diphtheria, gonorrhea, or pertussis.
- Assist in the diagnosis of upper respiratory infections resulting in bronchitis, pharyngitis, croup, and influenza.
- Isolate and identify group A β-hemolytic streptococci as the cause of strep throat, acute glomerulonephritis, scarlet fever, or rheumatic fever.

Urine
- Assist in the diagnosis of suspected UTI.
- Determine the sensitivity of significant organisms to antibiotics.
- Monitor the response to UTI treatment.

Wound
- Detect abscess or deep-wound infectious process.
- Determine if an infectious organism is the cause of wound redness, warmth, or edema with drainage at a site.
- Determine presence of infectious organisms in a stage 3 and stage 4 decubitus ulcer.
- Isolate and identify organisms responsible for the presence of pus or other exudate in an open wound.

INTERFERING FACTORS
Contraindications
◈ *Blood:* If the patient has a history of severe allergic reaction to any of the materials in the iodine disinfectant solution, care should be taken to avoid the use of iodine disinfectant solutions.

◈ *Throat/nasopharyngeal:* Patients with epiglottitis. In cases of acute epiglottitis, the throat culture may need to be obtained in the operating room or other appropriate location where the required emergency equipment and trained personnel can safely perform the procedure.

Factors that may alter the results of the study
General
- Pretest antimicrobial therapy will delay or inhibit growth of pathogens.
- Testing specimens more than 1 hr after collection may result in decreased growth or no growth of organisms. Delay in transport of specimen to the laboratory may result in specimen rejection. Verify submission requirements with the laboratory prior to specimen collection.
- Improper collection techniques may result in specimen contamination and invalidate interpretation of test results.
- Failure to collect adequate specimen, improper collection or storage technique, and failure to transport specimen in a timely fashion are causes for specimen rejection.

Blood
- An inadequate amount of blood or number of blood specimens drawn for examination may invalidate interpretation of results.
- Collection of the specimen in an expired media tube will result in specimen rejection.

Sputum, Throat/Nasopahryngeal
- Contamination with oral flora may invalidate results.

Stool

- A rectal swab does not provide an adequate amount of specimen for evaluating the carrier state and should be avoided in favor of a standard stool specimen.
- A rectal swab should never be submitted for *Clostridium* toxin studies. Specimens for *Clostridium* toxins should be refrigerated if they are not immediately transported to the laboratory because toxins degrade rapidly.
- A rectal swab should never be submitted for *Campylobacter* culture. Excessive exposure of the sample to air or room temperature may damage this bacterium so that it will not grow in the culture.
- Barium and laxatives used less than 1 wk before the test may reduce bacterial growth.

Urine

- Specimen storage for longer than 2 hr at room temperature or 24 hr at refrigerated temperature may result in overgrowth of bacteria and false-positive results. Such specimens may be rejected for analysis.
- Results of urine culture are often interpreted along with routine urinalysis findings.
- Discrepancies between culture and urinalysis may be reason to recollect the specimen.
- Specimens submitted in expired urine transport tubes will be rejected for analysis.

POTENTIAL MEDICAL DIAGNOSIS: CLINICAL SIGNIFICANCE OF RESULTS
Positive findings in
Anal/Endocervical/Genital

Infections or carrier states are caused by the following organisms: *Chlamydia trachomatis*, obligate intracellular bacteria without a cell wall, gram-variable *Gardnerella vaginalis*, gram-negative *Neisseria gonorrhoeae*, *Treponema pallidum*, and toxin-producing strains of gram-positive *Staphylococcus aureus* and gram-positive GBS

Blood

- Bacteremia or septicemia: Gram-negative organisms such as *Aerobacter, Bacteroides, Brucella, Escherichia coli* and other coliform bacilli, *Haemophilus influenzae, Klebsiella, Pseudomonas aeruginosa,* and *Salmonella*
- Bacteremia or septicemia: Gram-positive organisms such as *Clostridium perfringens, Enterococci, Listeria monocytogenes, Staphylococcus aureus, Staphylococcus epidermidis,* and β-hemolytic streptococci
- Plague
- Malaria (by special request, a stained capillary smear would be examined)
- Typhoid fever

Note: Candida albicans is a yeast that can cause disease and can be isolated by blood culture.

Ear

Commonly identified gram-negative organisms: *Escherichia coli, Proteus* spp., *Pseudomonas aeruginosa,* gram-positive *Staphylococcus aureus,* and β-hemolytic streptococci

Eye

Commonly identified organisms: *Chlamydia trachomatis* (transmitted to newborns from infected mothers), gram-negative *Haemophilus influenzae* (transmitted to newborns from infected mothers), *Haemophilus aegyptius, Neisseria gonorrhoeae* (transmitted to newborns from infected mothers), *Pseudomonas aeruginosa,* gram-positive *Staphylococcus aureus,* and *Streptococcus pneumoniae*

Skin

Commonly identified gram-negative organisms: *Bacteroides, Pseudomonas,* gram-positive *Clostridium, Corynebacterium,* staphylococci, and group A streptococci

Sputum

- The major difficulty in evaluating results is in distinguishing organisms infecting the lower respiratory tract from organisms that have colonized but not infected the lower respiratory tract. Review of the Gram stain assists in this process. The presence of greater than 25 squamous epithelial cells per low-power field indicates oral contamination, and the specimen should be rejected. The presence of many polymorphonuclear neutrophils and few squamous epithelial cells indicates that the specimen was collected from an area of infection and is satisfactory for further analysis.
- Bacterial pneumonia can be caused by *Streptococcus pneumoniae, Haemophilus influenzae,* staphylococci, and some gram-negative bacteria. Other pathogens that can be identified by culture are *Corynebacterium diphtheriae, Klebsiella pneumoniae,* and *Pseudomonas aeruginosa.* Some infectious agents, such as *Corynebacterium diphtheriae,* are more fastidious in their growth requirements and cannot be cultured and identified without special treatment. Suspicion of infection by less commonly identified and/or fastidious organisms must be communicated to the laboratory to ensure selection of the proper procedure required for identification.

Sterile Fluids

Commonly identified pathogens: gram-negative *Bacteroides, Escherichia coli, Pseudomonas aeruginosa,* gram-positive *Enterococcus* spp., and *Peptostreptococcus* spp.

Stool

- Bacterial infection: Gram-negative organisms such as *Aeromonas* spp., *Campylobacter, Escherichia coli* including serotype 0157: H7, *Plesiomonas shigelloides, Salmonella, Shigella, Vibrio,* and *Yersinia*
- Bacterial infection: Gram-positive organisms such as *Bacillus cereus, Clostridium difficile,* and *Listeria* (Isolation of *Staphylococcus aureus* may indicate infection or a carrier state.)
- Botulism: *Clostridium botulinum* (The bacteria must also be isolated from the food or the presence of toxin confirmed in the stool specimen.)
- Parasitic enterocolitis

Throat/Nasopharyngeal

Reports on cultures that are positive for group A β-hemolytic streptococci are generally available within 24 to 48 hr. Cultures that report on normal respiratory flora are issued after 48 hr. Culture results of no growth for *Corynebacterium* require 72 hr to report; 48 hr are required to report negative *Neisseria* cultures.

Urine

- UTIs

Wound

Aerobic and anaerobic microorganisms can be identified in wound culture specimens. Commonly identified gram-negative organisms include *Klebsiella, Proteus,* and *Pseudomonas* and gram-positive *Clostridium perfringens, Staphylococcus aureus,* and group A streptococci.

Negative findings in

- Negative findings do not ensure the absence of infection.

NURSING IMPLICATIONS

BEFORE THE STUDY: PLANNING AND IMPLEMENTATION

Teaching the Patient What to Expect

▸ Inform the patient this test can assist in identification of the organism causing infection.

▸ Explain that a blood, other body fluid, or site specific swab sample is needed for the test. Address concerns about pain, and explain there may be some discomfort during the invasive types of collection methods (venipuncture, sterile fluids).

▸ Instruct female patients not to douche for 24 hr before a cervical or vaginal specimen is to be obtained.

▸ Refer to related body fluid studies (i.e., amniotic fluid, cerebrospinal fluid, pericardial fluid, peritoneal fluid, pleural fluid, synovial fluid, urine) or to the general guidelines regarding the appropriate collection instructions. Additional information regarding specimen collection is presented with other general guidelines in Appendix A: Patient Preparation and Specimen Collection. The collection instructions, type of transport material, and applicator used to obtain swabs should be verified by consultation with the testing laboratory personnel. Specify the exact specimen source/origin (e.g., vaginal lesion or ear, left or right, as appropriate), patient age and gender, date and time of collection, and any medication the patient is taking that may interfere with the test results (e.g., antibiotics). Do not freeze the specimen or allow it to dry.

Chlamydia is an intracellular obligate pathogen. Culture of infected epithelial cells is considered the gold standard for the identification of chlamydia because of the higher sensitivity of nucleic acid amplification or DNA probe assays relative to antibody assays. Therefore, culture should always be the test of choice in cases of suspected or known child abuse.

Anal

▸ Specimen collection will require the patient be placed in a lithotomy or side-lying position and draped for privacy. A swab will be inserted 1 in. into the anal canal and rotated, moving it from side to side to allow it to come into contact with the microorganisms. The swab will be removed and placed in the Culturette tube. The bottom of the tube will be squeezed to release the transport medium. Specimen collectors should ensure that the end of the swab is immersed in the medium. Repeat with a clean swab if the swab is pushed into feces.

Blood

▸ Review the procedure with the patient. Inform the patient that specimen collection takes approximately 5 min. Inform the patient that multiple specimens may be required at timed intervals. Address concerns about pain and explain to the patient that there may be some discomfort during the venipuncture. Consider the use of pediatric culture tubes, if appropriate for the patient's age.

▸ The high risk for contamination of blood cultures by skin and other flora can be dramatically reduced by careful preparation of the puncture site and collection containers before specimen collection. Cleanse the rubber stoppers of the collection containers with the appropriate disinfectant as recommended by the laboratory, allow to air-dry, and cleanse with 70% alcohol. Once the vein has been located by palpation, it is cleansed with 70% alcohol followed by swabbing with an iodine disinfectant solution. The iodine disinfectant solution should be swabbed in a circular, concentric motion, moving outward or away from the puncture site. The iodine disinfectant solution should be allowed to completely dry before the sample is collected. If the patient is sensitive to iodine disinfectant solutions, a double alcohol scrub or green soap may be substituted.

▸ If collection is performed by directly drawing the sample into a culture tube, the aerobic culture tube should be filled first.

C

▶ If collection is performed using a syringe, the blood sample should be transferred directly into each culture bottle.

▶ More than three sets of cultures per day do not significantly add to the likelihood of pathogen capture. Capture rates are more likely affected by obtaining a sufficient volume of blood per culture.

▶ The use of antimicrobial removal devices (ARDs) or resin bottles is costly and controversial with respect to their effectiveness versus standard culture techniques. They may be useful in selected cases, such as when septicemia or bacteremia is suspected after antimicrobial therapy has been initiated.

Disease Suspected	Recommended Collection
Bacterial pneumonia, fever of unknown origin, meningitis, osteomyelitis, sepsis	Two sets of cultures, each collected from a separate site, 30 min apart
Acute or subacute endocarditis	Three sets of cultures, each collected from a separate site, 30–40 min apart. If cultures are negative after 24–48 hr, repeat collections
Septicemia, fungal or mycobacterial infection in immunocompromised patient	Two sets of cultures, each collected from a separate site, 30–60 min apart (laboratory may use a lysis concentration technique to enhance recovery)
Septicemia, bacteremia after therapy has been initiated, or request to monitor effectiveness of antimicrobial therapy	Two sets of cultures, each collected from a separate site, 30–60 min apart (consider use of ARD to enhance recovery)

General Information

▶ *Culturette Swab/Tubes:* Culturette swab/tubes are used to collect culture specimens from the *ear; skin; female external genitalia and perineum; male urethra; throat;* and *wound*, as well as other body sites. When obtaining a culture specimen, the swab is placed in the Culturette tube. The bottom of the tube should be squeezed to release the transport medium. Specimen collectors should ensure that the end of the swab is immersed in the medium.

▶ *Culturette or Gen-Probe Swab/ Tubes:* Culturette or Gen-Probe swab/ tubes can be used to collect culture specimens from the *eye* and *female vaginal and endocervical* areas. As with the Culturette swab/tubes, the bottom tube should be squeezed to release the transport medium. Specimen collectors using these tubes should also ensure that the end of the swab is immersed in the medium.

Ear

▶ The area surrounding the site is cleansed with a swab containing cleaning solution to remove any contaminating material or flora that have collected in the ear canal. If needed, assist the appropriate HCP in removing any cerumen that has collected.

▶ A Culturette swab is inserted approximately 1/4 in. into the external ear canal and rotated in the area containing the exudate. Once a specimen is obtained, the swab is carefully removed, ensuring that it does not touch the side or opening of the ear canal, and placed in the Culturette tube.

Eye

▶ A moistened swab is passed over the appropriate site, avoiding eyelid and eyelashes unless those areas are selected for study. Any visible pus or other exudate is collected. The swab is placed in the Culturette or Gen-Probe transport tube.

▶ An appropriate HCP should perform procedures requiring eye culture.

Genital
Female Patient

▶ The patient is positioned on the gynecological examination table with the feet up in stirrups and with the legs draped to provide privacy and reduce chilling.

▶ The external genitalia and perineum are cleansed from front to back with towelettes provided in culture kit. A Culturette swab is used to obtain a sample of the lesion or discharge from the urethra or vulva.

▶ To obtain a vaginal and endocervical culture, a water-lubricated vaginal speculum is inserted into the cervical orifice and then a swab is inserted and rotated along the surface of the endocervix to collect the secretions containing the microorganisms. The swab is removed and placed in the appropriate culture medium or Gen-Probe transport tube. Material from the vagina can be collected by moving a swab along the sides of the vaginal mucosa. Once the swab is removed, it is placed in a tube of saline medium.

Male Patient

▶ To obtain a urethral culture, the penis is cleansed (retracting the foreskin) and the patient is asked to milk the penis to express discharge from the urethra. A swab is inserted into the urethral orifice and rotated to obtain a sample of the discharge. The swab is placed in the Culturette or Gen-Probe transport tube.

Skin

▶ It may be necessary to assist the appropriate HCP in obtaining a skin sample from several areas of the affected site. If indicated, the dark, moist areas of the folds of the skin and outer growing edges of the infection where microorganisms are most likely to flourish should be selected. Scrapings should be placed in a collection container or spread on a slide. Any fluid from a pustule or vesicle is aspirated using a sterile needle and tuberculin syringe. The exudate is flushed into a sterile collection tube. If the lesion is not fluid filled, the lesion is opened with a scalpel and the area swabbed with a sterile cotton-tipped swab, which is then placed in the Culturette tube.

Sputum
Specimen Collection by Expectoration

▶ Additional liquids the night before may assist in liquefying secretions during expectoration the following morning.

▶ Assist the patient with oral cleaning before sample collection to reduce the amount of sample contamination by organisms that normally inhabit the mouth.

▶ Instruct the patient not to touch the edge or inside of the container with the hands or mouth.

▶ Emphasize that sputum and saliva are not the same. Inform the patient that multiple specimens may be required at timed intervals.

▶ Inform the patient that three samples may be required, on three separate mornings.

▶ Ask the patient to sit upright, with assistance and support (e.g., with an overbed table) as needed.

▶ Ask the patient to take two or three deep breaths and cough deeply. Any sputum raised should be expectorated directly into a sterile sputum collection container.

▶ If the patient is unable to produce the desired amount of sputum, several strategies may be attempted. One approach is to have the patient drink two glasses of water, and then assume the position for postural drainage of the upper and middle lung segments. Effective coughing may be assisted by placing either the hands or a pillow over the diaphragmatic area and applying slight pressure.

▶ Another approach is to place a vaporizer or other humidifying device at the bedside. After sufficient exposure to adequate humidification, postural drainage of the upper and middle lung segments may be repeated before attempting to obtain the specimen.

C

▶ Other methods may include obtaining an order for an expectorant to be administered with additional water approximately 2 hr before attempting to obtain the specimen. Chest percussion and postural drainage of all lung segments may also be employed. If the patient is still unable to raise sputum, the use of an ultrasonic nebulizer ("induced sputum") may be necessary; this is usually done by a respiratory therapist.

Specimen Collection by Suction

▶ Address concerns about pain related to the procedure. Reassure the patient that he or she will be able to breathe during the procedure if specimen is collected via suction method.

▶ Ensure that oxygen has been administered 20 to 30 min before the procedure if the specimen is to be obtained by tracheal suctioning. Explain that a sedative and/or analgesia may be administered to promote relaxation and reduce discomfort prior to the procedure. Lidocaine is sprayed in the patient's throat to reduce discomfort caused by the presence of the tube.

▶ Obtain the necessary equipment, including a suction device, suction kit, and Lukens tube or in-line trap.

▶ Position the patient with head elevated as high as tolerated.

▶ Put on sterile gloves. Maintain the dominant hand as sterile and the nondominant hand as clean.

▶ Using the sterile hand, attach the suction catheter to the rubber tubing of the Lukens tube or in-line trap. Then attach the suction tubing to the male adapter of the trap with the clean hand. Lubricate the suction catheter with sterile saline.

▶ Ask patients who are nonintubated to protrude the tongue and to take a deep breath as the suction catheter is passed through the nostril. When the catheter enters the trachea, a reflex cough is stimulated; immediately advance the catheter into the trachea and apply suction. Maintain suction for approximately 10 sec, but never longer than 15 sec. Withdraw the catheter

without applying suction. Separate the suction catheter and suction tubing from the trap, and place the rubber tubing over the male adapter to seal the unit.

▶ For patients who are intubated or patients with a tracheostomy, the previous procedure is followed except that the suction catheter is passed through the existing endotracheal or tracheostomy tube rather than through the nostril. The patient should be hyperoxygenated before and after the procedure in accordance with standard protocols for suctioning these patients.

▶ Generally, a series of three to five early-morning sputum samples are collected in sterile containers.

Specimen Collection by Bronchoscopy

▶ Review the procedure with the patient. Address concerns about pain related to the procedure. Atropine is usually given before bronchoscopy examinations to reduce bronchial secretions and prevent vagally induced bradycardia. A sedative may be given to promote relaxation. Lidocaine is sprayed in the patient's throat to reduce discomfort caused by the presence of the tube. Refer to study titled "Bronchoscopy" for description of specimen collection during bronchoscopy.

Sterile Fluid

▶ Refer to related body fluid studies (i.e., amniotic fluid, cerebrospinal fluid, pericardial fluid, peritoneal fluid, pleural fluid, synovial fluid, urine) for specimen collection.

Stool

▶ Collect a stool specimen directly into a clean container. If the patient requires a bedpan, make sure it is clean and dry, and use a tongue blade to transfer the specimen to the container. Make sure representative portions of the stool are sent for analysis. Note specimen appearance on collection container label.

Throat/Nasopharyngeal

▶ To collect the throat culture, tilt the patient's head back. Swab both tonsillar pillars and oropharynx with the sterile Culturette. A tongue depressor can be used to ensure that contact with the tongue and uvula is avoided.

▶ A nasopharyngeal specimen is collected through the use of a flexible probe inserted through the nose and directed toward the back of the throat.

▶ Place the swab in the Culturette tube and squeeze the bottom of the Culturette tube to release the liquid transport medium. Ensure that the end of the swab is immersed in the liquid transport medium.

Urine

▶ Information regarding specimen collection (clean-catch, pediatric, indwelling catheter, urinary catheterization, and suprapubic aspiration) is presented with other general guidelines in Appendix A: Patient Preparation and Specimen Collection.

▶ If a delay in transport is expected, an aliquot of the specimen into a special tube containing a preservative is recommended. Urine transport tubes can be requested from the laboratory.

Wound

▶ The patient is placed in a comfortable position and the site to be cultured is draped. The area around the wound is cleansed to remove flora indigenous to the skin.

▶ A Culturette swab is placed in a superficial wound where the exudate is the most excessive without touching the wound edges. Once a specimen is obtained and placed in a Culturette tube. It many be necessary to use more than one swab and Culturette tube to obtain specimens from other areas of the wound.

▶ To obtain a deep wound specimen, a sterile syringe and needle must be inserted into the wound to aspirate the drainage. Following aspiration, the material is injected into a tube containing an anaerobic culture medium.

Potential Nursing Actions

✦ *Make sure a written and informed consent has been*

signed prior to the bronchoscopy/ biopsy procedure and before administering any medications.

▶ *Blood Culture:* Avoid the use of iodine solutions if the patient has a history of severe allergic reaction to any of the materials in the iodine solution.

▶ Before any procedure involving anesthesia, have the patient remove dentures, contact lenses, eyeglasses, and jewelry. Notify the HCP before bronchoscopy if the patient has permanent crowns on teeth.

AFTER THE STUDY: POTENTIAL NURSING ACTIONS

Avoiding Complications

▶ *Throat/Nasopharyngeal:* In cases of epiglottitis, do not swab the throat. This can cause a laryngospasm resulting in a loss of airway. Symptoms associated with epiglottitis include sore throat, difficulty swallowing, difficulty breathing *(related to blocked airway)*, blue skin (especially around the lips), confusion, irritability, and sluggishness *(related to decreased oxygen levels)*. Potential interactions include stabilizing the airway, monitoring vital signs, and administering the appropriate medications which may include antibiotics. Antibiotics may be administered before the results of the culture are obtained.

Treatment Considerations

▶ Advise the patient that test results for cultures may take 24 to 72 hr depending on the method used and organism suspected but that antibiotic therapy may be started immediately. Test results for PCR methods are generally available a few hours after testing is completed. Instruct the patient in the importance of completing the entire course of antibiotic therapy even if no symptoms are present. *Note:* Antibiotic therapy is frequently contraindicated for *Salmonella* infection unless the infection has progressed to a systemic state.

▶ Instruct the patient to resume usual medication as directed by the HCP and in the use of any ordered

C

medications. Explain the importance of adhering to the therapy regimen. As appropriate, instruct the patient in significant adverse effects and systemic reactions associated with the prescribed medication. Encourage him or her to review corresponding literature provided by a pharmacist.
◗ Instruct the patient to report symptoms such as pain related to tissue inflammation or irritation, fever, chills, and other signs and symptoms of acute infection to the HCP.
◗ Inform the patient that a repeat culture may be needed in 1 wk after completion of the antimicrobial regimen.

Anal/Endocervical/Genital
◗ Advise the patient to avoid sexual contact until test results are available and that all sexual partners must be tested for the microorganism.
◗ Instruct the female patient in vaginal suppository and medicated cream installation and administration of topical medication to treat specific conditions, as indicated.
◗ Inform the patient that positive culture findings for certain organisms must be reported to a local health department official, who will question him or her regarding sexual partners.

Blood
◗ Cleanse the iodine solution from the collection site.

Sputum Obtained by Bronchoscopy or Tracheal Suctioning
◗ *Bronchoscopy:* Assess the patient's ability to swallow before allowing the patient to attempt liquids or solid foods.
◗ Inform the patient that he or she may experience some throat soreness and hoarseness. Instruct patient to treat throat discomfort with lozenges and warm gargles when the gag reflex returns. Inform the patient of smoking cessation programs as appropriate.
◗ Monitor vital signs and compare with baseline values every 15 min for 1 hr, then every 2 hr for 4 hr, and then as ordered by the HCP. Monitor temperature every 4 hr for 24 hr. Evaluate the patient for symptoms of empyema, such as fever, tachycardia, malaise, or elevated white blood cell count. Notify the HCP if temperature is elevated. Protocols may vary among facilities.
◗ *Special Considerations:* Tracheal suctioning may occasionally cause trauma due to the frailty of the patient's condition, trauma, or the aggressiveness of the suctioning technique. After a bronchoscopy, emergency resuscitation equipment should be readily available if the vocal cords become spastic after intubation. The patient should be evaluated for symptoms indicating the development of pneumothorax, such as dyspnea, tachypnea, anxiety, decreased breathing sounds, or restlessness. A chest x-ray may be ordered to check for the presence of this complication. For tracheal suction or bronchoscopy, the patient should be observed for hemoptysis, dyspnea, cough, air hunger, excessive coughing, pain, or absent breathing sounds over the affected area. Report any symptoms to the HCP.

Throat/Nasopharyngeal
◗ Assess the patient's ability to swallow before allowing the patient to attempt liquids or solid foods.
◗ Instruct the patient to notify the HCP immediately if difficulty in breathing or swallowing occurs or if bleeding occurs.
◗ Instruct the patient to perform mouth care after the specimen has been obtained.
◗ Provide comfort measures and treatment such as antiseptic gargles; inhalants; and warm, moist applications as needed. A cool beverage may aid in relieving throat irritation caused by coughing or suctioning.

Urine
◗ Instruct the patient to report pain from inflammation when voiding, bladder spasms, alterations in urinary elimination, or symptoms of infection.
◗ Observe for signs of inflammation if the specimen is obtained by suprapubic aspiration.
◗ Prevention of UTIs includes increasing daily water consumption,

urinating when urge occurs, wiping the perineal area from front to back after urination/defecation, and urinating immediately after intercourse. Prevention also includes maintaining the normal flora of the body. Patients should avoid using spermicidal creams with diaphragms or condoms (when recommended by an HCP), becoming constipated, douching, taking bubble baths, wearing tight-fitting garments, and using deodorizing feminine hygiene products that alter the body's normal flora and increase susceptibility to UTIs.

Wound

▶ Instruct the patient in wound care and nutritional requirements (e.g., protein, vitamin C) to promote wound healing.

Nutritional Considerations

▶ *Sputum:* Malnutrition is commonly seen in patients with severe respiratory disease for numerous reasons, including fatigue, lack of appetite, and gastrointestinal distress. Adequate intake of vitamins A and C is also important to prevent pulmonary infection and to decrease the extent of lung tissue damage.

▶ *Throat/Nasopharyngeal:* Dehydration can been seen in patients with a bacterial throat infection due to pain with swallowing. Pain medications reduce patient's dysphagia and allow for adequate intake of fluids and foods.

▶ *Urine:* Instruct the patient to increase water consumption by drinking 8 to 12 glasses of water to assist in flushing the urinary tract. Instruct the patient to avoid alcohol, caffeine, and carbonated beverages, which can cause bladder irritation.

Follow-Up, Evaluation, and Desired Outcomes

▶ Acknowledges information provided regarding vaccine-preventable diseases (e.g. diphtheria H1N1 flu, *Haemophilus influenza,* seasonal influenza, pneumococcal disease, cervical cancer, hepatitis A and B, human papillomavirus) for the CDC (www.cdc.gov/vaccines/vpd/vaccines-diseases.html) for guidelines on vaccine-preventable diseases.

▶ Victims of sexual assault accept offered support and access to counseling services.

▶ Recognizes the importance of taking and completing any ordered medications (oral, topical, drops). Acknowledges provided information regarding significant adverse effects associated with the prescribed medication and agrees to review corresponding literature provided by a pharmacist.

▶ Demonstrates the proper use of sterile technique for cleansing the affected site and application of dressings.

Culture, Fungal

SYNONYM/ACRONYM: N/A

RATIONALE: To identify the pathogenic fungal organisms causing infection.

PATIENT PREPARATION: There are no food, fluid, or activity restrictions unless by medical direction.

NORMAL FINDINGS: (Method: Culture on selective media; macroscopic and microscopic examination) No presence of fungi.

CRITICAL FINDINGS AND POTENTIAL INTERVENTIONS
• Positive findings in any sterile body fluid such as blood or cerebrospinal fluid.

Timely notification to the requesting health-care provider (HCP) of any critical findings and related symptoms is a role expectation of the professional nurse. Lists of specific organisms may vary among facilities; specific organisms are required to be reported to local, state, and national departments of health.

OVERVIEW: (Study type: Blood, urine, body fluid [cerebrospinal fluid (CSF) and other sterile fluids], fecal, tissue, or other [hair, nail, pus, sputum] collected in a sterile plastic, tightly capped container; related body system: Circulatory, Digestive, Immune, Integumentary, Nervous, Reproductive, Respiratory, and Urinary systems. Instructions regarding specimen collection and the appropriate transport materials for blood, bone marrow, bronchial washings, sputum, sterile fluids, stool, and tissue samples should be obtained from the laboratory.) Fungi, organisms that normally live in soil, can be introduced into humans through the accidental inhalation of spores or inoculation of spores into tissue through trauma. Yeast are classified as single-celled fungi. Individuals most susceptible to fungal infection usually are debilitated by chronic disease, are receiving prolonged antibiotic therapy, or have impaired immune systems. Fungal diseases may be classified according to the involved tissue type: Dermatophytoses involve superficial and cutaneous tissue; there are also subcutaneous and systemic mycoses. Culture is a method commonly used to identify the cause of a fungal infection. However, fungal growth occurs slowly, and it can take days to weeks before culture and susceptibility results are

available. Systemic fungal infections, especially those caused by fluconazole-resistant fungi, can be life threatening. Identification of the infectious agent and effective therapeutic treatment can be more time sensitive than what is required for the natural course of growth by culture. Rapid, direct testing platforms are not yet widely available, but molecular-based blood assays are being developed and approved for use in clinical situations. For example, the T2Candida panel employs a combination of molecular technology (DNA amplification) with magnetic resonance technology to identify five common yeast species from a single blood sample in 3 to 5 hr.

INDICATIONS
• Determine antimicrobial sensitivity of the organism.
• Isolate and identify organisms responsible for neonatal thrush.
• Isolate and identify organisms responsible for nail infections or abnormalities.
• Isolate and identify organisms responsible for skin eruptions, drainage, or other evidence of infection.
• Isolate and identify organisms responsible for systemic infection and sepsis.

INTERFERING FACTORS
• Prompt and proper specimen processing, storage, and

analysis are important to achieve accurate results.

POTENTIAL MEDICAL DIAGNOSIS: CLINICAL SIGNIFICANCE OF RESULTS

Positive findings in

- Blood
  Candida albicans
  Histoplasma capsulatum
- Cerebrospinal fluid
  Coccidioides immitis
  Cryptococcus neoformans
  Members of the order Mucorales
  Paracoccidioides brasiliensis
  Sporothrix schenckii
- Hair
  Epidermophyton
  Microsporum
  Trichophyton
- Nails
  Candida albicans
  Cephalosporium
  Epidermophyton
  Trichophyton
- Skin
  Actinomyces israelii
  Candida albicans
  Coccidioides immitis
  Epidermophyton
  Microsporum
  Trichophyton
- Tissue
  Actinomyces israelii
  Aspergillus
  Candida albicans
  Nocardia
  Paracoccidioides brasiliensis

NURSING IMPLICATIONS

BEFORE THE STUDY: PLANNING AND IMPLEMENTATION

Teaching the Patient What to Expect

- Inform the patient this test can assist in identification of the organism causing infection.
- Explain that a blood, body fluid, hair, tissue, or other type of sample is needed for the test. Address concerns about pain, and explain there may be some discomfort during the invasive types of collection methods. For further information regarding the various collection procedures refer to the specific studies (bronchoscopy, tissue biopsy, bone marrow aspiration, CFS by lumbar puncture).

Skin

- The site is cleansed with 70% alcohol. The peripheral margin of the collection site is scraped with a sterile scalpel or wooden spatula and the specimen placed in a sterile collection container.

Hair

- Fungi usually grow at the base of the hair shaft. Infected hairs can be identified by using a Wood lamp in a darkened room. A Wood lamp provides rays of ultraviolet light at a wavelength of 366 nm, or 3,660 Å. Infected hairs fluoresce a bright yellow-green when exposed to light from the Wood lamp. Once infected hair is identified, a tweezer is used to pluck the hair from the skin.

Nails

- Ideally, a sample of softened material can be obtained from the nailbed beneath the nail plate. Alternatively, shavings from the deeper portions of the nail itself can be collected.

General

- Results of a conventional fungal culture may take up to 4 wk. Results of fungal antibody tests are available within a few days of collection and may be ordered when there is a strong suspicion of a particular pathogen. Most often, results indicating the presence or absence of fungi can be obtained in moments by looking at small amounts of the specimen under a microscope. A portion of the sample or swab is placed in sterile saline, and a drop from the diluted sample is placed on a glass slide, also called a *wet prep*. Another portion of the sample or a second swab is mixed with 15% potassium hydroxide (KOH), and a drop from the KOH sample is placed on a glass slide. A coverslip is placed over each specimen on the slide. The slides are examined under a

C

microscope for the presence of fungal elements: mycelium, mycelial fragments, spores, or budding yeast cells. The KOH test is used in conjunction with the wet prep because the KOH destroys bacterial and epithelial cells while leaving fungal elements clearly visible, if present.

Potential Nursing Actions
▶ Note any recent medications, especially antifungals, that can interfere with test results.

AFTER THE STUDY: POTENTIAL NURSING ACTIONS

Treatment Considerations
▶ Instruct patient to begin antifungal therapy, as prescribed. Instruct the patient in the importance of completing the entire course of antifungal therapy even if no symptoms are present.

Follow-Up, Evaluation, and Desired Outcomes
▶ Acknowledges the importance of good hand hygiene, especially for all who

come in contact with the infant/child whose immune system is still developing and may be at higher risk for infection.
▶ Demonstrates good oral and personal hygiene. Educate the parents or caregivers of infants or children with thrush (oral *Candida* infection) regarding the mechanism for transmission of the infection; stress the importance of keeping bottle-feeding equipment (especially nipples), pacifiers, and toys cleaned and disinfected or sterilized, as appropriate, on a regular basis.
▶ Understands that the presence of diaper rash, or diaper candidiasis, may be instigated by changes in diet or frequent stools that affect the integrity of the infant's or child's delicate skin and allow an opportunity for infection to occur. Agrees that frequent diaper changes and proper cleansing of the genital area is important for infants or children with diaper rash.

Culture, Mycobacteria

SYNONYM/ACRONYM: Acid-fast bacilli (AFB) culture and smear, tuberculosis (TB) culture and smear, *Mycobacterium* culture and smear.

RATIONALE: To assist in the diagnosis of tuberculosis.

PATIENT PREPARATION: Instruct the patient undergoing a procedure requiring anesthesia, and during which cultures may be collected, that to reduce the risk of aspiration related to nausea and vomiting, solid food and milk or milk products are restricted for at least 6 hr, and clear liquids are restricted for at least 2 hr prior to general anesthesia, regional anesthesia, or sedation/analgesia (monitored anesthesia). The patient may be required to be NPO at midnight. The American Society of Anesthesiologists has fasting guidelines for risk levels according to patient status. More information can be located at www.asahq.org. Regarding the collection of most other specimen types (e.g., urine or stool), there are no food, fluid, or activity restrictions unless by medical direction. Whenever possible, specimens for culture should be collected before antimicrobial therapy begins, as these medications will delay or inhibit growth of pathogens.

Ensure that oxygen has been administered 20 to 30 min before the procedure if the specimen is to be obtained by tracheal suction.

Regarding the patient's risk for bleeding, the patient should be instructed to avoid taking natural products and medications with known anticoagulant, antiplatelet, or thrombolytic properties or to reduce dosage, as ordered, prior to the procedure. Number of days to withhold medication is dependent on the type of anticoagulant.

Patients on beta blockers before the surgical procedure should be instructed to take their medication as ordered during the perioperative period. Protocols may vary among facilities.

NORMAL FINDINGS: (Method: Culture on selected media, microscopic examination of sputum by acid-fast or auramine-rhodamine fluorochrome stain) Rapid methods include: chemiluminescent-labelled DNA probes that target ribosomal RNA of the *Mycobacterium* radiometric carbon dioxide detection from ^{14}C-labelled media, polymerase chain reaction/amplification techniques.

Culture: No growth
Smear: Negative for AFB
Rapid Testing Method: Mycobacterium

CRITICAL FINDINGS AND POTENTIAL INTERVENTIONS
- *Smear:* Positive for AFB
- *Rapid Testing Method:* Positive for *Mycobacterium*
- *Culture:* Growth of pathogenic bacteria

Timely notification to the requesting health-care provider (HCP) of any critical findings and related symptoms is a role expectation of the professional nurse. Lists of specific organisms may vary among facilities; specific organisms are required to be reported to local, state, and national departments of health.

OVERVIEW: (**Study type:** Blood, urine, body fluid [semen, CSF, gastric, and sterile fluids from other sites], fecal, tissue; **related body system:** Immune and Respiratory systems.) A culture and smear test is used primarily to detect *Mycobacterium tuberculosis,* which is a tubercular bacillus. The cell wall of this mycobacterium contains complex lipids and waxes that do not take up ordinary stains. Cells that resist decolorization by acid alcohol are termed *acid-fast.* There are only a few groups of AFB; this characteristic is helpful in rapid identification so that therapy can be initiated in a timely manner. Smears may be negative 50% of the time even though the culture develops positive growth 3 to 8 wk later. AFB cultures are used to confirm positive and negative AFB smears. *M. tuberculosis* grows in culture slowly. Automated liquid culture systems, such as the Bactec and MGIT, have a turnaround time of approximately 10 days. Results of tests by polymerase chain reaction culture methods are available in 24 to 72 hr. The QuantiFERON-TB Gold (QFT-G), QuantiFERON-TB Gold In-Tube (QFT-GIT), and T-SPOT interferon gamma release assays are approved for blood specimens by the U.S. Food and Drug Administration for all applications in which the TB skin test is used. The blood test is a procedure in which a sample of whole blood from the patient is incubated with a reagent cocktail of peptides known to be present in individuals infected by *M. tuberculosis* but not found in the blood of previously vaccinated individuals or individuals who do not have the disease. The blood test offers the advantage of eliminating many of the false reactions encountered with skin testing, only a single patient visit is required, and results can be available within 24 hr. The blood tests and skin tests are approved as indirect tests for *M. tuberculosis*, and the Centers for Disease Control and Prevention recommends their use in conjunction with risk assessment, chest x-ray, and other appropriate medical and diagnostic evaluations. Detailed information is found in the study titled "Tuberculosis: Skin and Blood Tests."

   M. tuberculosis is transmitted via the airborne route to the lungs. It causes areas of granulomatous inflammation, cough, fever, and hemoptysis. It can remain dormant in the lungs for long periods. The incidence of TB has increased since the late 1980s in depressed inner-city areas, among prison populations, and among HIV-positive patients. Of great concern is the increase in antibiotic-resistant strains. HIV-positive patients often become ill from concomitant infections caused by *M. tuberculosis* and *M. avium intracellulare*. *M. avium intracellulare* is acquired via the gastrointestinal (GI) tract through ingestion of contaminated food or water.

The organism's waxy cell wall protects it from acids in the human digestive tract. Isolation of mycobacteria in the stool does not mean the patient has tuberculosis of the intestines because mycobacteria in stool are most often present in sputum that has been swallowed.

INDICATIONS
- Assist in the diagnosis of mycobacteriosis.
- Assist in the diagnosis of suspected pulmonary tuberculosis secondary to AIDS.
- Assist in the differentiation of tuberculosis from cancer or bronchiectasis.
- Investigate suspected pulmonary tuberculosis.
- Monitor the response to treatment for pulmonary tuberculosis.

INTERFERING FACTORS
Factors that may alter the results of the study
- Specimen collection after initiation of treatment with antituberculosis drug therapy may result in inhibited or no growth of organisms.
- Contamination of the sterile container with organisms from an exogenous source may produce misleading results.
- Specimens received on a dry swab should be rejected: A dry swab indicates that the sample is unlikely to have been collected properly or unlikely to contain a representative quantity of significant organisms for proper evaluation.
- Inadequate or improper (e.g., saliva) samples should be rejected.

POTENTIAL MEDICAL DIAGNOSIS: CLINICAL SIGNIFICANCE OF RESULTS

Identified Organism	Primary Specimen Source	Condition
M. avium intracellulare	CSF, lymph nodes, semen, sputum, urine	Opportunistic pulmonary infection
M. fortuitum	Bone, body fluid, sputum, surgical wound, tissue	Opportunistic infection (usually pulmonary)
M. leprae	CSF, skin scrapings, lymph nodes	Hanson's disease (leprosy)
M. kansasii	Joint, lymph nodes, skin, sputum	Pulmonary tuberculosis
M. marinum	Joint	Granulomatous skin lesions
M. tuberculosis	CSF, gastric washing, sputum, urine	Pulmonary tuberculosis
M. xenopi	Sputum	Pulmonary tuberculosis

NURSING IMPLICATIONS

BEFORE THE STUDY: PLANNING AND IMPLEMENTATION

Teaching the Patient What to Expect

- Inform the patient this test can assist in diagnosing respiratory disease.
- Explain that a blood, other body fluid, or tissue sample is needed for the test. Address concerns about pain, and explain there may be some discomfort during the invasive types of collection methods. For further information regarding the various collection procedures, refer to the specific studies (bronchoscopy, cytology sputum, tissue biopsy or fine-needle aspiration various sites, bone marrow aspiration, CSF by lumbar puncture, gastric fluid aspiration).
- Review the procedure with the patient. Explain the procedure that best fits the process selected for your patient.
- Explain to the patient that the time it takes to collect a proper specimen varies according to the level of cooperation of the patient and the specimen collection site. Inform the patient that multiple specimens may be required at timed intervals. Inform the patient that the culture results will not be reported for 3 to 8 wk.

Potential Nursing Actions

- Make sure a written and informed consent has been signed prior to the procedure and before administering any medications.
- Obtain a history of the patient's exposure to TB.
- Before any procedure involving anesthesia, have the patient remove dentures, contact lenses, eyeglasses, and jewelry. Notify the HCP before bronchoscopy if the patient has permanent crowns on teeth.

AFTER THE STUDY: POTENTIAL NURSING ACTIONS

Avoiding Complications

- For detailed information regarding complications related to the various collection procedures refer to the specific studies (bronchoscopy, cytology sputum, tissue biopsy or fine-needle aspiration various sites, bone marrow aspiration, CFS by lumbar puncture, gastric fluid aspiration).

Treatment Considerations

- Monitor patient as appropriate for the specimen collection protocol.
- Evaluate the patient for symptoms indicating any adverse developments related to the specimen collection procedure.

▶ Administer antibiotic therapy if ordered. Remind the patient of the importance of completing the entire course of antibiotic therapy, even if signs and symptoms disappear before completion of therapy.

Nutritional Considerations
▶ Malnutrition is commonly seen in patients with severe *Mycoplasma* associated respiratory disease for numerous reasons, including fatigue, lack of appetite, and GI distress. The importance of adequate intake of vitamins and following the prescribed diet should be stressed to the patient/caregiver.

Follow-Up, Evaluation, and Desired Outcomes
▶ Understands to use lozenges or gargle for throat discomfort. Smoking cessation programs should be adhered to as appropriate.
▶ Acknowledges the importance of adhering to the therapeutic regimen. Understands the significant adverse effects associated with the prescribed medication and recognizes the importance of reviewing corresponding literature provided by a pharmacist.

Culture, Viral

SYNONYM/ACRONYM: N/A

RATIONALE: To identify infection caused by pathogenic viral organisms as evidenced by ocular, genitourinary, intestinal, or respiratory symptoms. Commonly identified are cytomegalovirus (CMV), Epstein-Barr virus, herpes simplex virus (HSV), H1N1 (swine flu), HIV, human papillomavirus (HPV), respiratory syncytial virus (RSV), and severe acute respiratory syndrome (SARS)–associated coronavirus, varicella zoster virus.

PATIENT PREPARATION: There are no food, fluid, or activity restrictions unless by medical direction.

NORMAL FINDINGS: (Method: Culture in special media, enzyme-linked immunoassays, direct fluorescent antibody techniques, latex agglutination, immunoperoxidase, polymerase chain reaction [PCR] techniques) No virus isolated.

CRITICAL FINDINGS AND POTENTIAL INTERVENTIONS
Timely notification to the requesting health-care provider (HCP) of any critical findings and related symptoms is a role expectation of the professional nurse. A listing of these findings varies among facilities. Positive RSV, influenza, and varicella zoster cultures should be reported immediately to the requesting HCP. Lists of specific organisms may vary among facilities; specific organisms are required to be reported to local, state, and national departments of health.

OVERVIEW: (Study type: Blood, urine, body fluid [semen, cerebrospinal fluid (CSF) and other sterile fluids], fecal, tissue, or swabs from the affected site; related body system: to include Digestive, Immune, Integumentary, Nervous, Reproductive, Respiratory, and Urinary systems. Instructions regarding the appropriate transport materials for blood, bronchial washings, sputum, sterile fluids, stool, and tissue samples should be obtained from the laboratory.

The type of applicator used to obtain swabs should be verified by consultation with the testing laboratory personnel. The appropriate viral transport material should be obtained from the laboratory. Nasopharyngeal washings or swabs for RSV testing should be immediately placed in cold viral transport media.) Viruses, the most common cause of human infection, are submicroscopic organisms that invade living cells. They can be classified as either RNA- or DNA-type viruses. Viral titers are highest in the early stages of disease before the host has begun to manufacture significant antibodies against the invader. Specimens need to be collected as early as possible in the disease process. The subspecialty of microbiology has been revolutionized by molecular diagnostics. Molecular diagnostics involves the identification of specific sequences of DNA. The application of molecular diagnostics techniques, such as PCR, has led to the development of automated instruments that can identify a single pathogen or multiple pathogens from a small amount of specimen in less than 2 hr. The instruments can detect the presence of bacteria and viruses commonly associated with viral infections.

INDICATIONS
Assist in the identification of viral infection.

INTERFERING FACTORS
Factors that may alter the results of the study
- Viral specimens are unstable. Prompt and proper specimen processing, storage, and analysis are important to achieve accurate results.

POTENTIAL MEDICAL DIAGNOSIS: CLINICAL SIGNIFICANCE OF RESULTS
Positive findings in
- AIDS
  HIV
- Acute respiratory failure
  Hantavirus
- Anorectal infections
  HSV
  HPV
- Bronchitis
  Parainfluenza virus
  RSV
- Cervical cancer
  HPV
- Condylomata
  HPV
- Conjunctivitis/keratitis
  Adenovirus
  Epstein-Barr virus
  HSV
  Measles virus
  Parvovirus
  Rubella virus
  Varicella zoster virus (shingles)
- Croup
  Parainfluenza virus
  RSV
- Cutaneous infection with rash
  Enteroviruses
  HSV
  Varicella zoster virus
- Encephalitis
  Enteroviruses
  Flaviviruses
  HSV
  HIV
  Measles virus
  Rabies virus
  Togaviruses
  West Nile virus (mosquito-borne arbovirus)
- Febrile illness with rash
  Coxsackieviruses
  Echovirus
- Gastroenteritis
  Norwalk virus
  Rotavirus
- Genital herpes
  HSV-1
  HSV-2

- **Genital warts**
  HPV
- **Hemorrhagic cystitis**
  Adenovirus
- **Hemorrhagic fever**
  Ebola virus
  Hantavirus
  Lassa virus
  Marburg virus
- **Herpangina**
  Coxsackievirus (group A)
- **Infectious mononucleosis**
  CMV
  Epstein-Barr virus
- **Meningitis**
  Coxsackieviruses
  Echovirus
  HSV-2
  Lymphocytic choriomeningitis
  virus
- **Myocarditis/pericarditis**
  Coxsackievirus
  Echovirus
- **Parotitis**
  Mumps virus
  Parainfluenza virus
- **Pharyngitis**
  Adenovirus
  Coxsackievirus (group A)
  Epstein-Barr virus
  HSV
  H1N1 influenza virus (swine flu)
  Influenza virus
  Parainfluenza virus
  Rhinovirus
- **Pleurodynia**
  Coxsackievirus (group B)
- **Pneumonia**
  Adenovirus
  H1N1 influenza virus (swine flu)
  Influenza virus
  Parainfluenza virus
  RSV
  SARS-associated corona virus
- **Upper respiratory tract infection**
  Adenovirus
  Coronavirus
  H1N1 influenza virus (swine flu)
  Influenza virus
  Parainfluenza virus
  RSV
  Rhinovirus

NURSING IMPLICATIONS

BEFORE THE STUDY: PLANNING AND IMPLEMENTATION

Teaching the Patient What to Expect

▶ Inform the patient this test can assist in identification of the organism causing infection.

▶ Explain that a blood, other body fluid, or tissue sample is needed for the test. Address concerns about pain, and explain there may be some discomfort during the invasive types of collection methods (venipuncture, bronchial washings, sterile fluids, and tissue samples).

▶ Instructions regarding the appropriate collection instructions and transport materials for blood, bronchial washings, sputum, stool, and tissue samples should be obtained from the laboratory. The type of applicator used to obtain swabs should be verified by consultation with the testing laboratory personnel.

▶ The appropriate viral transport material should be obtained from the laboratory. Nasopharyngeal washings or swabs for RSV testing should be immediately placed in cold viral transport media.

Potential Nursing Actions

▶ Note any recent medications, especially antivirals, that can interfere with test results.

AFTER THE STUDY: POTENTIAL NURSING ACTIONS

Treatment Considerations

▶ Provide a nonjudgmental, nonthreatening atmosphere for discussing the risks of sexually transmitted infections to victims of sexual assault. It is also important to address problems the patient may experience (e.g., guilt, depression, anger).

Nutritional Considerations

▶ Dehydration can been seen in patients with viral infections due to loss of fluids through fever, diarrhea, and/or vomiting. Antipyretic medication includes acetaminophen to decrease fever and allow for adequate intake of fluids and foods. Do not give acetylsalicylic acid to pediatric patients with a viral illness because it increases the risk of Reye syndrome.

Follow-Up, Evaluation, and Desired Outcomes

▶ Acknowledges contact information provided for the Centers for Disease Control and Prevention (www.cdc.gov/vaccines/vpd/vaccines-diseases.html) for guidelines on vaccine-preventable diseases.

▶ Understands that multiple specimens may be required during the course of the infection. The timeframe for serial sample collection may vary depending on the viral organism involved. Acknowledges provided information regarding vaccine-preventable diseases where indicated (e.g., encephalitis, H1N1 flu, seasonal influenza).

▶ Victims of sexual assault accept offered support and access to counseling services.

Cystometry

SYNONYM/ACRONYM: Cystometrography (CMG), urodynamic testing of bladder function.

RATIONALE: To assess bladder function related to obstruction, neurogenic pathology, and infection including evaluation of surgical, and medical management.

PATIENT PREPARATION: There are no food, fluid, activity, or medication restrictions unless by medical direction.

NORMAL FINDINGS

- Normal filling pattern
- Normal sensory perception of bladder fullness, desire to void, and ability to inhibit urination; appropriate response to temperature (hot and cold)
- Normal bladder capacity: 250 to 450 mL. Bladder size and corresponding capacity vary with gender and age; in the pediatric patient, the normal bladder stretches to maximum capacity without an increase in pressure
- Amount of postvoid residual urine is less than 30 to 50 mL
- Normal functioning bladder pressure: 8 to 15 cm H_2O
- Normal bladder pressure increases 30 to 40 cm H_2O during voiding
- Normal detrusor pressure: Less than 10 cm H_2O
- Normal first urge to void: 175 to 250 mL; sensation of fullness and need to empty the bladder: 350 to 450 mL
- Urethral pressure that is higher than bladder pressure, ensuring continence.

CRITICAL FINDINGS AND POTENTIAL INTERVENTIONS: N/A

OVERVIEW: (Study type: Manometry; related body system: Urinary system.) Cystometry evaluates the motor and sensory function of the bladder when incontinence is present or neurological bladder dysfunction is suspected and monitors the effects of treatment for the abnormalities. This manometric study measures the bladder pressure and volume characteristics in milliliters of water (cm H_2O) during the filling and emptying phases. The test provides information about bladder structure and function that can lead to uninhibited bladder contractions, sensations of bladder fullness and need to void, and ability to inhibit voiding. These abnormalities cause incontinence and other impaired patterns of micturition. Cystometry can be performed with electroencephalography (EEG) (sleep studies for nocturnal incontinence), cystoscopy, and electromyography pelvic floor sphincter.

A postvoid residual measurement can also be done at the bedside to measure how much urine is left in the bladder after the patient voids. Completion of this test requires catheterization of the patient directly after voiding. The amount of urine remaining is measured and reported as the postvoid or residual urine. Normal postvoid residual is less than 30 to 50 mL of urine. This may be adjusted to less than 100 mL for those over the age of 65.

INDICATIONS

• Detect congenital urinary abnormalities.
• Determine cause of bladder dysfunction and pathology.
• Determine cause of recurrent urinary tract infection (UTI).
• Determine cause of urinary retention.
• Determine type of incontinence: *Functional* (involuntary and unpredictable), *reflex* (involuntary when a specific volume is reached), *stress* (weak pelvic muscles), *total* (continuous and unpredictable), *urge* (involuntary when urgency is sensed),

and *psychological* (e.g., dementia, confusion affecting awareness).
• Determine type of neurogenic bladder (motor or sensory).
• Evaluate the management of neurological bladder before surgical intervention.
• Evaluate postprostatectomy incontinence.
• Evaluate signs and symptoms of urinary elimination pattern dysfunction.
• Evaluate urinary obstruction in male patients experiencing urinary retention.
• Evaluate the usefulness of drug therapy on detrusor muscle function and tonicity and on internal and external sphincter function.
• Evaluate voiding disorders associated with spinal cord injury.

INTERFERING FACTORS
Contraindications

Patients with acute UTI, because the study can cause infection to spread to the kidneys.

Patients with urethral obstruction.

Patients who are unable to be catheterized.

Patients with cervical cord lesions, *because they may exhibit autonomic dysreflexia, as seen by bradycardia, flushing, hypertension, diaphoresis, and headache.*

Factors that may alter the results of the study
• Inability of the patient to void in a supine position or straining to void during the study.
• A high level of patient anxiety or embarrassment, which may interfere with the study, making it difficult to distinguish whether the results are due to stress or organic pathology.
• Administration of drugs that affect bladder function, such as muscle relaxants or antihistamines.

POTENTIAL MEDICAL DIAGNOSIS: CLINICAL SIGNIFICANCE OF RESULTS

Abnormal findings related to

Bladder Dysfunction Related to Disorders of the Nervous System

- Diabetic neuropathy
- Multiple sclerosis
- Parkinson disease
- Spinal cord injury
- Stroke
- Tabes dorsalis

Bladder Dysfunction Related to Urinary Incontinence

- Emotional or psychological origin
- Hyperreflexia
- Urinary tract infection

Bladder Dysfunction Related to Urinary Retention

- Bladder obstruction (e.g., congenital origin, tumor)
- Enlarged prostate
- UTI

C

NURSING IMPLICATIONS

POTENTIAL NURSING PROBLEMS: ASSESSMENT & NURSING DIAGNOSIS

Problems	Signs and Symptoms
Altered urination (*related to obstruction, neurogenic bladder, infection*)	Decreased urinary output less than 30 mL/hr, distended bladder, loss of sensation for full bladder, high residual urine, urinary retention, urinary dribbling
Pain (*related to blockage, tumor infection, inflammation*)	Self-report of pain; facial grimace; crying; restlessness; diaphoresis; nausea; vomiting; guarding; social withdrawal; elevated blood pressure, heart rate, respiratory rate; pallor

BEFORE THE STUDY: PLANNING AND IMPLEMENTATION

Teaching the Patient What to Expect

- Inform the patient this procedure can assist in assessing bladder function.
- Review the procedure with the patient. Address concerns about pain and explain that there may be moments of discomfort experienced during the procedure. Instruct the patient to report pain, sweating, nausea, headache, and the urge to void during the study.
- Explain that the procedure is performed in a special urology room or in a clinic setting by the health-care provider (HCP), with support staff, and takes approximately 30 to 45 min.
- Positioning for the study will be in a supine or lithotomy position on the examination table. If spinal cord injury is present, the patient can remain on

a stretcher in a supine position and be draped appropriately.
- Advise the patient that he or she will be asked to void. During voiding, characteristics such as start time; force and continuity of the stream; volume voided; presence of dribbling, straining, or hesitancy; and stop time will be noted.
- Residual urine will be measured and recorded by inserting a catheter into the bladder under sterile conditions. A test for sensory response to temperature is done by instilling 30 mL of room-temperature sterile water followed by 30 mL of warm sterile water. Sensations are assessed and recorded.
- Fluid is removed from the bladder, and the catheter is connected to a cystometer that measures the pressure. Sterile normal saline, distilled water, or carbon dioxide gas is instilled

in controlled amounts into the bladder. When the patient indicates the urge to void, the bladder is considered full. The patient is instructed to void, and urination amounts as well as start and stop times are then recorded.

▶ Pressure and volume readings are recorded and graphed for response to heat, full bladder, urge to void, and ability to inhibit voiding. The patient is requested to void without straining, and pressures are taken and recorded during this activity.

▶ After completion of voiding, the bladder is emptied of any other fluid, and the catheter is withdrawn, unless further testing is planned.

▶ Further testing may be done to determine if abnormal bladder function is being caused by muscle incompetence or interruption in innervation; anticholinergic medication (e.g., atropine) or cholinergic medication (e.g., bethanechol [Urecholine]) can be administered and the study repeated in 20 or 30 min.

Potential Nursing Actions

✴ *Make sure a written and informed consent has been signed prior to the procedure and before administering any medications.*

Avoiding Complications
▶ UTI *related to use of a catheter.* Elevated temperature may indicate infection. Notify the HCP if temperature is elevated.

Treatment Considerations
▶ Monitor vital signs after the procedure every 15 min for 2 hr or as directed. Monitor intake and output at least every 8 hr for 24 hr after the procedure. Protocols may vary among facilities.

▶ Altered Urination: Assess for bladder distention every 4 hr or as appropriate. Assess urinary pattern, palpate the lower abdomen for urine retention, measure residual urine directly after voiding with catheter or with bladder scanner, insert ordered indwelling urinary catheter, schedule voiding for every 4 hr. Perform strict intake and output. Administer ordered medication to facilitate urination and antibiotics. Send ordered urine specimen for culture and sensitivity.

▶ Pain: Use a pain rating scale appropriate to age, mental status, and language. Administer ordered pain medications and identify alternative methods of pain management that work for the patient (imagery, diversion, etc.). Evaluate response to pain management and adjust as appropriate. Anticipate the need for pain relief to prevent ups and downs in pain management. Assure the patient that pain needs will be met in a timely manner to decrease anxiety.

▶ Inform the patient that he or she may experience burning or discomfort on urination for a few voidings after the procedure. Persistent flank or suprapubic pain, fever, chills, blood in the urine, difficulty urinating, or change in urinary pattern must be reported immediately to the HCP.

Follow-Up, Evaluation, and Desired Outcomes
▶ Understands symptoms that would indicate bladder distention.
▶ Acknowledges both medical and surgical treatment options related to urinary retention.

Cystoscopy

SYNONYM/ACRONYM: Cystoureterography, prostatography.

RATIONALE: To assess the urinary tract for bleeding, cancer, polyps, stones (calculi), tumor, and prostate health.

PATIENT PREPARATION: Instruct the patient that to reduce the risk of aspiration related to nausea and vomiting, solid food and milk or milk products have been restricted for at least 6 hr, and clear liquids have been restricted for at least 2 hr prior to general anesthesia, regional anesthesia, or sedation/analgesia (monitored anesthesia). The patient may be required to be NPO after midnight. The American Society of Anesthesiologists has fasting guidelines for risk levels according to patient status. More information can be located at www.asahq.org.

Note: If iodinated contrast medium is scheduled to be used in patients receiving metformin or drugs containing metformin for type 2 diabetes, the drug may be discontinued on the day of the test and continue to be withheld for 48 hr after the test.

Regarding the patient's risk for bleeding, the patient should be instructed to avoid taking natural products and medications with known anticoagulant, antiplatelet, or thrombolytic properties or to reduce dosage, as ordered, prior to the procedure. Number of days to withhold medication is dependent on the type of anticoagulant. Note the last time and dose of medication taken.

Patients on beta blockers before the surgical procedure should be instructed to take their medication as ordered during the perioperative period. Protocols may vary among facilities.

NORMAL FINDINGS
• Normal ureter, bladder, and urethral structure.

CRITICAL FINDINGS AND POTENTIAL INTERVENTIONS: N/A

OVERVIEW: (Study type: Endoscopy; related body system: Urinary system. Laboratory specimens should be placed in the appropriate containers, properly labelled, and immediately transported to the laboratory.) Cystoscopy provides direct visualization of the urethra, urinary bladder, and ureteral orifices—areas not usually visible with x-ray procedures. This procedure is also used to obtain specimens and treat pathology associated with the aforementioned structures. Cystoscopy is accomplished by transurethral insertion of a cystoscope into the bladder. Rigid cystoscopes contain an obturator and a telescope with a lens and light system; there are also flexible cystoscopes, which use fiberoptic technology. The procedure may be performed during or after ultrasonography or radiography or performed during retrograde urethrography (visualization of the urethra using contrast medium) or retrograde ureteropyelography (visualization of the ureters and kidneys using contrast medium). Ureteroscopes are used to examine the interior of the ureters and kidneys.

INDICATIONS
• Coagulate bleeding areas.
• Determine the possible source of persistent urinary tract infections.
• Determine the source of hematuria of unknown cause.
• Differentiate, through tissue biopsy, between benign and cancerous lesions involving the bladder.
• Dilate the urethra and ureters.
• Evacuate blood clots and perform fulguration of bleeding sites within the lower urinary tract.
• Evaluate changes in urinary elimination patterns.

- Evaluate the extent of prostatic hyperplasia and degree of obstruction.
- Evaluate the function of each kidney by obtaining urine samples via ureteral catheters.
- Evaluate urinary tract abnormalities such as dysuria, frequency, retention, inadequate stream, urgency, and incontinence.
- Identify and remove polyps and small tumors (including by fulguration) from the bladder.
- Identify and remove foreign body.
- Identify congenital anomalies, such as duplicate ureters, ureteroceles, urethral or ureteral strictures, diverticula, and areas of inflammation or ulceration.
- Implant radioactive seeds.
- Place ureteral catheters to drain urine from the renal pelvis or for retrograde pyelography.
- Place ureteral stents and resect prostate gland tissue (transurethral resection of the prostate).
- Remove kidney stones from the bladder or ureters.
- Resect small tumors

INTERFERING FACTORS
Contraindications

Patients who are pregnant or suspected of being pregnant, unless the potential benefits of a procedure using radiation far outweigh the risk of radiation exposure to the fetus and mother.

Patients with bleeding disorders, *because instrumentation may lead to excessive bleeding from the lower urinary tract.*

Patients with acute cystitis or urethritis, *because instrumentation could allow bacteria to enter the bloodstream, resulting in septicemia.*

POTENTIAL MEDICAL DIAGNOSIS: CLINICAL SIGNIFICANCE OF RESULTS
Abnormal findings related to

- Bladder cancer
- Diverticulum of the bladder, fistula, stones, and strictures
- Foreign body
- Inflammation or infection
- Obstruction
- Polyps
- Prostatic hyperplasia
- Prostatitis
- Renal calculi (kidney stones)
- Tumors
- Ureteral calculi
- Ureteral reflux
- Ureteral or urethral stricture
- Ureterocele
- Urinary fistula
- Urinary tract malformation and congenital anomalies

NURSING IMPLICATIONS

POTENTIAL NURSING PROBLEMS: ASSESSMENT & NURSING DIAGNOSIS

Problems	Signs and Symptoms
Altered urination *(related to obstruction, bladder infection, tumor, cancer)*	Decreased urinary output less than 30 mL/hr, distended bladder, high residual urine, urinary retention, urinary dribbling, incontinence, urgency, difficulty in starting and stopping urine flow
Infection *(related to inflammation, urine retention, invasive interventions)*	Fever, chills, elevated white blood cell (WBC) count, hematuria, urgency, frequency, burning with urination, odorous urine, cloudy urine, flank pain or tenderness, tachycardia, increased respiratory rate

BEFORE THE STUDY: PLANNING AND IMPLEMENTATION

Teaching the Patient What to Expect

▶ Inform the patient this procedure can assist in assessing the urinary tract.

▶ Explain that prior to the procedure, laboratory testing may be required to determine the possibility of bleeding risk (coagulation testing) or to assess for impaired kidney function (creatinine level and estimated glomerular filtration rate) if use of iodinated contrast medium is anticipated.

▶ Pregnancy is a general contraindication to procedures involving radiation. Explain to the female patient that she will be asked the date of her last menstrual period. Pregnancy testing may be performed to determine the possibility of pregnancy before exposure to radiation if iodinated contrast medium is used.

▶ Review the procedure with the patient. Address concerns about pain and explain that there may be moments of discomfort or pain experienced when the IV line or catheter is inserted to allow infusion of fluids such as saline, anesthetics, sedatives, contrast medium, medications used in the procedure, or emergency medications.

▶ Inform the patient that the procedure is usually performed in a special cystoscopy suite near or in the surgery department by a health-care provider (HCP), with support staff, and takes approximately 10 to 30 min. The procedure can also be performed in a urologist's office; pediatric cystoscopy is performed in the surgery unit.

▶ The patient will be asked to void before being assisted to the examination table where he or she will be draped and positioned with legs in stirrups. If general or spinal anesthesia is to be used, it is administered before positioning the patient on the table.

▶ Advise the patient that the external genitalia will be cleansed with antiseptic solution. If local anesthetic is used, it is instilled into the urethra and retained for 5 to 10 min. A penile clamp may be used for male patients to aid in retention of anesthetic.

▶ A cystoscope or a urethroscope will be inserted by the HCP to examine the urethra before cystoscopy. The urethroscope has a sheath that may be left in place, and the cystoscope is inserted through it, avoiding multiple instrumentations.

▶ After insertion of the cystoscope, a sample of residual urine may be obtained for culture or other analysis.

▶ The bladder is irrigated via an irrigation system attached to the scope. The irrigation fluid aids in bladder visualization.

▶ If a prostatic tumor is found, a biopsy specimen may be obtained by means of a cytology brush or biopsy forceps inserted through the scope. If the tumor is small and localized, it can be excised and fulgurated. This procedure is termed *transurethral resection of the bladder.* Polyps can also be identified and excised.

▶ Ulcers or bleeding sites can be fulgurated using electrocautery.

▶ Renal calculi can be crushed and removed from the ureters and bladder.

▶ Ureteral catheters can be inserted via the scope to obtain urine samples from each kidney for comparative analysis and radiographic studies.

▶ Ureteral and urethral strictures can also be dilated during this procedure.

▶ Upon completion of the examination and related procedures, the cystoscope is withdrawn.

Potential Nursing Actions

Make sure a written and informed consent has been signed prior to the procedure and before administering any medications.

Safety Considerations

▶ Anticoagulants, aspirin, and other salicylates should be discontinued by medical direction for the appropriate number of days prior to a procedure where bleeding is a potential complication.

AFTER THE STUDY: POTENTIAL NURSING ACTIONS

Avoiding Complications

▶ **Infection** *related to the use of the endoscope* or bleeding. Encourage the patient to drink increased amounts of fluids (125 mL/hr for 24 hr) after the procedure to help prevent stasis and bacterial overgrowth. Monitor the patient for delayed allergic reaction to contrast if contrast is used in the procedure.

Treatment Considerations

‣ Instruct the patient to resume usual diet and medications, as directed by the HCP.

‣ Monitor vital signs and neurological status every 15 min for 1 hr, then every 2 hr for 4 hr, and then as ordered by the HCP. Take the temperature every 4 hr for 24 hr. Monitor intake and output at least every 8 hr. Compare with baseline values. Notify the HCP if temperature is elevated. Protocols may vary among facilities.

‣ Altered Urination: Assess for bladder distention every 4 hr or as appropriate, urinary pattern, palpate the lower abdomen for urine retention, measure residual urine directly after voiding with a catheter or bladder scanner. Insert ordered indwelling urinary catheter. Schedule voiding for every 4 hr. Perform strict intake and output. Administer ordered medication to facilitate urination and antibiotics. Monitor

laboratory studies: BUN, Cr, PSA. Limit evening fluids after 1800.

‣ Infection: Obtain an ordered urine culture and sensitivity. Monitor urine characteristics (blood, color, odor, amount). Monitor and trend WBC count. Assess and monitor vital signs: blood pressure, pulse, temperature, and heart rate. Administer ordered antibiotics and antipyretics. Ensure aseptic technique in the presence of an indwelling catheter with good hand hygiene and perineal care.

‣ Inform the patient that burning or discomfort on urination can be experienced for a few voidings after the procedure and that the urine may be blood-tinged for the first and second voidings after the procedure. Persistent flank or suprapubic pain, fever, chills, blood in the urine, difficulty urinating, or change in urinary pattern must be reported immediately to the HCP.

Follow-Up, Evaluation, and Desired Outcomes

‣ Acknowledges the importance of taking all prescribed medications to support health maintenance.

‣ Understands the importance of emptying the bladder every 3 to 4 hr.

Cystourethrography, Voiding

SYNONYM/ACRONYM: Voiding cystourethrography (VCU), voiding cystourethrogram (VCUG), micturating cystourethrogram (MCUG).

RATIONALE: To visualize and assess the bladder during voiding for evaluation of chronic urinary tract infections.

PATIENT PREPARATION: There are no food, fluid, activity, or medication restrictions unless by medical direction. The patient may be instructed to increase fluid intake the day before the test and to have only clear fluids 8 hr before the test.

Note: If iodinated contrast medium is scheduled to be used in patients receiving metformin or drugs containing metformin for type 2 diabetes, the drug may be discontinued on the day of the test and continue to be withheld for 48 hr after the test.

Regarding the patient's risk for bleeding, the patient should be instructed to avoid taking natural products and medications with known anticoagulant, antiplatelet, or thrombolytic properties or to reduce dosage, as ordered, prior to the procedure. Number of days to withhold medication is dependent on the type of anticoagulant. Note the last time and dose of medication taken. Protocols may vary among facilities.

Ensure that this procedure is performed before an upper gastrointestinal (GI) or barium study.

NORMAL FINDINGS
• Normal bladder and urethra structure and function.

CRITICAL FINDINGS AND POTENTIAL INTERVENTIONS: N/A

OVERVIEW: (Study type: X-ray, special/contrast; related body system: Urinary system.) Voiding cystourethrography involves visualization of the bladder filled with contrast medium instilled through a catheter by use of a syringe or gravity, and, after the catheter is removed, the excretion of the contrast medium. Excretion or micturition is recorded and reviewed by the health-care provider (HCP) for confirmation or exclusion of ureteral reflux and evaluation of the urethra. Fluoroscopic or plain images may also be taken to record bladder filling and emptying. This procedure is often used to evaluate chronic urinary tract infections (UTIs).

INDICATIONS
• Assess the degree of compromise of a stenotic prostatic urethra.
• Assess hypertrophy of the prostate lobes.
• Assess ureteral stricture.
• Confirm the diagnosis of congenital lower urinary tract anomaly.
• Evaluate abnormal bladder emptying and incontinence.
• Evaluate the effects of bladder trauma.
• Evaluate possible cause of frequent UTIs.
• Evaluate the presence and extent of ureteral reflux.

• Evaluate the urethra for obstruction and strictures.

INTERFERING FACTORS
Contraindications

✷ Patients who are pregnant or suspected of being pregnant, unless the potential benefits of a procedure using radiation far outweigh the risk of radiation exposure to the fetus.

✷ Patients with conditions associated with adverse reactions to contrast medium (e.g., asthma, food allergies, or allergy to contrast medium). Although patients are asked specifically if they have a known allergy to iodine or shellfish (shellfish contain high levels of iodine), it has been well established that the reaction is not to iodine; an actual iodine allergy would be problematic because iodine is required for the production of thyroid hormones. In the case of shellfish, the reaction is to a muscle protein called *tropomyosin*; in the case of iodinated contrast medium, the reaction is to the noniodinated part of the contrast molecule. Patients with a known hypersensitivity to the medium may benefit from premedication with corticosteroids and diphenhydramine; the use of nonionic contrast or an alternative noncontrast imaging study, if available, may be considered for patients who have severe asthma or who have experienced moderate to severe reactions to ionic contrast medium.

C

✳ Patients with conditions associated with preexisting renal insufficiency (e.g., chronic kidney disease, single kidney transplant, nephrectomy, diabetes, multiple myeloma, treatment with aminoglycosides and NSAIDs), *because iodinated contrast is nephrotoxic.*

✳ Patients who are chronically dehydrated before the test, especially older adults and patients whose health is already compromised, *because of their risk of contrast-induced acute kidney injury.*

✳ Patients with bleeding disorders, *because the puncture site may not stop bleeding.*

✳ Patients with an active UTI, obstruction, or injury.

Factors that may alter the results of the study
• Gas or feces in the GI tract resulting from inadequate cleansing or failure to restrict food intake before the study.
• Metallic objects (e.g., jewelry, body rings) within the examination field, which may inhibit organ visualization and cause unclear images.
• Inability of the patient to cooperate or remain still during the procedure, because movement can produce blurred or otherwise unclear images.

POTENTIAL MEDICAL DIAGNOSIS: CLINICAL SIGNIFICANCE OF RESULTS
Abnormal findings related to
• Bladder trauma
• Bladder tumors
• Hematomas
• Neurogenic bladder
• Pelvic tumors
• Prostatic enlargement
• Ureteral stricture
• Ureterocele
• Urethral diverticula
• Vesicoureteral reflux

NURSING IMPLICATIONS

BEFORE THE STUDY: PLANNING AND IMPLEMENTATION

Teaching the Patient What to Expect
▶ Inform the patient this procedure can assist in assessing the urinary tract.
▶ Explain that prior to the procedure, laboratory testing may be required to assess for impaired kidney function (creatinine level and estimated glomerular filtration rate) if use of iodinated contrast medium is anticipated.
▶ Pregnancy is a general contraindication to procedures involving radiation. Explain to the female patient that she will be asked the date of her last menstrual period. Pregnancy testing may be performed to determine the possibility of pregnancy before exposure to radiation.
▶ Review the procedure with the patient. Address concerns about pain and explain that there may be moments of discomfort or pain experienced when the IV line or catheter is inserted to allow infusion of fluids such as saline, anesthetics, sedatives, contrast medium, medications used in the procedure, or emergency medications.
▶ Inform the patient that the procedure is usually performed in the radiology department by an HCP, with support staff, and takes approximately 30 to 60 min.
▶ **Pediatric Considerations:** There is no specific pediatric patient preparation for cystourethrography. Encourage parents to be truthful about unpleasant sensations (pinching or pushing) the child may experience during catheter insertion and to use words that they know their child will understand. Toddlers and preschool-age children have a very short attention span, so the best time to talk about the test is right before the procedure. The pediatric patient should be assured that he or she will be allowed to bring a favorite comfort item into the examination

room, and if appropriate, that a parent will be with the child during the procedure. Infants and small children may be wrapped tightly in a blanket to assist in keeping them still during the procedure.

▶ Explain that immediately prior to the procedure, the patient will be asked to remove all external metallic objects and to void, before being assisted to an examination table and placed either in a supine or lithotomy position. A kidney, ureter, and bladder radiograph is taken to ensure that no barium or stool obscures visualization of the urinary system.

▶ Assure the patient or the parents of the pediatric patient that the patient will be monitored for complications (e.g., allergic reaction, anaphylaxis, bronchospasm) before, during, and after the procedure.

▶ A catheter is used to inject approximately 300 mL of contrast medium (air or iodinated contrast); the volume used is adjusted lower for pediatric patients. When three-fourths of the contrast medium has been injected, an x-ray is taken while the remainder of the contrast medium is injected and the catheter is clamped. When the patient is able to void, the catheter is removed and the patient is asked to urinate while images of the bladder and urethra are recorded.

Potential Nursing Actions

✦ *Make sure a written and informed consent has been signed prior to the procedure and before administering any medications.*

▶ If iodinated contrast medium is scheduled to be used in patients receiving metformin or drugs containing metformin for type 2 diabetes, the drug may be discontinued on the day of the test and continue to be withheld for 48 hr after the test. Protocols may vary among facilities

Safety Considerations

▶ Advise diabetic patients to avoid all medications containing metformin for 48 hr following a procedure with iodinated contrast. Iodinated contrast

can temporarily impair kidney function, and failure to withhold metformin may indirectly result in drug-induced lactic acidosis, a dangerous and sometimes fatal adverse effect of metformin (related to renal impairment that does not support sufficient excretion of metformin).

Avoiding Complications

▶ Establishing an IV site and injection of contrast medium are invasive procedures. Complications are rare but include risk for allergic reaction *(related to contrast reaction),* dysuria, infection *related to use of a catheter,* and injury to the urethra. Monitor the patient for complications related to the procedure (e.g., allergic reaction, anaphylaxis, bronchospasm, infection, injury). Immediately report symptoms such as difficulty breathing, chest pain, fever, hyperpnea, hypertension, nausea, palpitations, pruritus, rash, tachycardia, urticaria, or vomiting to the appropriate HCP. Observe/assess the needle/catheter insertion site for bleeding, inflammation, or hematoma formation. Administer ordered antihistamines or prophylactic steroids if the patient has an allergic reaction. Encourage the patient to increase fluid intake after the procedure to prevent stasis and bacterial buildup; increased fluids will help eliminate contrast medium.

Treatment Considerations

▶ Instruct the patient to resume usual diet, fluids, medications, or activity, as directed by the HCP. Kidney function should be assessed before metformin is resumed.

▶ Monitor vital signs and neurological status every 15 min for 1 hr, then every 2 hr for 4 hr, and then as ordered by the HCP. Take the temperature every 4 hr for 24 hr. Monitor intake and output at least every 8 hr. Compare with baseline values. Notify the HCP if temperature is elevated. Protocols may vary among facilities.

C

Follow-Up, Evaluation, and Desired Outcomes

♦ Understands the importance of reporting to HCP symptoms such as persistent bladder spasms, fast heart rate, difficulty breathing, skin rash, itching, chest pain, or abdominal pain.

♦ Acknowledges that the urine may be slightly pink (tinges of blood) and there may be some discomfort when urinating for 24 to 48 hr after the test related to irritation from the catheter. Prolonged pain, fever, or bright red urine should be immediately reported to the HCP.

Cytology, Sputum

SYNONYM/ACRONYM: N/A

RATIONALE: To identify cellular changes associated with tumors or organisms that result in respiratory tract infections, such as *Pneumocystis jiroveci*.

PATIENT PREPARATION: For specimens collected by suctioning or expectoration without bronchoscopy, there are no food, fluid, activity, or medication restrictions unless by medical direction. Instruct patients who will undergo bronchoscopy or biopsy that to reduce the risk of aspiration related to nausea and vomiting, solid food and milk or milk products are restricted for at least 6 hr, and clear liquids are restricted for at least 2 hr prior to general anesthesia, regional anesthesia, or sedation/analgesia (monitored anesthesia). Patients may be required to be NPO after midnight. The American Society of Anesthesiologists has fasting guidelines for risk levels according to patient status. More information can be located at www.asahq.org.

Regarding the patient's risk for bleeding, the patient should be instructed to avoid taking natural products and medications with known anticoagulant, antiplatelet, or thrombolytic properties or to reduce dosage, as ordered, prior to the procedure. Number of days to withhold medication is dependent on the type of anticoagulant. Note the last time and dose of medication taken.

Patients on beta blockers before the surgical procedure should be instructed to take their medication as ordered during the perioperative period. Protocols may vary among facilities.

NORMAL FINDINGS: (Method: Macroscopic and microscopic examination) Negative for abnormal cells, fungi, ova, and parasites.

CRITICAL FINDINGS AND POTENTIAL INTERVENTIONS

• Identification of malignancy

Timely notification to the requesting health-care provider (HCP) of any critical findings and related symptoms is a role expectation of the professional nurse. A listing of these findings varies among facilities.

If the patient becomes hypoxic or cyanotic, remove catheter immediately and administer oxygen.

If patient has asthma or chronic bronchitis, watch for aggravated bronchospasms with use of normal saline or acetylcysteine in an aerosol.

OVERVIEW: (Study type: Tissue and cell microscopy from sputum collected on three to five consecutive first-morning, deep-cough expectorations; **related body system:** Immune and Respiratory systems. Cytology specimens may also be collected during bronchoscopy, expressed onto a glass slide, and sprayed with a fixative or 95% alcohol.) Cytology is the study of the origin, structure, function, and pathology of cells. In clinical practice, cytological examinations are generally performed to detect cell changes resulting from neoplastic or inflammatory conditions. Sputum specimens for cytological examinations may be collected by expectoration alone, by suctioning, by lung biopsy, during bronchoscopy, or by expectoration after bronchoscopy.

INDICATIONS
- Assist in the diagnosis of lung cancer.
- Assist in the identification of *Pneumocystis jiroveci* in persons with AIDS.
- Detect known or suspected fungal or parasitic infection involving the lung.
- Detect known or suspected viral disease involving the lung.
- Screen cigarette smokers for neoplastic (nonmalignant) cellular changes.
- Screen patients with history of acute or chronic inflammatory or infectious lung disorders, which may lead to benign atypical or metaplastic changes.

INTERFERING FACTORS
Factors that may alter the results of the study
- Improper specimen fixation may be cause for specimen rejection.
- Improper technique used to obtain bronchial washing may be cause for specimen rejection.
- Medication, such as antibiotics, that the patient is taking may interfere with test results.

POTENTIAL MEDICAL DIAGNOSIS: CLINICAL SIGNIFICANCE OF RESULTS
(Method: Microscopic examination) The method of reporting results of cytology examinations varies according to the laboratory performing the test. Terms used to report results may include *negative* (no abnormal cells seen), *inflammatory, benign atypical, suspect for tumor,* and *positive for tumor.*

Positive findings in
- Infections caused by fungi, ova, or parasites
- Lipoid or aspiration pneumonia, as seen by lipid droplets contained in macrophages
- Tumors
- Viral infections and lung disease

NURSING IMPLICATIONS

BEFORE THE STUDY: PLANNING AND IMPLEMENTATION

Teaching the Patient What to Expect
▸ Inform the patient this test can assist in identification of the organism causing infection.
▸ There are several ways that a sputum specimen can be obtained for evaluation. Explain the procedure that best fits the process selected for your patient.

C

▶ Review the procedure with the patient. If the laboratory has provided a container with fixative, instruct the patient that the fixative contents of the specimen collection container should not be ingested or otherwise removed.

▶ Refer to study titled "Culture, Bacterial, Various Sites (Anal/Genital, Ear, Eye, Skin, Wound, Blood, Sputum, Stool, Throat/Nasopharyngeal, Urine)" for description of sputum specimen collection.

Potential Nursing Actions

✤ *Make sure a written and informed consent has been signed prior to the bronchoscopy or biopsy procedure and before administering any medications.*

▶ Have patient remove dentures, contact lenses, eyeglasses, and jewelry. Notify the HCP if the patient has permanent crowns on teeth. Assist with mouth care (brushing teeth or rinsing mouth with water), if needed, before collection so as not to contaminate the specimen by oral secretions.

▶ Assist in providing extra fluids, unless contraindicated, and proper humidification to loosen tenacious secretions. Inform the patient that increasing fluid intake before retiring on the night before the test aids in liquefying secretions and may make it easier to expectorate in the morning. Also explain that humidifying inspired air also helps to liquefy secretions.

AFTER THE STUDY: POTENTIAL NURSING ACTIONS

Avoiding Complications

▶ Bleeding *(related to a bleeding disorder or the effects of natural products and medications with known anticoagulant, antiplatelet, or thrombolytic properties),* bronchospasm, hemoptysis, infection, or pneumothorax. Monitor the patient for complications related to the procedure (e.g., bleeding, bronchospasm, infection, pneumothorax). Immediately report to the appropriate HCP symptoms such as absent breathing sounds, air hunger, excessive coughing, or dyspnea (indications

of hemoptysis); elevated white blood cell count, fever, malaise, or tachycardia (indications of infection), dyspnea, tachypnea, anxiety, decreased breathing sounds, or restlessness (symptoms of developing pneumothorax). A chest x-ray may be ordered to check for the presence of pneumothorax. Observe/assess the needle/catheter insertion site for bleeding, inflammation, or hematoma formation. Administer ordered antihistamines or prophylactic steroids if the patient has an allergic reaction. The use of morphine sulfate in those with asthma or other pulmonary disease should be avoided. This drug can further exacerbate bronchospasms and respiratory impairment. Emergency resuscitation equipment should be readily available in the case of respiratory impairment or laryngospasm after intubation or after the procedure.

Treatment Considerations

▶ Instruct the patient to resume usual diet, as directed by the HCP.

▶ Assess the patient's ability to swallow before allowing the patient to attempt liquids or solid foods. Inform the patient that he or she may experience some throat soreness and hoarseness. Instruct patient to treat throat discomfort with lozenges and warm gargles when the gag reflex returns.

▶ Monitor vital signs and compare with baseline values every 15 min for 1 hr, then every 2 hr for 4 hr, and then as ordered by the HCP. Monitor temperature every 4 hr for 24 hr. Notify the HCP if temperature is elevated. Protocols may vary among facilities.

▶ Administer antibiotic therapy if ordered. Remind the patient of the importance of completing the entire course of antibiotic therapy, even if signs and symptoms disappear before completion of therapy.

Nutritional Considerations

▶ Malnutrition is commonly seen in patients with severe respiratory disease for numerous reasons including fatigue, lack of appetite, and gastrointestinal distress. Adequate intake of vitamins A and C are also important to prevent pulmonary infection and to decrease the extent of lung tissue damage.

Follow-Up, Evaluation, and Desired Outcomes
▶ Acknowledges the importance of adhering to the chosen therapeutic regimen. As appropriate, instruct the patient in significant adverse effects

associated with the prescribed medication and encourage the patient to read the literature provided by a pharmacist.
▶ Agrees to attend smoking cessation programs, as appropriate. Acknowledges contact information provided for the American Lung Association (www.lungusa.org)

Cytology, Urine

SYNONYM/ACRONYM: N/A

RATIONALE: To identify the presence of tumors of the urinary tract and assist in the diagnosis of urinary tract infections.

PATIENT PREPARATION: There are no food, fluid, activity, or medication restrictions unless by medical direction.

NORMAL FINDINGS: (Method: Microscopic examination) No abnormal cells or inclusions seen.

CRITICAL FINDINGS AND POTENTIAL INTERVENTIONS
• Identification of malignancy

Timely notification to the requesting health-care provider (HCP) of any critical findings and related symptoms is a role expectation of the professional nurse. A listing of these findings varies among facilities.

OVERVIEW: (Study type: Tissue and cell microscopy from urine collected in a clean wide-mouth plastic container; related body system: Immune and Urinary systems.) Cytology is the study of the origin, structure, function, and pathology of cells. In clinical practice, cytological examinations are generally performed to detect cell changes resulting from neoplastic or inflammatory conditions. Cells from the epithelial lining of the urinary tract can be found in the urine. Examination of these cells for abnormalities is useful with suspected

infection, inflammatory conditions, or malignancy.

INDICATIONS
• Assist in the diagnosis of urinary tract diseases, such as cancer, cytomegalovirus infection, and other inflammatory conditions.

INTERFERING FACTORS: N/A

POTENTIAL MEDICAL DIAGNOSIS: CLINICAL SIGNIFICANCE OF RESULTS
Positive findings in
• Cancer of the urinary tract
• Cytomegalic inclusion disease
• Inflammatory disease of the urinary tract

Negative findings in: N/A

NURSING IMPLICATIONS

BEFORE THE STUDY: PLANNING AND IMPLEMENTATION

Teaching the Patient What to Expect

▶ Inform the patient this test can assist in identification of the organism causing infection or the presence of a tumor in the urinary tract.
▶ Explain that a urine sample is needed for the test. If a catheterized specimen is to be collected, explain this procedure to the patient and obtain a catheterization tray. Address concerns about pain and explain that there may be some discomfort during the catheterization.
▶ Information regarding specimen collection (clean-catch, pediatric, indwelling catheter, urinary catheterization, and suprapubic aspiration) is presented with other general guidelines in Appendix A: Patient Preparation and Specimen Collection.

AFTER THE STUDY: POTENTIAL NURSING ACTIONS

Treatment Considerations

▶ Instruct the patient to report symptoms such as pain related to tissue inflammation, pain or irritation during void, bladder spasms, or alterations in urinary elimination.
▶ Observe for signs of inflammation if the specimen is obtained by suprapubic aspiration.
▶ Administer antibiotic therapy as ordered. Remind the patient of the importance of completing the entire course of antibiotic therapy, even if signs and symptoms disappear before completion of therapy.

Cytomegalovirus Testing

SYNONYM/ACRONYM: CMV.

RATIONALE: To assist in diagnosing cytomegalovirus infection.

PATIENT PREPARATION: There are no food, fluid, activity, or medication restrictions unless by medical direction.

NORMAL FINDINGS: Method: Enzyme immunoassay.

	IgM and IgG	Interpretation
Negative	0.9 index or less	No significant level of detectable antibody
Indeterminate	0.91–1.09 index	Equivocal results; retest in 10–14 d
Positive	1.1 index or greater	Antibody detected; indicative of recent immunization, current or recent infection

CRITICAL FINDINGS AND POTENTIAL INTERVENTIONS: N/A

OVERVIEW: (Study type: Blood collected in a plain red-top tube; related body system: Immune system.) Cytomegalovirus (CMV) is a double-stranded DNA herpesvirus. The Centers for Disease Control and Prevention estimates that 50% to 85% of adults are infected by age 40. The incubation period for primary infection is 4 to 8 wk. Transmission may occur by direct contact with oral, respiratory, or venereal secretions and excretions. CMV infection is of primary concern in pregnant or immunocompromised patients or patients who have recently received an organ transplant. Blood units are sometimes tested for the presence of CMV if patients in these high-risk categories are the transfusion recipients. CMV serology is part of the TORCH (*t*oxoplasmosis, *o*ther [congenital syphilis and viruses], *r*ubella, *C*MV, and *h*erpes simplex type 2) panel used to test pregnant women. CMV, as well as these other infectious organisms, can cross the placenta and result in congenital malformations, abortion, or stillbirth. The presence of immunoglobulin (Ig) M antibodies indicates acute infection. The presence of IgG antibodies indicates current or past infection. There are numerous methods for detection of CMV. The methodology selected is based on both the test purpose and specimen type. Other types of assays used to detect CMV include direct fluorescent assays used to identify CMV in tissue, sputum, and swab specimens; hemagglutination assays, cleared by the Food and Drug Administration for testing blood prior to transfusion; polymerase chain reaction, used to test a wide variety of specimen types, including amniotic fluid, plasma, urine, cerebrospinal fluid, and whole blood; and cell tissue culture, which remains the gold standard for the identification of CMV.

INDICATIONS

- Assist in the diagnosis of congenital CMV infection in newborns.
- Determine susceptibility, particularly in pregnant women, immunocompromised patients, and patients who recently have received an organ transplant.
- Screen blood for high-risk-category transfusion recipients.

INTERFERING FACTORS

Factors that may alter the results of the study

- False-positive results may occur in the presence of rheumatoid factor.
- False-negative results may occur if treatment was begun before antibodies developed or if the test was done less than 6 days after exposure to the virus.

POTENTIAL MEDICAL DIAGNOSIS: CLINICAL SIGNIFICANCE OF RESULTS

Positive findings in

- CMV infection

Negative findings in: N/A

NURSING IMPLICATIONS

BEFORE THE STUDY: PLANNING AND IMPLEMENTATION

Teaching the Patient What to Expect

▸ Inform the patient this test can assist in identification of the organism causing infection.

▶ Explain that a blood sample is needed for the test. Inform the patient that multiple specimens may be required.

▶ Any individual positive result should be repeated in 7 to 14 days to monitor a change in titer.

Potential Nursing Actions

▶ Instruct the patient in isolation precautions during time of communicability or contagion.

AFTER THE STUDY: POTENTIAL NURSING ACTIONS

Follow-Up, Evaluation, and Desired Outcomes

▶ Understands the importance of returning to have a convalescent blood sample taken in 7 to 14 days.

▶ Recognizes that once CMV virus is identified as present, it will remain present for the rest of his or her life.

D-Dimer

SYNONYM/ACRONYM: Dimer, fibrin degradation fragment.

RATIONALE: To assist in diagnosing a diffuse state of hypercoagulation as seen in disseminated intravascular coagulation (DIC), acute myocardial infarction (MI), deep venous thrombosis (DVT), and pulmonary embolism (PE).

PATIENT PREPARATION: There are no food, fluid, activity, or medication restrictions unless by medical direction.

NORMAL FINDINGS: Method: Immunoturbidimetric.

Conventional Units (FEU = Fibrinogen Equivalent Units)	SI Units (Conventional Units × 5.476)
0–0.5 mcg/mL FEU	0–2.7 nmol/L

Levels increase with age.

CRITICAL FINDINGS AND POTENTIAL INTERVENTIONS: N/A

OVERVIEW: (Study type: Blood collected in a completely filled blue-top (3.2% sodium citrate) tube; **related body system:** Circulatory/Hematopoietic and Respiratory systems. If the patient's hematocrit exceeds 55%, the volume of citrate in the collection tube must be adjusted. *Important note:* When multiple specimens are drawn, the blue-top tube should be collected after sterile [i.e., blood culture] tubes. Otherwise, when using a standard vacutainer system, the blue top is the first tube collected. When a butterfly is used, and due to the added tubing, an extra red-top tube should be collected before the blue-top tube to ensure complete filling of the blue-top tube. The recommendation for processed and unprocessed samples stored in unopened tubes is that testing should be completed within 1 to 4 hr of collection.) Activated factor II (thrombin) serves two functions. It helps convert fibrinogen to fibrin during the process of hemostasis and simultaneously activates the fibrinolytic system to provide a balance between blood clotting and vessel occlusion. D-dimers are cross-linked fragments of fibrin produced during fibrinolysis or dissolution of a clot. For this reason, increased D-dimers are utilized as an indication of the presence of a thrombus or clot. The test is not specific to the presence of a clot, as other factors, including infection, inflammation, and pregnancy, can increase D-dimer concentration. A negative test can largely rule out the presence of a new blood clot. A positive test is presumptive evidence of DIC, DVT, or PE, which must be confirmed using other tests. The D-dimer is specific to secondary fibrinolysis because it involves fibrin rather than fibrinogen. This test may be used in combination with fibrinogen split or fibrinogen degradation products to differentiate primary fibrinolysis from secondary fibrinolysis. The treatment for primary fibrinolysis would require antifibrinolytic therapy, whereas the treatment for secondary fibrinolysis (DIC) might include transfusion to replace consumed coagulation factors and platelets and anticoagulant therapy to prevent recurrent clot formation.

INDICATIONS
- Assist in the detection of DIC and DVT.
- Assist in the evaluation of MI and unstable angina.
- Assist in the evaluation of possible veno-occlusive disease associated with sequelae of bone marrow transplant.
- Assist in the evaluation of PE.

INTERFERING FACTORS
Factors that may alter the results of the study
- Drugs and other substances that may cause an increase in plasma D-dimer include those administered for antiplatelet therapy.
- Drugs and other substances that may cause a decrease in plasma D-dimer include pravastatin and warfarin.
- High rheumatoid factor titers can cause a false-positive result.
- Increased CA 125 levels can cause a false-positive result; patients with cancer may demonstrate increased levels.
- Placement of tourniquet for longer than 1 min can result in venous stasis and changes in the concentration of plasma proteins to be measured. Platelet activation may also occur under these conditions, causing erroneous results.
- Vascular injury during phlebotomy can activate platelets and coagulation factors, causing erroneous results.
- Hemolyzed specimens must be rejected because hemolysis is an indication of platelet and coagulation factor activation.
- Hematocrit greater than 55% may cause falsely prolonged results because of anticoagulant excess relative to plasma volume.
- Incompletely filled collection tubes, specimens contaminated with heparin, clotted specimens, or unprocessed specimens not delivered to the laboratory within 1 to 2 hr of collection should be rejected.
- Icteric or lipemic specimens interfere with optical testing methods, producing erroneous results.

POTENTIAL MEDICAL DIAGNOSIS: CLINICAL SIGNIFICANCE OF RESULTS
The sensitivity and specificity of the assay varies among test kits and between test methods.

Increased in
D-Dimers are formed in inflammatory conditions where plasmin carries out its fibrinolytic action on a fibrin clot.

- Arterial or venous thrombosis
- DVT
- DIC
- Neoplastic disease
- Pre-eclampsia
- Pregnancy (late and postpartum)
- PE
- Recent surgery (within 2 days)
- Secondary fibrinolysis
- Thrombolytic or fibrinolytic therapy

Decreased in: N/A

NURSING IMPLICATIONS

Problems	Signs and Symptoms
Bleeding *(related to alerted clotting factors secondary to anticoagulant therapy, depleted clotting factors)*	Altered level of consciousness, hypotension, increased heart rate, decreased hemoglobin (Hgb) and hematocrit (Hct), capillary refill greater than 3 sec, cool extremities
Tissue perfusion (cerebral, peripheral, renal) *(related to altered blood flow associated with platelet clumping)*	Hypotension, dizziness, cool extremities, capillary refill greater than 3 sec, weak pedal pulses, altered level of consciousness

BEFORE THE STUDY: PLANNING AND IMPLEMENTATION

Teaching the Patient What to Expect

▸ Inform the patient this test can assist in diagnosing and evaluating conditions affecting normal blood clot formation.

▸ Explain that a blood sample is needed for the test.

AFTER THE STUDY: POTENTIAL NURSING ACTIONS

Treatment Considerations

▸ Bleeding: Increase frequency of vital sign assessment; note and trend variances in results. Administer ordered blood or blood products, and stool softeners. Evaluate stool for blood. monitor and trend Hgb and Hct. Assess skin for petechiae, purpura, or hematoma; monitor for blood in emesis or sputum; and administer prescribed medications (recombinant human activated protein C; epsilon amino-caproic acid).

▸ Tissue Perfusion: Monitor blood pressure and assess for dizziness. Check skin temperature for warmth. Assess capillary refill and pedal pulses, and monitor level of consciousness. Administer prescribed vasodilators and inotropic drugs; provide oxygen as required.

Safety Considerations

▸ Institute bleeding precautions; prevent unnecessary venipuncture, avoid intramuscular injections, prevent trauma, be gentle with oral care, and avoid use of a sharp razor.

Nutritional Considerations

▸ Encourage intake of foods rich in vitamin K such as green leafy vegetables, brussels sprouts, asparagus, cucumbers, and dried prunes.

Follow-Up, Evaluation, and Desired Outcomes

▸ Understands that following bleeding precautions can decrease injury risk.

Dehydroepiandrosterone Sulfate

SYNONYM/ACRONYM: DHEAS.

RATIONALE: To assist in identifying the cause of infertility, amenorrhea, or hirsutism.

PATIENT PREPARATION: There are no food, fluid, activity, or medication restrictions unless by medical direction.

NORMAL FINDINGS: Method: Immunochemiluminometric assay (ICMA).

Age	Male Conventional Units mcg/dL	Male SI Units micromol/L (Conventional Units × 0.027)	Female Conventional Units mcg/dL	Female SI Units micromol/L (Conventional Units × 0.027)
Newborn	108–607	2.9–16.4	108–607	2.9–16.4
7–30 d	32–431	0.9–11.6	32–431	0.9–11.6
1–5 mo	3–124	0.1–3.3	3–124	0.1–3.3
6–35 mo	0–30	0–0.8	0–30	0–0.8
3–6 yr	0–50	0–1.4	0–50	0–1.4
7–9 yr	5–115	0.1–3.1	5–94	0.1–2.5
10–14 yr	22–332	0.6–9	22–255	0.6–6.9
15–19 yr	88–483	2.4–13	63–373	1.7–10
20–29 yr	280–640	7.6–17.3	65–380	1.8–10.3
30–39 yr	120–520	3.2–14	45–270	1.2–7.3
40–49 yr	95–530	2.6–14.3	32–240	0.9–6.5
50–59 yr	70–310	1.9–8.4	26–200	0.7–5.4
60–69 yr	42–290	1.1–7.8	13–130	0.4–3.5
70 yr and older	28–175	0.8–4.7	10–90	0.3–2.4

CRITICAL FINDINGS AND POTENTIAL INTERVENTIONS: N/A

OVERVIEW: (**Study type:** Blood collected in a red-, red/gray-, or lavender-[EDTA] top tube; **related body system:** Endocrine and Reproductive systems.) Dehydroepiandrosterone sulfate (DHEAS) is the major precursor of 17-ketosteroids. DHEAS is a metabolite of dehydroepiandrosterone, the principal adrenal androgen. DHEAS is primarily synthesized in the adrenal gland, with a small amount secreted by the testes. DHEAS is a weak androgen and can be converted into more potent androgens (e.g., testosterone) as well as estrogens (e.g., estradiol). It is secreted in concert with cortisol, under the control of adrenocorticotropic hormone (ACTH) and prolactin. Excessive production causes masculinization in women and children. DHEAS has replaced measurement of urinary 17-ketosteroids in the estimation of adrenal androgen production.

INDICATIONS
• Assist in the evaluation of androgen excess, including congenital adrenal hyperplasia, adrenal tumor, and Stein-Leventhal syndrome.
• Evaluate women with infertility, amenorrhea, or hirsutism.

INTERFERING FACTORS
Factors that may alter the results of the study
• Drugs and other substances that may increase DHEAS levels include aloin, benfluorex, clomiphene,

corticotropin, danazol, exemestane, gemfibrozil, metformin, mifepristone, and nitrendipine.

- Drugs and other substances that may decrease DHEAS levels include aspirin, carbamazepine, dexamethasone, exemestane, finasteride, ketoconazole, leuprolide, oral contraceptives, phenobarbital, phenytoin, and tamoxifen.

POTENTIAL MEDICAL DIAGNOSIS: CLINICAL SIGNIFICANCE OF RESULTS

Increased in

DHEAS is produced by the adrenal cortex and testis; therefore, any condition stimulating these organs or associated feedback mechanisms will result in increased levels.

- Anovulation
- Cushing syndrome
- Ectopic ACTH-producing tumors
- Hirsutism
- Hyperprolactinemia
- Polycystic ovary (Stein-Leventhal syndrome)
- Virilizing adrenal tumors

Decreased in

DHEAS is produced by the adrenal cortex and testis; therefore, any condition suppressing the normal function of these organs or associated feedback mechanisms will result in decreased levels.

- Addison disease
- Adrenal insufficiency (primary or secondary)

- Aging adults *(related to natural decline in production with age)*
- Hyperlipidemia
- Pregnancy *(related to DHEAS produced by fetal adrenals and converted to estrogens in the placenta)*
- Psoriasis *(some potent topical medications used for long periods of time can result in chronic adrenal insufficiency)*
- Psychosis *(related to acute adrenal insufficiency)*

NURSING IMPLICATIONS

BEFORE THE STUDY: PLANNING AND IMPLEMENTATION

Teaching the Patient What to Expect

- Inform the patient this test can assist in diagnosing the cause of hormonal fluctuations.
- Explain that a blood sample is needed for the test.

AFTER THE STUDY: POTENTIAL NURSING ACTIONS

Follow-Up, Evaluation, and Desired Outcomes

- Acknowledges that depending on the results of this procedure, additional testing may be performed to evaluate or monitor the progression of the disease process and determine the need for a change in therapy.

Delta-Aminolevulinic Acid

SYNONYM/ACRONYM: δ-ALA, δ-aminolevulinic acid.

RATIONALE: To assist in diagnosing lead poisoning in children, or porphyria, a disorder that disrupts heme synthesis, primarily affecting the liver.

PATIENT PREPARATION: There are no food, fluid, activity, or medication restrictions unless by medical direction. Usually, a 24-hr urine collection is ordered.

As appropriate, provide the required urine collection container and specimen collection instructions.

NORMAL FINDINGS: Method: Spectrophotometry.

Conventional Units	SI Units (Conventional Units × 7.626)
1.5–7.5 mg/24 hr	11.4–57.2 micromol/24 hr

D

CRITICAL FINDINGS AND POTENTIAL INTERVENTIONS

Signs and symptoms of an acute porphyria attack include pain (commonly in the abdomen, arms, and legs), nausea, vomiting, muscle weakness, rapid pulse, and high blood pressure. Possible interventions include medication for pain, nausea, and vomiting, and, if indicated, respiratory support. Initial treatment following a moderate to severe attack may include identification and cessation of harmful drugs the patient may be taking, IV infusion of glucose, and IV heme therapy (hematin, heme arginate) if indicated by markedly elevated urine δ-ALA and porphyrins.

OVERVIEW: (**Study type:** Urine from a timed specimen collected in a dark plastic container with glacial acetic acid as a preservative; **related body system:** Circulatory/Hematopoietic system.) δ-ALA is involved in the formation of porphyrins, which ultimately leads to hemoglobin synthesis. Toxins including alcohol, lead, and other heavy metals can inhibit porphyrin synthesis. Accumulated δ-ALA is excreted in urine. Symptoms of the acute phase of intermittent porphyrias include abdominal pain, nausea, vomiting, neuromuscular signs and symptoms, constipation, and occasionally psychotic behavior. Hemolytic anemia may also exhibit during the acute phase. δ-ALA is a test of choice in the diagnosis of acute intermittent porphyria, ALA dehydratase deficiency porphyria, and δ-ALA dehydratase deficiency. Analysis of porphobilinogen and porphyrins may also be requested to assist in differential diagnosis of the porphyrias. Although lead poisoning can cause increased urinary excretion, the measurement of δ-ALA is not useful to indicate lead toxicity because it is not detectable in the urine until the blood lead level approaches and exceeds 45 mcg/dL (SI = 2.17 micromol/L), the level at which children should be evaluated to determine the need for chelation therapy.

INDICATIONS

- Assist in the diagnosis of porphyrias.

INTERFERING FACTORS

Factors that may alter the results of the study

- Drugs and other substances that may increase δ-ALA levels include penicillins.
- Cimetidine may decrease δ-ALA levels.
- Numerous drugs and other substances are suspected as potential initiators of attacks of acute porphyria, but those classified as unsafe for high-risk individuals include barbiturates, chlordiazepoxide, chlorpropamide, diazepam, ergot preparations, griseofulvin, hydantoin derivatives,

meprobamate, methyldopa, methy-prylone, oral contraceptives, pen-tazocine, phenytoin, progestogens, succinimide, sulfonmethane, and tolbutamide.

- All urine voided for the timed collection period must be included in the collection, or else falsely decreased values may be obtained. Compare output records with volume collected to verify that all voids were included in the collection.

POTENTIAL MEDICAL DIAGNOSIS: CLINICAL SIGNIFICANCE OF RESULTS

Increased in

Related to inhibition of the enzymes involved in porphyrin synthesis; results in accumulation of δ-ALA and is evidenced by exposure to medications, toxins, diet, or infection that can precipitate an attack.

- Acute porphyrias
- Aminolevulinic acid dehydrase deficiency *(related to the inability to convert δ-ALA to porphobilinogen, leading to accumulation of δ-ALA)*
- Hereditary tyrosinemia
- Lead poisoning

Decreased in: N/A

NURSING IMPLICATIONS

BEFORE THE STUDY: PLANNING AND IMPLEMENTATION

Teaching the Patient What to Expect

- Inform the parent/patient this test can assist with identification of a disease that interrupts the normal formation of hemoglobin.
- Explain that a urine sample is needed for the test. Information regarding specimen collection is presented with other general guidelines in Appendix A: Patient Preparation and Specimen Collection.

Potential Nursing Actions

- Include on the collection container's label urine total volume, test start and stop times/dates, and any medications that may interfere with test results.
- Unless contraindicated, encourage oral fluid intake during the collection period.

AFTER THE STUDY: POTENTIAL NURSING ACTIONS

Avoiding Complications

- Avoid herbal or traditional folk remedies that contain lead.
- Compare the quantity of urine with the urinary output record for the collection at the conclusion of the test. If the specimen contains less than what was recorded as output, some urine may have been discarded, invalidating the test.

Treatment Considerations

- Assess the environment for lead exposure, which can cause pediatric developmental delay; old leaded paint; contaminated soil of older homes; lead pipes; leaded ceramics or pottery used for food preparation and dining; old toys with lead.
- Assess for lead exposure related to adult hobbies, which may disrupt mental acuity; the use of products containing lead; restoration that includes sanding or removal of old leaded paint; work-related lead exposure (mining, battery manufacturing, construction).
- Modify diet and food purchasing habits to ensure absence of lead-contaminated kitchen cookware (ceramics), utensils, and foods; decrease environmental exposure by removing all decorative ceramics, toys, loose paint that contain lead.

Safety Considerations

- Slow exposure to lead-based environment or products can cause irreversible damage over time to brain, kidneys, and nervous system and can lead to death.

Nutritional Considerations

- Increased δ-ALA levels may be associated with an acute porphyria attack. Patients prone to attacks should eat a normal or high-carbohydrate diet. Dietary recommendations may be indicated and will vary depending on the condition and its severity; however, wide variations or restrictions in dietary carbohydrate content should be avoided, even for short periods of time. After recovering from an attack, the patient's daily intake of carbohydrates should be 300 g or more per day.

▶ Some canned goods and candies imported from other countries may have been produced using lead-contaminated ingredients (e.g., tamarind products packed in lead-glazed pots, minimally refined chili powder), lead-contaminated ink used to label candy packaging, or by poor manufacturing and storage processes.

As appropriate, health-care providers should provide culturally sensitive education and discuss the safety issues related to consuming imported canned foods and candies.

Follow-Up, Evaluation, and Desired Outcomes

▶ Acknowledges contact information provided for the American Porphyria Foundation (www.porphyriafoundation .com).

▶ Understands that further testing may be necessary to evaluate or monitor progression of the disease process and determine the need for a change in therapy.

▶ Agrees to institute environmental and dietary changes to prevent further lead exposure.

Drug Monitoring, Therapeutic

SYNONYM/ACRONYM: N/A

RATIONALE: To monitor specific drugs for subtherapeutic, therapeutic, or toxic levels in evaluation of treatment and to detect toxic levels in suspected overdose.

PATIENT PREPARATION: There are no food, fluid, activity, or medication restrictions unless by medical direction; note the time and date of the last dose of medication taken. Obtain a culture, if ordered, before the first dose of aminoglycosides. Other considerations prior to medication administration include documentation of adequate renal function with creatinine (Cr) and blood urea nitrogen (BUN) levels, documentation of adequate hepatic function with alanine aminotransferase (ALT) and bilirubin levels, and documentation of adequate hematological and immune function with platelet and white blood cell (WBC) count. Patients receiving methotrexate must be well hydrated and, depending on the therapy, may be treated with sodium bicarbonate for urinary alkalinization to enhance drug excretion. Leucovorin calcium rescue therapy may also be part of the protocol.

Drug* (Anticonvulsants)	Route of Administration
Carbamazepine	Oral
Ethosuximide	Oral
Lamotrigine	Oral

Drug* (Anticonvulsants)	Route of Administration
Phenobarbital	Oral
Phenytoin	Oral
Primidone	Oral
Valproic acid	Oral

*Recommended collection time = trough: Immediately before next dose (at steady state) or at a consistent sampling time.

Drug (Antidepressants)	Route of Administration	Recommended Collection Time
Amitriptyline	Oral	Trough: Immediately before next dose (at steady state)
Nortriptyline	Oral	Trough: Immediately before next dose (at steady state)
Protriptyline	Oral	Trough: Immediately before next dose (at steady state)
Doxepin	Oral	Trough: Immediately before next dose (at steady state)
Imipramine	Oral	Trough: Immediately before next dose (at steady state)

Drug (Antidysrhythmics)	Route of Administration	Recommended Collection Time
Amiodarone	Oral	Trough: Immediately before next dose
Digoxin	Oral	Trough: 12–24 hr after dose Never draw peak samples
Disopyramide	Oral	Trough: Immediately before next dose Peak: 2–5 hr after dose
Flecainide	Oral	Trough: Immediately before next dose Peak: 3 hr after dose
Lidocaine	IV	15 min, 1 hr, then every 24 hr
Procainamide	IV	15 min; 2, 6, 12 hr; then every 24 hr
Procainamide	Oral	Trough: Immediately before next dose Peak: 75 min after dose
Quinidine sulfate	Oral	Trough: Immediately before next dose Peak: 1 hr after dose
Quinidine gluconate	Oral	Trough: Immediately before next dose Peak: 5 hr after dose
Quinidine polygalacturonate	Oral	Trough: Immediately before next dose Peak: 2 hr after dose

Drug (Antimicrobials)	Route of Administration	Recommended Collection Time*
Amikacin	IV, IM	Trough: Immediately before next dose Peak: 30 min after the end of a 30-min IV infusion
Gentamicin	IV, IM	Trough: Immediately before next dose Peak: 30 min after the end of a 30-min IV infusion
Tobramycin	IV, IM	Trough: Immediately before next dose Peak: 30 min after the end of a 30-min IV infusion
Tricyclic glycopeptide and vancomycin	IV, PO	Trough: Immediately before next dose Peak: 30–60 min after the end of a 60-min IV infusion

*Usually after fifth dose if given every 8 hr or third dose if given every 12 hr.
IM = intramuscular; PO = by mouth.

Drug (Antipsychotics, Antimanics)	Route of Administration	Recommended Collection Time
Haloperidol	Oral	Peak: 3–6 hr
Lithium	Oral	Trough: at least 12 hr after last dose; steady state occurs at 90–120 hr

Drug (Immunosuppressants)	Route of Administration	Recommended Collection Time
Cyclosporine	Oral or IV	12 hr after dose or immediately prior to next dose
Methotrexate	Oral or IM	Varies according to dosing protocol
Everolimus	Oral	Immediately prior to next dose
Sirolimus	Oral	Immediately prior to next dose
Tacrolimus	Oral	Immediately prior to next dose

Leucovorin therapy, also called *leucovorin rescue,* is used in conjunction with administration of methotrexate. Leucovorin, a fast-acting form of folic acid, protects healthy cells from the toxic effects of methotrexate.

NORMAL FINDINGS: Method: Immunoassay for acetaminophen, amikacin, amiodarone, carbamazepine, cyclosporine, digoxin, disopyramide, ethosuximide, flecainide, gentamicin, imipramine, lidocaine, methotrexate, phenobarbital, phenytoin, primidone, procainamide, quinidine, salicylate, tobramycin, valproic acid, and vancomycin. Chromatography for amitriptyline, doxepin, haloperidol, nortriptyline, and protriptyline. Ion-selective electrode for lithium. Liquid chromatography/tandem mass spectrometry for everolimus, lamotrigine, sirolimus, and tacrolimus.

Drug/Class (Analgesics, Anti-inflammatories, and Antipyretics)	Therapeutic Range Conventional Units	Conversion to SI units	Therapeutic Range SI Units	Half-Life	Protein Binding	Metabolism	Excretion	Crosses Placenta/ Enters Breast Milk
Acetaminophen	5–20 mcg/mL	SI units = Conventional Units × 6.62	33–132 micromol/L	1–3 hr	10%–25% (dose dependent)	1° hepatic (CYP2E1, CYP1A2, CYP2D6, UGT)	1° renal	Yes/Yes (small amounts)
Salicylate	10–30 mg/ dL (anti-inflammatory); 2–10 mg/dL (antipyretic/ analgesic)	SI units = Conventional Units × 0.073	0.7–2.2 mmol/L (anti-inflammatory); 0.15–0.7 mmol/L (antipyretic/ analgesic)	2–3 hr (low dose)	80%–90%	1° hepatic (CYP2C19)	1° renal	Yes/Yes

It should be noted that acetaminophen and acetylsalicylic acid are contained in many other medications, such as cold and cough medicines.

D

Drug/Class (Anticonvulsants)	Therapeutic Range Conventional Units	Conversion to SI Units	Therapeutic Range SI Units	Half-Life	Protein Binding	Metabolism	Excretion	Crosses Placenta/ Enters Breast Milk
Carbamazepine	4–12 mcg/mL	SI units = Conventional units × 4.23	16.9–50.8 micromol/L	15–40 hr (single dose); 16–24 hr (repeated dosing)	70%–80%	Hepatic (CYP3A4)	1° renal; 2° fecal	Yes/Yes
Ethosuximide	40–100 mcg/mL	SI units = Conventional units × 7.08	283.2–708 micromol/L	25–70 hr	0%–5%	Hepatic (CYP3A4, CYP2E1)	Renal (20%)	Yes/Yes
Lamotrigine	1–14 mcg/mL	SI units = Conventional units × 3.9	3.9–54.6 micromol/L	25–33 hr (monotherapy)	50%–55%	Hepatic (UGT1A4)	1° renal; 2° fecal	No information/Yes (Note: Significant binding to tissues containing melanin)
Phenobarbital	*Adult:* 15–40 mcg/mL	SI units = Conventional units × 4.31	*Adult:* 64.6–172.4 micromol/L	*Adult:* 50–140 hr	50%–60%	Hepatic (CYP2C19)	1° renal; 2° fecal	Yes/Unknown
	Child: 15–30 mcg/mL	SI units = Conventional units × 4.31	*Child:* 64.6–129.3 micromol/L	*Child:* 60–180 hr	50%–60%	Hepatic (CYP2C19)	1° renal; 2° fecal	Yes/Unknown
Phenytoin	10–20 mcg/mL	SI units = Conventional units × 3.96	40–79 micromol/L	7–42 (avg 22) hr	85%–95%	Hepatic (CYP2C9, CYPC219)	1° renal and biliary	Yes/Yes
Primidone	*Adult:* 5–12 mcg/mL	SI units = Conventional units × 4.58	*Adult:* 22.9–55 micromol/L	4–12 hr	0%–20%	Hepatic (CYPC219)	1° renal	Yes/No information
	Child: 7–10 mcg/mL	SI units = Conventional units × 4.58	*Child:* 32.1–45.8 micromol/L					
Valproic acid	50–125 mcg/mL	SI units = Conventional units × 6.93	346.5–866.2 micromol/L	8–15 hr	85%–95%	Hepatic (not CYP450 dependent)	1° renal	Yes/Yes

D

Drug/Class (Antidepressants)	Therapeutic Range Conventional Units	Conversion to SI Units	Therapeutic Range SI Units	Half-Life	Protein Binding	Metabolism	Excretion	Crosses Placenta/ Enters Breast Milk
Amitriptyline	125–250 ng/mL	SI units = Conventional units × 3.6	450–900 nmol/L	10–50 hr	85%–95%	Hepatic (CYP2D6)	1° renal	Yes/Yes
Nortriptyline	50–150 ng/mL	SI units = Conventional units × 3.8	190–570 nmol/L	16–90 hr	90%–95%	Hepatic (CYP2D6)	Renal	Probable/Yes
Protriptyline	70–250 ng/mL	SI units = Conventional units × 3.8	266–950 nmol/L	60–90 hr	91%–93%	Hepatic (CYP2D6)	Renal	No information/ Probable
Doxepin	110–250 ng/mL	SI units = Conventional units × 3.58	393.8–895 nmol/L	10–25 hr	75%–85%	Hepatic (CYP2D6, CYP2C19, CYP1A2, CYP3A4)	Renal	Probable/Yes
Imipramine	180–240 ng/mL	SI units = Conventional units × 3.57	642.6–856.8 nmol/L	8–20 hr	86%–95%	Hepatic (CYP1A2, CYP2C19, CYP2D6)	1° renal; 2° fecal	Probable/Yes

D

Drug/Class (Antidysrhythmics)	Therapeutic Range Conventional Units	Conversion to SI Units	Therapeutic Range SI Units	Half-Life	Protein Binding	Metabolism	Excretion	Crosses Placenta/ Enters Breast Milk
Amiodarone	0.5–2.5 mcg/mL	SI units = Conventional units × 1.55	0.8–3.9 micromol/L	15–142 (58 avg) days	90%–95%	1° hepatic (CYP3A, CYP2C8)	1° biliary	Yes/Yes
Digoxin	0.5–2 ng/mL	SI units = Conventional units × 1.28	0.6–2.6 nmol/L	36–48 hr	20%–30%	Hepatic (16%) (not CYP450 dependent)	Renal	Yes/Yes
Disopyramide	2.8–7 mcg/mL	SI units = Conventional units × 2.95	8.3–20.6 micromol/L	4–10 hr	50%–65%	Hepatic (CYP3A4)	Renal	Yes/Yes
Flecainide	0.2–1 mcg/mL	SI units = Conventional units × 2.41	0.5–2.4 micromol/L	11–27 hr	40%–50%	Hepatic (CYP2D6)	Renal	Probable/ Yes
Lidocaine	1.5–5 mcg/mL	SI units = Conventional units × 4.27	6.4–21.4 micromol/L	1.5–2 hr	60%–80%	1° hepatic (CYP3a4)	Renal	Yes/Yes
Procainamide	4–10 mcg/mL	SI units = Conventional units × 4.25	17–42.5 micromol/L	2–6 hr	10%–20%	Hepatic (CYP2D6)	Renal	Yes/Yes
N-acetyl procainamide	10–20 mcg/mL	SI units = Conventional units × 4.25	42.5–85 micromol/L	4–15 hr	10%–20%	Hepatic (CYP2D6)	Renal	Yes/Yes
Quinidine	2–5 mcg/mL	SI units = Conventional units × 3.08	6.2–15.4 micromol/L	6–8 hr	70%–90%	Hepatic (CYP3A4)	Hepatic (20% unchanged in urine)	Yes/Yes

Drug/Class (Antimicrobials)	Therapeutic Range Conventional Units	Conversion to SI Units	Therapeutic Range SI Units	Half-Life	Protein Binding	Metabolism	Excretion	Crosses Placenta/ Enters Breast Milk
Amikacin	Peak: 15–30 mcg/mL Trough: 4–8 mcg/mL	SI units = Conventional units × 1.71	Peak: 26–51 micromol/L Trough: 7–14 micromol/L	2–4 hr	50%	Renal	1° renal	Yes/Yes (small amts)
Gentamicin (standard dosing)	Peak: 5–10 mcg/mL Trough: Less than 2 mcg/ mL	SI units = Conventional units × 2.09	Peak: 10.4–20.9 micromol/L Trough: Less than 4.2 micromol/L	2–4 hr	50%	Renal	1° renal	Yes/Yes (small amts)
Tobramycin (standard dosing)	Peak: 4–8 mcg/mL Trough: Less than 1 mcg/ mL	SI units = Conventional units × 2.09	Peak: 8.4–16.7 micromol/L Trough: Less than 2.09 micromol/L	2–4 hr	50%	Renal	1° renal	Yes/Yes (small amts)
Tobramycin (once daily dosing)	Peak: 8–12 mcg/mL Trough: Less than 0.5 mcg/ mL	SI units = Conventional units × 2.09	Peak: 16.7–25 micromol/L Trough: Less than 1 micromol/L					
Vancomycin	Trough (general) values vary with indication: 5–15 mcg/mL	SI units = Conventional units × 0.69	3–10 micromol/L	5–8 hr	55%	Renal	1° renal (IV); feces (oral)	Yes/No information

D

Drug/Class (Antipsychotics and Antimanics)	Therapeutic Range Conventional Units	Conversion to SI Units	Therapeutic Range SI Units	Half-Life	Protein Binding	Metabolism	Excretion	Crosses Placenta/ Enters Breast Milk, Protein Binding (%)
Haloperidol	6–24 ng/mL	SI units = Conventional units × 2.66	16–63.8 nmol/L	21–24 hr	90%	Hepatic (CYP3A4)	Hepatic	Yes/Yes
Lithium (chronic)	0.6–1.2 mEq/L	SI units = Conventional units × 1	0.6–1.2 mmol/L	18–24 hr	0%	None	Renal	Yes/Yes

D

Drug/Class (Immunosuppressants)	Therapeutic Range Conventional Units	Conversion to SI Units	Therapeutic Range SI Units	Half-Life	Protein Binding	Metabolism	Excretion	Crosses Placenta/ Enters Breast Milk
Cyclosporine	100–300 ng/mL kidney transplant	SI units = Conventional units × 0.832	83.2–249.6 nmol/L	8–24 hr	90%–98%	Hepatic (CYP3A4)	Biliary	Yes/Yes
	200–350 ng/mL cardiac, hepatic, pancreatic transplant	SI units = Conventional units × 0.832	166.4–291.2 nmol/L	8–24 hr	90%–98%	Hepatic (CYP3A4)	Biliary	Yes/Yes
	100–300 ng/mL bone marrow transplant	SI units = Conventional units × 0.832	83.2–249.6 nmol/L	8–24 hr	90%–98%	Hepatic (CYP3A4)	Biliary	Yes/Yes
Methotrexate	Low dose: Less than 0.5 micromol/L after 48 hr	SI units = Conventional units × 1	Low dose: Less than 0.5 micromol/L after 48 hr	3–10 hr (low dose)	35%–50% (dosage dependent/ varies individually)	Hepatic and intracellular	1° renal; 2° fecal	Yes (embryotoxic)/ Yes
	High dose: Less than 5 micromol/L at 24 hr; less than 0.5 micromol/L at 48 hr; less than 0.1 micromol/L at 72 hr	SI units = Conventional units × 1	High dose: Less than 5 micromol/L at 24 hr; less than 0.5 micromol/L at 48 hr; less than 0.1 micromol/L at 72 hr	8–15 hr (high dose)	35%–50% (dosage dependent/ varies individually)	Hepatic and intracellular	1° renal; 2° fecal	Yes (embryotoxic)/ Yes
Everolimus	Transplant: 3–8 ng/mL	SI units = Conventional units × 1.04	Transplant: 3.1–8.3 nmol/L	18–35 hr (kidney); 30–35 hr (liver)	75%	Hepatic (CYP3A4)	1° fecal; 2° renal	Yes/Yes

(table continues on page 490)

D

Drug/Class (Immunosuppressants)	Therapeutic Range Conventional Units	Conversion to SI Units	Therapeutic Range SI Units	Half-Life	Protein Binding	Metabolism	Excretion	Crosses Placenta/ Enters Breast Milk
	Oncology: 5–10 ng/mL	SI units = Conventional units × 1	Oncology: 5–10 nmol/L	18–35 hr	75%	Hepatic (CYP3A4)	1° fecal; 2° renal	Yes/Yes
Sirolimus	Maintenance phase: kidney transplant: 4–12 ng/mL; liver transplant: 12–20 ng/mL	SI units = Conventional units × 1.1	Kidney transplant: 4.4–13.2 nmol/L; liver transplant: 13.2–22 nmol/L	57–78 hr	92%	Hepatic (CYP3A4)	1° fecal	No information
Tacrolimus	Maintenance phase: kidney transplant: 6–12 ng/mL; liver transplant: 4–10 ng/mL; pancreas transplant: 10–18 ng/mL; bone marrow transplant: 10–20 ng/mL	SI units = Conventional units × 1.24	Kidney transplant: 7.4–14.9 nmol/L; liver transplant: 5–12.4 nmol/L; pancreas transplant: 12.4–22.3 nmol/L; bone marrow transplant: 12.4–24.8 nmol/L	10–14 hr	99%	Hepatic (CYP3A4, CYP3A5)	1° fecal	Yes/Yes

Therapeutic targets for the initial phase post-transplantation are slightly higher than during the maintenance phase and are influenced by the specific therapy chosen for each patient with respect to coordination of treatment for other conditions and corresponding therapies. Therapeutic ranges for everolimus, sirolimus, and tacrolimus assume concomitant administration of cyclosporine and steroids.

D

CRITICAL FINDINGS AND POTENTIAL INTERVENTIONS

Note: The adverse effects of subtherapeutic levels are also important. Care should be taken to investigate signs and symptoms of too little and too much medication.

Timely notification to the requesting health-care provider (HCP) of any critical findings and related symptoms is a role expectation of the professional nurse. A listing of these findings varies among facilities.

Analgesics, Anti-inflammatories, and Antipyretics

Acetaminophen: Greater than 200 mcg/mL (4 hr Postingestion): (SI: Greater than 1,324 micromol/L [4 hr Postingestion])

Signs and symptoms of acetaminophen intoxication occur in stages over a period of time. In stage I (0 to 24 hr after ingestion), symptoms may include gastrointestinal (GI) irritation, pallor, lethargy, diaphoresis, metabolic acidosis, and possibly coma. In stage II (24 to 48 hr after ingestion), signs and symptoms may include right upper quadrant abdominal pain; elevated liver enzymes, aspartate aminotransferase (AST), and alanine aminotransferase (ALT); and possible decreased kidney function. In stage III (72 to 96 hr after ingestion), signs and symptoms may include nausea, vomiting, jaundice, confusion, coagulation disorders, continued elevation of AST and ALT, decreased kidney function, and coma. Intervention may include GI decontamination (stomach pumping) if the patient presents within 6 hr of ingestion or administration of *N*-acetylcysteine (Mucomyst) in the case of an acute intoxication.

Acetylsalicylic Acid (ASA): Greater than 40 mg/dL: (SI: Greater than 2.9 mmol/L)

Signs and symptoms of salicylate intoxication include ketosis, convulsions, dizziness, nausea, vomiting, hyperactivity, hyperglycemia, hyperpnea, hyperthermia, respiratory arrest, and tinnitus. Possible interventions include administration of activated charcoal as vomiting ceases, alkalinization of the urine with bicarbonate, and a single dose of vitamin K (for rare instances of hypoprothrombinemia).

Anticonvulsants

Carbamazepine: Greater than 20 mcg/mL (SI: Greater than 85 micromol/L)

Signs and symptoms of carbamazepine toxicity include respiratory depression, seizures, leukopenia, hyponatremia, hypotension, stupor, and possible coma. Possible interventions include gastric lavage (contraindicated if ileus is present); airway protection; administration of fluids and vasopressors for hypotension; treatment of seizures with diazepam, phenobarbital, or phenytoin; cardiac monitoring; monitoring of vital signs; and discontinuing the medication. Emetics are contraindicated.

Ethosuximide: Greater than 200 mcg/mL (SI: Greater than 1,416 micromol/L)

Signs and symptoms of ethosuximide toxicity include nausea, vomiting, and lethargy. Possible interventions include administration of activated charcoal, administration of saline cathartic and gastric lavage (contraindicated if ileus is present), airway protection, hourly assessment of neurological function, and discontinuing the medication.

Lamotrigine: Greater than 20 mcg/mL (SI: Greater than 78 micromol/L)
Signs and symptoms of lamotrigine toxicity include severe skin rash, nausea, vomiting, ataxia, decreased levels of consciousness, coma, increased seizures, nystagmus. Possible interventions include administration of activated charcoal, administration of saline cathartic and gastric lavage (contraindicated if ileus is present), airway protection, hourly assessment of neurologic function, and discontinuing the medication.

Phenobarbital: Greater than 60 mcg/mL (SI: Greater than 259 micromol/L)
Signs and symptoms of phenobarbital toxicity include cold, clammy skin; ataxia; central nervous system (CNS) depression; hypothermia; hypotension; cyanosis; Cheyne-Stokes respiration; tachycardia; possible coma; and possible renal impairment. Possible interventions include gastric lavage, administration of activated charcoal with cathartic, airway protection, possible intubation and mechanical ventilation (especially during gastric lavage if there is no gag reflex), monitoring for hypotension, and discontinuing the medication.

Phenytoin (Adults): Greater than 40 mcg/mL (SI: Greater than 158 micromol/L)
Signs and symptoms of phenytoin toxicity include double vision, nystagmus, lethargy, CNS depression, and possible coma. Possible interventions include airway support, electrocardiographic monitoring, administration of activated charcoal, gastric lavage with warm saline or tap water, administration of saline or sorbitol cathartic, and discontinuing the medication.

Primidone: Greater than 15 mcg/mL (SI: Greater than 69 micromol/L)
Signs and symptoms of primidone toxicity include ataxia, anemia, CNS depression, lethargy, somnolence, vertigo, and visual disturbances. Possible interventions include airway protection, treatment of anemia with vitamin B_{12} and folate, and discontinuing the medication.

Valproic acid: Greater than 200 mcg/mL (SI: Greater than 1,386 micromol/L)
Signs and symptoms of valproic acid toxicity include loss of appetite, mental changes, numbness, tingling, and weakness. Possible interventions include administration of activated charcoal and naloxone and discontinuing the medication.

Antidepressants

Amitriptyline: Greater than 500 ng/mL (SI: Greater than 1,800 nmol/L)

Nortriptyline: Greater than 500 ng/mL (SI: Greater than 1,900 nmol/L)

Protriptyline: Greater than 500 ng/mL (SI: Greater than 1,900 nmol/L)

Doxepin: Greater than 500 ng/mL (SI: Greater than 1,790 nmol/L)

Imipramine: Greater than 500 ng/mL (SI: Greater than 1,785 nmol/L)
Signs and symptoms of cyclic antidepressant toxicity include agitation, drowsiness, hallucinations, confusion, seizures, dysrhythmias, hyperthermia, flushing, dilation of the pupils, and possible coma. Possible interventions include administration of activated charcoal; emesis; gastric lavage with

saline; administration of physostigmine to counteract seizures, hypertension, or respiratory depression; administration of bicarbonate, propranolol, lidocaine, or phenytoin to counteract dysrhythmias; and electrocardiographic monitoring.

Antidysrhythmics

Amiodarone: Greater than 2.5 mcg/mL (SI: Greater than 3.9 micromol/L)
Signs and symptoms of pulmonary damage related to amiodarone toxicity include bronchospasm, wheezing, fever, dyspnea, cough, hemoptysis, and hypoxia. Possible interventions include discontinuing the medication, monitoring pulmonary function with chest x-ray, monitoring liver function tests to assess for liver damage, monitoring thyroid function tests to assess for thyroid damage (related to the high concentration of iodine contained in the medication), and electrocardiographic (ECG) monitoring for worsening of dysrhythmia.

Digoxin: Greater than 2.5 ng/mL (SI: Greater than 3.2 nmol/L)
Signs and symptoms of digoxin toxicity include dysrhythmias, anorexia, hyperkalemia, nausea, vomiting, diarrhea, changes in mental status, and visual disturbances (objects appear yellow or have halos around them). Possible interventions include discontinuing the medication, continuous ECG monitoring (prolonged P-R interval, widening QRS interval, lengthening Q-Tc interval, and atrioventricular block), transcutaneous pacing, administration of activated charcoal (if the patient has a gag reflex and CNS function), support and treatment of electrolyte disturbance, and administration of Digibind or DigiFab (digoxin immune Fab). The amount of Digibind or DigiFab given depends on the level of digoxin to be neutralized. Digoxin levels must be measured before the administration of Digibind or DigiFab. Digoxin levels should not be measured for several days after administration of Digibind or DigiFab in patients with normal kidney function (1 wk or longer in patients with decreased kidney function). Digibind or DigiFab cross-reacts in the digoxin assay and may provide misleading elevations or decreases in values depending on the particular assay in use by the laboratory.

Disopyramide: Greater than 7 mcg/mL (SI: Greater than 20.6 micromol/L)
Signs and symptoms of disopyramide toxicity include prolonged Q-T interval, ventricular tachycardia, hypotension, and heart failure. Possible interventions include discontinuing the medication, airway support, and ECG and blood pressure monitoring.

Flecainide: Greater than 1 mcg/mL (SI: Greater than 2.41 micromol/L)
Signs and symptoms of flecainide toxicity include exaggerated pharmacological effects resulting in dysrhythmia. Possible interventions include discontinuing the medication as well as continuous ECG, respiratory, and blood pressure monitoring.

Lidocaine: Greater than 6 mcg/mL (SI: Greater than 25.6 micromol/L)
Signs and symptoms of lidocaine toxicity include slurred speech, CNS depression, cardiovascular depression, convulsions, muscle twitches, and possible coma. Possible interventions include continuous ECG monitoring, airway support, and seizure precautions.

Procainamide: Greater than 10 mcg/mL (SI: Greater than 42.5 micromol/L); *N*-Acetyl Procainamide: Greater than 40 mcg/mL (SI: Greater than 170 micromol/L)

The active metabolite of procainamide is *N*-acetyl procainamide (NAPA). Signs and symptoms of procainamide toxicity include torsade de pointes (ventricular tachycardia), nausea, vomiting, agranulocytosis, and hepatic disturbances. Possible interventions include airway protection, emesis, gastric lavage, and administration of sodium lactate.

Quinidine: Greater than 6 mcg/mL (SI: Greater than 18.5 micromol/L)

Signs and symptoms of quinidine toxicity include ataxia, nausea, vomiting, diarrhea, respiratory system depression, hypotension, syncope, anuria, dysrhythmias (heart block, widening of QRS and Q-T intervals), asystole, hallucinations, paresthesia, and irritability. Possible interventions include airway support, emesis, gastric lavage, administration of activated charcoal, administration of sodium lactate, and temporary transcutaneous or transvenous pacemaker.

Antimicrobials

Amikacin: Greater than 10 mcg/mL (SI: Greater than 17 micromol/L)

Gentamicin: Peak Greater than 12 mcg/mL, Trough Greater than 2 mcg/mL (SI: Peak Greater than 25 micromol/L, Trough Greater than 4 micromol/L)

Tobramycin: Peak Greater than 12 mcg/mL, Trough Greater than 2 mcg/mL (SI: Peak Treater than 25 micromol/L, Trough Greater than 4 micromol/L)

Vancomycin: Trough Greater than 30 mcg/mL (SI: Trough Greater than 21 micromol/L)

Signs and symptoms of toxic levels of the antibiotics gentamicin and tobramycin are similar and include loss of hearing and decreased renal function. Suspected hearing loss can be evaluated by audiometry testing. Impaired renal function may be identified by monitoring blood urea nitrogen and creatinine levels as well as intake and output. The most important intervention is accurate therapeutic drug monitoring so the medication can be discontinued before irreversible damage is done.

Antipsychotics and Antimanics

Haloperidol: Greater than 42 ng/mL (SI: Greater than 112 nmol/L)

Signs and symptoms of haloperidol toxicity include hypotension, myocardial depression, respiratory depression, and extrapyramidal neuromuscular reactions. Possible interventions include emesis (contraindicated in the absence of gag reflex or central nervous system depression or excitation) and gastric lavage followed by administration of activated charcoal.

Lithium: Greater than 2 mEq/L (SI: Greater than 2 mmol/L)

Signs and symptoms of lithium toxicity include ataxia, coarse tremors, muscle rigidity, vomiting, diarrhea, confusion, convulsions, stupor, T-wave flattening, loss of consciousness, and possible coma. Possible interventions include administration of activated charcoal, gastric lavage, and administration of intravenous fluids with diuresis.

Immunosuppressants

Cyclosporine: Greater than 500 ng/mL (SI: Greater than 416 nmol/L)

Signs and symptoms of cyclosporine toxicity include increased severity of expected adverse effects, which include nausea, stomatitis, vomiting, anorexia, hypertension, infection, fluid retention, hypercalcemic metabolic acidosis, tremor, seizures, headache, and flushing. Possible interventions include close monitoring of blood levels to make dosing adjustments, inducing emesis (if orally ingested), performing gastric lavage (if orally ingested), withholding the drug, and initiating alternative therapy for a short time until the patient is stabilized.

Methotrexate: Greater than 5 micromol/L

Signs and symptoms of methotrexate toxicity include increased severity of expected adverse effects, which include nausea, stomatitis, vomiting, anorexia, bleeding, infection, bone marrow depression, and, over a prolonged period of use, hepatotoxicity. The effect of methotrexate on normal cells can be reversed by administration of 5-formyltetrahydrofolate (citrovorum or leucovorin). 5-Formyltetrahydrofolate allows higher doses of methotrexate to be given.

Everolimus: Greater than 15 ng/mL (SI: Greater than 15 mcg/L)

Signs and symptoms of everolimus pulmonary toxicity include hypoxia, pleural effusion, cough, and dyspnea. Possible interventions include dosing adjustments, administration of corticosteroids, and monitoring of pulmonary function with chest x-ray. Use of everolimus is contraindicated in patients with severe hepatic impairment. Concomitant administration of strong CYP3A4 inhibitors may significantly increase everolimus levels.

Sirolimus: Greater than 25 ng/mL (SI: Greater than 28 mcg/L)

Signs and symptoms of sirolimus pulmonary toxicity include cough, shortness of breath, chest pain, and rapid heart rate. Possible interventions include dosing adjustments, administration of corticosteroids, and monitoring of pulmonary function with chest x-ray.

Tacrolimus: Greater than 25 ng/mL (SI: Greater than 31 mcg/L)

Signs and symptoms of tacrolimus toxicity include tremors, seizures, headache, high blood pressure, hyperkalemia, tinnitus, nausea, and vomiting. Possible interventions include treatment of hypertension, administration of antiemetics for nausea and vomiting, and dosing adjustments.

OVERVIEW: (Study type: Blood collected in a red-top tube **except** for cyclosporine, everolimus, sirolimus, and tacrolimus which are collected in a lavender-top [EDTA] tube; related body system: Multisystem.)

The metabolism of many commonly prescribed medications is driven by the cytochrome P450 (CYP450) family of enzymes.

Genetic variants can alter enzymatic activity that results in a spectrum of effects ranging from the total absence of drug metabolism to ultrafast metabolism. Impaired drug metabolism can prevent the intended therapeutic effect or even lead to serious adverse drug reactions. *Poor metabolizer* (PM) are at increased risk for drug-induced adverse effects due to accumulation of drug in the blood, and *ultra rapid metabolizer* (UM) require a higher than normal dosage because the drug is metabolized over a shorter duration than intended. In the case of prodrugs, which require activation prior to metabolism, the opposite occurs: PM may require a higher dose because the activated drug becomes available more slowly than intended, and UM requires less because the activated drug becomes available sooner than intended. Other genetic phenotypes used to report CYP450 results are intermediate metabolizer (IM) and extensive metabolizer (EM). Testing for specific CYP450 genotype defects can be performed in some laboratories on blood and buccal specimens. The test method commonly used is polymerase chain reaction. Counseling and informed written consent are generally required for genetic testing. Testing allows for the possibility of personalized adjustments to the medication regimen or decisions to seek alternative drugs, which in turn results in safer, more effective treatment. CYP2C9 is a gene in the CYP450 family that metabolizes phenytoin as well as other drugs, such as the antihypertensive drug losartan and the anticoagulant drug warfarin. CYP2D6 is a gene in the CYP450 family that metabolizes tricyclic antidepressants such as nortriptyline, antipsychotics such as haloperidol, and beta blockers. Testing for the most common genetic variants of CYP2D6 and CYP2C9 is used to predict altered enzyme activity and anticipate the most effective therapeutic plan.

Analgesics, Anti-inflammatories, and Antipyretics

Acetaminophen is used for headache, fever, and pain relief, especially for individuals unable to take salicylate products or who have bleeding conditions. It is the analgesic of choice for children less than 13 yr old; salicylates are avoided in this age group because of the association between aspirin and Reye syndrome. Acetaminophen is rapidly absorbed from the GI tract and reaches peak concentration within 30 to 60 min after administration of a therapeutic dose. It can be a silent killer because by the time symptoms of intoxication appear 24 to 48 hr after ingestion, the antidote is ineffective. ASA is also used for headache, fever, inflammation, and pain relief. Some patients with cardiovascular disease take small prophylactic doses. The main site of toxicity for both drugs is the liver, particularly in the presence of liver disease or decreased drug metabolism and excretion. Other medications indicated for use in controlling neuropathic pain include amitriptyline and nortriptyline.

Anticonvulsants

Anticonvulsants are used to reduce the frequency and severity of seizures for patients with epilepsy. Carbamazepine is also used for controlling neurogenic pain in trigeminal neuralgia and diabetic neuropathy and for treating bipolar disease and other neurological and psychiatric conditions. Valproic acid is also used for some psychiatric conditions, such as bipolar disorder, and for prevention of migraine headache.

Antidepressants

Cyclic antidepressants are used in the treatment of major depression. They have also been used effectively to treat bipolar disorder, panic disorder, attention deficit-hyperactivity disorder, obsessive-compulsive disorder, enuresis, eating disorders (bulimia nervosa in particular), nicotine dependence (tobacco), and cocaine dependence. Numerous drug interactions occur with the cyclic antidepressants.

Antidysrhythmics

Cardiac glycosides are used in the prophylactic management and treatment of heart failure and ventricular and atrial dysrhythmias. Because these drugs have narrow therapeutic windows, they must be monitored closely. The signs and symptoms of toxicity are often difficult to distinguish from those of cardiac disease. Patients with toxic levels may show GI, ocular, and CNS effects and disturbances in potassium balance.

Antimicrobials

The aminoglycoside antibiotics amikacin, gentamicin, and tobramycin are used against many gram-negative (*Acinetobacter, Citrobacter, Enterobacter, Escherichia coli, Klebsiella, Proteus, Providencia, Pseudomonas, Raoultella, Salmonella, Serratia, Shigella,* and *Stenotrophomonas*) and some gram-positive (*Staphylococcus aureus*) pathogenic microorganisms. Aminoglycosides are poorly absorbed through the GI tract and are most frequently administered IV. Peak and trough collection times should be documented carefully in relation to the time of medication administration. Creatinine levels should be monitored every 2 to 3 days to detect renal impairment due to toxic drug levels.

Vancomycin is a tricyclic glycopeptide antibiotic used against many gram-positive microorganisms, such as staphylococci, *Streptococcus pneumoniae,* group A β-hemolytic streptococci, enterococci, *Corynebacterium,* and *Clostridium.* Vancomycin has also been used in an oral form for the treatment of pseudomembranous colitis resulting from *Clostridium difficile* infection. This approach is less frequently used because of the emergence of vancomycin-resistant enterococci (VRE).

Antipsychotics and Antimanics

Haloperidol is an antipsychotic tranquilizer used for treatment of acute and chronic psychotic disorders, Tourette syndrome, and hyperactive children with severe behavioral problems. Frequent monitoring is important due to the unstable relationship between dosage and circulating steady-state concentration. Lithium is used in the treatment of bipolar disorder. Daily monitoring of lithium levels is important until the proper dosage is achieved. Lithium is cleared and reabsorbed by the kidneys. Clearance is increased when sodium levels are increased and decreased in conditions associated with low sodium levels; therefore, patients receiving lithium therapy should try to maintain a balanced daily intake of sodium. Lithium levels affect other organ systems. A high incidence of pulmonary complications is associated with lithium toxicity. Lithium can also affect cardiac conduction, producing T-wave depressions. These ECG changes are usually insignificant and reversible and are seen in 10% to 20% of patients on lithium therapy. Chronic lithium therapy has been shown to result in enlargement of the thyroid gland in a small percentage of patients. Other medications indicated for use as mood stabilizers include carbamazepine, lamotrigine, and valproic acid.

Immunosuppressants

Cyclosporine is an immunosuppressive drug used in the management of organ rejection, especially rejection of heart, liver, pancreas, and kidney transplants. Its most serious adverse effect is renal impairment or chronic kidney disease. Cyclosporine is often administered in conjunction with corticosteroids (e.g., prednisone) for its anti-inflammatory or immune-suppressing properties and with other drugs (e.g., everolimus, sirolimus, tacrolimus) to reduce graft-versus-host disease. Methotrexate is a highly toxic drug that causes cell death by disrupting DNA synthesis. Methotrexate is also used in the treatment of rheumatoid arthritis, psoriasis, polymyositis, and Reiter syndrome. Cyclosporine, sirolimus, and tacrolimus are metabolized by the cytochrome enzyme CYP3A4, which is essential to achieve the desired therapeutic effect.

Many factors must be considered in interpreting drug levels, including patient age, patient ethnicity, patient weight, interacting medications, electrolyte balance, protein levels, water balance, conditions that affect absorption and excretion, and the ingestion of substances (e.g., foods and dietary supplements) that can potentiate or inhibit the intended target concentration.

These medications are metabolized and excreted by the kidneys and are therefore contraindicated in patients with kidney disease and cautiously advised in patients with kidney impairment. Information regarding medications must be clearly and accurately communicated to avoid misunderstanding of the dose time in relation to the collection time. Miscommunication between the individual administering the medication and the individual collecting the specimen is the most frequent cause of subtherapeutic levels, toxic levels, and misleading information used in the calculation of future doses. Some pharmacies use a computerized pharmacokinetics approach to dosing that eliminates the need to be concerned about peak and trough collections; random specimens are adequate. If administration of the drug is delayed, notify the appropriate department(s) to reschedule the blood draw and notify the requesting HCP if the delay has caused any real or perceived therapeutic harm.

INDICATIONS

- Monitor some patients who have a pacemaker, who have impaired kidney or liver function, who have had an organ transplant, or who are taking interacting drugs.
- Suspected overdose/misuse.
- Suspected subtherapeutic levels.
- Suspected toxicity.
- Therapeutic monitoring for adherence to and effectiveness of treatment.

INTERFERING FACTORS

Factors that may alter the results of the study

Analgesics, Anti-inflammatories, and Antipyretics

- Drugs and other substances that may increase acetaminophen levels include diflunisal, metoclopramide, and probenecid.
- Drugs and other substances that may decrease acetaminophen levels include carbamazepine, cholestyramine, iron, oral contraceptives, and propantheline.
- Drugs and other substances that increase ASA levels include choline magnesium trisalicylate, cimetidine, furosemide, and sulfinpyrazone.
- Drugs and other substances that decrease ASA levels include activated charcoal, antacids (aluminum hydroxide), corticosteroids, and iron.

Anticonvulsants

- Drugs and other substances that may increase carbamazepine levels or increase risk of toxicity include acetazolamide, azithromycin, bepridil, cimetidine, danazol, diltiazem, erythromycin, felodipine, fluoxetine, flurithromycin, fluvoxamine, gemfibrozil, isoniazid, itraconazole, josamycin, ketoconazole, loratadine, macrolides, niacinamide, nicardipine, nifedipine, nimodipine, nisoldipine, ritonavir, troleandomycin, valproic acid, verapamil, and viloxazine.
- Drugs and other substances that may decrease carbamazepine levels include phenobarbital, phenytoin, and primidone.
- Carbamazepine may affect other body chemistries, as seen by a decrease in calcium, sodium, T_3, T_4 levels, and WBC count and increase in ALT, alkaline phosphatase, ammonia, AST, and bilirubin levels.
- Drugs and other substances that may increase ethosuximide levels include isoniazid, ritonavir, and valproic acid.
- Drugs and other substances that may decrease ethosuximide levels include phenobarbital, phenytoin, and primidone.
- Drugs and other substances that may increase lamotrigine levels include valproic acid.
- Drugs and other substances that may decrease lamotrigine levels include acetaminophen, carbamazepine, hydantoins (e.g., phenytoin), oral contraceptives, orlistat, oxcarbazepine, phenobarbital, primidone, protease inhibitors (e.g., ritonavir), rifamycins (e.g., rifampin), and succinimides (e.g., ethosuximide).
- Drugs and other substances that may increase phenobarbital levels or increase risk of toxicity include barbital drugs, furosemide, primidone, salicylates, and valproic acid.
- Phenobarbital may affect the metabolism of other drugs, such as β-blockers, chloramphenicol, corticosteroids, doxycycline, griseofulvin, haloperidol, methylphenidate, phenothiazines, phenylbutazone, quinidine, theophylline, tricyclic antidepressants, and valproic acid, increasing their effectiveness.
- Phenobarbital may affect the metabolism of other drugs, such as chloramphenicol, cyclosporine, ethosuximide, oral anticoagulants, oral contraceptives, phenytoin, theophylline, vitamin D, and vitamin K, decreasing their effectiveness.
- Phenobarbital is an active metabolite of primidone, and both drug levels should be monitored while

the patient is receiving primidone to avoid either toxic or subtherapeutic levels of both medications.

• Phenobarbital may affect other body chemistries, as seen by a decrease in bilirubin and calcium levels and increase in alkaline phosphatase, ammonia, and gamma glutamyl transferase levels.

• Drugs and other substances that may increase phenytoin levels or increase the risk of phenytoin toxicity include amiodarone, azapropazone, carbamazepine, chloramphenicol, cimetidine, disulfiram, ethanol, fluconazole, halothane, ibuprofen, imipramine, levodopa, metronidazole, miconazole, nifedipine, phenylbutazone, sulfonamides, trazodone, tricyclic antidepressants, and trimethoprim. Small changes in formulation (i.e., changes in brand) also may increase phenytoin levels or increase the risk of phenytoin toxicity.

• Drugs and other substances that may decrease phenytoin levels include bleomycin, carbamazepine, cisplatin, disulfiram, folic acid, IV fluids containing glucose, nitrofurantoin, oxacillin, rifampin, salicylates, and vinblastine.

• Primidone decreases the effectiveness of carbamazepine, ethosuximide, felbamate, lamotrigine, oral anticoagulants, oxcarbazepine, topiramate, and valproic acid.

• Primidone may affect other body chemistries, as seen by a decrease in calcium levels and increase in alkaline phosphatase levels.

• Drugs and other substances that may increase valproic acid levels or increase risk of toxicity include dicumarol, phenylbutazone, and high doses of salicylate.

• Drugs and other substances that may decrease valproic acid levels include carbamazepine, phenobarbital, phenytoin, and primidone.

Antidysrhythmics
• Drugs and other substances that may increase amiodarone levels include cimetidine.

• Drugs and other substances that may decrease amiodarone levels include cholestyramine and phenytoin.

• Drugs and other substances that may increase digoxin levels or increase risk of toxicity include amiodarone, amphotericin B, diclofenac, diltiazem, erythromycin, ibuprofen, indomethacin, nifedipine, nisoldipine, propafenone, propantheline, quinidine, spironolactone, tetracycline, tiapamil, troleandomycin, and verapamil.

• Drugs and other substances that may decrease digoxin levels include albuterol, aluminum hydroxide (antacids), carbamazepine, cholestyramine, colestipol, digoxin immune Fab, hydralazine, hydroxychloroquine, iron, kaolinpectin, magnesium hydroxide, magnesium trisilicate, metoclopramide, neomycin, nitroprusside, paroxetine, phenytoin, rifabutin, sulfasalazine, and ticlopidine.

• Drugs and other substances that may increase disopyramide levels or increase risk of toxicity include amiodarone, atenolol, ritonavir, and troleandomycin.

• Drugs and other substances that may decrease disopyramide levels include phenobarbital, phenytoin, rifabutin, and rifampin.

• Drugs and other substances that may increase flecainide levels or increase risk of toxicity include amiodarone and cimetidine.

• Drugs and other substances that may decrease flecainide levels include carbamazepine, charcoal, phenobarbital, and phenytoin.

• Drugs and other substances that may increase lidocaine levels or increase risk of toxicity include beta blockers, cimetidine,

metoprolol, nadolol, propranolol, and ritonavir.
- Drugs and other substances that may decrease lidocaine levels include phenytoin.
- Drugs and other substances that may increase procainamide levels or increase risk of toxicity include amiodarone, cimetidine, quinidine, ranitidine, and trimethoprim.
- Drugs and other substances that may increase quinidine levels or increase risk of toxicity include acetazolamide, amiodarone, cimetidine, itraconazole, nifedipine, nisoldipine, quinidine, ranitidine, thiazide diuretics, and verapamil.
- Drugs and other substances that may decrease quinidine levels include kaolin-pectin, ketoconazole, phenobarbital, phenytoin, rifabutin, and rifampin.
- Concomitant administration of amiodarone with other medications may result in toxic levels of the other medications related to the suppression of enzyme activity required to metabolize many other medications by amiodarone. It may also potentiate the anticoagulating effects of warfarin, resulting in increased PT values.
- Digitalis-like immunoreactive substances are found in the serum of some patients who are not taking digoxin, causing false-positive results. Patients whose serum contains digitalis-like immunoreactive substances usually have a condition related to salt and fluid retention, such as kidney disease, hepatic failure, low-renin hypertension, and pregnancy.
- Unexpectedly low digoxin levels may be found in patients with thyroid disease.
- Disopyramide may cause a decrease in glucose levels. It may also potentiate the anticoagulating effects of warfarin, resulting in increased PT values.

- Long-term administration of procainamide can cause false-positive antinuclear antibody results and development of a lupus-like syndrome in some patients.
- Quinidine may potentiate the effects of neuromuscular blocking medications and warfarin anticoagulants.
- Concomitant administration of quinidine and digoxin can rapidly raise digoxin to toxic levels. If both drugs are to be given together, the digoxin level should be measured before the first dose of quinidine and again in 4 to 6 days.

Antimicrobials
- Drugs and other substances that may decrease aminoglycoside efficacy include penicillins (e.g., carbenicillin, piperacillin).

Antipsychotics and Antimanics
- Haloperidol may increase levels of tricyclic antidepressants and increase the risk of lithium toxicity.
- Drugs and other substances that may increase lithium levels include angiotensin-converting enzyme inhibitors, some NSAIDs, and thiazide diuretics.
- Drugs and other substances that may decrease lithium levels include acetazolamide, osmotic diuretics, theophylline, and caffeine.

Immunosuppressants
- Numerous drugs and other substances interact with cyclosporine and either increase cyclosporine levels or increase the risk of toxicity. These include acyclovir, aminoglycosides, amiodarone, amphotericin B, anabolic steroids, cephalosporins, cimetidine, danazol, erythromycin, furosemide, ketoconazole, melphalan, methylprednisolone, miconazole, NSAIDs, oral contraceptives, and trimethoprim-sulfamethoxazole.

- Drugs and other substances that may decrease cyclosporine levels include carbamazepine, ethotoin, phenobarbital, phenytoin, primidone, and rifampin.
- Drugs and other substances that may increase methotrexate levels or increase the risk of toxicity include NSAIDs, probenecid, salicylate, and sulfonamides.
- Antibiotics may decrease the absorption of methotrexate.
- Drugs and other substances that may increase everolimus levels include ketoconazole, amprenavir, aprepitant, atazanavir, clarithromycin, delavirdine, diltiazem, erythromycin, fluconazole, fosamprenavir, grapefruit juice, indinavir, itraconazole, nefazodone, nelfinavir, ritonavir, saquinavir, telithromycin, verapamil, and voriconazole.
- Drugs and other substances that may decrease everolimus levels include carbamazepine, dexamethasone, phenobarbital, phenytoin, rifabutin, rifampin, and St. John's wort.
- Drugs and other substances that may increase sirolimus levels include bromocriptine, cimetidine, cisapride, clotrimazole, danazol, diltiazem, fluconazole, indinavir, metoclopramide, nicardipine, ritonavir, troleandomycin, and verapamil.
- Drugs and other substances that may increase sirolimus levels include carbamazepine, phenobarbital, phenytoin, rifapentine, and St. John's wort.
- Drugs and other substances that may increase tacrolimus levels include bromocriptine, chloramphenicol, cimetidine, cisapride, clarithromycin, clotrimazole, cyclosporine, danazol, diltiazem, erythromycin, fluconazole, grapefruit juice, itraconazole, ketoconazole, methylprednisolone, metoclopramide, nelfinavir, nicardipine, nifedipine, troleandomycin, verapamil, and voriconazole.

- Drugs and other substances that may decrease tacrolimus levels include carbamazepine, ethotoin, octreotide, phenobarbital, primidone, rifabutin, rifampin, sirolimus, and St. John's wort.

Other considerations
- Blood drawn in serum separator tubes (gel tubes) is not acceptable; interference with test methods may occur.
- Cyclic antidepressants may potentiate the effects of oral anticoagulants.

POTENTIAL MEDICAL DIAGNOSIS: CLINICAL SIGNIFICANCE OF RESULTS

Level	Response
Normal levels	Therapeutic effect
Subtherapeutic levels	Adjust dose as indicated
Toxic levels (especially in the presence of hepatic or renal impairment)	Adjust dose as indicated

NURSING IMPLICATIONS

BEFORE THE STUDY: PLANNING AND IMPLEMENTATION

Teaching the Patient What to Expect
- Inform the patient this test can assist with evaluation of how much medication is in his or her system in order to provide effective treatment.
- Explain that a blood sample is needed for the test.

AFTER THE STUDY: POTENTIAL NURSING ACTIONS

Avoiding Complications
- Lack of consideration for the proper collection time relative to the dosing schedule can provide misleading

information that may result in erroneous interpretation of levels, creating the potential for a medication error–related injury to the patient.

Treatment Considerations

▶ Administer antibiotic therapy if ordered. Remind the patient of the importance of completing the entire course of antibiotic therapy, even if signs and symptoms disappear before completion of therapy.

▶ Teach patients receiving anticonvulsants the importance of immediately reporting any unusual sensations (e.g., ataxia, dizziness, dyspnea, lethargy, rash, tremors, mental changes, weakness, or visual disturbances) to his or her HCP.

▶ Teach patients receiving antidepressants to immediately report any unusual sensations (e.g., severe headache, vomiting, sweating, visual disturbances) to his or her HCP. Blood pressure should be monitored regularly.

▶ Instruct the patient receiving antidysrhythmics to immediately report any unusual sensations (e.g., dizziness, changes in vision, loss of appetite, nausea, vomiting, diarrhea, weakness, or irregular heartbeat) to his or her HCP. Instruct the patient not to take medicine within 1 hr of food high in fiber *(as the fiber may decrease absorption by binding some of the medication, reducing its bioavailability)*. Testing for aspirin responsiveness/resistance may be a consideration for patients, especially women, on low-dose aspirin therapy.

▶ Instruct the patient receiving aminoglycosides to immediately report any unusual symptoms (e.g., hearing loss, decreased urinary output) to his or her HCP. Instruct the patient receiving lithium to immediately report any unusual symptoms (e.g., anorexia, nausea, vomiting, diarrhea, dizziness, drowsiness, dysarthria, tremor, muscle twitching, visual disturbances) to his or her HCP.

Safety Considerations

▶ Make sure that all therapeutic drug levels are drawn within the correct time period in relation to when the medication is administered (peak and trough).

Collaborate with the pharmacist to make adjustments as necessary to ensure proper results.

Nutritional Considerations

▶ Discuss the reasons for avoidance of alcohol consumption while taking hepatotoxic medications.

▶ Antiepileptic drugs antagonize folic acid, and there is a corresponding slight increase in the incidence of fetal malformations in children of epileptic mothers. Women of childbearing age who are taking antiepileptic drugs should also be prescribed supplemental folic acid to reduce the incidence of neural tube defects. Newborns of women who have epilepsy may demonstrate a temporary deficiency of vitamin K–dependent blood clotting factors at birth. The deficiency is drug induced and can be avoided by administering vitamin K to the mother in the last weeks of pregnancy and to the neonate at birth. Phenobarbital has been associated with low folate and B-vitamin levels in all patient populations; supplementation may be ordered, if needed. Phenobarbital also decreases biologically active levels of vitamin D and reduces calcium absorption; dietary recommendations may include increased consumption of vitamin D–fortified foods and supplementation may be ordered, if needed.

▶ Patients taking immunosuppressant therapy tend to have decreased appetites due to the adverse effects of the medication. Instruct patients to consume a variety of foods within the basic food groups, maintain a healthy weight, be physically active, limit salt intake, limit alcohol intake, and be a nonsmoker.

Follow-Up, Evaluation, and Desired Outcomes

▶ Recognizes the importance of following the medication regimen and instructions regarding food and drug interactions.

▶ Participates in medication reconciliation to ensure accurate collaboration between prescribing HCPs related to medication type, dose, and frequency.

Drug Screen

Amphetamines	Cocaine
Opiates	Cannabinoids
Ethanol (Alcohol)	Phencyclidine

SYNONYM/ACRONYM: Amphetamines, cannabinoids (THC), cocaine, ethanol (alcohol, ethyl alcohol, ETOH), phencyclidine (PCP), opiates (heroin).

RATIONALE: To assist in rapid identification of commonly misused drugs in suspected drug overdose or for workplace drug screening.

PATIENT PREPARATION: There are no food, fluid, activity, or medication restrictions unless by medical direction. Workplace drug-screening programs, because of the potential medicolegal consequences associated with them, require collection of urine and blood specimens using a *chain of custody protocol.* Analysis is performed in laboratories that are specially certified to perform workplace drug testing. The protocol provides securing the sample in a sealed transport device in the presence of the donor and a representative of the donor's employer, such that tampering would be obvious. The protocol also provides a written document of specimen transfer from donor to specimen collection personnel, to storage, to analyst, and to disposal.

NORMAL FINDINGS: Method: Spectrophotometry for ethanol; immunoassay for drugs of abuse.
Ethanol: None detected
Drug screen: None detected

CRITICAL FINDINGS AND POTENTIAL INTERVENTIONS

Timely notification to the requesting health-care provider (HCP) of any critical findings and related symptoms is a role expectation of the professional nurse. A listing of these findings varies among facilities.

The legal limit for ethanol intoxication varies by state, but in most places, greater than 80 mg/dL (0.08%) is considered impaired for driving. Levels greater than 300 mg/dL are associated with amnesia, vomiting, double vision, and hypothermia. Levels of 80 to 400 mg/dL are associated with coma and may be fatal. Possible interventions for ethanol toxicity include administration of tap water or 3% sodium bicarbonate lavage, breathing support, and hemodialysis (usually indicated only if levels exceed 300 mg/dL).

Amphetamine intoxication (greater than 200 ng/mL) causes psychoses, tremors, convulsions, insomnia, tachycardia, dysrhythmias, impotence, cerebrovascular accident, and respiratory failure. Possible interventions include emesis (if orally ingested and if the patient has a gag reflex and normal central nervous system [CNS] function), administration of activated charcoal followed by magnesium citrate cathartic, acidification of the urine to promote excretion, and administration of liquids to promote urinary output.

Cocaine intoxication (greater than 1,000 ng/mL) causes short-term symptoms of CNS stimulation, hypertension, tachypnea, mydriasis, and tachycardia. Possible interventions include emesis (if orally ingested and if the patient has a gag reflex and normal CNS function), gastric lavage (if orally ingested), whole-bowel irrigation (if packs of the drug were ingested), airway protection, cardiac support, and administration of diazepam or phenobarbital for convulsions. The use of beta blockers is contraindicated.

Heroin and morphine are opiates that at toxic levels (greater than 200 ng/mL) cause bradycardia, flushing, itching, hypotension, hypothermia, and respiratory depression. Possible interventions include airway protection and the administration of naloxone (Narcan).

PCP (phencyclidine) intoxication (greater than 100 ng/mL) causes a variety of symptoms depending on the stage of intoxication. Stage I includes psychiatric signs, muscle spasms, fever, tachycardia, flushing, small pupils, salivation, nausea, and vomiting. Stage II includes stupor, convulsions, hallucinations, increased heart rate, and increased blood pressure. Stage III includes further increases of heart rate and blood pressure that may culminate in cardiac and respiratory failure. Possible interventions may include providing respiratory support, administration of activated charcoal with a cathartic such as sorbitol, gastric lavage and suction, administration of IV nutrition and electrolytes, and acidification of the urine to promote PCP excretion.

OVERVIEW: (Study type: Blood, for ethanol, collected in a red-, or gray-top [sodium fluoride/potassium oxalate] tube; related body system: Multisystem. Urine for drug screen, collected in a clean plastic container. Gastric contents may also be submitted for testing.) Drug misuse continues to be a significant social and economic problem in the workforce. The Substance Abuse and Mental Health Services Administration (SAMHSA) has identified opiates, cocaine, cannabinoids, amphetamines, and PCP as the most commonly misused illicit drugs. Alcohol is the most commonly encountered misused legal substance. Chronic alcohol misuse can lead to liver disease, high blood pressure, cardiac disease, and birth defects. Regulations relating to workplace drug and alcohol testing are defined at the federal and state levels by the Drug-Free Workplace Act (DFWA), Americans with Disabilities Act, Family and Medical Leave Act, and Fair Credit Reporting Act. The DFWA pertains to some federal contractors and all federal grantees who receive a contract or grant from a federal source. The U.S. Department of Transportation (DOT) also has stipulations regarding which of its agencies must participate in a workplace screening program and at defined levels of employee participation. Employers not covered by DFWA or DOT regulations may be covered by the laws of their particular state(s) and by their individual company's human resources policies. Federal and state laws often coexist, and when applicable, employers need to follow the legislation that best benefits their employees.

INDICATIONS

- Differentiate alcohol intoxication from diabetic coma, cerebral trauma, or drug overdose.
- Investigate suspected drug misuse.
- Investigate suspected drug overdose.
- Investigate suspected nonaderence with drug or alcohol treatment program.
- Monitor ethanol levels when administered to treat methanol intoxication.
- Routine workplace screening.

	Screening Cutoff Concentrations for Misused Drugs Recommended by SAMHSA	Confirmatory Cutoff Concentrations for Misused Drugs Recommended by SAMHSA	Detectable Duration After Last Single-Use Dose	Detectable Duration After Last Dose: Prolonged Use
Hallucinogens				
Cannabinoids	50 ng/mL	15 ng/mL	2–7 d	1–2 mo
Phencyclidine	25 ng/mL	25 ng/mL	1 wk	2–4 wk
Opiates	2,000 ng/mL	2,000 ng/mL	1–3 d	1–3 d
6–Acetylmorphine	10 ng/mL	10 ng/mL	20 hr	1–7 d
Stimulants				
Amphetamines (either amphetamine or methamphetamine)[a]	500 ng/mL	250 ng/mL	48 hr	7–10 d
Cocaine	150 ng/mL	100 ng/mL	3 d	4 d
MDMA (either methylenedioxymethamphetamine, methylenedioxyamphetamine, or methylenedioxyethylamphetamine)	500 ng/mL	250 ng/mL	24 hr	24 hr

[a]To be reported as positive for methamphetamine, the specimen must also contain amphetamine at a concentration of 100 ng/mL or greater.

INTERFERING FACTORS
Factors that may alter the results of the study

- Codeine-containing cough medicines and antidiarrheal preparations, as well as ingestion of large amounts of poppy seeds, may produce a false-positive opiate result.
- Alcohol is a volatile substance, and specimens should be stored in a tightly stoppered containers to avoid falsely decreased values.
- An approved non–alcohol-containing solution should be used to cleanse the venipuncture site before specimen collection for alcohol levels; otherwise, the specimen may be falsely increased. Contamination of an alcohol specimen related to improper venipuncture preparation would lead to rejection of the specimen; this situation might create serious repercussions if the specimen was collected for workplace or medicolegal purposes.

POTENTIAL MEDICAL DIAGNOSIS: CLINICAL SIGNIFICANCE OF RESULTS
A urine screen merely identifies the presence of these substances in urine; it does not indicate time of exposure, amount used, quality of the source used, or level of impairment. Positive screens should be considered presumptive. Drug-specific confirmatory methods should be used to investigate questionable results of a positive urine screen.

NURSING IMPLICATIONS

BEFORE THE STUDY: PLANNING AND IMPLEMENTATION

Teaching the Patient What to Expect
- Inform the patient this test can assist with identification of drugs in the body.
- Explain that a blood and/or urine sample is needed for the test. Information regarding specimen collection is presented with other general guidelines in Appendix A: Patient Preparation and Specimen Collection.

Potential Nursing Actions
If appropriate or required: *Make sure a written and informed consent has been signed prior to the procedure.*

AFTER THE STUDY: POTENTIAL NURSING ACTIONS

Treatment Considerations
- Ensure that required chain of custody protocol for the specimen has been strictly adhered to.

Follow-Up, Evaluation, and Desired Outcomes
- Agrees to attend detoxification programs, as appropriate. Ensure that results are communicated to the proper individual, as indicated in the chain-of-custody protocol.
- Acknowledges contact information provided for the National Institute on Drug Abuse (www.drugabuse.gov).

Ductography

SYNONYM/ACRONYM: Breast ductoscopy, fiberoptic ductoscopy, galactography.

RATIONALE: To visualize and assess the breast ducts for disease and malignancy in women with nipple discharge.

PATIENT PREPARATION: There are no food, fluid, activity, or medication restrictions unless by medical direction. Inform the patient not to apply deodorant, body creams, or powders on the day of the procedure, as they may interfere with the mammography.

NORMAL FINDINGS
• Normal breast tissue

CRITICAL FINDINGS AND POTENTIAL INTERVENTIONS
• Ductal cancer in situ
• Invasive breast cancer

Timely notification to the requesting health-care provider (HCP) of any critical findings and related symptoms is a role expectation of the professional nurse. A listing of these findings varies among facilities.

OVERVIEW: (Study type: Endoscopy with x-ray imaging; *related body system:* Immune and Reproductive systems.) The female breast is composed mostly of fatty tissue and a specialized type of glandular tissue, which is organized into 12 to 20 lobes. Each lobe contains clusters of smaller lobules that produce milk. The milk is transported to the breast nipple through a network of ductules connected to the lobes and lobules. Ductography is an imaging procedure used to visualize the ductal system of the breast and to investigate reasons for production of nipple discharge in the anatomical area of interest. The majority of both benign and malignant breast disease originates from the cells that line the ductal-lobular unit. In ductography, the lactiferous duct is identified, cannulated, and injected with a small amount of radiopaque contrast medium such as Conray (a solution containing iothalamate meglumine) followed by mammographic imaging. Ductography is not indicated in patients with bilateral discharge because this is generally caused by hormonal changes. Biopsy and ablation techniques can also be performed during ductoscopy with correlation between visual findings and histopathology.

INDICATIONS
• Evaluate for breast cancer.
• Determine the severity of normal breast examination with high risk of developing breast cancer.
• Determine the severity of unilateral nipple discharge, bloody or clear and watery.

INTERFERING FACTORS
Contraindications

Patients who are pregnant or suspected of being pregnant, unless the potential benefits of a procedure using radiation far outweigh the risk of radiation exposure to the fetus and mother.

Patients younger than age 25, *because the density of the breast tissue is such that diagnostic x-rays are of limited value.*

Patients with conditions associated with adverse reactions to contrast medium (e.g., asthma, food allergies, or allergy to contrast medium). Although patients are asked specifically if they have a known allergy to iodine or shellfish (shellfish contain high levels of iodine), it has been well established that the reaction is not to iodine; an actual iodine allergy would be problematic because iodine is required for the production of thyroid hormones. In the case of shellfish, the reaction is to a muscle protein called *tropomyosin;* in the case of iodinated contrast medium, the reaction is to the noniodinated part of the contrast molecule. Patients with a known hypersensitivity to the medium may benefit from premedication with corticosteroids and diphenhydramine; the use of nonionic contrast or an alternative noncontrast imaging study, if available, may be considered for patients who have severe asthma or who have experienced moderate to severe reactions to ionic contrast medium.

✸ Patients with bleeding disorders receiving an arterial or venous puncture, *because the site may not stop bleeding.*

Factors that may alter the results of the study
• Metallic objects within the examination field (e.g., jewelry, body rings), which may inhibit organ visualization and can produce unclear images.
• Application of substances such as talcum powder, deodorant, or creams to the skin of breasts or underarms, which may alter test results.
• Previous breast surgery, breast augmentation, or the presence of breast implants, which may decrease the readability of the examination.

POTENTIAL MEDICAL DIAGNOSIS: CLINICAL SIGNIFICANCE OF RESULTS
Abnormal findings related to
• Ductal thickening
• Papillary lesions (cancerous or noncancerous)

NURSING IMPLICATIONS

BEFORE THE STUDY: PLANNING AND IMPLEMENTATION

Teaching the Patient What to Expect
♦ Inform the patient this procedure can assist in evaluating the breast and mammary ducts for disease.

♦ Pregnancy is a general contraindication to procedures involving radiation. Explain to the female patient that she will be asked the date of her last menstrual period and pregnancy testing may be performed to determine the possibility of pregnancy before she is exposed to radiation.
♦ Review the procedure with the patient. Address concerns about pain and explain that there may be moments of discomfort experienced during the test.
♦ Inform the patient that the procedure is usually performed in a mammography department by an HCP, with support staff, and takes approximately 30 to 60 min.
♦ Positioning for the study will be in the supine position on an examination table. Prior to the examination, the nipple will be cleansed with an appropriate disinfectant material.
♦ Gentle manual periareolar pressure will be placed on the area of interest to identify the duct with the discharge by squeezing a small amount of fluid from the duct. A warm towel may be used to help visualize the location of the duct prior to cannulation.
♦ Once the duct is identified it will be cannulated until it passes beyond the sphincter of the orifice.
♦ Afterwards, a small amount of radiopaque contrast will be injected into the duct, allowing gravity to move it.
♦ The cannula will be taped to the breast, and the patient will be assisted to the mammography unit for mammographic images.
♦ When the study is completed, the cannula will be removed and a dressing applied over the nipple.

Safety Considerations
✸ *Make sure a written and informed consent has been signed prior to the procedure and before administering any medications.*

AFTER THE STUDY: POTENTIAL NURSING ACTIONS

Avoiding Complications
♦ Infection or bleeding. Observe/assess the cannula insertion site for bleeding, inflammation, or hematoma formation.

Treatment Considerations

▶ Instruct the patient in the care and assessment of the injection site.

Follow-Up, Evaluation, and Desired Outcomes

▶ Understands that decisions regarding the need for and frequency of breast self-examination, mammography, magnetic resonance imaging or ultrasound of the breast, or other cancer screening procedures should be made after consultation between the patient and HCP. Acknowledges that the most current guidelines for breast cancer screening of the general population as well as of individuals with increased risk are available from the American Cancer Society (ACS) (www.cancer.org), the American College of Obstetricians and Gynecologists (www.acog.org), and the American College of Radiology (www.acr.org). Screening guidelines vary depending on the age and health history of those at average risk and those at high risk for breast cancer. Guidelines may not always agree between organizations; therefore, it is important for patients to participate in their health care, be informed, ask questions, and follow their HCP's recommendations regarding frequency and type of screening. For additional information regarding screening guidelines, refer to the study titled "Mammography."

▶ Instruct the patient in the use of any ordered medications. Explain the importance of adhering to the therapy regimen. As appropriate, instruct the patient in significant adverse effects associated with the prescribed medication. Encourage the patient to review corresponding literature provided by a pharmacist.

▶ Understands the pathophysiology associated with breast cancer as well as ongoing treatment, screenings, and medical versus surgical options.

D-Xylose Tolerance Test

SYNONYM/ACRONYM: N/A

RATIONALE: To assist in the differential diagnosis of small intestine malabsorption syndromes such as celiac, tropical sprue, and Crohn diseases.

PATIENT PREPARATION: Instruct the patient to fast for at least 12 hr before the test. In addition, the patient should refrain from eating foods containing high amounts of pentose sugars, such as fruits, jams, jellies, and pastries, for 24 hr before the test (D-xylose is a pentose sugar). Some medications (e.g., acetylsalicylic acid, atropine, indomethacin, metformin, nalidixic acid, and neomycin) interfere with the test and should be withheld, by medical direction, for 24 hr before testing. Activity should be restricted for the duration of the test. Protocols may vary among facilities. The test should be started between 0600 and 0800, if possible. As appropriate, provide the required urine collection container and specimen collection instructions.

NORMAL FINDINGS: Method: Spectrophotometry.

Dose Given	Conventional Units	SI Units (Conventional Units × 0.0666)
	Plasma	*Plasma*
Infant dose 0.5 g/kg (max. 25 g)	Greater than 15 mg/dL after 2 hr	Greater than 1 mmol/L
Pediatric dose 0.5 g/kg (max. 25 g)	Greater than 20 mg/dL after 2 hr	Greater than 1.3 mmol/L
Adult dose		
25 g	Greater than 25 mg/dL after 2 hr	Greater than 1.7 mmol/L
5 g (given if patient is known or expected to have severe symptoms)	Greater than 20 mg/dL after 2 hr	Greater than 1.3 mmol/L

	Urine
Children	Greater than 16%–40% of dose in 5-hr urine sample
Adults	Greater than 16% or greater than 4 g of dose in 5-hr urine sample
Older adults (65 yr and older)	Greater than 14% or greater than 3.5 g of dose in 5-hr urine sample

CRITICAL FINDINGS AND POTENTIAL INTERVENTIONS: N/A

OVERVIEW: (Study type: Blood collected in a gray-top [fluoride/oxalate] tube and urine [from a 5-hr collection] in a clean amber plastic container; **related body system:** Digestive system.) The D-xylose tolerance test is used to screen for intestinal malabsorption of carbohydrates. D-Xylose is a pentose sugar not normally present in the blood in significant amounts. It is partially absorbed when ingested and normally passes unmetabolized in the urine.

INDICATIONS
Assist in the diagnosis of malabsorption syndromes.

INTERFERING FACTORS
Factors that may alter the results of the study
• Drugs and other substances that may increase urine D-xylose levels include phenazopyridine.
• Drugs and other substances that may decrease urine D-xylose levels include acetylsalicylic acid, aminosalicylic acid, arsenicals, colchicine, ethionamide, gold, indomethacin, isocarboxazid, kanamycin, monoamine oxidase inhibitors, neomycin, and phenelzine.
• Dehydration *related to vomiting or impaired kidney function* may cause low urine values.
• Exercise and the rate of gastric emptying may affect test results.

POTENTIAL MEDICAL DIAGNOSIS: CLINICAL SIGNIFICANCE OF RESULTS

Increased in: N/A

Decreased in

Conditions that involve defective mucosal absorption of carbohydrates and other nutrients.

- Amyloidosis
- Bacterial overgrowth *(sugar is consumed by bacteria)*
- Eosinophilic gastroenteritis
- Lymphoma
- Nontropical sprue (celiac disease, gluten-induced enteropathy)
- Parasitic infestations (*Giardia,* schistosomiasis, hookworm)
- Postoperative period after massive resection of the intestine
- Radiation enteritis
- Scleroderma
- Small bowel ischemia
- Tropical sprue
- Whipple disease
- Zollinger-Ellison syndrome

NURSING IMPLICATIONS

BEFORE THE STUDY: PLANNING AND IMPLEMENTATION

Teaching the Patient What to Expect

- Inform the patient this test can assist in assessing the ability of the small intestine to absorb carbohydrates.
- Explain that blood and urine samples are needed for the test. Information regarding specimen collection is presented with other general guidelines in Appendix A: Patient Preparation and Specimen Collection.
- Review the procedure with the patient. Inform the patient that multiple blood specimens may be collected during the test. Obtain the pediatric patient's weight to calculate dose of D-xylose to be administered.
- Advise the patient that he or she will be asked to void and discard the

urine before the administration of the D-xylose. Inform the patient that once the test has begun, all urine for a 5-hr period must be saved.

- Adults are given a 25-g dose of D-xylose dissolved in 250 mL of water to take orally. The dose for pediatric patients is calculated by weight up to a maximum of 25 g. The patient should drink an additional 250 mL of water as soon as the D-xylose solution has been taken. Some adult patients with severe symptoms may be given a 5-g dose, but the test results are less sensitive at the lower dose.

Blood

- Blood samples are collected 1 hr postdose for pediatric patients and 2 hr postdose for adults.

Urine

- Refer to the general guidelines section at the front of the book for detailed instructions regarding urine specimen collection.

Potential Nursing Actions

- Remind the patient to remain supine and at rest throughout the duration of the test. Instruct the patient to collect all urine for a 5-hr period after administration of the D-xylose.
- Include on the collection container's label the specimen collection type (e.g., clean catch, catheter), date and time of collection, and any medications that may interfere with test results.

AFTER THE STUDY: POTENTIAL NURSING ACTIONS

Treatment Considerations

- Instruct the patient to resume usual medications, as directed by the HCP.

Nutritional Considerations

- Decreased D-xylose levels may be associated with gastrointestinal disease. Nutritional therapy may be indicated in the presence of malabsorption disorders.
- Encourage the patient, as appropriate, to consult with a registered dietitian to plan a lactose- and gluten-free diet. This dietary planning is complex because patients are often

malnourished and have related nutritional problems.

▶ Malabsorption can cause vitamin deficiency because the vitamins cannot be absorbed normally and because fat-soluble vitamins such as A, E, K, and D can be "trapped" in and eliminated with fat in fatty stools.

Follow-Up, Evaluation, and Desired Outcomes

▶ Acknowledges the importance of nutritional therapy for disease management. Agrees to adhere to dietary recommendations and make lactose- and gluten-free food selections.

Echocardiography

SYNONYM/ACRONYM: Doppler echo, Doppler ultrasound of the heart, echo, sonogram of the heart, transthoracic echocardiogram (TTE).

RATIONALE: To assist in diagnosing cardiovascular disorders such as defect, heart failure, tumor, infection, and bleeding.

PATIENT PREPARATION: There are no food, fluid, activity, or medication restrictions unless by medical direction.

NORMAL FINDINGS

- Normal appearance in the size, position, structure, and movements of the heart valves visualized and recorded in a combination of ultrasound modes, and normal heart muscle walls of both ventricles and left atrium, with adequate blood filling. Established values for the measurement of heart activities obtained by the study may vary by health-care provider (HCP) and institution.

CRITICAL FINDINGS AND POTENTIAL INTERVENTIONS

- Aortic aneurysm
- Infection
- Obstruction
- Tumor with significant mass effect (rare)

Timely notification to the requesting HCP of any critical findings and related symptoms is a role expectation of the professional nurse. A listing of these findings varies among facilities.

OVERVIEW: (Study type: Ultrasound; related body system: Circulatory system.) Echocardiography, a noninvasive ultrasound (US) procedure, uses high-frequency sound waves of various intensities to assist in diagnosing cardiovascular disorders. The procedure records the echoes created by the deflection of an ultrasonic beam off the cardiac structures and allows visualization of the size, shape, position, thickness, and movement of all four valves, atria, ventricular and atria septa, papillary muscles, chordae tendineae, and ventricles. This study can also determine blood-flow velocity and direction and the presence of pericardial effusion during the movement of the transducer over areas of the chest. Electrocardiography and phonocardiography can be done simultaneously to correlate the findings with the cardiac cycle.

These procedures can be done at the bedside or in a specialized department, HPC's office, or clinic.

Included in the study are the M-mode method, which produces a linear tracing of timed motions of the heart, its structures, and associated measurements over time; and the two-dimensional grayscale method, or two-dimensional real-time Doppler color-flow imaging with pulsed and continuous-wave Doppler spectral tracings, which produces a cross section of the structures of the heart and their relationship to one another, including changes in the coronary vasculature, velocity and direction of blood flow, and areas of eccentric blood flow. Red and blue colors are assigned to represent the direction of blood flow, and the intensity of the color is an indication of velocity. Doppler color-flow imaging may also be helpful in depicting the function of biological and prosthetic valves.

Echocardiography has become the method of choice for cardiac stress testing and evaluation of chest pain. Congenital heart disease such as atrial or ventricular septal defects are frequently evaluated with echocardiography. Cardiac contrast medium, composed of noniodinated lipid microspheres, such as DEFINITY or Optison, may be used to improve the visualization of the heart. For additional information regarding screening guidelines for *atherosclerotic cardiovascular disease* (ASCVD), refer to the study titled "Cholesterol, Total and Fractions."

INDICATIONS

- Detect atrial tumors (myxomas).
- Detect subaortic stenosis *(evidenced either by displacement of the anterior atrial leaflet or by a reduction in aortic valve flow, depending on the obstruction).*
- Detect ventricular or atrial mural thrombi and evaluate cardiac wall motion after myocardial infarction.
- Determine the presence of pericardial effusion, tamponade, and pericarditis.
- Determine the severity of valvular abnormalities such as stenosis, prolapse, and regurgitation.
- Evaluate congenital heart disorders.
- Evaluate endocarditis.
- Evaluate or monitor prosthetic valve function.
- Evaluate the presence of shunt flow and continuity of the aorta and pulmonary artery.
- Evaluate unexplained chest pain, electrocardiographic changes, and abnormal chest x-ray *(evidenced by an enlarged cardiac silhouette).*
- Evaluate ventricular aneurysms and/or thrombus.

- Measure the size of the heart's chambers and determine if hypertrophic cardiomyopathy or heart failure is present.

INTERFERING FACTORS

Factors that may alter the results of the study

- Incorrect placement of the transducer over the desired test site.
- Patients who are dehydrated, resulting in failure to demonstrate the boundaries between organs and tissue structures.
- Metallic objects (e.g., jewelry, body rings) within the examination field, which may inhibit organ visualization and cause unclear images.
- The presence of chronic obstructive pulmonary disease or use of mechanical ventilation, which increases the air between the heart and chest wall (hyperinflation) and can attenuate the ultrasound waves.
- Obese patients, because of the enlarged space between the transducer and the heart and because fatty tissue may distort the sound waves.
- The presence of dysrhythmias.

POTENTIAL MEDICAL DIAGNOSIS: CLINICAL SIGNIFICANCE OF RESULTS

Abnormal findings related to

- Aortic aneurysm
- Aortic valve abnormalities
- Cardiac tumor
- Cardiomyopathy
- Congenital heart defect
- Coronary artery disease (CAD)
- Endocarditis
- Heart failure
- Mitral valve abnormalities
- Myxoma
- Pericardial effusion, tamponade, and pericarditis
- Pulmonary hypertension
- Pulmonary valve abnormalities
- Septal defects
- Ventricular hypertrophy
- Ventricular or atrial mural thrombi

E

E

NURSING IMPLICATIONS

POTENTIAL NURSING PROBLEMS: ASSESSMENT & NURSING DIAGNOSIS

Problems	Signs and Symptoms
Activity *(related to excess fluid, decreased cardiac function, diminished oxygenation)*	Unsteady, weak gait; self-report of fatigue; inability to successfully perform activities of daily living; increased heart rate, blood pressure, and respiratory rate associated with activity; shortness of breath with activity
Excess fluid volume (water) *(related to damaged or diseased cardiac muscle contractility resulting in diminished renal perfusion)*	Weight gain, edema, decreased urinary output, adventitious breath sounds, shortness of breath, cyanosis, positive jugular vein distention, hypertension, tachycardia, restlessness, anxiety, fear
Inadequate cardiac output *(related to damaged or diseased cardiac muscle affecting contractility, increased cardiac preload or afterload, decreased cardiac preload)*	Decreased peripheral pulses; slow capillary refill; shortness of breath; confusion; pallor; diminishing urinary output; hypotension (postural); changes in heart rate (tachycardia); cyanosis; cool, clammy skin; decreased oxygen saturation; peripheral edema; weight gain; fatigue; impaired activity tolerance

BEFORE THE STUDY: PLANNING AND IMPLEMENTATION

Teaching the Patient What to Expect

▶ Inform the patient this procedure can assist in assessing heart function.
▶ Review the procedure with the patient. Address concerns about pain and explain that there may be some moments of discomfort or pain experienced when the IV line is inserted to allow infusion of fluids such as saline, anesthetics, sedatives, contrast, medications used in the procedure, or emergency medications.
▶ Inform the patient the procedure is performed in a US or cardiology department, usually by an HCP, and takes approximately 30 to 45 min.
▶ Instruct the patient to remove jewelry and other metallic objects from the area to be examined.
▶ Positioning for this study is in a supine position on a flat table with foam wedges to help maintain position and immobilization.

▶ Explain that the chest will be exposed to allow attachment of electrocardiogram leads for simultaneous tracings, if desired.
▶ A conductive gel is applied to the chest. A transducer is then placed on the chest surface along the left sternal border, the subxiphoid area, suprasternal notch, and supraclavicular areas to obtain views and tracings of the portions of the heart. These areas are scanned by systematically moving the probe in a perpendicular position to direct the ultrasound waves to each part of the heart.
▶ Different views or information can be obtained about heart function by positioning the patient on the left side and/or sitting up, or requesting the patient breathe slowly or hold his or her breath during the procedure. To evaluate heart function changes, the patient may be asked to inhale amyl nitrate (vasodilator).
▶ Contrast medium may be administered if ordered. A second series of images is obtained.

▶ Once the study is completed, the needle is removed and a pressure dressing is applied over the puncture site.

Potential Nursing Actions

▶ Evaluate for the presence of other risk factors, such as family history of heart disease, smoking, obesity, diet, lack of physical activity, hypertension, diabetes, previous myocardial infarction (MI), and previous vascular disease, which should be investigated.

▶ Understanding genetics assists in identifying those who may benefit from additional education, risk assessment, and counseling.

AFTER THE STUDY: POTENTIAL NURSING ACTIONS

Treatment Considerations

▶ Activity: Pace activities to match energy stores and provide assistance to complete activities of daily living. Assess current level of activity to determine a baseline, and assess response to activity. Evaluate oxygen needs in relation to activity. Encourage the use of assistive devices.

▶ Excess Fluid Volume: Administer ordered diuretics and weigh every day at the same time. Evaluate for edema in the extremities; assess breath sounds for congestion (crackles), shortness of breath, use of accessory muscles, and nasal flare. Limit fluid as ordered.

▶ Inadequate Cardiac Output: Monitor vital signs: heart rate, blood pressure, and respiratory rate. Monitor for ECG changes, decreased urinary output, changes in level of consciousness, shortness of breath, cyanosis, pallor, and cool skin. Complete a daily weight, pace activities, use pulse oximetry to monitor oxygenation and administer oxygen as ordered. Monitor electrolytes and B-type natriuretic peptide. Administer prescribed medications: angiotensin-converting enzyme inhibitor, diuretic, beta blockers, aldosterone agonists, and vasodilators. Appropriate fluid management.

Nutritional Considerations

▶ Discuss ideal body weight and the purpose of and relationship between ideal weight and caloric intake to support cardiac health. Review ways to decrease intake of saturated fats and increase intake of polyunsaturated fats. Discuss limiting intake of refined processed sugar and sodium; discuss limiting cholesterol intake to less than 300 mg per day. Encourage the intake of fresh fruits and vegetables, unprocessed carbohydrates, poultry, and grains.

▶ *Sensitivity to Social and Cultural Issues:* Numerous studies point to the prevalence of excess body weight in American children and adolescents. Findings from the 2015–2016 National Health and Nutrition Examination Survey (NHANES), regarding the prevalence of obesity in younger members of the population, estimate that obesity is present in 13.9% of the population ages 2 to 5 yrs, 18.4% ages 6 to 11 yrs, and 20.6% ages 12 to 19 yrs. The medical, social, and emotional consequences of excess body weight are significant. Special attention should be given to instructing the pediatric patient and caregiver regarding health risks and weight control education.

▶ Nutritional therapy is recommended for those with identified CAD risk, especially for those with elevated low-density lipoprotein cholesterol levels, other lipid disorders, diabetes, insulin resistance, or metabolic syndrome. Always consider cultural influences with dietary choices to ensure better adherence to a change in lifestyle. A variety of dietary patterns is beneficial for people with ASCVD. For additional information regarding nutritional guidelines. refer to the study titled "Cholesterol, Total and Fractions."

▶ Other changeable risk factors warranting education include strategies to encourage regular participation of moderate aerobic physical activity three to four times per week, eliminate tobacco use, and adhere to a heart-healthy diet.

▶ Those with elevated triglycerides should be advised to eliminate or reduce alcohol.

Follow-Up, Evaluation, and Desired Outcomes

▶ Acknowledges contact information provided for the American Heart Association (www.americanheart.org/HEARTORG), National Heart, Lung, and Blood Institute (www.nhlbi.nih.gov), Legs for Life (www.legsforlife.org), and the U.S. Department of Agriculture's resource for nutrition (www.choosemyplate.gov).

▶ Understands risk factors for CAD, necessary lifestyle changes (diet, smoking, alcohol use), the importance of weight control, and reportable signs and symptoms of heart attack.

▶ Agrees to limit fluids as recommend by the HCP.

▶ Recognizes that weight gain is an indicator of fluid retention that should be reported to the HCP.

Echocardiography, Transesophageal

SYNONYM/ACRONYM: Echo, TEE.

RATIONALE: To assess and visualize cardiovascular structures toward diagnosing disorders such as tumors, congenital defects, valve disorders, chamber disorders, and bleeding.

PATIENT PREPARATION: There are no activity restrictions unless by medical direction. Instruct the patient that to reduce the risk of aspiration related to nausea and vomiting, solid food and milk or milk products are restricted for at least 6 hr, and clear liquids are restricted for at least 2 hr prior to general anesthesia, regional anesthesia, or sedation/analgesia (monitored anesthesia). The patient may be required to be NPO after midnight. The American Society of Anesthesiologists has fasting guidelines for risk levels according to patient status. More information can be located at www.asahq.org.

Regarding the patient's risk for bleeding, the patient should be instructed to avoid taking natural products and medications with known anticoagulant, antiplatelet, or thrombolytic properties or to reduce dosage, as ordered, prior to the procedure. Number of days to withhold medication is dependent on the type of anticoagulant. Note the last time and dose of medication taken.

Patients on beta blockers before the surgical procedure should be instructed to take their medication as ordered during the perioperative period. Protocols may vary among facilities.

NORMAL FINDINGS

• Normal appearance of the size, position, structure, movements of the heart valves and heart muscle walls, and chamber blood filling; no evidence of valvular stenosis or insufficiency, cardiac tumor, foreign bodies, or coronary artery disease (CAD). The established values for the measurement of heart activities obtained by the study may vary by health-care provider (HCP) and institution.

CRITICAL FINDINGS AND POTENTIAL INTERVENTIONS

• Aortic aneurysm
• Aortic dissection

Timely notification to the requesting HCP of any critical findings and related symptoms is a role expectation of the professional nurse. A listing of these findings varies among facilities.

OVERVIEW: (Study type: Ultrasound; related body system: Cardiovascular system.) Transesophageal echocardiography (TEE) is performed to assist in the diagnosis of cardiovascular disorders when noninvasive echocardiography is contraindicated or does not reveal enough information to confirm a diagnosis. Noninvasive echocardiography may be an inadequate procedure for patients who are obese, have chest wall structure abnormalities, or have chronic obstructive pulmonary disease (COPD). TEE provides a better view of the posterior aspect of the heart, including the atrium and aorta. It is done with a transducer attached to a gastroscope that is inserted into the esophagus. The transducer and the ultrasound (US) instrument allow the beam to be directed to the back of the heart. The echoes are amplified and recorded on a screen for visualization and recorded on graph paper or videotape. The depth of the endoscope and movement of the transducer is controlled to obtain various images of the heart structures. TEE is usually performed during surgery; it is also used on patients who are in the intensive care unit, in whom the transmission of waves to and from the chest has been compromised and more definitive information is needed. The images obtained by TEE have better resolution than those obtained by routine transthoracic echocardiography because TEE uses higher frequency sound waves and offers closer proximity of the transducer to the cardiac structures. Cardiac contrast medium, composed of noniodinated lipid microspheres, such as DEFINITY or Optison, is used to improve the visualization of viable myocardial tissue within the heart. For additional information regarding screening guidelines for *atherosclerotic cardiovascular disease* (ASCVD) refer to the study titled "Cholesterol, Total and Fractions."

INDICATIONS

- Confirm diagnosis if conventional echocardiography does not correlate with other findings.
- Detect and evaluate congenital heart disorders.
- Detect atrial tumors (myxomas).
- Detect or determine the severity of valvular abnormalities and regurgitation.
- Detect subaortic stenosis as evidenced by displacement of the anterior atrial leaflet and reduction in aortic valve flow, depending on the obstruction.
- Detect thoracic aortic dissection and CAD.
- Detect ventricular or atrial mural thrombi and evaluate cardiac wall motion after myocardial infarction.
- Determine the presence of pericardial effusion.
- Evaluate aneurysms and ventricular thrombus.
- Evaluate or monitor biological and prosthetic valve function.
- Evaluate septal defects.
- Measure the size of the heart's chambers and determine if

hypertrophic cardiomyopathy or heart failure is present.

• Monitor cardiac function during open heart surgery (most sensitive method for monitoring ischemia).

• Reevaluate after inadequate visualization with conventional echocardiography as a result of obesity, trauma to or deformity of the chest wall, or lung hyperinflation associated with COPD.

INTERFERING FACTORS
Contraindications: N/A

◆ A variety of circumstances that may be considered absolute or relative depending on the facility's providers:

• Barrett esophagus
• Bleeding disorders
• Esophageal obstruction (e.g., spasm, stricture, tumor)
• Esophageal trauma (e.g., laceration, perforation)
• Esophageal varices
• Known upper esophagus disease
• Tracheoesophageal fistula
• Recent esophageal surgery (e.g., esophagectomy or esophagogastrectomy)
• Unstable cardiac or respiratory status
• Zenker diverticulum

Factors that may alter the results of the study
• Incorrect placement of the transducer over the desired test site.
• Patients who are dehydrated, resulting in failure to demonstrate the boundaries between organs and tissue structures.
• Large diaphragmatic hernia.
• Unknown upper esophageal pathology.
• Conditions such as esophageal dysphagia and irradiation of the mediastinum *related to difficulty manipulating the US probe once it has been inserted in the esophagus.*

• The presence of COPD or use of mechanical ventilation, which increases the air between the heart and chest wall (hyperinflation) and can attenuate the US waves.

• Obese patients because of the enlarged space between the transducer and the heart and because fatty tissue can distort the sound waves.

• The presence of dysrhythmias.

POTENTIAL MEDICAL DIAGNOSIS: CLINICAL SIGNIFICANCE OF RESULTS
Abnormal findings related to
• Aortic aneurysm
• Aortic valve abnormalities
• CAD
• Cardiomyopathy
• Congenital heart defects
• Heart failure
• Mitral valve abnormalities
• Myocardial infarction
• Myxoma
• Pericardial effusion
• Pulmonary hypertension
• Pulmonary valve abnormalities
• Septal defects
• Shunting of blood flow
• Thrombus
• Ventricular hypertrophy
• Ventricular or atrial mural thrombi

NURSING IMPLICATIONS

BEFORE THE STUDY: PLANNING AND IMPLEMENTATION

Teaching the Patient What to Expect
▶ Inform the patient this procedure can assist in assessing cardiac (heart) function.
▶ Review the procedure with the patient. Address concerns about pain and explain that there may be some moments of discomfort or pain experienced when the IV line is inserted to allow infusion of fluids such as saline, anesthetics, sedatives, contrast, medications used in the procedure,

or emergency medications. There may also be some discomfort during insertion of the endoscope. Explain that lidocaine is sprayed in the patient's throat to reduce discomfort caused by the presence of the endoscope.

▶ Inform the patient that the procedure is performed in a US or cardiology department, usually by an HCP, and takes approximately 20 to 30 min.

▶ Ensure the patient has removed jewelry and other metallic objects from the area to be examined.

▶ Baseline vital signs and neurological status will be recorded. Protocols may vary among facilities.

▶ During the procedure, the patient will be monitored with pulse oximetry to determine oxygen saturation in sedated patients.

▶ The chest will be exposed and electrocardiogram leads attached for simultaneous tracings, if desired.

▶ Explain that the throat will be swabbed or sprayed with a local anesthetic, and an oral bridge device will be placed in the mouth to protect the mouth and teeth from accidental damage as well as to prevent damage to the endoscope from biting.

▶ Positioning for the study is in a left side-lying position (Sims) on a flat table with foam wedges to help maintain position and immobilization. The pharyngeal area is anesthetized, and the endoscope with the US device attached to its tip is inserted 30 to 50 cm to the posterior area of the heart, as in any esophagogastroduodenoscopy procedure.

▶ The patient is asked to swallow as the scope is inserted. When the transducer is in place, the scope is manipulated by controls on the handle to obtain scanning that provides real-time images of the heart motion and recordings of the images for viewing. Actual scanning is usually limited to 15 min or until the desired number of image planes is obtained at different depths of the scope.

▶ Contrast medium will be administered if ordered. A second series of images is obtained.

▶ Once the study is completed, the needle is removed and a pressure dressing is applied over the puncture site.

Potential Nursing Actions

✦ *Make sure a written and informed consent has been signed prior to* the procedure and before administering any medications.

▶ Ask the patient, as appropriate, to remove his or her dentures or oral prosthetics.

Safety Considerations

▶ Anticoagulants, aspirin, and other salicylates should be discontinued by medical direction for the appropriate number of days prior to a procedure where bleeding is a potential complication.

AFTER THE STUDY: POTENTIAL NURSING ACTIONS

Avoiding Complications

▶ While complications are rare, trauma to the upper GI tract (e.g., esophageal bleeding, perforation, or rupture) may occur. Other potential complications include undiagnosed esophageal pathology, laryngospasm, or bronchospasm.

Treatment Considerations

▶ Do not allow the patient to eat or drink until the gag reflex returns due to aspiration risk.

▶ Monitor vital signs and neurological status every 15 min for 1 hr, then every 2 hr for 4 hr, and as ordered. Take temperature every 4 hr for 24 hr. Monitor intake and output at least every 8 hr. Compare with baseline values. Notify the HCP if temperature is elevated. Protocols may vary among facilities.

▶ Instruct the patient to treat throat discomfort with lozenges and warm gargles when the gag reflex returns.

Safety Considerations

▶ Assess the patient's ability to swallow before allowing the patient to attempt liquids or solid foods. Instruct the patient to resume diet, as directed by the HCP.

Nutritional Considerations

▶ Discuss ideal body weight and the purpose of and relationship between ideal weight and caloric intake to support cardiac health. Review ways to decrease intake of saturated fats and increase intake of polyunsaturated fats. Discuss limiting intake of refined processed sugar and sodium; discuss limiting cholesterol intake to less than 300 mg per day. Encourage the intake of fresh fruits and vegetables, unprocessed carbohydrates, poultry, and grains.

▶ Nutritional therapy is recommended for those with identified CAD risk, especially for those with elevated low-density lipoprotein cholesterol levels, other lipid disorders, diabetes, insulin resistance, or metabolic syndrome. Always consider cultural influences with dietary choices to ensure better adherence to a change in lifestyle. A variety of dietary patterns are beneficial for people with ASCVD. For additional information regarding nutritional guidelines refer to the study titled "Cholesterol, Total and Fractions."

▶ Other changeable risk factors warranting education include strategies to encourage regular participation of moderate aerobic physical activity three to four times per week, eliminate tobacco use, and adhere to a heart-healthy diet.

▶ Those with elevated triglycerides should be advised to eliminate or reduce alcohol.

Follow-Up, Evaluation, and Desired Outcomes

▶ Acknowledges provided contact information for the American Heart Association (www.americanheart.org/HEARTORG), National Heart, Lung, and Blood Institute (www.nhlbi.nih.gov), and Legs for Life (www.legsforlife.org).

▶ Understands that restlessness, sleeplessness, and irritability can be symptoms of poor oxygenation that should be reported to the HCP.

▶ Recognizes that shortness of breath and activity intolerance are symptoms of diminished cardiac output that should be reported to the HCP.

Electrocardiogram

SYNONYM/ACRONYM: ECG, EKG.

RATIONALE: To evaluate the electrical impulses generated by the heart during the cardiac cycle to assist with diagnosis of cardiac dysrhythmias, blocks, damage, infection, or enlargement.

PATIENT PREPARATION: There are no food, fluid, activity, or medication restrictions unless by medical direction.

NORMAL FINDINGS

Normal Resting Heart Rate by Age

Age	Beats/Min
Newborns (0–1 mo)	70–180
Infants (2–11 mo)	80–160
1–2 yr	80–130
3–4 yr	75–140
5–7 yr	70–130
8–9 yr	70–120
10 yrs and older, adults, older adults	60–100

- Normal resting heart rate for trained athletes is in the range of 40 to 60 beats/min.
- Normal, regular rhythm and wave deflections with normal measurement of ranges of cycle components and height, depth, and duration of complexes are as follows:

P wave: 0.12 sec, or three small blocks with amplitude of 2.5 mm
Q wave: Less than 0.04 mm
R wave: 5 to 27 mm amplitude, depending on lead
T wave: 1 to 13 mm amplitude, depending on lead
QRS complex: 0.1 sec or two and a half small blocks
ST segment: 1 mm

CRITICAL FINDINGS AND POTENTIAL INTERVENTIONS

Adult
- Acute changes in ST elevation are usually associated with acute myocardial infarction (MI) or pericarditis
- Asystole
- Heart block, second- and third-degree with bradycardia less than 60 beats/min
- Pulseless electrical activity
- Pulseless ventricular tachycardia
- Premature ventricular contractions greater than three in a row, pauses greater than 3 sec, or identified blocks
- Unstable tachycardia
- Ventricular fibrillation

Pediatric
- Asystole
- Bradycardia less than 60 beats/min
- Pulseless electrical activity
- Pulseless ventricular tachycardia
- Supraventricular tachycardia
- Ventricular fibrillation

Timely notification to the requesting health-care provider (HCP) of any critical findings and related symptoms is a role expectation of the professional nurse. A listing of these findings varies among facilities.

OVERVIEW: (Study type: Electrophysiologic; **related body system:** Circulatory system.) The cardiac muscle consists of three layers of cells: the inner *endocardium,* the middle *myocardium,* and the outer *epicardium*. The systolic phase of the cardiac cycle reflects the contraction of the myocardium, whereas the diastolic phase takes place when the heart relaxes to allow blood to rush in. All muscle cells have a characteristic rate of contraction called *depolarization*. Therefore, the heart will maintain a predetermined heart rate unless other stimuli are received.

The monitoring of pulse and blood pressure evaluates only the mechanical activity of the heart. The ECG, a noninvasive study, measures the electrical currents or impulses that the heart generates during a cardiac cycle (see figure of a normal ECG at end of study). Electrical impulses travel through a conduction system beginning with the sinoatrial (SA) node, moving to the atrioventricular (AV) node via internodal pathways. From the AV node, the impulses travel to the bundle of His and onward to the right and left bundle branches. These bundles are located within the right and left ventricles. The impulses continue to the cardiac muscle cells by terminal fibers called *Purkinje fibers* The ECG is a graphic display of the electrical activity of the heart, which is analyzed by time intervals and segments. Continuous tracing of the cardiac cycle activity is captured as heart cells are electrically stimulated, causing depolarization and movement of the activity through the cells of the myocardium.

The ECG study is completed by using 12, 15, or 18 electrodes attached to the skin surface to obtain the total electrical activity of the heart. Each lead records the electrical potential between the limbs or between the heart and limbs. The ECG machine records and marks the 12 leads (most common system used) on the strip of paper in the machine in proper sequence, usually 6 in. of the strip for each lead. Leads I, II, and III, known as *extremity leads* in a 12-lead ECG, form a triangle known as the *Einthoven triangle* when placed on the body. The ECG pattern, called a *heart rhythm,* is recorded by a machine as a series of waves, intervals, and segments, each of which pertains to a specific occurrence during the contraction of the heart. The ECG tracings are recorded on graph paper using vertical and horizontal lines for analysis and calculations of time, measured by the vertical lines (1 mm apart and 0.04 sec per line), and of voltage,

measured by the horizontal lines (1 mm apart and 0.5 mV per 5 squares). A pulse rate can be calculated from the ECG strip to obtain the beats per minute. The P wave represents the depolarization of the atrial myocardium; the QRS complex represents the depolarization of the ventricular myocardium; the PR interval represents the time from beginning of the excitation of the atrium to the beginning of the ventricular excitation; the ST segment, which represents the time between the end of depolarization and initiation of repolarization, has no deflection from baseline but in an abnormal state may be elevated or depressed; and the T wave represents the repolarization of the ventricular myocardium. An abnormal rhythm is called a *dysrhythmia.*

Microvolt T wave alternans (MTWA) is a type of noninvasive testing that identifies variations or alterations in electrical activity of the T wave. These alterations are associated with sudden cardiac death from ventricular dysrhythmias. Specialized electrodes are used to reduce background noise from natural internal movement such as respirations or external movement such as caused by the friction of electrodes on skin. Research has shown that the extent of MTWA becomes more demonstrable as heart rate increases, which is why the test includes a period of controlled exercise. MTWA occurs at a rate that is specific to each individual and is reproducible at a rate above the initial threshold for an individual. The two main methods of interpreting the beat-to-beat data, or ECG T-wave data, collected from electrodes placed on the patient's chest at rest prior to a period of activity, during an interval of controlled exercise, and during the recovery period after exercise are the spectral and modified moving average methods. Either of the two methods can be combined with a computer program to produce printable reports from the study results, which are interpreted by a cardiologist as positive, negative, or indeterminate. Spectral analysis is considered the preferred method for measurement and comparison of T wave activity based on the availability of documented studies using spectral analysis.

Another modification of the ECG, used to evaluate for ventricular dysrhythmias, is the *signal-averaged ECG*. Heart rhythms in patients who have coronary artery disease (CAD), nonischemic dilated cardiomyopathy, left ventricular aneurysm, ventricular tachycardia, or healed ventricular incisions or who are recovering from an MI may demonstrate abnormally slow electrical conduction, called *late potentials*, through the heart. The late potentials are believed to be the result of delayed conduction through areas of plaque, fibrous scarring, or inflammation and can reliably predict significant and sudden ventricular dysrhythmias. The abnormal changes in conduction are too small to be detected by standard ECG equipment and require specially designed computer software. The test takes 15 to 20 min and analyzes hundreds of cardiac cycles to detect the presence of late potentials.

The ankle-brachial index (ABI) can also be assessed during this study. This noninvasive, simple comparison of blood pressure measurements in the arms and legs can be used to detect peripheral arterial disease (PAD). A Doppler stethoscope is used to obtain the systolic pressure in either the dorsalis pedis or the posterior tibial artery. This ankle pressure is then divided by the highest brachial systolic pressure acquired after taking the blood pressure in both arms of the patient. This index should be greater than 1. When the index falls below 0.5, blood flow impairment is considered significant. Patients should be scheduled for a vascular consult for an abnormal ABI. Patients with diabetes or kidney disease, as well as some older adult patients, may have a falsely elevated ABI due to calcifications of the vessels in the ankle causing an increased systolic pressure. The ABI test approaches 95% accuracy in detecting PAD. However, a normal ABI value does not absolutely rule out the possibility of PAD for some individuals, and additional tests should be done to evaluate symptoms.

For additional information regarding screening guidelines for *atherosclerotic cardiovascular disease* (ASCVD) refer to the study titled "Cholesterol, Total and Fractions."

INDICATIONS
- Assess the extent of congenital heart disease.
- Assess the extent of MI or ischemia, as indicated by abnormal ST segment, interval times, and amplitudes.
- Assess the function of heart valves.
- Assess global cardiac function.
- Detect dysrhythmias, as evidenced by abnormal wave deflections.
- Detect PAD.

- Detect pericarditis, shown by ST segment changes or shortened PR interval.
- Determine electrolyte imbalances, as evidenced by short or prolonged QT interval.
- Determine hypertrophy of the heart chamber, as evidenced by P- or R-wave deflections, atrial biphasic P waves in V1, and ventricular exaggerated R waves in V leads.
- Evaluate and monitor cardiac pacemaker function.
- Evaluate and monitor the effect of drugs, such as digoxin, antidysrhythmics, or vasodilating drugs.
- Monitor ECG changes during an exercise test.
- Monitor rhythm changes during the recovery phase after MI.

INTERFERING FACTORS
Factors that may alter the results of the study
- Anatomic variation of the heart (i.e., the heart may be rotated in both the horizontal and frontal planes).
- Distortion of cardiac cycles due to age, gender, weight, or a medical condition (e.g., infants, women [may exhibit slight ST segment depression], patients who are obese, patients who are pregnant, patients with ascites).
- High intake of carbohydrates or electrolyte imbalances of potassium or calcium.
- Increased patient anxiety, resulting in hyperventilation or deep respirations.
- Medications such as barbiturates and digoxin.
- Strenuous exercise before the procedure.
- Improper placement of electrodes or inadequate contact between skin and electrodes because of insufficient conductive gel or poor

placement, which can cause ECG tracing problems.
- ECG machine malfunction or interference from electromagnetic waves in the vicinity.

POTENTIAL MEDICAL DIAGNOSIS: CLINICAL SIGNIFICANCE OF RESULTS
Abnormal findings related to
- Atrial or ventricular hypertrophy
- Bundle branch block
- Dysrhythmias
- Electrolyte imbalances
- Heart rate of 40 to 60 beats/min in adults
- Ischemia or MI
- PAD
- Pericarditis
- Pulmonary infarction
- P wave: An enlarged P-wave deflection could indicate atrial enlargement; an absent or altered P wave could suggest that the electrical impulse did not come from the SA node
- PR interval: An increased interval could imply a conduction delay in the AV node
- QRS complex: An enlarged Q wave may indicate an old infarction; an enlarged deflection could indicate ventricular hypertrophy; increased time duration may indicate a bundle branch block
- ST segment: A depressed ST segment indicates myocardial ischemia; an elevated ST segment may indicate an acute MI or pericarditis; a prolonged ST segment (or prolonged QT) may indicate hypocalcemia. A shortened ST segment may indicate hypokalemia
- Tachycardia greater than 120 beats/min
- T wave: A flat or inverted T wave may indicate myocardial ischemia, infarction, or hypokalemia; a tall, peaked T wave with a shortened QT interval may indicate hyperkalemia

NURSING IMPLICATIONS

POTENTIAL NURSING PROBLEMS: ASSESSMENT & NURSING DIAGNOSIS

Problems	Signs and Symptoms
Inadequate tissue perfusion *(related to interrupted blood flow, blockage, narrowed carotid arteries, ischemia secondary to oxygen supply and demand mismatch)*	Elevated heart rate, shortness of breath, chest pain, elevated blood pressure
Pain *(related to cardiac ischemia, poor cardiac oxygenation)*	Chest pain, radiating pain (arm, jaw, back); self-report of pain; facial grimace; moan; groan

E

BEFORE THE STUDY: PLANNING AND IMPLEMENTATION

Teaching the Patient What to Expect

▶ Inform the patient this procedure can assist in assessing cardiac (heart) function.

▶ Review the procedure with the patient. Inform the patient that it may be necessary to remove hair from the site before the procedure. Address concerns about pain related to the procedure and explain that there should be no discomfort related to the procedure.

▶ Inform the patient that the procedure is performed by an ECG technician or HCP and takes approximately 15 min.

▶ Ensure the patient has removed jewelry and other metallic objects from the area to be examined.

▶ Baseline vital signs will be recorded and monitored throughout the procedure. Protocols may vary among facilities.

▶ Positioning for this study is in a supine position. The chest, arms, and legs are exposed and appropriately draped. Remind the patient to remain still throughout the procedure because movement produces unreliable results.

▶ The skin surface is prepared with alcohol, and excess hair is removed. Clippers can be used to remove hair from the site, if appropriate. Skin sites are dried before electrodes are placed.

▶ Electrodes are applied in the proper positions. When placing the six unipolar chest leads, place V_1 at the fourth intercostal space at the border of the right sternum, V_2 at the fourth intercostal space at the border of the left sternum, V_3 between V_2 and V_4, V_4 at the fifth intercostal space at the midclavicular line, V_5 at the left anterior axillary line at the level of V_4 horizontally, and V_6 at the level of V_4 horizontally and at the left midaxillary line. The wires are connected to the matched electrodes and the ECG machine. Chest leads (V_1, V_2, V_3, V_4, V_5, and V_6) record data from the horizontal plane of the heart.

▶ Three limb bipolar leads (two electrodes combined for each) are placed on the arms and legs. Lead I is the combination of two arm electrodes, lead II is the combination of right arm and left leg electrodes, and lead III is the combination of left arm and left leg electrodes. Limb leads (I, II, III, aVL, aVF, and aVR) record data from the frontal plane of the heart.

▶ The machine is set and turned on after the electrodes, grounding, connections, paper supply, computer, and data storage device are checked.

▶ Vectorcardiography is a variation of the ECG and provides another way of looking at the electrical currents of the heart by focusing on the moment to moment magnitude (vector) and direction of cardiac electrical currents in the form of vector loops on an oscilloscope during a complete cardiac cycle. Benefits to this type of evaluation are the ability to monitor cardiac activity and damage, monitor contraction and relaxation, and diagnose conditions such as hypertrophy, MI, hyperfunction, and bundle branch blocks.

◗ Once the procedure is completed, the electrodes are removed and the skin is cleaned where the electrodes were applied.

Potential Nursing Actions

◗ Evaluate for the presence of other risk factors, such as family history of heart disease, smoking, obesity, diet, lack of physical activity, hypertension, diabetes, previous MI, and previous vascular disease, which should be investigated.

◗ Understanding genetics assists in identifying those who may benefit from additional education, risk assessment, and counseling. Genetics is the study and identification of genes, genetic mutations, and inheritance. For example, genetics provides some insight into the likelihood of inheriting a medical condition such as CAD. Genomic studies evaluate the interaction of groups of genes. The combined activity or combined expression of groups of genes allows assumptions or predictions to be made. As an example, genomic studies measure the levels of activity in multiple genes to predict how they, along with environmental and lifestyle decisions, influence the development of type 2 diabetes, CAD, MI, or ischemic stroke.

Safety Considerations

◗ If the patient has any chest discomfort or pain during the procedure, that area on the ECG strip should be marked indicating that occurrence.

AFTER THE STUDY: POTENTIAL NURSING ACTIONS

Treatment Considerations

◗ Inadequate Tissue Perfusion: Assess chest pain for duration, intensity, and location. Perform vital signs every 15 min with trends and comparison to baseline. Evaluate respiratory status for shortness of breath, poor oxygenation, or cyanosis. Use continuous pulse oximetry and ECG monitoring to monitor health status. Trend cardiac-specific laboratory studies: creatine phosphokinase (CK), CK-MB fraction, troponin, and myoglobin. Administer ordered medications (beta blockers) and oxygen. Teach the patient the importance of wearing oxygen to decrease cardiac ischemia. Teach the patient to rest with the head of the bed elevated to improve oxygenation.

◗ Pain: Assess pain location, intensity, duration; administer ordered medication (morphine sulfate, nitroglycerin, beta blockers); administer ordered oxygen. Instruct the patient to immediately notify an HCP of chest pain, changes in pulse rate, or shortness of breath.

◗ Recognize anxiety related to the test results and be supportive of perceived loss of independence and fear of shortened life expectancy. Discuss the implications of abnormal test results for the patient's lifestyle. Provide teaching and information regarding the clinical implications of the test results, as appropriate.

Safety Considerations

◗ Monitor vital signs and compare with baseline values. Protocols may vary among facilities.

◗ Evaluate the results in relation to previously performed ECGs. Denote cardiac rhythm abnormalities on the strip.

Nutritional Considerations

◗ Discuss ideal body weight and the purpose of and relationship between ideal weight and caloric intake to support cardiac health. Review ways to decrease intake of saturated fats and increase intake of polyunsaturated fats. Discuss limiting intake of refined processed sugar and sodium; discuss limiting cholesterol intake to less than 300 mg per day. Encourage the intake of fresh fruits and vegetables, unprocessed carbohydrates, poultry, and grains.

◗ *Sensitivity to Social and Cultural Issues:* Numerous studies point to the prevalence of excess body weight in American children and adolescents. Findings from the 2015–2016 National

Health and Nutrition Examination Survey (NHANES), regarding the prevalence of obesity in younger members of the population, estimate that obesity is present in 13.9% of the population ages 2 to 5 yrs, 18.4% ages 6 to 11 yrs, and 20.6% ages 12 to 19 yrs. The medical, social, and emotional consequences of excess body weight are significant. Special attention should be given to instructing the pediatric patient and caregiver regarding health risks and weight control education.

▶ Nutritional therapy is recommended for those with identified CAD risk, especially for those with elevated low-density lipoprotein cholesterol levels, other lipid disorders, diabetes, insulin resistance, or metabolic syndrome. Always consider cultural influences with dietary choices to ensure better adherence to a change in lifestyle. A variety of dietary patterns are beneficial for people with ASCVD. For additional information regarding nutritional guidelines refer to the study titled "Cholesterol, Total and Fractions."

▶ Other changeable risk factors warranting education include strategies to encourage regular participation of moderate aerobic physical activity three to four times per wk, eliminate tobacco use, and adhere to a heart-healthy diet.

▶ Those with elevated triglycerides should be advised to eliminate or reduce alcohol.

Follow-Up, Evaluation, and Desired Outcomes

▶ Acknowledges contact information provided for the American Heart Association (www.americanheart.org/HEARTORG), National Heart, Lung, and Blood Institute (www.nhlbi.nih.gov), Legs for Life (www.legsforlife.org), and the U.S. Department of Agriculture's resource for nutrition (www.choosemyplate.gov).

▶ Understands risk factors for CAD, necessary lifestyle changes (diet, smoking, alcohol use), the importance of weight control, and reportable signs and symptoms of heart attack.

▶ Agrees to attend a cardiac rehabilitation program as part of overall treatment plan.

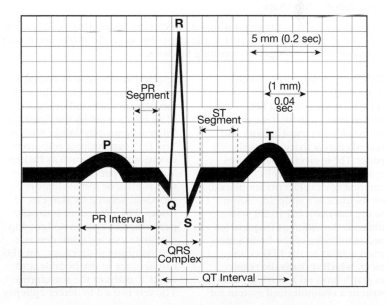

Electroencephalography

SYNONYM/ACRONYM: Electrical activity (for sleep disturbances), EEG.

RATIONALE: To assess the electrical activity in the brain toward assisting in diagnosis of brain death, injury, infection, and bleeding.

PATIENT PREPARATION: Instruct the patient to eat a meal before the study and to avoid stimulants such as caffeine and nicotine for 8 hr prior to the procedure. Under medical direction, the patient should avoid sedatives, anticonvulsants, anxiolytics, and alcohol for 24 to 48 hr before the test. Instruct the patient to clean the hair and to refrain from using hair sprays, creams, or solutions before the test. Instruct the patient to limit sleep to 5 hr for an adult and 7 hr for a child the night before the study. Young infants and children should not be allowed to nap before the study.

NORMAL FINDINGS
- Normal occurrences of alpha, beta, delta, and theta waves (rhythms varying depending on the patient's age).
- Normal amplitude, frequency, and characteristics of brain waves.

CRITICAL FINDINGS AND POTENTIAL INTERVENTIONS
- Abscess
- Brain death
- Head injury
- Hemorrhage
- Intracranial hemorrhage

Timely notification to the requesting health-care provider (HCP) of any critical findings and related symptoms is a role expectation of the professional nurse. A listing of these findings varies among facilities.

OVERVIEW: (Study type: Electrophysiologic; related body system: Nervous system.) EEG is a noninvasive study that measures the brain's electrical activity and records that activity on graph paper. These electrical impulses arise from the brain cells of the cerebral cortex. Electrodes, placed on the patient's scalp according to the International 10/20 system, transmit the different frequencies and amplitudes of the brain's electrical activity to the EEG equipment, which records the results in graph form on a moving paper strip or a computerized system for retrieval and review or comparison at a later date. Guidelines for the performance and evaluation of an EEG are set by the American Clinical Neurophysiology Society. The EEG can evaluate responses to various stimuli, such as flickering light, hyperventilation, auditory signals, or somatosensory signals generated by skin electrodes. The procedure is usually performed in a room designed to eliminate electrical interference and minimize distractions. An EEG can be done at the bedside, and an HCP analyzes the waveforms. The test is used to detect epilepsy, intracranial abscesses, or tumors; to evaluate cerebral involvement due to head injury or meningitis; and to monitor for cerebral tissue ischemia during surgery when cerebral vessels must be occluded (e.g., carotid endarterectomy). EEG is also used to confirm brain death, which can be defined as absence of electrical activity in the brain. To evaluate abnormal EEG waves further, the patient may be connected to an ambulatory EEG system similar to a Holter monitor for the heart.

INDICATIONS
• Confirm brain death.
• Confirm suspicion of increased intracranial pressure caused by trauma or disease.
• Detect cerebral ischemia during endarterectomy.
• Detect intracranial cerebrovascular lesions, such as hemorrhages and infarcts.
• Detect seizure disorders and identify focus of seizure and seizure activity, as evidenced by abnormal spikes and waves recorded on the graph.
• Determine the presence of tumors, abscesses, or infection.
• Evaluate the effect of drug intoxication on the brain.
• Evaluate sleeping disorders, such as sleep apnea and narcolepsy.
• Identify area of abnormality in dementia.

INTERFERING FACTORS
Factors that may alter the results of the study
• Drugs and other substances such as sedatives, anticonvulsants, anxiolytics, alcohol, and stimulants such as caffeine and nicotine.
• Hypoglycemic or hypothermic states.

• Hair that is dirty, oily, or sprayed or treated with hair preparations.

POTENTIAL MEDICAL DIAGNOSIS: CLINICAL SIGNIFICANCE OF RESULTS
Abnormal findings related to
• Abscess
• Alzheimer disease
• Brain death
• Cerebral infarct
• Encephalitis
• Glioblastoma and other brain tumors
• Head injury
• Hematoma
• Hypocalcemia or hypoglycemia
• Infarct
• Intracranial hemorrhage
• Meningitis
• Migraine headaches
• Narcolepsy
• Parkinson disease
• Seizure disorders (epilepsy, grand mal, focal, temporal lobe, myoclonic, petit mal)
• Sleep apnea

NURSING IMPLICATIONS

BEFORE THE STUDY: PLANNING AND IMPLEMENTATION

Teaching the Patient What to Expect
▶ Inform the patient/family this procedure can assist in measuring the electrical activity in the brain.
▶ Review the procedure with the patient. Address concerns about pain related to the procedure and assure the patient there is no discomfort during the procedure, but if needle electrodes are used, a slight pinch may be felt.
▶ Explain that electricity flows from the patient's body, not into the body, during the procedure. Also explain that the procedure reveals brain activity only, not thoughts, feelings, or intelligence.

E

E

▶ Inform the patient the procedure is performed in a neurodiagnostic department, usually by an HCP and support staff, and takes approximately 30 to 120 min, depending on the purpose of the study.

▶ Inform the patient that he or she may be asked to alter breathing pattern; be asked to follow simple commands such as opening or closing eyes, blinking, or swallowing; be stimulated with bright light; or be given a drug to induce sleep during the study.

▶ Positioning for this study is in the supine position in a bed or in a semi-Fowler position on a recliner in a special room protected from any noise or electrical interferences that could affect the tracings.

▶ Remind the patient to relax and not to move any muscles or parts of the face or head. The HCP should be able to observe the patient for movements or other interferences through a window into the test room.

▶ The electrodes are prepared and applied to the scalp. Electrodes are applied to the prefrontal, frontal, temporal, parietal, and occipital areas of both sides of the head, and amplifier wires are attached. An electrode is also attached to each earlobe as grounding electrodes. At this time, a baseline recording can be made with the patient at rest.

▶ Recordings are made with the patient at rest and with eyes closed. Recordings are stopped about every 5 min to allow the patient to move. Recordings are also made during a drowsy and sleep period, depending on the patient's clinical condition and symptoms.

▶ Procedures (e.g., stroboscopic light stimulation, hyperventilation to induce alkalosis, and sleep induction by administration of sedative to detect abnormalities that occur only during sleep) may be done to bring out abnormal electrical activity or other brain abnormalities.

▶ Observations for seizure activity are carried out during the study, and a description and time of activity is noted by the HCP.

Potential Nursing Actions

❖ *Make sure a written and informed consent has been signed prior to the procedure and before administering any medications.*

AFTER THE STUDY: POTENTIAL NURSING ACTIONS

Treatment Considerations
▶ Once the procedure is complete, the electrodes are removed from the hair, and the paste is removed by cleansing with oil or witch hazel.

▶ Allow the patient to recover if a sedative was given during the test. Bedside rails are put in the raised position for safety.

▶ Instruct the patient to resume medications, as directed by the HCP.

▶ Instruct the patient to report any seizure activity.

Safety Considerations
▶ Ensure seizure activity *(related to cerebral laceration, hypoxia; bleeding; contusions; penetrating injury)* precautions: padded side rails; observe for seizure activity; remain with the patient during a seizure; assess for obstructed airway, maintain open airway; suction as appropriate; administer ordered antiseizure medications (e.g., phenytoin).

Follow-Up, Evaluation, and Desired Outcomes
▶ Acknowledges contact information provided for the Epilepsy Foundation (www.epilepsy.com), Alzheimer's Association of America (alzfdn.org), or U.S. Government Information on Organ and Tissue Donation and Transplantation (www.organdonor.gov/index.html).

▶ Recognizes that there may be personality changes, speech deficits, or physical deficits with brain injury.

Electromyography

SYNONYM/ACRONYM: Electrodiagnostic study, EMG, neuromuscular junction testing.

RATIONALE: To assess the electrical activity within the skeletal muscles to assist in diagnosing diseases such as muscular dystrophy, Guillain-Barré, polio, and other myopathies.

PATIENT PREPARATION: There are no food or activity restrictions unless by medical direction. Under medical direction, the patient should avoid muscle relaxants, cholinergics, and anticholinergics for 3 to 6 days before the test. Instruct the patient to abstain from smoking and drinking caffeine-containing beverages for 3 hr before the procedure. Protocols may vary among facilities.

NORMAL FINDINGS
• Normal muscle electrical activity during rest and contraction states.

CRITICAL FINDINGS AND POTENTIAL INTERVENTIONS: N/A

OVERVIEW: (Study type: Electrophysiologic; related body system: Musculoskeletal system.) EMG measures skeletal muscle activity during rest, voluntary contraction, and electrical stimulation. Percutaneous extracellular needle electrodes containing fine wires are inserted into selected muscle groups to detect neuromuscular abnormalities and measure nerve and electrical conduction properties of skeletal muscles. The electrical potentials are amplified, displayed on a screen in waveforms, and electronically recorded, similar to electrocardiography. Comparison and analysis of the amplitude, duration, number, and configuration of the muscle activity provide diagnostic information about the extent of nerve and muscle involvement in the detection of primary muscle diseases, including lower motor neuron, anterior horn cell, or neuromuscular junction diseases; defective transmission at the neuromuscular junction; and peripheral nerve damage or disease. The responses of a relaxed muscle are electrically silent, but spontaneous muscle movement such as fibrillation and fasciculation can be detected in a relaxed, denervated muscle. Muscle action potentials are detected with minimal or maximal muscle contractions, and the differences in the size and numbers of activity potentials during voluntary contractions determine whether the muscle weakness is a disease of the striated muscle fibers or cell membranes (myogenic) or a disease of the lower motor neuron (neurogenic). Nerve conduction studies (electroneurography) are commonly done in conjunction with electromyelography; the combination of the procedures is known as *electromyoneurography*. The major use of the examination lies in differentiating among the following disease classes: primary myopathy, peripheral motor neuron disease, and disease of the neuromuscular junction.

EMG can aid with the diagnosis of nerve compression or injury such as carpal tunnel syndrome, nerve root injury such as sciatica, or other problems on the muscles or nerves. An EMG uses tiny devices called *electrodes,* which are inserted directly into a muscle, to transmit or detect electrical signals. A nerve conduction study or nerve conduction velocity test, which is another part of an EMG, uses electrodes taped to the skin to measure the strength and speed of the signals traveling between two or more points.

INDICATIONS

- Assess primary muscle diseases affecting striated muscle fibers or cell membrane, such as muscular dystrophy or myasthenia gravis.
- Detect muscle disorders caused by diseases of the lower motor neuron involving the motor neuron on the anterior horn of the spinal cord, such as anterior poliomyelitis, amyotrophic lateral sclerosis, amyotonia, and spinal tumors.
- Detect muscle disorders caused by diseases of the lower motor neuron involving the nerve root, such as Guillain-Barré syndrome, herniated disk, or spinal stenosis.
- Detect neuromuscular disorders, such as peripheral neuropathy caused by diabetes or alcohol misuse, and locate the site of the abnormality.
- Determine if a muscle abnormality is caused by the toxic effects of drugs (e.g., antibiotics,

chemotherapy) or toxins (e.g., *Clostridium botulinum*, snake venom, heavy metals).
- Differentiate between primary and secondary muscle disorders or between neuropathy and myopathy.
- Differentiate secondary muscle disorders caused by polymyositis, sarcoidosis, hypocalcemia, thyroid toxicity, tetanus, and other disorders.
- Monitor and evaluate progression of myopathies or neuropathies, including confirmation of diagnosis of carpal tunnel syndrome.

INTERFERING FACTORS
Contraindications

Patients with extensive skin infection or with an infection at the sites of electrode placement, *to avoid risk of spreading infection into the muscle,* or patients who are receiving anticoagulant therapy, *to avoid bleeding.*

Factors that may alter the results of the study
- Age-related decreases in electrical activity.
- Medications such as muscle relaxants, cholinergics, and anticholinergics.
- Improper placement of surface or needle electrodes.

POTENTIAL MEDICAL DIAGNOSIS: CLINICAL SIGNIFICANCE OF RESULTS
Abnormal findings related to
- Evidence of neuromuscular disorders or primary muscle disease (*Note:* Findings must be correlated with the patient's history, clinical features, and results of other neurodiagnostic tests.):
Amyotrophic lateral sclerosis
Bell palsy
Beriberi
Carpal tunnel syndrome
Dermatomyositis
Diabetic peripheral neuropathy

Eaton-Lambert syndrome
Guillain-Barré syndrome
Multiple sclerosis
Muscular dystrophy
Myasthenia gravis

Myopathy
Polymyositis as indicated by fast, small
  spontaneous waveforms
Radiculopathy
Traumatic injury

NURSING IMPLICATIONS

POTENTIAL NURSING PROBLEMS: ASSESSMENT & NURSING DIAGNOSIS

Problems	Signs and Symptoms
Mobility *(related to spasticity, weakness, tremors)*	Unsteady gait, uncoordinated movement, unable to perform purposeful movement, limited range of motion, avoidance of movement.
Self-care deficit *(related to loss of cognitive or motor function)*	Unable to complete the activities of daily living (eating, bathing, dressing, toileting) without assistance

BEFORE THE STUDY: PLANNING AND IMPLEMENTATION

Teaching the Patient What to Expect

▶ Inform the patient this procedure can assist in measuring the electrical activity of the muscles.

▶ Review the procedure with the patient. Address concerns about pain related to the procedure and warn the patient the procedure may be uncomfortable, but an analgesic or sedative will be administered.

▶ Inform the patient that as many as 10 electrodes may be inserted at various locations on the body. Inform the patient the procedure is performed in a special laboratory by a health-care provider (HCP) and takes approximately 1 to 3 hr to complete, depending on the patient's condition.

▶ Assess for the ability to adhere to directions given for exercising during the test.

▶ Instruct the patient to remove jewelry and other metallic objects from the area to be examined.

▶ Positioning for the study is in a supine or sitting position depending on the location of the muscle to be tested. Ensure that the area or room

is protected from noise or metallic interference that may affect the test results.

▶ The patient will be asked to remain still and relaxed and to cooperate with instructions given to contract muscles during the procedure.

▶ Ensure a mild analgesic (adult) or sedative (children) has been administered, as ordered, to promote a restful state before the procedure.

▶ The skin is thoroughly cleansed with alcohol pads, as necessary.

▶ A small needle is inserted into the muscle being examined and acts as a recording electrode. A second electrode, a reference electrode, is placed on the skin surface near the recording electrode. An oscilloscope displays any spontaneous electrical activity while the patient keeps the muscle at rest. The electrical waves produced are examined for the number, amplitude, and form.

▶ The patient is asked to alternate between a relaxed and a contracted muscle state or to perform progressive muscle contractions while the potentials are being measured.

▶ Note that this sequence may be repeated up to four times.

◗ When the procedure is complete, the electrodes are removed, and the skin is cleansed where the electrodes were applied. Pressure may need to be applied for 1 to 2 min to control any bleeding. Observe electrode sites for bleeding, hematoma, or inflammation.

Potential Nursing Actions

✦ Make sure a written and informed consent has been signed prior to the procedure and before administering any medications.

AFTER THE STUDY: POTENTIAL NURSING ACTIONS

Avoiding Complications

◗ EMG is a low-risk procedure, and complications are rare. There is a small risk of bleeding and infection or nerve injury where the needle electrodes are inserted. Monitor electrode sites for inflammation.

Treatment Considerations

◗ If residual pain is noted after the procedure, instruct the patient to apply warm compresses and to take analgesics, as ordered.

◗ Mobility: Assess current functional level and facilitate physical therapy evaluation and treatment. Encourage active or passive range of motion to maintain

muscle strength. Teach proper turning and assisting techniques.

◗ Self-Care Deficit: Assess self-care deficits and identify areas where the patient can provide own care or requires assistance. Evaluate the family's ability to assist with self-care needs; complete a home health evaluation and provide assistive devices to assist with self-care (commode, special utensils). Alter diet to accommodate swallowing ability (thick liquids, puree, small bites, etc.) and remind the patient to chew and swallow slowly.

Safety Considerations

◗ Facilitate the appropriate use of assistive devices and provide assistance with activities to decrease fall risk (gait belt, walker, etc.).

Nutritional Considerations

◗ Consider recommending swallow evaluation to decrease aspiration risk.

◗ Collaborate with HCP and dietitian to alter diet to meet swallowing capabilities.

Follow-Up, Evaluation, and Desired Outcomes

◗ Acknowledges that additional testing may be performed to evaluate or monitor progression of the disease process and determine the need for a change in therapy.

Electromyography, Pelvic Floor Sphincter

SYNONYM/ACRONYM: Electrodiagnostic study, rectal electromyography.

RATIONALE: To assess urinary sphincter electrical activity to assist with diagnosis of urinary incontinence.

PATIENT PREPARATION: There are no food or activity restrictions unless by medical direction. Under medical direction, the patient should avoid muscle relaxants, cholinergics, and anticholinergics for 3 to 6 days before the test. Instruct the patient to abstain from smoking and drinking caffeine-containing beverages for 3 hr before the procedure. Protocols may vary among facilities.

NORMAL FINDINGS
- Normal urinary and anal sphincter muscle function; increased electromyographic signals during the filling of the urinary bladder and at the conclusion of voiding; absence of signals during the actual voiding; no incontinence.

CRITICAL FINDINGS AND POTENTIAL INTERVENTIONS: N/A

OVERVIEW: (**Study type:** Electrophysiologic; **related body system:** Neuromuscular and Urinary systems.) Pelvic floor sphincter electromyography, also known as rectal electromyography, is performed to measure electrical activity of the external urinary sphincter. This procedure, often done in conjunction with cystometry and voiding urethrography as part of a full urodynamic study, helps to diagnose neuromuscular dysfunction and incontinence.

measured by the electrodes. Pelvic muscle weakness is commonly seen in older females as a result of muscles that become overstretched during pregnancy and childbirth; muscle weakness can also occur as a result of neurologic injury.

- Anal incontinence
- Urinary incontinence
- Uterine prolapse

INDICATIONS
Evaluate neuromuscular dysfunction and incontinence.

INTERFERING FACTORS
Contraindications
   Patients with bleeding disorders, *because the puncture sites may not stop bleeding.*

Factors that may alter the results of the study
- Age-related decreases in electrical activity.
- Medications such as muscle relaxants, cholinergics, and anticholinergics.

POTENTIAL MEDICAL DIAGNOSIS: CLINICAL SIGNIFICANCE OF RESULTS
Abnormal findings related to
Neuromuscular dysfunction of lower urinary sphincter, pelvic floor muscle, or anal sphincter is evidenced by diminished electrical activity as

NURSING IMPLICATIONS

BEFORE THE STUDY: PLANNING AND IMPLEMENTATION

Teaching the Patient What to Expect
- Inform the patient this procedure can assist in measuring the electrical activity of the pelvic floor muscles.
- Review the procedure with the patient. Address concerns about pain related to the procedure. Explain that the procedure may be uncomfortable during the catheter insertion.
- Inform the patient the procedure is performed in a special laboratory by a health-care provider (HCP) and takes about 30 min to complete.
- Instruct the patient to remove jewelry and other metallic objects from the area to be examined.
- Positioning for the study is in a supine position on the examining table; a drape is placed over the patient, exposing the perianal area.
- Baseline vital signs will be recorded and monitored throughout the procedure. Protocols may vary among facilities.

E

▶ The patient will be reminded to remain very still and relaxed and to cooperate when instructed to contract muscles during the procedure.

▶ Explain that two skin electrodes will be positioned slightly to the left and right of the perianal area and a grounding electrode is placed on the thigh.

▶ If needle electrodes are used, they are inserted into the muscle surrounding the urethra.

▶ Muscle activity signals are recorded as waves, which are interpreted for number and configurations in diagnosing urinary abnormalities.

▶ An indwelling urinary catheter is inserted, and the bulbocavernosus reflex is tested; the patient is instructed to cough while the catheter is gently pulled.

▶ Voluntary control is tested by requesting the patient to contract and relax the muscle. Electrical activity is recorded during this period of relaxation with the bladder empty.

▶ The bladder is filled with sterile water at a rate of 100 mL/min while the electrical activity during filling is recorded.

▶ The catheter is removed; the patient is then placed in a position to void and is asked to urinate and empty the full bladder. This voluntary urination is then recorded until completed. The complete procedure includes recordings of electrical signals before, during, and at the end of urination.

Potential Nursing Actions

Make sure a written and informed consent has been signed prior to the procedure and before administering any medications.

Avoiding Complications

▶ Complications are rare but include bleeding *related to a bleeding disorder or the effects of natural products and medications with known anticoagulant, antiplatelet, or thrombolytic properties* and urinary infection *related to use of a catheter.*

Treatment Considerations

▶ Monitor vital signs and neurological status every 15 min for 1 hr, then every 2 hr for 4 hr, and as ordered. Take temperature every 4 hr for 24 hr. Monitor intake and output at least every 8 hr. Compare with baseline values. Protocols may vary among facilities.

▶ Instruct the patient to increase fluid intake unless contraindicated.

▶ If tested with needle electrodes, warn female patients to expect hematuria after the first voiding.

▶ Advise the patient to report symptoms of urethral irritation, such as dysuria, persistent or prolonged hematuria, and urinary frequency.

Follow-Up, Evaluation, and Desired Outcomes

▶ Acknowledges that based on the results of the procedure, additional testing may be performed to evaluate or monitor the progression of the disease process and determine the need for a change in therapy.

Electroneurography

SYNONYM/ACRONYM: Electrodiagnostic study, nerve conduction study.

RATIONALE: To assess peripheral nerve conduction to assist in the diagnosis of diseases such as diabetic neuropathy and muscular dystrophy.

PATIENT PREPARATION: There are no food, fluid, activity, or medication restrictions unless by medical direction.

NORMAL FINDINGS
- No evidence of peripheral nerve injury or disease. Variable readings depend on the nerve being tested. For patients aged 3 yr and older, the maximum conduction velocity is 40 to 80 milliseconds; for infants and older adults, the values are divided by 2.

CRITICAL FINDINGS AND POTENTIAL INTERVENTIONS: N/A

OVERVIEW: (Study type: Electrophysiologic; related body system: Nervous system.) Electroneurography is performed to identify peripheral nerve injury, to differentiate primary peripheral nerve pathology from muscular injury, and to monitor response of the nerve injury to treatment. A stimulus is applied through a surface electrode over a nerve. After a nerve is electrically stimulated proximally, the time for the impulse to travel to a second or distal site is measured. Because the conduction study of a nerve can vary from nerve to nerve, it is important to compare the results of the affected side to those of the contralateral side. The results of the stimulation are shown on a monitor, but the actual velocity must be calculated by dividing the distance in meters between the stimulation point and the response point by the time between the stimulus and response. Traumatic nerve transection, contusion, or neuropathy will usually cause maximal slowing of conduction velocity in the affected side compared with that in the normal side. A velocity that is greater than normal does not indicate a pathological condition. This test is usually performed in conjunction with electromyography in a combined test called *electromyoneurography.*

INDICATIONS
Confirm diagnosis of peripheral nerve damage or trauma.

INTERFERING FACTORS
Contraindications
◈ Patients with a bleeding disorder when performed in addition to electromyography.

Factors that may alter the results of the study
- Age-related decreases in electrical activity.
- Poor electrode conduction or failure to obtain contralateral values for comparison.

POTENTIAL MEDICAL DIAGNOSIS: CLINICAL SIGNIFICANCE OF RESULTS
Abnormal findings related to
- Carpal tunnel syndrome
- Diabetic neuropathy
- Guillain-Barré syndrome
- Herniated disk disease
- Muscular dystrophy
- Myasthenia gravis
- Poliomyelitis
- Tarsal tunnel syndrome indicated by decreased conduction time
- Thoracic outlet syndrome

NURSING IMPLICATIONS

BEFORE THE STUDY: PLANNING AND IMPLEMENTATION

Teaching the Patient What to Expect
▶ Inform the patient this procedure is performed to measure the electrical activity of the muscles.

- Review the procedure with the patient. Address concerns about pain related to the procedure and inform the patient the procedure may be uncomfortable because of a mild electrical shock. Advise the patient that the electrical shock is brief and is not harmful.
- Inform the patient that it may be necessary to remove hair from the site before the procedure.
- Inform the patient the procedure is performed in a special laboratory by a health-care provider (HCP) and takes approximately 15 min to complete but can take longer depending on the patient's condition.
- Instruct the patient to remove jewelry and other metallic objects from the area to be examined.
- Positioning for this study is in a supine or sitting position, depending on the location of the muscle to be tested.
- Clippers may be used to remove hair from the site if appropriate. The skin is cleansed thoroughly with alcohol pads.
- Electrode gel is applied, and a recording electrode is placed at a known distance from the stimulation point. The distance between the stimulation point and the site of the recording electrode is measured in centimeters.
- A reference electrode is placed nearby on the skin surface.
- The nerve is electrically stimulated by a shock-emitter device; the time between nerve impulse and electrical contraction, measured in milliseconds (distal latency), is shown on a monitor.

- The nerve is also electrically stimulated at a location proximal to the area of suspected injury or disease.
- The time required for the impulse to travel from the stimulation site to the location of the muscle contraction (total latency) is recorded in milliseconds.
- Conduction velocity is calculated and converted to meters per second (m/sec) and computed using the following equation:

Conduction velocity (m/sec) = [distance (m)]/[total latency – distal latency]

- When the procedure is complete, the electrodes are removed and the skin is cleansed where the electrodes were applied.

Potential Nursing Actions

Make sure a written and informed consent has been signed prior to the procedure and before administering any medications.

AFTER THE STUDY: POTENTIAL NURSING ACTIONS

Avoiding Complications
- Monitor electrode sites for inflammation.

Treatment Considerations
- If residual pain is noted after the procedure, instruct the patient to apply warm compresses and to take analgesics, as ordered.

Follow-Up, Evaluation, and Desired Outcomes
- Acknowledges that based on the results of the procedure, additional testing may be performed to evaluate or monitor the progression of the disease process and determine the need for a change in therapy.

Endoscopy, Sinus

SYNONYM/ACRONYM: N/A

RATIONALE: To facilitate diagnosis and treatment of recurring sinus infections or infections resulting from unresolved sinus infection, including incursion into the brain, eye orbit, or eyeball.

PATIENT PREPARATION: There are no food, fluid, activity, or medication restrictions unless by medical direction.

NORMAL FINDINGS
• Normal soft tissue appearance.

CRITICAL FINDINGS AND POTENTIAL INTERVENTIONS: N/A

OVERVIEW: (Study type: Endoscopy; related body system: Respiratory system.) Sinus endoscopy, done with a narrow flexible tube, is used to help diagnose damage to the sinuses, nose, and throat. The tube contains an optical device with a magnifying lens with a bright light; the tube is inserted through the nose and threaded through the sinuses to the throat. A camera, monitor, or other viewing device is connected to the endoscope to record areas being examined. Sinus endoscopy helps to diagnose structural defects (e.g., polyps or other abnormal growths), damage, and acute or recurring infection to the nose, sinuses, and throat. Cultures can be obtained during the procedure to assist in the identification of infectious organisms and to determine appropriate treatments. Therapeutic applications include drainage of infected sinuses and administration of medications directly to the site of infection. The procedure is usually done in a health-care provider's (HCP's) office, but if done as a surgical procedure, the endoscope may be used to remove polyps from the nose or throat.

INDICATIONS
• Identify nasal obstruction.
• Assess recurrent sinusitis.

INTERFERING FACTORS
Contraindications: N/A

POTENTIAL MEDICAL DIAGNOSIS: CLINICAL SIGNIFICANCE OF RESULTS
Abnormal findings related to
• Foreign bodies in the nose
• Growths in the nasal passages
• Polyps
• Sinusitis

NURSING IMPLICATIONS

BEFORE THE STUDY: PLANNING AND IMPLEMENTATION

Teaching the Patient What to Expect
◗ Inform the patient this procedure can assist in locating and treating infection of the sinus or surrounding areas.
◗ Review the procedure with the patient. Address concerns about pain and explain that a local anesthetic spray or liquid may be applied to the throat to ease with insertion of the endoscope.
◗ Inform the patient that the procedure is usually performed in the office of an HCP, is usually done with the patient awake and seated upright in a chair, and takes about 10 min.
◗ Prior to the study, the patient is seated comfortably and ordered topical anesthetic is instilled in the throat and allowed time to work.
◗ The endoscope is inserted, and the structures inside the nose are examined.
◗ A specimen container is labelled with the corresponding patient demographics, initials of the person collecting the specimen, date, and time of collection, if cultures are to be obtained on aspirated sinus material.

Potential Nursing Actions
✦ *Make sure a written and informed consent has been signed prior to the procedure and before administering any medications.*

E

AFTER THE STUDY: POTENTIAL NURSING ACTIONS

Avoiding Complications
▶ Bleeding; cerebrospinal fluid leakage from the ethmoid sinus

Treatment Considerations
▶ Instruct the patient to wait until the numbness in the throat wears off

before attempting to eat or drink following the procedure.

Follow-Up, Evaluation, and Desired Outcomes
▶ Acknowledges that based on the results of the procedure, further testing or additional procedures may be needed to resolve conditions identified by endoscopy.

Eosinophil Count

SYNONYM/ACRONYM: Eos count, total eosinophil count.

RATIONALE: To assist in diagnosing conditions related to immune response such as asthma, dermatitis, and hay fever. Also used to assist in identification of parasitic infections.

PATIENT PREPARATION: There are no food, fluid, activity, or medication restrictions unless by medical direction.

NORMAL FINDINGS: Method: Manual count using eosinophil stain and hemocytometer or automated analyzer.
   Absolute count: 50 to 500 cells/microL [SI units (0.05–0.5 × 10⁹/L)]
   Relative percentage: 1% to 4%

CRITICAL FINDINGS AND POTENTIAL INTERVENTIONS: N/A

OVERVIEW: (**Study type:** Blood collected in a lavender-top [EDTA] tube or a swab containing nasal secretions; **related body system:** Circulatory/Hematopoietic and Immune systems.) Eosinophils are white blood cells whose function is phagocytosis of antigen-antibody complexes and response to allergy-inducing substances and parasites. Eosinophils have granules that contain histamine used to kill foreign cells in the body. Eosinophils also contain proteolytic substances that damage parasitic worms. The binding of histamine to receptor sites on cells results in smooth muscle contraction in the bronchioles and upper respiratory tract, constriction of pulmonary vessels,

increased mucus production, and secretion of acid by the cells that line the stomach. The contents of eosinophilic granules are very effective in neutralizing allergens. However, the substances released by the eosinophils can also damage normal cells in the area where the histamine and other enzymes are released. Eosinophil counts can increase to greater than 30% of normal in parasitic infections; however, a significant percentage of children with visceral larva migrans infestations have normal eosinophil counts.

A nasal smear can be examined for the presence of eosinophils to screen for allergic conditions. Either a single smear or smears of nasal secretions from each side of the nose should be submitted, at room temperature, for Hansel staining and evaluation. Normal findings vary by laboratory, but generally, greater than 10% to 15% is considered eosinophilia, or increased presence of eosinophils.

INDICATIONS
Assist in the diagnosis of conditions such as allergies, parasitic infections, drug reactions, collagen diseases, and myeloproliferative disorders.

INTERFERING FACTORS
Factors that may alter the results of the study
- Numerous drugs and other substances can cause an increase in eosinophil levels as a result of an allergic response or hypersensitivity reaction. These include acetophenazine, allopurinol, aminosalicylic acid, ampicillin, butaperazine, capreomycin, carisoprodol, cephaloglycin, cephaloridine, cephalosporins, cephapirin, cephradine, chloramphenicol, clindamycin, cloxacillin, dapsone, epicillin, erythromycin, fluorides, gold salts, imipramine, iodides, kanamycin, mefenamic acid, methicillin, methyldopa, minocycline, nalidixic acid, niridazole, nitrofurans (including nitrofurantoin), NSAIDs, nystatin, oxamniquine, penicillin, penicillin G, procainamide, ristocetin, streptokinase, streptomycin, tetracycline, triamterene, tryptophan, and viomycin.
- Drugs and other substances that can cause a decrease in eosinophil levels include acetylsalicylic acid, amphotericin B, corticotropin, desipramine, glucocorticoids, hydrocortisone, interferon, niacin, prednisone, and procainamide.

Other considerations
- Clotted specimens should be rejected for analysis.
- Specimens more than 4 hr old should be rejected for analysis.
- There is a diurnal variation in eosinophil counts. The count is lowest in the morning and continues to rise throughout the day until midnight. Therefore, serial measurements should be performed at the same time of day for purposes of continuity.

POTENTIAL MEDICAL DIAGNOSIS: CLINICAL SIGNIFICANCE OF RESULTS
Increased in
Eosinophils are released and migrate to inflammatory sites in response to numerous environmental, chemical/ drug, or immune-mediated triggers. T cells, mast cells, and macrophages release cytokines, such as interlukin-3 (IL3), interlukin-5 (IL5), granulocyte/ macrophage colony–stimulating factor, and chemokines such as the eotaxins, which can result in the activation of eosinophils.

- Addison disease *(most commonly related to autoimmune destruction of adrenal glands)*
- Allergy
- Asthma
- Cancer
- Dermatitis
- Drug reactions
- Eczema
- Hay fever
- Hodgkin disease
- Hypereosinophilic syndrome (rare and idiopathic)
- Löffler syndrome *(pulmonary eosinophilia due to allergic reaction or infection from a fungus or parasite)*
- Myeloproliferative disorders *(related to abnormal changes in the bone marrow)*
- Parasitic infection (visceral larva migrans)
- Rheumatoid arthritis *(possibly related to medications used in therapy)*
- Rhinitis
- Sarcoidosis

E

- Splenectomy
- Tuberculosis

Decreased in
- Aplastic anemia *(bone marrow failure)*
- Eclampsia *(shift to the left; relative to significant production of neutrophils)*
- Infections *(shift to the left; relative to significant production of neutrophils)*
- Stress *(release of cortisol suppresses eosinophils)*

NURSING IMPLICATIONS

BEFORE THE STUDY: PLANNING AND IMPLEMENTATION

Teaching the Patient What to Expect
▶ Inform the patient this test can assist in diagnosing immune response conditions and parasitic infections.

▶ Explain that a blood sample is needed for the test.

AFTER THE STUDY: POTENTIAL NURSING ACTIONS

Treatment Considerations
▶ Instruct the patient with an elevated eosinophil count to report any signs or symptoms of infection, such as fever.
▶ Instruct the patient with an elevated count to rest and take medications as prescribed, to increase fluid intake as appropriate, and to monitor temperature.

Nutritional Considerations
▶ Consideration should be given to diet if food allergies are present.

Follow-Up, Evaluation, and Desired Outcomes
▶ Acknowledges the correlation between an elevated eosinophil count and signs and symptoms of infection or allergic response.

Erythrocyte Protoporphyrin, Free

SYNONYM/ACRONYM: Free erythrocyte protoporphyrin (FEP).

RATIONALE: To assist in diagnosing anemias related to chronic disease, hemolysis, iron deficiency, and lead toxicity.

PATIENT PREPARATION: There are no food, fluid, activity, or medication restrictions unless by medical direction.

NORMAL FINDINGS: Method: Fluorometry.

Conventional Units	SI Units (Conventional Units × 0.0178)
Adult	
Male	
Less than 30 mcg/dL	Less than 0.534 micromol/L
Female	
Less than 40 mcg/dL	Less than 0.712 micromol/L

CRITICAL FINDINGS AND POTENTIAL INTERVENTIONS: N/A

OVERVIEW: (Study type: Blood collected in a lavender-top [EDTA], royal blue-top [EDTA], or a pink-top [EDTA] tube; **related body system:** Circulatory/Hemato-poietic system.) The FEP test measures the concentration of nonheme protoporphyrin in red blood cells. Protoporphyrin comprises the predominant porphyrin in red blood cells, which combines with iron to form the heme portion of hemoglobin. Protoporphyrin converts to bilirubin, combines with albumin, and remains unconjugated in the circulation after hemoglobin breakdown. Increased amounts of protoporphyrin can be detected in erythrocytes, urine, and stool in conditions interfering with heme synthesis. Protoporphyria is an autosomal dominant disorder in which increased amounts of protoporphyrin are secreted and excreted; the disorder is thought to be the result of an enzyme deficiency. Protoporphyria causes photosensitivity and may lead to cirrhosis of the liver and cholelithiasis as a result of protoporphyrin deposits. FEP is elevated in cases of lead toxicity or chronic exposure.

INDICATIONS
- Assist in the diagnosis of erythropoietic protoporphyria.
- Assist in the differential diagnosis of iron deficiency in pediatric patients.
- Evaluate lead poisoning.

INTERFERING FACTORS
Factors that may alter the results of the study
- Drugs and other substances that may increase FEP levels include erythropoietin.

Other considerations
- The test is unreliable in infants less than 6 mo of age.

POTENTIAL MEDICAL DIAGNOSIS: CLINICAL SIGNIFICANCE OF RESULTS
Increased in
- Anemia of chronic disease *(related to accumulation of protoporphyrin in the absence of available iron)*
- Conditions with marked erythropoiesis (e.g., hemolytic anemias) *(related to increased cell destruction)*
- Erythropoietic protoporphyria *(related to abnormal increased secretion)*
- Iron-deficiency anemias *(related to accumulation of protoporphyrin in the absence of available iron)*
- Lead poisoning *(possibly related to inactivation of enzymes involved in iron binding or transfer)*
- Some sideroblastic anemias

Decreased in: N/A

NURSING IMPLICATIONS

BEFORE THE STUDY: PLANNING AND IMPLEMENTATION

Teaching the Patient What to Expect
- Inform the patient this test can assist in diagnosing specific types of anemias and lead toxicity as well as monitor chronic lead exposure.
- Explain that a blood sample is needed for the test.

AFTER THE STUDY: POTENTIAL NURSING ACTIONS

Follow-Up, Evaluation, and Desired Outcomes
- Acknowledges contact information provided for the American Porphyria Foundation (www.porphyriafoundation.com).

Erythrocyte Sedimentation Rate

SYNONYM/ACRONYM: Sed rate, ESR.

RATIONALE: To assist in diagnosing acute infection in diseases such as tissue necrosis, chronic infection, and acute inflammation.

PATIENT PREPARATION: There are no food, fluid, activity, or medication restrictions unless by medical direction.

NORMAL FINDINGS: Method: Westergren or modified Westergren.

Age	Male	Female
Newborn	0–2 mm/hr	0–2 mm/hr
Less than 50 yr	0–15 mm/hr	0–25 mm/hr
50 yr and older	0–20 mm/hr	0–30 mm/hr

CRITICAL FINDINGS AND POTENTIAL INTERVENTIONS: N/A

OVERVIEW: (**Study type:** Blood collected in a completely filled lavender-top [EDTA] tube for the modified Westergren method or a completely filled gray-top [3.8% sodium citrate] tube for the original Westergren method; **related body system:** Circulatory/Hematopoietic and Immune systems.) The ESR is a measure of the rate of sedimentation of red blood cells (RBCs) in an anticoagulated whole blood sample over a specified period of time. The basis of the ESR test is the alteration of blood proteins by inflammatory and necrotic processes that cause the RBCs to stick together, become heavier, and rapidly settle at the bottom of a vertically held, calibrated tube over time. The most common promoter of rouleaux is an increase in circulating fibrinogen or globulin levels. In general, relatively little settling occurs in normal blood because normal RBCs do not form rouleaux and would not stack together. The sedimentation rate is proportional to the size or mass of the falling RBCs and is inversely proportional to plasma viscosity. The test is a nonspecific indicator of disease but is fairly sensitive and is frequently the earliest indicator of widespread inflammatory reaction due to infection or autoimmune disorders. Prolonged elevations are also present in malignant disease. The ESR can also be used to monitor the course of a disease and the effectiveness of therapy. The most commonly used method to measure the ESR is the Westergren (or modified Westergren) method.

INDICATIONS
- Assist in the diagnosis of acute infection, such as tuberculosis or tissue necrosis.
- Assist in the diagnosis of acute inflammatory processes.
- Assist in the diagnosis of chronic infections.

- Assist in the diagnosis of rheumatoid or autoimmune disorders.
- Assist in the diagnosis of temporal arthritis and polymyalgia rheumatica.
- Monitor inflammatory and malignant disease.

INTERFERING FACTORS
Factors that may alter the results of the study
- Some drugs and other substances cause an SLE-like syndrome that results in a physiological increase in ESR. These include anticonvulsants, hydrazine derivatives, nitrofurantoin, procainamide, and quinidine. Other drugs and substances that may cause an increased ESR include acetylsalicylic acid, cephalothin, cyclosporin A, dextran, and oral contraceptives.
- Drugs and other substances that may cause a decrease in ESR include aurothiomalate, corticotropin, cortisone, dexamethasone, methotrexate, minocycline, NSAIDs, penicillamine, prednisolone, prednisone, quinine, sulfasalazine, tamoxifen, and trimethoprim.
- Menstruation may cause falsely increased test results.
- Prolonged tourniquet constriction around the arm may cause hemoconcentration and falsely low values.
- The Westergren and modified Westergren methods are affected by heparin, which causes a false elevation in values.
- Bubbles in the Westergren tube or pipette, or tilting the measurement column more than 3 degrees from vertical, will falsely increase the values.

Other considerations
- Movement or vibration of the surface on which the test is being conducted will affect the results.

- Inaccurate timing or a delay in performing the test once the specimen has been collected will invalidate test results.
- Specimens that are clotted, hemolyzed, or insufficient in volume should be rejected for analysis.
- The test should be performed within 4 hr of collection when the specimen has been stored at room temperature; delays in testing may result in decreased values. If a delay in testing is anticipated, refrigerate the sample at 2°C to 4°C; stability at refrigerated temperature is reported to be extended up to 12 hr. Refrigerated specimens should be brought to room temperature before testing.

POTENTIAL MEDICAL DIAGNOSIS: CLINICAL SIGNIFICANCE OF RESULTS
Increased in

Increased rouleaux formation is associated with increased levels of fibrinogen and/or production of cytokines and other acute-phase reactant proteins in response to inflammation. Anemia of chronic disease as well as acute anemia influence the ESR because the decreased number of RBCs falls faster with the relatively increased plasma volume.

- Acute myocardial infarction
- Anemia *(RBCs fall faster with increased plasma volume)*
- Cancer
- Cat scratch fever (*Bartonella henselae*)
- Collagen diseases, including systemic lupus erythematosus (SLE)
- Crohn disease *(due to anemia or related to acute-phase reactant proteins)*
- Elevated blood glucose *(hyperglycemia in older adult patients can induce production of cytokines responsible for the inflammatory response; hyperglycemia related to insulin resistance can cause*

hepatocytes to shift protein synthesis from albumin to production of acute-phase reactant proteins)

- Endocarditis
- Heavy metal poisoning *(related to anemia affecting size and shape of RBCs)*
- Increased plasma protein level *(RBCs fall faster with increased plasma viscosity)*
- Infections (e.g., pneumonia, syphilis)
- Inflammatory diseases
- Lymphoma
- Lymphosarcoma
- Multiple myeloma *(RBCs fall faster with increased plasma viscosity)*
- Nephritis
- Pregnancy *(related to anemia)*
- Pulmonary embolism
- Rheumatic fever
- Rheumatoid arthritis
- Subacute bacterial endocarditis
- Temporal arteritis
- Toxemia
- Tuberculosis
- Waldenström macroglobulinemia *(RBCs fall faster with increased plasma viscosity)*

Decreased in

- Conditions resulting in high hemoglobin and RBC count

NURSING IMPLICATIONS

BEFORE THE STUDY: PLANNING AND IMPLEMENTATION

Teaching the Patient What to Expect

▶ Inform the patient this test can assist in identification of inflammation.
▶ Explain that a blood sample is needed for the test.

AFTER THE STUDY: POTENTIAL NURSING ACTIONS

Treatment Considerations

▶ Teach how to perform hand hygiene to decrease infection risk.
▶ Teach how to take and document temperature. Remind the patient that elevations are to be reported to the health-care provider.
▶ Explain the importance of follow-up ESR to monitor the effectiveness of therapeutic interventions.

Follow-Up, Evaluation, and Desired Outcomes

▶ Acknowledges contact information provided for the American College of Rheumatology (www.rheumatology .org) or the Arthritis Foundation (www .arthritis.org).
▶ Describes reportable signs and symptoms of infection.

Erythropoietin

SYNONYM/ACRONYM: EPO.

RATIONALE: To evaluate the effectiveness of EPO administration as a treatment for anemia, especially related to chemotherapy and kidney disease.

PATIENT PREPARATION: There are no food, fluid, activity, or medication restrictions unless by medical direction.

NORMAL FINDINGS: Method: Immunochemiluminometric assay.

Age	Conventional and SI Units	Conventional and SI Units
	Male	*Female*
0–3 yr	1.7–17.9 milli-international units/mL	2.1–15.9 milli-international units/mL
4–6 yr	3.5–21.9 milli-international units/mL	2.9–8.5 milli-international units/mL
7–9 yr	1.1–13.5 milli-international units/mL	2.1–8.2 milli-international units/mL
10–12 yr	1.1–14.1 milli-international units/mL	1.1–9.1 milli-international units/mL
13–15 yr	2.2–14.4 milli-international units/mL	3.8–20.5 milli-international units/mL
16–18 yr	1.5–15.2 milli-international units/mL	2.1–14.2 milli-international units/mL
Adult	4.2–27.8 milli-international units/mL	4.2–27.8 milli-international units/mL

Based on normal hemoglobin and hematocrit. Values may be decreased in older adults due to the effects of medications and the presence of multiple chronic or acute diseases with or without muted symptoms.

CRITICAL FINDINGS AND POTENTIAL INTERVENTIONS: N/A

OVERVIEW: (**Study type:** Blood collected in a gold-, red-, or red/gray-top tube; **related body system:** Circulatory/Hematopoietic system.) EPO is a glycoprotein produced mainly by the kidney. Its function is to stimulate the bone marrow to make red blood cells (RBCs). EPO levels fall after removal of the kidney but do not disappear completely. Small amounts of EPO are produced by the liver. Erythropoiesis is regulated by EPO and tissue Po_2. When Po_2 is normal, EPO levels decrease; when Po_2 falls, EPO secretion occurs and EPO levels increase.

INDICATIONS
- Assist in assessment of anemia of chronic kidney disease.
- Assist in the diagnosis of EPO-producing tumors.

- Evaluate the possibility of EPO misuse by athletes.
- Evaluate the presence of rare anemias.
- Monitor patients receiving EPO therapy.

INTERFERING FACTORS
Factors that may alter the results of the study
- Drugs and other substances that may increase EPO levels include adrenocorticotropic hormone, anabolic steroids, androgens, angiotensin, epinephrine, daunorubicin, fenoterol, growth hormone, thyroid-stimulating hormone, and xenon (gas).
- Phlebotomy may increase EPO levels.
- Drugs and other substances that may decrease EPO levels include amphotericin B, cisplatin, enalapril, estrogens, furosemide, and theophylline.

• Blood transfusions may also decrease EPO levels.

POTENTIAL MEDICAL DIAGNOSIS: CLINICAL SIGNIFICANCE OF RESULTS

Increased in

• After moderate bleeding in an otherwise healthy patient *(related to loss of RBCs, which stimulates production)*
• AIDS *(related to anemia, which stimulates production)*
• Anemias (e.g., hemolytic, iron deficiency, megaloblastic) *(related to low RBC count, which stimulates production)*
• Blood doping *(enhancement of athletic performance and stamina, related to increased production of RBCs)*
• Hepatoma *(related to EPO-producing tumors)*
• Kidney transplant rejection *(15% of cases respond with an exaggerated secretion of EPO and a transient post-transplantation erythrocytosis)*
• Nephroblastoma *(related to EPO-producing tumors)*
• Pheochromocytoma *(related to EPO-producing tumors)*
• Polycystic kidney disease *(related to EPO-producing tumors or cysts)*
• Pregnancy *(related to anemia of pregnancy, which stimulates production)*
• Secondary polycythemia where low oxygen levels stimulate production *(high-altitude hypoxia,*

chronic obstructive pulmonary disease, pulmonary fibrosis)

Decreased in

• Chemotherapy *(related to therapy, which can be toxic to the kidney)*
• Chronic kidney disease *(related to decreased production and excessive loss through excretion by damaged kidneys)*
• Primary polycythemia *(related to feedback loop response to elevated RBC count)*

NURSING IMPLICATIONS

BEFORE THE STUDY: PLANNING AND IMPLEMENTATION

Teaching the Patient What to Expect

▶ Inform the patient this test can assist in evaluation of anemia.
▶ Explain that a blood sample is needed for the test.

AFTER THE STUDY: POTENTIAL NURSING ACTIONS

Treatment Considerations

▶ Teach the patient reportable symptoms of anemia.

Follow-Up, Evaluation, and Desired Outcomes

▶ Acknowledges that based on the results of the procedure, additional testing may be performed to evaluate or monitor the progression of the disease process and determine the need for a change in therapy.

Esophageal Manometry

SYNONYM/ACRONYM: Esophageal function study, esophageal acid study (Tuttle test), acid reflux test, Bernstein test (acid perfusion), esophageal motility study.

RATIONALE: To evaluate potential ineffectiveness of the esophageal muscle and structure in swallowing, vomiting, and regurgitation in diseases such as scleroderma, infection, and gastric esophageal reflux.

PATIENT PREPARATION: There are no activity restrictions unless by medical direction. Under medical direction, the patient should withhold medications for 24 hr before the study. Instruct the patient to fast and restrict fluids for 6 hr prior to the procedure to reduce the risk of aspiration related to nausea and vomiting. Patient may be required to be NPO after midnight. The American Society of Anesthesiologists has fasting guidelines for risk levels according to patient status. More information can be located at www.asahq.org.

Regarding the patient's risk for bleeding, the patient should be instructed to avoid taking natural products and medications with known anticoagulant, antiplatelet, or thrombolytic properties or to reduce dosage, as ordered, prior to the procedure. Number of days to withhold medication is dependent on the type of anticoagulant. Protocols may vary among facilities.

Ensure that barium studies were performed more than 4 days before the esophageal manometry (EM).

E

NORMAL FINDINGS
- Acid clearing: Fewer than 10 swallows
- Acid perfusion: No gastroesophageal reflux disease (GERD)
- Acid reflux: No regurgitation into the esophagus
- Bernstein test: Negative (no discomfort or pain following instillation of hydrochloric acid)
- Esophageal secretions: pH 5 to 6
- Esophageal sphincter pressure: 10 to 20 mm Hg.

CRITICAL FINDINGS AND POTENTIAL INTERVENTIONS: N/A

OVERVIEW: (Study type: Manometric; related body system: Digestive system.) EM consists of a group of invasive studies performed to assist in diagnosing abnormalities of esophageal muscle function and esophageal structure. These studies measure esophageal pressure, the effects of gastric acid in the esophagus, lower esophageal sphincter pressure, and motility patterns that result during swallowing. EM can be used to document and quantify GERD. It is indicated when a patient is experiencing difficulty swallowing, heartburn, regurgitation, or vomiting or has chest pain for which no diagnosis has been found. Tests performed in combination with EM include the acid reflux, acid clearing, and acid perfusion (Bernstein) tests.

INDICATIONS
- Aid in the diagnosis of achalasia, *evidenced by increased pressure in EM.*
- Aid in the diagnosis of achalasia in children, *evidenced by decreased pressure in EM.*
- Aid in the diagnosis of esophageal scleroderma, *evidenced by decreased pressure in EM.*
- Aid in the diagnosis of esophagitis, *evidenced by decreased motility.*
- Aid in the diagnosis of GERD, *evidenced by low pressure in EM, decreased pH in acidity test, and pain in acid reflux and perfusion tests.*
- Differentiate between esophagitis or cardiac condition as the cause of epigastric pain.
- Evaluate pyrosis and dysphagia to determine if the cause is GERD or esophagitis.

INTERFERING FACTORS
Contraindications
◈ Patients with unstable cardiopulmonary status, blood coagulation defects, recent gastrointestinal surgery, esophageal varices, or bleeding.

Factors that may alter the results of the study
- Administration of medications (e.g., sedatives, antacids, anticholinergics, cholinergics, corticosteroids) that can change pH or relax the sphincter muscle, causing inaccurate results.

POTENTIAL MEDICAL DIAGNOSIS: CLINICAL SIGNIFICANCE OF RESULTS
Abnormal findings related to
- Achalasia (sphincter pressure of 50 mm Hg)
- Chalasia
- Esophageal scleroderma
- Esophagitis
- GERD (sphincter pressure of 0–5 mm Hg, pH of 1–3)
- Hiatal hernia
- Progressive systemic sclerosis (scleroderma)
- Spasms

NURSING IMPLICATIONS

BEFORE THE STUDY: PLANNING AND IMPLEMENTATION

Teaching the Patient What to Expect
- Inform the patient this procedure can assist in assessing the esophagus.
- Pregnancy is a general contraindication to procedures involving radiation. Explain to the female patient that she will be asked the date of her last menstrual period and pregnancy testing may be performed to determine the possibility of pregnancy before she is exposed to radiation.
- Review the procedure with the patient. Address concerns about pain and explain that there may be moments of discomfort or pain experienced when the IV line is inserted to allow infusion of fluids such as saline, anesthetics, sedatives, contrast medium, medications used in the procedure, or emergency medications; there may be moments of discomfort and gagging when the scope is inserted, but there are no complications resulting from the procedure; and the throat will be anesthetized with a spray or swab. Inform the patient that he or she will not be able to speak during the procedure but breathing will not be affected.
- Instruct the patient to remove dentures and eyewear.
- Inform the patient that the procedure is performed in an endoscopy suite by a health-care provider (HCP), under local anesthesia, and takes approximately 30 to 45 min.
- Baseline vital signs will be recorded and monitored throughout the procedure. Protocols may vary among facilities.
- The oropharynx will be sprayed or swabbed with a topical local anesthetic.
- An emesis basin will be provided so the patient can spit out the increased saliva, since the gag reflex may be impaired.
- During the procedure, the patient will be monitored for complications related to the procedure.
- Suctioning of the mouth, pharynx, and trachea will be performed as necessary, and oxygen will be administered as ordered.

Esophageal Manometry
- One or more small tubes are inserted through the nose into the esophagus and stomach.
- A small transducer is attached to the ends of the tubes to measure lower esophageal sphincter pressure, intraluminal pressures, and regularity and duration of peristaltic contractions.
- The patient is instructed to swallow small amounts of water or flavored gelatin.

Esophageal Acid and Clearing (Tuttle Test)
- With the tube in place, a pH electrode probe is inserted into the esophagus

with Valsalva maneuvers performed to stimulate reflux of stomach contents into the esophagus.
- If acid reflux is absent, 100 mL of 0.1% hydrochloric acid is instilled into the stomach during a 3-min period, and the pH measurement is repeated.
- To determine acid clearing, hydrochloric acid is instilled into the esophagus and the patient is asked to swallow while the probe measures the pH.

Acid Perfusion (Bernstein Test)
- A catheter is inserted through the nose into the esophagus, and the patient is asked to inform the HCP when pain is experienced.
- Normal saline solution is allowed to drip into the catheter at about 10 mL/min. Then hydrochloric acid is allowed to drip into the catheter.
- Pain experienced when the hydrochloric acid is instilled determines the presence of an esophageal abnormality. If no pain is experienced, symptoms are the result of some other condition.

Potential Nursing Actions
Make sure a written and informed consent has been signed prior to the procedure and before administering any medications.

Safety Considerations
- Avoid using morphine sulfate in patients with asthma or other pulmonary disease. This drug can further exacerbate bronchospasms and respiratory impairment.
- Anticoagulants, aspirin, and other salicylates should be discontinued by medical direction for the appropriate number of days prior to a procedure in which bleeding is a potential complication.

AFTER THE STUDY: POTENTIAL NURSING ACTIONS

Avoiding Complications
- Potential complications related to the procedure include aspiration of stomach contents into the lungs, dyspnea, tachypnea, or adventitious sounds.
- Establishing an IV site is an invasive procedures. Complications are rare but include risk for bleeding from the

puncture site *related to a bleeding disorder or the effects of natural products and medications with known anticoagulant, antiplatelet, or thrombolytic properties;* hematoma *related to blood leakage into the tissue following needle insertion;* or infection *that might occur if bacteria from the skin surface is introduced at the puncture site.* Observe/assess the needle insertion site for bleeding, inflammation, or hematoma formation.

Treatment Considerations
- Instruct the patient not to eat or drink until the gag reflex returns and then to eat lightly for 12 to 24 hr.
- Instruct the patient to resume usual activity, medication, and diet 24 hr after the examination or as tolerated, as directed by the HCP.
- Monitor the patient for signs of respiratory depression (less than 15 respirations/min) every 15 min for 2 hr. Resuscitation equipment should be available.
- Inform the patient to expect some throat soreness and possible hoarseness. Advise the patient to use warm gargles, lozenges, or ice packs to the neck and to drink cool fluids to alleviate throat discomfort.
- Emphasize that any severe pain, fever, difficulty breathing, or expectoration of blood must be reported to the HCP immediately.
- Teach the patient and family symptoms of low hemoglobin and hematocrit associated with anemia and blood loss.

Safety Considerations
- *Observe the patient for indications of perforation:* painful swallowing with neck movement, substernal pain with respiration, shoulder pain, dyspnea, abdominal or back pain, cyanosis, and fever.

Follow-Up, Evaluation, and Desired Outcomes
- Understands treatment options for anemia, including the purpose, risks, and benefits of blood transfusion.
- Recognizes the importance of reporting symptoms of anemia and blood loss to the HCP.

E

Esophagogastroduodenoscopy

SYNONYM/ACRONYM: Esophagoscopy, gastroscopy, upper GI endoscopy, EGD.

RATIONALE: To visualize and assess the esophagus, stomach, and upper portion of the duodenum to assist in diagnosis of bleeding, ulcers, inflammation, tumor, and cancer.

PATIENT PREPARATION: There are no activity restrictions unless by medical direction. The patient may be given additional instructions about following a special diet for 1 or 2 days before the procedure. Instruct the patient to fast and restrict fluids for 6 to 8 hr prior to the procedure to reduce the risk of aspiration related to nausea and vomiting. The patient may be required to be NPO after midnight. The American Society of Anesthesiologists has fasting guidelines for risk levels according to patient status. More information can be located at www.asahq.org.

The patient may be instructed to take a laxative, an enema, or a rectal laxative suppository.

Regarding the patient's risk for bleeding, the patient should be instructed to avoid taking natural products and medications with known anticoagulant, antiplatelet, or thrombolytic properties or to reduce dosage, as ordered, prior to the procedure. Number of days to withhold medication is dependent on the type of anticoagulant. Note the last time and dose of medication taken.

Patients on beta blockers before the surgical procedure should be instructed to take their medication as ordered during the perioperative period.

Ensure that barium studies were performed more than 4 days before the esophagogastroduodenoscopy (EGD). Protocols may vary among facilities.

NORMAL FINDINGS

- Esophageal mucosa is normally yellow-pink. At about 9 in. from the incisor teeth, a pulsation indicates the location of the aortic arch. The gastric mucosa is orange-red and contains rugae. The proximal duodenum is reddish and contains a few longitudinal folds, whereas the distal duodenum has circular folds lined with villi. No abnormal structures or functions are observed in the esophagus, stomach, or duodenum.

CRITICAL FINDINGS AND POTENTIAL INTERVENTIONS

- Presence and location of acute gastrointestinal (GI) bleed

Timely notification to the requesting health-care provider (HCP) of any critical findings and related symptoms is a role expectation of the professional nurse. A listing of these findings varies among facilities.

OVERVIEW: (Study type: Endoscopy; related body system: Digestive system.) EGD allows direct visualization of the upper GI tract mucosa, which includes the esophagus, stomach, and upper portion of the duodenum, by means of a flexible endoscope. The standard flexible fiberoptic endoscope contains three channels that allow passage of the instruments needed to perform therapeutic or diagnostic procedures, such as biopsies or cytology washings. The endoscope, a multichannel instrument, allows visualization of the GI tract linings, insufflation of air, aspiration of fluid, removal of foreign bodies by suction or by snare or forceps, and passage of a laser beam for obliteration of abnormal tissue or control of bleeding. Direct visualization yields greater diagnostic data than is possible through radiological procedures, and therefore EGD is rapidly replacing upper GI series as the diagnostic procedure of choice.

INDICATIONS

- Assist in differentiating between benign and neoplastic tumors.
- Detect gastric or duodenal ulcers.
- Detect upper GI inflammatory disease.
- Determine the presence and location of acute upper GI bleeding.
- Evaluate the extent of esophageal injury after ingestion of chemicals.
- Evaluate stomach or duodenum after surgical procedures.
- Evaluate suspected gastric outlet obstruction.
- Identify tissue abnormalities and obtain biopsy specimens.
- Investigate the cause of dysphagia, dyspepsia, and epigastric pain.

INTERFERING FACTORS

Contraindications

✺ Patients who have had surgery involving the stomach or duodenum, which can make locating the duodenal papilla difficult.

✺ Patients with a bleeding disorder.

✺ Patients with unstable cardiopulmonary status, blood coagulation defects, or cholangitis, unless the patient received prophylactic antibiotic therapy before the test (otherwise the examination must be rescheduled).

✺ Patients with known aortic arch aneurysm, large esophageal Zenker diverticulum, recent GI surgery, esophageal varices, or known esophageal perforation.

Factors that may alter the results of the study
- Gas or food in the GI tract resulting from inadequate cleansing or failure to restrict food intake before the study.
- Retained barium from a previous radiological procedure.

POTENTIAL MEDICAL DIAGNOSIS: CLINICAL SIGNIFICANCE OF RESULTS

Abnormal findings related to
- Acute and chronic gastric and duodenal ulcers
- Diverticular disease
- Duodenitis
- Esophageal varices
- Esophageal or pyloric stenosis
- Esophagitis or strictures
- Gastritis
- Hiatal hernia
- Mallory-Weiss syndrome
- Tumors (benign or malignant)

E

NURSING IMPLICATIONS

POTENTIAL NURSING PROBLEMS: ASSESSMENT & NURSING DIAGNOSIS

Problems	Signs and Symptoms
Inadequate nutrition *(related to pain, bleeding, nausea, vomiting, excessive alcohol intake, anorexia)*	Weight loss, emaciation, malabsorption, poor intake

(table continues on page 556)

Problems	Signs and Symptoms
Pain *(related to gastric irritation associated with the use of acetylsalicylic acid and NSAIDs, cramping, distention)*	Weight loss, self-report of pain, nausea, vomiting, relief of pain with the use of antacids, intermittent pain located in the abdomen

BEFORE THE STUDY: PLANNING AND IMPLEMENTATION

Teaching the Patient What to Expect

◗ Inform the patient this procedure can assist in assessing the esophagus and GI tract.

◗ Pregnancy is a general contraindication to procedures involving anesthesia and other medications. Explain to the female patient that she will be asked the date of her last menstrual period and pregnancy testing may be performed to determine the possibility of pregnancy before she receives anesthetics.

◗ Review the procedure with the patient. Address concerns about pain and explain that there may be moments of discomfort or pain experienced when the IV line or catheter is inserted to allow infusion of fluids such as saline, anesthetics, sedatives, medications used in the procedure, or emergency medications; there may be moments of discomfort or pain experienced when the endoscope is inserted, but the throat will be anesthetized with a spray or swab. Inform the patient that he or she will not be able to speak during the procedure, but breathing will not be affected.

◗ Inform the patient that the procedure is performed in a GI laboratory or radiology department, usually by an HCP and support staff, and takes approximately 30 to 60 min.

◗ Instruct the patient to remove dentures, eyewear, jewelry, and other metallic objects before the test.

◗ Baseline vital signs will be recorded and monitored throughout the procedure. Protocols may vary among facilities.

◗ An emesis basin will be provided for the increased saliva. The patient will be encouraged to spit out the saliva because the gag reflex may be impaired.

◗ Positioning for this study will be on an examination table in the left lateral decubitus position with the neck slightly flexed forward.

◗ The endoscope is passed through the mouth with a dental suction device in place to drain secretions. A side-viewing flexible, fiberoptic endoscope is advanced, and visualization of the GI tract is started.

◗ Air is insufflated to distend the upper GI tract, as needed. Biopsy specimens are obtained and/or endoscopic surgery is performed.

◗ Specimens are promptly transported to the laboratory for processing and analysis.

◗ At the end of the procedure, excess air and secretions are aspirated through the scope and the endoscope is removed.

◗ The needle or catheter is removed, and a pressure dressing is applied over the puncture site.

Potential Nursing Actions

✷ *Make sure a written and informed consent has been signed prior to the procedure and before administering any medications.*

Safety Considerations

◗ Anticoagulants, aspirin, and other salicylates should be discontinued by medical direction for the appropriate number of days prior to a procedure in which bleeding is a potential complication.

AFTER THE STUDY: POTENTIAL NURSING ACTIONS

Avoiding Complications

◗ May include bleeding and cardiac dysrhythmias. Monitor the patient's vital signs. Observe/assess the needle/

catheter insertion site for bleeding, inflammation, or hematoma formation and instruct the patient in its care. Observe the patient for indications of esophageal perforation (i.e., painful swallowing with neck movement, substernal pain with respiration, shoulder pain or dyspnea, abdominal or back pain, cyanosis, or fever). Instruct the patient to immediately report symptoms such as excessive bleeding, difficulty breathing, expectoration of blood, or fever to the HCP.

Treatment Considerations
- Do not allow the patient to eat or drink after the procedure until the gag reflex returns; then allow the patient to eat lightly for 12 to 24 hr.
- Instruct the patient to resume usual activity and diet in 24 hr or as tolerated after the examination, as directed by the HCP.
- Monitor vital signs and neurological status every 15 min for 1 hr, then every 2 hr for 4 hr, and as ordered by the HCP. Take temperature every 4 hr for 24 hr. Monitor intake and output at least every 8 hr. Compare with baseline values. Notify the HCP if temperature is elevated. Protocols may vary among facilities.
- Advise the patient to report pain that occurs within 1 to 4 hr of eating or in the middle of the night. Administer prescribed medications (antibiotics, antacids, H_2 receptor antagonist, proton pump inhibitor) for pain management.
- Explain there may be some throat soreness and hoarseness and to treat throat discomfort with lozenges and warm gargles when the gag reflex returns.
- Inform the patient that any belching, bloating, or flatulence is the result of air insufflation and is temporary.

Nutritional Considerations
- Recommendations to improve nutritional status are to complete a daily weight, calorie count, and dietary consult. Complete a good nutritional history, monitor and trend albumin, and avoid caffeinated drinks (coffee, tea).

Follow-Up, Evaluation, and Desired Outcomes
- Acknowledges the value of avoiding foods that cause gastric upset (e.g., caffeine, alcohol).

Estradiol

SYNONYM/ACRONYM: E2.

RATIONALE: To assist in diagnosing female fertility problems that may occur from tumor or ovarian failure.

PATIENT PREPARATION: There are no food, fluid, activity, or medication restrictions unless by medical direction.

NORMAL FINDINGS: Method: Liquid chromatography/mass spectrometry.

Age	Conventional Units	SI Units (Conventional Units × 3.67)
12 mo–10 yr		
Male and female	Less than 7 pg/mL	Less than 25.7 pmol/L
11–15 yr		
Male	Less than 40 pg/mL	Less than 147 pmol/L
Female	Less than 300 pg/mL	Less than 1,100 pmol/L

(table continues on page 558)

Age	Conventional Units	SI Units (Conventional Units × 3.67)
Adult male	Less than 50 pg/mL	Less than 184 pmol/L
Adult female		
Early follicular phase	20–150 pg/mL	73–551 pmol/L
Late follicular phase	40–350 pg/mL	147–1,285 pmol/L
Midcycle peak	150–750 pg/mL	551–2,753 pmol/L
Luteal phase	30–450 pg/mL	110–1,652 pmol/L
Postmenopause	Less than 20 pg/mL	Less than 73 pmol/L

CRITICAL FINDINGS AND POTENTIAL INTERVENTIONS: N/A

OVERVIEW: (Study type: Blood collected in a gold-, red-, red/gray-, or green-top [heparin] tube; **related body system:** Endocrine and Reproductive systems.) Estrogens are steroid hormones named for their role in the female estrous cycle. Estrogens are responsible for the development of secondary female sex characteristics (development of breasts, appearance of pubic hair), maintenance of the menstrual cycle, maintenance of the placenta during pregnancy, and initiation of lactation (via a feedback loop involving prolactin). The three types of estrogen commonly measured are estrone (E1), estradiol (E2), and estriol (E3). Estrogens are produced by the ovaries, liver, adrenal glands, and in fatty tissue (e.g., breast tissue). Ovarian estrogen hormone formation begins with the conversion of cholesterol into androstendione in the theca interna cells, followed by conversion to estradiol in ovarian granulosa cells. Estradiol, the most powerful of the estrogens, is the main estrogen produced in women who are not pregnant during the period between puberty and menopause. Estriol is the primary estrogen secreted during pregnancy, and it is provided by the placenta. Secretion of estrogens is influenced by the pituitary gonadotropins follicle-stimulating hormone (FSH) and luteinizing hormone (LH). After menopause, the ovaries stop producing estrogens, and the secondary sources (liver, adrenal glands, and breast tissue) provide estrogens mostly in the form of estrone.

INDICATIONS
- Assist in determining the presence of gonadal dysfunction.
- Evaluate menstrual abnormalities, fertility problems, estrogen-producing tumors in women, and testicular or adrenal tumors and feminization disorders in men.
- Monitor menotropins (Pergonal) therapy; menotropins is a preparation of FSH and LH used to induce ovulation and increase the chance of pregnancy.

INTERFERING FACTORS
Factors that may alter the results of the study
- Drugs and other substances that may increase estradiol levels include cimetidine, clomiphene, dehydroepiandrosterone, diazepam, estrogen/progestin therapy, ketoconazole, mifepristone (some

patients with meningiomas and not receiving any other drugs), nafarelin, nilutamide, phenytoin, tamoxifen, and troleandomycin.

- Drugs and other substances that may decrease estradiol levels include chemotherapy drugs, cimetidine, danazol, fadrozole, formestane, goserelin, leuprolide, megestrol, mepartricin, mifepristone (pregnant women with expulsion of fetus), nafarelin (women being treated for endometriosis), and oral contraceptives.

Other considerations
- Estradiol is secreted in a biphasic pattern during normal menstruation. Knowledge of the phase of the menstrual cycle may assist interpretation of estradiol levels.

POTENTIAL MEDICAL DIAGNOSIS: CLINICAL SIGNIFICANCE OF RESULTS
Increased in
- Adrenal tumors *(related to overproduction by tumor cells)*
- Estrogen-producing tumors
- Feminization in children *(related to increased production)*
- Gynecomastia *(newborns may demonstrate swelling of breast tissue in response to maternal estrogens; somewhat common and transient in pubescent males)*
- Hepatic cirrhosis *(accumulation occurs due to lack of liver function)*

- Hyperthyroidism *(related to primary increases in estrogen or response to increased levels of sex hormone–binding globulin)*

Decreased in
- Ovarian failure *(resulting in lack of estrogen synthesis)*
- Primary and secondary hypogonadism *(related to lack of estrogen synthesis)*
- Turner syndrome *(genetic abnormality in females in which there is only one X chromosome, resulting in varying degrees of underdeveloped sexual characteristics)*

E

NURSING IMPLICATIONS

BEFORE THE STUDY: PLANNING AND IMPLEMENTATION
Teaching the Patient What to Expect
- Inform the patient this test can assist in assessing hormone level.
- Explain that a blood sample is needed for the test.

AFTER THE STUDY: POTENTIAL NURSING ACTIONS
Follow-Up, Evaluation, and Desired Outcomes
- Explain that study results may indicate the need for additional testing to evaluate or monitor progression of the disease process and determine the need for a change in therapy.

Evoked Brain Potentials

SYNONYM/ACRONYM: Brainstem auditory evoked potentials (BAEP), brainstem auditory evoked responses (BAER), EP studies.

RATIONALE: To assist in diagnosing sensory deficits related to nervous system lesions manifested by visual defects, hearing defects, neuropathies, and cognitive disorders.

PATIENT PREPARATION: There are no food, fluid, activity, or medication restrictions unless by medical direction. Instruct the patient to clean the hair and to refrain from using hair sprays, creams, or solutions before the test.

NORMAL FINDINGS

- *Visual evoked response (VER) and auditory brainstem response (ABR):* Normal latency in recorded cortical and brainstem waveforms depending on age, gender, and stature
- *Event-related potential (ERP):* Normal recognition and attention span
- *Somatosensory evoked response (SER):* No loss of consciousness or presence of weakness.

CRITICAL FINDINGS AND POTENTIAL INTERVENTIONS: N/A

E

OVERVIEW: (**Study type:** Electrophysiologic; **related body system:** Nervous system.) Evoked brain potentials, also known as evoked potential (EP) responses, are electrophysiological studies performed to measure the brain's electrical responses to various visual, auditory, and somatosensory stimuli. EP studies help diagnose lesions of the nervous system by evaluating the integrity of the visual, somatosensory, and auditory nerve pathways. Three response types are measured: VER, ABR, and SER. The stimuli activate the nerve tracts that connect the stimulated (receptor) area with the cortical (visual and somatosensory) or midbrain (auditory) sensory area. A number of stimuli are given, and then responses are electronically displayed in waveforms, recorded, and computer analyzed. Abnormalities are determined by a delay in time, measured in milliseconds, between the stimulus and the response. This is known as *increased latency.* VER provides information about visual pathway function to identify lesions of the optic nerves, optic tracts, and demyelinating diseases such as multiple sclerosis. ABR provides information about auditory pathways to identify hearing loss and lesions of the brainstem. SER provides information about the somatosensory pathways to identify lesions at various levels of the central nervous system (spinal cord and brain) and peripheral nerve disease. EP studies are especially useful in patients with problems related to the nervous system and those unable to speak or respond to instructions during the test, because these studies do not require voluntary cooperation or participation in the activity. This allows collection of objective diagnostic information about visual or auditory disorders affecting infants and children and allows differentiation between organic brain and psychological disorders in adults. EP studies are also used to monitor the progression of or the effectiveness of treatment for deteriorating neurological diseases such as multiple sclerosis.

INDICATIONS

VER (Potentials)
- Detect cryptic or past retrobulbar neuritis.
- Detect lesions of the eye or optic nerves.
- Detect neurological disorders such as multiple sclerosis, Parkinson disease, and Huntington chorea.

- Evaluate binocularity in infants.
- Evaluate optic pathway lesions and visual cortex defects.

ABR (Potentials)
- Detect abnormalities or lesions in the brainstem or auditory nerve areas.
- Detect brainstem tumors and acoustic neuromas.
- Screen or evaluate neonates, infants, children, and adults for auditory problems.
- EP studies may be indicated when a child falls below growth chart norms.
- Evaluate patients in comatose states.

SER (Potentials)
- Detect multiple sclerosis and Guillain-Barré syndrome.
- Detect sensorimotor neuropathies and cervical pathology.
- Evaluate spinal cord and brain injury and function.
- Monitor sensory potentials to determine spinal cord function during a surgical procedure or medical regimen.

ERP (Potentials)
- Detect suspected psychosis or dementia.
- Differentiate between organic brain disorder and cognitive function abnormality.

INTERFERING FACTORS
Factors that may alter the results of the study
- Inability of the patient to cooperate or remain still during the procedure because of age, significant pain, or mental status. (*Note:* Significant behavioral problems may limit the ability to complete the test.)
- Improper placement of electrodes.
- Patient stress, which can affect brain chemistry, thus making it difficult to distinguish whether the results are due to the patient's emotional reaction or to organic pathology.

- Extremely poor visual acuity, which can hinder accurate determination of VER.
- Severe hearing loss, which can interfere with accurate determination of ABR.

POTENTIAL MEDICAL DIAGNOSIS: CLINICAL SIGNIFICANCE OF RESULTS
Abnormal findings related to
- VER (extended latencies):
  Absence of biocular vision
  Amblyopias
  Blindness
  Demyelinating diseases such as multiple sclerosis
  Huntington chorea
  Lesions or disease of the optic nerve and eye (e.g., anterior optic chiasm, neuritis)
  Lesions or disease of the optic tract
  Optic nerve neuritis
  Parkinson disease
  Visual field defects
- ABR (extended latencies):
  Acoustic neuroma
  Auditory nerve or brain stem damage or disease
  Cerebrovascular accidents
  Demyelinating diseases such as multiple sclerosis
- SER (extended latencies):
  Abnormal upper limb latencies suggest cervical spondylosis or intracerebral lesions.
  Abnormal lower limb latencies suggest peripheral nerve root disease such as Guillain-Barré syndrome, multiple sclerosis, transverse myelitis, or traumatic spinal cord injuries.

E

NURSING IMPLICATIONS

BEFORE THE STUDY: PLANNING AND IMPLEMENTATION

Teaching the Patient What to Expect
- Inform the patient this procedure measures electrical activity in the nervous system.
- Review the procedure with the patient. Address concerns about pain related

to the procedure and explain that the procedure is painless and harmless.

▶ Inform the patient that the procedure is performed in a special laboratory by a health-care provider (HCP) and takes approximately 30 min to 2 hr, depending on the type of studies required.

▶ Instruct the patient to remove jewelry and other metallic objects from the area to be examined.

Potential Nursing Actions

※ *Make sure a written and informed consent has been signed prior to the procedure and before administering any medications.*

▶ Ensure the patient is able to relax; report any extreme anxiety or restlessness.

Visual Evoked Potentials

▶ The patient is placed in a comfortable position about 1 m from the stimulation source. Electrodes are attached to the occipital and vertex lobe areas, and a reference electrode is attached to the ear. Placement of electrodes for VER generally follows the International 10/20 system. A light-emitting stimulation or a checkerboard pattern is projected on a screen at a regulated speed. This procedure is done for each eye (with the opposite eye covered) as the patient looks at a dot on the screen without any change in the gaze while the stimuli are delivered. A computer interprets the brain's responses to the stimuli and records them in waveforms.

Auditory Evoked Potentials

▶ The patient is placed in a comfortable position, and the electrodes are placed on the scalp at the vertex lobe area and on each earlobe. Earphones are placed on the patient's ears, and a clicking noise stimulus is delivered into one ear while a continuous tone is delivered to the opposite ear. Responses to the stimuli are recorded as waveforms for analysis.

Somatosensory Evoked Potentials

▶ The patient is placed in a comfortable position. Electrodes placed at the nerve sites of the wrist, knee, and ankle and on the scalp at the sensory cortex of the hemisphere on the opposite side (the electrode that picks up the response and delivers it to the recorder). Additional electrodes can be positioned at the cervical or lumbar vertebrae for upper or lower limb stimulation. The rate at which the electric shock stimulus is delivered to the nerve electrodes and travels to the brain is measured, computer analyzed, and recorded in waveforms for analysis. Both sides of the area being examined can be tested by switching the electrodes and repeating the procedure.

Event-Related Potentials

▶ Positioning for this study is in a sitting position in a chair in a quiet room. Earphones are placed on the patient's ears and auditory cues administered. The patient is asked to push a button when the tones are recognized. Flashes of light are also used as visual cues, with the patient pushing a button when cues are noted. Results are compared to normal EP waveforms for correct, incorrect, or absent responses.

AFTER THE STUDY: POTENTIAL NURSING ACTIONS

Treatment Considerations

▶ When the procedure is complete, the electrodes are removed and the skin is cleaned where the electrodes were applied.

Follow-Up, Evaluation, and Desired Outcomes

▶ Acknowledges contact information provided for the National Multiple Sclerosis Society (www.nationalms society.org).

Fecal Analysis

SYNONYM/ACRONYM: Stool evaluation and examination for ova and parasites, rotavirus antigen, *Clostridium difficile* toxin.

RATIONALE: To assess for indication of disease in the gastrointestinal (GI) tract evidenced in stool samples (e.g., presence of blood, white blood cells [WBCs], parasites, or other pathogens) toward diagnosing GI bleeding, cancer, inflammation, and infection.

PATIENT PREPARATION: There are no fluid or activity restrictions unless by medical direction. Instruct the patient to follow a normal diet unless instructed otherwise. If the test is being performed to identify blood, instruct the patient to follow a special diet that includes small amounts of chicken, turkey, and tuna (no red meats), raw and cooked vegetables and fruits, and bran cereal for several days before the test. Foods to avoid with the special diet include beets, turnips, cauliflower, broccoli, bananas, parsnips, and cantaloupe, because these foods can interfere with the occult blood test. Instruct the patient not to use laxatives, enemas, or suppositories for 3 days before the test. As appropriate, provide the required stool collection container and specimen collection instructions.

NORMAL FINDINGS: Method: Macroscopic examination, for appearance and color; microscopic examination for presence of parasites, larvae, or eggs, for cell count, and presence of meat fibers; leukocyte esterase for leukocytes; Benedict solution (copper sulfate) for reducing substances; guaiac for occult blood; x-ray paper for trypsin; enzyme immunoassay (EIA) for rotavirus antigen; immunoassay or molecular methods for *Clostridium* glutamate dehydrogenase (GDH), toxin A or toxin B.

Characteristic	Normal Result
Appearance	Solid and formed
Color	Brown
Epithelial cells	Few to moderate
Fecal fat	See "Fecal Fat" study
Leukocytes (WBCs)	Negative
Meat fibers	Negative
Occult blood	Negative
Reducing substances	Negative
Trypsin	2+ to 4+
Ova and parasites (O&P)	No presence of parasites, ova, or larvae
Rotavirus	Negative
Clostridium GDH, toxin A or toxin B	Negative

CRITICAL FINDINGS AND POTENTIAL INTERVENTIONS: N/A

OVERVIEW: (Study type: Fecal analysis; related body system: Digestive and Immune systems.) Feces consist mainly of cellulose and other undigested foodstuffs, bacteria, and water. Other substances normally found in feces include epithelial cells shed from the GI tract, small amounts of fats, bile pigments in the form of urobilinogen, GI and pancreatic secretions, electrolytes, and trypsin. Trypsin is a proteolytic enzyme produced in the pancreas. The average adult excretes 100 to 300 g of fecal material per day, the residue of approximately 10 L of liquid material that enters the GI tract each day. The laboratory analysis of feces includes macroscopic examination (volume, odor, shape, color, consistency, presence of mucus), microscopic examination (leukocytes, epithelial cells, ova and parasites, meat fibers), and chemical tests for specific substances (occult blood, trypsin, estimation of carbohydrate). Detection of occult blood is the most common test performed on stool. The prevalence of colorectal adenoma is greater than 30% in people aged 60 and older. Progression from adenoma to cancer occurs over a period of 5 to 12 yr and from cancer to metastatic disease in 2 to 3 yr. Routine fecal analysis also evaluates stool for the presence of intestinal parasites and their eggs. Some parasites are nonpathogenic; others, such as protozoa and worms, can cause serious illness.

Rotavirus, a double-stranded RNA virus in the family Reoviridae, has more than 40 known serotypes worldwide; 6 of which are prevalent in the United States. The two structural proteins, protease-cleaved protein (P protein) and glycoprotein (G protein), make up the outermost layer of the virus's capsid. The gene segments that produce P and G proteins are known to assort independently, and the protein recombinations are used to define the different serotypes and to develop vaccines against the virus. The name *rotavirus* is a Latin derivation of *rota*, or "wheel," that describes the wheel-like appearance of the virus as seen by electron microscopy. Rotavirus gastroenteritis (RGE) is the major cause of severe GI inflammation in children under 2 yr of age; studies have predicted that all children will be infected by rotavirus by age 5 yr. Older adults, especially those living in long-term residential facilities and patients of any age who are immunocompromised, are also susceptible to infection. The disease is highly contagious. It is transmitted by the fecal-oral route through direct person-person contact or handling of fomites (inanimate objects, such as toys, magazines, etc., that can transmit disease). Symptoms begin to appear within 1 to 3 days after exposure. Symptoms include fever, vomiting, and severe diarrhea, which lasts about 7 days; some patients also experience abdominal pain. Infections generally peak in the cooler, dryer months of the year. Vulnerable individuals can be reinfected multiple times during their lives, most likely by different viral serotypes. The development of natural immunity over time makes subsequent infections less severe, which is why healthy adults are rarely affected.

There are two oral rotavirus vaccines currently licensed for use in the United States. The Centers for Disease Control and Prevention recommends that all doses of vaccine be given before age 8 mo; RotaTeq (RV5) is given in three doses at ages 2 mo, 4 mo, and 6 mo; Rotarix (RV1) is given in two doses at ages 2 mo and 4 mo. Childhood vaccinations can be somewhat controversial. As with other preventive health-care practices, all patients, parents, or caregivers should discuss the benefits and risks of this vaccine with their health-care provider (HCP) before making a decision. Health situations that warrant a decision to forgo vaccination include allergic reaction to any given dose of the oral vaccine, known allergy to any component of the vaccine, diseases that affect the immune system (HIV/AIDS, severe combined immunodeficiency), or intussusception. Consideration to withhold the vaccine should be given to infants being treated with steroids or who are undergoing cancer treatment. Infants who are mildly ill may be given the vaccine, but vaccination for significantly affected individuals should be postponed until after recovery. Laboratory methods used to obtain results from stool specimens include EIA and molecular methods (multiplexed reverse transcriptase polymerase chain reaction [RT-PCR], semi-nested RT-PCR, nucleotide sequencing).

Clostridium difficile is a gram-positive, spore-forming bacterium that can cause a life-threatening bowel infection in patients who are susceptible or are receiving broad-spectrum antibiotic therapy (e.g., clindamycin, ampicillin, cephalosporins). *C. difficile* infection (CDI) is a major concern with respect to hospital-acquired infection (HAI) surveillance efforts. Older adults, especially those living in long-term health-care or residential facilities, children aged 1 to 3 yr, and those who are immunocompromised are most susceptible to infection. The bacteria release a toxin that causes necrosis of the colon tissue. The organism can be identified from a stool culture (see the study titled "Culture, Bacterial, Various Sites"). It is important to distinguish *C. difficile* colonization from cytogenic *C. difficile* infection in patients with diarrhea of unknown cause. Colonization is often asymptomatic, so in these patients the cause of diarrhea would warrant further investigation and different treatment than that administered for CDI. The presence of *C. difficile* in watery stool without evidence of the toxin or genes associated with toxin production does not provide the basis for diagnosis of CDI. Two toxins, A and B, are associated with toxigenic strains of *C. difficile* and can be identified more rapidly by using methods that do not involve stool culture.

Summary of Methods That Can Be Used to Assess for CID (With Their Strengths and Weaknesses)

Stool culture	Can detect the presence of any *C. difficile* regardless of whether toxin is produced—false-positive results are reported due to lack of specificity, lengthy time to obtain culture results, and difficulty of anaerobic culture; use of culture alone is not recommended.
GDH antigen testing*	GDH is produced by all *C. difficile* organisms regardless of whether toxin is produced—false-positive results are reported; time to obtain results is fairly quick, but due to lack of specificity, these assays are not recommended for use to independently confirm toxigenic infection.

(table continues on page 566)

Summary of Methods That Can Be Used to Assess for CID (With Their Strengths and Weaknesses)

Toxin immunoassays (A and/or B)*	Toxin assays have a rapid turnaround time to result and are easy to perform—false-negative results are reported due to specimen integrity issues (the toxin is very unstable, and specimens are subject to wide variations in handling, transportation, and storage temperatures), and not all kits detect both toxin A and toxin B. Significant variability in test results between kits from different manufacturers has also been demonstrated. These assays are less sensitive than other methods (e.g., tissue culture cytotoxicity, polymerase chain reaction [PCR]). They are not recommended for use to independently confirm toxigenic infection.
Molecular nucleic acid amplification test (NAAT; PCR or other NAAT) assays for the toxin B gene*	PCR assays are rapid and sensitive methods that can confirm the presence of the gene for the *C. difficile* B toxin; however, molecular testing is expensive and unavailable in most hospital laboratories.
Tissue culture cytotoxicity assay	Identifies the presence of toxin based on the cytotoxic effects of bacteria cultured from a stool sample and incubated in a human cell culture medium. Drawbacks include a high level of technical expertise required to perform; costliness; lengthy turnaround for results; and although it provides specific and sensitive results, it is less sensitive than PCR or toxigenic culture for detecting the organism in patients with diarrhea.
Toxigenic *C. difficile* culture	Toxigenic stool culture is a two-step process by which a routine stool culture for *C. difficile* is accomplished and then followed by NAAT to identify the presence of toxin genes. Main drawback is the length of time to results.

*Indicates tests preferred for use in the two-step algorithm.

Guidelines have been developed by the American College of Gastroenterology www.gi.org, American Society of Microbiology www.asm.org, CDC (www.cdc.gov), Infectious Disease Society of America (www.idsociety.org), and Society for Healthcare Epidemiology for America (www.shea-online.org); the most current information is available on their respective Web sites. There is some general overlap in recommendations regarding testing for toxin-producing *C. difficile*. A two-step algorithm has been recommended that combines the rapid screen for GDH and toxins with confirmation by NAAT. The combination of test methods provides highly sensitive and specific results produced in a clinically relevant timeframe. Screening test results that are all positive are interpreted as CDI infection likely. Screening test results that are all negative are interpreted as CDI infection unlikely. Screening test results that are mixed (GDH pos/Toxin neg or GDH neg/Toxin pos) are confirmed by NAAT.

INDICATIONS

- Assist in diagnosing disorders associated with GI bleeding or drug therapy that leads to bleeding.
- Assist in the diagnosis of pseudo-membranous enterocolitis after use of broad-spectrum antibiotic therapy.
- Assist in the diagnosis of suspected inflammatory bowel disorder.
- Detect altered protein digestion.
- Detect intestinal parasitic, viral, or bacterial infection, as indicated by diarrhea of unknown cause.
- Monitor effectiveness of therapy for intestinal malabsorption or pancreatic insufficiency.
- Screen for colorectal cancer.
- Screen for cystic fibrosis.

INTERFERING FACTORS

Factors that may alter the results of the study

- Drugs that can cause positive results for occult blood include acetylsalicylic acid, anticoagulants, colchicine, corticosteroids, iron preparations, and phenylbutazone.
- Drugs and other substances such as antacids, antibiotics, antidiarrheal compounds, bismuth, castor oil, iron, magnesia, or psyllium fiber (Metamucil) may interfere with analysis for O&P.
- Ingestion of a diet high in red meat, certain vegetables, and bananas can cause false-positive results for occult blood.
- Large doses of vitamin C can cause false-negative occult blood.
- Constipated stools may not indicate any trypsin activity owing to extended exposure to intestinal bacteria.
- Failure to test a fresh specimen may yield a false-negative O&P result.
- Antimicrobial or antiamebic therapy within 10 days of test may yield a false-negative O&P result.

- Failure to wait 1 wk after a GI study using barium or after laxative use can affect O&P test results.

POTENTIAL MEDICAL DIAGNOSIS: CLINICAL SIGNIFICANCE OF RESULTS

Unusual Appearance

- **Bloody:** *Excessive intestinal wall irritation or malignancy*
- **Bulky or frothy:** *Malabsorption*
- **Mucous:** *Inflammation of intestinal walls*
- **Slender or ribbonlike:** *Obstruction*

Unusual Color

- **Black:** *Bismuth (antacid) or charcoal ingestion, iron therapy, upper GI bleeding*
- **Grayish white:** *Barium ingestion, bile duct obstruction*
- **Green:** *Antibiotics, biliverdin, green vegetables*
- **Red:** *Beets and food coloring, lower GI bleed, phenazopyridine hydrochloride compounds, rifampin*
- **Yellow:** *Rhubarb*

Increased

- **Blood:** *Related to bleeding in the digestive tract*
- **Carbohydrates/reducing substances:** *Malabsorption syndromes, inability to digest some sugars*
- **Epithelial cells:** *Inflammatory bowel disorders*
- **Fat:** *Pancreatitis, sprue (celiac disease), cystic fibrosis related to malabsorption*
- **Leukocytes:** *Inflammation of the intestines related to bacterial infections of the intestinal wall, salmonellosis, shigellosis, or ulcerative colitis*
- **Meat fibers:** *Altered protein digestion, pancreatitis*
- **Occult blood:** *Anal fissure, diverticular disease, esophageal varices, esophagitis, gastritis, hemorrhoids, infectious diarrhea, inflammatory bowel disease, Mallory-Weiss tears, polyps, tumors, ulcers*

F

- pH: *Related to inflammation in the intestine from colitis, cancer, or antibiotic use*

Decreased
- Carbohydrates/reducing substances: *Sprue, cystic fibrosis, malnutrition, medications such as colchicine (gout) or birth control pills*
- Leukocytes: *Amebic colitis, cholera, disorders resulting from toxins, parasites, viral diarrhea*
- pH: *Related to poor absorption of carbohydrate or fat*
- Trypsin: *Cystic fibrosis, malabsorption syndromes, pancreatic deficiency*

O&P
Positive findings in
- Amebiasis—*Entamoeba histolytica* infection
- Ascariasis—*Ascaris lumbricoides* infection
- Blastocystis—*Blastocystis hominis* infection
- Cryptosporidiosis—*Cryptosporidium parvum* infection

- Enterobiasis—*Enterobius vermicularis* (pinworm) infection
- Giardiasis—*Giardia lamblia* infection
- Hookworm disease—*Ancylostoma duodenale, Necator americanus* infection
- Isospora—*Isospora belli* infection
- Schistosomiasis—*Schistosoma haematobium, S. japonicum, S. mansoni* infection
- Strongyloidiasis—*Strongyloides stercoralis* infection
- Tapeworm disease—*Diphyllobothrium, Hymenolepiasis, Taenia saginata, Taenia solium* infection
- Trematode disease—*Clonorchis sinensis, Fasciola hepatica, Fasciolopsis buski* infection
- Trichuriasis—*Trichuris trichiura* infection

Other
- Rotavirus infection
- Toxogenic *C. difficile* infection

NURSING IMPLICATIONS

POTENTIAL NURSING PROBLEMS: ASSESSMENT & NURSING DIAGNOSIS

Problems	Signs and Symptoms
Bleeding *(related to bowel inflammation, irritation, infection, chronic disease)*	Altered level of consciousness, hypotension, increased heart rate, decreased hemoglobin (Hgb) and hematocrit (Hct), capillary refill greater than 3 sec, cool extremities
Fluid volume (water) *(related to nausea, vomiting, diarrhea)*	Hypotension, decreased cardiac output, decreased urinary output, dry skin/mucous membranes, poor skin turgor, sunken eyeballs, increased urine specific gravity, hemoconcentration
Infection (tapeworm) *(related to drinking contaminated water, eating food contaminated with fecal matter infested with larva, eating raw or uncooked meat from an infected animal)*	Nausea, poor appetite, weakness, abdominal pain, diarrhea, weight loss secondary to inadequate nutrient absorption, fever, the presence of a cystic mass or lumps, allergic reactions to the larvae, bacterial infections, neurologic symptoms, seizures; in some cases, there are no symptoms

F

Problems	Signs and Symptoms
Infection (Giardiasis) *(related to contact with infected fecal contaminated food, water, or soil; swallowing infected water while swimming [lakes, rivers, streams]; eating uncooked food containing Giardiasis)*	Diarrhea, greasy stools, gas, nausea, abdominal pain/cramps, dehydration
Nutrition *(related to inadequate absorption, decreased caloric intake, nausea, diarrhea with nitrogen loss, ingestion of parasitic contaminated food or water)*	Decreased weight; poor wound healing; pedal edema; decreased calcium, potassium, vitamins, zinc, folic acid; skin lesions; muscle wasting
Pain *(related to infection, inflammation, contractions of diseased bowel, diarrhea)*	Colicky, intermittent abdominal pain; bloating; cramping; distention; self-report of pain; abdominal tenderness; hyperactive bowel sounds; increased pain and cramping with eating; disturbed sleep; diaphoresis; altered blood pressure and heart rate; nausea; vomiting

F

BEFORE THE STUDY: PLANNING AND IMPLEMENTATION

Teaching the Patient What to Expect

▶ Inform the patient this test can assist in the diagnosis of intestinal disorders or infection.

▶ Explain that a fresh stool sample is needed for the test.

▶ Review the procedure with the patient. Inform the patient of the procedure for collecting a stool sample, including the importance of good hand-washing techniques.

▶ Emphasize that if an infection is present, it may be contagious.

▶ Ask the patient to place the stool sample in a tightly covered container and not to contaminate the specimen with urine, water, or toilet tissue.

▶ Collect the specimen in a waterproof container with a tight-fitting lid; if the patient is not ambulatory, collect it in a clean, dry bedpan.

▶ Collect specimens from the first, middle, and last portion of the stool.

▶ Use a tongue blade to transfer the specimen to the container, and include any mucoid and bloody portions.

▶ The specimen should be refrigerated if it will not be transported to the laboratory within 4 hr after collection.

▶ To collect specimen by rectal swab, insert the swab past the anal sphincter, rotate gently, and withdraw. Place the swab in the appropriate container.

▶ Specimens to be examined for the presence of pinworms are collected by the "Scotch tape" method in the morning before bathing or defecation. A small paddle with a piece of cellophane tape (sticky side facing out) is pressed against the perianal area. The tape is placed in a collection container and submitted to determine if ova are present. Sometimes adult worms are observed protruding from the rectum.

Potential Nursing Actions

▶ Document any travel to foreign countries if parasitic infection is suspected.

▶ *Ensure that the risks and benefits of blood transfusion have been discussed and signed informed consent has been obtained prior to administration of blood and blood products.*

AFTER THE STUDY: POTENTIAL NURSING ACTIONS

Treatment Considerations

▶ Bleeding: Monitor and trend Hgb/Hct and platelet count. Increase the frequency of vital sign assessment, trend and note variances in results. Administer ordered blood or blood products, assess for cultural or religious barriers to blood transfusion. Assess the diet for iron-rich and vitamin K–rich foods. Explain the importance of reporting black or tarry stools that are indicative of GI bleeding.

▶ Fluid Volume: Assess current hydration status: skin turgor, dry mucous membranes, decreased urine output or dark urine, hypotension, or tarry or black stools (indicative of bleeding). Administer ordered IV fluids, blood, and blood products.

▶ Giardia Infection: Administer prescribed IV fluids and antibiotics, and encourage oral liquids. Explain observable symptoms of dehydration (especially in children). Educate on prevention of infection reoccurrence. Explain the importance of staying away from those infected with Giardiasis. Emphasize the value of vigilant hand washing.

▶ Tapeworm Infection: Administer prescribed tapeworm medication (praziquantel [Biltricide], albendazole, nitazoxanide). Educate on how to prevent an infection reoccurrence. Emphasize the value of vigilant hand washing.

▶ Rotavirus: Monitor vomiting and diarrhea; it may be necessary to seek medical attention to prevent dehydration that could be life threatening in children and older adults. Rehydration may be completed orally if able to keep fluid down or by replacement intravenous fluids. Monitor color and consistency of the stool (bloody, black and tarry) or pus, take the temperature every 4 hr (can get up to 104°F). Explain the importance of ensuring

that areas or items of exposure are cleansed (toys, toilets, counters) to prevent additional exposure of other family members. Emphasize vigilant handwashing.

▶ *Clostridium difficile*: Monitor for symptoms of infection, which will vary in severity based on patient age and condition. Classic symptoms include dehydration, nausea, bloody stools or pus in the stools, appetite loss, fever, abdominal cramping. Dehydration is a primary concern, as diarrhea may occur up to 15 times a day. Oral or IV fluid replacement should be facilitated. Monitor intake and output, as kidney injury or damage is a risk. Emphasize vigilant hand washing with soap and water. Explain that all contaminated surfaces should be cleansed with bleach, as other cleansers may not kill this organism.

▶ Pain: Auscultate bowel sounds and evaluate the severity of crampy, colicky abdominal pain and bloating when eating. Assess the tolerance of dietary products and collaborate to make necessary dietary alterations that will decrease bowel irritation. Identify successful pain management strategies and administer prescribed medications (sulfasalazine, corticosteriods, immunosuppressants, immunomodulators, anticholinergics, antidiarrheal). Attempt diversional activities as a pain management modality.

Nutritional Considerations

▶ Monitor and trend serum calcium, potassium, vitamin K and B$_{12}$, zinc, and folic acid. Perform an accurate actual weight daily (not verbally reported or estimated). Assess for skin lesions, current dietary habits and caloric intake, and collaborate with the dietitian to develop an appropriate diet. Administer ordered vitamin supplements, and discuss the possibility of using total parenteral nutrition if oral intake is insufficient. Teach the patient to abstain from eating raw food. Teach the patient and family to use vigilant hand washing before meals. Emphasize the importance of using clean water for food preparation and drinking.

Follow-Up, Evaluation, and Desired Outcomes

▶ Recognizes colon cancer screening options and understands that decisions regarding the need for and frequency of occult blood testing, colonoscopy, or other cancer screening procedures may be made after consultation between the patient and HCP. Colonoscopy should be used to follow up abnormal findings obtained by any of the screening tests. The most current guidelines for colon cancer screening of the general population as well as of individuals with increased risk are available from the American Cancer Society (www.cancer.org), U.S. Preventive Services Task Force (www.uspreventiveservicestaskforce.org), and American College of Gastroenterology (http://gi.org). For additional information regarding screening guidelines, refer to the study titled "Colonoscopy."

O&P

▶ Understands the importance of good hand hygiene to decrease risk of parasitic infection. Recognizes that nighttime anal itching could indicate an enterobiasis (pinworm) infection.

▶ Acknowledges changes in food and water handling, including the use of clean surfaces to prevent parasitic infection.

F

Fecal Fat

SYNONYM/ACRONYM: Stool fat, fecal fat stain.

RATIONALE: To assess for the presence of fat in the stool toward diagnosing malabsorption disorders such as Crohn disease and cystic fibrosis.

PATIENT PREPARATION: There are no fluid or activity restrictions unless by medical direction. Instruct the patient to ingest a diet containing 50 to 150 g of fat for at least 3 days before beginning specimen collection. This approach does not work well with children; instruct the caregiver to record the child's dietary intake to provide a basis from which an estimate of fat intake can be made. Instruct the patient not to use laxatives, enemas, or suppositories for 3 days before the test. As appropriate, provide the required stool collection container and specimen collection instructions; the test may require either a random specimen or a 72-hr collection. A large, clean, preweighed container should be used for the timed test. A smaller, clean container can be used for the collection of the random sample. Ensure specimen collection for this study is accomplished before any barium procedures are performed.

NORMAL FINDINGS: Method: Stain with Sudan black or oil red O. Treatment with ethanol identifies neutral fats; treatment with acetic acid identifies fatty acids.

	Random, Semiquantitative
Neutral fat	Less than 60 fat globules/hpf*
Fatty acids	Less than 100 fat globules/hpf

(table continues on page 572)

	72-hr, Quantitative
Age (normal diet)	
Infant (breast milk)	Less than 1 g/24 hr
0–6 yr	Less than 2 g/24 hr
Adult	Less than 7 g/24 hr; less than 20% of total solids
Adult (fat-free diet)	Less than 4 g/24 hr

*hpf = high-power field.

CRITICAL FINDINGS AND POTENTIAL INTERVENTIONS: N/A

OVERVIEW: (**Study type:** Fecal analysis, stool aliquot from an unpreserved and homogenized 24- to 72-hr timed collection; **related body system:** Digestive system. Random specimens may also be submitted.) Fecal fat consists primarily of triglycerides (neutral fats), fatty acids, and fatty acid salts. Through microscopic examination, the number and size of fat droplets as well as the type of fat present can be determined. Excretion of more than 7 g of fecal fat in a 24-hr period is abnormal but nonspecific for disease. Increases in excretion of neutral fats are associated with pancreatic exocrine insufficiency, whereas decreases are related to small bowel disease. An increase in triglycerides indicates that insufficient pancreatic enzymes are available to convert the triglycerides into fatty acids. Patients with malabsorption conditions have normal amounts of triglycerides but an increase in total fecal fat because the fats are not absorbed through the intestine. Malabsorption disorders (e.g., cystic fibrosis) cause blockage of the pancreatic ducts by mucus, which prevents the enzymes from reaching the duodenum and results in lack of fat digestion. Without digestion, the fats cannot be absorbed, and steatorrhea results. The appearance and odor of stool from patients with steatorrhea is typically foamy, greasy, soft, and foul-smelling. The semiquantitative test is used to screen for the presence of fecal fat. The quantitative method, which requires a 72-hr stool collection, measures the amount of fat present in grams.

INDICATIONS
• Assist in the diagnosis of malabsorption or pancreatic insufficiency, as indicated by elevated fat levels.
• Monitor the effectiveness of therapy.

INTERFERING FACTORS
Factors that may alter the results of the study
• Cimetidine has been associated with decreased fecal fat in some patients with cystic fibrosis who are also receiving pancreatic enzyme therapy.
• Some drugs cause steatorrhea as a result of mucosal damage. These include colchicine, kanamycin, lincomycin, methotrexate, and neomycin. Drugs and other substances that can cause an increase in fecal fat include aminosalicylic acid, bisacodyl and phenolphthalein (observed in individuals who misuse laxatives), and cholestyramine (in high doses).
• Use of suppositories, oily lubricants, or mineral oil in the perianal area for 3 days before the test can falsely increase neutral fats.
• Use of herbals with laxative effects, including cascara, psyllium, and senna, for 3 days before the test can falsely increase neutral fats.

- Barium interferes with test results.
- Failure to collect all stools may reflect falsely decreased results.
- Ingestion of a diet too high or low in fats may alter the results.

POTENTIAL MEDICAL DIAGNOSIS: CLINICAL SIGNIFICANCE OF RESULTS

Increased in

- Abetalipoprotein deficiency *(related to lack of transport proteins for absorption)*
- Addison disease *(related to impaired transport)*
- Amyloidosis *(increased rate of excretion related to malabsorption)*
- Bile salt deficiency *(related to lack of bile salts required for proper fat digestion)*
- Carcinoid syndrome *(increased rate of excretion related to malabsorption)*
- Celiac disease *(increased rate of excretion related to malabsorption)*
- Crohn disease *(increased rate of excretion related to malabsorption)*
- Cystic fibrosis *(related to insufficient digestive enzymes)*
- Diabetes *(abnormal motility related to primary condition)*
- Enteritis *(increased rate of excretion related to malabsorption)*
- Malnutrition *(related to detrimental effects on organs and systems responsible for digestion, transport, and absorption)*
- Multiple sclerosis *(abnormal motility related to primary condition)*
- Pancreatic insufficiency or obstruction *(related to insufficient digestive enzymes)*
- Peptic ulcer disease *(related to improper digestion due to low pH)*
- Pernicious anemia *(related to bacterial overgrowth that decreases overall absorption and results in vitamin B_{12} deficiency)*

- Progressive systemic sclerosis *(abnormal motility related to primary condition)*
- Thyrotoxicosis *(abnormal motility related to primary condition)*
- Tropical sprue *(increased rate of excretion related to malabsorption)*
- Viral hepatitis *(related to insufficient production of digestive enzymes and bile)*
- Whipple disease *(increased rate of excretion related to malabsorption)*
- Zollinger-Ellison syndrome *(related to improper digestion due to low pH)*

Decreased in: N/A

NURSING IMPLICATIONS

BEFORE THE STUDY: PLANNING AND IMPLEMENTATION

Teaching the Patient What to Expect

- Inform the patient this test can assist in the diagnosis of intestinal disorders.
- Explain that a stool sample is needed for the test.
- Review the procedure with the patient. Stress the importance of collecting all stools for the quantitative test, including diarrhea, over the timed specimen-collection period. Inform the patient not to urinate in the stool-collection container and not to put toilet paper in the container.
- For the timed, quantitative procedure, instruct the patient to collect each stool and place it in the 500-mL container during the timed collection period. Keep the container refrigerated in the plastic bag throughout the entire collection period.

Potential Nursing Actions

- Investigate the patient's health concerns that indicate a gastrointestinal (GI) disorder, diarrhea related to GI dysfunction, pain related to tissue inflammation or irritation, alteration in diet resulting from an inability to

F

digest certain foods, or fluid volume deficit related to active loss.

Treatment Considerations
▶ Instruct the patient with abnormal values on the importance of fluid intake and proper diet specific to his or her condition. Help the patient and caregiver cope with long-term implications.

Follow-Up, Evaluation, and Desired Outcomes
▶ Acknowledges contact information provided for the American Diabetes Association (www.diabetes.org), the Celiac Disease Foundation (https://celiac.org), the Crohn's and Colitis Foundation of America (www.crohnscolitisfoundation.org), or the Cystic Fibrosis Foundation (www.cff.org).

Ferritin

SYNONYM/ACRONYM: N/A

RATIONALE: To assist in diagnosing and monitoring various forms of anemia related to ferritin levels such as iron-deficiency anemia, anemia of malnourishment related to alcohol misuse, hemolytic anemia, chronic anemia of inflammation, and anemia related to long-term kidney dialysis.

PATIENT PREPARATION: There are no food, fluid, activity, or medication restrictions unless by medical direction.

NORMAL FINDINGS: Method: Immunoassay.

Age	Conventional Units	SI Units (Conventional Units × 1)
Newborn	25–200 ng/mL	25–200 mcg/L
1 mo	200–600 ng/mL	200–600 mcg/L
2–5 mo	50–200 ng/mL	50–200 mcg/L
6 mo–15 yr	7–140 ng/mL	7–140 mcg/L
Adult		
Males	20–250 ng/mL	20–250 mcg/L
Females (18–39 yr)	10–120 ng/mL	10–120 mcg/L
Females (40 yr and older)	12–263 ng/mL	12–263 mcg/L

CRITICAL FINDINGS AND POTENTIAL INTERVENTIONS: N/A

OVERVIEW: (**Study type:** Blood collected in a gold-, red-, or red/gray-top tube; **related body system:** Circulatory/Hematopoietic system.) Ferritin, a protein manufactured in the liver, spleen, and bone marrow, consists of a protein shell, apoferritin, and an iron core.

The amount of ferritin in the circulation is usually proportional to the amount of stored iron (ferritin and hemosiderin) in body tissues. Levels vary according to age and gender, but they are not affected by exogenous iron intake or subject to diurnal variations.

Compared to iron and total iron-binding capacity, ferritin is a more sensitive and specific test for diagnosing iron-deficiency anemia. Iron-deficiency anemia in adults is indicated at ferritin levels less than 10 ng/mL (SI = 10 mcg/L); hemochromatosis or hemosiderosis is indicated at levels greater than 400 ng/mL (SI = 400 mcg/L).

INDICATIONS
- Assist in the diagnosis of iron-deficiency anemia.
- Assist in the differential diagnosis of microcytic, hypochromic anemias.
- Monitor hematological responses during pregnancy, when serum iron is usually decreased and ferritin may be decreased.
- Support diagnosis of hemochromatosis or other disorders of iron metabolism and storage.

INTERFERING FACTORS
Factors that may alter the results of the study
- Drugs and other substances that may increase ferritin levels include ethanol, ferric polymaltose, iron, and oral contraceptives.
- Drugs and other substances that may decrease ferritin levels include erythropoietin and methimazole.
- Recent transfusion can elevate serum ferritin.

POTENTIAL MEDICAL DIAGNOSIS: CLINICAL SIGNIFICANCE OF RESULTS
Increased in
- **Alcohol misuse** *(active misuse, as evidenced by release of ferritin into the circulation from damaged hepatocytes and red blood cells [RBCs])*
- **Breast cancer** *(acute, related to release of ferritin as an acute-phase reactant protein; chronic, pathophysiology is uncertain)*
- **Hemochromatosis** *(related to increased iron deposits in the liver, which stimulate ferritin production)*
- **Hemolytic anemia** *(related to increased iron levels from hemolyzed RBCs, which stimulate ferritin production)*
- **Hemosiderosis** *(related to increased iron levels, which stimulate ferritin production)*
- **Hepatocellular disease** *(acute, related to release of ferritin as an acute-phase reactant protein; chronic, related to release of ferritin into the circulation from damaged hepatocytes)*
- **Hodgkin disease** *(acute, related to release of ferritin as an acute-phase reactant protein; chronic, pathophysiology is uncertain)*
- **Hyperthyroidism** *(possibly related to the stimulating effect of thyroid-stimulating hormone on ferritin production)*
- **Infection** *(acute, related to release of ferritin as an acute-phase reactant protein; chronic, pathophysiology is uncertain)*
- **Inflammatory diseases** *(related to release of ferritin as an acute-phase reactant protein)*
- **Leukemias** *(acute, related to release of ferritin as an acute-phase reactant protein; chronic, pathophysiology is uncertain)*
- **Oral or parenteral administration of iron** *(evidenced by an increased circulating iron level, which stimulates ferritin production)*
- **Thalassemia** *(related to increased iron levels from hemolyzed RBCs, which stimulate ferritin production)*

Decreased in
Conditions that decrease iron stores result in corresponding low levels of ferritin.

- Hemodialysis
- Iron-deficiency anemia

NURSING IMPLICATIONS

BEFORE THE STUDY: PLANNING AND IMPLEMENTATION

Teaching the Patient What to Expect
▶ Inform the patient this test can assist in the diagnosis of anemia.
▶ Explain that a blood sample is needed for the test.

AFTER THE STUDY: POTENTIAL NURSING ACTIONS

Nutritional Considerations
▶ Nutritional therapy may be indicated for patients with decreased ferritin

values because this may indicate corresponding iron deficiency. Instruct these patients in the dietary inclusion of iron-rich foods and in the administration of iron supplements, including adverse effects, as appropriate.

Follow-Up, Evaluation, and Desired Outcomes
▶ Acknowledges that based on the results of the procedure, additional testing may be performed to evaluate or monitor the progression of the disease process and determine the need for a change in therapy.

F

Fetal Fibronectin

SYNONYM/ACRONYM: fFN.

RATIONALE: To assist in assessing for premature labor.

PATIENT PREPARATION: There are no food, fluid, activity, or medication restrictions unless by medical direction.

NORMAL FINDINGS: (Method: Immunoassay) Negative (Less than 0.05 mcg/mL).

CRITICAL FINDINGS AND POTENTIAL INTERVENTIONS: N/A

OVERVIEW: (Study type: Body fluid, swab of vaginal secretions; **related body system:** Reproductive system. The specimen should be promptly delivered to the laboratory.) Fibronectin is a protein found in fetal connective tissue, amniotic fluid, and the placenta of pregnant women. Placental fetal fibronectin (fFN) is concentrated in the area where the placenta and its membranes are in contact with the uterine wall. It is first secreted early in pregnancy and is believed to help implantation of the fertilized egg to the uterus. Fibronectin is not detectable again until just

before delivery, at approximately 37 wk. If it is detected in vaginal secretions at 22 to 34 wk of gestation, delivery may happen prematurely. The test is a useful marker for impending membrane rupture within 7 to 14 days if the level rises to greater than 0.05 mcg/mL.

INDICATIONS
Investigate signs of premature labor.

INTERFERING FACTORS
Other considerations
If signs and symptoms persist in light of negative test results, repeat testing may be necessary.

POTENTIAL MEDICAL DIAGNOSIS: CLINICAL SIGNIFICANCE OF RESULTS

Positive findings in

- Premature labor *(possibly initiated by mechanical or infectious processes, the membranes pull away from the uterine wall and amniotic fluid containing fFN leaks into endocervical fluid)*

NURSING IMPLICATIONS

BEFORE THE STUDY: PLANNING AND IMPLEMENTATION

Teaching the Patient What to Expect

- Inform the patient this test can assess for risk of preterm delivery.
- Explain that a vaginal swab sample is needed for the test.
- Review the procedure with the patient. Address concerns about pain and explain that there should be no discomfort during the procedure.
- Positioning for this study is on the gynecological examination table with the feet up in stirrups. The patient's legs are draped to provide privacy and to reduce chilling. A small amount of vaginal secretion is collected using a special swab from an fFN kit.

Potential Nursing Actions

- Ensure that the patient knows the symptoms of premature labor, which include uterine contractions (with or without pain) lasting 20 sec or longer or increasing in frequency, menstrual-like cramping (intermittent or continuous), pelvic pressure, lower back pain that does not dissipate with a change in position, persistent diarrhea, intestinal cramps, changes in vaginal discharge, or a feeling that something is wrong.
- Emphasize the importance of notifying the health-care provider (HCP) if contractions occur more frequently than four times per hour.

AFTER THE STUDY: POTENTIAL NURSING ACTIONS

Treatment Considerations

- Discuss the implications of abnormal test results on the patient's lifestyle. Provide teaching and information regarding the clinical implications of the test results, as appropriate. Educate the patient regarding access to counseling services.
- Reinforce education on signs and symptoms of labor, as appropriate. Inform the patient that hospitalization or more frequent prenatal checks may be ordered.
- Explain that other therapies may also be administered, such as antibiotics, corticosteroids, and IV tocolytics. Advise on the importance of completing the entire course of antibiotic therapy, if ordered, even if no symptoms are present.

Follow-Up, Evaluation, and Desired Outcomes

- Acknowledges information given by the HCP regarding further testing, treatment, or referral to another HCP, including the possible causes and increased risks associated with premature labor and delivery.

Fetoscopy

SYNONYM/ACRONYM: Endoscopic fetal surgery, fetal endoscopy.

RATIONALE: To facilitate diagnosis and treatment of the fetus, evaluate for disorders such as neural tube defects and congenital blood disorders, and assist with fetal karyotyping.

PATIENT PREPARATION: Instruct the patient to withhold food and fluid for 8 hr prior to the endoscopic procedure. There are no activity or medication restrictions unless by medical direction.

NORMAL FINDINGS
• Absence of birth defects or findings that suggest presence of a birth defect

CRITICAL FINDINGS AND POTENTIAL INTERVENTIONS: N/A

OVERVIEW: (Study type: Endoscopy; related body system: Reproductive system.) Fetoscopy is usually performed around the 18th week of pregnancy or later when the fetus is developed sufficiently for diagnosis of potential problems. It is done to evaluate or treat the fetus during pregnancy. Fetoscopy can be accomplished externally using a stethoscope with an attached headpiece, which is placed on the mother's abdomen to assess the fetal heart tones. Endoscopic fetoscopy is accomplished using an instrument called a *fetoscope,* a thin, 1-mm flexible scope, which is placed with the aid of sonography. The fetoscope is inserted into the uterus through a thin incision in the abdominal wall (transabdominally) or through the cervix (transcervically) in earlier stages of pregnancy. Fetal tissue and blood samples can be obtained through the fetoscope. In addition, fetal surgery can be performed for such procedures as the repair of a fetal congenital diaphragmatic hernia, enlarged bladder, and spina bifida.

INDICATIONS
• Assess the fetus for birth defects during pregnancy; areas examined include the amniotic fluid, umbilical cord, and fetal side of the placenta.

INTERFERING FACTORS
Factors that may alter the results of the study
• Activity of fetus.
• Amniotic fluid that is extremely cloudy.

POTENTIAL MEDICAL DIAGNOSIS: CLINICAL SIGNIFICANCE OF RESULTS
Abnormal findings related to
• Acardiac twin
• Congenital diaphragmatic hernia
• Hemophilia
• Neural tube defects
• Spinal bifida

NURSING IMPLICATIONS

BEFORE THE STUDY: PLANNING AND IMPLEMENTATION

Teaching the Patient What to Expect
◗ Inform the patient this procedure can assist in locating and treating fetal abnormalities.
◗ Review the procedure with the patient. Address concerns about pain and explain that a local anesthetic will be applied to the abdomen to ease with insertion of the fetoscope.
◗ Inform the patient that the procedure is performed in an ultrasound department, by a health-care provider (HCP) specializing in this procedure, with support staff, and takes approximately 60 min.
◗ The patient will be instructed to lie on her back for this procedure.

Endoscopic Procedure
◗ The lower abdomen area is cleaned, and a local anesthetic is administered

in the area where the incision will be made. Label the appropriate specimen container with the corresponding patient demographics, initials of the person collecting the specimen, date, and time of collection if samples are to be obtained on aspirated amniotic fluid or fetal material.

- Conductive gel is applied to the skin, and a Doppler transducer is moved over the skin to locate the position of the fetus.
- The patient will be asked to breathe normally during the examination. If necessary for better fetal visualization, the patient will be asked to inhale deeply and hold her breath.
- When the study is completed, the gel is removed from the skin.

Potential Nursing Actions

 Make sure a written and informed consent has been signed prior to *the procedure and before administering any medications.*

AFTER THE STUDY: POTENTIAL NURSING ACTIONS

Avoiding Complications

- Instruct the patient in the care of the incision and to contact her HCP immediately if she is experiencing chills, fever, dizziness, moderate or severe abdominal cramping, or fluid or blood loss from the vagina or incision.

Treatment Considerations

- Observe/assess the incision for redness or leakage of fluid or blood following the endoscopic procedure.

Follow-Up, Evaluation, and Desired Outcomes

- Understands that a follow-up ultrasound will be completed the next day to assess the fetus and placenta.

Fibrinogen

SYNONYM/ACRONYM: Factor I.

RATIONALE: Commonly used to evaluate fibrinolytic activity as well as identify congenital deficiency, disseminated intravascular coagulation (DIC), and severe liver disease.

PATIENT PREPARATION: There are no food, fluid, activity, or medication restrictions unless by medical direction.

NORMAL FINDINGS: Method: Photo-optical clot detection.

Age	Conventional Units	SI Units (Conventional Units × 0.0294)
Newborn	200–500 mg/dL	5.9–14.7 micromol/L
Adult	200–400 mg/dL	5.9–11.8 micromol/L

Values are higher in older adults.

CRITICAL FINDINGS AND POTENTIAL INTERVENTIONS
- Less than 80 mg/dL (SI: Less than 2.4 micromol/L).
- Greater than 800 mg/dL (SI: Greater than 23.5 micromol/L).

Timely notification to the requesting health-care provider (HCP) of any critical findings and related symptoms is a role expectation of the professional nurse. A listing of these findings varies among facilities.

Signs and symptoms of microvascular thrombosis include cyanosis, ischemic tissue necrosis, hemorrhagic necrosis, tachypnea, dyspnea, pulmonary emboli, venous distention, abdominal pain, and oliguria. Possible interventions include identification and treatment of the underlying cause, support through administration of required blood products (cryoprecipitate or fresh frozen plasma), and administration of heparin. Cryoprecipitate may be a more effective product than fresh frozen plasma in cases where the fibrinogen level is less than 100 mg/dL (SI = 2.94 micromol/L), the minimum level required for adequate hemostasis, because it delivers a concentrated amount of fibrinogen without as much plasma volume.

OVERVIEW: (**Study type:** Blood collected in a completely filled blue-top [3.2% sodium citrate] tube; **related body system:** Circulatory/Hematopoietic system. If the patient's hematocrit exceeds 55%, the volume of citrate in the collection tube must be adjusted. The collection tube should be completely filled. *Important note:* When multiple specimens are drawn, the blue-top tube should be collected after sterile [i.e., blood culture] tubes. Otherwise, when using a standard vacutainer system, the blue-top tube is the first tube collected. When a butterfly is used, due to the added tubing, an extra red-top tube should be collected before the blue-top tube to ensure complete filling of the blue top tube. Promptly transport the specimen to the laboratory for processing and analysis. The recommendation for processed and unprocessed samples stored in unopened tubes is that testing should be completed within 1 to 4 hr of collection.) Fibrinogen (factor I) is an acute-phase reactant protein synthesized in the liver. It is an essential component in the process of hemostasis or clot formation. In the common final pathway of the coagulation process, thrombin converts fibrinogen to fibrin, which then becomes crosslinked fibrin monomers and ultimately a stable fibrin clot. The use of fibrinogen levels is not limited to coagulation studies. The role of fibrinogen in the inflammatory response has also established an association between elevated levels and vascular diseases such as coronary heart disease, myocardial infarction, stroke, and peripheral arterial disease.

INDICATIONS

- Assist in the diagnosis of suspected DIC, as indicated by decreased fibrinogen levels.
- Evaluate congenital or acquired dysfibrinogenemias.
- Monitor hemostasis in disorders associated with low fibrinogen levels or elevated levels that can predispose patients to excessive thrombosis.

INTERFERING FACTORS

Factors that may alter the results of the study

- Drugs and other substances that may increase fibrinogen levels include acetylsalicylic acid and oral contraceptives.
- Drugs and other substances that may decrease fibrinogen levels include anabolic steroids, asparaginase, bezafibrate, danazol, dextran, fenofibrate, fish oils, gemfibrozil, lovastatin, pentoxifylline, phosphorus, and ticlopidine.
- Placement of tourniquet for longer than 60 sec can result in venous

stasis and changes in the concentration of plasma proteins to be measured. Platelet activation may also occur under these conditions, causing erroneous results.

- Vascular injury during phlebotomy can activate platelets and coagulation factors, causing erroneous results.
- Hemolyzed specimens must be rejected because hemolysis is an indication of platelet and coagulation factor activation.
- Hematocrit greater than 55% may cause falsely prolonged results because of anticoagulant excess relative to plasma volume.
- Incompletely filled collection tubes, specimens contaminated with heparin, clotted specimens, or unprocessed specimens not delivered to the laboratory within 1 to 2 hr of collection should be rejected.
- Icteric or lipemic specimens interfere with optical testing methods, producing erroneous results.
- Traumatic venipuncture and excessive agitation of the sample can alter test results.

Other considerations

- Considerations for draw times after transfusion include the type of product, the amount of product transfused, and the patient's clinical situation. The circulating half-life of fibrinogen is 3 to 5 days. Generally, specimens are collected 30 to 60 min after a massive transfusion to provide guidance regarding the need for administration of additional units.

POTENTIAL MEDICAL DIAGNOSIS: CLINICAL SIGNIFICANCE OF RESULTS
Increased in
Fibrinogen is an acute-phase reactant protein and will be increased in inflammatory conditions.

- Acute myocardial infarction
- Cancer
- Eclampsia
- Hodgkin disease
- Inflammation
- Multiple myeloma
- Nephrotic syndrome
- Pregnancy
- Stroke
- Tissue necrosis

Decreased in
- Congenital fibrinogen deficiency (rare) *(related to deficient synthesis)*
- DIC *(related to rapid consumption as fibrinogen is converted to fibrin)*
- Dysfibrinogenemia *(related to an inherited abnormality in fibrinogen synthesis)*
- Liver disease (severe) *(related to decreased synthesis)*
- Primary fibrinolysis *(related to rapid conversion during fibrinolysis; plasmin breaks down fibrinogen and fibrin)*

NURSING IMPLICATIONS

BEFORE THE STUDY: PLANNING AND IMPLEMENTATION

Teaching the Patient What to Expect
- Inform the patient that this laboratory study can assist in diagnosing diseases associated with clotting disorders.
- Explain that a blood sample is needed for the test.

AFTER THE STUDY: POTENTIAL NURSING ACTIONS

Treatment Considerations
- Instruct the patient to report bruising, petechiae, and bleeding from mucous membranes, hematuria, and occult blood.

Follow-Up, Evaluation, and Desired Outcomes
- Acknowledges the correlation between abnormal clotting of the importance of

taking precautions against bruising and bleeding.
▶ Acknowledges examples of taking precautions against bruising and bleeding to include the use of a soft bristle toothbrush, use of an electric razor, avoidance of constipation, avoidance of acetylsalicylic acid and similar products, and avoidance of intramuscular injections.

Fibrinogen Degradation Products

SYNONYM/ACRONYM: Fibrin split products, fibrin breakdown products, FDP, FSP, FBP.

RATIONALE: To evaluate conditions associated with abnormal fibrinolytic and fibrinogenolytic activity such as disseminated intravascular coagulation (DIC), deep vein thrombosis (DVT), and pulmonary embolism (PE).

PATIENT PREPARATION: There are no food, fluid, activity, or medication restrictions unless by medical direction.

NORMAL FINDINGS: Method: Latex agglutination.

Conventional Units	SI Units (Conventional Units x 1)
Less than 5 mcg/mL	Less than 5 mg/dL

CRITICAL FINDINGS AND POTENTIAL INTERVENTIONS: N/A

OVERVIEW: (Study type: Blood collected in a completely filled blue-top [3.2% sodium citrate] tube; **related body system:** Circulatory/Hematopoietic system. If the patient's hematocrit [Hct] exceeds 55%, the volume of citrate in the collection tube must be adjusted. Blood collected in a completely filled blue-top [3.2% sodium citrate] tube. If the patient's Hct exceeds 55%, the volume of citrate in the collection tube must be adjusted. The collection tube should be completely filled. *Important note:* When multiple specimens are drawn, the blue-top tube should be collected after sterile [i.e., blood culture] tubes. Otherwise, when using a standard vacutainer system, the blue-top tube is the first tube collected. When a butterfly is used, due to the added tubing, an extra red-top tube should be collected before the blue-top tube to ensure complete filling of the blue top tube. Promptly transport the specimen to the laboratory for processing and analysis. The recommendation for processed and unprocessed samples stored in unopened tubes is that testing should be completed within 1 to 4 hr of collection.) This coagulation test evaluates fibrin split products or fibrin/fibrinogen degradation products (FDPs) that interfere with normal coagulation and formation of the hemostatic platelet plug. As thrombin initiates the formation of the fibrin clot, it also activates the fibrinolytic system to limit the size of clot formation and prevent venous occlusion. The D-dimer is specific to secondary fibrinolysis because it detects the disintegration of fibrin rather than fibrinogen. The FDP test detects degradation products of primary fibrinolysis generated by the action of thrombin on fibrinogen as well as degradation products of secondary fibrinolysis by the action of plasmin on fibrin. The two tests together can be useful for differentiation and treatment of suspected cases of fibrinolysis. In the case of primary fibrinolysis, the FDP will be positive while the D-dimer is normal. In DIC, or secondary fibrinolysis, both will be elevated. FDPs are normally cleared rapidly from circulation; however, increased circulating levels can interfere with hemostasis by interfering with fibrin polymerization and adhering to platelet cell membranes, thereby inhibiting their normal function.

INDICATIONS
• Assist in the diagnosis of suspected DIC.
• Evaluate response to therapy with fibrinolytic drugs.
• Monitor the effects on hemostasis of trauma, extensive surgery, obstetric complications, and disorders such as liver or kidney disease.

INTERFERING FACTORS
Factors that may alter the results of the study
• Drugs and other substances that may increase fibrin degradation product levels include heparin and fibrinolytic drugs such as streptokinase and urokinase.

• The presence of rheumatoid factor may falsely elevate results with some test kits.
• Hct greater than 55% may cause falsely prolonged results because of anticoagulant excess relative to plasma volume.
• Incompletely filled collection tubes, specimens contaminated with heparin, clotted specimens, or unprocessed specimens not delivered to the laboratory within 1 to 2 hr of collection should be rejected.
• Traumatic venipunctures and excessive agitation of the sample can alter test results.

Other considerations
• The test should not be ordered on patients receiving heparin therapy.

POTENTIAL MEDICAL DIAGNOSIS: CLINICAL SIGNIFICANCE OF RESULTS
Increased in
• DIC *(FDP can be positive in a number of conditions in which the coagulation system has been excessively stimulated as a result of tissue injury and fibrin and/or fibrinogen is being degraded by plasmin)*
• Excessive bleeding *(clot formation related to depletion of platelets and clotting factors will stimulate fibrinolysis and increase circulation of fibrin breakdown products)*
• Kidney disease *(FDP can be positive in a number of conditions in which the coagulation system has been excessively stimulated as a result of tissue injury and fibrin and/ or fibrinogen is being degraded by plasmin)*
• Kidney transplant rejection
• Liver disease *(related to decreased hepatic clearance)*
• Myocardial infarction *(FDP can be positive in a number of conditions in which the coagulation system has been excessively stimulated as a result of tissue injury and fibrin*

and/or fibrinogen is being degraded by plasmin)

- Obstetric complications, such as pre-eclampsia, abruptio placentae, intrauterine fetal death *(excessive stimulation of the coagulation system; microthrombi are formed and plasminogen is released to dissolve the fibrin clots)*
- Post-cardiothoracic surgery period *(FDP can be positive in a number of conditions in which the coagulation system has been excessively stimulated as a result of tissue injury and fibrin and/or fibrinogen is being degraded by plasmin)*
- Pulmonary embolism *(FDP can be positive in a number of conditions in which the coagulation system has been excessively stimulated as a result of tissue injury and fibrin and/or fibrinogen is being degraded by plasmin)*

Decreased in: N/A

NURSING IMPLICATIONS

BEFORE THE STUDY: PLANNING AND IMPLEMENTATION

Teaching the Patient What to Expect
▶ Inform the patient this test can assist in diagnosing diseases associated with clotting disorders.
▶ Explain that a blood sample is needed for the test.

Potential Nursing Actions
▶ Ensure that laboratory draws are bundled to prevent unnecessary venipuncture.

AFTER THE STUDY: POTENTIAL NURSING ACTIONS

Treatment Considerations
▶ When bleeding is a concern, increase the frequency of vital sign assessment and note result variances with trends. Monitor for blood in stool, emesis, and sputum. Assess skin for petechiae, purpura, or hematoma, and institute bleeding precautions. Instruct the patient to report bleeding from skin or mucous membranes, ecchymosis, petechiae, hematuria, and occult blood. Monitor and trend Hgb and Hct. Administer ordered blood or blood products, and stool softeners. Administer prescribed medications: recombinant human activated protein C, epsilon aminocaproic acid.
▶ Gas exchange can become an issue with blood loss. Monitor and trend ABG results, vital signs, respiratory rate and effort, and pulse oximetry. Teach patient that crossing legs increases DVT risk, and ensure patient does not cross legs while lying or sitting. Assess lung sounds frequently. Use pulse oximetry to monitor oxygen saturation and collaborate with health-care provider (HCP) to administer oxygen as needed. Elevate the head of the bed 30 degrees, assess for hypoxia, and administer prescribed anticoagulant therapy.
▶ Tissue perfusion can be affected when a DVT occurs. Assess for symptoms of DVT and for contributing factors: trauma, recent surgery, smoking, varicose veins, age, venous stasis, obesity, pregnancy, or oral contraceptive use. Monitor diagnostic test results: D-dimer, ultrasound, impedance plethysmography. Monitor and trend coagulation studies: prothrombin time, international normalized ratio, and partial thromboplastin time. Encourage bedrest with leg elevation, administer prescribed anticoagulant therapy, and institute bleeding precautions. Apply leg compression devices as prescribed and prepare for potential adjunct therapy: thrombolytic, vena cava filter, or thrombectomy.

Safety Considerations
▶ Inform the patient with increased levels of fibrin degradation products of the importance of taking precautions against bruising and bleeding, including gentle oral care with the use of a soft bristle toothbrush, use

of an electric razor, avoidance of constipation, avoidance of acetyl-salicylic acid and similar products, and avoidance of intramuscular injections.

Nutritional Considerations
▶ Encourage intake of foods rich in vitamin K, such as dark leafy green vegetables such as kale, spinach, collard greens, and brussels sprouts.

Follow-Up, Evaluation, and Desired Outcomes
▶ Demonstrates proficiency in self-administration of ordered anticoagulant therapy.
▶ Adheres to the request to maintain bedrest until the HCP deems it is safe to resume activity.
▶ Adheres to the request to refrain from risky activities to prevent injury.

Fluorescein Angiography

SYNONYM/ACRONYM: FA.

RATIONALE: To assist in detecting vascular changes in the eyes affecting vision related to diseases such as diabetic retinopathy and macular degeneration.

PATIENT PREPARATION: There are no food, fluid, or activity restrictions unless by medical direction. Instruct the patient to avoid eye medications (particularly miotic eye drops which may constrict the pupil preventing a clear view of the fundus and mydriatic eyedrops in order to avoid instigation of an acute open angle attack in patients with narrow angle glaucoma) for at least 1 day prior to the test.

NORMAL FINDINGS
• No leakage of dye from retinal blood vessels
• Normal retina and retinal and choroidal vessels
• No evidence of vascular abnormalities, such as hemorrhage, retinopathy, aneurysms, or obstructions caused by stenosis and resulting in collateral circulation.

CRITICAL FINDINGS AND POTENTIAL INTERVENTIONS: N/A

OVERVIEW: (Study type: Sensory (ocular); related body system: Nervous system.) Fluorescein angiography (FA) involves the color radiographic examination of the retinal vasculature following rapid IV injection of a sodium fluorescein contrast medium. A special camera allows images to be taken in sequence and manipulated by a computer to provide views of the retinal vessels during filling and emptying of the dye. The camera allows only light waves in the blue range to strike the fundus of the eye. When the fluorescein reaches the blood vessels in the eye, blue light excites the dye molecules to a higher state of activity and causes them to emit a greenish-yellow fluorescence that is recorded.

INDICATIONS
• Detect arterial or venous occlusion evidenced by the reduced, delayed, or absent flow of the

contrast medium through the vessels or possible vessel leakage of the medium.

- Detect possible vascular disorders affecting visual acuity.
- Detect presence of microaneurysms caused by hypertensive retinopathy.
- Detect the presence of tumors, retinal edema, or inflammation, as evidenced by abnormal patterns or degree of fluorescence.
- Diagnose and manage diabetic retinopathy. For additional information regarding screening guidelines and management of diabetes, refer to the study titled "Glucose."
- Diagnose past reduced flow or patency of the vascular circulation of the retina, as evidenced by neovascularization.
- Diagnose presence of macular degeneration and any other degeneration and any associated hemorrhaging.
- Observe ocular effects resulting from the long-term use of high-risk medications.

INTERFERING FACTORS

Contraindications

✺ Patients with a past history of hypersensitivity to radiographic dyes. Address concerns about nausea and vomiting, as appropriate.

✺ Patients with narrow-angle glaucoma if pupil dilation is performed; dilation can initiate a severe and sight-threatening open-angle attack.

✺ Patients with allergies to mydriatics if pupil dilation using mydriatics is performed.

Factors that may alter the results of the study

- Presence of cataracts may interfere with fundal view.
- Ineffective dilation of the pupils may impair clear imaging.

Other considerations

- Allergic reaction to radiographic dye, including nausea and vomiting, may interrupt the procedure.

POTENTIAL MEDICAL DIAGNOSIS: CLINICAL SIGNIFICANCE OF RESULTS

Abnormal findings related to

- Aneurysm
- Arteriovenous shunts
- Diabetic retinopathy
- Macular degeneration
- Neovascularization
- Obstructive disorders of the arteries or veins that lead to collateral circulation
- Ocular histoplasmosis
- Retinal vascular occlusion

NURSING IMPLICATIONS

BEFORE THE STUDY: PLANNING AND IMPLEMENTATION

Teaching the Patient What to Expect

▸ Inform the patient this procedure can assist in detecting changes in the eye that affect vision. It may also be used as a preoperative assessment tool prior to retinal laser procedures.

▸ Explain that prior to the procedure, laboratory testing may be required to determine the possibility of bleeding risk (coagulation testing) or to assess for impaired kidney function (creatinine level and estimated glomerular filtration rate). The effects of fluorescein sodium on kidney function are not well understood, and the health-care provider (HCP) may choose to assess kidney function if warranted.

▸ Review the procedure with the patient. Explain that the patient will be requested to fixate the eyes during the procedure. Address concerns about pain and explain that mydriatics, if used, may cause blurred vision and sensitivity to light. There may also be a brief stinging sensation when the drop is put in the eye. Also explain that

some discomfort may be experienced during the insertion of the IV to allow intermittent infusion of dye. Inform the patient that when fluorescein dye is injected, it may cause facial flushing or nausea and vomiting.
▶ Inform the patient that an HCP performs the test, in a quiet, darkened room, and that to dilate and evaluate both eyes, the test can take up to 60 min.
▶ Instruct the patient to remove contact lenses or glasses, as appropriate, and that it is important to keep the eyes open for the test.
▶ The patient is seated in a chair that faces the camera and is instructed to look at a directed target while the eyes are examined.
▶ The ordered mydriatic is administered to each eye and repeated in 5 to 15 min if dilation is to be performed. Drops are placed in the eye with the patient looking up and the solution directed at the six o'clock position of the sclera (white of the eye) near the limbus (gray, semitransparent area of the eyeball where the cornea and sclera meet). Neither dropper nor bottle should touch the eyelashes.
▶ An intermittent infusion device is inserted, as ordered, for subsequent injection of the contrast media or emergency medications.
▶ After the eyedrops are administered but before the dye is injected, color fundus photographs are taken.
▶ The patient is instructed to place the chin in the chin rest and gently press the forehead against the support bar. Instruct the patient to open his or her eyes wide and look at the desired target.
▶ Fluorescein dye is injected into the brachial vein using the intermittent infusion device, and a rapid sequence of photographs is taken and repeated after the dye has reached the retinal vascular system. Follow-up photographs are taken in 20 to 30 min.
▶ At the conclusion of the procedure, the IV is removed and direct pressure is applied with a dry gauze to stop bleeding. Observe venipuncture site for bleeding or hematoma formation

and secure gauze with adhesive bandage.

Potential Nursing Actions
▶ Investigate the patient's known or suspected vision loss; changes in visual acuity, including type and cause; use of glasses or contact lenses; and eye conditions with treatment regimens.

✧ *Make sure a written and informed consent has been signed prior to the procedure and before administering any medications.*

Safety Considerations
▶ Ensure that the patient understands that he or she must refrain from driving until the pupils return to normal (about 4 hr) after the test and has made arrangements to have someone else be responsible for transportation after the test.

AFTER THE STUDY: POTENTIAL NURSING ACTIONS

Avoiding Complications
▶ Observe for hypersensitive reaction to the dye. Anaphylaxis, bronchospasm, cardiac arrest, laryngeal edema, myocardial infarction, nausea, pruritus, urticaria, or vomiting can occur in response to the dye, and extravasation of the dye can occur during injection. Dilation can initiate a severe and sight-threatening open-angle attack in patients with narrow-angle glaucoma if pupil dilation is performed.

Treatment Considerations
▶ Inform the patient that visual acuity and responses to light may change. Suggest that the patient wear dark glasses after the test until the pupils return to normal size. Inform the patient that yellow discoloration of the skin and urine from the radiographic dye is normally present for up to 2 days.

Nutritional Considerations
▶ Abnormal FA findings may be associated with diabetes. There is no "diabetic diet"; however, many meal-planning approaches with nutritional goals are endorsed by the American Diabetes Association. Patients who adhere to dietary recommendations report a better general feeling of health, better

weight management, greater management of glucose and lipid values, and improved use of insulin. Instruct the patient, as appropriate, in nutritional management of diabetes. A variety of dietary patterns are beneficial for people with diabetes. Encourage consultation with a registered dietitian who is a certified diabetes educator.

Follow-Up, Evaluation, and Desired Outcomes
▶ Accepts that vision loss may impair independent activity and percipitate

the loss of driving privileges. Acknowledges contact information regarding vision aids provided for the American Heart Association (www.heart.org/HEARTORG), American Macular Degeneration Foundation (www.macular.org), Glaucoma Research Foundation (www.glaucoma.org), ADA (www.diabetes.org), National Heart, Lung, and Blood Institute (www.nhlbi.nih.gov), or the US Department of Agriculture's resource for nutrition (www.choosemyplate.gov).

F

Folic Acid

SYNONYM/ACRONYM: Folate, vitamin B_9.

RATIONALE: To assist in evaluation of diagnoses that are related to fluctuations in folate levels such as vitamin B_{12} deficiency and malabsorption.

PATIENT PREPARATION: There are no food, fluid, activity, or medication restrictions unless by medical direction.

NORMAL FINDINGS: Method: Immunochemiluminometric assay (ICMA).

	Conventional Units	SI Units (Conventional Units × 2.265)
Child	Greater than 7 ng/mL	
Adult		
Normal	Greater than 5.4 ng/mL	Greater than 12.2 nmol/L
Intermediate	3.4–5.4 ng/mL	7.7–12.2 nmol/L
Deficient	Less than 3.4 ng/mL	Less than 7.7 nmol/L

Values may be slightly decreased in older adults due to the effects of medications and the presence of multiple chronic or acute diseases with or without muted symptoms.

CRITICAL FINDINGS AND POTENTIAL INTERVENTIONS: N/A

OVERVIEW: (**Study type:** Blood collected in a gold-, red-, or red/gray-top tube; **related body system:** Circulatory/Hematopoietic and Digestive systems.) Folate, a water-soluble vitamin, is produced by bacteria in the intestines and stored in small amounts in the liver. Dietary folate is absorbed through the intestinal mucosa and stored in the liver. Folate is necessary for normal red blood cell (RBC) and white blood cell function, DNA replication, and cell division. Folate levels are often measured in association with serum vitamin B_{12} determinations because vitamin B_{12} is required for folate to enter tissue cells. Folate is an essential coenzyme in the conversion of homocysteine to methionine. Hyperhomocysteinemia resulting from folate deficiency in pregnant women is believed to increase the risk of neural tube defects. Hyperhomocysteinemia related to low folic acid levels is also associated with increased risk for cardiovascular disease.

INDICATIONS

- Assist in the diagnosis of megaloblastic anemia resulting from deficient folate intake or increased folate requirements, such as in pregnancy and hemolytic anemia.
- Monitor the effects of prolonged parenteral nutrition.
- Monitor response to disorders that may lead to folate deficiency or decreased absorption and storage.

INTERFERING FACTORS

Factors that may alter the results of the study

- Drugs and other substances that may decrease folate levels include aminopterin, ampicillin, antacids, anticonvulsants, barbiturates, chloramphenicol, chloroguanide, erythromycin, ethanol, lincomycin, metformin, methotrexate, nitrofurans, oral contraceptives, penicillins, pentamidine, phenytoin, pyrimethamine, tetracycline, and triamterene.
- Hemolysis may falsely increase folate levels.

POTENTIAL MEDICAL DIAGNOSIS: CLINICAL SIGNIFICANCE OF RESULTS

Increased in

- Blind loop syndrome *(related to malabsorption in a segment of the intestine due to competition for absorption of folate produced by bacterial overgrowth)*
- Excessive dietary intake of folate or folate supplements

- Pernicious anemia *(related to inadequate levels of vitamin B_{12} due to impaired absorption, resulting in increased circulating folate levels)*
- Vitamin B_{12} deficiency *(related to vitamin B_{12} levels inadequate to metabolize folate, resulting in increased circulating folate levels)*

Decreased in

- Chronic alcohol misuse *(related to insufficient intake combined with malabsorption)*
- Crohn disease *(related to malabsorption)*
- Exfoliative dermatitis *(related to increased demand)*
- Hemolytic anemias *(related to increased demand due to shortened RBC life span caused by folate deficiency)*
- Liver disease *(related to increased excretion)*
- Malnutrition *(related to insufficient intake)*
- Megaloblastic anemia *(related to folate deficiency, which affects development of RBCs and results in anemia)*
- Myelofibrosis *(related to increased demand)*
- Tumors *(related to increased demand)*
- Pregnancy *(related to increased demand possibly combined with insufficient dietary intake)*
- Regional enteritis *(related to malabsorption)*
- Scurvy *(related to insufficient intake)*
- Sideroblastic anemias *(evidenced by an acquired anemia resulting from folate deficiency; iron enters and accumulates in the RBCs but cannot become incorporated in hemoglobin)*
- Sprue *(related to malabsorption)*
- Ulcerative colitis *(related to malabsorption)*
- Whipple disease *(related to malabsorption)*

F

NURSING IMPLICATIONS

POTENTIAL NURSING PROBLEMS: ASSESSMENT & NURSING DIAGNOSIS

Problems	Signs and Symptoms
Confusion; altered sensory perception *(related to hepatic disease and encephalopathy, acute alcohol consumption, hepatic metabolic insufficiency)*	Disorganized thinking, restlessness, irritability, altered concentration and attention span, changeable mental function over the day, hallucinations; unable to follow directions; disoriented to person, place, time, and purpose; inappropriate affect
Fatigue *(related to hepatic disease process, malnutrition, anemia, chemotherapy, radiation therapy)*	Decreased concentration, increased physical complaints, unable to restore energy with sleep, reports being tired, unable to maintain normal routine
Gas exchange *(related to deficient oxygen capacity of the blood)*	Irregular breathing pattern, use of accessory muscles; altered chest excursion; adventitious breath sounds (crackles, rhonchi, wheezes, diminished breath sounds); signs of hypoxia; altered blood gas results; confusion; lethargy; cyanosis
Nutrition *(related to poor eating habits, excessive alcohol use, altered liver function, nausea, vomiting)*	Known inadequate caloric intake, weight loss, muscle wasting in arms and legs, stool that is pale or gray colored, skin that is flaky with loss of elasticity

BEFORE THE STUDY: PLANNING AND IMPLEMENTATION

Teaching the Patient What to Expect

▶ Inform the patient this test can assist in detecting folate deficiency and monitoring folate therapy.

▶ Explain that a blood sample is needed for the test.

Potential Nursing Actions

▶ Observe the patient for oral lesions or complaints of pain when swallowing. The patient may complain of a sore tongue which may appear red, shiny, or swollen at the tip or around the edges.

▶ Investigate the patient's history when evaluating for the underlying cause of suspected folate deficiency in order to prepare an effective treatment plan. Examples might be history of alcohol misuse accompanied by poor nutrition; deficiency related to pregnancy or lactation; prescription drugs associated with a decrease in folate levels, such as certain anticonvulsants (e.g., phenytoin), sulfonamides, or methotrexate; chronic hemolytic anemia; or malabsorption syndromes.

AFTER THE STUDY: POTENTIAL NURSING ACTIONS

Treatment Considerations

▶ Fatigue: Assess for the physical cause of fatigue. Pace activities to preserve energy stores. Rate fatigue on a numeric scale to trend degree of fatigue over time, identify what aggravates and decreases fatigue, and assess for related emotional factors such as depression. Evaluate current medications in relation to fatigue and assess for physiologic factors such as anemia.

▶ Gas Exchange: Monitor respiratory rate and effort based on assessment of patient condition. Assess lung sounds frequently, use pulse oximetry to monitor oxygen saturation, and collaborate with health-care provider to administer oxygen as needed. Elevate the head of the bed 30 degrees or higher to facilitate ease of breathing. Monitor IV fluids and avoid aggressive fluid resuscitation. Assess level of consciousness and anticipate the need for possible intubation.

▶ Nutrition: Document food intake with possible calorie count. Assess barriers to eating, consider using a food diary, and monitor continued alcohol use because it is a barrier to adequate nutrition. Monitor glucose levels, daily weight, and food selections. Provide dietary consult with assessment of cultural food selections. Administer multivitamin as prescribed and provide parenteral and enteral nutrition as needed. Assess and trend liver function tests (alanine aminotransferase [ALT], aspartate aminotransferase [AST], alkaline phosphatase [ALP], protein, albumin, bilirubin), folic acid, glucose, thiamine, and electrolytes.

Safety Considerations

▶ Confusion: Treat the medical condition and evaluate medications. Prevent falls and injury through appropriate use of postural support, bed alarm, or restraints and protect from physical harm. Consider pharmacological interventions and administer prescribed medication. Record accurate intake and output to assess fluid status. Monitor and trend blood ammonia level and electrolytes. Determine last alcohol use and assess for symptoms of hepatic encephalopathy, sleep disturbances, or incoherence. Administer ordered blood or blood products to treat the disease.

Nutritional Considerations

▶ Instruct the patient who is folate-deficient (especially pregnant women), as appropriate, to eat foods rich in folate, such as liver, salmon, eggs, asparagus, green leafy vegetables, broccoli, sweet potatoes, beans, and whole wheat.

▶ Educate the patient regarding access to nutritional counseling services with a registered dietitian.

Follow-Up, Evaluation, and Desired Outcomes

▶ Acknowledges contact information provided for the U.S. Department of Agriculture's resource for nutrition (www.choosemyplate.gov).

Follicle-Stimulating Hormone

SYNONYM/ACRONYM: Follitropin, FSH.

RATIONALE: To distinguish primary causes of gonadal failure from secondary causes, evaluate menstrual disturbances, and assist in infertility evaluations.

PATIENT PREPARATION: There are no food, fluid, activity, or medication restrictions unless by medical direction.

NORMAL FINDINGS: Method: Immunoassay.

Age	Conventional Units and SI Units
Child	
Prepuberty	Less than 10 international units/mL
Adult	
Male	1.4–15.5 international units/mL

Age	Conventional Units and SI Units
Female	
Follicular phase	1.4–9.9 international units/mL
Ovulatory peak	6.2–17.2 international units/mL
Luteal phase	1.1–9.2 international units/mL
Postmenopause	19–100 international units/mL

CRITICAL FINDINGS AND POTENTIAL INTERVENTIONS: N/A

OVERVIEW: (**Study type:** Blood collected in a gold-, red-, or red/gray-top tube; **related body system:** Endocrine and Reproductive systems.) Follicle-stimulating hormone (FSH) is produced and stored in the anterior portion of the pituitary gland. In women, FSH promotes maturation of the graafian (germinal) follicle, causing estrogen secretion and allowing the ovum to mature. In men, FSH partially controls spermatogenesis, but the presence of testosterone is also necessary. Gonadotropin-releasing hormone secretion is stimulated by a decrease in estrogen and testosterone levels. Gonadotropin-releasing hormone secretion stimulates FSH secretion. FSH production is inhibited by an increase in estrogen and testosterone levels. FSH production is pulsatile, episodic, and cyclic and is subject to diurnal variation. Serial measurement is often required.

INDICATIONS
- Assist in distinguishing between primary and secondary (pituitary or hypothalamic) gonadal failure.
- Define menstrual cycle phases as a part of infertility testing.
- Evaluate ambiguous sexual differentiation in infants.
- Evaluate early sexual development in girls younger than age 9 or boys younger than age 10 (precocious puberty associated with elevated levels).
- Evaluate failure of sexual maturation in adolescence.
- Evaluate testicular dysfunction.
- Investigate impotence, gynecomastia, and menstrual disturbances.

INTERFERING FACTORS
Factors that may alter the results of the study
- Drugs and other substances that may increase FSH levels include bicalutamide, bombesin, cimetidine, clomiphene, digoxin, erythropoietin, exemestane, finasteride, gonadotropin-releasing hormone, ketoconazole, levodopa, metformin, nafarelin, naloxone, nilutamide, oxcarbazepine, pravastatin, and tamoxifen.
- Drugs and other substances that may decrease FSH levels include anabolic steroids, anticonvulsants, buserelin, estrogens, corticotropin-releasing hormone, danazol, diethylstilbestrol, goserelin, megestrol, mestranol, oral contraceptives, phenothiazine, pravastatin, progesterone, tamoxifen, toremifene, and valproic acid.

Other considerations
- In women who are menstruating, values vary in relation to the phase of the menstrual cycle. Values are higher in women who are postmenopausal.

POTENTIAL MEDICAL DIAGNOSIS: CLINICAL SIGNIFICANCE OF RESULTS

Increased in

- Castration *(oversecretion related to feedback mechanism involving decreased testosterone levels)*
- Gonadal failure *(oversecretion related to feedback mechanism involving decreased estrogen or testosterone levels)*
- Gonadotropin-secreting pituitary tumors *(related to oversecretion by tumor cells)*
- Klinefelter syndrome *(oversecretion related to feedback mechanism involving decreased estrogen or testosterone levels)*
- Menopause *(oversecretion related to feedback mechanism involving decreased estrogen levels)*
- Orchitis *(oversecretion related to feedback mechanism involving decreased testosterone levels)*
- Precocious puberty in children *(related to oversecretion from the pituitary gland)*
- Primary hypogonadism *(oversecretion related to feedback mechanism involving decreased estrogen or testosterone levels; failure of testes or ovaries to produce sex hormones)*
- Reifenstein syndrome *(oversecretion related to feedback mechanism involving familial partial resistance to testosterone levels)*
- Turner syndrome *(oversecretion related to feedback mechanism involving decreased estrogen or testosterone levels)*

Decreased in

- Anorexia nervosa *(related to suppressive effects of severe caloric restriction on the hypothalamic-pituitary axis)*
- Anterior pituitary hypofunction *(underproduction resulting from dysfunctional pituitary gland)*
- Hemochromatosis *(hypogonadotropic hypogonadism related to absence of the gonadal-stimulating pituitary hormones, estrogen, and testosterone; iron deposits in pituitary may affect normal production of FSH)*
- Hyperprolactinemia *(related to suppressive effect on estrogen production)*
- Hypothalamic disorders *(decreased production in response to lack of hypothalamic stimulators)*
- Polycystic ovary disease (Stein-Leventhal syndrome) *(suppressed secretion related to feedback mechanism involving increased estrogen levels)*
- Pregnancy *(related to elevated estrogen levels)*
- Sickle cell anemia *(although primary testicular dysfunction is mainly associated with sickle cell disease, related to testicular micro-infarcts, hypogonadotropic hypogonadism has been reported in some men with sickle cell disease)*

F

NURSING IMPLICATIONS

BEFORE THE STUDY: PLANNING AND IMPLEMENTATION

Teaching the Patient What to Expect
- Inform the patient this test can assist in evaluating disturbances in hormone levels.
- Explain that a blood sample is needed for the test. Inform the patient that multiple specimens may be required.

Potential Nursing Actions
- Obtain information regarding the patient's phase of menstrual cycle.

AFTER THE STUDY: POTENTIAL NURSING ACTIONS

Follow-Up, Evaluation, and Desired Outcomes
- Female patients acknowledge teaching regarding the potential effects of FSH deficiency, which may include an absence of menstrual cycles, infertility,

decreased sex drive, and vaginal dryness. Male patients acknowledge teaching regarding the potential effects of FSH deficiency, which may include decreased sex drive, erectile dysfunction, and infertility.

▶ Acknowledges information regarding the potential for development of osteoporosis with a resulting tendency to develop bone fractures, which can occur in both female and male patients with this hormone deficiency.

Fructosamine

SYNONYM/ACRONYM: Glycated albumin.

RATIONALE: To assist in assessing long-term glucose management in diabetes.

PATIENT PREPARATION: There are no food, fluid, activity, or medication restrictions unless by medical direction.

NORMAL FINDINGS: Method: Spectrophotometry.

Status	Conventional Units	SI Units (Conventional Units × 0.01)
Nondiabetic	174–286 micromol/L	1.74–2.86 mmol/L
Diabetic (values vary with degree of management)	210–563 micromol/L	2.10–5.63 mmol/L

CRITICAL FINDINGS AND POTENTIAL INTERVENTIONS: N/A

OVERVIEW: (**Study type:** Blood collected in a gold-, red-, or red/gray-top tube; **related body system:** Endocrine system.) Fructosamine is the result of a covalent linkage between glucose and albumin or other proteins. Similar to glycated hemoglobin, fructosamine can be used to monitor long-term management of glucose in patients with diabetes. It has a shorter half-life than glycated hemoglobin and is thought to be more sensitive to short-term fluctuations in glucose concentrations. Some glycated hemoglobin methods are affected by hemoglobin variants. Fructosamine is not subject to this interference. For additional information

regarding screening guidelines and management of diabetes, refer to the study titled "Glucose."

INDICATIONS
• Evaluate management of diabetes.

INTERFERING FACTORS
Factors that may alter the results of the study
• Drugs and other substances that may increase fructosamine levels include bendroflumethiazide and captopril.
• Drugs and other substances that may decrease fructosamine levels include ascorbic acid, pyridoxine, and terazosin.
• Decreased albumin levels may result in falsely decreased fructosamine levels.

POTENTIAL MEDICAL DIAGNOSIS: CLINICAL SIGNIFICANCE OF RESULTS

Increased in
- Patients with diabetes with poor glucose management

Decreased in
- Severe hypoproteinemia

NURSING IMPLICATIONS

BEFORE THE STUDY: PLANNING AND IMPLEMENTATION

Teaching the Patient What to Expect
▶ Inform the patient this test can assist in evaluating blood sugar management.
▶ Explain that a blood sample is needed for the test.

AFTER THE STUDY: POTENTIAL NURSING ACTIONS

Treatment Considerations
▶ Instruct the patient and caregiver to report signs and symptoms of hypoglycemia (weakness, confusion, diaphoresis, rapid pulse) or hyperglycemia (thirst, polyuria, hunger, lethargy).

Nutritional Considerations
▶ Increased levels of fructosamine may be associated with diabetes. There is no "diabetic diet"; however, many meal-planning approaches with nutritional goals are endorsed by the American Diabetes Association (ADA). Patients who adhere to dietary recommendations report a better general feeling of health, better weight management, greater management of glucose and lipid values, and improved use of insulin. Instruct the patient, as appropriate, in nutritional management of diabetes. A variety of dietary patterns are beneficial for people with diabetes. Encourage consultation with a registered dietitian who is a certified diabetes educator.

Follow-Up, Evaluation, and Desired Outcomes
▶ Acknowledges contact information provided for the American Heart Association (www.heart.org/ HEARTORG), ADA (www.diabetes .org), National Heart, Lung, and Blood Institute (www.nhlbi.nih.gov), or U.S. Department of Agriculture's resource for nutrition (www.choosemyplate .gov).

Fundoscopy With or Without Photography

SYNONYM/ACRONYM: Funduscopy, ophthalmoscopy.

RATIONALE: To evaluate vascular and structural changes in the eye in assessing the progression of diseases such as glaucoma, diabetic retinopathy, and macular degeneration.

PATIENT PREPARATION: There are no food, fluid, or activity, restrictions unless by medical direction. Instruct the patient to avoid eye medications (particularly miotic eyedrops, which may constrict the pupil, preventing a clear view of the fundus, and mydriatic eyedrops in order to avoid instigation of an acute open-angle attack in patients with narrow-angle glaucoma) for at least 1 day prior to the test.

NORMAL FINDINGS
- Normal optic nerve and vessels
- No evidence of other ocular abnormalities.

CRITICAL FINDINGS AND POTENTIAL INTERVENTIONS
• Detached retina

Flashers, floaters, or a veil that moves across the field of vision may indicate detached retina or retinal tear. This condition requires immediate examination by an ophthalmologist. Untreated, full retinal detachment can result in irreversible and complete loss of vision in the affected eye.

Timely notification to the requesting health-care provider (HCP) of any critical findings and related symptoms is a role expectation of the professional nurse. A listing of these findings varies among facilities.

OVERVIEW: (Study type: Sensory (ocular); related body system: Nervous system.) Fundoscopy is performed as part of a routine eye examination. This test involves the examination of the structures of the eye to document the condition of the eye, detect abnormalities, and assist in following the progress of treatment. The fundus is the inner lining of the eye. The retina, optic disc, and macula can be visualized directly or indirectly by fundoscopic examination. Photographic images may be taken through dilated pupils to document findings for review and comparison. The Amsler grid is an additional test that may be included in the eye examination, especially if macular degeneration is suspected. This simple test for central vision can be performed using a grid with instructions printed from a home computer.

INDICATIONS
• Detect the presence of choroidal nevus.
• Detect various types and stages of glaucoma.
• Document the presence of diabetic retinopathy. For additional information regarding screening guidelines and management of diabetes, refer to the study titled "Glucose."

• Document the presence of macular degeneration and any other degeneration and any associated hemorrhaging.
• Observe ocular effects resulting from the long-term use of high-risk medications.

INTERFERING FACTORS
Contraindications

⬥ Patients with acute narrow-angle glaucoma if pupil dilation is performed; dilation can initiate a severe and sight-threatening open-angle attack.

⬥ Patients with allergies to mydriatics if pupil dilation using mydriatics is performed.

Factors that may alter the results of the study
• Presence of cataracts may interfere with fundal view.
• Ineffective dilation of the pupils may impair clear imaging.
• Rubbing or squeezing the eyes may affect results.

POTENTIAL MEDICAL DIAGNOSIS: CLINICAL SIGNIFICANCE OF RESULTS
Abnormal findings related to
• Aneurysm
• Atrial hypertension
• Benign intracranial hypertension from brain tumor
• Choroidal nevus
• Color vision deficiencies
• Diabetic retinopathy
• Disorders of the optic nerve
• Glaucoma
• Histoplasmosis

- Macular degeneration
- Obstructive disorders of the arteries or veins that lead to collateral circulation
- Papilledema
- Raised intracranial pressure associated with hydrocephalus
- Retinal detachment or tear
- Sickle cell anemia
- Stroke

NURSING IMPLICATIONS

BEFORE THE STUDY: PLANNING AND IMPLEMENTATION

Teaching the Patient What to Expect

▶ Inform the patient this procedure assists in detecting changes in the eye that effect vision.
▶ Review the procedure with the patient. Address concerns about pain and explain that mydriatics, if used, may cause blurred vision and sensitivity to light. There may also be a brief stinging sensation when the drop is put in the eye, but no discomfort will be experienced during the examination.
▶ Inform the patient that an HCP performs the test, in a quiet, darkened room, and that to dilate and evaluate both eyes, the test can take up to 60 min or longer if photographs are included.
▶ The patient will be seated in a chair that faces the camera and asked to look at a directed target while the eyes are examined.
▶ The ordered mydriatic will be administered to each eye and repeated in 5 to 15 min if dilation is to be performed. Drops are placed in the eye with the patient looking up and the solution directed at the six o'clock position of the sclera (white of the eye) near the limbus (gray, semitransparent area of the eyeball where the cornea and sclera meet). Neither dropper nor bottle should touch the eyelashes.
▶ The patient will be instructed to place the chin in the chin rest and gently press the forehead against the support

bar. The patient will be asked to open the eyes wide and look at desired target while the HCP examines the fundus, with or without dilation. The examination is performed at a variety of prescribed levels of gaze. The patient should be encouraged to maintain a constant gaze but informed that it is alright to blink as needed. The direct examination is performed using an instrument called an *ophthalmoscope*. The instrument is about the size of a penlight through which a beam of light is directed into the pupil while the HCP uses magnifying lenses to visualize the interior of the fundus. The indirect examination is carried out using either a binocular indirect ophthalmoscope, a slit-lamp microscope and hand lens, or a hand lens with the light source affixed to the HCP's head.

Potential Nursing Actions

▶ Investigate the patient's known or suspected vision loss; changes in visual acuity, including type and cause; use of glasses or contact lenses; and eye conditions with treatment regimens. Inquire about known allergens, especially allergies or sensitivities to latex or mydriatics (if dilation is to be performed).
▶ Ask the patient to remove contact lenses or glasses, as appropriate.
▶ Ensure that the patient understands that he or she must refrain from driving until the pupils return to normal (about 4 hr) after the test and has made arrangements to have someone else be responsible for transportation after the test.

AFTER THE STUDY: POTENTIAL NURSING ACTIONS

Avoiding Complications

▶ Dilation can initiate a severe and sight-threatening open-angle attack in patients with narrow-angle glaucoma.

Treatment Considerations

▶ Instruct the patient to resume usual medications, as directed by the HCP.
▶ Teach how to perform a self-check glucose accurately and to correctly self-administer insulin or to take oral

antihyperglycemic drugs. Ensure the patient understands to report signs and symptoms of hypoglycemia (weakness, confusion, diaphoresis, rapid pulse) or hyperglycemia (thirst, polyuria, hunger, lethargy) to the HCP.

▶ Emphasize, as appropriate, that good glycemic management delays the onset of and slows the progression of diabetic retinopathy, nephropathy, and neuropathy.

Safety Considerations

▶ Instruct the patient to avoid strenuous physical activities, such as lifting heavy objects, that may increase pressure in the eye, as ordered.

▶ Inform the patient that visual acuity and responses to light may change. Suggest that the patient wear dark glasses after the test until the pupils return to normal size.

▶ Discuss the possibility of a change in lifestyle, independence, and driving privileges based on loss of visual acuity.

Nutritional Considerations

▶ Abnormal findings may be associated with diabetes. There is no "diabetic diet"; however, many meal-planning approaches with nutritional goals are

endorsed by the ADA. Patients who adhere to dietary recommendations report a better general feeling of health, better weight management, greater management of glucose and lipid values, and improved use of insulin. Instruct the patient, as appropriate, in nutritional management of diabetes. A variety of dietary patterns are beneficial for people with diabetes. Encourage consultation with a registered dietitian who is a certified diabetes educator.

Follow-Up, Evaluation, and Desired Outcomes

▶ Acknowledges contact information provided regarding vision aids provided for the American Macular Degeneration Foundation (www.macular.org), American Heart Association (www.heart.org/HEARTORG), ADA (www.diabetes.org), National Heart, Lung, and Blood Institute (www.nhlbi.nih.gov), or U.S. Department of Agriculture's resource for nutrition (www.choosemyplate.gov).

▶ Acknowledges that The American Optometric Association's recommendations for the frequency of eye examinations can be accessed at (www.aoa.org).

Gallium Scan

SYNONYM/ACRONYM: Ga scan.

RATIONALE: To assist in diagnosing, evaluating, and staging tumors and in detecting areas of infection, inflammation, and abscess.

PATIENT PREPARATION: There are no food, fluid, activity, or medication restrictions unless by medical direction. If an abdominal abscess or infection is suspected, laxatives or enemas may be ordered before imaging at 48 or 72 hr after the injection. No other radionuclide scans should be scheduled within 24 to 48 hr before this procedure. Protocols may vary among facilities.

NORMAL FINDINGS
- Normal distribution of gallium; some localization of the radionuclide within the liver, spleen, bone, nasopharynx, lacrimal glands, breast, and bowel is expected.

CRITICAL FINDINGS AND POTENTIAL INTERVENTIONS: N/A

OVERVIEW: (Study type: Nuclear scan; **related body system:** Multisystem.) Gallium imaging is a nuclear medicine study that assists in diagnosing tumor and inflammation activity. Gallium, which has 90% sensitivity for inflammatory disease, is readily distributed throughout plasma and body tissues. Gallium imaging is sensitive in detecting abscesses, pneumonia, pyelonephritis, active sarcoidosis, and active tuberculosis. In immunocompromised patients, such as patients with AIDS, gallium imaging can detect complications such as *Pneumocystis jiroveci* pneumonitis. Gallium imaging is useful but less commonly performed in the diagnosis and staging of some tumors, including Hodgkin disease, lymphoma, melanoma, and leukemia. Imaging can be performed 6 to 72 hr after injection of the gallium, and a gamma camera detects the radiation emitted from the injected radioactive material. A representative image of the distribution of the radioactive material is then obtained. Single-photon emission computed tomography (SPECT) has significantly improved the resolution and accuracy of gallium scanning and may or may not be included as part of the examination. SPECT enables images to be recorded from multiple angles around the body and reconstructs them by a computer to produce images, or *slices,* representing the area of interest at different levels. Generally, the nonspecificity of gallium imaging requires correlation with other diagnostic studies, such as computed tomography (CT), CT/PET (positron emission tomography), magnetic resonance imaging, and ultrasonography.

INDICATIONS
- Aid in the diagnosis of infectious or inflammatory diseases.
- Evaluate lymphomas.
- Evaluate recurrent lymphomas or tumors after radiation therapy or chemotherapy.
- Perform as a screening examination for fever of undetermined origin.

INTERFERING FACTORS
Contraindications

Patients who are pregnant or suspected of being pregnant, unless the potential benefits of a procedure using radiation far outweigh the risk of radiation exposure to the fetus and mother.

Factors that may alter the results of the study
• Administration of certain medications (e.g., gastrin, cholecystokinin), which may interfere with gastric emptying.
• Metallic objects (e.g., jewelry, body rings) within the examination field, other nuclear scans done within the previous 24 to 48 hr, or retained barium from a previous radiological procedure, which may inhibit organ visualization and cause unclear images.

• Improper injection of the radionuclide that allows the tracer to seep deep into the muscle tissue can produce erroneous hot spots.
• Inability of the patient to cooperate or remain still during the procedure because movement can produce blurred or otherwise unclear images.

POTENTIAL MEDICAL DIAGNOSIS: CLINICAL SIGNIFICANCE OF RESULTS
Abnormal findings related to
• Abscess
• Infection
• Inflammation
• Lymphoma
• Tumor

NURSING IMPLICATIONS

POTENTIAL NURSING PROBLEMS: ASSESSMENT & NURSING DIAGNOSIS

Problems	Signs and Symptoms
Fatigue *(related to infection, abscess, tumor)*	Difficulty sleeping, disease progression, inadequate nutrition, emotional withdrawal, anxiety, pain, self-report of fatigue
Infection *(related to abscess, inflammation)*	Fever, chills, changes in laboratory studies (white blood cell count, C-reactive protein), diaphoresis, increased heart rate

BEFORE THE STUDY: PLANNING AND IMPLEMENTATION

Teaching the Patient What to Expect
◗ Inform the patient this procedure can assist in identifying infection or other disease.
◗ Pregnancy is a general contraindication to procedures involving radiation. Explain to the female patient that she will be asked the date of her last menstrual period and pregnancy testing may be performed to determine the possibility of pregnancy before she is exposed to radiation.
◗ Review the procedure with the patient. Address concerns about pain and explain that there may be moments of discomfort or pain experienced when the IV line is inserted to allow infusion of fluids such as saline, anesthetics, sedatives, radionuclides, medications used in the procedure, or emergency medications.
◗ Inform the patient that the procedure is performed in a nuclear medicine department by a health-care provider (HCP) specializing in this procedure, with support staff, and takes approximately 60 min.
◗ **Pediatric Considerations:** Preparing children for a gallium scan depends on the age of the child. Encourage parents to be truthful about what the child may experience during the procedure (e.g., the child may feel a pinch or

minor discomfort when the IV needle is inserted) and to use words that they know their child will understand. Toddlers and preschool-age children have a very short attention span, so the best time to talk about the test is right before the procedure. The child should be assured that he or she will be allowed to bring a favorite comfort item into the examination room, and if appropriate, that a parent will be with the child during the procedure.

▶ Reassure the patient that the radionuclide poses no radioactive hazard and rarely produces adverse effects.

▶ Instruct the patient to remove jewelry and other metallic objects from the area to be examined.

▶ Baseline vital signs and neurological status will be recorded. Protocols may vary among facilities.

▶ Positioning for this procedure is in a supine position on a flat table with foam wedges, which help maintain position and immobilization.

▶ IV radionuclide is administered, and the patient is instructed to return for scanning at a designated time after injection. Typical scanning occurs at 6, 24, 48, 72, 96, and/or 120 hr postinjection depending on diagnosis.

▶ Explain that once the study is completed, the needle or catheter will be removed and a pressure dressing applied over the puncture site.

Potential Nursing Actions

✳ *Make sure a written and informed consent has been signed prior to the procedure and before administering any medications.*

AFTER THE STUDY: POTENTIAL NURSING ACTIONS

Avoiding Complications

▶ Establishing an IV site and injection of radionuclides are invasive procedures. Complications are rare but include risk for allergic reaction *(related to contrast reaction)*, hematoma *(related to blood leakage into the tissue following needle insertion)*, bleeding from the puncture site *(related to a bleeding disorder or the effects of natural products and medications with known anticoagulant,*

antiplatelet, or thrombolytic properties), or infection *(which might occur if bacteria from the skin surface is introduced at the puncture site)*. Monitor the patient for complications related to the procedure (e.g., allergic reaction, anaphylaxis, bronchospasm). Observe/assess the needle/catheter insertion site for bleeding, inflammation, or hematoma formation.

Treatment Considerations

▶ Explain that the radionuclide is eliminated from the body within 6 to 24 hr. Advise the patient to drink increased amounts of fluids for 24 to 48 hr to eliminate the radionuclide from the body, unless contraindicated.

▶ Instruct the patient to resume usual medication or activity, as directed by the HCP.

▶ Fatigue: Assess the patient's stated level of fatigue. Assess nutritional status, emotional status, level of anxiety, withdrawal, and sleep pattern. Monitor and trend hemoglobin and hematocrit, and administer ordered medications to facilitate rest and decrease anxiety.

▶ Infection: Administer ordered antibiotics and antipyretics. Monitor and trend laboratory results (WBC, CRP) and vital signs.

▶ Instruct the patient in the care and assessment of the injection site.

▶ Explain that application of cold compresses to the puncture site may reduce discomfort or edema.

Safety Considerations

▶ The patient who is breastfeeding should consult with the requesting HCP regarding alternate testing that does not involve radiation. In general, if a woman who is breastfeeding must have a nuclear scan, she should not breastfeed the infant for 72 hr after the scan, until the radionuclide has been eliminated. She should be instructed to express the milk in order to prevent cessation of milk production; the milk can be stored and used after the 3-day period.

▶ Refer to organizational policy for additional precautions that may include instructions on handwashing, toilet flushing, limited contact with others,

G

and other aspects of nuclear medicine safety.

Follow-Up, Evaluation, and Desired Outcomes
♦ Acknowledges that depending on the results of this procedure, additional

testing and HCP referral may be needed to evaluate or monitor progression of the disease process and determine the need for a change in therapy.

γ-Glutamyltranspeptidase

SYNONYM/ACRONYM: Serum γ-glutamyltransferase, γ-glutamyl transpeptidase, GGT, SGGT.

RATIONALE: To assist in diagnosing and monitoring liver disease.

PATIENT PREPARATION: There are no food, fluid, activity, or medication restrictions unless by medical direction.

NORMAL FINDINGS: Method: Enzymatic spectrophotometry.

Age	Conventional and SI Units
Newborn–6 mo	12–122 units/L
7 mo and older	
Male	0–30 units/L
Female	0–24 units/L

Values may be elevated in older adults due to the effects of medications and the presence of multiple chronic or acute diseases with or without muted symptoms.

CRITICAL FINDINGS AND POTENTIAL INTERVENTIONS: N/A

OVERVIEW: (**Study type:** Blood collected in a gold-, red-, red/gray-, or green-top [heparin] tube; **related body system:** Digestive system.) Glutamyltransferase (GGT) assists with the reabsorption of amino acids and peptides from the glomerular filtrate and intestinal lumen. Hepatobiliary, renal tubular, and pancreatic tissues contain large amounts of GGT. Other sources include the prostate gland, brain, and heart. GGT is elevated in all types of liver disease and is more responsive to biliary obstruction, cholangitis, or cholecystitis than any of the other enzymes used as markers for liver disease.

INDICATIONS
• Assist in the diagnosis of obstructive jaundice in neonates.
• Detect the presence of liver disease.
• Evaluate and monitor patients with known or suspected alcohol misuse (levels rise after ingestion of small amounts of alcohol).

INTERFERING FACTORS
Factors that may alter the results of the study
• Drugs and other substances that may increase GGT levels include acetaminophen, alcohol, aminoglutethimide, anticonvulsants, aurothioglucose, barbiturates,

captopril, cetirizine, dactinomycin, dantrolene, estrogens, flucytosine, halothane, labetalol, medroxyprogesterone, meropenem, methyldopa, naproxen, niacin, nortriptyline, oral contraceptives, pegaspargase, phenothiazines, piroxicam, probenecid, rifampin, streptokinase, tocainide, and trifluoperazine.

- Drugs and other substances that may decrease GGT levels include clofibrate, conjugated estrogens, and ursodiol.

POTENTIAL MEDICAL DIAGNOSIS: CLINICAL SIGNIFICANCE OF RESULTS

Increased in

GGT is released from any damaged cell in which it is stored, so conditions that affect the liver, kidneys, or pancreas and cause cellular destruction demonstrate elevated GGT levels.

- Cirrhosis
- Diabetes with hypertension
- Hepatitis
- Hepatobiliary tract disorders
- Hepatocellular cancer
- Hyperthyroidism *(there is a strong association with concurrent liver abnormalities)*
- Infectious mononucleosis
- Kidney transplantation
- Obstructive liver disease
- Pancreatitis
- Significant alcohol ingestion

Decreased in
- Hypothyroidism *(related to decreased enzyme production by the liver)*

NURSING IMPLICATIONS

BEFORE THE STUDY: PLANNING AND IMPLEMENTATION

Teaching the Patient What to Expect
♦ Inform the patient this test can assist in assessing liver function.

♦ Explain that a blood sample is needed for the test.

AFTER THE STUDY: POTENTIAL NURSING ACTIONS

Treatment Considerations
♦ Fluid excess or deficit can occur. Each situation requires strict attention to fluid and electrolyte balance with monitoring and trending of laboratory values (potassium, BUN, Cr, calcium, Hgb, and Hct), that reflect alterations in fluid status. Pertinent actions for fluid management include daily weight, accurate intake and output, administration or limitation of fluids both oral and IV as the clinical picture requires, identifying the underlying cause of fluid alteration, and monitoring and tending urine characteristics and respiratory status. Collaborate with health-care provider (HCP) to support hydration.
♦ The patient who is misusing alcohol should be encouraged to avoid alcohol and to seek appropriate counseling for alcohol misuse.
♦ Fatigue can be a serious roadblock for patient care. Assess the degree of fatigue over time using a numeric scale. Observe for physical causes of fatigue, identify what aggravates and decreases fatigue, how to pace activities to preserve energy stores, or if there any related emotional factors such as depression. Evaluate current medications in relation to fatigue and assess for physiologic factors such as anemia.
♦ Jaundice, if noted, can impact skin integrity. Simple interventions include applying lotion to keep the skin moisturized, avoiding alkaline soaps that may irritate, discouraging scratching, and applying mittens if patient is not able to follow direction to avoid scratching. Administer ordered antihistamines.

Safety Considerations
♦ Confusion is a reason for serious concern. Correlate confusion with the need to reverse altered electrolytes. When researching for a cause, consider the patient's medications as well

G

as physical changes. Prevent falls and injury through appropriate use of postural support, bed alarm, or restraints as well as pharmacological interventions. Monitor blood ammonia level, determine last alcohol use, and assess for symptoms of hepatic encephalopathy. Administer ordered lactulose as prescribed.

Nutritional Considerations
♦ Increased GGT levels may be associated with liver disease. In general, patients should be encouraged to eat a well-balanced diet that includes foods high in fiber. Dietary recommendations will vary depending on the condition and its severity. For example, a diet of soft foods is recommended if esophageal varices develop, fat substitutes are recommended for bile duct disease, and limiting salt intake is recommended if ascites develop. Treatment of cirrhosis is different because a low-protein diet may be in order if the patient's liver has lost the ability to process the end products of protein metabolism. Currently, specific drugs are used to treat different types of viral hepatitis. For example, a number of drugs are used

to treat hepatitis B, such as pegylated interferon (adults only), interferon alpha (adults and children), and lamivudine (adults and children); ledipasvir/sofosbuvir and sofusbuvir are examples of drugs used to treat hepatitis C. There are also drugs that can be given to treat and reverse the symptoms of nonviral hepatitis once the primary cause of hepatic inflammation is identified. Elimination of alcohol ingestion and a diet optimized for convalescence are commonly included in the treatment plan.
♦ Administer ordered enteral or parenteral nutrition; monitor laboratory values (albumin, protein, potassium), and collaborate with the HCP on replacement strategies; correlate laboratory values with IV fluid infusion, and collaborate with the HCP and pharmacist to adjust to patient needs; ensure adequate pain control; monitor vital signs for alterations associated metabolic imbalances.

Follow-Up, Evaluation, and Desired Outcomes
♦ Acknowledges information provided regarding access to nutritional and counseling services.

Gastric Analysis and Gastric Acid Stimulation Test

SYNONYM/ACRONYM: N/A

RATIONALE: To evaluate gastric fluid and the amount of gastric acid secreted toward diagnosing gastrointestinal disorders such as ulcers, cancers, and inflammation.

PATIENT PREPARATION: There are no activity restrictions unless by medical direction. Instruct the patient to fast from food after the evening meal the night before the test and not to drink water for 1 hr before the test. Instruct the patient to refrain from the use of chewing gum or tobacco products for at least 12 hr prior to and for the duration of the test. Drugs and substances that may alter gastric secretions (e.g., alcohol, histamine, nicotine, adrenocorticotropic steroids, insulin, parasympathetic drugs, belladonna alkaloids, anticholinergic drugs, histamine receptor antagonists) should be restricted by medical direction for 72 hr before the test. Protocols may vary among facilities.

NORMAL FINDINGS: Method: Volume measurement and pH by ion-selective electrode.

Basal acid output (BAO)	Male: 0–10.5 mmol/hr
	Female: 0–5.6 mmol/hr
Peak acid output (PAO)	Male: 12–60 mmol/hr
	Female: 8–40 mmol/hr
Peak response time	Pentagastrin, intramuscular: 15–45 min
	Pentagastrin, subcutaneous: 10–30 min
BAO/PAO ratio	Less than 0.2

CRITICAL FINDINGS AND POTENTIAL INTERVENTIONS: N/A

OVERVIEW: (**Study type:** Body fluid, gastric fluid collected in eight plastic tubes at 15-min intervals; **related body system:** Digestive system.) Gastric fluid is evaluated macroscopically for general physical and chemical characteristics, such as color, presence of mucus or blood, and pH; gastric fluid is also evaluated microscopically for the presence of organisms and abnormal cells. The normal appearance of gastric fluid is a translucent, pale gray, slightly viscous fluid containing some mucus but not usually blood. pH is usually less than 2 and not greater than 6. Organisms are usually absent in gastric fluid owing to the acidic pH.

The gastric acid stimulation test is performed to determine the response to substances administered to induce increased gastric acid production. Pentagastrin is the usual drug of choice to induce gastric secretion because it has no major adverse effects. The samples obtained from gastric acid stimulation tests are examined for volume, pH, and amount of acid secreted. First, BAO is determined by averaging the results of gastric samples collected before the administration of a gastric stimulant. Then a gastric stimulant is administered and PAO is determined by adding together the gastric acid output of the highest two consecutive 15-min stimulation samples. Finally, BAO and PAO are compared as a ratio, which is normally less than 0.2.

INDICATIONS
• Detect duodenal ulcer.
• Detect gastric cancer.
• Detect pernicious anemia.
• Detect Zollinger-Ellison syndrome.
• Evaluate effectiveness of vagotomy in the treatment of peptic ulcer disease.

INTERFERING FACTORS
Contraindications
　　Patients with esophageal varices, diverticula, stenosis, malignant tumor of the esophagus, aortic aneurysm, severe gastric hemorrhage, and congenital heart failure.
　　Patients with a history of asthma, paroxysmal hypertension, urticaria, or other allergic conditions should not be administered histamine diphosphate.

Factors that may alter the results of the study
• Drugs and other substances that may increase gastric volume include atropine, diazepam,

ganglionic blocking drugs, and insulin.

• Drugs and substances that may increase gastric pH include caffeine, calcium salts, corticotropin, ethanol, rauwolfia, reserpine, and tolazoline.

• Drugs and other substances that may decrease gastric pH include atropine, cimetidine, diazepam, famotidine, ganglionic blocking drugs, glucagon, nizatidine, omeprazole, oxmetidine, propranolol, prostaglandin F_{2a}, ranitidine, and secretin.

• Exposure to the sight, smell, or thought of food immediately before and during the test may result in stimulation of gastric secretions.

POTENTIAL MEDICAL DIAGNOSIS: CLINICAL SIGNIFICANCE OF RESULTS

Increased in

Any alteration in the balance between the digestive and protective functions of the stomach that increases gastric acidity, such as hypersecretion of gastrin, use of NSAIDs, or Helicobacter pylori infection.

Appearance

• Color

Yellow to green indicates the presence of bile *(related to obstruction in the small intestine distal to the ampulla of Vater)*

Pink, red, brown indicates the presence of blood *(related to some type of gastric lesion evidenced by ulcer, gastritis, or cancer)*

• Microscopic evaluation

Red blood cells *(related to trauma or active bleeding)*

White blood cells *(related to inflammation of the gastric mucosa, mouth, paranasal sinuses, or respiratory tract)*

Epithelial cells *(related to inflammation of the gastric mucosa)*

Malignant cells *(related to gastric cancer)*

Bacteria and yeast *(related to conditions such as pyloric obstruction, pulmonary tuberculosis)*

Parasites *(related to parasitic infestation such as Giardia, H. pylori, Ancylostoma duodenale or Necator americanus, the most common infectious hookworms or, Strongyloides, the genus of commonly infectious roundworms)*

Increased Gastric Acid Output

• BAO

Basophilic leukemia

Duodenal ulcer

G-cell hyperplasia

Recurring peptic ulcer

Retained antrum syndrome

Systemic mastocytosis

Vagal hyperfunction

Zollinger-Ellison syndrome

• PAO

Duodenal ulcer

Zollinger-Ellison syndrome

Decreased in

Conditions that result in the gradual loss of function of the antrum and G cells, where gastrin is produced, will reflect decreased gastrin levels.

Decreased Gastric Acid Output

• BAO

Gastric ulcer

• PAO

Chronic gastritis

Gastric cancers

Gastric polyps

Gastric ulcer

Myxedema

Pernicious anemia

NURSING IMPLICATIONS

BEFORE THE STUDY: PLANNING AND IMPLEMENTATION

Teaching the Patient What to Expect

▶ Inform the patient this procedure can assist in diagnosing disease and inflammation in the stomach and upper intestine.

- Pregnancy is a general contraindication to procedures involving radiation. Explain to the female patient that she will be asked the date of her last menstrual period. Pregnancy testing may be performed to determine the possibility of pregnancy before exposure to radiation if an x-ray is expected to be ordered.
- Review the procedure with the patient. Explain that a sample of gastric fluid is needed for the test and that specimen collection takes approximately 60 to 120 min. Address concerns about pain and explain that some discomfort is experienced from insertion of the nasogastric tube.
- Baseline vital signs will be obtained and recorded.
- Positioning for this procedure is sitting or reclining on the left side.
- Explain that study completion requires a gastric tube with a radiopaque tip be inserted. Nasal insertion may be preferred for patients who have a hyperactive gag reflex.
- Gastric tube placement will be confirmed by fluoroscopy or x-ray before the start of the test.
- Gastric contents will be obtained through the use of constant gentle suction. Specimens obtained during the first 15 to 30 min of suctioning are discarded and not used for testing.
- Once the gastric stimulant is administered, four 15-min peak specimens will be obtained over 60 min. Specimen tubes are numbered in the order in which they are collected.

Potential Nursing Actions

Make sure a written and informed consent has been signed prior to the procedure and before administering any medications.

- Explain that dentures will need to be removed.
- If histamine diphosphate is being used for the test, verify there is no history of asthma, paroxysmal hypertension, urticaria, or other allergic conditions.

AFTER THE STUDY: POTENTIAL NURSING ACTIONS

Avoiding Complications

- Complications may include improper insertion of the gastric tube, bleeding, esophageal perforation, and laryngospasm. Monitor the patient for complications related to the procedure. Instruct the patient to immediately report to the appropriate health-care provider (HCP) any chest pain, upper abdominal pain, pain on swallowing, difficulty breathing, or expectoration of blood.

Treatment Considerations

- Unless otherwise advised by the HCP, resume usual diet and medications.
- Vital signs and neurological status should be checked every 15 min for 1 hr, then every 2 hr for 4 hr, and then as ordered by the HCP for evaluation. Protocols may vary among facilities.
- Monitor for adverse effects of drugs administered to induce gastric secretion (e.g., flushing, headache, nasal stuffiness, dizziness, faintness, nausea).

Nutritional Considerations

- Nutritional support with calcium, iron, and vitamin B_{12} supplementation may be ordered, as appropriate. Dietary modifications may include encouraging liquids and low-residue foods, eating multiple small meals throughout the day, and avoidance of foods that slow digestion, such as foods high in fat and fiber. Severe cases of gastroparesis may require temporary treatments that include total parenteral nutrition or use of jejunostomy tubes.

Follow-Up, Evaluation, and Desired Outcomes

- Acknowledges that depending on the results of this procedure, additional testing and HCP referral may be needed to evaluate or monitor progression of the disease process and determine the need for a change in therapy.

G

Gastric Emptying Scan

SYNONYM/ACRONYM: Gastric emptying quantitation, gastric emptying scintigraphy.

RATIONALE: To visualize and assess the timeframe for gastric emptying to assist in the diagnosis of diseases such as gastroenteritis and dumping syndrome.

PATIENT PREPARATION: There are no activity or medication restrictions unless by medical direction. Instruct the patient to restrict food and fluids for 8 hr before the scan. Inquire about allergic reactions to eggs. No other radionuclide scans or procedures using barium contrast medium should be scheduled within 24 to 48 hr before this procedure. Protocols may vary among facilities.

NORMAL FINDINGS
- Mean time emptying of liquid phase: 30 min (range, 11–49 min)
- Mean time emptying of solid phase: 40 min (range, 28–80 min)
- No delay in gastric emptying rate.

CRITICAL FINDINGS AND POTENTIAL INTERVENTIONS: N/A

OVERVIEW: (Study type: Nuclear scan; related body system: Digestive system.) A gastric emptying scan quantifies gastric emptying physiology. The procedure is indicated for patients with gastric motility symptoms, including diabetic gastroparesis, anorexia nervosa, gastric outlet obstruction syndromes, postvagotomy and postgastrectomy syndromes, and assessment of medical and surgical treatments for diseases known to affect gastric motility. A radionuclide is administered, and the clearance of solids and liquids may be evaluated. The images are recorded electronically, showing the gastric emptying function over time.

INDICATIONS
- Investigate the cause of rapid or slow rate of gastric emptying.
- Measure gastric emptying rate.

INTERFERING FACTORS
Contraindications

✦ Patients who are pregnant or suspected of being pregnant, unless the potential benefits of a procedure using radiation far outweigh the risks to the fetus and mother.

✦ Patients with esophageal motor disorders or swallowing difficulties.

Factors that may alter the results of the study
- Administration of certain medications (e.g., gastrin, cholecystokinin), which may interfere with gastric emptying.
- Metallic objects (e.g., jewelry, body rings) within the examination field, other nuclear scans done within the previous 24 to 48 hr, or retained barium from a previous radiological procedure, which may inhibit organ visualization and cause unclear images.
- Inability of the patient to cooperate or remain still during the procedure,

because movement can produce blurred or otherwise unclear images.

POTENTIAL MEDICAL DIAGNOSIS: CLINICAL SIGNIFICANCE OF RESULTS

Abnormal findings related to

- Decreased rate of gastric emptying:
  Amyloidosis
  Anorexia nervosa
  Gastric outlet obstruction
  Gastric ulcer
  Gastroenteritis
  Gastroesophageal reflux
  Gastroparesis (e.g., damage to nerves
    that control stomach muscles related to
    diabetes or as a result of surgery)
  Hypokalemia, hypomagnesemia
  Postoperative ileus
  Post–radiation therapy period
  Scleroderma
- Increased rate of gastric emptying:
  Dumping syndrome
  Post–gastric surgery period
  Zollinger-Ellison syndrome

NURSING IMPLICATIONS

BEFORE THE STUDY: PLANNING AND IMPLEMENTATION

Teaching the Patient What to Expect

- Inform the patient this procedure can assist in evaluating the time it takes for the stomach to empty.
- Pregnancy is a general contraindication to procedures involving radiation. Explain to the female patient that she will be asked the date of her last menstrual period and pregnancy testing may be performed to determine the possibility of pregnancy before she is exposed to radiation.
- Review the procedure with the patient. Address concerns about pain related to the procedure and explain that no pain should be experienced during the test.
- Inform the patient that the procedure is performed in a nuclear medicine department by an health-care provider

(HCP) specializing in this procedure, with support staff, and takes approximately 30 to 120 min.

- **Pediatric Considerations:** Preparing children for a gastric emptying scan depends on the age of the child. Encourage parents to be truthful about what the child may experience during the procedure (e.g., length of time the examination will take and the need to intermittently have scans performed), stressing the importance of eating as much of the "breakfast" as possible so the test is successful, and to use words that they know their child will understand. Toddlers and preschool-age children have a short attention span, so the best time to talk about the test is right before the procedure. The child should be assured that he or she will be allowed to bring a favorite comfort item into the examination room, and if appropriate, that a parent will be with the child during the procedure. Explain the importance of remaining still while the images are taken.
- Reassure the patient that the radionuclide poses no radioactive hazard and rarely produces adverse effects.
- Instruct the patient to remove jewelry and other metallic objects from the area to be examined.
- Record baseline vital signs and neurological status. Protocols may vary among facilities.
- Place the patient in an upright or supine position in front of the gamma camera; positioning protocols may vary among facilities.
- Ask the patient to orally take the radionuclide mixed with water or other liquid or combined with eggs for a solid study. **Pediatric Considerations:** If the patient is an infant, a small amount of radionuclide will be added to the patient's feeding.
- Images are recorded over a period of time (30–60 min) and evaluated with regard to the amount of time the stomach takes to empty its contents.

Potential Nursing Actions

 Make sure a written and informed consent has been signed prior to

G

the procedure and before administering any medications.

❖ *Ensure that the patient does not have a known allergy to eggs if the radionuclide will be administered in eggs.*

AFTER THE STUDY: POTENTIAL NURSING ACTIONS

Avoiding Complications

▶ Although it is rare, there is the possibility of allergic reaction to the radionuclide. Have emergency equipment and medications readily available. If the patient has a history of allergic reactions to any substance or drug, administer ordered prophylactic steroids or antihistamines before the procedure. Monitor the patient for complications related to the procedure (e.g., allergic reaction, anaphylaxis, bronchospasm). Immediately report symptoms such as fast heart rate, difficulty breathing, skin rash, itching, or chest pain to the appropriate HCP.

Treatment Considerations

▶ Explain that the radionuclide is eliminated from the body within 6 to 24 hr. Advise the patient to drink increased amounts of fluids for 24 to 48 hr to eliminate the radionuclide from the body, unless contraindicated.
▶ Instruct the patient to resume usual medication or activity, as directed by the HCP.

▶ Monitor vital signs every 15 min for 1 hr, then every 2 hr for 4 hr, and then as ordered by the HCP. Monitor intake and output at least every 8 hr. Compare with baseline values. Protocols may vary among facilities.

Safety Considerations

▶ The patient who is breastfeeding should consult with the requesting HCP regarding alternate testing that does not involve radiation. In general, if a woman who is breastfeeding must have a nuclear scan, she should not breastfeed the infant for 72 hr after the scan, until the radionuclide has been eliminated. She should be instructed to express the milk in order to prevent cessation of milk production; the milk can be stored and used after the 3-day period.
▶ Refer to organizational policy for additional precautions that may include instructions on handwashing, toilet flushing, limited contact with others, and other aspects of nuclear medicine safety.

Follow-Up, Evaluation, and Desired Outcomes

▶ Acknowledges that depending on the results of this procedure, additional testing and HCP referral may be needed to evaluate or monitor progression of the disease process and determine the need for a change in therapy.

Gastrin and Gastrin Stimulation Test

SYNONYM/ACRONYM: N/A

RATIONALE: To evaluate gastric production to assist in diagnosis of gastric disease such as Zollinger-Ellison syndrome and gastric cancer.

PATIENT PREPARATION: There are no fluid or activity restrictions unless by medical direction. Instruct the patient to fast for 12 hr before the test. Instruct the patient to refrain from the use of chewing gum or tobacco products for at least 4 hr prior to and for the duration of the test. Instruct the patient to withhold medications and alcohol for 12 to 24 hr, as ordered by the health-care provider (HCP). Protocols may vary among facilities.

NORMAL FINDINGS: Method: Immunoassay.

Age	Conventional Units	SI Units (Conventional Units × 0.481)
Child	Less than 65 pg/mL	Less than 31 pmol/L
Adult	Less than 100 pg/mL	Less than 48.1 pmol/L

Values represent fasting levels.

Stimulation Tests	
Gastrin stimulation test with secretin; 0.4 mcg/kg by IV bolus	No response or slight increase over baseline; increase of greater than 200 pg/ml (SI units: 96 pmol/L) above baseline is considered abnormal

Calcium may also be used as a stimulant.

CRITICAL FINDINGS AND POTENTIAL INTERVENTIONS: N/A

OVERVIEW: (**Study type:** Blood collected in a red- or red/gray-top tube; **related body system:** Digestive system.) Gastrin is a peptide hormone produced by the G cells of the duodenum and pyloric antrum of the stomach. Gastrin is released into the blood in response to certain stimuli, including vagal stimulation from the sight, smell, or taste of food; the presence of proteins and amino acids from partially digested food; alcohol; stomach distention; and hypercalcemia (as the main site of dietary calcium absorption is the duodenum). As blood levels of gastrin rise, gastrin is returned to the stomach to stimulate the parietal cells to secrete hydrochloric acid (gastric acid) for further digestion of food. At this point in the digestive process, gastrin also stimulates the chief cells of the stomach to secrete pepsinogen, increases antral muscle mobility, and promotes stomach contractions to stimulate gastric emptying. Gastrin also induces pancreatic secretions, gallbladder emptying, and release of intrinsic factor. Gastrin release is inhibited by the presence of acid in the stomach, somatostatin, glucagon and calcitonin. When enough gastric acid has been produced by the stomach, gastrin levels in the blood decrease. Gastrin stimulation tests can be performed after a test meal or IV infusion of calcium or secretin.

INDICATIONS
- Assist in the diagnosis of gastric cancer, pernicious anemia, or G-cell hyperplasia.
- Assist in the diagnosis of Zollinger-Ellison syndrome.
- Assist in the differential diagnosis of ulcers from other gastrointestinal peptic disorders.

INTERFERING FACTORS
Factors that may alter the results of the study
- Drugs and other substances that may increase gastrin levels include amino acids, calcium products,

G

catecholamines, cimetidine, coffee, insulin, morphine, omeprazole, pantoprazole, sufotidine, and terbutaline.

• Drugs and other substances that may decrease gastrin levels include atropine, enprostil, glucagon, secretin, streptozocin, and tolbutamide.

• In some cases, protein ingestion elevates serum gastrin levels.

POTENTIAL MEDICAL DIAGNOSIS: CLINICAL SIGNIFICANCE OF RESULTS

Increased in

• Chronic gastritis *(related to hypersecretion of gastrin, use of NSAIDs, or Helicobacter pylori infection)*
• Chronic kidney disease *(related to inadequate renal excretion)*
• Gastric and duodenal ulcers *(related to hypersecretion of gastrin, use of NSAIDs, or H. pylori infection)*
• Gastric cancer *(related to disturbance in pH favoring alkalinity, which stimulates gastrin production)*
• G-cell hyperplasia *(hyperplastic G cells produce excessive amounts of gastrin)*
• Hyperparathyroidism *(related to hypercalcemia; calcium is a potent stimulator for the release of gastrin)*
• Pernicious anemia *(related to antibodies against gastric intrinsic factor [66% of cases] and parietal cells [80% of cases that affect the stomach's ability to secrete acid; achlorhydria is a strong stimulator of gastrin production])*
• Pyloric obstruction *(related to gastric distention, which stimulates gastrin production)*
• Retained antrum *(remaining tissue stimulates gastrin production)*
• Zollinger-Ellison syndrome *(gastrin-producing tumor)*

Decreased in

• Hypothyroidism *(related to hypocalcemia)*
• Vagotomy *(vagus nerve impulses stimulate secretion of digestive secretions; interruptions in these nerve impulses result in decreased gastrin levels)*

NURSING IMPLICATIONS

BEFORE THE STUDY: PLANNING AND IMPLEMENTATION

Teaching the Patient What to Expect

❱ Inform the patient this test can assist in diagnosing stomach disease.
❱ Review the procedure with the patient. Explain that a blood sample is needed for the test.
❱ Inform the patient that multiple specimens will be collected. Explain that pretest samples will be collected at 10 min and 1 min before administration of the stimulant. Poststimulation samples will be collected at 2, 5, 10, 15, 20, and 30 min.

Potential Nursing Actions

✦ *Make sure a written and informed consent has been signed prior to the procedure and before administering any medications.*
❱ Administer gastrin stimulators as appropriate.

AFTER THE STUDY: POTENTIAL NURSING ACTIONS

Treatment Considerations

❱ Instruct the patient to resume usual diet and medications, as directed by the HCP.
❱ Instruct the patient in the use of any ordered medications and potential significant adverse effects, and encourage a literature review provided by a pharmacist.

Nutritional Considerations

❱ Nutritional support with calcium, iron, and vitamin B_{12} supplementation may be ordered, as appropriate. Dietary modifications may include encouraging liquids and low-residue foods, eating multiple small meals throughout the day, and avoidance of foods that slow digestion, such as foods high in fat and fiber. Severe cases of gastroparesis may require temporary treatments that include total parenteral nutrition or use of jejunostomy tubes.

Follow-Up, Evaluation, and Desired Outcomes
▶ Acknowledges that depending on the results of this procedure, additional testing and HCP referral may be needed to evaluate or monitor progression of the disease process and determine the need for a change in therapy.

Gastroesophageal Reflux Scan

SYNONYM/ACRONYM: Aspiration scan, GER scan, GERD scan, milk scan (pediatric patients).

RATIONALE: To assess for gastric reflux in relation to heartburn, difficulty swallowing, vomiting, and aspiration.

PATIENT PREPARATION: There are no food, fluid, activity, or medication restrictions unless by medical direction. No other radionuclide scans or procedures using barium contrast medium should be scheduled within 24 to 48 hr before this procedure. Protocols may vary among facilities.

NORMAL FINDINGS
• Reflux less than or equal to 4% across the esophageal sphincter.

CRITICAL FINDINGS AND POTENTIAL INTERVENTIONS: N/A

OVERVIEW: (**Study type:** Nuclear scan; **related body system:** Digestive system.) The GER scan assesses gastric reflux across the esophageal sphincter. Symptoms of GER can include heartburn, regurgitation, vomiting, dysphagia, and a bitter taste in the mouth. This procedure may be used to evaluate the medical or surgical treatment of pediatric and adult patients with GER and to detect aspiration of gastric contents into the lungs. A radionuclide such as technetium-99m sulfur colloid is ingested orally in orange juice, and scanning studies are done immediately to assess the amount of liquid that has reached the stomach. An abdominal binder

is applied and then tightened gradually to obtain images at increasing degrees of abdominal pressure: 0, 20, 40, 60, 80, and 100 mm Hg. A computer calculates the amount of reflux into the esophagus at each of these abdominal pressures as recorded on the images. For aspiration scans, images are taken over the lungs to detect possible tracheo-esophageal aspiration of the radionuclide.

In infants, the study distinguishes between vomiting and reflux. Reflux occurs predominantly in infants younger than age 2 who are mainly on a milk diet. This procedure is indicated when an infant has symptoms such as failure to thrive, feeding problems, and episodes of wheezing with chest infection. The radionuclide is added to the infant's milk, images are obtained of the gastric and esophageal area, and the images are evaluated visually and by computer.

INDICATIONS

• Aid in the diagnosis of GER in patients with unexplained nausea and vomiting.
• Distinguish between vomiting and reflux in infants with failure to thrive, feeding problems, and wheezing combined with chest infection.

INTERFERING FACTORS

Contraindications

Patients who are pregnant or suspected of being pregnant, unless the potential benefits of a procedure using radiation far outweigh the risk of radiation exposure to the fetus and mother.

Patients with hiatal hernia, esophageal motor disorders, or swallowing difficulties.

Factors that may alter the results of the study

• Metallic objects (e.g., jewelry, body rings) within the examination field, other nuclear scans done within the previous 24 to 48 hr, or retained barium from a previous radiological procedure, which may inhibit organ visualization and cause unclear images.
• Improper injection of the radionuclide that allows the tracer to seep deep into the muscle tissue can produce erroneous hot spots.
• Inability of the patient to cooperate or remain still during the procedure, because movement can produce blurred or otherwise unclear images.

POTENTIAL MEDICAL DIAGNOSIS: CLINICAL SIGNIFICANCE OF RESULTS

Abnormal findings related to

• Reflux of greater than 4% at any pressure level
• Pulmonary aspiration

NURSING IMPLICATIONS

POTENTIAL NURSING PROBLEMS: ASSESSMENT & NURSING DIAGNOSIS

Problems	Signs and Symptoms
Inadequate gas exchange *(related to aspiration of gastric fluids, ineffective swallowing, inflammation, consolidation secondary to aspiration)*	Shortness of breath, cyanosis, lethargy, fatigue, adventitious breath sounds (crackles, wheeze), increased heart rate, activity intolerance, decreased oxygen saturation, confusion, altered level of consciousness, diminished breath sounds, fever
Inadequate nutrition *(related to diet choices that stimulate gastric reflux, fear of eating, pain, fear of aspiration)*	Gastric reflux after eating foods, heartburn, dry cough, sense of a lump in the throat
Pain *(related to acid reflux)*	Heartburn, dry cough, hoarse voice

Teaching the Patient What to Expect

▶ Inform the patient this procedure can assist in evaluating stomach reflux.

▶ Pregnancy is a general contraindication to procedures involving radiation. Explain to the female patient that she will be asked the date of her last menstrual period and pregnancy testing may be performed to determine the possibility of pregnancy before she is exposed to radiation.

▶ Review the procedure with the patient. Address concerns about pain related to the procedure and explain that no pain should be experienced during the test.

▶ Inform the patient that the procedure is performed in a nuclear medicine department by a health-care provider (HCP) specializing in this procedure, with support staff, and takes approximately 30 to 60 min.

▶ **Pediatric Considerations:** Preparing children for a gastroesophageal reflux scan depends on the age of the child. Encourage parents to be truthful about what the child may experience during the procedure (e.g., the child may feel an upset stomach), stressing the importance of drinking as much of the "juice" as possible so the test is successful, and to use words that they know their child will understand. Toddlers and preschool-age children have a short attention span, so the best time to talk about the test is right before the procedure. The child should be assured that he or she will be allowed to bring a favorite comfort item into the examination room, and if appropriate, that a parent will be with the child during the procedure. Explain the importance of remaining still while the images are taken.

▶ Reassure the patient that the radionuclide poses no radioactive hazard and rarely produces adverse effects.

▶ Instruct the patient to remove jewelry and other metallic objects from the area to be examined prior to the procedure.

▶ Baseline vital signs and neurological status will be recorded. Protocols may vary among facilities.

▶ Patients will be placed in an upright position and instructed to ingest the radionuclide combined with orange juice. **Pediatric Considerations:** If the patient is an infant, a small amount of radionuclide will be added to the patient's feeding.

▶ Positioning for this procedure is in a supine position on a flat table 15 min after ingestion of radionuclide.

▶ An abdominal binder with an attached sphygmomanometer is applied, and scans are taken as the binder is tightened at various pressures.

▶ If reflux occurs at lower pressures, an additional 30 mL of water may be given to clear the esophagus.

▶ Patients who become nauseated during the procedure will be asked to take slow, deep breaths. An ordered antiemetic drug may be given and an emesis basin will be available for use.

Potential Nursing Actions

✸ *Make sure a written and informed consent has been signed prior to the procedure and before administering any medications.*

Avoiding Complications

▶ Although it is rare, there is the possibility of allergic reaction to the radionuclide. Have emergency equipment and medications readily available. If the patient has a history of allergic reactions to any substance or drug, administer ordered prophylactic steroids or antihistamines before the procedure. Monitor the patient for complications related to the procedure (e.g., allergic reaction, anaphylaxis, bronchospasm). Immediately report symptoms such as fast heart rate, difficulty breathing, skin rash, itching, or chest pain to the appropriate HCP.

Treatment Considerations

▶ Explain that the radionuclide is eliminated from the body within 6 to 24 hr. Advise the patient to drink increased

G

amounts of fluids for 24 to 48 hr to eliminate the radionuclide from the body, unless contraindicated.

▶ Instruct the patient to resume usual diet, fluids, medication, and activity, as directed by the HCP.

▶ After the procedure. monitor vital signs and neurological status every 15 min for 1 hr, then every 2 hr for 4 hr, and then as ordered by the HCP. Monitor intake and output at least every 8 hr. Compare with baseline values. Protocols may vary among facilities.

▶ Inadequate Gas Exchange: Decrease aspiration risk by maintaining NPO status while waiting for adequate swallowing to be restored or reflux controlled. Administer ordered antibiotics, antiemetics, and oxygen to maintain adequate oxygenation. Monitor and trend heart and respiratory rate, breath sounds, level of consciousness and confusion. Elevate the head of the bed to relieve dyspnea and provide assistance with activity.

▶ Inadequate Nutrition: Avoid trigger foods such as chocolate, spicy foods, high-fat foods (red meat, whole milk, cream, cheese), alcohol, citrus fruits (orange, lemons, grapefruit), raw onions, and very hot liquids.

▶ Pain: Administer prescribed H_2 receptor blockers, antacids, and proton pump inhibitors.

Safety Considerations
▶ The patient who is breastfeeding should consult with the requesting HCP regarding alternate testing that does not involve radiation. In general, if a woman who is breastfeeding must have a nuclear scan, she should not breastfeed the infant for 72 hr after the scan, until the radionuclide has been eliminated. She should be instructed to express the milk in order to prevent cessation of milk production; the milk can be stored and used after the 3-day period.

▶ Refer to organizational policy for additional precautions that may include instructions on handwashing, toilet flushing, limited contact with others, and other aspects of nuclear medicine safety.

Nutritional Considerations
▶ A low-fat, low-cholesterol, and low-sodium diet should be consumed to reduce current disease processes. High fat consumption increases the amount of bile acids in the colon and should be avoided.

Follow-Up, Evaluation, and Desired Outcomes
▶ Acknowledges the value of following the established therapeutic regime to improve overall health, including specific dietary and lifestyle changes.

Gastrointestinal Blood Loss Scan

SYNONYM/ACRONYM: Gastrointestinal bleed localization study, GI scintigram, GI bleed scintigraphy, lower GI blood loss scan.

RATIONALE: To detect areas of active GI bleeding or hemorrhage to facilitate surgical intervention or medical treatment. Usefulness is limited in emergency situations because of time constraints in performing the scan.

PATIENT PREPARATION: There are no food, fluid, activity, or medication restrictions unless by medical direction. No other radionuclide scans or procedures using barium contrast medium should be scheduled within 24 to 48 hr before this procedure. Protocols may vary among facilities.

NORMAL FINDINGS
- Normal distribution of radionuclide in the large vessels with no extravascular activity

CRITICAL FINDINGS AND POTENTIAL INTERVENTIONS
- GI bleed

Timely notification to the requesting health-care provider (HCP) of any critical findings and related symptoms is a role expectation of the professional nurse. A listing of these findings varies among facilities.

OVERVIEW: (Study type: Nuclear scan; related body system: Digestive system.) GI blood loss is a symptom of medical conditions involving the GI system. The studies used to investigate GI blood loss depend on whether the origin of the bleed is proximal (above) or distal (below) to the ligament of Treitz. The GI blood loss scan (red blood cell [RBC] scintigraphy) is a nuclear medicine study that assists in detecting active lower GI tract bleeding. It is commonly used in conjunction with endoscopic (colonoscopy) or angiographic studies. Depending on the location of the bleed and rate of blood loss, the scan can detect bleeding across a range of blood loss rates from 0.04 mL/min and greater, but it is not specific for site localization or cause of bleeding. Esophagogastroduodenoscopy is the procedure of choice for diagnosing upper GI bleeding.

The radionuclide used in the GI blood loss scan is commonly prepared by adding a radioactive tracer, technetium-99m, to a sample of the patient's blood and reinjecting the labelled blood after approximately 30 minutes. Imaging of the abdomen begins immediately after injection, and images are taken over the next 1 to 2 hr. The radionuclide remains in the circulation long enough to extravasate and accumulate within the bowel lumen at the site of active bleeding. Delayed images may be taken to identify slow, continuous, or intermittent bleeding. A gamma camera detects the radiation emitted from the injected radioactive material. Single-photon emission computed tomography (SPECT) may or may not be included as part of the examination. SPECT enables images to be recorded from multiple angles around the body and reconstructed by a computer to produce images or "slices" representing the area of interest at different levels.

INDICATIONS
- Diagnose unexplained abdominal pain and GI bleeding.

INTERFERING FACTORS
Contraindications

Patients who are pregnant or suspected of being pregnant, unless the potential benefits of a procedure using radiation far outweigh the risk of radiation exposure to the fetus and mother.

Factors that may alter the results of the study
- Metallic objects (e.g., jewelry, body rings) within the

examination field, other nuclear scans done within the previous 24 to 48 hr, or retained barium from a previous radiological procedure, which may inhibit organ visualization and cause unclear images.

• Improper injection of the radionuclide that allows the tracer to seep deep into the muscle tissue can produce erroneous hot spots.

• Inability of the patient to cooperate or remain still during the procedure, because movement can produce blurred or otherwise unclear images.

Other considerations
• The examination detects only active or intermittent bleeding.

• The scan is less accurate for localization of bleeding sites in the upper GI tract.

POTENTIAL MEDICAL DIAGNOSIS: CLINICAL SIGNIFICANCE OF RESULTS
Abnormal findings related to
The radioactive tracer will accumulate in areas of active bleeding, and hot spots will identify specific areas of concern.

• Angiodysplasia
• Aortoduodenal fistula
• Diverticulosis
• Inflammatory bowel disease
• Meckel diverticulum
• Polyps
• Rectal bleeding *(e.g., related to hemorrhoids, radiation proctitis)*
• Tumor
• Ulcer *(e.g., related to colitis, NSAID use)*

NURSING IMPLICATIONS

POTENTIAL NURSING PROBLEMS: ASSESSMENT & NURSING DIAGNOSIS

Problems	Signs and Symptoms
Inadequate cardiac output *(related to decreased vascular volume secondary to blood loss)*	Decreased oxygenation, increased heart rate, cool skin and peripheral cyanosis, decreased peripheral pulses, slow capillary refill, diminished urine output, altered level of consciousness, confusion, shortness of breath
Insufficient fluid volume *(related to blood loss secondary to ulcer, tumor, fistula, inflammation)*	Agitation; dizziness; altered level of consciousness; hypotension; tachycardia; cool, clammy skin; pallor; slow capillary refill; diminished urinary output

BEFORE THE STUDY: PLANNING AND IMPLEMENTATION

Teaching the Patient What to Expect
▶ Inform the patient this procedure can assist in evaluating for stomach and intestinal bleeding.
▶ Pregnancy is a general contraindication to procedures involving radiation. Explain to the female patient that she will be asked the date of her last menstrual period and pregnancy testing may be performed to determine the possibility of pregnancy before she is exposed to radiation.
▶ Review the procedure with the patient. Address concerns about pain and explain that there may be moments of discomfort or pain experienced when the IV line is inserted to allow infusion

of fluids such as saline, anesthetics, sedatives, radionuclides, medications used in the procedure, or emergency medications.

▶ Inform the patient that the procedure is performed in a nuclear medicine department by a health-care provider (HCP) specializing in this procedure, with support staff, and takes approximately 60 min to complete, with additional images taken periodically over 24 hr as needed.

▶ Reassure the patient that the radionuclide poses no radioactive hazard and rarely produces adverse effects.

▶ Instruct the patient to remove jewelry and other metallic objects from the area to be examined.

▶ Positioning for the study is in a supine position on a flat table with foam wedges to help maintain position and immobilization.

▶ Baseline vital signs and neurological status will be assessed. Protocols may vary among facilities.

▶ Once the radionuclide is administered IV, images are recorded immediately by and every 5 min over a period of 60 min in various positions. Additional images may be taken up to 24 hr after injection if initial images do not indicate active bleeding in the presence of clinical signs or symptoms of bleeding.

▶ Once the scan is completed, the needle or catheter is removed and a pressure dressing is applied over the puncture site.

Potential Nursing Actions

✦ *Make sure a written and informed consent has been signed prior to the procedure and before administering any medications.*

AFTER THE STUDY: POTENTIAL NURSING ACTIONS

Avoiding Complications

▶ Establishing an IV site and injection of radionuclides are invasive procedures. Complications are rare but include risk for allergic reaction *(related to contrast reaction)*, hematoma *(related to blood leakage into the tissue following needle*

insertion)*, bleeding from the puncture site *(related to a bleeding disorder or the effects of natural products and medications with known anticoagulant, antiplatelet, or thrombolytic properties)*, or infection *(which might occur if bacteria from the skin surface is introduced at the puncture site)*. Monitor the patient for complications related to the procedure (e.g., allergic reaction, anaphylaxis, bronchospasm). Immediately report symptoms such as fast heart rate, difficulty breathing, skin rash, itching, or chest pain to the appropriate HCP. Observe/assess the needle/catheter insertion site for bleeding, inflammation, or hematoma formation.

Treatment Considerations

▶ Explain that the radionuclide is eliminated from the body within 6 to 24 hr. Advise the patient to drink increased amounts of fluids for 24 to 48 hr to eliminate the radionuclide from the body, unless contraindicated.

▶ Instruct the patient to resume usual diet, fluids, medication, and activity, as directed by the HCP.

▶ Inadequate Cardiac Output: Adhere to strict intake and output and monitor for urine less than 30 mL/hr. Monitor skin temperature and color, peripheral pulses, capillary refill, level of consciousness, confusion, oxygen saturation, shortness of breath, and adventitious breath sounds. Administer ordered oxygen and emphasize the importance of wearing oxygen to support oxygenation until blood volume is restored.

▶ Monitor vital signs and neurological status every 15 min for 1 hr, then every 2 hr for 4 hr, and then as ordered by the HCP. Monitor intake and output at least every 8 hr. Compare with baseline values. Protocols may vary among facilities.

▶ Insufficient Fluid Volume: Teach the patient the purpose of blood or blood product transfusion and possible reportable reactions. Consider cultural and religious

objections to transfusion. Provide education related to alternatives to blood transfusion and transfusion reaction. Verify informed consent. Administer ordered blood or blood products. Monitor and trend vital signs, hemoglobin and hematocrit, pallor, capillary refill, urinary output, skin warmth, blood urea nitrogen, and electrolytes. Administer ordered normal saline or other fluids.
▶ Instruct the patient in the care and assessment of the injection site.
▶ Explain that application of cold compresses to the puncture site may reduce discomfort or edema.

Safety Considerations
▶ The patient who is breastfeeding should consult with the requesting HCP regarding alternate testing that does not involve radiation. In general, if a woman who is breastfeeding must have a nuclear scan, she should not breastfeed the infant for 72 hr after the scan, until the radionuclide has been eliminated. She should be instructed to express the milk in order to prevent

cessation of milk production; the milk can be stored and used after the 3-day period.
▶ Refer to organizational policy for additional precautions that may include instructions on handwashing, toilet flushing, limited contact with others, and other aspects of nuclear medicine safety.

Nutritional Considerations
▶ A low-fat, low-cholesterol, and low-sodium diet should be consumed to reduce current disease processes. High fat consumption increases the amount of bile acids in the colon and should be avoided.

Follow-Up, Evaluation, and Desired Outcomes
▶ Teach the patient regarding medications that irritate the GI tract and should be avoided (NSAIDs, salicylates).
▶ Acknowledges the importance of avoiding taking medications that could contribute to GI bleeding (NSAIDs, acetylsalicylic acid).

Genetic Testing

SYNONYM/ACRONYM: Related terms include personalized medicine, precision medicine, companion diagnostics, molecular diagnostics.

RATIONALE: To assist in the identification of genetic mutations in humans with implications regarding health and treatment decisions; to assist in the identification of pathogenic organisms.

PATIENT PREPARATION: There are no food, fluid, activity, or medication restrictions unless by medical direction.

NORMAL FINDINGS: Method: Methods are specific to the study of interest and preferred specimen type. Methods include polymerase chain reaction (PCR), immunohistochemical assay, DNA probe using fluorescence in situ hybridization (FISH), gene amplification using chromogenic in situ hybridization (CISH), and cell culture with karyotyping. Absence of findings consistent with genetic abnormalities related to disease or the ability to metabolize medications normally.

CRITICAL FINDINGS AND POTENTIAL INTERVENTIONS: N/A

OVERVIEW: (Study type: The facility or testing laboratory should be contacted regarding specimen collection requirements. Possible specimen types include whole blood, buccal samples, and tissue samples; related body system: Multisystem.) Genetic testing has become an important piece of the continuously evolving healthcare model. It is now possible to identify diseases before symptoms appear, predict the likelihood of disease development, and implement lifestyle or therapeutic interventions that will reduce or eliminate the effects of disease. Closer investigation into the nature of disease has sometimes revealed a more complex set of interactions than what was previously understood. While human DNA has similarities, there are also many individual differences. Additionally, numerous factors, such as diet, activity, environment, and stress levels, contribute to variations between one individual and another. These factors in combination with our genetic makeup impact our tendency toward the development of illnesses. Technologies made possible through the accomplishments of the Human Genome Project and a multitude of findings from other collaborative research efforts have resulted in an explosion of diagnostic and prognostic information. The subspecialty of microbiology has been revolutionized by molecular diagnostics. Molecular diagnostics involves the identification of specific sequences of DNA. Molecular methods are used to help identify pathogens that were previously undetectable or inconsistently identified by the culture and biochemical methods available at the time. Molecular methods are also used to examine human samples for genetic disorders that are the result of both simple and complex mutations. Areas of great interest and active development related to genetic testing are in microbiology, virology, oncology, and the development of pharmaceuticals. Diagnostic and biotechnology companies are developing assays to identify gene sequences that code for proteins associated with a specific disease. Notable examples include the following:

- Mutations in the epidermal growth factor receptor (EGFR) gene: The gene encodes a protein (EGFR) associated with many types of cancer, including lung, breast, and colorectal cancer.
- Mutations in the KRAS gene: If mutations are present, specific medications used to treat lung, breast, and colorectal cancers will be rendered ineffective; therefore, other options can more immediately be considered.
- Mutations in the HER2-NEU gene associated with breast cancer: If mutations are present, the cancer risk can be stratified, survival can be predicted, and selection of treatment options can be made.
- Mutations in the BRAF gene: If present, the mutations are used to identify patients, with cancers such as melanoma, who might benefit from treatment with specific drugs that are known to be effective.
- Mutations in the P450 cytochrome series: If present, the mutations are used to predict response to specific drugs—some people are poor metabolizers (requiring adjustments to higher doses), and some people

are ultrasensitive metabolizers (requiring adjustments to smaller doses).

• Factor V Leiden mutation: If present, this mutation indicates the person has a higher than normal risk for thromboembolism.

• Mutations in the BRCA1 and BRCA2 genes: If present, this mutation indicates the person has a high risk for development of hereditary breast or ovarian cancer. This knowledge provides the opportunity to make informed decisions regarding prophylactic mastectomy or oophorectomy.

New assays are being developed either after an effective therapy for the disease has also been developed or at the same time the treatment is being developed, as companion diagnostics. The cost-benefit analysis for the development of companion diagnostics makes a clear case for the simultaneous development of tests and targeted therapies rather than application by trial and error. The companion diagnostics model is based on the development of tests that identify diseases or their related pathways, from genetic expression to production and interaction of proteins, and then to development of specific related therapies that are predicted with confidence to be effective.

Precision medicine is the combination of identifying specific knowledge about an individual's genetic makeup with customized therapeutics or adjustments in lifestyle, for example, genotyping for single nucleotide polymorphisms (SNPs). An SNP, or variation of a single nucleic acid in a DNA sequence, has been identified that causes malfunction of an enzyme needed for the metabolism of warfarin. Identification of this genotype has led to the development of algorithms for safe, tailored dosing and administration based on a patient's genotype, age, weight or body mass index, and gender. Personalization can also be achieved in the customized production or compounding of pharmaceuticals with respect to the strength or formulation of the medication. Customized pharmaceuticals are being used to address dosing issues revealed by the presence of mutations in the CYP 450 series; adverse drug reactions either by undermedication or overmedication are sometimes the result of genetic programming rather than a medication error.

Knowledge of genetics assists in identifying those who may benefit from additional education, risk assessment, and counseling. Genetics is the study and identification of genes, genetic mutations, and inheritance. For example, genetics provides some insight into the likelihood of inheriting a medical condition such as sickle cell anemia. Genes are segments of DNA arranged on chromosomes and are inherited from each parent. Humans normally have 46 chromosomes, or 23 pairs of chromosomes, in each cell: 23 chromosomes are inherited from the mother, and 23 chromosomes are inherited from the father. Twenty-two of the 23 chromosomes inherited from each parent are called *autosomes*. The 23rd pair of chromosomes is called the *sex chromosomes*: two X chromosomes (an XX pair) are found in females (one X chromosome from each parent) and an X and a Y chromosome (an XY pair) are found in males (one X from the mother and one Y from the father).

Variations in number or structure can be congenital or acquired. Variations can range from a small, single-gene mutation to abnormalities in an entire chromosome or set of chromosomes due to duplication, deletion, substitution, translocation, or other rearrangement. Molecular probe techniques are used to detect smaller, more subtle changes in chromosomes. Chromosomes vary in size and may contain hundreds to thousands of genes. Every gene has a specific location on each of its paired chromosomes. Gene sequences on paired chromosomes are also referred to as *alleles,* and they may be identical or varied. Identical alleles for a gene are termed *homozygous;* variable alleles are termed *heterozygous.* An allele can be demonstrated as either a *dominant* (represented by a capital letter) or a *recessive* (represented by a lowercase letter) trait. Since one allele comes from each parent, the possible combinations are DD, Dd, and dd. Expression of an *autosomal dominant* trait would occur with either DD or Dd; expression of an *autosomal recessive* trait would occur with dd. Expression of a recessive X chromosome–linked trait would always occur in male offspring because there is only a single X chromosome (the father will have contributed a Y chromosome); expression in female offspring would depend on whether the trait was D or d in the X chromosome contributed by the father. Recessive genes are not weaker than dominant genes; rather, expression of the recessive gene is masked by expression of the dominant gene. Some conditions are the result of mutations involving a single gene, and other conditions may involve multiple genes and/or multiple chromosomes. Sickle cell anemia and cystic fibrosis are examples of autosomal recessive, single-gene disorders. Down syndrome is an example of a chromosome disorder in which the cells have three copies of chromosome 21 (trisomy) instead of the normal two copies. Hemophilia is an example of a recessive sex-linked genetic disorder passed from a mother to male children.

Genomic studies evaluate the interaction of groups of genes. The combined activity or combined expression of groups of genes allows assumptions or predictions to be made. As an example, genomic studies measure the levels of activity in multiple genes to predict how they, along with environmental and lifestyle decisions, influence the development of coronary artery disease, type 2 diabetes, or development and growth of a tumor.

INDICATIONS

- Assist in confirming the diagnosis of conditions associated with genetic disorders before or after associated symptoms are manifested.
- Assist in determining drug selection and appropriate dosing on an individual basis.
- Assist in forensic identifications or paternity determinations.
- Assist in monitoring the efficacy of therapeutic interventions.
- Determine the probability of passing a heritable disease to unborn children; discuss prenatal planning.

- Establish a predisposition for the development of certain diseases.
- Identify matches for organ donation.
- Identify the cause of an infectious disease.
- Provide an explanation of death (e.g., miscarriage, stillbirth).
- Screen for a genetic disease or condition that may affect an embryo, fetus, or neonate.

INTERFERING FACTORS
Contraindications

✷ Patients who are not capable of comprehending information presented in the pre- and post-testing genetic counseling sessions. The test should not be performed if the parents of an affected born or unborn child, or if the patient himself or herself, is not emotionally capable of understanding the test results and managing the ramifications of the test results. Written and informed consent, in combination with additional education and a support system, are crucial in order to prepare the patient to make life-altering decisions.

Other considerations

- Proper specimen handling and transport are crucial in order to provide accurate results. The laboratory should be consulted regarding specific instructions prior to specimen collection, especially since tissue specimens are considered irretrievable.

POTENTIAL MEDICAL DIAGNOSIS: CLINICAL SIGNIFICANCE OF RESULTS

- Identification of a condition or disease based on the results of specific genetic testing.
- Identification or disqualification of therapies related to a condition or disease based on the results of specific genetic testing.

NURSING IMPLICATIONS

BEFORE THE STUDY: PLANNING AND IMPLEMENTATION

Teaching the Patient What to Expect

- Inform the patient this test can assist in assessing for infection or disease using genetic testing.
- Review the procedure with the patient. Inform the patient that several tests may be necessary to confirm the diagnosis.
- Explain the type of sample needed for the test and inform the patient that the specimen collection process depends on the type of specimen required for testing.
- Address concerns about pain and explain that there may be some discomfort during specimen collection. (See related studies for specific information.)

Potential Nursing Actions

✷ *Make sure a written and informed consent, if required, has been signed prior to specimen collection.*
- Contact the testing laboratory prior to specimen collection in order to obtain accurate information regarding specimen collection containers, sample volumes, and specific transport instructions.

AFTER THE STUDY: POTENTIAL NURSING ACTIONS

Treatment Considerations

- Assist in coping with anxiety associated with test results and provide emotional support if results are positive.
- Provide teaching and information regarding the clinical implications of the test results, as appropriate.

Follow-Up, Evaluation, and Desired Outcomes

- Acknowledges contact information provided for counseling services and emotional support.

Glucagon

SYNONYM/ACRONYM: N/A

RATIONALE: To evaluate the amount of circulating glucagon toward diagnosing diseases such as hypoglycemia, glucagon secreting tumor, pancreatic cancer, or inflammation.

PATIENT PREPARATION: There are no fluid, activity, or medication restrictions unless by medical direction. Instruct the patient to fast for at least 12 hr before specimen collection for baseline values. Patients with diabetes should have good glycemic management before testing.

NORMAL FINDINGS: Method: Radioimmunoassay.

Age	Conventional Units	SI Units (Conventional Units × 1)
Cord blood	0–215 pg/mL	0–215 ng/L
Newborn	0–1,750 pg/mL	0–1,750 ng/L
Child	0–148 pg/mL	0–148 ng/L
Adult	20–100 pg/mL	20–100 ng/L

CRITICAL FINDINGS AND POTENTIAL INTERVENTIONS: N/A

OVERVIEW: (**Study type:** Blood collected in chilled, lavender-top [EDTA] tube; **related body system:** Endocrine system. Specimen should be transported tightly capped and in an ice slurry.) Glucagon is a peptide hormone secreted by the alpha cells of the islets of Langerhans in the pancreas in response to hypoglycemia. This hormone acts primarily on the liver and muscles to release glucose from glycogen stores and if needed, to activate a pathway, called gluconeogenesis, by which the liver converts amino acids to glucose. Glucagon, along with other hormones, such as catecholamines, adrenocorticotropic hormone, growth hormone, and corticosteroids, stimulate release of an enzyme called *hormone-sensitive lipase*, which participates in the oxidation of stored fatty acids such as triglycerides to basic glycerol components used to produce glucose. Insulin works in opposition to glucagon by decreasing circulating glucose levels.

People with type 1 diabetes may use injectable glucagon to raise the blood sugar when a severe hypoglycemic emergency occurs, such that they are rendered unable to swallow liquid or food containing glucose due to sleepiness, loss of consciousness, or related to seizure activity.

Patients with glucagonoma, a tumor almost always localized in the pancreas, have values greater than 500 pg/mL. Values greater than 1,000 pg/mL are diagnostic for this condition. Glucagonoma causes three different syndromes:

Syndrome 1: A characteristic skin rash, diabetes or impaired glucose tolerance, weight loss, anemia, and venous

G

thrombosis (For additional information regarding screening guidelines and management of diabetes, refer to the study titled "Glucose.")

Syndrome 2: Severe diabetes
Syndrome 3: Multiple endocrine neoplasia

A dramatic increase in glucagon occurring soon after kidney transplantation may indicate organ rejection. In the case of kidney transplant rejection, glucagon levels increase several days before an increase in creatinine levels.

Glucagon deficiency can be confirmed by measuring glucagon levels before and after IV infusion of arginine 0.5 g/kg. Glucagon deficiency is confirmed when levels fail to rise 30 to 60 min after infusion. Newborn infants of mothers with diabetes have impaired glucagon secretion, which may play a role in their hypoglycemia.

INDICATIONS
- Assist in confirming glucagon deficiency.
- Assist in the diagnosis of suspected glucagonoma (alpha islet-cell neoplastic tumor).
- Assist in the diagnosis of suspected chronic kidney disease or kidney transplant rejection.

INTERFERING FACTORS
Factors that may alter the results of the study
- Drugs and other substances that may increase glucagon levels include amino acids (e.g., arginine), cholecystokinin, danazol, gastrin, glucocorticoids, insulin, and nifedipine.
- Drugs and other substances that may decrease glucagon levels include atenolol, pindolol, propranolol, secretin, and verapamil.

- Recent radioactive scans or radiation within 1 wk before the test can interfere with test results when radioimmunoassay is the test method.

POTENTIAL MEDICAL DIAGNOSIS: CLINICAL SIGNIFICANCE OF RESULTS
Increased in
Glucagon is produced in the pancreas and excreted by the kidneys; conditions that affect the pancreas and cause cellular destruction or conditions that impair the ability of the kidneys to remove glucagon from circulation will result in elevated glucagon levels.

- **Acromegaly** *(related to stimulated production of glucagon in response to growth hormone)*
- **Acute pancreatitis** *(related to decreased pancreatic function)*
- **Burns** *(related to stress-induced release of catecholamines, which stimulates glucagon production)*
- **Chronic kidney disease** *(related to decreased renal excretion)*
- **Cirrhosis** *(pathophysiology is not well established)*
- **Cushing syndrome** *(evidenced by overproduction of cortisol, which stimulates glucagon production)*
- **Diabetes (unmanaged)** *(pathophysiology is not well established)*
- **Glucagonoma** *(related to excessive production by the tumor)*
- **Hyperlipoproteinemia** *(pathophysiology is not well established)*
- **Hypoglycemia** *(related to response to decreased glucose level)*
- **Infection** *(related to feedback loop in response to stress)*
- **Kidney transplant rejection** *(related to decreased renal excretion)*
- **Pheochromocytoma** *(excessive production of catecholamines stimulates increased glucagon levels)*
- **Stress** *(related to stress-induced release of catecholamines, which stimulates glucagon production)*

G

- Trauma *(related to stress-induced release of catecholamines, which stimulates glucagon production)*

Decreased in
Low glucagon levels are related to decreased pancreatic function.

- Chronic pancreatitis
- Cystic fibrosis
- Postpancreatectomy period

NURSING IMPLICATIONS

BEFORE THE STUDY: PLANNING AND IMPLEMENTATION

Teaching the Patient What to Expect
▶ Inform the patient this test can assist in evaluating the hormone that participates in regulating blood sugar.
▶ Explain that a blood sample is needed for the test.

Potential Nursing Actions
▶ It is important that patients with diabetes have good glycemic management before the study. Identify the degree of glycemic management before the study.

AFTER THE STUDY: POTENTIAL NURSING ACTIONS

Treatment Considerations
▶ Provide teaching and information regarding the clinical implications of the test results. Emphasize that good glycemic management delays the onset and slows the progression of diabetic retinopathy, nephropathy, and neuropathy.

▶ Instruct the patient to resume usual diet, as directed by the health-care provider.
▶ Increased glucagon levels may be associated with diabetes. Instruct the patient and caregiver to report signs and symptoms of hypoglycemia (weakness, confusion, diaphoresis, rapid pulse) or hyperglycemia (thirst, polyuria, hunger, lethargy).

Nutritional Considerations
▶ Abnormal results may be associated with diabetes. There is no "diabetic diet"; however, many meal-planning approaches with nutritional goals are endorsed by the American Diabetes Association. Patients who adhere to dietary recommendations report a better general feeling of health, better weight management, greater management of glucose and lipid values, and improved use of insulin. Instruct the patient, as appropriate, in nutritional management of diabetes. A variety of dietary patterns are beneficial for people with diabetes. Encourage consultation with a registered dietitian who is a certified diabetes educator.

Follow-Up, Evaluation, and Desired Outcomes
▶ Acknowledges contact information provided for the ADA (www.diabetes .org), American Heart Association (www.heart.org/HEARTORG), National Heart, Lung, and Blood Institute (www .nhlbi.nih.gov), National Institute of Diabetes and Digestive and Kidney Disease (NIDDK) (www.niddk.nih.gov), and U.S. Department of Agriculture's resource for nutrition (www.choosemy plate.gov).

Glucose

SYNONYM/ACRONYM: Blood sugar, fasting blood sugar (FBS), postprandial glucose, 2-hr PC (post cibum).

RATIONALE: To assist in the diagnosis of diabetes and to evaluate disorders of carbohydrate metabolism such as malabsorption syndrome.

PATIENT PREPARATION: There are no activity or medication restrictions unless by medical direction. There are no restrictions for the random glucose test. Instruct the patient to fast for at least 8 hr before specimen collection for the fasting glucose test and not to consume any caffeinated products or chew any type of gum before specimen collection; these factors are known to elevate glucose levels. Instruct the patient to follow the instructions given for 2-hr postprandial glucose test. Some health-care providers (HCPs) may order administration of a standard glucose solution, whereas others may instruct the patient to eat a meal with a known carbohydrate composition.

NORMAL FINDINGS: Method: Spectrophotometry.

Age	Conventional Units	SI Units (Conventional Units × 0.0555)
Nondiabetic, fasting		
Cord blood	45–96 mg/dL	2.5–5.3 mmol/L
Premature infant	20–80 mg/dL	1.1–4.4 mmol/L
Newborn 2 days–2 yr	30–100 mg/dL	1.7–5.6 mmol/L
Child	60–100 mg/dL	3.3–5.6 mmol/L
Adult–older adult	Less than 100 mg/dL	Less than 5.6 mmol/L
Nondiabetic, 2-hr postprandial	65–139 mg/dL	3.6–7.7 mmol/L
Nondiabetic, random	Less than 200 mg/dL	Less than 11.1 mmol/L
Prediabetic, fasting	100–125 mg/dL	5.6–6.9 mmol/L
Prediabetic, 2-hr postprandial	140–199 mg/dL	7.8–11 mmol/L

Fasting means no caloric intake for 8 hr or longer. Values tend to increase in older adults.

CRITICAL FINDINGS AND POTENTIAL INTERVENTIONS

Glucose
Adults & children
• Less than 40 mg/dL (SI: Less than 2.22 mmol/L)
• Greater than 400 mg/dL (SI: Greater than 22.2 mmol/L)

Newborns
• Less than 32 mg/dL (SI: Less than 1.8 mmol/L)
• Greater than 328 mg/dL (SI: Greater than 18.2 mmol/L)

Timely notification to the requesting HCP of any critical findings and related symptoms is a role expectation of the professional nurse. A listing of these findings varies among facilities.

Consideration may be given to verification of critical findings before action is taken. Policies vary among facilities and may include requesting immediate recollection and retesting by the laboratory or retesting using a rapid point-of-care testing instrument at the bedside, if available.

Glucose monitoring is an important measure in achieving tight glycemic management. The enzymatic GDH-PQQ test method may produce falsely elevated results in patients who are receiving products that contain other sugars (e.g., oral xylose, parenterals containing maltose or galactose, and peritoneal dialysis solutions that contain icodextrin). The GDH-NAD, glucose oxidase, and glucose hexokinase methods can distinguish between glucose and other sugars.

Symptoms of decreased glucose levels include headache, confusion, polyphagia, irritability, nervousness, restlessness, diaphoresis, and weakness. Possible interventions include oral or IV administration of glucose, IV or intramuscular injection of glucagon, and continuous glucose monitoring.

Symptoms of elevated glucose levels include abdominal pain, fatigue, muscle cramps, nausea, vomiting, polyuria, polyphagia, and polydipsia. Possible interventions include fluid replacement in addition to subcutaneous or IV injection of insulin with continuous glucose monitoring.

OVERVIEW: (Study type: Blood collected in a gray- [sodium fluoride] or green-top [heparin] tube; *plasma is recommended for diagnosis*. Serum collected in a gold-, red-, or red/gray-top tube is also acceptable. It is important to use the same type of collection container throughout the entire test; related body system: Endocrine system.) Glucose, a simple six-carbon sugar (monosaccharide), enters the diet as part of the sugars sucrose, lactose, and maltose and from the complex polysaccharide, dietary starch. The body acquires most of its energy from the oxidative metabolism of glucose. Excess glucose is stored in the liver or in muscle tissue as glycogen. Glucose levels in plasma (one of the components of blood) are generally 10% to 15% higher than glucose measurements in whole blood (and even more after eating). This is important because home blood glucose meters measure the glucose in whole blood, whereas most laboratory tests measure the glucose in either plasma or serum.

Diabetes is a group of diseases characterized by hyperglycemia, or elevated glucose levels. Hyperglycemia can result from a defect in insulin secretion due to destruction of the beta cells of the pancreas (type 1 diabetes), a defect in insulin action, or a combination of defects in secretion and action (type 2 diabetes), or from a specific cause such as gestational diabetes, neonatal hyperglycemia, cystic fibrosis, or hyperglycemia induced by drugs used to treat other medical conditions (e.g., corticosteroids). The chronic hyperglycemia of diabetes over time may lead to damage, dysfunction, and eventually failure of the eyes (retinopathy), kidneys (nephropathy), nerves (neuropathy), heart (cardiovascular disease), and blood vessels (micro- and macrovascular conditions). The American Diabetes Association (ADA) and National Institute of Diabetes and Digestive and Kidney Disease (NIDDK) have established criteria for diagnosing diabetes.

Diagnostic Criteria for Diabetes: Any Combination of the Following Findings or Confirmation of Any of the Individual Findings by Repetition of the Same Test on a Subsequent Day

Glucose	Conventional Units	SI Units (Conventional Units × 0.0555)
Fasting	Equal to or greater than 126 mg/dL	Equal to or greater than 7 mmol/L
2-hr post-challenge with standardized 75-mg load	Greater than 200 mg/dL	Greater than 11.1 mmol/L
Random	Greater than 200 mg/dL **with** symptoms of diabetes (e.g., polyuria, polydipsia, polyphagia, unexplained weight loss)	Greater than 11.1 mmol/L **with** symptoms of diabetes (e.g., polyuria, polydipsia, polyphagia, unexplained weight loss)
A$_{1c}$	6.5% or greater	6.5% or greater

Glucose measurements have been used for many years as an indicator of short-term glycemic management to identify diabetes and assist in management of the disease. Glycated hemoglobin, or hemoglobin A$_{1c}$, is used to indicate long-term glycemic management over a period of 3 to 4 mo and is used as a diagnostic tool in the diagnosis of type 2 diabetes. The estimated average glucose (eAG) is a mathematical relationship between hemoglobin A$_{1c}$ and glucose levels expressed by the formula

$$eAG = (mg/dL)$$
$$= [(A_{1c} \times 28.7) - 46.7]$$

For example, eAG for a patient with an A$_{1c}$ of 6% would be calculated as $[(6 \times 28.7) - 46.7] = 125.5$ mg/dL. Studies have documented the need for markers that reflect intermediate glycemic management, or the period of time between 2 to 4 wk as opposed to hr or months. Many patients who appear to be well managed according to glucose and A$_{1c}$ values actually have significant postprandial hyperglycemia. Management of postprandial hyperglycemia is considered to be extremely important in preventing or delaying the development of diabetes-related complications. The GlycoMark assay measures serum 1,5-anhydroglucitol, a validated marker of short-term glycemic management, and can be used in combination with glucose and hemoglobin A$_{1c}$ measurements to provide a more complete picture of glucose levels over time. Glyco-Mark values greater than 8 mcg/mL are considered normal for adults. Serum 1,5-anhydroglucitol is a naturally occurring monosaccharide found in most foods. It is not normally metabolized by the body and is excreted by the kidneys. During periods of normal glucose levels, there is an equilibrium between glucose and 1,5-anhydroglucitol concentrations. When blood glucose concentration rises above 180 mg/dL (SI = 10 mmol/L), the renal threshold for glucose, levels of circulating serum 1,5-anhydroglucitol decrease due to competitive inhibition of renal tubular absorption favoring glucose over serum 1,5-anhydroglucitol. As glucose is retained in the circulating blood and levels of glucose increase, correspondingly higher amounts of 1,5-anhydroglucitol are excreted in the urine, resulting in lower serum concentrations. The change in serum 1,5-anhydroglucitol levels is directly proportional to the severity and frequency of hyperglycemic episodes. Serum 1,5-anhydroglucitol concentration

returns to normal after 2 wk with no recurrence of hyperglycemia. The Centers for Disease Control and Prevention releases a National Diabetes Statistics Report about every other year (www.cdc.gov/diabetes/data/index.html). The report provides up-to-date statistical information on diabetes and prediabetes in the United States. The combined use of available markers of glycemic management will greatly improve the ability to achieve tighter, more timely glycemic management.

Comparison of Markers of Glycemic Management to Approximate Blood Glucose Concentration

1,5-Anhydroglucitol Measured Using the GlycoMark Assay	Hemoglobin A_{1c}	Estimated Blood Glucose (mg/dL)	Degree of Glycemic Management
14 mcg/mL or greater	4%–5%	68–97 mg/dL	Normal/nondiabetic
10–12 mcg/mL	4%–6%	68–126 mg/dL	Well managed
5–10 mcg/mL	6%–8%	126–183 mg/dL	Moderately well managed
2–5 mcg/mL	8%–10%	183–240 mg/dL	Poorly managed
Less than 2 mcg/mL	Greater than 10% (11%–14%)	269–355 mg/dL	Very poorly managed

Assessment of medications used to manage diabetes is an important facet of managing the disease and its health-related complications. Drug response is an active area of study to ensure that the medications prescribed are meeting the needs of the patients who are taking them. Insulin and metformin are two commonly prescribed medications for the treatment of diabetes. See the "Insulin Antibodies" study for more detailed information. The AccuType Metformin Assay is a genetic test that identifies individuals who may not respond appropriately or who

have a suboptimal response to metformin related to a genetic mutation in the proteins responsible for transporting metformin.

INDICATIONS
- Assist in the diagnosis of diabetes.
- Assist in the diagnosis of insulinoma.
- Assist in the management of glucose levels in individuals with diabetes.
- Determine insulin requirements.
- Evaluate disorders of carbohydrate metabolism.
- Identify hypoglycemia.

INTERFERING FACTORS

Factors that may alter the results of the study

- Drugs and other substances that may increase glucose levels include acetazolamide, alanine, albuterol, anesthetic drugs, antipyrine, atenolol, betamethasone, cefotaxime, chlorpromazine, chlorprothixene, clonidine, clorexolone, corticotropin, cortisone, cyclic AMP, cyclopropane, dexamethasone, dextroamphetamine, diapamide, epinephrine, enflurane, ethacrynic acid, ether, fludrocortisone, furosemide, glucagon, glucocorticoids, homoharringtonine, hydrochlorothiazide, hydroxydione, isoniazid, maltose, meperidine, meprednisone, methyclothiazide, metolazone, niacin, nifedipine, nortriptyline, octreotide, oral contraceptives, oxyphenbutazone, pancreozymin, phenelzine, phenylbutazone, piperacetazine, polythiazide, prednisone, quinethazone, reserpine, rifampin, ritodrine, secretin, somatostatin, thiazides, thyroid hormone, and triamcinolone.
- Drugs and other substances that may decrease glucose levels include acarbose, acetylsalicylic acid, acipimox, alanine, allopurinol, antimony compounds, arsenicals, ascorbic acid, benzene, buformin, cannabis, captopril, chloroform, clofibrate, enalapril, enprostil, erythromycin, gemfibrozil, glibornuride, glyburide, guanethidine, niceritrol, nitrazepam, oral contraceptives, phentolamine, phosphorus, promethazine, ramipril, rotenone, sulfonylureas, thiocarlide, tolbutamide, tromethamine, and verapamil.
- Elevated urea levels and uremia can lead to falsely elevated glucose levels.
- Extremely elevated white blood cell counts can lead to falsely decreased glucose values.
- Administration of insulin or oral hypoglycemic drugs within 8 hr of a fasting blood glucose can lead to falsely decreased values.
- Specimens should never be collected above an IV line because of the potential for dilution when the specimen and the IV solution combine in the collection container, falsely decreasing the result. There is also the potential of contaminating the sample with the substance of interest, if it is present in the IV solution, falsely increasing the result.
- Failure to follow dietary restrictions before the fasting test can lead to falsely elevated glucose values.

POTENTIAL MEDICAL DIAGNOSIS: CLINICAL SIGNIFICANCE OF RESULTS

Increased in

- Acromegaly, gigantism *(growth hormone [GH] stimulates the release of glucagon, which in turn increases glucose levels)*
- Acute stress reaction *(hyperglycemia is stimulated by the release of catecholamines and glucagon)*
- Cerebrovascular accident *(possibly related to stress)*
- Chronic kidney disease *(glucagon is degraded by the kidneys; when damaged kidneys cannot metabolize glucagon, glucagon levels in blood rise and result in hyperglycemia)*
- Cushing syndrome *(related to elevated cortisol)*
- Diabetes *(glucose intolerance and elevated glucose levels define diabetes)*
- Glucagonoma *(glucagon releases stored glucose; glucagon-secreting tumors will increase glucose levels)*
- Hemochromatosis *(related to iron deposition in the pancreas; subsequent damage to pancreatic tissue releases cell contents, including glucagon, resulting in hyperglycemia)*
- Liver disease (severe) *(damaged liver tissue releases cell contents,*

G

including stored glucose, into circulation)

- Metabolic syndrome *(related to the development of diabetes)*
- Myocardial infarction *(related to stress and/or preexisting diabetes)*
- Pancreatic adenoma *(damage to pancreatic tissue releases cell contents, including glucagon, resulting in hyperglycemia)*
- Pancreatitis (acute and chronic) *(damage to pancreatic tissue releases cell contents, including glucagon, resulting in hyperglycemia)*
- Pancreatitis due to mumps *(damage to pancreatic tissue releases cell contents, including glucagon, resulting in hyperglycemia)*
- Pheochromocytoma *(related to increased catecholamines, which increase glucagon; glucagon increases glucose levels)*
- Shock, trauma *(hyperglycemia is stimulated by the release of catecholamines and glucagon)*
- Somatostatinoma *(somatostatin-producing tumor of pancreatic delta cells, associated with diabetes)*
- Strenuous exercise *(hyperglycemia is stimulated by the release of catecholamines and glucagon)*
- Thyrotoxicosis *(related to loss of kidney function)*
- Vitamin B$_1$ deficiency *(thiamine is involved in the metabolism of glucose; deficiency results in accumulation of glucose)*

Decreased in

- Acute alcohol ingestion *(most glucose metabolism occurs in the liver; alcohol inhibits the liver from making glucose)*
- Addison disease *(cortisol affects glucose levels; insufficient levels of cortisol result in diminished glucose levels)*
- Ectopic insulin production from tumors (adrenal cancer, cancer of the stomach, fibrosarcoma)
- Excess insulin by injection
- Galactosemia *(inherited enzyme disorder that results in accumulation of galactose in excessive proportion to glucose levels)*
- Glucagon deficiency *(glucagon controls glucose levels; hypoglycemia occurs in the absence of glucagon)*
- Glycogen storage diseases *(deficiencies in enzymes involved in conversion of glycogen to glucose)*
- Hereditary fructose intolerance *(inherited disorder of fructose metabolism; phosphates needed for intermediate steps in gluconeogenesis are trapped from further action by the enzyme deficiency responsible for fructose metabolism)*
- Hypopituitarism *(decreased levels of hormones such as adrenocorticotropic hormone [ACTH] and GH result in decreased glucose levels)*
- Hypothyroidism *(thyroid hormones affect glucose levels; decreased thyroid hormone levels result in decreased glucose levels)*
- Insulinoma *(the function of insulin is to decrease glucose levels)*
- Malabsorption syndromes *(insufficient absorption of carbohydrates)*
- Maple syrup urine disease *(inborn error of amino acid metabolism; accumulation of leucine is believed to inhibit the rate of gluconeogenesis, independently of insulin, and thereby diminish release of hepatic glucose stores)*
- Poisoning resulting in severe liver disease *(decreased liver function correlates with decreased glucose metabolism)*
- Postgastrectomy *(insufficient intake of carbohydrates)*
- Starvation *(insufficient intake of carbohydrates)*
- von Gierke disease *(most common glycogen storage disease; G6PD deficiency)*

G

NURSING IMPLICATIONS

POTENTIAL NURSING PROBLEMS: ASSESSMENT & NURSING DIAGNOSIS

Problems	Signs and Symptoms
Blood glucose *(related to sedentary lifestyle, circulating insulin deficiency secondary to pancreatic insufficiency, excessive dietary intake, insulin resistance)*	**Excess:** Fatigue, mild dehydration, elevated blood glucose, weight loss, weakness, polyuria, polydipsia, polyphagia, blurred vision, headache, paresthesia, poor skin turgor, dry mouth, nausea, vomiting, abdominal pain, Kussmaul respirations **Deficit:** Tremor, diaphoresis, decreased concentration, elevated blood pressure, palpitations, headache, polyphagia, restlessness, lethargy, altered mental status, combativeness, altered speech, altered coordination
Nutrition *(related to excessive dietary intake more than body requirements, insulin deficiency, stress, anxiety, depression, cultural lifestyle, unhealthy food sources, financial restrictions)*	Polydipsia, polyuria, weight loss, fatigue, elevated blood glucose levels, inadequate glucose management, polyphagia

BEFORE THE STUDY: PLANNING AND IMPLEMENTATION

Teaching the Patient What to Expect

◆ Inform the patient this test can assist in evaluating blood sugar levels.
◆ Explain that a blood sample is needed for the test.

Potential Nursing Actions

◆ Verify adherence to dietary restrictions for the specified study prior to study completion.

AFTER THE STUDY: POTENTIAL NURSING ACTIONS

Treatment Considerations

◆ Instruct the patient to resume usual diet, as directed by the HCP, once the laboratory draw is completed.
◆ Comparative studies demonstrate that certain populations are disproportionately affected by type 2 diabetes and complications of type 2 diabetes as compared to the general population.

Nonmodifiable risk factors include age, ethnicity, and family history of diabetes or metabolic syndrome. The risk of developing type 2 diabetes increases with age. In the United States, affected populations include African Americans, Asian Americans, Hispanics, native Hawaiians and Pacific Islanders, American Indians, and Alaska natives. Modifiable risk factors include lifestyle choices related to making healthy dietary choices, maintaining a healthy body weight, and meeting recommended levels of physical activity. The financial and emotional burdens of diabetes and related complications continue to grow at an alarming rate. A system for the prevention, management, and support of patients with type 2 diabetes should be provided through the coordinated efforts of multidisciplinary partners using strategies that are culturally appropriate.

◆ Blood Glucose: Educate and encourage the patient to participate in glucose self-checks. Instruct the patient in the use of home testing strips or meters approved for glucose, ketones, or A_{1c} by the U.S. Food and Drug Administration, if prescribed. Check blood glucose before meals and at bedtime. Administer prescribed insulin or oral drugs. Explain that long-term use of metformin can lead to deficiencies in folate and/or vitamin B_{12}, which can affect memory.

‣ Monitor blood glucose results and administer ordered insulin or oral anti-hyperglycemic drugs.

‣ Assess the cultural aspects of diet selection.

‣ Correlate dietary intake with blood glucose.

‣ Monitor laboratory studies that may be impacted by altered glucose and trend results (Hemoglobin A_{1c}, blood urea nitrogen, creatinine, electrolytes, arterial pH, magnesium, urine ketones, urine microalbumin, white blood cell count, amylase, hemoglobin/hematocrit, C-reactive protein, liver enzymes). Correlate blood glucose with other laboratory values and medical conditions, address the psychosocial aspects of the disease, and monitor serum insulin levels. Instruct the patient and caregiver to report signs and symptoms of hypoglycemia (weakness, confusion, diaphoresis, rapid pulse) or hyperglycemia (thirst, polyuria, hunger, lethargy).

‣ Collaborate with the HCP to develop a plan of exercise commensurate with the patient's physical abilities and discuss lifestyle alterations necessary to support positive health management.

‣ Nutrition: Inadequate nutritional management can be a barrier to good glycemic management. Monitor blood glucose results, collaborate with the dietitian to correlate dietary intake with blood glucose, and evaluate the effectiveness of administered insulin or oral antihyperglycemic drugs. Collaborate with the HCP and a registered dietitian (who is a certified diabetes educator) to develop a cultural- and age-appropriate diet plan. Ensure the patient understands the relationship between caloric intake, ordered medication, and glucose results.

‣ Individuals with poor glycemic management have a greater infection risk. Provide standard precautions in the provision of care. Educate the patient in vigilant hand hygiene and the correlation between poor hygiene and infection risk. Adequate rest and avoiding exposure to opportunistic hosts can minimize infection risk.

‣ Nonadherence to medication, diet, and activity therapeutic goals can make glycemic management problematic. Assess the patient's ability and prior efforts to manage the disease process, including blood glucose self-checks, dietary management, exercise, and medication self-administration. Evaluate for personal factors that may limit the patient's ability to self-perform, such as visual, cognitive, or hearing deficits or lack of financial resources. Emphasize, if indicated, that good glycemic management delays the onset and slows the progression of diabetic retinopathy, nephropathy, and neuropathy.

‣ Discuss the implications of abnormal test results on the patient's lifestyle.

Nutritional Considerations

‣ Increased glucose levels may be associated with diabetes. There is no "diabetic diet"; however, many meal-planning approaches with nutritional goals are endorsed by the ADA. Patients who adhere to dietary recommendations report a better general feeling of health, better weight management, better management of glucose and lipid values, and improved use of insulin. Instruct the patient, as appropriate, in nutritional management of diabetes. A variety of dietary patterns are beneficial for people with diabetes. Encourage consultation with a registered dietitian who is a certified diabetes educator.

‣ *Sensitivity to Social and Cultural Issues:* Numerous studies point to the prevalence of excess body weight in American children and adolescents. Findings from the 2015–2016 National

G

Health and Nutrition Examination Survey (NHANES), regarding the prevalence of obesity in younger members of the population, estimate that obesity is present in 13.9% of the population ages 2 to 5 years, 18.4% ages 6 to 11 years, and 20.6% ages 12 to 19 years. The medical, social, and emotional consequences of excess body weight are significant. Special attention should be given to instructing the pediatric patient and caregiver regarding health risks and weight management education.

Follow-Up, Evaluation, and Desired Outcomes

▶ Acknowledges contact information provided for the ADA (www.diabetes.org), American Heart Association (www.heart.org/HEARTORG), National Heart, Lung, and Blood Institute (www.nhlbi.nih.gov), NIDDK (www.niddk.nih.gov), and

U.S. Department of Agriculture's resource for nutrition (www.choosemyplate.gov).

▶ Understands that the ADA recommends A_{1c} testing four times a year for insulin-dependent type 1 or type 2 diabetes when glycemic targets are not being met or when therapy has changed and twice a year when treatment goals are being met for non–insulin-dependent type 2 diabetes. The ADA also recommends that testing for diabetes commence at age 45 for asymptomatic individuals, be considered for adults of any age who are overweight and have additional risk factors, and continue every 3 yr in the absence of symptoms.

▶ Understands the link between good glycemic management and a delay in the onset of and in slowing the progression of diabetic retinopathy, nephropathy, and neuropathy.

Glucose-6-Phosphate Dehydrogenase

SYNONYM/ACRONYM: G6PD.

RATIONALE: To identify an enzyme deficiency that can result in hemolytic anemia.

PATIENT PREPARATION: There are no food, fluid, activity, or medication restrictions unless by medical direction.

NORMAL FINDINGS: (Method: Enzymatic) 7–15 units/G hemoglobin; SI Units (Conventional Units × 0.0645) = 0.45–0.97 micro units/mol hemoglobin.

CRITICAL FINDINGS AND POTENTIAL INTERVENTIONS: N/A

OVERVIEW: (Study type: Blood collected in a lavender-top [EDTA] tube; related body system: Circulatory system.) G6PD is a red blood cell (RBC) enzyme. It is involved in the hexose monophosphate shunt, and its function is to protect hemoglobin from oxidation. G6PD deficiency is the most common enzyme

abnormality and affects over 400 million people worldwide. This deficiency results in hemolysis of varying degrees and acuity depending on the severity of the abnormality. Globin chains from the oxidized hemoglobin attach to the RBC membrane and can be seen in stained peripheral smears; the round inclusions are called

Heinz bodies and are associated with hemolytic anemias such as G6PD deficiency. The deficiency is passed on as a sex-linked recessive (X chromosome) mutation expressed more frequently in males than in females. There are numerous G6PD variants, and of these three have a high frequency in specific ethnic groups. G6PD A is more common in males of African descent (10%) than in other populations. G6PD Mediterranean is especially common in Iraqis, Kurds, Sephardic Jews, and Lebanese and less common in Greeks, Italians, Turks, North Africans, Spaniards, Portuguese, and Ashkenazi Jews. G6PD Mahidol is common in Southeast Asians (22% of males). Polymerase chain reaction (PCR) methods that can detect gene mutations for the enzyme in whole blood are also available. Counseling and written, informed consent are recommended and sometimes required before genetic testing.

Knowledge of genetics assists in identifying those who may benefit from additional education, risk assessment, and counseling. Genetics is the study and identification of genes, genetic mutations, and inheritance. For example, genetics provides some insight into the likelihood of inheriting a medical condition such as G6PD deficiency. Some conditions are the result of mutations involving a single gene, whereas other conditions may involve multiple genes and/or multiple chromosomes. G6PD is an example of a recessive sex-linked genetic disorder passed from a mother to male children. Further information regarding inheritance of genes can be found in the study titled "Genetic Testing."

INDICATIONS
- Assist in identifying the cause of hemolytic anemia resulting from drug sensitivity, metabolic disorder, or infection
- Assist in identifying the cause of hemolytic anemia resulting from enzyme deficiency

INTERFERING FACTORS
Factors that may alter the results of the study
- Drugs and other substances that may increase G6PD levels include fluorouracil.
- Drugs and other substances that may precipitate hemolysis in G6PD-deficient individuals include acetylsalicylic acid, ascorbic acid (large doses), chloramphenicol, dapsone, doxorubicin, furazolidone, methylene blue, nalidixic acid, naphthalene, niridazole, nitrofurantoin, pentaquine, phenazopyridine, phenylhydrazine, primaquine, quinidine, quinine, sulfacetamide, sulfamethoxazole, sulfanilamide, sulfapyridine, sulfisoxazole, thiazolsulfone, toluidine blue, uricase (rasburicase), and vitamin K.
- G6PD levels are increased in reticulocytes; the test results may be falsely positive when a patient is in a period of acute hemolysis. G6PD levels can also be affected by the presence of large numbers of platelets and white blood cells, which also contain significant amounts of the enzyme.

POTENTIAL MEDICAL DIAGNOSIS: CLINICAL SIGNIFICANCE OF RESULTS
Increased in
The pathophysiology is not well understood, but release of the enzymes from hemolyzed cells increases blood levels.

- Chronic blood loss *(related to reticulocytosis; replacement of RBCs)*
- Hepatic coma *(pathophysiology is unclear)*

- Hyperthyroidism *(possible response to increased basal metabolic rate and role of G6PD in glucose metabolism)*
- Idiopathic thrombocytopenic purpura
- Megaloblastic anemia *(related to reticulocytosis; replacement of RBCs)*
- Myocardial infarction *(medications [e.g., salicylates] may aggravate or stimulate a hemolytic crisis in G6PD-deficient patients)*
- Pernicious anemia *(related to reticulocytosis; replacement of RBCs)*
- Viral hepatitis *(pathophysiology is unclear)*

Decreased in
- Congenital nonspherocytic anemia
- G6PD deficiency
- Nonimmunological hemolytic disease of the newborn

NURSING IMPLICATIONS

BEFORE THE STUDY: PLANNING AND IMPLEMENTATION

Teaching the Patient What to Expect
▶ Inform the patient this test can assist in diagnosing anemia.
▶ Explain that a blood sample is needed for the test.

AFTER THE STUDY: POTENTIAL NURSING ACTIONS

Treatment Considerations
▶ Chronic fatigue related to anemia can be problematic for the patient in maintaining activities of daily living. Collaborate with the patient to prioritize activities and conserve energy. Discuss limiting daytime napping to facilitate nighttime sleeping. Correct anemia with ordered interventions such as blood transfusion.

Nutritional Considerations
▶ Educate the patient with G6PD deficiency, as appropriate, to avoid certain foods (e.g., fava beans), vitamins, and drugs that may precipitate an acute episode of intravascular hemolysis.

Follow-Up, Evaluation, and Desired Outcomes
▶ Acknowledges key signs and symptoms of hemolytic anemia that must be reported to the health-care provider to include back pain, fatigue, jaundice, rapid breathing, and rapid heart rate; knowledge of signs and symptoms is especially important for individuals in high-risk groups based on age (newborns with severe jaundice that does not resolve), ethnicity (African, Middle Eastern, or Asian descent with a family history of hemolytic anemia), and gender (males with a family history of jaundice, enlarged spleen or hemolytic anemia).

Glucose Tolerance Tests

SYNONYM/ACRONYM: Standard oral tolerance test, standard gestational screen, standard gestational tolerance test, GTT.

RATIONALE: To evaluate blood glucose levels to assist in diagnosing diabetes.

PATIENT PREPARATION: There are no activity or medication restrictions unless by medical direction; additionally, there are no fluid restrictions prior to the gestational screen (unless by medical direction). Instruct the patient to fast for at least 8 hr before the standard oral and standard gestational GTTs and not to consume any caffeinated products or chew any type of gum before specimen collection for the test; these factors are known to elevate glucose levels.

NORMAL FINDINGS: Method: Spectrophotometry.

Standard Oral Glucose Tolerance (Up to 75-g Glucose Load)

	Conventional Units	SI Units (Conventional Units × 0.0555)
Nondiabetic, fasting sample	Less than 100 mg/dL	Less than 5.6 mmol/L
Nondiabetic, 2-hr sample	Less than 140 mg/dL	Less than 7.8 mmol/L
Prediabetes, fasting sample	100–125 mg/dL	5.6–6.9 mmol/L
Prediabetes, 2-hr sample	140–199 mg/dL	7.8–11 mmol/L

Plasma glucose values are reported to be 10% to 20% higher than serum values.
A diagnosis of diabetes is made when the fasting glucose is equal to or greater than 126 mg/dL (7 mmol/L) or the 2-hr sample is equal to or greater than 200 mg/dL (11.1 mmol/L).

Tolerance Tests for Gestational Diabetes

One-Step Approach (75-g Glucose Load)	Conventional and SI Units (SI = Conventional Units × 0.0555)
Fasting sample	Less than 93 mg/dL (SI: Less than 5.1 mmol/L)
1-hr sample	Less than 181 mg/dL (SI: Less than 10 mmol/L)
2-hr sample	Less than 154 mg/dL (SI: Less than 8.5 mmol/L)

Plasma glucose values are reported to be 10% to 20% higher than serum values.
A diagnosis of gestational diabetes is made when any of the three thresholds are met or exceeded.

Tolerance Tests for Gestational Diabetes

	Two-Step Approach	Conventional and SI Units (SI = Conventional Units × 0.0555)	
Step 1	Standard Gestational Screen (50-g Glucose Load)		
1-hr sample performed while the patient is not fasting		Less than 141 mg/dL; if results exceed 140 mg/dL, the 100-g GTT should be performed (American College of Obstetricians and Gynecologists [ACOG])	Less than 7.8 mmol/L; if results exceed 7.7 mmol/L, the 75-g GTT should be performed
Step 2	Gestational GTT (100-g Glucose Load)	Carpenter and Coustan	National Diabetes Data Group

(table continues on page 640)

Tolerance Tests for Gestational Diabetes

	Two-Step Approach	Conventional and SI Units (SI = Conventional Units × 0.0555)	
Fasting sample		Less than 95 mg/dL (SI: Less than 5.3 mmol/L)	Less than 105 mg/dL (SI: Less than 5.8 mmol/L)
1-hr sample		Less than 180 mg/dL (SI: Less than 10 mmol/L)	Less than 190 mg/dL (SI: Less than 10.5 mmol/L)
2-hr sample		Less than 155 mg/dL (SI: Less than 8.6 mmol/L)	Less than 165 mg/dL (SI: Less than 9.2 mmol/L)
3-hr sample		Less than 140 mg/dL (SI: Less than 7.8 mmol/L)	Less than 145 mg/dL (SI: Less than 8 mmol/L)

Plasma glucose values are reported to be 10% to 20% higher than serum values.
GTT = glucose tolerance test.
A diagnosis of gestational diabetes is made when two or more of the four thresholds are met or exceeded.

CRITICAL FINDINGS AND POTENTIAL INTERVENTIONS

Glucose
Adults & Children
• Less than 40 mg/dL (SI: Less than 2.22 mmol/L)
• Greater than 400 mg/dL (SI: Greater than 22.2 mmol/L)

Newborns
• Less than 32 mg/dL (SI: Less than 1.8 mmol/L)
• Greater than 328 mg/dL (SI: Greater than 18.2 mmol/L)

Timely notification to the requesting health-care provider (HCP) of any critical findings and related symptoms is a role expectation of the professional nurse. A listing of these findings varies among facilities.

Consideration may be given to verification of critical findings before action is taken. Policies vary among facilities and may include requesting immediate recollection and retesting by the laboratory or retesting using a rapid point-of-care testing instrument at the bedside, if available.

Symptoms of decreased glucose levels include headache, confusion, polyphagia, irritability, nervousness, restlessness, diaphoresis, and weakness. Possible interventions include oral or IV administration of glucose, IV or intramuscular injection of glucagon, and continuous glucose monitoring.

Symptoms of elevated glucose levels include abdominal pain, fatigue, muscle cramps, nausea, vomiting, polyuria, polyphagia, and polydipsia. Possible interventions include fluid replacement in addition to subcutaneous or IV injection of insulin with continuous glucose monitoring.

OVERVIEW: (Study type: Blood collected in a gray- [sodium fluoride] or green-top [heparin] tube; *plasma is recommended for diagnosis.* Serum collected in a gold-, red-, or red/gray-top tube is also acceptable. It is important to use the same type of collection container throughout the entire test; related body system: Endocrine system.) The GTT measures glucose levels after administration of an oral or IV carbohydrate challenge. Patients with diabetes are unable to metabolize glucose at a normal rate. The oral glucose tolerance test (OGTT) is used for individuals who are able to eat and who are not known to have problems with gastrointestinal malabsorption. The IV GTT is used for individuals who are unable to tolerate oral glucose.

Glucose, a simple six-carbon sugar (monosaccharide), enters the diet as part of the sugars sucrose, lactose, and maltose and from the complex polysaccharide, dietary starch. The body acquires most of its energy from the oxidative metabolism of glucose. Excess glucose is stored in the liver or in muscle tissue as glycogen. Glucose levels in plasma (one of the components of blood) are generally 10% to 15% higher than glucose measurements in whole blood (and even more after eating). This is important because home blood glucose meters measure the glucose in whole blood, whereas most laboratory tests measure the glucose in either plasma or serum.

Diabetes is a group of diseases characterized by hyperglycemia, or elevated glucose levels. Hyperglycemia can result from a defect in insulin secretion due to destruction of the beta cells of the pancreas (type 1 diabetes), a defect in insulin action, or a combination of defects in secretion and action (type 2 diabetes), or from a specific cause such as gestational diabetes, neonatal hyperglycemia, cystic fibrosis, or hyperglycemia induced by drugs used to treat other medical conditions (e.g., corticosteroids). The chronic hyperglycemia of diabetes over time may lead to damage, dysfunction, and eventually failure of the eyes (retinopathy), kidneys (nephropathy), nerves (neuropathy), heart (cardiovascular disease), and blood vessels (micro- and macrovascular conditions). The American Diabetes Association (ADA) and National Institute of Diabetes and Digestive and Kidney Disease (NIDDK) have established criteria for diagnosing diabetes. For additional information regarding screening guidelines and management of diabetes, refer to the study titled "Glucose."

The ACOG and ADA recommend screening for all pregnant women at 24 to 28 wk of gestation using patient history, clinical risk factors, and carbohydrate challenge testing. Protocol recommendations may vary among requesting HCPs. The ADA and International Association of Diabetes and Pregnancy Study Groups recommend that all women not previously diagnosed with diabetes undergo a 75-g OGTT at 24 to 28 wk of gestation because unrecognized glucose intolerance may have existed prior to the pregnancy, glucose intolerance identified during pregnancy may have continued unmonitored

G

after pregnancy, and the frequency of diabetes in women of childbearing age has dramatically increased. The ADA also recommends a diagnosis of overt, rather than gestational, diabetes if test results meet the criteria for diabetes at the initial prenatal visit. For more information regarding diagnostic criteria for unrecognized diabetes, refer to the study titled "Glucose." There are a number of differences in carbohydrate metabolism between pregnant and nonpregnant women. Glucose levels in the pregnant female with normal glucose metabolism are lower than in the nonpregnant female with normal glucose metabolism *related to insulin-independent demand and uptake of glucose by the placenta and the developing fetus, insulin production by the fetal placenta (creating a higher demand for glucose), and the development of maternal insulin resistance induced by diabetogenic pregnancy hormones to meet the increasing demand for glucose by the fetus (e.g., progesterone, estrogens, and human placental lactogen). Hemoglobin A_{1c} goals are stricter for pregnant females especially in the second and third trimester related to hemodilution and increased RBC turnover, which has the effect of independently decreasing A_{1c}*

INDICATIONS
- Evaluate abnormal fasting or postprandial blood glucose levels that do not clearly indicate diabetes.
- Evaluate glucose metabolism in women of childbearing age, especially women who are pregnant and have (1) a history of previous fetal loss or birth of infants weighing 9 lb or more and/or (2) a family history of diabetes.

- Identify abnormal renal tubular function if glycosuria occurs without hyperglycemia.
- Identify impaired glucose metabolism without overt diabetes.
- Support the diagnosis of hyperthyroidism and liver disease related to alcohol misuse, which are characterized by a sharp rise in blood glucose followed by a decline to subnormal levels.

INTERFERING FACTORS
Contraindications: N/A

Factors that may alter the results of the study
- Drugs and other substances that may increase GTT values include acetylsalicylic acid, atenolol, bendroflumethiazide, caffeine, clofibrate, glyburide, guanethidine, lisinopril, metoprolol, niceritrol, nifedipine, nitrendipine, norethisterone, phenformin, phenobarbital, prazosin, and terazosin.
- Drugs and other substances that may decrease GTT values include acebutolol, beclomethasone, bendroflumethiazide, betamethasone, calcitonin, catecholamines, chlorothiazide, chlorpromazine, chlorthalidone, cimetidine, corticotropin, cortisone, danazol, deflazacort, dexamethasone, diapamide, diethylstilbestrol, ethacrynic acid, fludrocortisone, furosemide, glucagon, glucocorticosteroids, heroin, hydrochlorothiazide, mestranol, methadone, methylprednisolone, muzolimine, niacin, nifedipine, norethindrone, norethynodrel, oral contraceptives, paramethasone, perphenazine, phenolphthalein, phenothiazine, phenytoin, pindolol, prednisolone, prednisone, propranolol, quinethazone, thiazides, triamcinolone, triamterene, and verapamil.
- The test should be performed on ambulatory patients. Impaired

physical activity can lead to falsely increased values.

- Excessive physical activity before or during the test can lead to falsely decreased values.
- Failure of the patient to ingest a diet with sufficient carbohydrate content (e.g., 150 g/day) for at least 3 days before the test can result in falsely decreased values.
- Smoking before or during the test can lead to falsely increased values.

Other considerations

- The patient may have difficulty drinking the extremely sweet glucose beverage and become nauseous. Vomiting during the course of the test will cause the test to be canceled.
- The patient should not be under recent or current physiological stress during the test. If the patient has had recent surgery (less than 2 wk previously), an infectious disease, or a major illness (e.g., myocardial infarction), the test should be delayed or rescheduled.

POTENTIAL MEDICAL DIAGNOSIS: CLINICAL SIGNIFICANCE OF RESULTS

Tolerance Increased in

- Decreased absorption of glucose:
  Adrenal insufficiency (Addison disease, hypopituitarism)
  Hypothyroidism
  Intestinal diseases, such as celiac disease and tropical sprue
  Whipple disease
- Increased insulin secretion:
  Pancreatic islet cell tumor

Tolerance Impaired in

- Increased absorption of glucose:
  Excessive intake of glucose
  Gastrectomy
  Gastroenterostomy
  Hyperthyroidism
  Vagotomy

- Decreased usage of glucose:
  Central nervous system lesions
  Cushing syndrome
  Diabetes
  Hemochromatosis
  Hyperlipidemia
- Decreased glycogenesis:
  Hyperthyroidism
  Infections
  Liver disease (severe)
  Pheochromocytoma
  Pregnancy
  Stress
  Von Gierke disease

NURSING IMPLICATIONS

BEFORE THE STUDY: PLANNING AND IMPLEMENTATION

Teaching the Patient What to Expect

- Inform the patient this test can assist in evaluating blood sugar levels.
- Explain that a blood sample is needed for the test and multiple samples may be required over the course of the test.

Standard OGTT

- The standard OGTT takes 2 hr. A fasting blood glucose is determined before administration of an oral glucose load. If the fasting blood glucose is less than 126 mg/dL, the patient is given an oral glucose load.
- An oral glucose load should not be administered before the value of the fasting specimen has been received. If the fasting blood glucose is greater than 126 mg/dL, the standard glucose load is not administered and the test is canceled.
- The laboratory will follow its protocol as far as notifying the patient of his or her glucose level and the reason the test was canceled.
- The requesting HCP will be issued a report indicating the glucose level and the cancellation of the test.
- A fasting glucose greater than 126 mg/dL indicates diabetes; therefore, the glucose load would never be

administered before allowing the requesting HCP to evaluate the clinical situation.

▶ Adults receive 75 g and children receive 1.75 g/kg ideal weight, not to exceed 75 g. The glucose load should be consumed within 5 min, and time 0 begins as soon as the patient begins to ingest the glucose load.

▶ A second specimen is collected at 2 hr, concluding the test. The test is discontinued if the patient vomits before the second specimen has been collected.

Gestational Screen or Challenge Test

▶ The gestational screen is performed on pregnant women, usually at their first prenatal visit. If results from the screen are abnormal, a gestational GTT is performed.

▶ The gestational screen does not require a fast. The patient is given a 50-g oral glucose load. The glucose load should be consumed within 5 min, and time 0 begins as soon as the patient begins to ingest the glucose load.

▶ A specimen is collected 1 hr after ingestion. The test is discontinued if the patient vomits before the 1-hr specimen has been collected. If the result is normal, the test may be repeated between 24 and 28 wk gestation.

Gestational GTT

▶ The gestational GTT takes 3 hr. A fasting blood glucose is determined before administration of a 75-g or 100-g oral glucose load, depending on the order. If the fasting blood glucose is less than 126 mg/dL, the patient is given an oral glucose load.

▶ An oral glucose load should not be administered before the value of the fasting specimen has been received. *If the fasting blood glucose is greater than 126 mg/dL, the Glucola is not administered and the test is canceled* (see previous explanation).

▶ The glucose load should be consumed within 5 min, and time 0 begins as soon as the patient begins to ingest the glucose load. Subsequent specimens are collected at 1, 2, and 3 hr, concluding the test. The test is discontinued if the patient vomits before all specimens have been collected.

AFTER THE STUDY: POTENTIAL NURSING ACTIONS

Avoiding Complications

▶ Note that the patient may have difficulty drinking the extremely sweet glucose beverage and become nauseous. Vomiting during the course of the test will cause the test to be canceled.

Treatment Considerations

▶ Studies comparing risk for developing diabetes demonstrate that certain populations are disproportionately affected by type 2 diabetes and complications of type 2 diabetes as compared to the general population. Nonmodifiable risk factors include age, ethnicity, and family history of diabetes or metabolic syndrome. The risk of developing type 2 diabetes increases with age. In the United States, affected populations include African Americans, Asian Americans, Hispanics, native Hawaiians and Pacific Islanders, American Indians, and Alaska natives. Modifiable risk factors include lifestyle choices related to making healthy dietary choices, maintaining a healthy body weight, and meeting recommended levels of physical activity. The financial and emotional burdens of diabetes and related complications continue to grow at an alarming rate. A system for the prevention, management, and support of patients with type 2 diabetes should be provided through the coordinated efforts of multidisciplinary partners using strategies that are culturally appropriate.

▶ Provide diabetic education and information regarding the clinical implications of the test results, as appropriate.

▶ Explain to the pregnant patient that untreated gestational diabetes can increase health risks to self and fetus and may resolve after the pregnancy is over but that diabetes may reoccur later in life.

▶ Instruct the patient in the use of home testing strips or meters approved for glucose, ketones, or A_{1c} by the U.S. Food and Drug Administration, if prescribed. Answer any questions or

address any concerns voiced by the patient or family.
- Advise reporting signs and symptoms of hypoglycemia (weakness, confusion, diaphoresis, rapid pulse) or hyperglycemia (thirst, polyuria, hunger, lethargy).
- Emphasize, if indicated, that good glycemic management delays the onset and slows the progression of diabetic retinopathy, nephropathy, and neuropathy.

Nutritional Considerations
- Impaired glucose tolerance may be associated with diabetes. There is no "diabetic diet"; however, many meal-planning approaches with nutritional goals are endorsed by the ADA. Patients who adhere to dietary recommendations report a better general feeling of health, better weight management, better management of glucose and lipid values, and improved

use of insulin. Instruct the patient, as appropriate, in nutritional management of diabetes. A variety of dietary patterns are beneficial for people with diabetes. Encourage consultation with a registered dietitian who is a certified diabetes educator.

Follow-Up, Evaluation, and Desired Outcomes
- Adheres to the recommended medication and dietary plan to manage blood glucose during pregnancy.
- Acknowledges contact information provided for the ADA (www .diabetes.org), American Heart Association (www.heart.org/ HEARTORG), National Heart, Lung, and Blood Institute (www.nhlbi.nih .gov), NIDDK (www.niddk.nih.gov), and U.S. Department of Agriculture's resource for nutrition (www .choosemyplate.gov).

Gonioscopy

SYNONYM/ACRONYM: N/A

RATIONALE: To detect abnormalities in the structure of the anterior chamber of the eye such as in glaucoma.

PATIENT PREPARATION: There are no food, fluid, activity, or medication restrictions unless by medical direction.

NORMAL FINDINGS
- Normal appearance of anterior chamber structures and wide, unblocked, normal angle.

CRITICAL FINDINGS AND POTENTIAL INTERVENTIONS: N/A

OVERVIEW: (Study type: Sensory (ocular); related body system: Nervous system.) Gonioscopy is a technique used for examination of the anterior chamber structures of the eye (i.e., the trabecular meshwork and the anatomical relationship of the trabecular meshwork to the iris). The trabecular meshwork is

the drainage system of the eye, and gonioscopy is performed to determine if the drainage angle is damaged, blocked, or clogged. Gonioscopy in combination with biomicroscopy is considered to be the most thorough basis to confirm a diagnosis of glaucoma and to differentiate between open-angle and angle-closure glaucoma. The angle structures of the anterior chamber are normally not visible because light entering the eye through the cornea is reflected back into the anterior chamber. Placement of a special contact lens (goniolens) over the cornea allows reflected light to pass back through the cornea and onto a reflective mirror in the contact lens. It is in this way that the angle structures can be visualized. There are two types of gonioscopy: indirect and direct. The more commonly used indirect technique employs a mirrored goniolens and biomicroscope. Direct gonioscopy is performed with a gonioscope containing a dome-shaped contact lens known as a *gonioprism*. The gonioprism eliminates internally reflected light, allowing direct visualization of the angle. Interpretation of visual examination is usually documented in a colored hand-drawn diagram. Scheie classification is used to standardize definition of angles based on appearance by gonioscopy. Shaffer classification is based on the angular width of the angle recess.

INDICATIONS

- Assess degenerative conditions of the anterior chamber.
- Assess for hyperpigmentation.
- Assess peripheral anterior synechiae (PAS).
- Assess for the presence of glaucoma (confirmation of normal structures and estimation of angle width).
- Assess for the presence of uveitis.
- Evaluate growth or tumor in the angle.
- Evaluate posttrauma evaluation for angle recession.
- Investigate conditions affecting the ciliary body.
- Investigate suspected neovascularization of the angle.

INTERFERING FACTORS: N/A

POTENTIAL MEDICAL DIAGNOSIS: CLINICAL SIGNIFICANCE OF RESULTS

Scheie Classification Based on Visible Angle Structures

Classification	Appearance
Wide open	All angle structures seen
Grade I narrow	Difficult to see over the iris root
Grade II narrow	Ciliary band obscured
Grade III narrow	Posterior trabeculae hazy
Grade IV narrow	Only Schwalbe line visible

Shaffer Classification Based on Angle Width

Classification	Appearance
Wide open (20°–45°)	Closure improbable
Moderately narrow (10°–20°)	Closure possible
Extremely narrow (less than 10°)	Closure possible
Partially/totally closed	Closure present

Abnormal findings related to
- Corneal endothelial disorders (Fuchs endothelial dystrophy, iridocorneal endothelial syndrome)
- Glaucoma
- Lens disorders (cataract, displaced lens)
- Malignant ocular tumor in angle
- Neovascularization in angle
- Ocular hemorrhage
- PAS
- Schwartz syndrome
- Trauma
- Tumors
- Uveitis

NURSING IMPLICATIONS

BEFORE THE STUDY: PLANNING AND IMPLEMENTATION

Teaching the Patient What to Expect

- Inform the patient this procedure can assist in evaluating the eye for disease.
- Review the procedure with the patient. Address concerns about pain and explain that no pain will be experienced during the test, but there may be moments of discomfort. Some discomfort may be experienced after the test when the numbness wears off from anesthetic drops administered prior to the test.
- Inform the patient that the test is performed by a health-care provider (HCP) specially trained to perform this procedure and takes about 5 min to complete.
- The patient is seated comfortably. Topical anesthetic drops are instilled in each eye and allowed time to work.

- The chin is placed in the chin rest and the forehead gently pressed against the support bar. The patient is asked to open the eyes wide and look at desired target. The ophthalmologist or optometrist places a lens on the eye while a narrow beam of light is focused on the eye.

Potential Nursing Actions

- Investigate health concerns related to known or suspected vision loss or changes in visual acuity, including type and cause, use of glasses or contact lenses, eye conditions with treatment regimens, and eye surgery.
- Instruct the patient to remove contact lenses or glasses, as appropriate, and explain the importance of keeping the eyes open for the test.

AFTER THE STUDY: POTENTIAL NURSING ACTIONS

Treatment Considerations

- Provide information on glaucoma treatment and information regarding the clinical implications of the test results.
- Review implications of abnormal test results on the patient's lifestyle, such as impaired activity or anticipated loss of driving privileges due to loss of visual acuity.

Follow-Up, Evaluation, and Desired Outcomes

- Acknowledges that glaucoma is a leading cause of blindness in the United States. Agrees to seek additional information from the American Academy of Ophthalmology (www.aao.org), American Optometric Association (www.aoa.org/optometrists), National Eye Institute (https://nei.nih.gov/health/glaucoma), and All About Vision (www.allaboutvision.com/conditions/glaucoma.htm).

Gram Stain

SYNONYM/ACRONYM: N/A

RATIONALE: To provide a quick identification of gram-negative or gram-positive organisms to assist in medical management.

PATIENT PREPARATION: There are no food, fluid, activity, or medication restrictions unless by medical direction.

NORMAL FINDINGS: N/A

CRITICAL FINDINGS AND POTENTIAL INTERVENTIONS
• Any positive results in blood, cerebrospinal fluid, or any body cavity fluid.

Timely notification to the requesting health-care provider (HCP) of any critical findings and related symptoms is a role expectation of the professional nurse. A listing of these findings varies among facilities.

OVERVIEW: (Study type: Blood, biopsy specimen, or body fluid as collected for culture; related body system: Immune and Multi-system.) Gram stain is a technique commonly used to identify bacterial organisms on the basis of their specific staining characteristics. The method involves smearing a small amount of specimen on a slide, and then exposing it to gentian or crystal violet, iodine, alcohol, and safranin O. Gram-positive bacteria retain the gentian or crystal violet and iodine stain complex after a decolorization step and appear purple-blue in color. Gram-negative bacteria do not retain the stain after decolorization but can pick up the pink color of the safranin O counterstain. Gram stains provide information regarding the adequacy of a sample. For example, a sputum Gram stain showing greater than 25 squamous epithelial cells per low-power field, regardless of the number of polymorphonuclear white blood cells, indicates contamination of the specimen with saliva, and the specimen should be rejected for subsequent culture. Gram stains are reviewed over a number of fields for an impression of the quantity of organisms present, which reflects the extent of infection. For example, a Gram stain of unspun urine showing the occasional presence of bacteria per low-power field suggests a correlating colony count of 10,000 bacteria/mL, while the presence of bacteria in most fields is clinically significant and suggests greater than 100,000 bacteria/mL of urine. Gram stain results should be correlated with culture and sensitivity results to interpret the significance of isolated organisms and to select appropriate antibiotic therapy.

INDICATIONS
• Provide a rapid determination of the acceptability of the specimen for further analysis.
• Provide rapid, presumptive information about the type of potential pathogen present in the specimen (i.e., gram-positive bacteria, gram-negative bacteria, or yeast).

INTERFERING FACTORS
Factors that may alter the results of the study
• Very young, very old, or dead cultures may react atypically to the Gram stain technique.

POTENTIAL MEDICAL DIAGNOSIS: CLINICAL SIGNIFICANCE OF RESULTS

Gram Positive

Actinomadura	Actinomyces	Bacillus	Clostridium	Corynebacterium
Enterococcus	Erysipelothrix	Lactobacillus	Listeria	Micrococcus
Mycobacterium (gram variable)	Peptostreptococcus	Propionibacterium	Rhodococcus	Staphylococcus
Streptococcus				

Gram Negative

Acinetobacter	Aeromonas	Alcaligenes	Bacteroides	Bordetella
Borrelia	Brucella	Campylobacter	Citrobacter	Chlamydia
Enterobacter	Escherichia	Flavobacterium	Francisella	Fusobacterium
Gardnerella	Haemophilus	Helicobacter	Klebsiella	Legionella
Leptospira	Moraxella	Neisseria	Pasteurella	Plesiomonas
Porphyromonas	Prevotella	Proteus	Pseudomonas	Rickettsia
Salmonella	Serratia	Shigella	Vibrio	Xanthomonas
Yersinia				

Acid Fast or Partial Acid Fast

Nocardia   *Mycobacterium*

Note: *Treponema* species are classified as gram-negative spirochetes, but they are most often visualized using dark-field or silver-staining techniques.

NURSING IMPLICATIONS

BEFORE THE STUDY: PLANNING AND IMPLEMENTATION

Teaching the Patient What to Expect
◗ Inform the patient this test can assist in identifying the presence of pathogenic organisms.
◗ Review the procedure with the patient. Inform the patient that the time it takes to collect a proper specimen varies according to the patient's level of cooperation as well as the specimen collection site.

◗ Address concerns about pain and explain that there may be some discomfort during the procedure.
◗ Specific collection instructions are found in the associated culture studies.

AFTER THE STUDY: POTENTIAL NURSING ACTIONS

Treatment Considerations
◗ Administer antibiotics as ordered, and instruct the patient in the importance of completing the entire course of antibiotic therapy even if no symptoms are present.
◗ Address concerns about pain or fever and interventional options to address each issue.

Follow-Up, Evaluation, and Desired Outcomes
◗ Recognizes the importance of strict adherence to the HCP's therapeutic regime in order to resolve any identified infectious process.

Group A Streptococcal Screen

SYNONYM/ACRONYM: Strep screen, rapid strep screen, direct strep screen.

RATIONALE: To detect a group A streptococcal infection such as strep throat.

PATIENT PREPARATION: There are no food, fluid, activity, or medication restrictions unless by medical direction.

NORMAL FINDINGS: (Method: Enzyme immunoassay or latex agglutination) Negative.

CRITICAL FINDINGS AND POTENTIAL INTERVENTIONS: N/A

OVERVIEW: (Study type: Body fluid, throat swab [two swabs should be submitted so that a culture can be performed if the screen is negative]; **related body system:** Immune and Respiratory systems.) Rheumatic fever is a possible sequela to an untreated streptococcal infection. Early diagnosis and treatment appear to lessen the seriousness of symptoms during the acute phase and overall duration of the infection and sequelae. The onset of strep throat is sudden and includes symptoms such as chills, headache, sore throat, malaise, and exudative gray-white patches on the tonsils or pharynx. The group A streptococcal screen should not be ordered unless the results would be available within 1 to 2 hr of specimen collection to make rapid, effective therapeutic decisions. A positive result can be a reliable basis for the initiation of therapy. A negative result is presumptive for infection and should be backed up by culture results. In general, specimens showing growth of less than 10 colonies on culture yield negative results by the rapid screening method. Evidence of group A streptococci disappears rapidly after the initiation of antibiotic therapy. A nucleic acid probe method has also been developed for rapid detection of group A streptococci.

INDICATIONS
- Assist in the rapid determination of the presence of group A streptococci.

INTERFERING FACTORS
Factors that may alter the results of the study
- Polyester (rayon or Dacron) swabs are favored over cotton for best chance of detection. Fatty acids are created on cotton fibers during the sterilization process. Detectable target antigens on the streptococcal cell wall are destroyed without killing the organism when there is contact between the specimen and the fatty acids on the cotton collection swab. False-negative test results can be obtained on specimens collected with cotton tip swabs. Negative strep screens should always be followed with a traditional culture.

Other considerations
- Sensitivity of the method varies among manufacturers.
- Adequate specimen collection in children may be difficult to achieve, which explains the higher

percentage of false-negative results in this age group.

POTENTIAL MEDICAL DIAGNOSIS: CLINICAL SIGNIFICANCE OF RESULTS
Positive findings in
- Rheumatic fever
- Scarlet fever
- Strep throat
- Streptococcal glomerulonephritis
- Tonsillitis

NURSING IMPLICATIONS

BEFORE THE STUDY: PLANNING AND IMPLEMENTATION

Teaching the Patient What to Expect
- Inform the patient this test can assist in identifying a streptococcal infection.
- Explain that a throat swab is needed for the test. Address concerns about pain and explain that there may be some discomfort during the swabbing procedure.

Potential Nursing Actions
- Vigorous swabbing of both tonsillar pillars and the posterior throat enhances the probability of streptococcal antigen detection.
- Obtain a history of prior antibiotic therapy.

AFTER THE STUDY: POTENTIAL NURSING ACTIONS

Treatment Considerations
- Infection prevention and treatment are important during any illness. Emphasize the value of good hand hygiene and assist with hygiene as needed. Adhere to standard precautions and obtain ordered cultures. Monitor and trend temperatures and associated laboratory values (white blood cells, C-reactive protein).
- Serious throat infection and inflammation can impinge on airway patency. A key intervention to decrease this risk is to administer ordered antibiotics and emphasize the importance of completing the entire course of antibiotic

G

therapy even if no symptoms are present. Other potential interventions are to assess respiratory rate, rhythm, depth, and accessory muscle use and to administer prescribed oxygen with humidification and pulse oximetry to evaluate oxygenation.

Follow-Up, Evaluation, and Desired Outcomes
▶ Collaborates with health-care provider to develop a plan of care that supports health, including adherence to the recommended medication regime and adherence to follow-up appointments.

Growth Hormone, Stimulation and Suppression Tests

SYNONYM/ACRONYM: Somatotropic hormone, somatotropin, GH, hGH.

RATIONALE: To assess pituitary function and evaluate the amount of secreted growth hormone (GH) to assist in diagnosing diseases such as giantism and dwarfism.

PATIENT PREPARATION: There are no medication restrictions unless by medical direction. The patient should fast and avoid strenuous exercise for 12 hr before specimen collection. Protocols may vary depending on the type of induction used.

NORMAL FINDINGS: Method: Immunoassay.

Growth Hormone

Age	Conventional Units	SI Units (Conventional Units × 1)
Cord blood	8–40 ng/mL	8–40 mcg/L
1 d	5–50 ng/mL	5–50 mcg/L
1 wk	5–25 ng/mL	5–25 mcg/L
Child	2–10 ng/mL	2–10 mcg/L
Adult		
Male	0–5 ng/mL	0–5 mcg/L
Female	0–10 ng/mL	0–10 mcg/L
Male older than 60 yr	0–10 ng/mL	0–10 mcg/L
Female older than 60 yr	0–14 ng/mL	0–14 mcg/L
Stimulation Tests		
Rise above baseline	Greater than 5 ng/mL	Greater than 5 mcg/L
Peak response	Greater than 10 ng/mL	Greater than 10 mcg/L
Suppression Tests	0–2 ng/mL	0–2 mcg/L

CRITICAL FINDINGS AND POTENTIAL INTERVENTIONS: N/A

OVERVIEW: (Study type: Blood collected in a gold-, red-, or red/gray-top tube; related body system: Endocrine system.) GH is secreted in episodic bursts by the anterior pituitary gland; the highest level is usually secreted during deep sleep. Release of GH is modulated by three hypothalamic factors: GH-releasing hormone, GH-releasing peptide-6, and GH inhibitory hormone (also known as *somatostatin*). The effects of GH are carried out by insulin-like growth factors, formerly called *somatomedins*. GH plays an integral role in growth from birth to puberty. GH promotes skeletal growth by stimulating hepatic production of proteins; it also affects lipid and glucose metabolism. Random levels are rarely useful because secretion of GH is episodic and pulsatile. Stimulation tests with arginine, glucagon, insulin, or L-dopa, as well as suppression tests with glucose, provide useful information.

INDICATIONS

- Assist in the diagnosis of acromegaly in adults.
- Assist in establishing a diagnosis of dwarfism or growth delay in children with decreased GH levels, indicative of a pituitary cause.
- Assist in establishing a diagnosis of gigantism in children with GH increased levels, indicative of a pituitary cause.
- Detect suspected disorder associated with decreased GH.
- Monitor response to treatment of growth delay.

INTERFERING FACTORS

Factors that may alter the results of the study

- Drugs and other substances that may increase GH levels include alanine, anabolic steroids, angiotensin II, apomorphine, arginine, clonidine, corticotropin, cyclic AMP, desipramine, dexamethasone, dopamine, galanin, glucagon, GH-releasing hormone, hydrazine, levodopa, methamphetamine, methyldopa, metoclopramide, midazolam, niacin, oral contraceptives, phenytoin, propranolol, and vasopressin.
- Drugs and other substances that may decrease GH levels include corticosteroids, corticotropin, hydrocortisone, octreotide, and pirenzepine.

POTENTIAL MEDICAL DIAGNOSIS: CLINICAL SIGNIFICANCE OF RESULTS

Increased in

Production of GH is modulated by numerous factors, including stress, exercise, sleep, nutrition, and response to circulating levels of GH.

- Acromegaly
- Anorexia nervosa
- Chronic kidney disease
- Cirrhosis
- Diabetes (unmanaged)
- Ectopic GH secretion (tumors of stomach, lung)
- Exercise
- Gigantism (pituitary)
- Hyperpituitarism
- Laron dwarfism
- Malnutrition
- Stress

Decreased in

- Adrenocortical hyperfunction *(inhibits secretion of GH)*
- Dwarfism (pituitary) *(related to GH deficiency)*
- Hypopituitarism *(related to lack of production)*

G

NURSING IMPLICATIONS

BEFORE THE STUDY: PLANNING AND IMPLEMENTATION

Teaching the Patient What to Expect

◗ Inform the patient this test can assist in assessing the amount of GH secreted.
◗ Explain that a blood sample is needed for the test and multiple samples may be required.
◗ Test samples may be requested at baseline and 30-, 60-, 90-, and 120-min intervals after stimulation and at baseline and 60- and 120-min intervals after suppression.
◗ Patients may be allowed to walk around, or they may be required to be recumbent.

Potential Nursing Actions

◗ Record pertinent information related to diet, sleep pattern, and activity at the time of the test.

AFTER THE STUDY: POTENTIAL NURSING ACTIONS

Treatment Considerations

◗ Advise resumption of the usual diet, fluids, medications, and activity, as directed by the HCP.

Follow-Up, Evaluation, and Desired Outcomes

◗ Understands that additional testing may be necessary to evaluate or monitor disease progression and determine the need for a change in therapy.

G

Ham Test for Paroxysmal Nocturnal Hemoglobinuria

SYNONYM/ACRONYM: Acid hemolysis test for PNH.

RATIONALE: To assist in diagnosing a rare condition called *paroxysmal nocturnal hemoglobinuria* (PNH), wherein red blood cells (RBCs) undergo lysis during and after sleep with hemoglobin excreted in the urine.

PATIENT PREPARATION: There are no food, fluid, activity, or medication restrictions unless by medical direction.

NORMAL FINDINGS: (Method: Acidified hemolysis) No hemolysis seen.

CRITICAL FINDINGS AND POTENTIAL INTERVENTIONS: N/A

OVERVIEW: (Study type: Blood collected in lavender-top [EDTA] tube and serum collected in red-top tube; related body system: Circulatory system.) PNH is a rare condition in which the patient experiences nocturnal hemoglobinuria, chronic hemolytic anemia, diminished or absent generation of new RBCs, and a tendency to thrombose. It is not considered a primary disease in and of itself but rather a secondary condition caused by an acquired defect in hematopoietic stem cells. Specifically, PNH occurs through acquired mutations in the PIGA gene (phosphatidylinositol glycan anchor biosynthesis, class A) that eventually result in absence of glycosylphosphatidylinositol (GPI) anchor proteins on cell surfaces of damaged stem cell progeny. Normally, the GPI anchor proteins attach a numerous variety of proteins to the cell membrane so they are available when needed. It is believed that PNH is caused by complement-mediated cellular lysis that occurs in the absence of GPI-anchored complement inhibitors. The gene can have multiple mutations acquired throughout a person's lifetime and can occur in all three cell types (RBCs, white blood cells [WBCs], and platelets), although the type affecting the RBCs is the easiest to identify by the presence of corresponding symptoms. It was originally thought that the nighttime hemolysis was initiated by a state of acidosis that occurred during sleep. This theory was later disproved, and the prevailing logic is that hemolysis takes place continuously. The hematuria is more noticeable when the accumulated contents of the bladder are passed in the morning and the color of the concentrated urine is dramatically different than that seen during the day. The disease affects males and females equally because the mutations take place in somatic or body cells rather than in germ cells, which are then inherited. Symptoms of the disease usually manifest between the ages of 20 and 40 yr. PNH is frequently associated with aplastic anemia. It has also been associated with myelodysplasia, which may point to bone marrow failure syndromes as a condition that favors exposure of GPI anchor protein–deficient hematopoietic stem cells.

In patients with PNH, erythrocytes have an increased sensitivity to complement and will lyse when mixed with acidified control serum that contains complement. The patient's RBCs are also mixed with fresh, normal serum that is

H

ABO compatible with the patient's cells. Some of the control serum is acidified, and some is heated to inactivate the complement. The result is positive if 10% to 50% cell lysis occurs in the samples mixed with patient and control acidified serum. No hemolysis should occur in the heated control serum.

The sugar water or sucrose hemolysis test can also be performed to investigate the presence of PNH. Low-ionic-strength isotonic sucrose will cause serum globulin to fix complement on the RBC surface. When a small amount of type-specific serum and sucrose solution is added to a sample of the patient's washed RBCs, PNH RBCs will be lysed compared to type-specific serum and sucrose added to washed normal control RBCs. Platelet and granulocyte membranes are affected as well, but RBC hemolysis in a positive test is clear evidence of PNH. Greater than 5% hemolysis is considered positive for PNH.

Flow cytometry has replaced the Ham test as the definitive test for PNH. Levels of CD55 and CD59, membrane glycoproteins that regulate complement, on WBC and RBC surfaces are measured using flow cytometry. CD59 is more prevalent in the membrane than CD55, and the use of both is effective in identifying small and large clones of PNH cells. The findings are described as type I PNH cells, which have normal levels of both proteins; type II PNH cells, which have reduced levels; and type III PNH cells, which demonstrate an absence of CD55 and CD59 proteins. Testing is more accurately accomplished using WBCs, because the life of circulating WBCs is normal in PNH, whereas the life of PNH RBCs is

considerably shortened by chronic hemolysis, especially for PNH type III RBCs. Another advantage of WBC studies over RBC is that PNH RBCs are diluted by transfusion, one of the therapeutic modalities used to treat the anemia of PNH.

The treatment strategies for PNH depend on the type and degree of affect. Treatments are limited, and there is a need for improvement in treatment options. While transfusions are effectively used to treat the anemia of PNH, iron overload is a significant consideration in the administration of serial blood cell transfusions.

INDICATIONS
- Evaluate hemolytic anemia, especially with hemosiderinuria.
- Evaluate suspected congenital dyserythropoietic anemia, type II (also known as HEMPAS [*h*ereditary *e*rythroblastic *m*ultinuclearity with *p*ositive *a*cidified *s*erum test]).
- Evaluate suspected PNH.

INTERFERING FACTORS
Factors that may alter the results of the study
- False positives may occur in the presence of other disorders, such as aplastic anemia, HEMPAS, hereditary or acquired spherocytosis, leukemia, and myeloproliferative syndromes. False positives may also occur with aged RBCs. The sugar water test is negative in HEMPAS.
- False negatives can occur if the patient's serum sample contains a low level of complement.

POTENTIAL MEDICAL DIAGNOSIS: CLINICAL SIGNIFICANCE OF RESULTS
Increased in
- Congenital dyserythropoietic anemia, type II
- PNH

Decreased in: N/A

BEFORE THE STUDY: PLANNING AND IMPLEMENTATION

Teaching the Patient What to Expect

◗ Inform the patient this test can assist in testing for causes of anemia.

◗ Explain that a blood sample is needed for the test.

AFTER THE STUDY: POTENTIAL NURSING ACTIONS

Follow-Up, Evaluation, and Desired Outcomes

◗ Understands that additional testing may be necessary to evaluate or monitor disease progression and determine the need for a change in therapy.

Haptoglobin

SYNONYM/ACRONYM: Hapto, HP, Hp.

RATIONALE: To assist in evaluating for intravascular hemolysis related to transfusion reactions, chronic liver disease, hemolytic anemias, and tissue inflammation or destruction.

PATIENT PREPARATION: There are no food, fluid, activity, or medication restrictions unless by medical direction.

NORMAL FINDINGS: Method: Immunoturbidimetric.

Age	Conventional Units	SI Units (Conventional Units × 0.01)
Newborn	5–48 mg/dL (levels may be undetectable at birth)	0.05–0.48 g/L (levels may be undetectable at birth)
6 mo–16 yr	25–138 mg/dL (adult levels are reached by 1 yr)	0.25–1.38 g/L (adult levels are reached by 1 yr)
Adult	15–200 mg/dL	0.15–2 g/L

CRITICAL FINDINGS AND POTENTIAL INTERVENTIONS: N/A

OVERVIEW: (Study type: Blood collected in a gold-, red-, or red/gray-top tube; **related body system:** Circulatory/Hematopoietic and Digestive systems.) Haptoglobin is an α_2-globulin produced in the liver. It binds with the free hemoglobin released when red blood cells (RBCs) are lysed. The complexed hemoglobin is then removed from circulation by the spleen. Haptoglobin is used as a marker for intravascular hemolysis because the amount of free hemoglobin from a significant number of lysed RBCs will exceed the amount of haptoglobin normally available for binding. In conditions such as hemolytic anemia (e.g., drug induced, inherited, acute transfusion reaction), the liver is unable to compensate, so consumption exceeds production and haptoglobin levels are decreased.

INDICATIONS

- Assist in the investigation of suspected transfusion reaction.
- Evaluate known or suspected chronic liver disease, as indicated by decreased levels of haptoglobin.
- Evaluate known or suspected disorders characterized by excessive RBC hemolysis, as indicated by decreased levels of haptoglobin.
- Evaluate known or suspected disorders involving a diffuse inflammatory process or tissue destruction, as indicated by elevated levels of haptoglobin.

INTERFERING FACTORS

Factors that may alter the results of the study

- Drugs and other substances that may increase haptoglobin levels include anabolic steroids and danazol.
- Drugs and other substances that may decrease haptoglobin levels include aminosalicylic acid, chlorpromazine, dapsone, dextran, diphenhydramine, furazolidone, isoniazid, nitrofurantoin, norethindrone, oral contraceptives, quinidine, resorcinol, stibophen, tamoxifen, and tripelennamine.

POTENTIAL MEDICAL DIAGNOSIS: CLINICAL SIGNIFICANCE OF RESULTS

Increased in

Haptoglobin is an acute-phase reactant protein, and any condition that stimulates an acute-phase response will result in elevations of haptoglobin.

- Biliary obstruction
- Disorders involving tissue destruction, such as cancers, burns, and acute myocardial infarction
- Infection or inflammatory diseases, such as ulcerative colitis, arthritis, and pyelonephritis
- Tumors
- Steroid therapy

Decreased in

- Autoimmune hemolysis *(related to increased excretion rate of haptoglobin bound to free hemoglobin; rate of excretion exceeds the liver's immediate ability to replenish)*
- Hemolysis due to drug reaction *(related to increased excretion rate of haptoglobin bound to free hemoglobin; rate of excretion exceeds the liver's immediate ability to replenish)*
- Hemolysis due to mechanical destruction (e.g., artificial heart valves, contact sports, subacute bacterial endocarditis) *(related to increased excretion rate of haptoglobin bound to free hemoglobin; rate of excretion exceeds the liver's immediate ability to replenish)*
- Hemolysis due to RBC membrane or metabolic defects *(related to increased excretion rate of haptoglobin bound to free hemoglobin; rate of excretion exceeds the liver's immediate ability to replenish)*
- Hemolysis due to transfusion reaction *(related to increased excretion rate of haptoglobin bound to free hemoglobin; rate of excretion exceeds the liver's immediate ability to replenish)*
- Hypersplenism *(related to increased excretion rate of haptoglobin bound to free hemoglobin due to increased RBC destruction; rate of excretion exceeds the liver's immediate ability to replenish)*
- Ineffective hematopoiesis due to conditions such as folate deficiency or hemoglobinopathies *(related to decreased numbers of RBCs or dysfunctional binding in the presence of abnormal hemoglobins)*
- Liver disease *(related to decreased production)*
- Pregnancy *(related to effect of estrogen)*

NURSING IMPLICATIONS

BEFORE THE STUDY: PLANNING AND IMPLEMENTATION

Teaching the Patient What to Expect
◗ Inform the patient this test can assist with evaluating causes of RBC loss.
◗ Explain that a blood sample is needed for the test.

AFTER THE STUDY: POTENTIAL NURSING ACTIONS

Avoiding Complications
◗ Instruct the patient receiving blood products to immediately report symptoms of a transfusion reaction, including chills, fever, flushing, back pain, or rapid heartbeat, to the health-care provider.

Treatment Considerations
◗ RBC loss can contribute to anemia and associated nursing problems. Observe the patient closely for fatigue, changing oxygenation, altered level of consciousness, confusion, and fall and injury risk associated with these issues.

Follow-Up, Evaluation, and Desired Outcomes
◗ Understands that additional testing may be necessary to quickly evaluate, monitor, and treat a suspected transfusion reaction.

Helicobacter Pylori Testing

SYNONYM/ACRONYM: *H. pylori.* antibody test; *H. pylori* stool antigen test; *H. pylori* breath test; urea breath test (UBT) PY test; C-14 urea breath test; rapid urease test (RUT is also known as the CLO, or Campylobacter-like organism test).

RATIONALE: To assist in diagnosing a gastrointestinal infection and ulceration of the stomach or duodenum related to a *H. pylori* infection.

PATIENT PREPARATION: Instruct the patient to fast and restrict fluids for 6 to 8 hr prior to the UBT or tissue biopsy procedure. Additionally, patients scheduled for a UBT, stool antigen test, or tissue biopsy and culture may be instructed to avoid the use of proton pump inhibitors (e.g., omeprazole, lansoprazole, esomeprazole), antacids, antibiotics, or oral bismuth subsalicylate (Pepto-Bismol); instructions for withholding medications are by medical direction. Protocols may vary among facilities.

NORMAL FINDINGS: Method: Enzyme immunoassay for stool antigen test, negative. UBT: Less than 50 dpm (disintegrations per minute) is considered a negative finding. Tissue biopsy and culture, negative for *H. pylori*.

CRITICAL FINDINGS AND POTENTIAL INTERVENTIONS: N/A

OVERVIEW: (Study type: Stool for antigen testing; nuclear scan for urea breath analysis; endoscopy for stomach tissue biopsy with microscopic examination and culture of tissue; related body system: Digestive and Immune systems.) *H. pylori* is a bacterium that can infect the stomach lining and interfere with the ability of the stomach lining to produce mucous. There is a strong association between *H. pylori* infection and gastric cancer, duodenal and gastric ulcer, and chronic gastritis. Tests recommended for diagnosis and therapeutic monitoring of *H. pylori* infection include the stool antigen and urea breath tests. These two tests provide noninvasive, rapid results and are recommended by the American Gastroenterological Association and the American College of Gastroenterology as tests appropriate for diagnosis and confirmation that the infection has been effectively treated and the bacteria have been eliminated. The presence of *H. pylori* can also be demonstrated in endoscopic tissue biopsy samples or tissue cultures; drawbacks include the invasive specimen collection procedure, the time required to prepare and examine the tissue, and the time required to produce culture results. Blood tests for antibodies to *H. pylori* are available but seldom requested because they are no longer considered to be clinically useful. Patients with symptoms and evidence of *H. pylori* infection are considered to be infected with the organism; patients who demonstrate evidence of *H. pylori* but are without symptoms are said to be colonized.

The C-14 UBT is an accurate way to identify the presence of *H. pylori*. It is a simple, noninvasive diagnostic nuclear medicine procedure that requires the patient to swallow a small amount of radiopharmaceutical C-14–labelled urea in a capsule with lukewarm water. In the presence of urease, an enzyme secreted by *H. pylori* in the gut, the urea in the capsule is broken down into nitrogen and C-14– labelled carbon dioxide (CO_2). The labelled CO_2 is absorbed through the stomach lining into the blood and excreted by the lungs. Breath samples are collected 10 to 15 min after the capsule has been ingested and trapped in a Mylar balloon. The C-14 urea is counted and quantitated with a liquid scintillation counter. The UBT can also be used to indicate the elimination of *H. pylori* infection after treatment with antibiotics. When the organism has been effectively treated with antibiotics, the test changes from positive to negative.

A stool antigen test may be used to identify the presence of *H. pylori*. This is an accurate test and may be requested for patients who are unable to cooperate for the UBT.

Examination of tissue biopsy, obtained by endoscopy, from the lining of the stomach is another way to identify the presence of *H. pylori*. Biopsy specimens may be taken from multiple sites of the stomach lining, such as the lesser and greater curvatures of the antrum (each in close proximity to the pylorus), the lesser curvature of the corpus, the middle of the greater curvature of the corpus, and the incisura angularis. The samples are tested for urease activity and are histologically examined for the presence of inflammatory epithelial cells in the presence of the characteristically curve-shaped *H. pylori* bacteria. Additionally, tissue samples or brushings may be cultured for the presence of *H. pylori*. Sensitivity testing of positive cultures is helpful in identifying the most effective antibiotic, especially in patients who do not respond to therapy.

INDICATIONS

- Aid in detection of *H. pylori* infection in the stomach.
- Assist in differentiating between *H. pylori* infection and NSAID use as the cause of gastritis or peptic or duodenal ulcer.
- Assist in establishing a diagnosis of gastritis, gastric cancer, or peptic or duodenal ulcer.
- Monitor eradication of *H. pylori* infection following treatment regimen.
- Evaluate new-onset dyspepsia.

INTERFERING FACTORS

Contraindications

✷ Patients who are pregnant or suspected of being pregnant, unless the potential benefits far outweigh the risk of an endoscopic procedure or radiation exposure to the fetus and mother.

✷ Patients who have taken antibiotics, Pepto-Bismol, or bismuth in the past 30 days.

✷ Patients who have taken sucralfate in the past 14 days.

✷ Patients who have used a proton pump inhibitor within the past 14 days.

Other considerations

- Patients who have had resective gastric surgery have the potential for resultant bacterial overgrowth (non–*H. pylori* urease), which can cause a false-positive result.
- Achlorhydria can cause a false-positive result.

POTENTIAL MEDICAL DIAGNOSIS: CLINICAL SIGNIFICANCE OF RESULTS

Positive findings in

Stool Antigen Test, Direct Examination of Stomach Tissue, or Culture of Tissue Samples
- *H. pylori* infection
- *H. pylori* colonization

Urea Breath Test
- Indeterminate for *H. pylori:* 50 to 199 dpm.
- Positive for *H. pylori:* Greater than 200 dpm.

NURSING IMPLICATIONS

BEFORE THE STUDY: PLANNING AND IMPLEMENTATION

Teaching the Patient What to Expect

▶ Inform the patient that the test is used to assist in the diagnosis of *H. pylori* infection in patients with duodenal and gastric disease; it is also used for monitoring therapy and documentation that the infection has been healed.

▶ Explain that the sample required will depend on the health-care provider (HCP)'s choice of test (e.g. stool, tissue, or breath).

Stool Antigen Test

▶ Instruct the patient or caregiver to collect a solid stool sample in a clean, leakproof plastic container. Watery or diarrheal specimens are not acceptable.

Urea Breath Test

▶ Review the procedure with the patient. Address concerns about pain and explain that there should be no discomfort during the procedure.

▶ Explain that the procedure is done in the nuclear medicine department by technologists and support staff and usually takes approximately 30 to 60 min.

▶ Pregnancy is a general contraindication to procedures involving radiation. Explain to the female patient that she will be asked the date of her last menstrual period and pregnancy testing may be performed to determine the possibility of pregnancy before she is exposed to radiation.

▶ Reassure the patient that the radionuclide poses no radioactive hazard and rarely produces adverse effects.

▶ Explain that at the beginning of the procedure, a breath sample will be obtained by blowing into a balloon.

H

▶ Next, the patient will be instructed to swallow the C-14 capsule directly from a cup, followed by 20 mL of lukewarm water. An additional 20 mL of lukewarm water is to be drunk 3 min after the dose.

▶ Breath samples will be taken at different periods of time. Patients will be instructed to take in a deep breath and hold it for approximately 5 to 10 sec before exhaling through a straw into a Mylar balloon.

▶ Samples from the balloon are counted on a scintillation counter and recorded in disintegrations per minute.

Potential Nursing Actions

Endoscopic Biopsy Sample

▶ The laboratory should be consulted regarding the appropriate transport container, preservative, or culture medium for tissue samples.

AFTER THE STUDY: POTENTIAL NURSING ACTIONS

Treatment Considerations

▶ Chronic pain and emotional factors associated with illness can contribute to fatigue. When fatigue is present, pace activities to preserve energy stores, identify what aggravates and decreases fatigue, and assess for physiologic factors such as anemia. Monitor for black tarry stools that are indicative of bleeding, and facilitate

interventions such as blood transfusion or antiemetic and antidiarrheal medication.

▶ Facilitate adequate pain management to identify the best modality to provide relief. Administer ordered proton pump inhibitors, antibiotics, H_2 receptor antagonists, and antacids.

Safety Considerations

▶ The patient who is pregnant or breastfeeding should consult with the requesting HCP regarding alternate testing that does not involve radiation. The safety of some C-14 UBT methods for pregnant or lactating women is not well established. The C-13 test is nonradioactive and considered safe for pediatric patients, pregnant patients, or patients who are breastfeeding.

Nutritional Considerations

▶ Encourage the avoidance of alcoholic and caffeinated beverages. Consider consultation with a registered dietitian to assess cultural food selections and barriers to eating.

Follow-Up, Evaluation, and Desired Outcomes

▶ Acknowledges education provided regarding the disease, factors that can trigger symptoms, and possible treatment options that may include surgery.

▶ Understands that a positive test result constitutes an independent risk factor for gastric cancer.

Hemoglobin A_{1c}

SYNONYM/ACRONYM: A_{1c}, glycated hemoglobin (Hgb), glycohemoglobin.

RATIONALE: To identify individuals with diabetes and to monitor treatment in individuals with diabetes by evaluating their long-term glycemic management.

PATIENT PREPARATION: There are no food, fluid, activity, or medication restrictions unless by medical direction.

NORMAL FINDINGS: Method: Chromatography
Values vary widely by method. The recommended treatment goal assumes the use of a standardized test, as referenced to the National Glycohemoglobin Standardization Program—Diabetes Control and Complications Trial, and the absence of clinical conditions such as hemoglobinopathies, anemias, and kidney and liver diseases known to affect the accuracy of the test results.

Recommended Goals for Monitoring Glycemic Management Using Hgb A$_{1c}$

	A$_{1c}$%
Children and adolescents (applicable to all ages in the pediatric category; however, goals should be individualized especially for type 1 diabetes, and special consideration should be given to age-related lack of awareness for hypoglycemia when setting goals)	Less than 7.5%
Pregnant females without hypoglycemia (goals are stricter for pregnant females, especially in the second and third trimesters, *related to hemodilution and increased red blood cell (RBC) turnover which has the effect of independently decreasing A$_{1c}$*)	6%–6.5%
Nonpregnant adults with or without diabetes who do not experience significant hypoglycemia **(see table note)**	Less than 7%
Diabetes (stricter goals are reasonably recommended for certain individuals with diabetes, e.g., those who are otherwise healthy, are newly diagnosed, are type 2 diabetics being treated with lifestyle adjustments and limited oral antidiabetes medications such as metformin to lower glucose levels, have not yet developed complications related to diabetes, do not experience significant hypoglycemia)	6.5% or less
Diabetes (less strict goals are reasonably recommended for certain individuals with diabetes, e.g., those who have been diagnosed with diabetes for a lengthy period of time and have been unsuccessful achieving lower A$_{1c}$ goals; have complications related to diabetes; have one or more comorbidities; have a short life expectancy; are being treated with multiple antidiabetes medications, including insulin, to lower glucose levels; have a documented history of hypoglycemia)	Less than 8%

Age, ethnicity, and hemoglobinopathies are variables that independently affect blood glucose levels, thereby also affecting A$_{1c}$ levels and the approach to glycemic management. A$_{1c}$ goals for persons with diabetes are set and monitored by the health-care provider (HCP) in collaboration with the patient. Goals are based on a variety of factors that include the number of years diagnosed with diabetes, identification of complications related to diabetes, identification of comorbidities, evidence of hypoglycemia, life expectancy based on risk factors, recommended therapies, ability to access resources required to support the treatment plan, level of available and dependable support (e.g., for pediatric patients, patients with language barriers, or patients with intellectual, emotional, or physical impairments).

Abridged from American Diabetes Association. Standards of Medical Care in Diabetes. (2018). *Diabetes Care, 41*(Suppl. 1):S1–S159.

CRITICAL FINDINGS AND POTENTIAL INTERVENTIONS: N/A

OVERVIEW: (**Study type:** Blood collected in a lavender-top [EDTA] tube; **related body system:** Circulatory and Endocrine systems.) Hgb A$_{1c}$, also known as *glycosylated* or *glycated Hgb*, is the combination of glucose and Hgb into a ketamine; the rate at which this occurs is proportional to glucose concentration. The average life span of an RBC is approximately 120 days; measurement of glycated Hgb is a way to monitor long-term diabetic management. A change of 1% in the A$_{1c}$ is roughly equivalent to a change in glucose concentration of 29 mg/dL or 1.6 mmol/L. The average plasma glucose can be estimated using the formula (mg/dL) = [(A$_{1c}$ × 28.7) – 46.7].

The same formula can be used to convert the estimated average glucose (eAG) to glucose in SI units (after multiplying the eAG by 0.555 to convert from mg/dL to mmol/L). For example, an A_{1c} value of 6% would reflect an average plasma glucose of 125.5 mg/dL, or $[(6 \times 28.7) - 46.7]$. Expressed in SI units, $[(6 \times 28.7) - 46.7] = 125.5 \times 0.555 = 7$ mmol/L.

Hgb A_{1c} levels are not age dependent and are not affected by exercise, diabetic medications, or nonfasting state before specimen collection. The Hgb A_{1c} assay would not be useful for patients with hemolytic anemia, abnormal Hgb (e.g., Hgb S), or abnormal RBC turnover (e.g., sickle cell disease, pregnancy, hemodialysis, recent blood loss, recent blood transfusion, erythropoietin therapy). These patients would be screened, diagnosed, and managed using symptoms, clinical risk factors, short-term glycemic indicators (glucose), and intermediate glycemic indicators (1,5-anhydroglucitol or glycated albumin).

Diabetes is a group of diseases characterized by hyperglycemia, or elevated glucose levels. Hyperglycemia can result from a defect in insulin secretion due to destruction of the beta cells of the pancreas (type 1 diabetes), a defect in insulin action, or a combination of defects in secretion and action (type 2 diabetes), or from a specific cause such as gestational diabetes, neonatal hyperglycemia, cystic fibrosis, or hyperglycemia induced by drugs used to treat other medical conditions (e.g., corticosteroids). The chronic hyperglycemia of diabetes over time may lead to damage, dysfunction, and eventually failure of the eyes (retinopathy), kidneys (nephropathy), nerves (neuropathy), heart (cardiovascular disease), and blood vessels (micro- and macrovascular conditions). The American Diabetes Association (ADA) and National Institute of Diabetes and Digestive and Kidney Disease (NIDDK) have established criteria for diagnosing diabetes.

Diagnostic Criteria for Diabetes*

Glucose	Conventional Units	SI Units (Conventional Units × 0.0555)
Fasting	Greater than 126 mg/dL	Greater than 7 mmol/L
2-hr post challenge with standardized 75-mg load	Greater than 200 mg/dL	Greater than 11.1 mmol/L
Random	Greater than 200 mg/dL **with** symptoms of diabetes (e.g., polyuria, polydipsia, polyphagia, unexplained weight loss)	Greater than 11.1 mmol/L **with** symptoms of diabetes (e.g., polyuria, polydipsia, polyphagia, unexplained weight loss)
A_{1c}	6.5% or greater	6.5% or greater

*Any combination of the these findings or confirmation of any of the individual findings by repetition of the same test on a subsequent day is diagnostic for diabetes.

INDICATIONS

Assist in the diagnosis of diabetes and assess long-term management of glucose levels in individuals with diabetes.

INTERFERING FACTORS

Factors that may alter the results of the study

- Drugs and other substances that may increase glycated Hgb values include aspirin (large doses), atenolol, chronic use of opiates, drugs that increase glucose levels, propranolol, and sulfonylureas.
- Drugs and other substances that may decrease glycated Hgb values include antiretroviral drugs, aspirin (small doses), cholestyramine, drugs that cause RBC hemolysis (e.g., dapsone), drugs that decrease glucose levels (e.g., metformin), vitamin C, and vitamin E.
- Conditions involving abnormal Hgb (hemoglobinopathies) affect the reliability of glycated Hgb values, causing.
  (1) falsely increased values,
  (2) falsely decreased values, or
  (3) discrepancies in either direction depending on the method.

POTENTIAL MEDICAL DIAGNOSIS: CLINICAL SIGNIFICANCE OF RESULTS

Increased in

- Diabetes *(related to and evidenced by elevated glucose levels)*
- Pregnancy *(evidenced by gestational diabetes)*
- Splenectomy *(related to prolonged RBC survival, which extends the amount of time Hgb is available for glycosylation)*

Decreased in

- Chronic blood loss *(related to decreased concentration of RBC-bound glycated Hgb due to blood loss)*
- Chronic kidney disease *(low RBC count associated with this condition reflects corresponding decrease in RBC-bound glycated Hgb)*
- Conditions that decrease RBC life span *(evidenced by anemia and low RBC count, reflecting a corresponding decrease in RBC-bound glycated Hgb)*
- Hemolytic anemia *(evidenced by low RBC count due to hemolysis, reflecting a corresponding decrease in RBC-bound glycated Hgb)*
- Pregnancy *(evidenced by anemia and low RBC count due to increased RBC turnover, reflecting a corresponding decrease in RBC-bound glycated Hgb or related to hemodilution)*

NURSING IMPLICATIONS

H

BEFORE THE STUDY: PLANNING AND IMPLEMENTATION

Teaching the Patient What to Expect

- Inform the patient this test can assist in evaluating blood sugar management over approximately the past 3 mo.
- Explain that a blood sample is needed for the test.

AFTER THE STUDY: POTENTIAL NURSING ACTIONS

Avoiding Complications

- Emphasize, as appropriate, that good management of glucose levels delays the onset and slows the progression of diabetic retinopathy, nephropathy, and neuropathy.
- Explain that unmanaged diabetes can cause multiple health issues, including diabetic kidney disease, amputation of limbs, and ultimately in death.

Treatment Considerations

- Studies comparing risk for developing diabetes demonstrate that certain populations are disproportionately affected by type 2 diabetes and complications of type 2 diabetes as compared to the general population. Nonmodifiable risk factors include age, ethnicity, and family history of diabetes or metabolic syndrome. The risk of developing type 2 diabetes increases with age. In the United States, affected populations include African Americans, Asian Americans, Hispanics, native Hawaiians and Pacific Islanders, American Indians, and Alaska natives. Modifiable risk factors include lifestyle choices related to making healthy dietary choices, maintaining a healthy body weight, and meeting recommended levels of physical activity. The financial and emotional burdens of diabetes and related complications continue to grow at an alarming rate. A system for the prevention, management, and support of patients with type 2 diabetes should be provided through the coordinated efforts of multidisciplinary partners using strategies that are culturally appropriate.

- Instruct the patient in the use of home testing strips or meters approved for glucose, ketones, or A_{1c} by the U.S. Food and Drug Administration, if prescribed.
- Explain the importance of reporting signs and symptoms of hypoglycemia (weakness, confusion, diaphoresis, rapid pulse) or hyperglycemia (thirst, polyuria, hunger, lethargy).
- Monitor blood glucose results and administer ordered insulin or oral antihyperglycemic drugs.
- Assess the cultural aspects of diet selection.
- Correlate dietary intake with blood glucose.

Nutritional Considerations
- Increased levels of Hgb A_{1c} may be associated with diabetes. There is no "diabetic diet"; however, many meal-planning approaches with nutritional goals are endorsed by the ADA. Patients who adhere to dietary recommendations report a better general feeling of health, better weight management, better management of glucose and lipid values, and improved use of insulin. Instruct the patient, as appropriate, in nutritional management of diabetes. A variety of dietary patterns are beneficial for people with diabetes. Encourage consultation with a registered dietitian who is a certified diabetes educator.
- *Sensitivity to Social and Cultural Issues:* Numerous studies point to the prevalence of excess body weight in American children and adolescents. Findings from the 2015–2016 National Health and Nutrition Examination Survey (NHANES), regarding the prevalence of obesity in younger members of the population, estimate that obesity is present in 13.9% of the population ages 2–5 yr, 18.4% ages 6–11 yr, and 20.6% ages 12–19 yr. The medical, social, and emotional consequences of excess body weight are significant. Special attention should be given to instructing the pediatric patient and caregiver regarding health risks and weight management education.

Follow-Up, Evaluation, and Desired Outcomes
- Acknowledges contact information provided for the ADA (www.diabetes.org), American Heart Association (www.heart.org/HEARTORG), National Heart, Lung, and Blood Institute (www.nhlbi.nih.gov), NIDDK (www.niddk.nih.gov), and U.S. Department of Agriculture's resource for nutrition (www.choosemyplate.gov).
- Understands that the ADA recommends A_{1c} testing four times a year for insulin-dependent type 1 or type 2 diabetes when glycemic targets are not being met or when therapy has changed and twice a year when treatment goals are being met for non–insulin-dependent type 2 diabetes. The ADA also recommends that testing for diabetes commence at age 45 for asymptomatic individuals, be considered for adults of any age who are overweight and have additional risk factors, and continue every 3 yr in the absence of symptoms.
- Understands the link between good glycemic management and a delay in the onset of, and slowing the progression of, diabetic retinopathy, nephropathy, and neuropathy.
- Adheres to the request for periodic A_{1c} laboratory studies to better manage the disease process over time.

Hemoglobin Electrophoresis and Abnormal Hemoglobins

SYNONYM/ACRONYM: Hemoglobin F (fetal hemoglobin), hemoglobin S (sickle cell test), methemoglobin (hemoglobin M, MetHb, Hgb M).

RATIONALE: To assist in evaluating hemolytic anemias and identifying hemoglobin variants, diagnose thalassemias and sickle cell anemia. To assess for cyanosis and hypoxemia associated with pathologies affecting hemoglobin.

PATIENT PREPARATION: There are no food, fluid, activity, or medication restrictions unless by medical direction.

NORMAL FINDINGS: Method: Electrophoresis for hemoglobin (Hgb) electrophoresis. Spectrophotometry for methemoglobin. Hemoglobin high-salt solubility for sickle cell screen.

Hgb A	
Adult	Greater than 95%
Hgb A$_2$	
Adult	1.5%–3.7%
Hgb C	None
Hgb D	None
Hgb E	None
Hgb F	
Newborns and infants	
1 day–3 wk	70%–77%
6–9 wk	42%–64%
3–4 mo	7%–39%
6 mo	3%–7%
8–11 mo	0.6%–2.6%
Adult–older adult	Less than 2%
Hgb H	None
Methemoglobin (Hgb M)	Less than 1% of total Hgb
Hgb S (sickle cell screen)	None (negative screen)

CRITICAL FINDINGS AND POTENTIAL INTERVENTIONS

Methemoglobin

Cyanosis can occur at levels greater than 10%.

Dizziness, fatigue, headache, and tachycardia can occur at levels greater than 30%.

Signs of central nervous system depression can occur at levels greater than 45%.

Death may occur at levels greater than 70%.

Timely notification to the requesting health-care provider (HCP) of any critical findings and related symptoms is a role expectation of the professional nurse. A listing of these findings varies among facilities.

Possible interventions include airway protection, administration of oxygen, monitoring neurological status every hour, continuous pulse oximetry, hyperbaric oxygen therapy, and exchange transfusion. Administration of activated charcoal or gastric lavage may be effective if performed soon after the toxic material is ingested. Emesis should never be induced in patients with no gag reflex because of the risk of aspiration. Methylene blue may be used to reverse the process of methemoglobin formation, but it should be used cautiously when methemoglobin levels are greater than 30%. Use of methylene blue is contraindicated in the presence of glucose-6-phosphate dehydrogenase deficiency.

OVERVIEW: (**Study type:** Blood collected in a lavender-top [EDTA] tube; **related body system:** Circulatory/Hematopoietic system. The specimen should be placed in an ice slurry immediately after collection. Information on the specimen label should be protected from water in the ice slurry by first placing the specimen in a protective plastic bag. The specimen should be promptly transported to the laboratory for processing and analysis.) Hgb electrophoresis is a separation process used to identify normal and abnormal forms of Hgb. Electrophoresis and high-performance liquid chromatography as well as molecular genetics testing for mutations can also be used to identify abnormal forms of Hgb. Hgb A is the main form of Hgb in the healthy adult. Hgb F is the main form of Hgb in the fetus, the remainder being composed of Hgb A_1 and A_2. Small amounts of Hgb F are normal in the adult. Hgb C, D, E, H, and S result from abnormal amino acid substitutions during the formation of Hgb and are inherited hemoglobinopathies.

Hgb M is a congenital or acquired structural Hgb variant. It is formed when the heme portion of the deoxygenated Hgb is oxidized to a ferric state rather than to the normal ferrous state, rendering it incapable of combining with and transporting oxygen to tissues. Visible cyanosis can result as levels approach 10% to 15% of total Hgb.

The sickle cell screen is one of several screening tests for a group of hereditary hemoglobinopathies. The test is positive in the presence of rare sickling Hgb variants such as Hgb S and Hgb C Harlem. Electrophoresis and high-performance liquid chromatography as well as molecular genetics testing for beta-globin mutations can also be used to identify Hgb S. Hgb S results from an amino acid substitution during Hgb synthesis whereby valine replaces glutamic acid. Hgb C Harlem results from the substitution of lysine for glutamic acid. Individuals with sickle cell disease have chronic anemia because the abnormal Hgb is unable to carry oxygen. The red blood cells (RBCs) of affected individuals are also abnormal in shape, resembling a crescent or sickle rather than the normal disk shape. This abnormality, combined with cell-wall rigidity, prevents the cells from passing through smaller blood vessels. Blockages in blood vessels result in hypoxia, damage, and pain.

Knowledge of genetics assists in identifying those who may benefit from additional education, risk assessment, and counseling.

Genetics is the study and identification of genes, genetic mutations, and inheritance. For example, genetics provides some insight into the likelihood of inheriting a medical condition such as a hemoglobinopathy like sickle cell anemia. Some conditions are the result of mutations involving a single gene, whereas other conditions may involve multiple genes and/or multiple chromosomes. Sickle cell disease is an example of an autosomal recessive disorder in which the offspring inherits a copy of the defective gene from each parent. Individuals with the sickle cell trait do not have the clinical manifestations of the disease but may pass the disease on to children if the other parent has the trait (or the disease) as well. Further information regarding inheritance of genes can be found in the study titled "Genetic Testing."

INDICATIONS

Hgb Electrophoresis
- Assist in the diagnosis of Hgb C disease.
- Assist in the diagnosis of thalassemia, especially in patients with a family history positive for the disorder.
- Differentiate among thalassemia types.
- Evaluate hemolytic anemia of unknown cause.
- Evaluate a positive sickle cell screening test to differentiate sickle cell trait from sickle cell disease.

Methemoglobin
- Assist in the detection of acquired methemoglobinemia caused by the toxic effects of chemicals and drugs.

- Assist in the detection of congenital methemoglobinemia, indicated by deficiency of RBC nicotinamide adenine dinucleotide (NADH)-methemoglobin reductase or presence of methemoglobin.
- Evaluate cyanosis in the presence of normal blood gases.

Sickle Cell Screen
- Detect sickled RBCs.
- Evaluate hemolytic anemias.

INTERFERING FACTORS

Hgb Electrophoresis
Factors that may alter the results of the study
- High altitude *(related to a compensatory mechanism whereby RBC production is increased to increase availability of oxygen binding to Hgb)* and dehydration *(related to hemoconcentration)* may increase values.
- Iron deficiency may decrease Hgb A_2, C, and S *(related to decreased amounts of Hgb in smaller, iron-deficient RBCs).*
- In patients less than 3 mo of age, false-negative results for Hgb S occur in coincidental polycythemia *(related to technical limitations of the procedure where increased total Hgb levels reflect a small, possibly undetectable percentage of Hgb S when compared to large amounts of Hgb F).*
- RBC transfusion within 4 mo of test can mask abnormal Hgb levels.

Hgb S by Sickle Cell Screen
Factors that may alter the results of the study
- Drugs and other substances that may increase sickle cells in vitro include prostaglandins.
- A positive test does not distinguish between the sickle trait and sickle cell anemia; to make this determination, follow-up testing

by Hgb electrophoresis should be performed.

- False-negative results may occur in children younger than 3 mo of age.
- False-negative results may occur in patients who have received a recent blood transfusion before specimen collection, as a result of the dilutional effect.
- False-positive results may occur in patients without the trait or disease who have received a blood transfusion from a sickle cell–positive donor; this effect can last for 4 mo after the transfusion.

Other considerations
- Test results are unreliable if the patient has pernicious anemia or polycythemia.

Methemoglobin
Factors that may alter the results of the study
- Drugs and other substances that may increase methemoglobin levels include amyl nitrate, aniline derivatives, benzocaine, dapsone, glucosulfone, isoniazid, phenytoin, silver nitrate, and sulfonamides.

Other considerations
- Well water containing nitrate is the most common cause of methemoglobinemia in infants.
- Breastfeeding infants are capable of converting inorganic nitrate from common topical anesthetic applications containing nitrate to the nitrite ion, causing nitrite toxicity and increased methemoglobin.
- Prompt and proper specimen processing, storage, and analysis are important to achieve accurate results. Methemoglobin is unstable and should be transported on ice within a few hours of collection, or else the specimen should be rejected.

POTENTIAL MEDICAL DIAGNOSIS: CLINICAL SIGNIFICANCE OF RESULTS

Increased in
Hemoglobin Electrophoresis
Hgb A$_2$
- Hyperthyroidism
- Megaloblastic anemia
- β-Thalassemias
- Sickle trait

Hgb C
- Hgb C disease (one of the most common structural variants in the human population; has a higher prevalence among people of African ancestry)

Hgb D
- Hgb D (rare hemoglobinopathy that may also be found in combination with Hgb S or thalassemia)

Hgb E
- Hgb E disease; thalassemia-like condition (second-most common hemoglobinopathy in the world; occurs with the highest frequency in people of South Asian [India, Bangladesh], Southeast Asian [Thailand, Laos, Cambodia], and African ancestry, where it is common for individuals to inherit alleles for both Hgb E and β-thalassemia)

Hgb F
- Anemia (aplastic, associated with chronic disease or due to blood loss)
- Erythropoietic porphyria
- Hereditary elliptocytosis or spherocytosis
- Hereditary persistence of fetal Hgb
- Hyperthyroidism
- Leakage of fetal blood into maternal circulation
- Leukemia (acute or chronic)
- Myeloproliferative disorders

- Paroxysmal nocturnal hemoglobinuria
- Pernicious anemia
- Sickle cell disease
- Thalassemias
- Unstable hemoglobins

Hgb H
- α-Thalassemias
- Hgb Bart hydrops fetalis syndrome

Hgb S
- Sickle cell trait or disease (most common variant in the United States; occurs with a frequency of about 8% among people of African ancestry)

Methemoglobin
- Acquired methemoglobinemia (drugs, tobacco smoking, or ionizing radiation)
- Carbon monoxide poisoning (*carbon monoxide is a form of deoxygenated hemoglobin*)
- Hereditary methemoglobinemia (*evidenced by a deficiency of NADH-methemoglobin reductase or related to the presence of a hemoglobinopathy*)

Hgb S by Sickle Cell Screen
Deoxygenated Hgb S is insoluble in the presence of a high-salt solution and will form a cloudy turbid suspension when present.

- Combination of Hgb S with other hemoglobinopathies
- Hgb C Harlem anemia
- Sickle cell anemia
- Sickle cell trait
- Thalassemias

Decreased in
Hemoglobin Electrophoresis
Hgb A$_2$
- Erythroleukemia
- Hgb H disease
- Iron-deficiency anemia (untreated)
- Sideroblastic anemia

NURSING IMPLICATIONS

BEFORE THE STUDY: PLANNING AND IMPLEMENTATION

Teaching the Patient What to Expect
▶ Inform the patient this test can assist in diagnosing various types of anemias and identifying the cause of poor oxygenation.
▶ Explain that a blood sample is needed for the test.

AFTER THE STUDY: POTENTIAL NURSING ACTIONS

Treatment Considerations
▶ Teach patient and family the pathophysiology of sickle cell disease in understandable terms. Explain that the frequency of sickling crises is related to disease control and the need to review therapeutic management.
▶ Advise the patient with sickle cell disease to avoid situations in which hypoxia may occur, such as strenuous exercise, staying at high altitudes, or traveling in an unpressurized aircraft. Obstetric and surgical patients with sickle cell anemia are at risk for hypoxia and therefore require close observation: Obstetric patients are at risk for hypoxia during the stress of labor and delivery, and surgical patients may become hypoxic while under general anesthesia.
▶ Instruct the patient with methemoglobinemia to avoid carbon monoxide from firsthand or secondhand smoking, to have home gas furnace checked yearly for leaks, and to use gas appliances such as gas grills in a well-ventilated area.
▶ Pain management is a priority for those with sickle cell disease. Collaborate with the HCP and patient to identify the best ways to provide relief. Some of those strategies are judicious application of heat or cold and administration of morphine, hydromorphone, or NSAIDS. Other interventions are blood transfusion, joint support, and distraction.

H

◗ Mobility can become a problem in the presence of pain, fear of pain, and anxiety. Emotional support, activity premedication, and the implementation of assistive devices can facilitate mobility.

Follow-Up, Evaluation, and Desired Outcomes
◗ Acknowledges contact information provided for the Sickle Cell Disease Association of America (www.sicklecelldisease.org).

Hemoglobin and Hematocrit

SYNONYM/ACRONYM: Hgb and Hct, H&H.

RATIONALE: To evaluate anemia, polycythemia, hydration status, and monitor therapy such as transfusion.

PATIENT PREPARATION: There are no food, fluid, activity, or medication restrictions unless by medical direction.

NORMAL FINDINGS: Method: Spectrophotometry.

Age	Conventional Units	SI Units		
	Hgb (g/dL)	Hct (%)	Hgb: SI Units g/L (Conventional Units × 10)	Hct: SI Units Volume Fraction (Conventional Units × 0.01)
Cord blood	13.5–20.7	42–62	135–207	0.42–0.62
0–1 wk	15.2–23.6	46–68	152–236	0.46–0.68
2–3 wk	13.3–18.7	41–56	133–187	0.41–0.56
1–2 mo	10.7–18	39–59	107–180	0.39–0.59
3–6 mo	11.7–16.3	35–49	117–163	0.35–0.49
7 mo–15 yr	10.3–14.3	31–43	103–143	0.31–0.43
16–18 yr	11–15	33–45	110–150	0.33–0.45
Adult				
Male	14–17.3	42–52	140–173	0.42–0.52
Female	11.7–15.5	36–48	117–155	0.36–0.48
Pregnant female				
First trimester	11.6–13.9	35–42	116–139	0.35–0.42
Second and third trimesters	9.5–11	28–33	95–110	0.28–0.33

Values are slightly lower in older adults.
Reference range values may vary between laboratories.

CRITICAL FINDINGS AND POTENTIAL INTERVENTIONS

Hgb

Adults & Children
- Less than 6.6 g/dL (SI: Less than 66 mmol/L)
- Greater than 20 g/dL (SI: Greater than 200 mmol/L)

Newborns
- Less than 9.5 g/dL (SI: Less than 95 mmol/L)
- Greater than 22.3 g/dL (SI: Greater than 223 mmol/L)

Hct

Adults & Children
- Less than 19.8% (SI: Less than 0.2 volume fraction)
- Greater than 60% (SI: Greater than 0.6 volume fraction)

Newborns
- Less than 28.5% (SI: Less than 0.28 volume fraction)
- Greater than 66.9% (SI: Greater than 0.67 volume fraction)

Timely notification to the requesting health-care provider (HCP) of any critical findings and related symptoms is a role expectation of the professional nurse. A listing of these findings varies among facilities.

Consideration may be given to verifying the critical findings before action is taken. Policies vary among facilities and may include requesting immediate recollection and retesting by the laboratory.

Low Hgb/Hct leads to anemia. Anemia can be caused by blood loss, decreased blood cell production, increased blood cell destruction, and hemodilution. Causes of blood loss include menstrual excess or frequency, gastrointestinal bleeding, inflammatory bowel disease, and hematuria. Decreased blood cell production can be caused by folic acid deficiency, vitamin B$_{12}$ deficiency, iron deficiency, and chronic disease. Increased blood cell destruction can be caused by a hemolytic reaction, chemical reaction, medication reaction, and sickle cell disease. Hemodilution can be caused by heart failure, chronic kidney disease, polydipsia, and overhydration. Symptoms of anemia (due to these causes) include anxiety, dyspnea, edema, fatigue, hypertension, hypotension, hypoxia, jugular venous distention, pallor, rales, restlessness, and weakness. Treatment of anemia depends on the cause.

High Hgb/Hct leads to polycythemia. Polycythemia can be caused by dehydration, decreased oxygen levels in the body, and an overproduction of red blood cells (RBCs) by the bone marrow. Dehydration from diuretic use, vomiting, diarrhea, excessive sweating, severe burns, or decreased fluid intake decreases the plasma component of whole blood, thereby increasing the ratio of RBCs to plasma, and leads to a higher than normal Hgb. Causes of decreased oxygen include smoking, exposure to carbon monoxide, high altitude, and chronic lung disease, which leads to a mild hemoconcentration of blood in the body to carry more oxygen to the body's tissues. An overproduction of RBCs by the bone marrow leads to polycythemia vera, which is a rare chronic myeloproliferative disorder that results in a severe hemoconcentration of blood. Severe hemoconcentration can lead to thrombosis (spontaneous blood clotting).

Symptoms of hemoconcentration include decreased pulse pressure and volume, loss of skin turgor, dry mucous membranes, headaches, hepatomegaly, low central venous pressure, orthostatic hypotension, pruritus (especially after a hot bath), splenomegaly, tachycardia, thirst, tinnitus, vertigo, and weakness. Treatment of polycythemia depends on the cause. Possible interventions for hemoconcentration due to dehydration include IV fluids and discontinuance of diuretics if they are believed to be contributing to critically elevated Hgb. Polycythemia due to decreased oxygen states can be treated by removal of the offending substance, such as smoke or carbon monoxide. Treatment includes oxygen therapy in cases of smoke inhalation, carbon monoxide poisoning, and desaturating chronic lung disease. Symptoms of polycythemic overload crisis include signs of thrombosis, pain and redness in extremities, facial flushing, and irritability. Possible interventions for hemoconcentration due to polycythemia include therapeutic phlebotomy and IV fluids.

OVERVIEW: (**Study type:** Blood collected in a lavender-top [EDTA] tube, Microtainer, or capillary; **related body system:** Circulatory/Hematopoietic system. Whole blood from a green-top [lithium or sodium heparin] tube may also be submitted.) Blood consists of a liquid plasma portion and a solid cellular portion. The solid portion is comprised of RBCs, white blood cells (WBCs), and platelets. It is important to be able to assess whether the number of circulating RBCs is sufficient to transport the required amount of oxygen throughout the body. The Hgb and Hct levels are part of the complete blood count (CBC). Frequently, Hgb and Hct measures are requested together as an H&H. H&H levels parallel each other and are the best determinant of the degree of anemia or polycythemia. *Polycythemia* is a term used in conjunction with conditions resulting from an abnormal increase in Hgb, Hct, and RBC counts. *Anemia* is a term associated with conditions resulting from an abnormal decrease in Hgb, Hct, and RBC counts. Results of the Hgb, Hct, and RBC counts should be evaluated simultaneously because the same underlying conditions affect this triad of

tests similarly. The RBC count multiplied by 3 should approximate the Hgb concentration. The Hct should be within 3 times the Hgb if the RBC population is normal in size and shape. The Hct plus 6 should approximate the first two figures of the RBC count within 3 (e.g., Hct is 40%; therefore, 40 + 6 = 46, and the RBC count should be 4.6 or in the range of 4.3 to 4.9). There are some ethnic variations in H&H values. After the first decade of life, the mean Hgb in African Americans is 0.5 to 1 g lower than in individuals of European descent.

The Hct is a mathematical expression of the number of RBCs, or packed cell volume, expressed as a percentage of whole blood. For example, a packed cell volume, or Hct, of 45% means that a 100-mL sample of blood contains 45 mL of packed RBCs, which would reflect an acceptable level of RBCs for a patient of any given age. The Hct depends primarily on the number of RBCs; however, the average size of the RBCs influences Hct. Conditions that cause RBC size to be increased (e.g., swelling of the RBC due to change in osmotic pressure related to elevated sodium levels) may increase the Hct, whereas conditions that result in smaller than normal RBCs (e.g., microcytosis related to iron deficiency anemia) may decrease the Hct. Hct can be estimated directly by centrifuging a sample of whole blood for a specific time period. As the blood spins, it is separated into fractions. The RBC fraction is read against a scale. Most often, the Hct is measured indirectly by multiplying the RBC count and mean cell volume (MCV), using an automated cell counter. Hct can also be estimated by multiplying the Hgb by 3.

Hgb is the main intracellular protein of erythrocytes. It carries oxygen (O_2) to and removes carbon dioxide (CO_2) from RBCs. It also serves as a buffer to maintain acid-base balance in the extracellular fluid. Each Hgb molecule consists of heme and globulin. Copper is a cofactor necessary for the enzymatic incorporation of iron molecules into heme. Heme contains iron and porphyrin molecules that have a high affinity for O_2. The affinity of Hgb molecules for O_2 is influenced by 2,3-diphosphoglycerate (2,3-DPG), a substance produced by anaerobic glycolysis to generate energy for the RBCs. When Hgb binds with 2,3-DPG, O_2 affinity decreases. The ability of Hgb to bind and release O_2 can be graphically represented by an oxyhemoglobin dissociation curve. The term *shift to the left* describes an increase in the affinity of Hgb for O_2. Conditions that can cause this leftward shift include decreased body temperature, decreased 2,3-DPG, decreased CO_2 concentration, and increased pH. Conversely, a *shift to the right* represents a decrease in the affinity of Hgb for O_2. Conditions that can cause a rightward shift include increased body temperature, increased 2,3-DPG levels, increased CO_2 concentration, and decreased pH.

Hgb levels are a direct reflection of the O_2-combining capacity of the blood. It is the combination of heme and O_2 that gives blood its characteristic red color. RBC counts parallel the O_2-combining capacity of Hgb, but because some RBCs contain more Hgb than others, the relationship is not directly proportional. As CO_2 diffuses into RBCs, an enzyme called *carbonic anhydrase* converts the CO_2 into bicarbonate and hydrogen ions. Hgb that is not bound to O_2 combines with the free hydrogen ions, increasing pH. As this binding is occurring, bicarbonate is leaving the RBC in exchange for chloride ions. (For additional information about the relationship between the respiratory and renal components of this buffer system, see study titled "Blood Gases.")

INDICATIONS

- Detect hematological disorder, tumor, or immunological abnormality.
- Determine the presence of hereditary hematological abnormality.
- Evaluate known or suspected anemia and related treatment, in combination with Hct.
- Monitor blood loss and response to blood replacement, in combination with Hct.
- Monitor the effects of physical or emotional stress on the patient.
- Monitor fluid imbalances or their treatment.
- Monitor hematological status during pregnancy, in combination with Hct.
- Monitor the progression of non-hematological disorders, such as chronic obstructive pulmonary disease (COPD), malabsorption

syndromes, cancer, and kidney disease.

• Monitor response to drugs or chemotherapy and evaluate undesired reactions to drugs that may cause blood dyscrasias.

• Provide screening as part of a CBC in a general physical examination, especially upon admission to a health-care facility or before surgery.

INTERFERING FACTORS
Factors that may alter the results of the study

• Drugs and other substances that may cause a decrease in Hgb and Hct include those that induce hemolysis due to drug sensitivity or enzyme deficiency and those that result in anemia (see study titled "RBC Count, Indices, Morphology, and Inclusions").

• Some drugs and other substances may also affect Hgb and Hct values by increasing the RBC count (see study titled "RBC Count, Indices, Morphology, and Inclusions").

• A severe copper deficiency may result in decreased Hgb levels.

• Cold agglutinins may falsely increase the mean corpuscular Hgb concentration (MCHC) and decrease the RBC count, affecting Hgb values. This can be corrected by warming the blood or replacing the plasma with warmed saline and repeating the analysis.

• Elevated blood glucose or serum sodium levels may produce elevated Hct levels because of swelling of the erythrocytes.

• Leaving the tourniquet in place for longer than 60 sec can falsely increase Hgb and Hct levels by 2% to 5%.

• The results of RBC counts may vary depending on the patient's position: Hgb and Hct can decrease when the patient is recumbent as a result of hemodilution and can increase when the patient rises as a result of hemoconcentration.

POTENTIAL MEDICAL DIAGNOSIS: CLINICAL SIGNIFICANCE OF RESULTS
Increased in

• Burns *(related to dehydration; total blood volume is decreased, but RBC count remains the same)*

• COPD *(related to chronic hypoxia that stimulates production of RBCs and a corresponding increase in Hgb)*

• Dehydration *(total blood volume is decreased, but RBC count remains the same)*

• Erythrocytosis *(total blood volume remains the same, but RBC count is increased)*

• Heart failure *(when the underlying cause is anemia, the body responds by increasing production of RBCs with a corresponding increase in Hct)*

• Hemoconcentration *(same effect as seen in dehydration)*

• High altitudes *(related to hypoxia that stimulates production of RBCs and therefore increases Hgb)*

• Polycythemia vera *(abnormal bone marrow response resulting in overproduction of RBCs)*

• Shock

Decreased in

• Anemias *(overall decrease in RBCs and corresponding decrease in Hgb)*

• Blood loss (acute and chronic) *(overall decrease in RBC and corresponding decrease in Hct)*

• Bone marrow hyperplasia *(bone marrow failure that results in decreased RBC production)*

- Cancer *(anemia is often associated with chronic disease)*
- Chronic disease *(anemia is often associated with chronic disease)*
- Chronic kidney disease *(related to decreased levels of erythropoietin, which stimulates production of RBCs)*
- Cirrhosis *(related to accumulation of fluid)*
- Fluid retention *(dilutional effect of increased blood volume while RBC count remains stable)*
- Hemoglobinopathies *(reduced RBC survival with corresponding decrease in Hgb)*
- Hemolytic disorders (e.g., hemolytic anemias, prosthetic valves) *(reduced RBC survival with corresponding decrease in Hct)*
- Hemorrhage (acute and chronic) *(overall decrease in RBCs and corresponding decrease in Hgb)*

- Hodgkin disease *(bone marrow failure that results in decreased RBC production)*
- Incompatible blood transfusion *(reduced RBC survival with corresponding decrease in Hgb)*
- IV overload *(dilutional effect)*
- Leukemia *(bone marrow failure that results in decreased RBC production)*
- Lymphomas *(bone marrow failure that results in decreased RBC production)*
- Nutritional deficit *(anemia related to dietary deficiency in iron, vitamins, folate needed to produce sufficient RBCs; decreased RBC count with corresponding decrease in Hgb)*
- Pregnancy *(related to anemia)*
- Splenomegaly *(total blood volume remains the same, but spleen retains RBCs and Hgb reflects decreased RBC count)*

H

NURSING IMPLICATIONS

POTENTIAL NURSING PROBLEMS: ASSESSMENT & NURSING DIAGNOSIS

Problems	Signs and Symptoms
Activity *(related to decreased oxygen-carrying capacity of the blood secondary to anemia, decreased number of RBCs)*	Weakness, fatigue, shortness of breath with activity, dizziness, palpitations, headache, verbalization of difficulty with activity tolerance
Bleeding *(related to malfunction of bone marrow)*	Altered level of consciousness, hypotension, increased heart rate, decreased Hgb and Hct, capillary refill greater than 3 sec, cool extremities
Fatigue *(related to decreased oxygenation associated with a decreased number of RBCs)*	Verbalization of fatigue, altered ability to perform activities of daily living due to lack of energy, shortness of breath with exertion, increasingly frequent rest periods, presence of fatigue after sleep, inability to adhere to daily routine, altered level of concentration, reports of tiredness

BEFORE THE STUDY: PLANNING AND IMPLEMENTATION

Teaching the Patient What to Expect

▶ Inform the patient this test can assist in evaluating the amount of Hgb in the blood to assist in diagnosis and monitor therapy.
▶ Explain that a blood sample is needed for the test.

Potential Nursing Actions

✦ Ensure informed consent for blood transfusion has been given and the consent signed prior to administration of blood or blood products. Follow organization protocol.

Safety Considerations

✦ Ensure correct verification process by two licensed nurses prior to transfusion, or follow emergency protocol. Follow organization guidelines for safe administration.

AFTER THE STUDY: POTENTIAL NURSING ACTIONS

Treatment Considerations

▶ Activity: Assess for fall risk and implement strategies commensurate with level of risk. Administer prescribed oxygen and use pulse oximetry to evaluate effectiveness. Administer ordered blood and blood products and monitor for transfusion reaction. Coordinate episodes of activity with rest periods and increase activity gradually as anemia resolves.
▶ Bleeding: Monitor and trend platelet count. Increase frequency of vital sign assessment and monitor and trend results. Administer ordered blood or blood products and stool softeners. Monitor and assess stool, urine, sputum, gums, and nose for blood. Coordinate laboratory draws to decrease frequency of venipuncture. Institute bleeding precautions; avoid intramuscular injections, prevent trauma, be gentle with oral care and suctioning, and avoid use of a sharp razor. Administer prescribed medications and assess diet for iron- and vitamin K–rich foods.

▶ Fatigue: Monitor and trend CBC, Hgb, and Hct. Monitor for shortness of breath. Administer ordered oxygen and assesses effectiveness with pulse oximetry. Assess nutritional intake. Assess ability to perform self-care, encourage frequent rest periods, prioritize and bundle activities to decrease fatigue, and teach techniques for conserving energy expenditure. Administer blood and blood products. Assess for medical or psychological factors contributing to fatigue. Administer prescribed erythropoietin.
▶ Assess the color of the patient's skin, as pallor is an indication of poor tissue perfusion. Oxygen and blood or blood product administration may be necessary to alleviate some of the symptoms the patient is experiencing due to the effects of the anemia. Frequently assess vital signs and explain to the patient that elevating the head of the bed may reduce difficulty in breathing. Educate the patient regarding access to nutritional counseling services with a registered dietitian.
▶ The results of a CBC should be carefully evaluated during transfusion or acute blood loss because the body is not in a state of homeostasis and values may be misleading. Considerations for draw times after transfusion include the type of product, the amount of product transfused, and the patient's clinical situation. Generally, specimens collected an hour after transfusion will provide an acceptable reflection of the effects of the transfused product. Measurements taken during a massive transfusion are an exception, providing essential guidance for therapeutic decisions during critical care.

Safety Considerations

▶ Follow all safety precautions to ensure transfused blood is a correct match for the patient.

Nutritional Considerations

▶ Nutritional therapy may be indicated for patients with *increased Hgb and Hct* if iron levels are also elevated. Educate the patient with abnormally elevated iron values, as appropriate, on the importance of reading food labels. Patients with hemochromatosis or acute pernicious anemia should be educated to avoid foods rich in iron. Iron absorption is affected by numerous factors that may enhance or decrease absorption regardless of the original content of the iron-containing dietary source (see study titled "Iron Studies: Iron (Total), Iron-Binding Capacity (Total), Transferrin, and Iron Saturation"). Iron levels in foods can be increased if foods are cooked in cookware containing iron. Consumption of large amounts of alcohol damages the intestine and allows increased absorption of iron. A high intake of calcium and ascorbic acid also increases iron absorption. Iron absorption after a meal is also increased by factors in meat, fish, and poultry.

▶ Nutritional therapy may be indicated for patients with *decreased Hgb and Hct*, which may indicate corresponding iron deficiency. Iron deficiency is the most common nutrient deficiency in the United States. Patients at risk (e.g., children, pregnant women, women of childbearing age, and low-income populations) should be instructed to include in their diet foods that are high in iron, such as meats (especially liver), eggs, grains, green leafy vegetables,

and multivitamins with iron. Instruct these patients in the administration of iron supplements, including adverse effects, as appropriate. The Hgb level should increase by about 1 g/dL (SI: 10 g/L) after 3 to 4 wk of oral iron supplementation. Educate the patient with abnormally decreased Hgb values, as appropriate, about the importance of reading food labels and of dietary inclusion of iron-rich foods. Iron absorption is affected by numerous factors that may enhance or decrease absorption regardless of the original content of the iron-containing dietary source. Iron absorption is decreased by the absence (gastric resection) or diminished presence (use of antacids) of gastric acid.

Follow-Up, Evaluation, and Desired Outcomes

▶ Acknowledges contact information provided for the Institute of Medicine of the National Academies (www.iom.edu) or the U.S. Department of Agriculture's resource for nutrition (www.choosemyplate.gov).
▶ States understanding of the risks and benefits associated with blood transfusion.
▶ Adheres to the request to include dietary foods high in iron.

Hemosiderin

SYNONYM/ACRONYM: Hemosiderin stain, Pappenheimer body stain, iron stain.

RATIONALE: To assist in investigating recent intravascular hemolysis and in the diagnosis of unexplained anemias, hemochromatosis, and renal tube damage.

PATIENT PREPARATION: There are no food, fluid, activity, or medication restrictions unless by medical direction. As appropriate, provide the required urine collection container and specimen collection instructions.

NORMAL FINDINGS: (Method: Microscopic examination of Prussian blue–stained specimen) None seen.

CRITICAL FINDINGS AND POTENTIAL INTERVENTIONS: N/A

OVERVIEW: (**Study type:** Urine from a random first morning sample, collected in a clean plastic collection container; **related body system:** Circulatory system.) Hemosiderin stain is used to indicate the presence of iron storage granules called *hemosiderin* by microscopic examination of urine sediment. Granules of hemosiderin stain blue when potassium ferrocyanide is added to the sample. Hemosiderin is normally found in the liver, spleen, and bone marrow but not in the urine. Under normal conditions, hemosiderin is absorbed by the renal tubules; however, in extensive hemolysis, renal tubule damage, or an iron metabolism disorder, hemosiderin filters its way into the urine. The Prussian blue stain may also be used to identify siderocytes (iron-containing red blood cells [RBCs]) in peripheral blood. The presence of siderocytes in circulating RBCs is abnormal.

INDICATIONS
- Assist in the diagnosis of hemochromatosis (tissue damage caused by iron toxicity).
- Detect excessive RBC hemolysis within the systemic circulation.
- Evaluate renal tubule dysfunction.

INTERFERING FACTORS: N/A

POTENTIAL MEDICAL DIAGNOSIS: CLINICAL SIGNIFICANCE OF RESULTS
Increased in
Any condition that involves hemolysis will release hemoglobin from RBCs into circulation. Hemoglobin is converted to hemosiderin in the renal tubular epithelial cells.

- Burns
- Cold hemagglutinin disease

- Hemochromatosis
- Hemolytic transfusion reactions
- Mechanical trauma to RBCs
- Megaloblastic anemia
- Microangiopathic hemolytic anemia
- Paroxysmal nocturnal hemoglobinuria
- Pernicious anemia
- Sickle cell anemia
- Thalassemia major

Decreased in: N/A

NURSING IMPLICATIONS

BEFORE THE STUDY: PLANNING AND IMPLEMENTATION

Teaching the Patient What to Expect
- Inform the patient this test can assist in diagnosing various types of anemias.
- Explain that a urine sample is needed for the test. Information regarding specimen collection is presented with other general guidelines in Appendix A: Patient Preparation and Specimen Collection.

Potential Nursing Actions
- Include on the collection container's label the specimen collection type (e.g., clean catch, catheter), date and time of collection, and any medications that may interfere with test results.

AFTER THE STUDY: POTENTIAL NURSING ACTIONS

Treatment Considerations
- Provide disease-specific education to allow the patient to anticipate relevant reportable signs and symptoms.

Follow-Up, Evaluation, and Desired Outcomes
- Understands that additional testing may be necessary to evaluate or monitor disease progression and determine the need for a change in therapy.

Hepatitis Testing

SYNONYM/ACRONYM: Hepatitis A antibody: HAV, hepatitis B antigen and antibodies: HBV (HBeAg, HBeAb, HBcAb, HBsAb, HBsAg), hepatitis C antibody: HCV, hepatitis D antibody: HDV (delta hepatitis), hepatitis E antibody: HEV.

RATIONALE: To test blood for the presence of antibodies that would indicate a past or current hepatitis infection.

PATIENT PREPARATION: There are no food, fluid, activity, or medication restrictions unless by medical direction.

NORMAL FINDINGS: Method: Enzyme immunoassay for HAV, HBV, HDV, HEV; polymerase chain reaction (PCR) may also be used where indicated. Negative.

(Method: Enzyme immunoassay, chemiluminescent immunoassay, branched chain DNA [bDNA], PCR, recombinant immunoblot assay [RIBA], viral RNA RT [reverse transcription] PCR) for HCV. Negative.

CRITICAL FINDINGS AND POTENTIAL INTERVENTIONS: N/A

H

OVERVIEW: (Study type: Blood collected in a gold-, red-, or red/gray-top tube for HAV, HBV, HCV, HDV, or HEV enzyme immunoassay and chemiluminescent immunoassay; **related body system:** Digestive and Immune systems. Blood collected in lavender-top [EDTA] or white-top [PPT EDTA] tubes for HCV molecular testing of viral DNA or RNA.) *Hepatitis* is a term used to describe inflammation of the liver. There are a variety of causes of hepatitis that include exposure to hepatotoxic substances such as alcohol or drugs or infection by a hepatitis virus. The resulting illness can range from a mild, self-limiting condition to a life-threatening disease. The disease may present as an acute illness or develop into a chronic condition. This study reviews the viral sources of hepatitis infections.

HAV: The hepatitis A virus (HAV) is classified as a picornavirus. Its primary mode of transmission is by the fecal-oral route under conditions of poor personal hygiene or inadequate sanitation. The incubation period is about 28 days, with a range of 15 to 50 days. Onset is usually abrupt, with the acute disease lasting about 1 wk. Therapy is supportive, and there is no development of chronic or carrier states. Assays for total (immunoglobulin G [IgG] and immunoglobulin M [IgM]) hepatitis A antibody and IgM-specific hepatitis A antibody assist in differentiating recent infection from prior exposure. If results from the IgM-specific or from both assays are positive, recent infection is suspected. If the IgM-specific test results are negative and the total antibody test results are positive, past infection is indicated. The clinically significant assay—IgM-specific antibody—is often the only test requested. Jaundice occurs in 70% to 80% of adult cases of HAV infection and in 70% of pediatric cases.

HBV: The hepatitis B virus (HBV) is classified as a

double-stranded DNA retrovirus of the Hepadnaviridae family. Its primary modes of transmission are parenteral, perinatal, and sexual contact. Serological profiles vary with different scenarios (i.e., asymptomatic infection, acute/resolved infection, coinfection, and chronic carrier state). The formation and detectability of markers is also dose dependent. The following description refers to HBV infection that becomes resolved. The incubation period is generally 6 to 16 wk. The hepatitis B surface antigen (HBsAg) is the first marker to appear after infection. It is detectable 8 to 12 wk after exposure and often precedes symptoms. At about the time liver enzymes fall back to normal levels, the HBsAg titer has fallen to nondetectable levels. If the HBsAg remains detectable after 6 mo, the patient will likely become a chronic carrier who can transmit the virus. Hepatitis Be antigen (HBeAg) appears in the serum 10 to 12 wk after exposure. HBeAg can be found in the serum of patients with acute or chronic HBV infection and is a sign of active viral replication and infectivity. Levels of hepatitis Be antibody (HBeAb) appear about 14 wk after exposure, suggesting resolution of the infection and reduction of the patient's ability to transmit the disease. The more quickly HBeAg disappears, the shorter the acute phase of the infection. IgM-specific hepatitis B core antibody (HBcAb) appears 6 to 14 wk after exposure to HBsAg and continues to be detectable either until the infection is resolved or over the life span of patients who are in a chronic carrier state. In some cases, HBcAb may be the only detectable

marker; hence, its lone appearance has sometimes been referred to as the *core window*. HBcAb is not an indicator of recovery or immunity; however, it does indicate current or previous infection. Hepatitis B surface antibody (HBsAb) appears 2 to 16 wk after HBsAg disappears. Appearance of HBsAb represents clinical recovery and immunity to the virus.

Onset of HBV infection is usually insidious. Most infected children and half of infected adults are asymptomatic. During the acute phase of infection, symptoms range from mild to severe. Chronicity decreases with age. HBsAg and HBcAb tests are used to screen donated blood before transfusion. HBsAg testing is often part of the routine prenatal screen. Vaccination of infants, children, and young adults is becoming a standard of care and in some cases a requirement.

HCV: The hepatitis C virus (HCV) causes the majority of bloodborne non-A/non-B hepatitis cases. There are six main genotypes, or strains, of the virus, and 50 subtypes of the virus have been identified. It is possible to be infected with more than one genotype at a time. The virus is a flavivirus and contains a single-stranded RNA core. Its primary modes of transmission are parenteral, perinatal, and sexual contact. The incubation period varies widely, from 2 to 52 wk. Onset is insidious, and the risk of chronic liver disease after infection is high. On average, antibodies to hepatitis C are detectable in infected individuals within 4 to 10 wk of infection by enzyme immunoassay screening methods and as early as 2 to 3 wk of infection by PCR methods. Once infected with

HCV, 75% to 85% of patients will become chronic carriers. Infected individuals and carriers have a high frequency of chronic liver diseases such as cirrhosis and chronic active hepatitis, and they have a higher risk of developing hepatocellular cancer. The transmission of hepatitis C by blood transfusion has decreased dramatically since it became part of the routine screening panel for blood donors. The possibility of prenatal transmission exists, especially in the presence of HIV coinfection. Therefore, this test is often included in prenatal testing packages. The test sequence begins with a qualitative immunoassay screening test for viral antibodies. Indeterminate or suspected false-positive results may be confirmed by the RIBA assay, which also detects viral antibodies. Nucleic acid amplification testing is the method used to document the presence of ongoing infection. Viral genotype testing is used to identify HCV RNA by RT PCR. Genotype and viral load testing (bDNA or RT PCR) are used to select and guide therapeutic interventions.

Genotype	Geographic Prevalence
Genotype 1	North America (found throughout the world)
Genotype 2	Worldwide
Genotype 3	Worldwide
Genotype 4	Northern Africa
Genotype 5	South Africa
Genotype 6	Asia

HDV: Symptoms of hepatitis D virus (HDV) infection are similar but often more severe than those of hepatitis B virus (HBV) infection. As with HBV, the primary modes of HDV transmission are parenteral, perinatal, and sexual contact. The virus contains a single-stranded RNA core. Replication of this virus requires the presence of the hepatitis B outer coat. Therefore, HDV infection can occur only with hepatitis B coinfection or superinfection. Onset is abrupt, after an incubation period of 3 to 13 wk. Because of its dependence on HBV, prevention can be accomplished by using the same pre-exposure and postexposure protective measures used for HBV.

HEV: The hepatitis E virus (HEV) is classified as a single-stranded RNA hepevirus with five separate genotypes. HEV is a major cause of enteric non-A hepatitis worldwide; about 20% of the U.S. population demonstrates presence of IgG antibody. Its primary mode of transmission is the fecal-oral route under conditions of poor personal hygiene or inadequate sanitation. The incubation period is about 28 days. IgM and IgG are detectable within 1 mo after infection. Onset is usually abrupt, with the acute disease lasting several weeks. Therapy is supportive, and patients usually recover, although the disease is quite debilitating during the acute phase. Hepatitis E infection can occasionally develop into a severe liver disease and may cause chronic infection in organ transplant or other immunocompromised patients. Assays for total (IgG and IgM) hepatitis E antibody and IgM-specific hepatitis E antibody help differentiate recent infection from prior exposure. If results from the IgM-specific or from both assays are positive, recent infection is suspected.

H

If the IgM-specific test results are negative and the total antibody test results are positive, past infection is indicated. IgM remains detectable for about 2 mo; IgG levels persist for months to years after recovery.

INDICATIONS
- Detect possible carrier status.
- Determine therapeutic approach based on identification of viral genotype.
- Establish the presence of coinfection or superinfection in patients with HBV (clinical course of superinfection is more severe).
- Pre- and postvaccination testing.
- Routine prenatal testing.
- Screen donated blood before transfusion.
- Screen individuals with suspected viral hepatitis infection.
- Screen for individuals at high risk of exposure, such as patients on hemodialysis, persons with multiple sex partners, persons with a history of other sexually transmitted infections, individuals who misuse IV drugs, infants born to infected mothers, individuals residing in long-term residential facilities or correctional facilities, recipients of blood- or plasma-derived products, allied health-care workers, and public service employees who come in contact with blood and blood products.

INTERFERING FACTORS
- Drugs that may decrease HBeAb, HBsAb, hepatitis C antibody levels, and hepatitis D antibody levels include interferon alfa-2b.

POTENTIAL MEDICAL DIAGNOSIS: CLINICAL SIGNIFICANCE OF RESULTS
Positive findings in
- Individuals with current viral hepatitis infection
- Individuals with past or chronic viral hepatitis infection

NURSING IMPLICATIONS

POTENTIAL NURSING PROBLEMS: ASSESSMENT & NURSING DIAGNOSIS

Problems	Signs and Symptoms
Activity *(related to inadequate nutrient metabolism, increased basal metabolic rate associated with viral infection)*	Verbal report of weakness; inability to tolerate activity; shortness of breath with activity; altered heart rate, blood pressure, and respiratory rate with activity
Infection: **HAV, HEV** *(related to crowded living conditions with poor sanitation; poor personal hygiene; fecal-oral exposure; exposure to contaminated water, milk, food; raw shellfish);* **HBV, HCV, or HDV** *(related to unprotected sex, exposure to blood and body fluids of an infected person, sharing needles with an infected person)*	Fever, fatigue, loss of appetite, jaundice, nausea and vomiting, dark-colored urine, abdominal pain, stool that is clay colored, joint pain; it is possible to be infected and have no symptoms

H

Problems	Signs and Symptoms
Nutrition *(related to the inability to adequately store or metabolize foods, lack of appetite, refusal to eat, nausea and vomiting)*	Unintended weight loss; pale, dry skin; dry mucous membranes; documented inadequate caloric intake; subcutaneous tissue loss; hair pulls out easily; paresthesias

BEFORE THE STUDY: PLANNING AND IMPLEMENTATION

Teaching the Patient What to Expect
▶ Inform the patient this test can assist in detecting, evaluating, and monitoring hepatitis infection.
▶ Explain that a blood sample is needed for the test.

Potential Nursing Actions
▶ Obtain a history of IV drug use, high-risk sexual activity, and occupational exposure.

Safety Considerations
▶ Follow recommended precautions to decrease risk of staff exposure associated with blood, body fluids, and needle sticks.

AFTER THE STUDY: POTENTIAL NURSING ACTIONS

Avoiding Complications
▶ Counsel the patient and significant contacts, as appropriate, that hepatitis B immune globulin (HBIG) immunization is available (for HBV and HDV) and is in fact required in many places as part of childhood immunization and employee health programs. Parents may choose to sign a waiver preventing their newborns from receiving the vaccine; they may choose not to vaccinate on the basis of philosophical, religious, or medical reasons. Vaccination regulations vary by state.

Treatment Considerations
▶ It is important to teach patients how disease transmission occurs in order to avoid reinfection and to prevent ongoing medical problems.
▶ Victims of sexual assault, including children and older adults, may be at risk for developing hepatitis. Provide access to counseling services. Provide a nonjudgmental, nonthreatening atmosphere for a discussion during which the risks of sexually transmitted infections are explained. It is also important to discuss the problems that the patient may experience (e.g., guilt, depression, anger).
▶ Infection: The best treatment for infection is adequate rest, good nutrition, and adequate fluid intake. It is important to recommend both family and significant others receive the hepatitis vaccination. Explain that alcohol should be avoided to decrease risk of liver damage and that over-the-counter medication should be checked with the health-care provider (HCP) before taking to ensure there is no risk to the liver; explain that jaundice can last several months.
▶ Prevention and early treatment are key components of hepatitis therapeutic strategies. Immune globulin can be given before HAV exposure (in the case of individuals who may be traveling to a location where the disease is endemic) or after exposure, during the incubation period. Prophylaxis is most effective when administered 2 wk after exposure.
▶ *Hepatitis A* does not have a specific treatment. The best course of action is to treat the symptoms, such as nausea and fatigue. An adequate diet and rest are also very important to a full recovery.
▶ *HBIG* vaccination should be given immediately after situations in which there is a potential for HBV exposure (e.g., accidental needle stick, perinatal period, sexual contact) for temporary,

H

passive protection. Immune globulin can be given before exposure (in the case of individuals who may be traveling to a location where the disease is endemic) or after exposure, during the incubation period. Interferon alfa-2b may be useful in the treatment of hepatitis B. Antiviral drugs used to treat hepatitis B include lamivudine, adefovir, telbivudine, and entecavir. The specific course of treatment is decided through discussions between the patient and HCP.

▸ *Hepatitis C* does not have a designated vaccine; however, Interferon alfa-2b may be useful in the treatment of hepatitis C. Antiviral drugs used to treat hepatitis C include boceprevir, daclatasvir, ledipasvir, peginterferon, ribavirin, simeprevir, sofosbuvir, and telaprevir. The specific course of treatment is decided through discussions between the patient and HCP. Therapeutic interventions are based on factors that include the type of virus identified, the patient's complete health history (including any history of liver disease, kidney disease, HIV coinfection, and previous treatment), and the patient's response to treatment. It should be noted that the average treatment is over a period of 12 wk but may extend over a period of a year and may be financially prohibitive for some patients.

▸ *Hepatitis D* has limited options as far as treatment. The only drug found to be effective is pegylated interferon alpha. Duration of therapy is not clear, but it is estimated to be more than a year.

▸ *Hepatitis E* is not treated with specific interventions in most situations, as it will eventually run its course. However, patients who are immunosuppressed can be given the antiviral ribavirin or interferon with some positive effect. Hospitalization may be considered for pregnant women who are symptomatic.

▸ Counsel the patient, as appropriate, regarding the risk of transmission and proper prophylaxis. Stress the importance of hand hygiene to prevent transmission of the virus.

Discuss chronic infection in organ transplant or other patients who are immunocompromised.

Safety Considerations
▸ Activity: There are several assessment and intervention techniques that can assist in managing altered activity tolerance. Assess current level of activity and activity tolerance. Assist patient in setting realistic activity goals. Trend vital signs, including orthostatic blood pressure, with activity; monitor for oxygen desaturation and administer oxygen as necessary. Collaborate with physical therapy to support activity, pace activities to match energy stores, and collaborate with the patient to establish activity goals. As needed, assist with self-care and encourage long, uninterrupted periods of rest. Introduce the use of assistive devices as needed.

▸ Fatigue can be common with hepatitis. Some interventions to address fatigue are to pace activities to preserve energy stores, identify what aggravates and decreases fatigue, and assess for physiologic factors such as anemia. Observe for emotional factors such as depression, which can contribute to the presence of fatigue. Fall and injury risk precautions should be put in place.

Nutritional Considerations
▸ Adequate nutrition is important with all forms of hepatitis. In general, patients should be encouraged to eat a well-balanced diet. Dietary recommendations will vary depending on the condition and its severity. Valuable areas of inquiry are nutritional history, current eating habits, and attitude toward eating. Assess for the presence of ascites and nausea. Some potential strategies to address nutrition concerns are to monitor weight daily and administer ordered vitamins and antiemetics for nausea. Monitor nutritional laboratory values such as albumin, serum electrolytes, hemoglobin, red blood cells, transferrin, and white blood cells. Encourage cultural home foods.

▸ Explain the importance of providing an adequate daily fluid intake of at

H

least 4 L. Alcohol should be eliminated from the diet. As a general rule, small, frequent meals that are high in carbohydrates and low in fat will provide the required energy while not burdening the inflamed liver. There are some specific instances when hepatitis can affect the diet:

▶ Treatment with interferon, which may result in side effects such as loss of appetite, soreness in the mouth and throat, nausea and vomiting.

▶ Disease progression that results in further deterioration of health, which may result in loss of appetite or fatigue such that significant malnourishment occurs.

▶ Presence of additional medical conditions such as diabetes, hypercholesterolemia, hypertension, or kidney disease with specific dietary restrictions.

Follow-Up, Evaluation, and Desired Outcomes

▶ Acknowledges contact information provided for the Centers for Disease Control and Prevention (www.cdc.gov/ DiseasesConditions) for information regarding hepatitis.

▶ Acknowledges contact information provided regarding vaccine-preventable diseases (e.g., hepatitis A and B) for the Centers for Disease Control and Prevention (www.cdc .gov/vaccines/vpd/vaccines-diseases .html and www.cdc.gov/Diseases Conditions).

▶ Is aware that positive findings must be reported to local health department officials, who will question him or her regarding sexual partners.

Hepatobiliary Scan

SYNONYM/ACRONYM: Biliary tract radionuclide scan, cholescintigraphy, hepatobiliary imaging, hepatobiliary scintigraphy, gallbladder scan, HIDA or hepatobiliary iminodiacetic scan.

RATIONALE: To visualize and assess the cystic and common bile ducts of the gallbladder toward diagnosing obstructions, stones, inflammation, and tumor.

PATIENT PREPARATION: There are no activity restrictions unless by medical direction. Instruct the patient to restrict food and fluids for 4 to 6 hr prior to the procedure. Explain that fasting for more than 24 hr before the procedure or receiving total parenteral nutrition may produce a false-positive result. Instruct the patient, as ordered, to discontinue use of opiate-based or morphine-based drugs 2 to 6 hr before the procedure. No other radionuclide scans or procedures using barium contrast medium should be scheduled within 24 to 48 hr before this procedure. Protocols may vary among facilities.

NORMAL FINDINGS

• Normal shape, size, and function of the gallbladder with patent cystic and common bile ducts; radionuclide should pass through the biliary system, and a significant amount should be visualized in the gallbladder within 15 to 30 min.

CRITICAL FINDINGS AND POTENTIAL INTERVENTIONS: N/A

OVERVIEW: (Study type: Nuclear scan; related body system: Digestive system.) The hepatobiliary scan is a nuclear medicine study of the hepatobiliary excretion system. It is primarily used to determine the patency of the cystic and common bile ducts, but it can also be used to determine overall hepatic function, gallbladder function, presence of gallstones (indirectly), and sphincter of Oddi dysfunction. A technetium-99 (Tc-99m)–labelled iminodiacetic acid analogue (e.g., tribromoethyl) is administered by IV injection and excreted into the bile duct system. A gamma camera detects the radiation emitted from the injected contrast medium, and a representative image of the duct system is obtained. The results are correlated with other diagnostic studies, such as IV cholangiography, computed tomography (CT) scan of the gallbladder, and ultrasonography. Gallbladder emptying or ejection fraction can be determined by administering a fatty meal or cholecystokinin to the patient. This procedure can be used before and after surgery to determine the extent of bile reflux.

INDICATIONS
- Aid in the diagnosis of acute and chronic cholecystitis.
- Aid in the diagnosis of suspected gallbladder disorders, such as inflammation, perforation, or calculi.
- Assess enterogastric reflux.
- Assess obstructive jaundice when done in combination with radiography or ultrasonography.
- Determine common duct obstruction caused by tumors or choledocholithiasis.
- Evaluate biliary enteric bypass patency.
- Postoperatively evaluate gastric surgical procedures and abdominal trauma.

INTERFERING FACTORS
Contraindications

Patients who are pregnant or suspected of being pregnant, unless the potential benefits of a procedure using radiation far outweigh the risk of radiation exposure to the fetus and mother.

Factors that may alter the results of the study
- Bilirubin levels greater than or equal to 30 mg/mL, depending on the radionuclide used, indicate significant liver damage, which may decrease hepatic uptake.
- The use of opiate or morphine-based drugs 2 to 6 hr before the procedure may interfere with smooth muscle motility, affecting the passage of the radionuclide through the biliary system.
- Fasting for more than 24 hr before the procedure or receiving total parenteral nutrition may produce a false-positive result because *the absence of the digestive process prevents the gallbladder from filling.*
- Metallic objects (e.g., jewelry, body rings) within the examination field, other nuclear scans done within the previous 24 to 48 hr, or retained barium from a previous radiological procedure, which may inhibit organ visualization and cause unclear images.
- Improper injection of the radionuclide that allows the tracer to seep deep into the muscle tissue can produce erroneous hot spots.
- Inability of the patient to cooperate or remain still during the procedure, because movement

can produce blurred or otherwise unclear images.

POTENTIAL MEDICAL DIAGNOSIS: CLINICAL SIGNIFICANCE OF RESULTS

Abnormal findings related to

Uneven distribution of the radionuclide, deposited in concentrated "hot spots," indicates areas where lesions, trauma, abnormal anatomy, or obstructions in the biliary system are located. Delayed visualization or absence of the radionuclide within 60 min or more is abnormal.

- Cholecystitis (acalculous, acute, chronic) *(evidenced by visualization of the biliary tree and lack of visualization of the gallbladder related to obstruction of the cystic duct by gallstones)*
- Common bile duct obstruction secondary to gallstones, tumor, or stricture *(evidenced by visualization in the bile duct but absent visualization of the tracer in the small intestine, related to bile duct obstruction)*
- Congenital biliary atresia or choledochal cyst *(evidenced by delayed visualization of the tracer and low ejection fracture [less than 35%])*
- Postoperative biliary leak, fistula, or obstruction
- Trauma-induced bile leak or cyst

NURSING IMPLICATIONS

BEFORE THE STUDY: PLANNING AND IMPLEMENTATION

Teaching the Patient What to Expect

- Inform the patient this procedure can assist in detecting inflammation or obstruction of the gallbladder or ducts.
- Pregnancy is a general contraindication to procedures involving radiation. Explain to the female patient that she will be asked the date of her last menstrual period and pregnancy testing may be performed to determine the possibility of pregnancy before she is exposed to radiation.
- Review the procedure with the patient. Address concerns about pain and explain that there may be moments of discomfort or pain experienced when the IV line is inserted to allow infusion of fluids such as saline, anesthetics, sedatives, radionuclides, medications used in the procedure, or emergency medications.
- Inform the patient the procedure is performed in a nuclear medicine department by a health-care provider (HCP) specializing in this procedure, with support staff, and takes approximately 1 to 4 hr.
- Reassure the patient that the radionuclide poses no radioactive hazard and rarely produces adverse effects.
- Instruct the patient to remove jewelry and other metallic objects from the area to be examined prior to the procedure.
- Baseline vital signs and neurological status will be recorded. Protocols may vary among facilities.
- Positioning for the study is in the supine position on a flat table with foam wedges to help maintain position and immobilization.
- IV radionuclide is administered, and the upper right quadrant of the abdomen is scanned immediately, with images then taken every 5 min for the first 30 min and every 10 min for the next 30 min. If the gallbladder cannot be visualized, delayed views are taken in 2, 4, and 24 hr to differentiate acute from chronic cholecystitis or to detect the degree of obstruction.
- IV morphine may be administered during the study to initiate spasms of the sphincter of Oddi, forcing the radionuclide into the gallbladder, if the organ is not visualized within 1 hr of injection of the radionuclide. Imaging is then done 20 to 50 min later to determine delayed visualization or nonvisualization of the gallbladder.
- If gallbladder function or bile reflux is being assessed, the patient will be

H

given a fatty meal or cholecystokinin 60 min after the injection.

▶ Explain that once the study is completed, the needle or catheter will be removed and a pressure dressing applied over the puncture site.

Potential Nursing Actions

◈ *Make sure a written and informed consent has been signed prior to the procedure and before administering any medications.*

AFTER THE STUDY: POTENTIAL NURSING ACTIONS

Avoiding Complications
▶ Establishing an IV site and injection of radionuclides are invasive procedures. Complications are rare but include risk for allergic reaction *(related to contrast reaction)*, hematoma *(related to blood leakage into the tissue following needle insertion)*, bleeding from the puncture site *(related to a bleeding disorder or the effects of natural products and medications with known anticoagulant, antiplatelet, or thrombolytic properties)*, or infection *(which might occur if bacteria from the skin surface is introduced at the puncture site)*. Monitor the patient for complications related to the procedure (e.g., allergic reaction, anaphylaxis, bronchospasm). Immediately report symptoms such as fast heart rate, difficulty breathing, skin rash, itching, or chest pain to the appropriate HCP. Observe/assess the needle/catheter insertion site for bleeding, inflammation, or hematoma formation.

Treatment Considerations
▶ Inform the patient that radionuclide is eliminated from the body within 6 to 24 hr. Advise the patient to drink increased amounts of fluids for 24 to 48 hr to eliminate the radionuclide from the body, unless contraindicated.

▶ Administer ordered antiemetics as needed.

▶ Instruct the patient to resume usual diet, fluids, medications, and activity as directed by the HCP.

▶ Instruct the patient in the care and assessment of the injection site.

▶ Explain that application of cold compresses to the puncture site may reduce discomfort or edema.

▶ Evaluate pain and facilitate pain management with administration of ordered narcotics, anticholinergics, and alternative methods of pain management (relaxation, imagery, music, etc.)

Safety Considerations
▶ The patient who is breastfeeding should consult with the requesting HCP regarding alternate testing that does not involve radiation. In general, if a woman who is breastfeeding must have a nuclear scan, she should not breastfeed the infant for 72 hr after the scan, until the radionuclide has been eliminated. She should be instructed to express the milk in order to prevent cessation of milk production; the milk can be stored and used after the 3-day period.

▶ Refer to organizational policy for additional precautions that may include instructions on handwashing, toilet flushing, limited contact with others, and other aspects of nuclear medicine safety.

Follow-Up, Evaluation, and Desired Outcomes
▶ Acknowledges medical and surgical therapeutic options for disease management.

Hexosaminidase A and B

SYNONYM/ACRONYM: TSD (Tay-Sachs disease) testing.

RATIONALE: To assist in diagnosing Tay-Sachs disease by identifying a hexosaminidase enzyme deficiency.

PATIENT PREPARATION: There are no food, fluid, activity, or medication restrictions unless by medical direction.

NORMAL FINDINGS: Method: Fluorometry for enzyme assay, polymerase chain reaction (PCR)/primer extension for molecular assay.

Enzyme Assay

Total Hexosaminidase	Conventional Units	SI Units (Conventional Units × 0.0167)
Noncarrier	589–955 nmol/hr/mL	9.83–15.95 units/L
Heterozygote	465–675 nmol/hr/mL	7.77–11.27 units/L
Tay-Sachs homozygote	Greater than 1,027 nmol/hr/mL	Greater than 17.15 units/L

Hexosaminidase A	Conventional Units	SI Units (Conventional Units × 0.0167)
Noncarrier	456–592 nmol/hr/mL or 55–76% of total hexosaminidase	7.62–9.88 units/L or 55–76% of total hexosaminidase
Heterozygote	197–323 nmol/hr/mL	3.29–5.39 units/L
Tay-Sachs homozygote	0 nmol/hr/mL	0 units/L

Hexosaminidase B	Conventional Units	SI Units (Conventional Units × 0.0167)
Noncarrier	12–32 nmol/hr/mL	0.2–0.54 units/L
Heterozygote	21–81 nmol/hr/mL	0.35–1.35 units/L
Tay-Sachs homozygote	Greater than 305 nmol/hr/mL	Greater than 5.09 units/L

Molecular assay: Negative for HEXA 7 mutations (samples are evaluated for seven specific HEXA gene mutations).

CRITICAL FINDINGS AND POTENTIAL INTERVENTIONS: N/A

OVERVIEW: (Study type: Blood collected in a yellow-top [acid-citrate-dextrose (ACD)] or a red-top tube for hexosaminidase enzyme assay; lavender-top [EDTA], pink-top [K$_2$ EDTA] or yellow-top tube [ACD] for molecular PCR assay; related body system: Reproductive system. The specimen should be transported *immediately* to the laboratory for processing and analysis.) Hexosaminidase is a lysosomal enzyme, the deficiency of which results in accumulation of complex sphingolipids and gangliosides in the brain and spinal cord. The three predominant isoenzymes are hexosaminidase A, B, and S. There are more than 70 lysosomal enzyme disorders. Testing for hexosaminidase A deficiency is done to determine the presence of Tay-Sachs disease, a genetic autosomal recessive condition characterized by a progressive lack of physical and intellectual development that becomes noticeable between 3 and 6 mo of age. Tay-Sachs disease is also known as *GM2 gangliosidosis type 1*. Testing is also done to establish carrier status for this inherited trait. This enzyme deficiency is most common among Ashkenazi Jews, for whom the incidence is 1 in 3,000 and carrier rate is 1 in 30. Biochemical screening tests are used to measure enzyme activity in serum or in white blood cells (WBCs). Serum screening tests should be chosen for low-risk populations because molecular assays have less than 50% specificity in the low-risk and carrier populations. WBC screening tests should be chosen instead of serum screening tests for women who are pregnant, who are taking oral contraceptives, or who have severe liver or autoimmune disease because of the unreliability of test results in samples from these patients. Negative screening results may be further investigated for the presence of pseudodeficiency mutations, which are non–disease-causing mutations. Molecular testing should be ordered for confirmation when screening results are either inconclusive or indicative of carrier status. Genetic testing by DNA PCR analysis can identify as many as 94% of the gene mutations associated with Tay-Sachs disease in persons with Ashkenazi Jewish heritage, 80% of the mutations in persons with French-Canadian ancestry, and 25% of mutations in non-Jewish Caucasians. Genetic testing combined with enzyme screening analysis and correlation of clinical information provides the most reliable means of determining carrier status. The American College of Obstetricians and Gynecologists Committee on Genetics recommends that preconceptual or prenatal screening be offered to both persons in a couple if both are of Ashkenazi Jewish, French-Canadian, or Cajun ancestry or to any person with a family history of Tay-Sachs disease. Counseling and written, informed consent are recommended and sometimes required before genetic testing. Patients who are homozygous for this trait have no hexosaminidase A and have greatly elevated levels of hexosaminidase B; signs and symptoms include red spot in the retina, blindness, and muscular weakness. Tay-Sachs disease results in early death, usually by age 3 or 4. Sandhoff disease is caused by a deficiency of hexosaminidase A and hexosaminidase B.

Knowledge of genetics assists in identifying those who may benefit from additional education, risk assessment, and counseling. Genetics is the study and identification of genes, genetic mutations, and inheritance. For example, genetics provides some insight into the likelihood of inheriting a medical condition such as Tay-Sachs disease. Some conditions are the result of mutations involving a single gene, whereas other conditions may involve multiple genes and/or multiple chromosomes. Every person receives a copy of the HEXA gene from each parent. If each parent is a carrier, has one normal and one abnormal or mutated HEXA gene, the baby has a 25% chance of developing Tay-Sachs disease because the possible combinations are 25% normal (a normal gene provided from each parent), 50% normal/carrier (a normal gene from the father and an abnormal gene from the mother or a normal gene from the mother and an abnormal gene from the father), and 25% abnormal (an abnormal gene provided from each parent). Babies who inherit a normal and abnormal copy of the HEXA gene are also considered carriers because they provide the potential for transmitting the condition to the next generation. Further information regarding inheritance of genes can be found in the study titled "Genetic Testing."

Hereditary Disease	Estimated Incidence in Ashkenazim	Estimated Carrier Rate in Ashkenazim
Bloom syndrome	1:40,000	1 in 100
Canavan disease	1:10,000	1 in 50
Familial dysautonomia	1:3,600	1 in 32
Fanconi anemia group C	1:32,000	1 in 89
Gaucher disease	1:900	1 in 15
Mucolipidosis IV	1:63,000	1 in 127
Niemann-Pick disease type A	1:32,000	1 in 90
Tay-Sachs disease	1:3,000	1 in 30
Cystic fibrosis	1:3,000	1 in 25

INDICATIONS
• Assist in the diagnosis of Tay-Sachs disease.
• Identify carriers with hexosaminidase deficiency.

INTERFERING FACTORS
Contraindications

⬥ Parents who are not emotionally capable of understanding the test results and managing the ramifications of the test results.

Factors that may alter the results of the study
• Drugs and other substances that may increase hexosaminidase levels include ethanol, isoniazid, oral contraceptives, and rifampin.
• The serum specimen hexosaminidase assay should not be performed on women who are pregnant or who are taking oral contraceptives. Increases in enzyme activity during pregnancy occur in carriers and noncarriers of the Tay-Sachs gene. Enzyme activity is also notably increased in women taking oral contraceptives regardless of carrier status.

POTENTIAL MEDICAL DIAGNOSIS: CLINICAL SIGNIFICANCE OF RESULTS
Increased in
Alterations in lysosomal enzymes metabolism are associated with various conditions.

• Total
Gastric cancer
Hepatic disease
Myeloma
Myocardial infarction
Pregnancy
Symptomatic porphyria
Vascular complications of diabetes
• Hexosaminidase A
Diabetes
Pregnancy
• Hexosaminidase B
Tay-Sachs disease

Decreased in
• Total
Sandhoff disease *(inherited disorder of enzyme metabolism lacking both essential enzymes for metabolizing gangliosides)*
• Hexosaminidase A
Tay-Sachs disease *(inherited disorder of enzyme metabolism lacking only the hexosaminidase A enzyme for metabolizing gangliosides)*

Sandhoff disease *(inherited disorder of enzyme metabolism lacking both essential enzymes for metabolizing gangliosides)*
• Hexosaminidase B

Sandhoff disease

NURSING IMPLICATIONS

BEFORE THE STUDY: PLANNING AND IMPLEMENTATION

Teaching the Patient What to Expect
▶ Inform the patient this test can assist in diagnosing or identifying carrier status for Tay-Sachs disease.

▶ Explain that a blood sample is needed for the test.

AFTER THE STUDY: POTENTIAL NURSING ACTIONS

Treatment Considerations
▶ Encourage the family to seek genetic counseling if results are abnormal.
▶ Discuss feelings the mother and father may experience (e.g., guilt, depression, anger) if abnormalities are detected.

Follow-Up, Evaluation, and Desired Outcomes
▶ Acknowledges contact information provided for counseling services and for the National Tay-Sachs and Allied Diseases Association (www.ntsad.org).

H

Holter Monitor

SYNONYM/ACRONYM: Ambulatory electrocardiography, ambulatory monitoring, event recorder, Holter electrocardiography.

RATIONALE: To evaluate cardiac symptoms associated with activity to assist with diagnosis of dysrhythmias and cardiomegaly.

PATIENT PREPARATION: There are no food, fluid, activity, or medication restrictions unless by medical direction.

NORMAL FINDINGS
• Normal sinus rhythm.

CRITICAL FINDINGS AND POTENTIAL INTERVENTIONS: N/A

OVERVIEW: (**Study type:** Electrophysiologic; **related body system:** Circulatory system.) The Holter monitor records electrical cardiac activity on a continuous basis for 24 to 72 hr. This noninvasive study entails the use of a portable device worn around the waist or over the shoulder that records cardiac electrical impulses on a magnetic tape. The recorder has a clock that allows accurate time markings on the tape, and the patient is asked to keep a log or diary of daily activities and record any occurrence of cardiac symptoms. When the patient pushes a button indicating that symptoms (e.g., pain, palpitations, dyspnea, syncope) have occurred, an event marker is placed on the tape for later comparison with the cardiac activity recordings and the daily activity log. Some recorders allow the data to be transferred to the health-care provider (HCP)'s office by telephone, where the tape is interpreted by a computer to detect any significantly abnormal variations in the recorded waveform patterns.

INDICATIONS
- Detect dysrhythmias that occur during normal daily activities and correlate them with symptoms experienced by the patient.
- Evaluate activity intolerance related to oxygen supply and demand imbalance.
- Evaluate chest pain, dizziness, syncope, and palpitations.
- Evaluate the effectiveness of antidysrhythmic medications for dosage adjustment, if needed.
- Evaluate pacemaker function.
- Monitor for ischemia and dysrhythmias after myocardial infarction or cardiac surgery before changing rehabilitation and other therapy regimens.

INTERFERING FACTORS
Factors that may alter the results of the study
- Improper placement of the electrodes or movement of the electrodes.
- Failure of the patient to maintain a daily log of symptoms or to push the button to produce a mark on the strip when experiencing a symptom.

POTENTIAL MEDICAL DIAGNOSIS: CLINICAL SIGNIFICANCE OF RESULTS
Abnormal findings related to
- Dysrhythmias such as premature ventricular contractions, bradycardias, tachycardias, conduction defects, and bradycardia
- Cardiomyopathy
- Hypoxic or ischemic changes
- Mitral valve abnormality
- Palpitations

NURSING IMPLICATIONS

BEFORE THE STUDY: PLANNING AND IMPLEMENTATION

Teaching the Patient What to Expect
- Inform the patient this procedure can assist in evaluating the heart's response to exercise or medication.
- Review the procedure with the patient. Address concerns about pain related to the procedure and explain that no electricity is delivered to the body during this procedure and no discomfort is experienced during monitoring.
- Inform the patient that it may be necessary to remove hair from the site before the procedure.
- Explain that the electrocardiography (ECG) recorder is worn for 24 to 48 hr. Afterwards, the patient is to return to the laboratory with an activity log to have the monitor and strip removed for interpretation.
- Instruct the patient to wear loose-fitting clothing over the electrodes and not to disturb or disconnect the electrodes or wires.
- Advise the patient to avoid contact with magnetic or electrical devices that can affect the strip tracings (e.g., shavers, toothbrush, massager, blanket, microwave, metal detector) and to avoid showers and tub bathing.
- Explain the importance of performing normal activities, such as walking, sleeping, climbing stairs, sexual activity, bowel or urinary elimination, cigarette smoking, emotional upsets, and medications and of recording them in an activity log.
- Explain the importance of pressing the record button upon experiencing pain or discomfort.
- Positioning for electrode attachment will be in the supine position.
- The skin surface will be prepared with alcohol and excess hair removal. Clippers may be used to remove hair from the site if appropriate, then the skin will be cleansed thoroughly with alcohol and rubbed until red in color.

H

▶ Electropaste will be applied to the skin sites to provide conduction between the skin and electrodes. Alternatively, prelubricated disposable disk electrodes may be applied.

▶ Two negative electrodes will be applied on the manubrium, one in the V_1 position (fourth intercostal space at the border of the right sternum) and one at the V_5 position (level of the fifth intercostal space at the midclavicular line, horizontally and at the left axillary line). A ground electrode will also be placed and secured to the skin of the chest or abdomen.

▶ Electrodes will be checked to ensure they are secure, then the electrode cable will be attached to the monitor and the lead wires to the electrodes.

▶ The monitor will be checked for paper supply and battery, then the tape will be inserted and the recorder turned on. All wires are taped to the chest, and the belt or shoulder strap is placed in the proper position.

AFTER THE STUDY: POTENTIAL NURSING ACTIONS

Treatment Considerations
▶ Explain that after wearing the monitor for the required 24 to 48 hr, the tape and other items securing the electrodes will be gently removed.
▶ Explain that the activity log and tape recording will be compared for changes during the monitoring period.

Follow-Up, Evaluation, and Desired Outcomes
▶ Understands the importance of reporting symptoms such as fast heart rate or difficulty breathing.
▶ Accepts that additional testing may be needed to evaluate or monitor progression of the disease process and determine the need for a change in therapy.

Homocysteine and Methylmalonic Acid

SYNONYM/ACRONYM: N/A

RATIONALE: To assist in evaluating increased risk for blood clots, plaque formation, and platelet aggregations associated with atherosclerosis and stroke risk.

PATIENT PREPARATION: There are no food, fluid, activity, or medication restrictions unless by medical direction.

NORMAL FINDINGS: Method: Chromatography

	Conventional and SI Units
Homocysteine	4.6–11.2 micromol/L
Methylmalonic Acid	70–270 nmol/L

CRITICAL FINDINGS AND POTENTIAL INTERVENTIONS: N/A

OVERVIEW: (**Study type:** Blood collected in a gold-, red-, or red/gray-top tube if methylmalonic acid and homocysteine are to be measured together; **related body system:** Circulatory system. Alternatively, a lavender-top [EDTA] tube may be acceptable for the homocysteine measurement. The laboratory should be consulted before specimen collection because specimen type may be method dependent. Care must be taken to use the same type of collection container if serial measurements are to be taken.) Homocysteine is an amino acid formed from methionine. Normally, homocysteine is rapidly remetabolized in a biochemical pathway that requires vitamin B_{12} and folate, preventing the buildup of homocysteine in the blood. Excess levels damage the endothelial lining of blood vessels; change coagulation factor levels, increasing the risk of blood clot formation and stroke; prevent smaller arteries from dilating, increasing the risk of plaque formation; cause platelet aggregation; and cause smooth muscle cells lining the arterial wall to multiply, promoting atherosclerosis. For additional information regarding screening guidelines for *atherosclerotic cardiovascular disease* (ASCVD), refer to the study titled "Cholesterol, Total and Fractions."

Approximately one-third of patients with hyperhomocystinuria have normal fasting levels. Patients with a heterozygous biochemical enzyme defect in cystathionine B synthase or with a nutritional deficiency in vitamin B_6 can be identified through the administration of a methionine challenge or loading test. Specimens are collected while fasting and 2 hr later. An increase in homocysteine after 2 hr is indicative of hyperhomocystinuria. In patients with vitamin B_{12} deficiency, elevated levels of methylmalonic acid and homocysteine develop fairly early in the course of the disease. Unlike vitamin B_{12} levels, homocysteine levels will remain elevated for at least 24 hr after the start of vitamin therapy. This may be useful if vitamin therapy is inadvertently begun before specimen collection. Patients with

folate deficiency, for the most part, will only develop elevated homocysteine levels. A methylmalonic acid level can differentiate between vitamin B_{12} and folate deficiency, since it is increased in vitamin B_{12} deficiency but not in folate deficiency. Hyperhomocysteinemia due to folate deficiency in pregnant women is believed to increase the risk of neural tube defects. Elevated levels of homocysteine are thought to chemically damage the exposed neural tissue of the developing fetus.

INDICATIONS
- Evaluate inherited enzyme deficiencies that result in homocystinuria.
- Evaluate the risk for cardiovascular disease.
- Evaluate the risk for venous thrombosis.

INTERFERING FACTORS
Factors that may alter the results of the study
- Drugs and other substances that may increase plasma homocysteine levels include anticonvulsants, cycloserine, hydralazine, isoniazid, methotrexate, penicillamine, phenelzine, and procarbazine.
- Drugs and other substances that may decrease plasma homocysteine levels include folic acid.

Other considerations
- Specimens should be kept at a refrigerated temperature and delivered immediately to the laboratory for processing.

POTENTIAL MEDICAL DIAGNOSIS: CLINICAL SIGNIFICANCE OF RESULTS
Increased in
- Cerebrovascular disease *(there is a relationship, but the pathophysiology is unclear)*
- Chronic kidney disease *(pathophysiology is unclear)*

H

- Coronary artery disease (CAD) *(there is a relationship, but the pathophysiology is unclear)*
- Folic acid deficiency *(folate is required for completion of biochemical reactions involved in homocysteine metabolism)*
- Homocystinuria *(inherited disorder of methionine metabolism that results in accumulation of homocysteine)*
- Peripheral vascular disease *(related to vascular wall damage and formation of occlusive plaque)*
- Vitamin B$_{12}$ deficiency *(vitamin B$_{12}$ is required for completion of biochemical reactions involved in homocysteine metabolism)*

Decreased in: N/A

NURSING IMPLICATIONS

BEFORE THE STUDY: PLANNING AND IMPLEMENTATION

Teaching the Patient What to Expect
- Inform the patient this test can assist in screening for risk of cardiovascular disease and stroke.
- Explain that a blood sample is needed for the test.
- Obtain a history of the patient's health concerns (symptoms, surgical procedures) and results of previous laboratory and diagnostic studies.

Potential Nursing Actions
- Investigate for a family history of heart disease, smoking, obesity, poor diet, lack of physical activity, hypertension, diabetes, previous myocardial infarction, and previous vascular disease.
- Knowledge of genetics assists in identifying those who may benefit from additional education, risk assessment, and counseling. Evaluation of genetic factors can provide direction for risk assessment related to development of type 2 diabetes, CAD, myocardial infarction, or ischemic stroke.

AFTER THE STUDY: POTENTIAL NURSING ACTIONS

Treatment Considerations
- Evaluate homocysteine levels. Increased levels may be associated with atherosclerosis, CAD, or individuals who have specific risk factors and/or existing medical conditions (e.g., elevated low-density lipoprotein cholesterol levels, other lipid disorders, type 1 diabetes, type 2 diabetes, insulin resistance, or metabolic syndrome). A variety of dietary patterns are beneficial for people with ASCVD. For additional information regarding nutritional guidelines, refer to the study titled "Cholesterol, Total and Fractions."
- Educate the patient on changeable risk factors, especially those who are overweight and have high blood pressure.
- Explain that the following lifestyle choices can decrease risk: safely decrease sodium intake, achieve a normal weight, ensure regular participation of moderate aerobic physical activity three to four times per week, eliminate tobacco use, and adhere to a heart-healthy diet. Those with elevated triglycerides should be advised to eliminate or reduce alcohol.

Nutritional Considerations
- Dietary recommendations include foods rich in fruits, grains, and cereals. Adding a multivitamin containing B$_{12}$ and folate may be recommended for patients with elevated homocysteine levels related to a dietary deficiency. Processed and refined foods should be kept to a minimum.
- Instruct the folate-deficient patient (especially pregnant women), as appropriate, to eat foods rich in folate, such as liver, salmon, eggs, asparagus, green leafy vegetables, broccoli, sweet potatoes, beans, and whole wheat.
- Instruct the patient with vitamin B$_{12}$ deficiency, as appropriate, in the use of vitamin supplements. Inform the patient, as appropriate, that the best dietary sources of vitamin B$_{12}$ are meats, fish, poultry, eggs, and milk.

H

Follow-Up, Evaluation, and Desired Outcomes
▶ Acknowledges contact information provided for the American Heart Association (www.heart.org/ HEARTORG), National Heart, Lung, and Blood Institute (www.nhlbi.nih .gov), and U.S. Department of Agriculture's resource for nutrition (www .choosemyplate.gov).

Homovanillic Acid and Vanillylmandelic Acid

SYNONYM/ACRONYM: HVA.

RATIONALE: To assist in diagnosis of neuroblastoma, pheochromocytoma, and ganglioblastoma and to monitor therapy.

PATIENT PREPARATION: There are no food, fluid, or activity restrictions unless by medical direction. If possible, and with medical direction, patients should withhold acetylsalicylic acid, disulfiram, pyridoxine, and reserpine for 2 days before specimen collection. Levodopa should be withheld for 2 wk before specimen collection. The test should begin between 0600 and 0800 if possible. Usually, a 24-hr urine collection is ordered. As appropriate, provide the required urine collection container and specimen collection instructions.

NORMAL FINDINGS: Method: Chromatography.

Age	Conventional Units	SI Units
Homovanillic Acid		*(Conventional Units × 5.49)*
3–6 yr	1.4–4.3 mg/24 hr	8–24 micromol/24 hr
7–10 yr	2.1–4.7 mg/24 hr	12–26 micromol/24 hr
11–16 yr	2.4–8.7 mg/24 hr	13–48 micromol/24 hr
Adult–older adult	1.4–8.8 mg/24 hr	8–48 micromol/24 hr
Vanillylmandelic Acid		*(Conventional Units × 5.05)*
3–6 yr	1–2.6 mg/24 hr	5–13 micromol/24 hr
7–10 yr	2–3.2 mg/24 hr	10–16 micromol/24 hr
11–16 yr	2.3–5.2 mg/24 hr	12–26 micromol/24 hr
Adult–older adult	1.4–6.5 mg/24 hr	7–33 micromol/24 hr

CRITICAL FINDINGS AND POTENTIAL INTERVENTIONS: N/A

OVERVIEW: (Study type: Urine from a timed specimen collected in a clean plastic collection container with 6N HCl as a preservative; related body system: Endocrine system. Include on the collection container's label the amount of urine, test start and stop times, and ingestion of any foods or medications that can affect test results.) HVA is the main terminal metabolite of dopamine. Vanillylmandelic acid is a major metabolite of epinephrine and norepinephrine. Both of these tests should be evaluated together for the diagnosis of neuroblastoma, one of the most common tumors affecting pediatric patients. Excretion may be intermittent; therefore, a 24-hr specimen is preferred. Creatinine is usually measured simultaneously to ensure adequate collection and to calculate an excretion ratio of metabolite to creatinine.

INDICATIONS
- Assist in the diagnosis of pheochromocytoma, neuroblastoma, and ganglioblastoma.
- Monitor the course of therapy.

INTERFERING FACTORS
Factors that may alter the results of the study
- Drugs and other substances that may increase HVA levels include acetylsalicylic acid, disulfiram, levodopa, pyridoxine, and reserpine.
- Drugs and other substances that may decrease HVA levels include moclobemide.

Other considerations
- All urine voided for the timed collection period must be included in the collection, or else falsely decreased values may be obtained. Compare output records with volume collected to verify that all voids were included in the collection.

POTENTIAL MEDICAL DIAGNOSIS: CLINICAL SIGNIFICANCE OF RESULTS
Increased in
HVA is excreted in excessive amounts in the following conditions:

- Ganglioblastoma (tumor of the nervous system)

- Neuroblastoma (tumor usually originating in the adrenal gland)
- Pheochromocytoma (tumor usually originating in the adrenal gland)
- Riley-Day syndrome (inherited disorder of the nervous system; also known as *familial dysautonomia*)

Decreased in
- Schizotypal personality disorders

NURSING IMPLICATIONS

BEFORE THE STUDY: PLANNING AND IMPLEMENTATION

Teaching the Patient What to Expect
- Inform the patient this test can assist in screening for presence of a tumor.
- Explain that a urine sample is needed for the test. Information regarding specimen collection is presented with other general guidelines in Appendix A: Patient Preparation and Specimen Collection.

Potential Nursing Actions
- Include on the collection container's label urine total volume, test start and stop times/dates, and any medications that may interfere with test results.

AFTER THE STUDY: POTENTIAL NURSING ACTIONS

Treatment Considerations
- Advise resumption of usual medications, as directed by the health-care provider.

Follow-Up, Evaluation, and Desired Outcomes
- Understands that additional testing may be necessary to evaluate or monitor disease progression and determine the need for a change in therapy.

Human Chorionic Gonadotropin

SYNONYM/ACRONYM: Chorionic gonadotropin, pregnancy test, HCG, hCG, α-HCG, β-subunit HCG.

RATIONALE: To assist in verification of pregnancy, screen for neural tube defects, and evaluate human chorionic gonadotropin (HCG)–secreting tumors.

PATIENT PREPARATION: There are no food, fluid, activity, or medication restrictions unless by medical direction.

NORMAL FINDINGS: Method: Immunoassay

	Conventional Units	SI Units (Conventional Units × 1)
Males and nonpregnant females	Less than 5 milli-international units/mL	Less than 5 international units/L
Pregnant females by week of gestation:		
Less than 1 wk	5–50 milli-international units/mL	5–50 international units/L
2 wk	5–100 milli-international units/mL	5–100 international units/L
3 wk	200–3,000 milli-international units/mL	200–3,000 international units/L
4 wk	10,000–80,000 milli-international units/mL	10,000–80,000 international units/L
5–12 wk	10,000–200,000 milli-international units/mL	10,000–200,000 international units/L
13–24 wk	5,000–80,000 milli-international units/mL	5,000–80,000 international units/L
26–28 wk	3,000–15,000 milli-international units/mL	3,000–15,000 international units/L

CRITICAL FINDINGS AND POTENTIAL INTERVENTIONS: N/A

OVERVIEW: (**Study type:** Blood collected in a gold-, red-, red/gray, or green-top [heparin] tube; **related body system:** Immune and Reproductive systems.) HCG is a hormone secreted by the placenta beginning 8 to 10 days after conception, which coincides with implantation of the fertilized ovum. It stimulates secretion of progesterone by the corpus luteum. HCG levels peak at 8 to 12 wk of gestation and then fall to less than 10% of first trimester levels by the end of pregnancy. By postpartum week 2, levels are undetectable. HCG levels increase at a slower rate in ectopic pregnancy and spontaneous abortion than in normal pregnancy; a low rate of change between serial specimens

H

is predictive of a nonviable fetus. As assays improve in sensitivity over time, ectopic pregnancies are increasingly being identified before rupture. HCG is used along with α-fetoprotein, dimeric inhibin-A, and estriol in prenatal screening for neural tube defects. These prenatal measurements are also known as *triple* or *quad markers,* depending on which tests are included. Serial measurements are needed for an accurate estimate of gestational stage and determination of fetal viability. Triple- and quad-marker testing has also been used to screen for trisomy 21 (Down syndrome). (To correlate HCG with other tests used in the prenatal genetic screening procedure, see study titled "Maternal Markers.") HCG is also produced by some germ cell tumors and may indicate testicular cancer in males and ovarian or molar (hydatidiform) cancer in females (see study titled "Cancer Markers"). Most assays measure both the intact and free β-HCG subunit, but if HCG is to be used as a tumor marker, the assay must be capable of detecting both intact and free β-HCG. Pregnancy testing is performed in many settings: at home using over-the-counter test kits, in the health-care provider (HCP)'s office using Clinical Laboratory Improvement Amendments (CLIA)–approved test kits or point-of-care instruments, and in full-service laboratories. HCG can be reliably measured using urine or blood specimens. Blood specimens are preferred because HCG levels are detectable in blood earlier than in urine specimens; urine specimens are susceptible to false-negative results if the specific gravity is too low, which is not a factor for blood specimens.

INDICATIONS

- Assist in the diagnosis of suspected HCG-producing tumors, such as choriocarcinoma, germ cell tumors of the ovary and testes, or hydatidiform moles.
- Confirm pregnancy, assist in the diagnosis of suspected ectopic pregnancy, or determine threatened or incomplete abortion.
- Determine adequacy of hormonal levels to maintain pregnancy.
- Monitor effects of surgery or chemotherapy.
- Monitor ovulation induction treatment.
- Prenatally detect neural tube defects and trisomy 21.

INTERFERING FACTORS

Factors that may alter the results of the study

- Drugs and other substances that may decrease HCG levels include epostane and mifepristone.

Other considerations

- Results may vary widely depending on the sensitivity and specificity of the assay. Performance of the test too early in pregnancy may cause false-negative results. HCG is composed of an α and a β subunit. The structure of the α subunit is essentially identical to the α subunit of follicle-stimulating hormone, luteinizing hormone, and thyroid-stimulating hormone. The structure of the β subunit differentiates HCG from the other hormones. False-positive results can therefore be obtained if the HCG assay does not detect β subunit.

POTENTIAL MEDICAL DIAGNOSIS: CLINICAL SIGNIFICANCE OF RESULTS

Increased in

- Choriocarcinoma *(related to HCG-producing tumor)*
- Ectopic HCG-producing tumors (stomach, lung, colon, pancreas, liver, breast) *(related to HCG-producing tumor)*
- Erythroblastosis fetalis *(hemolytic anemia, as a result of fetal sensitization by incompatible maternal blood group antigens such as Rh, Kell, Kidd, and Duffy, is associated with increased HCG levels)*
- Germ cell tumors (ovary and testes) *(related to HCG-producing tumors)*
- Hydatidiform mole *(related to HCG-secreting mole)*
- Islet cell tumors *(related to HCG-producing tumors)*
- Multiple gestation pregnancy *(related to increased levels produced by the presence of multiple fetuses)*
- Pregnancy *(related to increased production by placenta)*

Decreased in

Any condition associated with diminished viability of the placenta will reflect decreased levels.

- Ectopic pregnancy *(HCG levels increase slower than in viable intrauterine pregnancies, plateau, and then decrease prior to rupture)*
- Incomplete abortion
- Intrauterine fetal demise
- Spontaneous abortion
- Threatened abortion

NURSING IMPLICATIONS

BEFORE THE STUDY: PLANNING AND IMPLEMENTATION

Teaching the Patient What to Expect

- Inform the patient this test can assist in screening for pregnancy, identifying tumors, and evaluating fetal health.
- Explain that a blood sample is needed for the test.

AFTER THE STUDY: POTENTIAL NURSING ACTIONS

Treatment Considerations

- Instruct the patient in the use of home pregnancy test kits approved by the U.S. Food and Drug Administration, as appropriate.
- Encourage participation in counseling if concerned with pregnancy termination or to seek genetic counseling if a chromosomal abnormality is determined.
- Facilitate conversations regarding elective abortion in the presence of both parents.
- Provide a supportive atmosphere to discuss the risks and difficulties of delivering and raising an infant who is developmentally challenged as well as to explore other options (termination of pregnancy or adoption).
- Validate feelings the mother and father may experience (e.g., guilt, depression, anger) if fetal abnormalities are detected.
- Provide emotional support to victims of rape or sexual assault. Ensure access to counseling services is available.
- Provide a supportive atmosphere to explain and discuss the risks of sexually transmitted infections. Recognize feelings such as guilt, depression, or anger if there is possibility of pregnancy related to the assault.

Follow-Up, Evaluation, and Desired Outcomes

- Acknowledges that surgical intervention may be necessary in the event of fetal demise to ensure all of the tissue is removed to prevent infection and facilitate future viable pregnancies.
- Understands that future laboratory studies may be required to monitor and verify the continuation of the pregnancy.

Human Immunodeficiency Virus Testing

SYNONYM/ACRONYM: HIV-1/HIV-2.

RATIONALE: Test blood for the presence of antibodies that would indicate a HIV infection.

PATIENT PREPARATION: There are no food, fluid, activity, or medication restrictions unless by medical direction.

NORMAL FINDINGS: (Method: Enzyme immunoassay) Negative.

CRITICAL FINDINGS AND POTENTIAL INTERVENTIONS: N/A

OVERVIEW: (Study type: Blood collected in a red-top tube; **related body system:** Circulatory/Hematopoietic and Immune systems.) HIV is the etiological agent of AIDS and is transmitted through bodily secretions, especially by blood or sexual contact. The virus preferentially binds to the T4 helper lymphocytes and replicates within the cells using viral reverse transcriptase, integrase, and protease enzymes. World Health Organization guidelines recommend that antiretroviral therapy (ART) should be offered to any person with HIV, regardless of CD4 test results or clinical stage, along with a discussion of the availability of daily oral pre-exposure prophylactic medications for patients considered to be at high risk for HIV infection. High-risk populations include gay and bisexual men, bisexual women, transgender people, sex workers, people who share IV needles contaminated with HIV-positive blood, people who receive HIV-positive blood products, and neonates who become infected in utero or during birth. Availability of postexposure prophylactic regimens should also be discussed as appropriate. The process for obtaining specimens and communicating test results has changed dramatically since the disease was first identified. However, confirmed positive HIV findings continue to have a significant medical, psychological, and social impact on affected individuals and their potentially infected contacts. Test methods and algorithms have been developed to include as many potentially infected people as possible. Testing is available in a variety of settings, including the traditional laboratory (generally from blood specimens), specialty laboratories by mail (generally oral, finger stick, or urine specimens collected at home and mailed to the testing facility), clinical settings (using approved rapid-test kits in labor and delivery for emergencies), and nonclinical community-based screening sites (using either approved rapid-test kits or mail-in test kits). Accuracy of test results varies depending on specimen type, quality of collection technique, and test method. In the traditional laboratory setting, initial HIV screening is generally performed using a combined immunoassay for HIV1 p24 antigen and antibodies to HIV1/HIV2. The antibody screening tests most commonly used do not distinguish between HIV1 and HIV2. A positive antigen/antibody screen may be followed by repeat testing by the same method, in duplicate, if recommended by the manufacturer. Otherwise, positive initial screens should be followed by an immunoassay that differentiates between HIV1 and HIV2 antibodies. A negative or indeterminate result for HIV1 obtained by HIV1/HIV2 differentiation testing could mean that the initial positive screen was related to the presence of HIV1 p24 antigen and the specimen was obtained after infection occurred but before the development of antibodies to the virus. Negative or indeterminate differentiation testing should be followed by a nucleic acid amplification test (NAAT or NAT) to determine whether HIV1 viral RNA is present. Positive HIV1 NAT results indicate acute HIV infection. The HIV screening test is routinely recommended as part of a prenatal work-up, unless the patient declines, and is required for evaluating donated blood units before release for transfusion. The Centers for Disease Control and Prevention (CDC) has structured its recommendations to increase identification of patients who are infected with HIV as early as possible; early identification increases treatment options, increases frequency of successful treatment, and can decrease further spread of disease. The CDC recommends the following:

- Include HIV testing in routine medical care, and screen all patients between the ages of 13 and 64 years of age as part of routine medical care unless the patient requests to opt out.

- Implement new models to diagnose HIV infections outside medical settings; promote availability of rapid waived test kits such as OraQuick.
- Prevent new infections by working with persons diagnosed with HIV and their partners; adapt a voluntary opt-out approach that includes elimination of pretest counseling and consent requirements specific for HIV. General consents should cover all aspects of care.
- Further decrease prenatal transmission of HIV by incorporating HIV testing as a routine part of prenatal medical care, and also perform third-trimester testing in areas with high rates of HIV infection among pregnant women.

HIV genotyping by polymerase chain reaction (PCR) methods may also be required to guide selection of medications for therapeutic regimens, assess potential for drug resistance, and monitor for transmission of drug-resistant HIV. Genotyping is also useful to determine eligibility for new medications once resistance to conventional drugs has been identified.

INDICATIONS
- Evaluate donated blood units before transfusion.
- Perform as part of prenatal screening.
- Screen organ transplant donors.
- Test individuals who have documented and significant exposure to other infected individuals.
- Test exposed high-risk individuals for detection of antibody (e.g., persons with multiple sex partners, persons with a history of other

H

sexually transmitted infections, people who use injection drugs, infants born to infected mothers, allied health-care workers, public service employees who have contact with blood and blood products).

INTERFERING FACTORS
Factors that may alter the results of the study
- Drugs and other substances that may decrease HIV antibody levels include didanosine, dideoxycytidine, zalcitabine, and zidovudine.
- Negative HIV test results occur during the acute stage of the disease, when the virus is present but antibodies have not sufficiently developed to be detected. It may take

up to 6 mo for the test to become positive. During this stage, the test for HIV antigen may not confirm an HIV infection.
- False-positive HIV test results can occur in patients who are immunocompromised due to conditions that include autoimmune disease, leukemias, and lymphomas.

Other considerations
- Test kits for HIV are very sensitive. As a result, nonspecific reactions may occur, leading to a false-positive result.

POTENTIAL MEDICAL DIAGNOSIS: CLINICAL SIGNIFICANCE OF RESULTS
Positive findings in
- HIV1 or HIV2 infection

H

NURSING IMPLICATIONS

POTENTIAL NURSING PROBLEMS: ASSESSMENT & NURSING DIAGNOSIS

Problems	Signs and Symptoms
Infection *(related to decreased CD4 cells, detectable viral load, confirmed HIV antibody secondary to HIV infection)*	Fever; swollen lymph glands in the armpit, neck, and groin; sore throat; rash; unexplained fatigue; achy muscles and joints with pain; headache; weight loss; fever and night sweats; diarrhea lasting more than a week; mouth, anal, and genital sores; pneumonia; blotches (red, brown, pink, or purplish) on or under the skin located in the mouth or nose; depression; memory loss; neurologic disorders
Nutrition *(related to fatigue, no appetite, oral candidiasis, nausea, vomiting, malabsorption, secondary to HIV infection)*	Weight loss; pale, dry skin; dry mucous membranes; documented inadequate caloric intake; loss of subcutaneous tissue, muscle, fat; hair pulls out easily; decreased body mass index

BEFORE THE STUDY: PLANNING AND IMPLEMENTATION

Teaching the Patient What to Expect
- Inform the patient that this laboratory test can assist in evaluating for HIV infection.

- Explain that a blood sample is needed for the test.
- Warn the patient that false-positive results occur and that the absence of antibody does not guarantee absence of infection, because the virus may be latent or may not have produced

detectable antibody at the time of testing.

Treatment Considerations

▶ Instruct the patient in the use of home test kits approved by the U.S. Food and Drug Administration, if prescribed. Answer any questions or address any concerns voiced by the patient or family.

▶ Understanding how best to manage a disease can be confusing. Explain the importance of receiving pre- or postexposure HIV prophylaxis, hepatitis B vaccine, annual influenza vaccine, and pneumococcal vaccine to protect health. Counsel the patient, as appropriate, regarding risk of transmission and proper prophylaxis, and reinforce the importance of strict adherence to the treatment regimen, including consultation with a pharmacist. Assist patient to identify at-risk behaviors such as sexual activities and IV drug use. Compromised individuals can avoid circumstances that would place them at a greater risk. Avoidance of raw foods can protect against infection from bacteria and protozoa. Those with cats should avoid emptying cat litter boxes to prevent organism exposure. Safe sex practices should be discussed along with the importance of using safe needles for recreational drug use. Encourage drug rehabilitation and explain the importance of refraining from blood donation.

▶ Infection: Monitor and trend vial load and CD4 laboratory results. Explain the purpose of antiviral medication and administer as ordered; options are nucleoside and nonnucleoside, reverse transcriptase inhibitors, protease inhibitors, integrase strand transfer inhibitors, or fusion inhibitors. Ensure legal regulations regarding testing are adhered to. Reinforce the necessity of strict adherence to the designated treatment plan.

▶ *Sensitivity to Social and Cultural Issues:* Offer support, as appropriate, to patients who may be the victims of sexual assault. Educate the patient regarding access to counseling services. Provide a nonjudgmental, nonthreatening atmosphere for a discussion during which risks of sexually transmitted infections are explained. It is also important to discuss problems the patient may experience (e.g., guilt, depression, anger).

Nutritional Considerations

▶ Emphasize the importance of an accurate daily weight at the same time each day with the same scale. Obtain a nutritional history, assess attitude toward eating, and promote a dietary consult to evaluate current eating habits and best method of nutritional supplementation. Inspect the mouth for oral candidiasis infection and assess for nausea. Administer ordered medications; antiemetics, antimonilial, anabolic steroids, testosterone supplements, human growth hormones, dronabinol, and medications to enhance nutrient absorption within the gastrointestinal tract. Discuss the possibility of using total parenteral nutrition to support caloric intake with the health-care provider. Monitor laboratory values that reflect nutritional status such as albumin, transferrin, red blood cells, white blood cell count, and serum electrolytes. Encourage cultural home foods.

Follow-Up, Evaluation, and Desired Outcomes

▶ Is aware that positive findings must be reported to local health department officials, who will ask about sexual partners.

▶ Acknowledges information provided regarding pre- and postexposure HIV prophylaxis and vaccine-preventable diseases (e.g., hepatitis B, human papillomavirus) for the CDC (www .cdc.gov/vaccines/vpd/vaccines-diseases.html) and (www.cdc.gov/ DiseasesConditions).

▶ Reviews information related to HIV prevention, infection, and treatment provided by the National Institutes of Health (https://aidsinfo.nih.gov/) or CDC (www.cdc.gov/HIV).

H

Human Leukocyte Antigen B27

SYNONYM/ACRONYM: HLA-B27.

RATIONALE: To assist in diagnosing juvenile rheumatoid arthritis, psoriatic arthritis, ankylosing spondylitis, and Reiter syndrome.

PATIENT PREPARATION: There are no food, fluid, activity, or medication restrictions unless by medical direction.

NORMAL FINDINGS: (Method: Flow cytometry) Negative (indicating absence of the antigen).

CRITICAL FINDINGS AND POTENTIAL INTERVENTIONS: N/A

OVERVIEW: (**Study type:** Blood collected in a green-top [heparin] or a yellow-top [acid-citrate-dextrose (ACD)] tube; **related body system:** Immune system.) The human leukocyte antigens (HLAs) are gene products of the major histocompatibility complex, derived from their respective loci on the short arm of chromosome 6. There are three general groups: HLA-A, HLA-B, and HLA-DR. Each group contains many different proteins. HLA-B27 is an allele (one of two or more genes for an inheritable trait that occupy the same location on each chromosome, paternal and maternal) of the HLA-B locus. There are a number of HLA-B27 subtypes, not all of which are associated with disease. The antigens are present on the surface of nucleated tissue cells as well as on white blood cells. HLA testing is used in determining histocompatibility for organ and tissue transplantation. Another application for HLA testing is in paternity investigations. The presence of HLA-B27 is associated with several specific autoimmune conditions, including ankylosing spondylitis, rheumatoid arthritis, psoriatic arthritis, undifferentiated oligoarthritis, uveitis, and inflammatory bowel disease. Although less than 10% of the population are carriers of HLA B-27, 20% of carriers will develop an autoimmune condition.

INDICATIONS
* Assist in diagnosing ankylosing spondylitis and Reiter syndrome (reactive arthritis).
* Determine compatibility for organ and tissue transplantation.

INTERFERING FACTORS
Other considerations
* The specimen should be stored at room temperature and should be received by the laboratory performing the assay within 24 hr of collection. It is highly recommended that the laboratory be contacted before specimen collection to avoid specimen rejection.

POTENTIAL MEDICAL DIAGNOSIS: CLINICAL SIGNIFICANCE OF RESULTS
Positive findings in
* Ankylosing spondylitis
* Inflammatory bowel disease
* Juvenile rheumatoid arthritis
* Psoriatic arthritis
* Reiter syndrome
* Sacroiliitis
* Uveitis

NURSING IMPLICATIONS

BEFORE THE STUDY: PLANNING AND IMPLEMENTATION

Teaching the Patient What to Expect

▶ Inform the patient this test can assist with investigation of specific leukocyte disorders and determine compatibility for organ and tissue transplantation.

▶ Explain that a blood sample is needed for the test.

AFTER THE STUDY: POTENTIAL NURSING ACTIONS

Treatment Considerations

▶ Recognize the fear of shortened life expectancy, as these diseases can be moderately to severely debilitating.

Follow-Up, Evaluation, and Desired Outcomes

▶ Acknowledges the clinical implications of the test results and the lifestyle changes that will need to be made.

Human T-Lymphotropic Virus Testing

SYNONYM/ACRONYM: HTLV-I/HTLV-II.

RATIONALE: To test the blood for the presence of antibodies that would indicate past or current human T-lymphocyte virus (HTLV) infection. Helpful in diagnosing certain types of leukemia.

PATIENT PREPARATION: There are no food, fluid, activity, or medication restrictions unless by medical direction.

NORMAL FINDINGS: (Method: Enzyme immunoassay) Negative.

CRITICAL FINDINGS AND POTENTIAL INTERVENTIONS: N/A

OVERVIEW: (**Study type:** Blood collected in a red-top tube; **related body system:** Circulatory/Hematopoietic and Immune systems.) Human T-lymphotropic virus type I (HTLV-I) and type II (HTLV-II) are two closely related retroviruses known to remain latent for extended periods before becoming reactive. The viruses are transmitted by sexual contact, contact with blood, placental transfer from mother to fetus, or ingestion of breast milk. As with HIV-1 and HIV-2, HTLV targets the T4 lymphocytes. HTLV-I has been associated with adult T-cell leukemia/lymphoma (ATL) and myelopathy/tropical spastic paraparesis (HAM/TSP). Although it is believed

HTLV-II may affect the immune system, it has been not been associated clearly with any particular disease or condition. Retrospective studies demonstrated that a small percentage of transfusion recipients became infected by HTLV-positive blood. The results of this study led to a requirement that all donated blood units be tested for HTLV-I/HTLV-II before release for transfusion.

INDICATIONS

- Distinguish HTLV-I/HTLV-II infection from spastic myelopathy.
- Establish HTLV-I as the causative organism in adult lymphoblastic (T-cell) leukemia.

- Evaluate donated blood units before transfusion.
- Evaluate HTLV-II as a contributing cause of chronic neuromuscular disease.

INTERFERING FACTORS: N/A

POTENTIAL MEDICAL DIAGNOSIS: CLINICAL SIGNIFICANCE OF RESULTS
Positive findings in
- HTLV-I/HTLV-II infection

NURSING IMPLICATIONS

BEFORE THE STUDY: PLANNING AND IMPLEMENTATION

Teaching the Patient What to Expect
▶ Inform the patient this test can assist with indicating a past or present HTLV infection.
▶ Explain that a blood sample is needed for the test.
▶ Warn that false-positive results occur and that the absence of antibody does not guarantee absence of infection, because the virus may be latent or not

have produced detectable antibody at the time of testing.
▶ Advise that subsequent retesting may be necessary.

AFTER THE STUDY: POTENTIAL NURSING ACTIONS

Treatment Considerations
▶ Be supportive of impaired activity related to weakness, perceived loss of independence, and fear of shortened life expectancy. Discuss the implications of positive test results on the patient's lifestyle.
▶ Explain the information regarding the clinical implications of the test results, as appropriate.
▶ Encourage and facilitate access to counseling services.
▶ Explain that the presence of HTLV-I/ HTLV-II antibodies precludes blood donation but does not mean that leukemia or a neurological disorder is present or will develop.

Follow-Up, Evaluation, and Desired Outcomes
▶ Understands the risk of transmission and importance of proper prophylaxis.
▶ Recognizes the value of strict adherence to the treatment regimen and collaboration with a pharmacist.

5-Hydroxyindoleacetic Acid

SYNONYM/ACRONYM: 5-HIAA.

RATIONALE: To assist in diagnosing carcinoid tumors.

PATIENT PREPARATION: There are no fluid or activity restrictions unless by medical direction. Inform the patient that foods and medications listed under "Interfering Factors" should be restricted by medical direction for at least 4 days before specimen collection. Usually, a 24-hr urine collection is ordered. As appropriate, provide the required urine collection container and specimen collection instructions.

NORMAL FINDINGS: Method: High-pressure liquid chromatography.

Conventional Units	SI Units (Conventional Units × 5.23)
2–7 mg/24 hr	10.5–36.6 micromol/24 hr

CRITICAL FINDINGS AND POTENTIAL INTERVENTIONS: N/A

OVERVIEW: (Study type: Urine from a timed specimen collected in a clean plastic collection container with boric acid as a preservative; related body system: Digestive, Endocrine, and Immune systems.) Because 5-HIAA is a metabolite of serotonin, 5-HIAA levels reflect plasma serotonin concentrations. 5-HIAA is excreted in the urine. Increased urinary excretion occurs in the presence of carcinoid tumors. This test, which replaces serotonin measurement, is most accurate when obtained from a 24-hr urine specimen.

INDICATIONS

Detect early, small, or intermittently secreting carcinoid tumors.

INTERFERING FACTORS

Factors that may alter the results of the study
- Drugs and other substances that may increase 5-HIAA levels include cisplatin, fluorouracil, cough syrups containing glyceryl guaiacolate, melphalan, rauwolfia alkaloids, and reserpine.
- Drugs and other substances that may decrease 5-HIAA levels include corticotropin, ethanol, imipramine, isocarboxazid, isoniazid, levodopa, methyldopa, monoamine oxidase inhibitors, and octreotide.
- Foods containing serotonin, such as avocados, bananas, chocolate, eggplant, pineapples, plantains, red plums, tomatoes, and walnuts, can falsely elevate levels if ingested within 4 days of specimen collection.

Other considerations
- Severe gastrointestinal disturbance or diarrhea can interfere with test results.
- All urine voided for the timed collection period must be included in the collection, or else falsely decreased values may be obtained.

Compare output records with volume collected to verify that all voids were included in the collection.

POTENTIAL MEDICAL DIAGNOSIS: CLINICAL SIGNIFICANCE OF RESULTS

Increased in

Serotonin is produced by the enterochromaffin cells of the small intestine and secreted ectopically by tumor cells. It is converted to 5-HIAA in the liver and excreted in the urine. Increased values are associated with malabsorption conditions, but the relationship is unclear.

- Celiac and tropical sprue
- Cystic fibrosis
- Foregut and midgut carcinoid tumors
- Oat cell cancer of the bronchus
- Ovarian carcinoid tumors
- Whipple disease

Decreased in

The documented relationship between decreased levels of serotonin, defective amino acid metabolism, and mental illness is not well understood.

- Chronic kidney disease *(related to decreased renal excretion)*
- Depressive illnesses
- Hartnup disease
- Mastocytosis
- Phenylketonuria
- Small intestine resection *(related to a decrease in enterochromaffin-producing cells)*

NURSING IMPLICATIONS

BEFORE THE STUDY: PLANNING AND IMPLEMENTATION

Teaching the Patient What to Expect
- Inform the patient this test can assist in diagnosing tumor.
- Explain that a urine sample is needed for the test. Information regarding specimen collection is presented with

H

other general guidelines in Appendix A: Patient Preparation and Specimen Collection.

Potential Nursing Actions
▶ Include on the collection container's label urine total volume, test start and stop times/dates, and any medications that may interfere with test results.

AFTER THE STUDY: POTENTIAL NURSING ACTIONS

Treatment Considerations
▶ Instruct the patient to resume usual diet, as directed by the health-care provider.

Nutritional Considerations
▶ Consideration may be given to niacin supplementation and increased protein, if appropriate, for patients with abnormal findings. In some cases, the tumor may divert dietary tryptophan to serotonin, resulting in pellagra.

Follow-Up, Evaluation, and Desired Outcomes
▶ Acknowledges that additional testing may be required to monitor progression of the disease process and evaluate the need for a change in therapy.

Hypersensitivity Pneumonitis Serology

SYNONYM/ACRONYM: Farmer's lung disease serology, extrinsic allergic alveolitis.

RATIONALE: To assist in identification of pneumonia related to inhaled allergens containing *Aspergillus* or actinomycetes (dust, mold, or chronic exposure to moist organic materials).

PATIENT PREPARATION: There are no food, fluid, activity, or medication restrictions unless by medical direction.

NORMAL FINDINGS: (Method: Immunodiffusion) Negative.

CRITICAL FINDINGS AND POTENTIAL INTERVENTIONS: N/A

OVERVIEW: (Study type: Blood collected in a red-top tube; **related body system:** Immune and Respiratory systems.) Hypersensitivity pneumonitis is a respiratory disease caused by the inhalation of organisms from an organic source. Affected and symptomatic individuals demonstrate acute bronchospastic reaction 4 to 6 hr after exposure to the offending antigen. Inhalation of the antigen stimulates the production of immunoglobulin G antibodies. The combination of immune complexing and cell-mediated immunopathogenesis results in a chronic granulomatous pneumonitis of the interstitial space of the lung. Hypersensitivity pneumonitis serology includes detection of antibodies to *Aspergillus fumigatus, Saccharopolyspora rectivirgula, Thermoactinomyces vulgaris, Thermoactinomyces sacchari,* and *Thermoactinomyces candidus*. A negative test result does not rule out hypersensitivity pneumonitis as a possible diagnosis, nor does a positive test result confirm the diagnosis. Also, individuals with a positive test result may not exhibit the typical symptoms, and patients with severe symptoms may not have detectable levels of antibody while their disease is inactive. To confirm the diagnosis, it is necessary to obtain a sputum culture and chest x-rays.

INDICATIONS

Assist in establishing a diagnosis of hypersensitivity pneumonitis in patients experiencing fever, chills, and dyspnea after repeated exposure to moist organic sources.

INTERFERING FACTORS: N/A

POTENTIAL MEDICAL DIAGNOSIS: CLINICAL SIGNIFICANCE OF RESULTS

Increased in
• Hypersensitivity pneumonitis

NURSING IMPLICATIONS

BEFORE THE STUDY: PLANNING AND IMPLEMENTATION

Teaching the Patient What to Expect
▶ Inform the patient this test can assist in diagnosing pneumonitis.
▶ Explain that a blood sample is needed for the test.

AFTER THE STUDY: POTENTIAL NURSING ACTIONS

Treatment Considerations
▶ Instruct the patient in deep breathing and pursed-lip breathing to enhance breathing patterns, as appropriate.
▶ Advise avoiding the use of tobacco, highly polluted areas, and work environments with hazards such as fumes, dust, and other respiratory pollutants.

Nutritional Considerations
▶ Positive test results may be associated with respiratory disease. Malnutrition is commonly seen in patients with severe respiratory disease related to fatigue and lack of appetite. Stressing the importance of following the prescribed diet may be necessary.

Follow-Up, Evaluation, and Desired Outcomes
▶ Acknowledges contact information provided for the American Lung Association (www.lungusa.org).
▶ Agrees to attend smoking cessation programs.
▶ Understands the importance of protecting the lungs by avoiding contact with individuals persons who have respiratory infections.

Hysterosalpingography

SYNONYM/ACRONYM: Hysterogram, uterography, uterosalpingography.

RATIONALE: To visualize and assess the uterus and fallopian tubes to assess for obstruction, adhesions, malformations, or injuries that may be related to infertility.

PATIENT PREPARATION: There are no food, fluid, or activity restrictions unless by medical direction. Instruct the patient to take a laxative or a cathartic, as ordered, on the evening before the examination.

Note: If iodinated contrast medium is scheduled to be used in patients receiving metformin or drugs containing metformin for type 2 diabetes, the drug may be discontinued on the day of the test and continue to be withheld for 48 hr after the test.

Regarding the patient's risk for bleeding, the patient should be instructed to avoid taking natural products and medications with known anticoagulant, antiplatelet, or thrombolytic properties or to reduce dosage, as ordered, prior to the procedure. Number of days to withhold medication is dependent on the type of anticoagulant. Note the last time and dose of medication taken.

Patients on beta blockers before the surgical procedure should be instructed to take their medication as ordered during the perioperative period. Protocols may vary among facilities.

Ensure that barium studies were performed more than 4 days before the hysterosalpingography.

NORMAL FINDINGS
- Contrast medium flowing freely into the fallopian tubes and from the uterus into the peritoneal cavity
- Normal position, shape, and size of the uterine cavity.

CRITICAL FINDINGS AND POTENTIAL INTERVENTIONS: N/A

OVERVIEW: (**Study type:** X-ray, special/contrast; **related body system:** Reproductive system.) Hysterosalpingography (HSG) is performed as part of an infertility study to identify anatomical abnormalities of the uterus or occlusion of the fallopian tubes. The procedure allows visualization of the uterine cavity, fallopian tubes, and peritubal area after the injection of iodinated contrast medium into the cervix. The contrast medium should flow through the uterine cavity, through the fallopian tubes, and into the peritoneal cavity, where it is absorbed if no obstruction exists. The procedure has therapeutic indications in that passage of the contrast medium through the tubes may clear mucous plugs, straighten kinked tubes, or break up adhesions, thus restoring fertility. This procedure is also used to evaluate the fallopian tubes after tubal ligation and to evaluate the results of reconstructive surgery.

INDICATIONS
- Assist in the investigation of abnormal uterine bleeding, amenorrhea, or recurrent abortion.

- Confirm the presence of fistulas, adhesions, polyps, or pelvic masses.
- Confirm tubal abnormalities such as adhesions and occlusions; evaluate the patency of the tubes.
- Confirm uterine abnormalities such as congenital malformation, traumatic injuries, missing or ectopic contraceptive devices, or indicate the presence of foreign bodies.
- Detect bicornate uterus.
- Evaluate adequacy of surgical tubal ligation and reconstructive surgery.

INTERFERING FACTORS
Contraindications

⬥ Patients who are pregnant or suspected of being pregnant, unless the potential benefits of a procedure using radiation far outweigh the risk of radiation exposure to the fetus and mother.

⬥ Conditions associated with adverse reactions to contrast medium (e.g., asthma, food allergies, or allergy to contrast medium). Although patients are asked specifically if they have a known allergy to iodine or shellfish (shellfish contain high levels of iodine), it has been well established that the reaction is not to iodine; an actual iodine allergy would be problematic because iodine is required for the production of thyroid hormones.

In the case of shellfish, the reaction is to a muscle protein called *tropomyosin*; in the case of iodinated contrast medium, the reaction is to the noniodinated part of the contrast molecule. Patients with a known hypersensitivity to the medium may benefit from premedication with corticosteroids and diphenhydramine; the use of nonionic contrast or an alternative noncontrast imaging study, if available, may be considered for patients who have severe asthma or who have experienced moderate to severe reactions to ionic contrast medium.

✳ Conditions associated with pre-existing renal insufficiency (e.g., chronic kidney disease, single kidney transplant, nephrectomy, diabetes, multiple mycloma, treatment with aminoglycosides and NSAIDs), *because iodinated contrast is nephrotoxic.*

✳ Patients who are chronically dehydrated before the test, especially older adults and patients whose health is already compromised, *because of their risk of contrast-induced acute kidney injury.*

✳ Patients with bleeding disorders, *because the puncture site may not stop bleeding.*

✳ Patients with menses, undiagnosed vaginal bleeding, or pelvic inflammatory disease.

Factors that may alter the results of the study
- Gas or feces in the gastrointestinal tract resulting from inadequate cleansing or failure to restrict food intake before the study.
- Retained barium from a previous radiological procedure.
- Insufficient injection of contrast medium.
- Excessive traction during the test or tubal spasm, which may cause the appearance of a stricture in an otherwise normal fallopian tube.

- Excessive traction during the test may displace adhesions, making the fallopian tubes appear normal.
- Metallic objects (e.g., jewelry, body rings) within the examination field, which may inhibit organ visualization and cause unclear images.
- Inability of the patient to cooperate or remain still during the procedure, because movement can produce blurred or otherwise unclear images.

POTENTIAL MEDICAL DIAGNOSIS: CLINICAL SIGNIFICANCE OF RESULTS
Abnormal findings related to
- Bicornate uterus
- Developmental abnormalities
- Extrauterine pregnancy
- Internal scarring
- Kinking of the fallopian tubes due to adhesions
- Partial or complete blockage of fallopian tube(s)
- Tumors
- Uterine cavity anomalies
- Uterine fistulas
- Uterine masses or foreign body
- Uterine fibroid tumors (leiomyomas)

H

NURSING IMPLICATIONS

BEFORE THE STUDY: PLANNING AND IMPLEMENTATION

Teaching the Patient What to Expect
- Inform the patient this procedure can assist in assessing the uterus and fallopian tubes.
- Explain that prior to the procedure, laboratory testing may be required to determine the possibility of bleeding risk (coagulation testing) or to assess for impaired kidney function (creatinine level and estimated glomerular filtration rate) if use of iodinated contrast medium is anticipated.

▶ Pregnancy is a general contraindication to procedures involving radiation. Explain to the female patient that she will be asked the date of her last menstrual period. Pregnancy testing may be performed to determine the possibility of pregnancy before exposure to radiation.

▶ Review the procedure with the patient. Address concerns about pain and explain that there may be temporary sensations of nausea, dizziness, slow heartbeat, and menstrual-like cramping during the procedure and shoulder pain from subphrenic irritation related to the contrast medium as it spills into the peritoneal cavity.

▶ Explain that the procedure is performed in a radiology department by a health-care provider (HCP), with support staff, and takes approximately 30 to 60 min.

▶ Instruct the patient to remove jewelry and other metallic objects from the area of examination.

▶ Positioning for the procedure is in the lithotomy position on the fluoroscopy table.

▶ A kidney, ureter, and bladder film will be taken to ensure that no stool, gas, or barium will obscure visualization of the uterus and fallopian tubes.

▶ A speculum will be inserted into the vagina, and contrast medium will be introduced into the uterus through the cervix via a cannula, after which both fluoroscopic and radiographic images are taken.

Potential Nursing Actions

✦ *Make sure a written and informed consent has been signed prior to the procedure and before administering any medications.*

▶ If iodinated contrast medium is scheduled to be used in patients receiving metformin or drugs containing metformin for type 2 diabetes, the drug may be discontinued on the day of the test and continue to be withheld for 48 hr after the test. Protocols may vary among facilities.

Safety Considerations

▶ Anticoagulants, aspirin and other salicylates should be discontinued by medical direction for the appropriate number of days prior to a procedure where bleeding is a potential complication.

AFTER THE STUDY: POTENTIAL NURSING ACTIONS

Avoiding Complications

▶ Establishing an IV site and injection of contrast medium are invasive procedures. Complications are rare but include risk for severe abdominal pain or cramping, allergic reaction *(related to contrast reaction),* heavy vaginal bleeding, infection (pelvic—uterine or of the fallopian tubes) *(related to use of a catheter),* pulmonary embolism, and uterine perforation. Monitor the patient for complications related to the procedure (e.g., allergic reaction, anaphylaxis, bronchospasm, infection, injury). Immediately report symptoms such as difficulty breathing, chest pain, fever, hyperpnea, hypertension, nausea, palpitations, pruritus, rash, tachycardia, urticaria, or vomiting to the appropriate HCP. Observe/assess the needle/catheter insertion site for bleeding, inflammation, or hematoma formation. Administer ordered antihistamines or prophylactic steroids if the patient has an allergic reaction.

Treatment Considerations

▶ Instruct the patient to resume usual medications and activity, as directed by the HCP. Kidney function should be assessed before metformin is resumed.

▶ Advise that vaginal discharge is common and that it may be bloody, lasting 1 to 2 days after the test.

▶ Dizziness and cramping may follow this procedure, and analgesia may be given if there is persistent cramping. Advise contacting the HCP in the event of severe cramping or profuse bleeding.

Safety Considerations

▶ Advise diabetic patients to avoid all medications containing metformin for 48 hr following a procedure with iodinated contrast. Iodinated contrast can temporarily impair kidney function, and failure to withhold metformin may indirectly result in drug-induced lactic acidosis, a dangerous and sometimes fatal adverse effect of metformin (related to renal impairment that does not support sufficient excretion of metformin).

Follow-Up, Evaluation, and Desired Outcomes

▶ Recognizes the importance of immediately reporting symptoms such as fast heart rate, difficulty breathing, skin rash, itching, chest pain, or abdominal pain to HCP.

▶ Understands that additional testing may be necessary to evaluate or monitor disease progression and determine the need for a change in therapy.

Hysteroscopy

SYNONYM/ACRONYM: N/A

RATIONALE: To visualize and assess the endometrial lining of the uterus to assist in diagnosing disorders such as fibroids, cancer, and polyps.

PATIENT PREPARATION: There are no activity or medication restrictions unless by medical direction. Instruct the patient not to douche or use tampons or vaginal medications for 24 hr prior to the procedure. The patient may be instructed to be NPO at midnight before the procedure. Otherwise, instruct the patient that to reduce the risk of aspiration related to nausea and vomiting, solid food and milk or milk products are restricted for at least 6 hr, and clear liquids are restricted for at least 2 hr prior to general anesthesia, regional anesthesia, or sedation/analgesia (monitored anesthesia). The American Society of Anesthesiologists has fasting guidelines for risk levels according to patient status. More information can be located at www.asahq.org.

Regarding the patient's risk for bleeding, the patient should be instructed to avoid taking natural products and medications with known anticoagulant, antiplatelet, or thrombolytic properties or to reduce dosage, as ordered, prior to the procedure. Number of days to withhold medication is dependent on the type of anticoagulant. Note the last time and dose of medication taken. Protocols may vary among facilities.

Patients on beta blockers before the surgical procedure should be instructed to take their medication as ordered during the perioperative period.

NORMAL FINDINGS
• Normal uterine appearance

CRITICAL FINDINGS AND POTENTIAL INTERVENTIONS: N/A

OVERVIEW: (**Study type:** Endoscopy; **related body system:** Reproductive system.) Hysteroscopy is a diagnostic or minor surgical procedure of the uterus. It is done using a thin telescope (hysteroscope), which is inserted through the cervix with minimal or no dilation. Normal saline, glycine, or carbon dioxide is used to fill and distend the uterus. The inner surface of the uterus is examined, and laser beam or electrocautery can be accomplished during the procedure. Diagnostic hysteroscopy is used to diagnose uterine abnormalities and may be completed in conjunction with a dilatation and curettage (D & C). This procedure is usually done to assess abnormal uterine bleeding or repeated miscarriages. An operative hysteroscopy is done instead of abdominal surgery to treat many uterine conditions such as septums or fibroids (myomas). A resectoscope (a hysteroscope that uses high-frequency electrical current to cut or coagulate tissue) may be used to remove any localized myomas. Local, regional, or general anesthesia can be used, but usually general anesthesia is needed. The procedure may done in a health-care provider (HCP)'s office, but if done as an outpatient surgical procedure, it is usually completed in a hospital setting.

INDICATIONS

- Confirm the presence of uterine fibroids.
- Aid in the diagnosis and/or treatment of intrauterine adhesions.
- Investigate abnormal uterine bleeding.
- Assist in the removal of intrauterine devices.
- Assist in the removal of uterine polyps.

INTERFERING FACTORS

Contraindications

✸ Patients with bleeding disorders or receiving anticoagulant therapy *(related to the potential for continued bleeding as a result of the procedure).*

POTENTIAL MEDICAL DIAGNOSIS: CLINICAL SIGNIFICANCE OF RESULTS

Abnormal findings related to
- Areas of active bleeding
- Adhesions
- Displaced intrauterine devices
- Fibroid tumors
- Polyps
- Uterine septum

NURSING IMPLICATIONS

BEFORE THE STUDY: PLANNING AND IMPLEMENTATION

Teaching the Patient What to Expect

◗ Inform the patient that this procedure can assist in assessing uterine health.

◗ Review the procedure with the patient. Address concerns about pain and explain that there may be moments of discomfort or pain experienced when the IV line or catheter is inserted to allow infusion of fluids such as saline, anesthetics, sedatives, medications used in the procedure, or emergency medications. Explain that a local anesthetic spray or liquid may be applied to the cervix to ease insertion of the hysteroscope if general anesthesia is not used.

◗ Explain to the patient that she will be asked the date of her last menstrual period and pregnancy testing may be performed to determine the possibility of pregnancy before she undergoes the procedure in order to prevent any harm in the event of an unsuspected pregnancy.

◗ Advise that the procedure is usually performed in the office of an HCP or a surgery suite and takes about 30 to 45 min.

◗ Baseline vital signs will be recorded and monitored throughout the procedure. Protocols may vary among facilities.

◗ The patient should be asked to void prior to the procedure to reduce the risk of perforating a distended bladder.

◗ Positioning for the procedure is in the lithotomy position on an examination table where the vaginal area will be cleansed and draped.

Potential Nursing Actions

✸ *Make sure a written and informed consent has been signed prior to the procedure and before administering any medications.*

Safety Considerations

▶ Anticoagulants, aspirin, and other salicylates should be discontinued by medical direction for the appropriate number of days prior to a procedure where bleeding is a potential complication.

AFTER THE STUDY: POTENTIAL NURSING ACTIONS

Avoiding Complications

▶ Complications of the procedure may include bleeding. Advise to immediately

report symptoms such as excessive uterine bleeding or fever.

Treatment Considerations

▶ Instruct the patient to resume usual diet, fluids, medications, and activity as directed by the HCP.

Follow-Up, Evaluation, and Desired Outcomes

▶ Understands that additional testing, treatment, or referral may be necessary to monitor and treat the disease process.

Immunofixation Electrophoresis, Blood and Urine

SYNONYM/ACRONYM: IFE.

RATIONALE: To identify the individual types of immunoglobulins, toward diagnosing diseases such as multiple myeloma, and to evaluate effectiveness of chemotherapy.

PATIENT PREPARATION: There are no food, fluid, medication, or activity restrictions unless by medical direction. As appropriate, provide the required urine collection container and specimen collection instructions.

NORMAL FINDINGS: (Method: Immunoprecipitation combined with electrophoresis) Test results are interpreted by a pathologist. Normal placement and intensity of staining provide information about the immunoglobulin bands.

CRITICAL FINDINGS AND POTENTIAL INTERVENTIONS: N/A

OVERVIEW: (Study type: Blood collected in a gold-, red-, or red/gray-top tube; related body system: Circulatory/Hematopoietic and Immune systems. Place separated serum in a standard transport tube within 2 hr of collection. Place urine from a random or timed collection in a clean plastic container.) Immunofixation electrophoresis (IFE) is a qualitative technique that provides a detailed separation of individual immunoglobulins according to their electrical charges followed by the application of specific antiserum (anti-IgM, anti-kappa, etc.) and a stain, to help visualize the patterns. It is usually requested when there is an abnormality in the gamma globulin fraction of a serum protein electrophoresis, either monoclonal or polyclonal. IFE is frequently used to identify the three main immunoglobulin groups (IgG, IgM, and IgA) and the light chain proteins (kappa and lambda). Antisera for IgE and IgD are available for use, if indicated. Abnormalities are revealed by changes produced in the individual bands, such as

displacement compared to a normal pattern; intense color, which reflects an increase; or absence of color, which reflects a decrease. Urine IFE has replaced the Bence Jones screening test for light chains. IFE has replaced immunoelectrophoresis because it is more sensitive and easier to interpret. IFE is used to help detect, diagnose, and monitor the course and treatment of conditions such as chronic kidney disease, multiple myeloma, and Waldenström macroglobulinemia.

INDICATIONS

- Assist in the diagnosis of multiple myeloma and amyloidosis.
- Assist in the diagnosis of suspected immunodeficiency.
- Assist in the diagnosis of suspected immunoproliferative disorders, such as multiple myeloma and Waldenström macroglobulinemia.
- Identify biclonal or monoclonal gammopathies.
- Identify cryoglobulinemia.
- Monitor the effectiveness of chemotherapy or radiation therapy.

INTERFERING FACTORS

Factors that may alter the results of the study

- Drugs and other substances that may increase immunoglobulin levels include asparaginase, cimetidine, and opioids.
- Drugs and other substances that may decrease immunoglobulin levels include dextran, oral contraceptives, methylprednisolone (high doses), and phenytoin.

Other considerations

- Chemotherapy and radiation treatments may alter the width of the bands and make interpretation difficult.
- All urine voided for the timed collection period must be included in the collection, or else falsely decreased values may be obtained. Compare output records with volume collected to verify that all voids were included in the collection.

POTENTIAL MEDICAL DIAGNOSIS: CLINICAL SIGNIFICANCE OF RESULTS

See the "Immunoglobulins A, D, E, G, and M" and "Protein, Blood, Total and Fractions" studies.

NURSING IMPLICATIONS

BEFORE THE STUDY: PLANNING AND IMPLEMENTATION

Teaching the Patient What to Expect

- Inform the patient this test can assist in assessing the immune system.
- Explain that a blood or urine sample is needed for the test. Information regarding specimen collection is presented with other general guidelines in Appendix A: Patient Preparation and Specimen Collection.

Potential Nursing Actions

- Assess whether the patient received any vaccinations or immunizations within the last 6 mo or any blood or blood components within the last 6 wk, as these might interfere with accurate interpretation of test results.
- Include on the timed collection container's label urine total volume, test start and stop times/dates, and any medications that may interfere with test results.

AFTER THE STUDY: POTENTIAL NURSING ACTIONS

Treatment Considerations

- Independent mobility can become a concern with some disease processes. Evaluate the patient's ability to perform movement. Encourage and assist the patient to move every 2 hr to relieve tissue pressure, assist with activities of daily living, and encourage use of assistive devices. If range of motion is necessary, encourage independent range-of-motion exercises and assist where needed.
- Discuss decreasing the risk of injury and trauma that could result in bleeding. Monitor and trend hemoglobin/hematocrit, platelets, and red blood cells. Institute bleeding precautions, provide soft toothbrush, avoid aspirin, avoid intramuscular and IV injections, and coordinate laboratory draws to minimize venipuncture. Administer prescribed steroids, erythropoietin, and ordered blood and blood products. Discuss exposure to microbes that could result in infection.

Nutritional Considerations

- The patient makes dietary selections that may include omitting fresh fruit to decrease exposure to bacteria.

Follow-Up, Evaluation, and Desired Outcomes

- Understands that additional testing may be necessary to evaluate or monitor disease progression and determine the need for a change in therapy.

Immunoglobulins A, D, E, G, and M

SYNONYM/ACRONYM: IgA, IgD, IgG, and IgM.

RATIONALE: To quantitate immunoglobulins A, D, G, and M as indicators of immune system function, to assist in the diagnosis of conditions that result in deficient or excessive production of immunoglobulins; to investigate immune system disorders such as multiple myeloma. To assess IgE levels in order to identify the presence of an allergic or inflammatory immune response.

PATIENT PREPARATION: There are no food, fluid, activity, or medication restrictions unless by medical direction.

NORMAL FINDINGS: Method: Nephelometry for IgA, IgD, IgG, and IgM. Immunoassay for IgE.

Age	Conventional Units	SI Units
IgA		*(Conventional Units × 0.01)*
Newborn	1–4 mg/dL	0.01–0.04 g/L
1–9 mo	2–80 mg/dL	0.02–0.8 g/L
10–12 mo	15–90 mg/dL	0.15–0.9 g/L
2–3 yr	18–150 mg/dL	0.18–1.5 g/L
4–5 yr	25–160 mg/dL	0.25–1.6 g/L
6–8 yr	35–200 mg/dL	0.35–2 g/L
9–12 yr	45–250 mg/dL	0.45–2.5 g/L
Older than 12 yr	40–350 mg/dL	0.40–3.5 g/L
IgD		*(Conventional Units × 10)*
Newborn	Greater than 2 mg/dL	Greater than 20 mg/L
Adult	Less than 15 mg/dL	Less than 150 mg/L
IgG		*(Conventional Units × 0.01)*
Newborn	650–1,600 mg/dL	6.5–16 g/L
1–9 mo	250–900 mg/dL	2.5–9 g/L
10–12 mo	290–1,070 mg/dL	2.9–10.7 g/L
2–3 yr	420–1,200 mg/dL	4.2–12 g/L
4–6 yr	460–1,240 mg/dL	4.6–12.4 g/L
Greater than 6 yr	650–1,600 mg/dL	6.5–16 g/L
IgM		*(Conventional Units × 0.01)*
Newborn	Less than 25 mg/dL	Less than 0.25 g/L
1–9 mo	20–125 mg/dL	0.2–1.25 g/L
10–12 mo	40–150 mg/dL	0.4–1.5 g/L
2–8 yr	45–200 mg/dL	0.45–2 g/L
9–12 yr	50–250 mg/dL	0.5–2.5 g/L
Greater than 12 yr	50–300 mg/dL	0.5–3 g/L

IgE	Conventional and SI Units
Less than 1 yr	Less than 20 units/mL
2–4 yr	Less than 85 units/mL
5–9 yr	Less than 1500 units/mL
10 yr and older	Less than 160 units/mL

Values vary by method and instrument.

CRITICAL FINDINGS AND POTENTIAL INTERVENTIONS: N/A

OVERVIEW: (Study type: Blood collected in a gold-, red-, or red/gray-top tube; **related body system:** Circulatory/Hematopoietic, Immune, and Respiratory [IgE] systems.) Immunoglobulins A, D, E, G, and M are made by plasma cells in response to foreign substances. Immunoglobulins neutralize toxic substances, support phagocytosis, and destroy invading microorganisms. They are made up of heavy and light chains. Immunoglobulins produced by the abnormal proliferation of a single plasma cell (clone) are called *monoclonal.* Polyclonal increases result when multiple cell lines produce excessive amounts of antibody. IgA is found mainly in secretions such as tears, saliva, and breast milk. It is believed to protect mucous membranes from viruses and bacteria. The function of IgD is not well understood, but it is believed to participate in the activation of B lymphocytes. IgG is the predominant serum immunoglobulin and is important in long-term defense against disease. It is the only antibody that crosses the placenta. IgM is the largest immunoglobulin, and it is the first antibody to react to an antigenic stimulus. IgM also forms natural antibodies, such as ABO blood group antibodies. The presence of IgM in cord blood is an indication of congenital infection.

IgE is an antibody whose primary response is to allergic reactions and parasitic infections. Most of the body's IgE is bound to specialized tissue cells; little is available in the circulating blood. IgE binds to the membrane of special granulocytes called *basophils* in the circulating blood and *mast cells* in the tissues. Basophil and mast cell membranes have receptors for IgE. Mast cells are abundant in the skin and the tissues lining the respiratory and alimentary tracts. When IgE antibody becomes cross-linked with antigen/allergen, the release of histamine, heparin, and other chemicals from the granules in the cells is triggered. A sequence of events follows activation of IgE that affects smooth muscle contraction, vascular permeability, and inflammatory reactions. The inflammatory response allows proteins from the bloodstream to enter the tissues. Helminths (worm parasites) are especially susceptible to immunoglobulin-mediated cytotoxic chemicals. The inflammatory reaction proteins attract macrophages from the circulatory system and granulocytes, such as eosinophils, from circulation and bone marrow. Eosinophils also contain enzymes effective against the parasitic invaders. A nasal smear can be examined for the presence of eosinophils to screen for allergic conditions. Either a single smear or smears of nasal secretions from each side of the nose should be submitted, at room temperature, for Hansel staining and evaluation. Normal findings vary by laboratory, but generally, greater than 10% to 15% is considered eosinophilia or increased presence of eosonophils. Results may be invalid for patients already taking local or systemic corticosteroids.

INDICATIONS

IgA, IgD, IgG, and IgM
- Assist in the diagnosis of multiple myeloma.
- Evaluate humoral immunity status.
- Monitor therapy for multiple myeloma.
- IgA: Evaluate patients suspected of IgA deficiency prior to transfusion. Evaluate anaphylaxis associated with the transfusion of blood and blood products (anti-IgA antibodies may develop in patients with low levels of IgA, possibly resulting in anaphylaxis when donated blood is transfused).

IgE
- Assist in the evaluation of allergy and parasitic infection.

INTERFERING FACTORS
Factors that may alter the results of the study

IgA, IgD, IgG, and IgM
- Drugs and other substances that may increase immunoglobulin levels include asparaginase, cimetidine, and narcotics.
- Drugs and other substances that may decrease immunoglobulin

levels include dextran, oral contraceptives, methylprednisolone (high doses), and phenytoin.
- Chemotherapy, immunosuppressive therapy, and radiation treatments decrease immunoglobulin levels.
- Specimens with macroglobulins, cryoglobulins, or cold agglutinins tested at cold temperatures may give falsely low values.

IgE
- Drugs and other substances that may cause a decrease in IgE levels include phenytoin and tryptophan.
- Penicillin G has been associated with increased IgE levels in some patients with drug-induced acute interstitial nephritis.

Other considerations
- Normal IgE levels do not eliminate allergic disorders as a possible diagnosis.

POTENTIAL MEDICAL DIAGNOSIS: CLINICAL SIGNIFICANCE OF RESULTS
Increased in

IgA
Polyclonal

- Chronic liver disease *(pathophysiology is unclear)*
- Immunodeficiency states, such as Wiskott-Aldrich syndrome *(inherited condition of lymphocytes characterized by increased IgA and IgE)*
- Inflammatory bowel disease *(IgG and/or IgA antibody positive for **Saccharomyces cerevisiae** with negative perinuclear-antineutrophil cytoplasmic antibody is indicative of Crohn disease)*
- Lower gastrointestinal (GI) cancer *(pathophysiology is unclear)*
- Rheumatoid arthritis *(pathophysiology is unclear)*

Monoclonal

- IgA-type multiple myeloma *(related to excessive production by a single clone of plasma cells)*

IgD

Polyclonal (*pathophysiology is unclear, but increases are associated with increases in IgM*)

- Chronic infections
- Connective tissue disorders

Monoclonal

- IgD-type multiple myeloma (*related to excessive production by a single clone of plasma cells*)

IgG

Conditions that involve inflammation and/or development of an infection stimulate production of IgG.

Polyclonal

- Autoimmune diseases, such as systemic lupus erythematosus, rheumatoid arthritis, and Sjögren syndrome
- Chronic liver disease
- Chronic or recurrent infections
- Intrauterine devices (*the IUD creates a localized inflammatory reaction that stimulates production of IgG*)
- Sarcoidosis

Monoclonal

- IgG-type multiple myeloma (*related to excessive production by a single clone of plasma cells*)
- Leukemias
- Lymphomas

IgM

Polyclonal (*humoral response to infections and inflammation; both acute and chronic*)

- Active sarcoidosis
- Chronic hepatocellular disease
- Collagen vascular disease
- Early response to bacterial or parasitic infection
- Hyper-IgM dysgammaglobulinemia
- Rheumatoid arthritis
- Variable in nephrotic syndrome
- Viral infection (hepatitis or mononucleosis)

Monoclonal

- Cold agglutinin hemolysis disease
- Malignant lymphoma
- Tumors (especially in GI tract)
- Reticulosis
- Waldenström macroglobulinemia (*related to excessive production by a single clone of plasma cells*)

IgE

Conditions involving allergic reactions or infections that stimulate production of IgE.

- Alcohol misuse (*alcohol may play a role in the development of environmentally instigated IgE-mediated hypersensitivity*)
- Allergy
- Asthma
- Bronchopulmonary aspergillosis
- Dermatitis
- Eczema
- Hay fever
- IgE myeloma
- Parasitic infestation
- Sinusitis
- Wiskott-Aldrich syndrome

Decreased in

IgA
- Ataxia-telangiectasia
- Chronic sinopulmonary disease
- Genetic IgA deficiency

IgD
- Genetic IgD deficiency
- Malignant melanoma of the skin
- Pre-eclampsia

IgG
- Burns
- Genetic IgG deficiency
- Nephrotic syndrome
- Pregnancy

IgM
- Burns
- Secondary IgM deficiency associated with IgG or IgA gammopathies

IgE

- **Advanced cancer** *(related to generalized decrease in immune system response)*
- **Agammaglobulinemia** *(related to decreased production)*
- **Ataxia-telangiectasia** *(evidenced by familial immunodeficiency disorder)*
- **IgE deficiency**

NURSING IMPLICATIONS

BEFORE THE STUDY: PLANNING AND IMPLEMENTATION

Teaching the Patient What to Expect

- Inform the patient that testing for IgA, IgD, IgG, and IgM can assess the immune system by evaluating the levels of immunoglobulins in the blood.
- Inform the patient that testing for IgE can assist in identification of an allergic or inflammatory response. Explain that a negative result does not necessarily preclude the presence of a sensitivity to an allergen.
- Explain that a blood sample is needed for the test.

AFTER THE STUDY: POTENTIAL NURSING ACTIONS

Treatment Considerations

- Explain to patients with an IgA deficiency that care will be taken to request and provide blood products that have either been collected from IgA deficient donors or have been specially prepared to remove even small amounts of IgA (e.g. washed RBCs). Depending on the severity of the deficiency, blood product infusion could initiate sensitization of the immune system or result in anaphylactic shock during a subsequent blood product transfusion, *related to instigation by donor IgA in the product.* IgA deficiency is a lifelong condition.

Nutritional Considerations

- Increased IgE levels may be associated with allergy. Consideration should be given to consultation with a registered dietitian if the patient has food allergies.

Follow-Up, Evaluation, and Desired Outcomes

- Understands that additional testing may be necessary to evaluate or monitor disease progression and determine the need for a change in therapy.

Insulin and Insulin Response to Glucose

SYNONYM/ACRONYM: N/A

RATIONALE: To assess the amount of insulin secreted in response to blood glucose to assist in diagnosis of types of hypoglycemia and insulin-resistant pathologies.

PATIENT PREPARATION: There are no fluid or activity restrictions unless by medical direction. If a single sample is to be collected, the patient should have fasted and refrained, with medical direction, from taking insulin or other oral hypoglycemic drugs for at least 8 hr before specimen collection. If serial specimens are to be collected, the patient should be prepared as for a standard oral glucose tolerance test over a 5-hr period. Protocols may vary among facilities.

NORMAL FINDINGS: Method: Immunoassay.

75-g Glucose Load	Insulin	SI Units (Conventional Units × 6.945)	Tolerance for Glucose (Hypoglycemia)
Fasting	Less than 17 micro-international units/L	Less than 118.1 pmol/L	Less than 110 mg/dL
30 min	6–86 micro-international units/L	41.7–597.3 pmol/L	Less than 200 mg/dL
1 hr	8–118 micro-international units/L	55.6–819.5 pmol/L	Less than 200 mg/dL
2 hr	5–55 micro-international units/L	34.7–382 pmol/L	Less than 140 mg/dL
3 hr	Less than 25 micro-international units/L	Less than 174 pmol/L	65–120 mg/dL
4 hr	Less than 15 micro-international units/L	Less than 104.2 pmol/L	65–120 mg/dL
5 hr	Less than 8 micro-international units/L	Less than 55.6 pmol/L	65–115 mg/dL

CRITICAL FINDINGS AND POTENTIAL INTERVENTIONS: N/A

OVERVIEW: (Study type: Blood collected in a red-top tube; related body system: Endocrine system.) Insulin is a hormone secreted by the beta cells of the pancreatic islets of Langerhans in response to elevated blood glucose levels. Its overall effect is to help regulate the metabolism of glucose. Specifically, insulin decreases blood levels of glucose by promoting transport of glucose into the liver and muscles to be stored as glycogen. Insulin also participates in regulation of the processes required for metabolism of fats, carbohydrates, and proteins. The insulin response test measures insulin response to a standardized dose of glucose, administered over a fixed period of time, and is useful in evaluating patients with hypoglycemia and suspected insulin-resistance.

INDICATIONS
- Assist in the diagnosis of early or developing type 2 diabetes, as indicated by excessive production of insulin in relation to blood glucose levels (best shown with glucose tolerance tests or 2-hr postprandial tests). For additional information regarding screening guidelines and management of diabetes, refer to the study titled "Glucose."
- Assist in the diagnosis of insulinoma, as indicated by sustained high levels of insulin and absence of blood glucose–related variations.
- Confirm functional hypoglycemia, as indicated by circulating insulin levels appropriate to changing blood glucose levels.
- Differentiate between type 1 diabetes, in which insulin levels are high, and type 2 diabetes, in which insulin levels are low.
- Evaluate fasting hypoglycemia of unknown cause.

- Evaluate postprandial hypoglycemia of unknown cause.
- Evaluate uncontrolled type 1 diabetes.

INTERFERING FACTORS
Contraindications: N/A

Factors that may alter the results of the study
- Drugs and other substances that may increase insulin levels include albuterol, amino acids, beclomethasone, betamethasone, broxaterol, calcium gluconate, cannabis, chlorpropamide, glibornuride, glipizide, glisoxepide, glucagon, glyburide, ibopamine, insulin, oral contraceptives, pancreozymin, prednisolone, prednisone, rifampin, terbutaline, tolazamide, tolbutamide, trichlormethiazide, and verapamil.
- Drugs and other substances that may decrease insulin levels include acarbose, calcitonin, cimetidine, clofibrate, diltiazem, doxazosin, enalapril, enprostil, ether, hydroxypropyl methylcellulose, metformin, niacin, nifedipine, nitrendipine, octreotide, phenytoin, propranolol, and psyllium.
- Administration of insulin or oral hypoglycemic drugs within 8 hr of the test can lead to falsely elevated levels.
- Hemodialysis destroys insulin and affects test results.

POTENTIAL MEDICAL DIAGNOSIS: CLINICAL SIGNIFICANCE OF RESULTS
Increased in
- **Acromegaly** *(related to excess production of growth hormone, which increases insulin levels)*
- **Alcohol use** *(related to stimulation of insulin production)*
- **Cushing syndrome** *(related to overproduction of cortisol, which increases insulin levels)*
- **Excessive administration of insulin**

- **Insulin- and proinsulin-secreting tumors (insulinomas)**
- **Obesity** *(related to development of insulin resistance; body does not respond to insulin being produced)*
- **Persistent hyperinsulinemic hypoglycemia** *(collection of hypoglycemic disorders of infants and children)*
- **Reactive hypoglycemia in developing diabetes**
- **Severe liver disease**

Decreased in
- **Beta cell failure** *(pancreatic beta cells produce insulin; therefore, damage to these cells will decrease insulin levels)*
- **Type 1 diabetes or type 2 diabetes** *(related to lack of endogenous insulin)*

NURSING IMPLICATIONS

BEFORE THE STUDY: PLANNING AND IMPLEMENTATION

Teaching the Patient What to Expect
- Inform the patient this test can assist in the evaluation of low blood sugar.
- Explain that a blood sample is needed for the test and that multiple specimens may be required.
- Hypoglycemia: Serial specimens for insulin levels are collected in conjunction with glucose levels after administration of a 75-g glucose load.

AFTER THE STUDY: POTENTIAL NURSING ACTIONS

Avoiding Complications
- Note that the patient may have difficulty drinking the extremely sweet glucose beverage and become nauseous.
- Emphasize, as appropriate, that good management of glucose levels delays the onset and slows the progression of diabetic retinopathy, nephropathy, and neuropathy.

- Explain that unmanaged diabetes can cause multiple health issues, including diabetic kidney disease, amputation of limbs, and ultimately in death.
- Emphasize the importance of adhering to the health-care provider–recommended therapeutic regime to manage diabetes.
- Discuss the advantages of attending support group meetings to learn how to manage the disease from other people with diabetes.

Treatment Considerations

- Demonstrate how to perform a self-check glucose accurately and to correctly self-administer insulin or to take oral antihyperglycemic drugs with return demonstration.
- Explain the importance of reporting signs and symptoms of hypoglycemia (weakness, confusion, diaphoresis, rapid pulse) or hyperglycemia (thirst, polyuria, hunger, lethargy).

Nutritional Considerations

- An abnormal insulin response and impaired glucose tolerance may be associated with diabetes. There is no "diabetic diet"; however, many meal-planning approaches with nutritional goals are endorsed by the American Diabetes Association (ADA). Patients who adhere to dietary recommendations report a better general feeling of health, better weight management, better management of glucose and lipid values, and improved use of insulin. Instruct the patient, as appropriate, in nutritional management of diabetes. A variety of dietary patterns are beneficial for people with diabetes. Encourage consultation with a registered dietitian who is a certified diabetes educator.

Follow-Up, Evaluation, and Desired Outcomes

- Acknowledges contact information provided for the ADA (www.diabetes .org), American Heart Association (www.heart.org/HEARTORG), National Heart, Lung, and Blood Institute (www.nhlbi.nih.gov), National Institute of Diabetes and Digestive and Kidney Disease (www.niddk.nih .gov), and U.S. Department of Agriculture's resource for nutrition (www .choosemyplate.gov).

Insulin Antibodies

SYNONYM/ACRONYM: Islet cell antibody, glutamic acid decarboxylase antibody.

RATIONALE: To assist in the prediction, diagnosis, and management of type 1 diabetes as well as insulin resistance and insulin allergy.

PATIENT PREPARATION: There are no food, fluid, activity, or medication restrictions unless by medical direction.

NORMAL FINDINGS: (Method: Radioimmunoassay) Less than 0.4 Units/mL.

CRITICAL FINDINGS AND POTENTIAL INTERVENTIONS: N/A

OVERVIEW: (Study type: Blood collected in a red-top tube; related body system: Endocrine and Immune systems.) The onset of type 1 diabetes has been shown to correspond to the development of a number of autoantibodies. The most common anti-insulin antibody is immunoglobulin G (IgG), but IgA, IgM, IgD, and IgE antibodies also have anti-insulin properties. IgM is thought to participate in insulin resistance and IgE in insulin allergy. Increased use of human insulin instead of purified animal insulin has resulted in a significant decrease in the incidence of insulin antibody formation as a result of treatment for diabetics using insulin. The presence of insulin antibodies has been demonstrated to be a strong predictor for development of type 1 diabetes in individuals who do not have diabetes but are genetically predisposed. For additional information regarding screening guidelines and management of diabetes, refer to the study titled "Glucose."

INDICATIONS
- Assist in confirming insulin resistance.
- Assist in determining if hypoglycemia is caused by insulin misuse.
- Assist in determining insulin allergy.

INTERFERING FACTORS
Other considerations
Recent radioactive scans or radiation can interfere with test results when radioimmunoassay is the test method.

POTENTIAL MEDICAL DIAGNOSIS: CLINICAL SIGNIFICANCE OF RESULTS
Increased in
- Factitious hypoglycemia *(assists in differentiating lack of response due to the presence of insulin antibodies from secretive self-administration of insulin)*
- Insulin allergy or resistance *(antibodies bind to insulin and decrease amount of free insulin available for glucose metabolism)*
- Polyendocrine autoimmune syndromes
- Steroid-induced diabetes *(an adverse effect of treatment for systemic lupus erythematosus)*

Decreased in: N/A

NURSING IMPLICATIONS

BEFORE THE STUDY: PLANNING AND IMPLEMENTATION
Teaching the Patient What to Expect
▶ Inform the patient this test can assist in the diagnosis and management of type 1 diabetes.
▶ Explain that a blood sample is needed for the test.

AFTER THE STUDY: POTENTIAL NURSING ACTIONS
Avoiding Complications
▶ Explain that good glucose management delays the onset and slows the progression of diabetic retinopathy, nephropathy, and neuropathy.
▶ Explain that unmanaged diabetes can cause multiple health issues including diabetic kidney disease, amputation of limbs, and ultimately in death.
▶ Emphasize the importance of adhering to the health-care provider–recommended therapeutic regime to manage diabetes.
▶ Discuss the advantages that attendance in support group meetings has to learn how to manage the disease process from other people with diabetes.

Treatment Considerations
▶ Demonstrate how to perform glucose self-check and correct self-administer insulin or oral antihyperglycemic drugs including return demonstration.
▶ Explain the importance of reporting signs and symptoms of hypoglycemia (weakness, confusion, diaphoresis, rapid pulse) or hyperglycemia (thirst, polyuria, hunger, lethargy).

Nutritional Considerations
▶ The presence of insulin antibodies may be associated with diabetes. There is no "diabetic diet"; however, many meal-planning approaches with nutritional goals are endorsed by the American Diabetes

Association (ADA). Patients who adhere to dietary recommendations report a better general feeling of health, better weight management, better management of glucose and lipid values, and improved use of insulin. Instruct the patient, as appropriate, in nutritional management of diabetes. A variety of dietary patterns are beneficial for people with diabetes. Encourage consultation with a registered dietitian who is a certified diabetes educator.

Follow-Up, Evaluation, and Desired Outcomes
♦ Acknowledges contact information provided for the ADA (www.diabetes .org), American Heart Association (www.heart.org/HEARTORG), National Heart, Lung, and Blood Institute (www.nhlbi.nih.gov), National Institute of Diabetes and Digestive and Kidney Disease (www.niddk.nih.gov), and U.S. Department of Agriculture's resource for nutrition (www.choose myplate.gov).

Intraocular Muscle Function

SYNONYM/ACRONYM: IOM function.

RATIONALE: To assess the function of the extraocular muscle to assist with diagnosis of strabismus, amblyopia, and other ocular disorders.

PATIENT PREPARATION: There are no food, fluid, activity, or medication restrictions unless by medical direction.

NORMAL FINDINGS
• Normal range of ocular movements in all gaze positions.

CRITICAL FINDINGS AND POTENTIAL INTERVENTIONS: N/A

OVERVIEW: (Study type: Sensory (ocular); **related body system:** Nervous system.) Evaluation of ocular motility is performed to detect and measure muscle imbalance in conditions classified as heterophorias or heterotropias. This evaluation is performed in a manner to assess fixation of each eye, alignment of both eyes in all directions, and the ability of both eyes to work together binocularly. Heterophorias are latent ocular deviations kept in check by the binocular power of fusion and made intermittent by disrupting fusion. Heterotropias are conditions that manifest constant ocular deviations. The prefixes *eso-* (tendency for the eye to turn in),

exo- (tendency for the eye to turn out), and *hyper-* (tendency for one eye to turn up) indicate the direction in which the affected eye moves spontaneously. *Strabismus* is the failure of both eyes to spontaneously fixate on the same object because of a muscular imbalance (crossed eyes). *Amblyopia,* or lazy eye, is a term used for loss of vision in one or both eyes that cannot be attributed to an organic pathological condition of the eye or optic nerve. There are six extraocular muscles in each eye; their movement is controlled by three nerves. The actions of the muscles vary depending on the position of the eye when they become innervated. The cover test is commonly used because it is reliable, easy to perform, and does not require special equipment. The cover test method is described in this study. Another method for evaluation of ocular muscle function is the corneal light reflex test. It is useful with patients who cannot cooperate for prism cover testing or for patients who have poor fixation.

INDICATIONS
- Detection and evaluation of extraocular muscle imbalance.

INTERFERING FACTORS
Factors that may alter the results of the study
- Rubbing or squeezing the eyes may affect results.

POTENTIAL MEDICAL DIAGNOSIS: CLINICAL SIGNIFICANCE OF RESULTS
The examiner should determine the range of ocular movements in all gaze positions, usually to include up and out, in, down and out, up and in, down and in, and out. Limited movements in gaze position can be recorded semi-quantitatively as –1 (minimal), –2 (moderate), –3 (severe), or –4 (total).

Abnormal findings related to
- Amblyopia
- Heterophorias
- Heterotropias
- Strabismus

NURSING IMPLICATIONS

BEFORE THE STUDY: PLANNING AND IMPLEMENTATION

Teaching the Patient What to Expect
- Inform the patient this procedure can assist in evaluating eye muscle function.

- Review the procedure with the patient. Address concerns about pain and explain that no discomfort will be experienced during the test.
- Inform the patient that a health-care provider (HCP) performs the test in a quiet room and that to evaluate both eyes, the test can take 2 to 4 min.
- The study is performed by testing one eye at a time. The patient is given a fixation point such as the testing personnel's index finger. For pediatric patients, an object, such as a small toy, can be used to ensure fixation.
- Instructions are given to gaze at and follow the fixation point as it moves. Then the procedure is repeated using the other eye.
- This procedure is performed first at a distance and then near with and then without corrective lenses. The examiner should determine the range of ocular movements in all gaze positions, usually to include up and out, in, down and out, up and in, down and in, and out.

Potential Nursing Actions
- Obtain a history of the patient's known or suspected vision loss; changes in visual acuity, including type and cause; use of glasses or contact lenses; eye conditions with treatment regimens; eye surgery.
- Advise removal of contact lenses or glasses and explain the importance of keeping the eyes open for the test.

AFTER THE STUDY: POTENTIAL NURSING ACTIONS

Treatment Considerations
- Explain that it may be necessary to be referred for special therapy to correct the anomaly, which may include glasses, prisms, eye exercises, eye patches, or chemical patching with drugs that modify the focusing power of the eye.
- Explain that the chosen mode of therapy involves the process of mental retraining but does not correct vision. It is the process by

which the brain becomes readapted to accept, receive, and store visual images received by the eye that results in vision correction. Therefore, the patient must be prepared to be alert, cooperative, and properly motivated.

Follow-Up, Evaluation, and Desired Outcomes
▶ Acknowledges the possibility of impaired activity related to vision loss, potential loss of driving privileges, and self-image adjustments related to wearing corrective lenses.

Intraocular Pressure

SYNONYM/ACRONYM: IOP.

RATIONALE: To evaluate changes in ocular pressure to assist in diagnosis of disorders such as glaucoma.

PATIENT PREPARATION: There are no food, fluid, activity, or medication restrictions unless by medical direction.

NORMAL FINDINGS
• Normal IOP is between 10 and 20 mm Hg.

CRITICAL FINDINGS AND POTENTIAL INTERVENTIONS: Increased IOP in the presence of sudden pain, sudden change in vision, a partially dilated and nonreactive pupil, and firm globe implies acute angle-closure glaucoma, which is an ocular emergency requiring immediate attention to avoid permanent vision loss. This condition requires immediate examination by an ophthalmologist. Iridotomy is the most likely intervention.

Timely notification to the requesting health-care provider (HCP) of any critical findings and related symptoms is a role expectation of the professional nurse. A listing of these findings varies among facilities.

OVERVIEW: (Study type: Sensory (ocular); related body system: Nervous system.) The intraocular pressure (IOP) of the eye depends on a number of factors. The two most significant are the amount of aqueous humor present in the eye and the circumstances by which it leaves the eye. Other physiological variables that affect IOP include respiration, pulse, and the degree of hydration of the body. Individual eyes respond to IOP differently. Some can tolerate high pressures (20–30 mm Hg), and some will incur optic nerve damage at lower pressures. With respiration, variations of up to 4 mm Hg in IOP can occur, and changes of 1 to 2 mm Hg occur with every pulsation of the central retinal artery. IOP is measured with a tonometer; normal values indicate the pressure at which no damage is done to the intraocular contents. The rate of fluid leaving the eye, or its ability to leave the eye unimpeded, is the most important factor regulating IOP. There are three primary conditions that result in occlusion of the outflow channels for fluid.

The most common condition is open-angle glaucoma, in which the diameter of the openings of the trabecular meshwork becomes narrowed, resulting in an increased IOP due to an increased resistance of fluid moving out of the eye. In secondary or angle-closure glaucoma, the trabecular meshwork becomes occluded by tumor cells, pigment, red blood cells in hyphema, or other material. Additionally, the obstructing material may cover parts of the meshwork itself, as with scar tissue or other types of adhesions that form after severe iritis, an angle-closure glaucoma attack, or a central retinal vein occlusion. The third condition impeding fluid outflow in the trabecular channels occurs with pupillary block, most commonly associated with primary angle-closure glaucoma. In eyes predisposed to this condition, dilation of the pupil causes the iris to fold up like an accordion against the narrow-angle structures of the eye. Fluid in the posterior chamber has difficulty circulating into the anterior chamber; therefore, pressure in the posterior chamber increases, causing the iris to bow forward and obstruct the outflow channels even more. Angle-closure attacks occur quite suddenly and therefore do not give the eye a chance to adjust itself to the sudden increase in pressure. The eye becomes very red, the cornea edematous (patient may report seeing halos), and the pupil fixed and dilated, accompanied by a complaint of moderate pain. Pupil dilation can be initiated by emotional arousal or fear, conditions in which the eye must adapt to darkness (movie theaters), or mydriatics. Acute angle-closure

glaucoma is an ocular emergency usually resolved by a peripheral iridotomy to allow movement of fluid between the anterior and posterior chambers. Iridotomy uses a laser to create a hole in the iris and is the preferred method of treatment. An iridectomy is a more invasive and less often used procedure that constitutes removal of a portion of the peripheral iris either by traditional surgery or by laser. Laser iridotomy is facilitated by the neodymium yttrium-aluminum-garnet laser, also known as the Nd:YAG laser. In some cases, an argon laser may be used alone or in combination with the YAG laser.

INDICATIONS
- Diagnosis or ongoing monitoring of glaucoma.
- Screening test included in a routine eye examination.

INTERFERING FACTORS
Factors that may alter the results of the study
- Rubbing or squeezing the eyes may affect results.

POTENTIAL MEDICAL DIAGNOSIS: CLINICAL SIGNIFICANCE OF RESULTS
Abnormal findings related to
- Open-angle glaucoma
- Primary angle-closure glaucoma
- Secondary glaucoma

NURSING IMPLICATIONS

BEFORE THE STUDY: PLANNING AND IMPLEMENTATION

Teaching the Patient What to Expect
- Inform the patient this procedure can assist in measuring eye pressure.
- Review the procedure with the patient and explain there will be a feeling

of coldness or a slight sting when the anesthetic/fluorescein drops are instilled at the beginning of the procedure but that no discomfort will be experienced during the test.
- Explain that during the procedure a tonometer tip will touch the tear film and not the eye directly.
- Explain that the test is performed by an HCP in a quiet, darkened room and may take 1 to 3 min to evaluate both eyes.
- During the test, the patient will be comfortably seated and asked to look at a directed target while the eyes are examined.
- Ordered topical anesthetic/fluorescein drops will be instilled in each eye and allowed time to work.
- The patient will be instructed to look straight ahead, keeping the eyes open and unblinking.
- Several techniques are used to measure IOP; by applanation at the slit lamp (Goldmann), with a handheld (Perkins) applanation tonometer, or with a non-touch airpuff tonometer.
- When the applanation tonometer is positioned on the patient's cornea, the instrument's headrest is placed against the patient's forehead and the tonometer at an angle with the handle slanted away from the patient's nose. The tonometer tip should not touch the eyelids.
- When the tip is properly aligned and in contact with the fluorescein-stained tear film, force is applied to the tip using an adjustment control to the desired endpoint. The tonometer is removed from the eye. The reading is taken a second time, and if the pressure is elevated, a third reading is taken. The procedure is repeated on the other eye.

- With the airpuff tonometer, an air pump blows air onto the cornea, and the time it takes for the air puff to flatten the cornea is detected by infrared light and photoelectric cells. This time is directly related to the IOP.

Potential Nursing Actions
- Obtain a history of the patient's known or suspected vision loss; changes in visual acuity, including type and cause; use of glasses or contact lenses; eye conditions with treatment regimens; or eye surgery.
- Advise removal of contact lenses or glasses as instructed and emphasize the importance of keeping the eyes open for the test.

AFTER THE STUDY: POTENTIAL NURSING ACTIONS

Treatment Considerations
- Provide instruction on the use of any ordered medications, usually eyedrops, that are intended to decrease IOP, including both the ocular adverse effects and systemic reactions associated with the prescribed medication.
- Explain the importance of adhering to the therapy regimen, especially since increased IOP does not present symptoms.
- Recommend review of corresponding literature provided by a pharmacist.

Follow-Up, Evaluation, and Desired Outcomes
- Acknowledges contact information provided for the Glaucoma Research Foundation (www.glaucoma.org).
- Understands there may be some impaired activity related to vision loss or potential loss of driving privileges.

Intravenous Pyelography

SYNONYM/ACRONYM: Antegrade pyelography, excretory urography (EUG), intravenous urography (IVU, IUG), IVP.

RATIONALE: To assess urinary tract dysfunction or evaluate progression of kidney disease such as stones, bleeding, and congenital anomalies.

PATIENT PREPARATION: There are no activity restrictions unless by medical direction. Instruct the patient to fast and restrict fluids for 8 hr, or as ordered, prior to the procedure. Fasting may be ordered as a precaution against aspiration related to possible nausea and vomiting. The American Society of Anesthesiologists has fasting guidelines for risk levels according to patient status. More information can be located at www.asahq.org.

Instruct the patient to take a laxative or a cathartic, as ordered, on the evening before the examination; the bowel must be cleansed to achieve good visualization of the kidneys. Ensure that barium studies were performed more than 4 days before the IVP.

Pediatric and Older Adult Considerations: Special considerations regarding fluid restrictions may apply to patients experiencing chronic dehydration, including older adult patients in whom dehydration is common; considerations may also be given to pediatric patients. Fluid restrictions for pediatric patients may be adjusted based on age and weight.

Note: If iodinated contrast medium is scheduled to be used in patients receiving metformin or drugs containing metformin for type 2 diabetes, the drug may be discontinued on the day of the test and continue to be withheld for 48 hr after the test.

Regarding the patient's risk for bleeding, the patient should be instructed to avoid taking natural products and medications with known anticoagulant, antiplatelet, or thrombolytic properties or to reduce dosage, as ordered, prior to the procedure. Number of days to withhold medication is dependent on the type of anticoagulant. Note the last time and dose of medication taken.

Patients on beta blockers before the surgical procedure should be instructed to take their medication as ordered during the perioperative period. Protocols may vary among facilities.

NORMAL FINDINGS
- Normal size and shape of kidneys, ureters, and bladder
- Normal bladder and absence of masses or renal calculi, with prompt visualization of contrast medium through the urinary system.

CRITICAL FINDINGS AND POTENTIAL INTERVENTIONS: N/A

OVERVIEW: (Study type: X-ray, special/contrast; related body system: Urinary system.) Intravenous pyelography (IVP) is most commonly performed to determine urinary tract dysfunction or kidney disease. IVP uses IV radiopaque contrast medium to visualize the kidneys, ureters, bladder, and renal pelvis. The contrast medium concentrates in the blood and is filtered out by the glomeruli passing out through the renal tubules and concentrated in the urine. Renal function is reflected by the length of time it takes the contrast medium to appear and to be excreted by each kidney. A series of images is performed over a 30-min period to view passage of the contrast through the kidneys and ureters into the bladder. Tomography may be employed during the IVP to permit the examination of an individual layer or plane of the organ that may be obscured by surrounding overlying structures. Many facilities have replaced the IVP with computed tomography (CT) studies.

CT provides detail of the anatomical structures in the urinary system and therefore greater sensitivity in the identification of renal pathology.

INDICATIONS

- Aid in the diagnosis of renovascular hypertension.
- Evaluate the cause of blood in the urine.
- Evaluate the effects of urinary system trauma.
- Evaluate function of the kidneys, ureters, and bladder.
- Evaluate known or suspected ureteral obstruction.
- Evaluate the presence of kidney, ureter, or bladder calculi.
- Evaluate space-occupying lesions or congenital anomalies of the urinary system.

INTERFERING FACTORS

Contraindications

Patients who are pregnant or suspected of being pregnant, unless the potential benefits of a procedure using radiation far outweigh the risk of radiation exposure to the fetus and mother.

Patients with conditions associated with adverse reactions to contrast medium (e.g., asthma, food allergies, or allergy to contrast medium). Although patients are asked specifically if they have a known allergy to iodine or shellfish (shellfish contain high levels of iodine), it has been well established that the reaction is not to iodine; an actual iodine allergy would be problematic because iodine is required for the production of thyroid hormones. In the case of shellfish, the reaction is to a muscle protein called *tropomyosin*; in the case of iodinated contrast medium, the reaction is to the noniodinated part of the contrast molecule. Patients with a known hypersensitivity to the medium may benefit from premedication with corticosteroids and diphenhydramine; the use of nonionic contrast or an alternative noncontrast imaging study, if available, may be considered for patients who have severe asthma or who have experienced moderate to severe reactions to ionic contrast medium.

Conditions associated with preexisting renal insufficiency (e.g., chronic kidney disease, single kidney transplant, nephrectomy, diabetes, multiple myeloma, treatment with aminoglycosides and NSAIDs), *because iodinated contrast is nephrotoxic.*

Patients who are chronically dehydrated before the test, especially older adults and patients whose health is already compromised, *because of their risk of contrast-induced acute kidney injury.*

Patients with bleeding disorders or receiving anticoagulant therapy, *because the puncture site may not stop bleeding.*

Factors that may alter the results of the study

- Gas or feces in the gastrointestinal tract resulting from inadequate cleansing or failure to restrict food intake before the study.
- Retained barium from a previous radiological procedure.
- Metallic objects (e.g., jewelry, body rings) within the examination field, which may inhibit organ visualization and cause unclear images.
- Inability of the patient to cooperate or remain still during the procedure because movement can produce blurred or otherwise unclear images.

POTENTIAL MEDICAL DIAGNOSIS: CLINICAL SIGNIFICANCE OF RESULTS

Abnormal findings related to

- Absence of a kidney (congenital malformation)
- Benign and malignant kidney tumors

- Bladder tumors
- Congenital kidney or urinary tract abnormalities
- Glomerulonephritis
- Hydronephrosis
- Prostatic enlargement

- Pyelonephritis
- Renal cysts
- Renal hematomas
- Renal or ureteral calculi
- Soft tissue masses
- Tumors of the collecting system

NURSING IMPLICATIONS

POTENTIAL NURSING PROBLEMS: ASSESSMENT & NURSING DIAGNOSIS

Problems	Signs and Symptoms
Infection *(related to stones, urinary stasis, invasive procedure, postoperative change in skin condition [incision])*	Fever; chills; changes in laboratory studies (white blood cell [WBC] count, C-reactive protein, urine culture); diaphoresis; increased heart rate; urine frequency and burning; cloudy, foul-smelling urine; red indurated incision; draining incision
Insufficient fluid volume (water) *(related to vomiting, nausea)*	Dry mucous membranes, low blood pressure, increased heart rate, slow capillary refill, diminished skin turgor, diminished urine output
Pain *(related to stones, obstruction and/or anomalies, spasm)*	Self-report of pain in flank area, facial grimace, moaning, crying, abdominal guarding

BEFORE THE STUDY: PLANNING AND IMPLEMENTATION

Teaching the Patient What to Expect

▶ Inform the patient this procedure can assist in assessing the kidneys, ureters, and bladder.

▶ Explain that prior to the procedure, laboratory testing may be required to determine the possibility of bleeding risk (coagulation testing) or to assess for impaired kidney function (creatinine level and estimated glomerular filtration rate) if use of iodinated contrast medium is anticipated.

▶ Pregnancy is a general contraindication to procedures involving radiation. Explain to the female patient that she will be asked the date of her last menstrual period. Pregnancy testing may be performed to determine the possibility of pregnancy before exposure to radiation.

▶ Review the procedure with the patient. Address concerns about pain and explain that there may be moments of discomfort or pain experienced when the IV line or catheter is inserted to allow infusion of fluids such as saline, anesthetics, sedatives, contrast medium, medications used in the procedure, or emergency medications.

▶ Explain that contrast medium will be injected, by catheter, at a separate site from the IV line.

▶ Advise that a burning and flushing sensation may be felt throughout the body during injection of the contrast medium and the patient may experience an urge to cough, flushing, nausea, or a salty or metallic taste.

▶ Explain that the procedure is performed in a radiology department by a health-care provider (HCP) and takes approximately 30 to 60 min.

▶ Instruct the patient to remove jewelry and other metallic objects from the area of examination.

▶ Baseline vital signs will be recorded and monitored throughout the procedure. Protocols may vary among facilities.

- Positioning for this study will be in the supine position on an examination table.
- A kidney, ureter, and bladder (KUB) or plain film is taken to ensure that no barium or stool obscures visualization of the urinary system.
- Advise taking slow, deep breaths if nausea occurs during the procedure. An ordered antiemetic drug can be administered as needed. An emesis basin can be ready for use.
- Explain to the patient he or she will be monitored for complications related to the procedure (e.g., allergic reaction, anaphylaxis, bronchospasm).
- Images will be taken at 1, 5, 10, 15, 20, and 30 min following injection of the contrast medium into the urinary system. The patient will be asked to exhale deeply and to hold his or her breath while each image is taken.
- Explain that once the study is completed, the needle or catheter is removed, and a pressure dressing is applied over the puncture site.
- Patients will be instructed to void if a postvoiding exposure is required to visualize the empty bladder.

Potential Nursing Actions

✴ *Make sure a written and informed consent has been signed prior to the procedure and before administering any medications.*

- If iodinated contrast medium is scheduled to be used in patients receiving metformin or drugs containing metformin for type 2 diabetes, the drug may be discontinued on the day of the test and continue to be withheld for 48 hr after the test. Protocols may vary among facilities.

Safety Considerations

- Anticoagulants, aspirin and other salicylates should be discontinued by medical direction for the appropriate number of days prior to a procedure in which bleeding is a potential complication.
- **Older Adult Considerations:** The combination of fluid restrictions and administration of laxatives may cause increased injury risk from falling for older adult patients, related to weakness. Additional monitoring and assistance while ambulating may be required.

Avoiding Complications

- Establishing an IV site and injection of contrast medium are invasive procedures. Complications are rare but include risk for allergic reaction *(related to contrast reaction).* Monitor the patient for complications related to the procedure (e.g., allergic reaction, anaphylaxis, bronchospasm, infection, injury). Immediately report symptoms such as difficulty breathing, chest pain, fever, hyperpnea, hypertension, nausea, palpitations, pruritus, rash, tachycardia, urticaria, or vomiting to the appropriate HCP. Observe/assess the needle/catheter insertion site for bleeding, inflammation, or hematoma formation. Administer ordered antihistamines or prophylactic steroids if the patient has an allergic reaction.

Treatment Considerations

- Instruct the patient to resume usual diet, fluids, medications, or activity, as directed by the HCP. Kidney function should be assessed before metformin is resumed.
- Infection: Treatment includes administration of ordered antibiotics and antipyretics. Monitor and trend laboratory results and vital signs. Monitor surgical site for redness, induration, and drainage. Assess urine characteristics, color, odor, and for the presence of blood.
- Monitor urinary output after the procedure. Decreased urine output may indicate acute kidney injury.
- Insufficient Fluid Volume: Observation and assessment for dehydration is important when fluids are insufficient. Applicable interventions are to monitor and trend vital signs, urine color, intake and output, and laboratory studies (uric acid, blood urea nitrogen [BUN], creatinine [Cr], electrolytes). Administer ordered parenteral fluids, encourage oral fluid intake, and administer ordered antiemetics.
- Pain: Management of pain should be individualized. Some interventions are

to assess pain character, location, duration, and intensity. Use an easily understood pain rating scale, consider alternate measures for pain management (imagery, relaxation, music, etc.), and place the patient in a position of comfort (knees to chest). Administer ordered analgesics and parenteral fluids, and encourage oral fluids. Monitor and trend laboratory studies (BUN, Cr, WBC count, uric acid, calcium, electrolytes), and strain urine.

◗ Instruct the patient in the care and assessment of the injection site and to apply cold compresses as needed, to reduce discomfort or edema.

Safety Considerations

◗ Advise diabetic patients to avoid all medications containing metformin for 48 hr following a procedure with iodinated contrast. Iodinated contrast can temporarily impair kidney function, and failure to withhold metformin may indirectly result in drug-induced lactic acidosis, a dangerous and sometimes fatal adverse effect of metformin (related to renal impairment that does not support sufficient excretion of metformin).

Follow-Up, Evaluation, and Desired Outcomes

◗ Collaborates with the HCP to devise a plan of care that supports renal health.

Intrinsic Factor Antibodies

SYNONYM/ACRONYM: IF antibodies, intrinsic factor blocking antibodies.

RATIONALE: To assist in the investigation of suspected pernicious anemia.

PATIENT PREPARATION: There are no food, fluid, or activity restrictions unless by medical direction. Administration of vitamin B_{12}, injected, ingested, or administered otherwise (e.g., absorbed by nasal gel or sublingual tablet), should be withheld within 2 wk before testing.

NORMAL FINDINGS: (Method: Immunoassay) Negative.

CRITICAL FINDINGS AND POTENTIAL INTERVENTIONS: N/A

OVERVIEW: (**Study type:** Blood collected in a gold-, red-, or red/gray-top tube; **related body system:** Circulatory/Hematopoietic, Digestive, and Immune systems.) Intrinsic factor (IF) is a glycoprotein produced by the parietal cells of the gastric mucosa. IF is required for the normal absorption of vitamin B_{12} and measurement of circulating antibodies to IF is used to evaluate conditions of vitamin B_{12} deficiency. There are two types of antibodies: type 1, the more commonly present blocking antibody, and type 2, the binding antibody. The blocking

antibody prevents attachment of vitamin B_{12} at the binding site of IF. Binding antibody combines with either free or complexed IF, inhibiting attachment of the vitamin B_{12}–intrinsic factor complex to ileal receptors. Autoantibodies may also form against parietal cells and can be detected by enzyme immunoassay.

INDICATIONS

• Assist in the diagnosis of pernicious anemia.
• Evaluate patients with decreased vitamin B_{12} levels.

INTERFERING FACTORS

Factors that may alter the results of the study

- Vitamin B_{12} injected or ingested within 48 hr of the test invalidates results.

Other considerations

- Recent treatment with methotrexate or another folic acid antagonist can interfere with test results.

POTENTIAL MEDICAL DIAGNOSIS: CLINICAL SIGNIFICANCE OF RESULTS

Increased in

Conditions that involve the production of these blocking and binding autoantibodies

- Megaloblastic anemia
- Pernicious anemia
- Some patients with hyperthyroidism
- Some patients with type 1 diabetes

Decreased in: N/A

NURSING IMPLICATIONS

BEFORE THE STUDY: PLANNING AND IMPLEMENTATION

Teaching the Patient What to Expect

- Inform the patient this test can assist in assessing for anemia.
- Explain that a blood sample is needed for the test.

Potential Nursing Actions

- Central nervous system changes have a strong association with pernicious and megaloblastic anemias. Onset of the anemia may occur over a prolonged period of time during which the patient may be unaware of the development of symptoms; ask the patient whether he or she has experienced alterations in sensory organ function, such as blurred or other changes in vision, loss of hearing, or changes in how foods taste. Ask the patient if he or she is experiencing dizziness,

disorientation, irritability, memory loss, numbness, tingling, or lack of coordination. Ask male patients if they are experiencing impotence.

AFTER THE STUDY: POTENTIAL NURSING ACTIONS

Treatment Considerations

- Explain that anemias associated with vitamin B_{12} deficiency produce a variety of signs and symptoms that may cause significant distress.
- Explain that neurological complications may cause personality changes such as irritability, paranoia, disorientation, or delirium. Depending on the family situation, arrangements for social service or home care referrals may be indicated.
- Discuss ways to help those with fine motor deficits feel greater independence. For example, the patient may have an easier time dressing if clothing without small buttons or hooks is chosen. If permanent neurological deficits are experienced, the health-care provider (HCP) may recommend a referral to physical therapy for rehabilitation.
- Demonstrate how to self-administer a vitamin B_{12} injection with return demonstration. Provide resources for education regarding adverse effects and interactions with other drugs.
- Since there is an association between pernicious anemia and increased risk for developing gastric cancer, encourage the patient to have regular complete physical examinations.

Safety Considerations

- Institute fall risk precautions related to the level of risk associated with the patient's condition.

Nutritional Considerations

- Discuss the need for a well-balanced diet with foods that contain vitamin B_{12}, including adequate daily fluid volume.

Follow-Up, Evaluation, and Desired Outcomes

- Acknowledges it may be necessary for further testing to be performed and that a referral to another HCP may be necessary for better therapeutic management.

Iron Studies: Iron (Total), Iron-Binding Capacity (Total), Transferrin, and Iron Saturation

SYNONYM/ACRONYM: Iron: Fe; iron-binding capacity and iron saturation: TIBC, Fe Sat; transferrin: siderophilin, TRF.

RATIONALE: To monitor and assess iron levels related to blood loss, dietary intake and metabolism, storage disorders, and replacement therapy. To assist in diagnosing types of anemia such as iron deficiency.

PATIENT PREPARATION: Instruct the patient to fast for at least 12 hr before specimen collection for iron or transferrin and, with medical direction, to refrain from taking iron-containing medicines before specimen collection. There are no food, fluid, activity, or medication restrictions unless by medical direction for the TIBC and iron saturation. Specimen collection for iron studies should be delayed for several days after blood transfusion. Protocols may vary among facilities.

NORMAL FINDINGS: Method: Spectrophotometry for iron and TIBC; nephelometry for transferrin.

Iron

Age	Conventional Units	SI Units (Conventional Units × 0.179)
Newborn	100–250 mcg/dL	17.9–44.8 micromol/L
Infant–9 yr	20–105 mcg/dL	3.6–18.8 micromol/L
10–14 yr	20–145 mcg/dL	3.6–26 micromol/L
Adult		
Male	65–175 mcg/dL	11.6–31.3 micromol/L
Female	50–170 mcg/dL	9–30.4 micromol/L

Values tend to decrease in older adults.

Test	Conventional Units	SI Units (Conventional Units × 0.179)
TIBC	250–450 mcg/dL	45–81 micromol/L
Transferrin-iron saturation %	10%–50%	10%–50%

The percentage of transferrin saturated with iron can be calculated as either (serum iron/TIBC value) × 100 or (serum iron × 100%)/TIBC.

Transferrin (Direct Measurement)		
Age	Conventional Units	SI Units (Conventional Units × 0.01)
Newborn	130–275 mg/dL	1.3–2.75 g/L
1–9 yr	180–330 mg/dL	1.8–3.3 g/L
10–19 yr	195–385 mg/dL	1.95–3.85 g/L

Transferrin (Direct Measurement)		
Age	Conventional Units	SI Units (Conventional Units × 0.01)
Adult		
Male	215–365 mg/dL	2.2–3.6 g/L
Female	250–380 mg/dL	2.5–3.8 g/L

CRITICAL FINDINGS AND POTENTIAL INTERVENTIONS

Iron

- Mild Toxicity: Greater than 350 mcg/dL (SI: Greater than 62.6 micromol/L)
- Serious Toxicity: Greater than 400 mcg/dL (SI: Greater than 71.6 micromol/L)
- Lethal: Greater than 1,000 mcg/dL (SI: Greater than 179 micromol/L).

Timely notification to the requesting health-care provider (HCP) of any critical findings and related symptoms is a role expectation of the professional nurse. A listing of these findings varies among facilities.

Intervention may include chelation therapy by administration of deferoxamine mesylate (Desferal).

OVERVIEW: (Study type: Blood collected in a gold-, red-, or red/gray-top tube; **related body system:** Circulatory system.) Iron plays a principal role in erythropoiesis, the formation and maturation of red blood cells (RBCs) and is required for hemoglobin (Hgb) synthesis. The human body contains between 4 and 5 grams of iron, about 65% of which is present in hemoglobin and 3% of which is present in myoglobin, the oxygen storage protein found in skeletal and cardiac muscle. A small amount is also found in cellular enzymes that catalyze the oxidation and reduction of iron. Excess iron is stored in the liver and spleen as ferritin and hemosiderin. Any iron present in the serum is in transit between the alimentary tract, the bone marrow, and available iron storage forms. Sixty to seventy percent of the body's iron is carried by its specific transport protein, transferrin.

TIBC and transferrin are sometimes referred to interchangeably, even though other proteins carry iron and contribute to the TIBC. Transferrin is a glycoprotein formed in the liver. Its role is the transportation of iron obtained from dietary intake or RBC breakdown; normally, one-third of available transferrin is saturated. Inadequate transferrin levels can lead to impaired Hgb synthesis and anemia. Transferrin is subject to diurnal variation, and it is responsible for the variation in levels of serum iron throughout the day. Normally, iron enters the body by oral ingestion; only 10% is absorbed, but as much as 20% to 30% can be absorbed in patients with iron-deficiency anemia. Unbound iron is highly toxic, but there is generally an excess of transferrin available to prevent the buildup of unbound iron in the circulation. Iron overload is as clinically significant as iron deficiency.

An example of acute iron overload is the accidental poisoning of children caused by excessive intake of iron-containing multivitamins. Chronic iron overload can occur in patients receiving serial therapeutic transfusions of RBCs over time for treatment of various cancers, hemoglobinopathies such as sickle cell anemia, the thalassemias, and other hemolytic anemias.

INDICATIONS

- Assist in the diagnosis of blood loss, as evidenced by decreased serum iron.
- Assist in the diagnosis of hemochromatosis or other disorders of iron metabolism and storage.
- Determine the differential diagnosis of anemia (e.g., between iron-deficiency anemia and anemia secondary to chronic disease).
- Determine the iron-binding capacity of the blood.
- Determine the presence of disorders that involve diminished protein synthesis or defects in iron absorption.
- Evaluate accidental iron poisoning.
- Evaluate iron metabolism in iron-deficiency anemia.
- Evaluate iron overload in dialysis patients or patients with transfusion-dependent anemias.
- Evaluate nutritional status.
- Evaluate thalassemia and sideroblastic anemia.
- Monitor hematological responses during pregnancy, when serum iron is usually decreased.
- Monitor response to treatment for anemia.

INTERFERING FACTORS

Factors that may alter the results of the study

- Drugs and other substances that may increase iron levels include blood transfusion products, chemotherapy drugs, iron (intramuscular), iron dextran, iron-protein-succinylate, methimazole, methotrexate, oral contraceptives, and rifampin.
- Failure to withhold iron-containing medications 24 hr before the test may falsely increase iron values.
- Drugs and other substances that may increase TIBC levels include mestranol and oral contraceptives.
- Drugs and other substances that may increase transferrin levels include carbamazepine, danazol, mestranol, and oral contraceptives.
- Drugs and other substances that may decrease iron levels include acetylsalicylic acid, allopurinol, cholestyramine, corticotropin, cortisone, deferoxamine mesylate, and metformin.
- Drugs and other substances that may decrease TIBC levels include asparaginase, chloramphenicol, corticotropin, cortisone, and testosterone.
- Drugs and other substances that may decrease transferrin levels include cortisone and dextran.

Other considerations

- Gross hemolysis can interfere with iron test results.
- Transferrin levels are subject to diurnal variation and should be collected in the morning, when levels are highest.

POTENTIAL MEDICAL DIAGNOSIS: CLINICAL SIGNIFICANCE OF RESULTS

Summary of the Relationship Between Serum Iron, TIBC, Transferrin, % Iron Saturation, and Ferritin in Select Circumstances

	Iron	TIBC	Transferrin	% Saturation	Ferritin (Stored Iron)
Iron-deficiency (anemia)	Decreased	Increased	Increased	Decreased	Decreased
Chronic etiology (cancer, infection, liver disease)	Decreased	Decreased	Decreased	Normal	Normal/ increased
Hemolytic (anemia)	Increased	Normal/ decreased	Normal/ decreased	Increased	Increased
Iron overload/ hemochromatosis	Increased	Decreased	Decreased	Increased	Increased
Iron overload/ therapy/poisoning	Increased	Normal/ decreased	Decreased	Increased	Normal

Increased in

Iron

- Acute iron poisoning (children) *(related to excessive intake)*
- Acute leukemia
- Acute liver disease *(possibly related to decrease in synthesis of iron storage proteins by damaged liver; iron accumulates and levels increase)*
- Aplastic anemia *(related to repeated blood transfusions)*
- Excessive iron therapy *(related to excessive intake)*
- Hemochromatosis *(inherited disorder of iron overload; the iron is not excreted in proportion to the rate of accumulation)*
- Hemolytic anemias *(related to release of iron from lysed RBCs)*
- Lead toxicity *(lead can biologically mimic iron, displace it, and release it into circulation where its concentration increases)*
- Nephritis *(related to decreased renal excretion; accumulation in blood)*
- Pernicious anemias (PA) *(achlorhydria associated with PA prevents absorption of dietary iron, and it accumulates in the blood)*
- Sideroblastic anemias *(enzyme disorder prevents iron from being incorporated into Hgb, and it accumulates in the blood)*
- Thalassemia *(treatment for some types of thalassemia include blood transfusions, which can lead to iron overload)*
- Transfusions (repeated)
- Vitamin B_6 deficiency *(this vitamin is essential to Hgb formation; deficiency prevents iron from being incorporated into Hgb, and it accumulates in the blood)*

TIBC and Transferrin

- Estrogen therapy *(estrogen stimulates the liver to produce transferrin)*

- Hypochromic (iron-deficiency) anemias *(insufficient circulating iron levels to saturate binding sites)*
- Pregnancy *(the liver produces transferrin in response to anemia of pregnancy)*

Decreased in

Iron

- Acute and chronic infection *(iron is a nutrient for invading organisms)*
- Cancer *(related to depletion of iron stores)*
- Chronic blood loss (gastrointestinal [GI], uterine) *(blood contains iron incorporated in Hgb)*
- Dietary deficiency
- Hypothyroidism *(pathophysiology is unclear)*
- Intestinal malabsorption
- Iron-deficiency anemia *(related to depletion of iron stores)*
- Nephrosis *(anemia is common in people with kidney disease; fewer RBCs are made because of a deficiency of erythropoietin related to the damaged kidneys, blood can be lost in dialysis, and iron intake may be lower due to lack of appetite)*
- Postoperative state
- Pregnancy *(related to depletion of iron stores by developing fetus)*
- Protein malnutrition (kwashiorkor) *(protein is required to form transport proteins, RBCs, and Hgb)*

TIBC and Transferrin

- Acute or chronic infection *(transferrin is a negative acute-phase reactant protein whose levels decrease in response to inflammation)*
- Cancer (especially of the gastrointestinal tract) *(related to malnutrition)*
- Hemochromatosis *(occurs early in the disease as intestinal absorption of iron available for binding increases)*

- Hemolytic anemias *(transferrin becomes saturated, and the iron-binding capacity is significantly decreased)*
- Kidney disease *(transferrin is a negative acute-phase reactant protein that demonstrates decreased levels during periods of inflammation)*
- Liver disease or damage *(related to decreased synthesis of transferrin in the liver)*
- Protein depletion *(transferrin contributes to the total protein concentration and will reflect a decrease in protein depletion)*
- Sideroblastic anemias *(transferrin becomes saturated, and the iron-binding capacity is significantly decreased)*
- Thalassemia *(transferrin becomes saturated, and the iron-binding capacity is significantly decreased)*

NURSING IMPLICATIONS

POTENTIAL NURSING PROBLEMS: ASSESSMENT & NURSING DIAGNOSIS

Problems	Signs and Symptoms
Blood loss *(related to heavy menses, disease process with chronic blood loss [GI ulcer, malignancy], overuse of NSAIDs)*	Altered level of consciousness, hypotension, increased heart rate, decreased Hgb and Hct, decreased serum iron, capillary refill greater than 3 sec, cool extremities, poor dietary selections
Fatigue *(related to decreased oxygenation associated with unhealthy RBCs secondary to inadequate iron)*	Verbalization of fatigue, altered ability to perform activities of daily living due to lack of energy, shortness of breath with exertion, increasingly frequent rest periods, presence of fatigue after sleep, inability to adhere to daily routine, altered level of concentration, complaints of tiredness
Nutrition *(related to inability to digest, metabolize, ingest foods; refusal to eat; increased metabolic needs associated with disease process; lack of understanding; unable to obtain healthy iron-rich foods)*	Unintended weight loss; current weight is 20% below ideal weight; pale, dry skin; dry mucous membranes; documented inadequate caloric intake; subcutaneous tissue loss; hair pulls out easily; paresthesia
Tissue perfusion (cerebral, peripheral, renal) *(related to inadequate cellular oxygen associated with unhealthy RBCs secondary to iron deficiency)*	Confusion, altered mental status, headaches, dizziness, visual disturbances, hypotension, dizziness, cool extremities, capillary refill greater than 3 sec, weak pedal pulses, altered level of consciousness, decreased urine output

BEFORE THE STUDY: PLANNING AND IMPLEMENTATION

Teaching the Patient What to Expect
▶ Inform the patient this test can assist in evaluating anemia and the amount of iron in the blood.
▶ Explain that a blood sample is needed for the test.

AFTER THE STUDY: POTENTIAL NURSING ACTIONS

Treatment Considerations
▶ Instruct the patient to resume usual diet, fluids, medications, or activity, as directed by the HCP.
▶ Blood Loss: Monitor the effects of blood loss by monitoring serum iron. Monitor and trend vital signs. Administer ordered blood or blood products and prescribed iron. Identify the cause of chronic blood loss, and assess stool for blood. Consider a dietary consult; assess for iron-rich foods and foods that inhibit absorption of iron.
▶ Fatigue: Monitor and trend complete blood count, Hgb, Hct, and iron. Monitor for shortness of breath and administer ordered oxygen with use of pulse oximetry. Assess for medical or psychological factors contributing to fatigue, prioritize and bundle activities to conserve energy, assess ability to perform self-care, encourage frequent rest periods, and assess nutritional intake of iron-rich foods. Administer ordered blood and blood products and prescribed iron supplements as ordered. Monitor urine, stool, and sputum for bleeding.
▶ Tissue Perfusion: Blood loss can contribute to poor tissue perfusion. Some valuable interventions are to monitor blood pressure, assess for dizziness, check skin temperature for warmth, and assess capillary refill and pulses. Monitor level of consciousness, monitor urine output (to be in excess of 30 mL/hr). Ensure adequate fluid intake or administer ordered IV fluids. Administer ordered iron supplements.

Nutritional Considerations
▶ There are numerous factors that affect the absorption of iron, enhancing or decreasing absorption, regardless of the original content of the iron-containing dietary source.
▶ Educate the patient with abnormally elevated iron values on the importance of reading food labels. Foods high in iron include meats (especially liver), eggs, grains, and green leafy vegetables. Also explain that iron levels in foods can be increased if foods are cooked in cookware containing iron.
▶ Explain to either increase or avoid intake of iron and iron-rich foods depending on the specific condition; for example, a patient with hemochromatosis or acute pernicious anemia should be educated to avoid foods rich in iron.
▶ Inform the patient that consumption of large amounts of alcohol damages the intestine and allows increased absorption of iron, as does a high intake of calcium and ascorbic acid.
▶ Explain that iron absorption after a meal is also increased by factors in meat, fish, and poultry. Iron absorption is decreased by the absence (gastric resection) or diminished presence (use of antacids) of gastric acid.
▶ Phytic acids from cereals, tannins from tea and coffee, oxalic acid from vegetables, and minerals such as copper, zinc, and manganese interfere with iron absorption.
▶ Obtain an accurate nutritional history, assess attitude toward eating, and promote a dietary consult to evaluate current eating habits and best method of nutritional supplementation focusing on iron-rich foods.
▶ Monitor serum iron, assess swallowing ability, and encourage iron-rich cultural home foods.

Follow-Up, Evaluation, and Desired Outcomes
▶ Acknowledges contact information provided for the U.S. Department of Agriculture's resource for nutrition (www.choosemyplate.gov).

Ketones, Blood and Urine

SYNONYM/ACRONYM: Ketone bodies, acetoacetate, acetone.

RATIONALE: To investigate diabetes as the cause of ketoacidosis and monitor therapeutic interventions.

PATIENT PREPARATION: There are no food, fluid, activity, or medication restrictions unless by medical direction. As appropriate, provide the required urine collection container and specimen collection instructions.

NORMAL FINDINGS: (Method: Colorimetric nitroprusside reaction) Negative.

CRITICAL FINDINGS AND POTENTIAL INTERVENTIONS
• Strongly positive test results for glucose and ketones.

Timely notification to the requesting health-care provider (HCP) of any critical findings and related symptoms is a role expectation of the professional nurse. A listing of these findings varies among facilities.

Consideration may be given to verification of critical findings before action is taken. Policies vary among facilities and may include requesting immediate recollection and retesting by the laboratory or retesting using a rapid point-of-care testing instrument at the bedside, if available.

An elevated level of ketone bodies is evidenced by fruity-smelling breath, acidosis, ketonuria, and decreased level of consciousness. Administration of insulin and frequent blood glucose measurement may be indicated.

OVERVIEW: (Study type: Blood collected from gold-, red-, or red/gray-top tube; **related body system:** Endocrine system. Urine, collected in a clean plastic collection container.) Ketone bodies refer to the three intermediate products of metabolism: acetone, acetoacetic acid, and β-hydroxybutyrate. Even though β-hydroxybutyrate is not a ketone, it is usually listed with the ketone bodies. In healthy individuals, ketones are produced and completely metabolized by the liver so that measurable amounts are not normally present in serum. Ketones appear in the urine before a significant serum level is detectable. If the patient has excessive fat metabolism, ketones are found in blood and urine. Excessive fat metabolism may occur if the patient has impaired ability to metabolize carbohydrates, inadequate carbohydrate intake, inadequate insulin levels, excessive carbohydrate loss, or increased carbohydrate demand. For additional information regarding screening guidelines and management of diabetes, refer to the study titled "Glucose." A strongly positive acetone result without severe acidosis, accompanied by normal glucose, electrolyte, and bicarbonate levels, is strongly suggestive of isopropyl alcohol poisoning. A low-carbohydrate or high-fat diet may cause a positive acetone test. Ketosis in people with diabetes is usually accompanied by increased glucose and decreased bicarbonate and pH. Extremely elevated levels of ketone bodies can result in coma. This situation is particularly life threatening in children younger than 10 yr. Ketones are qualitatively evaluated as part of the routine urinalysis.

INDICATIONS

- Assist in the diagnosis of starvation, stress, alcohol misuse, suspected isopropyl alcohol ingestion, glycogen storage disease, and other metabolic disorders.
- Detect and monitor treatment of diabetic ketoacidosis.
- Monitor the management of diabetes.
- Screen for ketonuria due to acute illness or stress in nondiabetic patients.
- Screen for ketonuria to assist in the assessment of inborn errors of metabolism.
- Screen for ketonuria to assist in the diagnosis of suspected isopropyl alcohol poisoning.

INTERFERING FACTORS

Factors that may alter the results of the study

- Drugs and other substances that may cause an increase in serum ketone levels include acetylsalicylic acid (if therapy results in acidosis, especially in children), albuterol, nifedipine, and rimiterol. Increases have been shown in hyperthyroid patients receiving propranolol hydrochloride and propylthiouracil.
- Drugs and other substances that may cause a decrease in serum ketone levels include acetylsalicylic acid and valproic acid.
- Drugs and other substances that may increase urine ketone levels include acetylsalicylic acid (if therapy results in acidosis, especially in children), ether, metformin, and niacin.
- Drugs and other substances that may decrease urine ketone levels include acetylsalicylic acid.
- Bacterial contamination of urine can cause false-negative results.
- Failure to keep reagent strip container tightly closed can cause false-negative results. Light and moisture affect the ability of the chemicals in the strip to perform as expected.

- False-negative or weakly false-positive test results can be obtained when β-hydroxybutyrate is the predominating ketone body in cases of lactic acidosis.

Other considerations

- Urine should be checked within 60 min of collection; specimen stability studies have shown that reliability and reproducibility of results begins to deteriorate in samples tested after longer periods.

POTENTIAL MEDICAL DIAGNOSIS: CLINICAL SIGNIFICANCE OF RESULTS

Increased in

Ketones are generated in conditions that involve the metabolism of carbohydrates, fatty acids, and protein.

- Acidosis
- Branched-chain ketonuria
- Carbohydrate deficiency
- Eclampsia
- Fasting or starvation
- Gestational diabetes
- Glycogen storage diseases
- High-fat or high-protein diet
- Hyperglycemia
- Ketoacidosis of alcohol misuse and diabetes
- Illnesses with marked vomiting and diarrhea
- Isopropyl alcohol ingestion
- Methylmalonic aciduria
- Postanesthesia period
- Propionyl coenzyme A carboxylase deficiency

Decreased in: N/A

NURSING IMPLICATIONS

BEFORE THE STUDY: PLANNING AND IMPLEMENTATION

Teaching the Patient What to Expect

▶ Inform the patient this test can assist in diagnosing metabolic disorders such as diabetes.

K

Explain that a blood or urine sample is needed for the test. Information regarding specimen collection is presented with other general guidelines in Appendix A: Patient Preparation and Specimen Collection.

AFTER THE STUDY: POTENTIAL NURSING ACTIONS

Avoiding Complications
▶ Emphasize, as appropriate, that good management of glucose levels delays the onset and slows the progression of diabetic retinopathy, nephropathy, and neuropathy.
▶ Explain that unmanaged diabetes can cause multiple health issues, including diabetic kidney disease, amputation of limbs, and ultimately in death.

Treatment Considerations
▶ Impaired glucose tolerance may be associated with diabetes.
▶ Advise reporting any signs and symptoms of hypoglycemia (weakness, confusion, diaphoresis, rapid pulse) or hyperglycemia (thirst, polyuria, hunger, lethargy).

Nutritional Considerations
▶ Increased levels of ketone bodies may be associated with poor carbohydrate intake in an unbalanced diet; therefore, the body breaks down fat instead of carbohydrate for energy. Increasing carbohydrate intake in the patient's diet reduces the levels of ketone bodies. Carbohydrates can be found in starches and sugars. Starch is a complex carbohydrate that can be found in foods such as grains (breads, cereals, pasta, rice) and starchy vegetables (corn, peas, potatoes). Sugar is a simple carbohydrate that can be found in natural foods (fruits and natural honey) and processed foods (desserts and candy).
▶ Increased glucose levels may be associated with diabetes. There is no "diabetic diet"; however, many meal-planning approaches with nutritional goals are endorsed by the American Diabetes Association (ADA). Patients who adhere to dietary recommendations report a better general feeling of health, better weight management, better management of glucose and lipid values, and improved use of insulin. Instruct the patient, as appropriate, in nutritional management of diabetes. A variety of dietary patterns are beneficial for people with diabetes. Encourage consultation with a registered dietitian who is a certified diabetes educator.

Follow-Up, Evaluation, and Desired Outcomes
▶ Acknowledges contact information provided for the ADA (www.diabetes.org), American Heart Association (www.heart.org/HEARTORG), National Heart, Lung, and Blood Institute (www.nhlbi.nih.gov), National Institute of Diabetes and Digestive and Kidney Disease (www.niddk.nih.gov), and U.S. Department of Agriculture's resource for nutrition (www.choosemyplate.gov).

Kidney Stone Evaluation

SYNONYM/ACRONYM: Kidney stone analysis, nephrolithiasis analysis, calculus panel.

RATIONALE: To identify the presence of kidney stones.

PATIENT PREPARATION: There are no food, fluid, activity, or medication restrictions unless by medical direction.

NORMAL FINDINGS: (Method: Infrared spectrometry) None detected.

CRITICAL FINDINGS AND POTENTIAL INTERVENTIONS: N/A

OVERVIEW: (Study type: Kidney stone evaluation; **related body system:** Urinary system.) Renal calculi (kidney stones) are formed by the crystallization of calcium oxalate (most common), magnesium ammonium phosphate, calcium phosphate, uric acid, and cystine. Formation of stones may be hereditary, related to diet or poor hydration, urinary tract infections (UTIs) caused by urease-producing bacteria, conditions resulting in reduced urine flow, or excessive amounts of the previously mentioned insoluble substances due to other predisposing conditions. The presence of stones is confirmed by diagnostic visualization or passing of the stones in the urine. The chemical nature of the stones is confirmed qualitatively. Analysis also includes a description of color, size, and weight.

INDICATIONS
• Identify substances present in renal calculi.

INTERFERING FACTORS
Factors that may alter the results of the study
• Drugs and other substances that may increase the formation of urine calculi include probenecid and vitamin D.

Other considerations
• Adhesive tape should not be used to attach stones to any transportation or collection container, because the adhesive interferes with infrared spectrometry.

POTENTIAL MEDICAL DIAGNOSIS: CLINICAL SIGNIFICANCE OF RESULTS
Positive findings in

Presence of Calcium Calculi (75%–85%)
• Decreased levels of citric acid, which creates an imbalance of mineral salts *(related to conditions such as enteric hyperoxaluria, enterocystoplasty, or small bowel resection)*
• Distal renal tubular acidosis *(related to accumulation of calcium in the kidneys)*
• Etiology unknown
• Increased levels of calcium with or without alkaline pH, which creates an imbalance of mineral salts *(related to conditions such as Cushing disease, Dent disease, enterocystoplasty, ileostomy, immobilization, medullary sponge kidney, metabolic syndrome, milk alkali syndrome, primary biliary cholangitis, primary hyperparathyroidism, sarcoidosis, Sjögren syndrome, use of calcium carbonate–containing antacids, use of corticosteroids, or vitamin D intoxication)*
• Increased levels of oxalic acid, which creates an imbalance of mineral salts *(related to conditions such as bariatric surgery, enteric hyperoxaluria, enterocystoplasty, hereditary hyperoxaluria, hypomagnesemia, jejunal-ileal bypass, metabolic syndrome, pancreatitis, or small bowel resection)*
• Increased levels of uric acid, which creates an imbalance of mineral salts (uric acid crystals sometimes provide the base upon which calcium oxalate crystals grow)

Presence of Magnesium Ammonium Phosphate (Struvite or Triple Phosphate) Calculi (10%–15%)
• UTI *(related to chronic indwelling catheter, neurogenic bladder dysfunction, obstruction, or urinary diversion)*
• Gram-positive bacteria associated with development of struvite calculi include *Bacillus* species, *Corynebacterium* species, *Peptococcus asaccharolyticus, Staphylococcus*

aureus, and *Staphylococcus epidermidis*

- Gram-negative bacteria associated with development of struvite calculi include *Bacteroides corrodens, Flavobacterium* species, *Klebsiella* species, *Pasteurella* species, *Proteus* species, *Providencia stuartii, Pseudomonas aeruginosa, Serratia marcescens, Ureaplasma urealyticum,* and *Yersinia enterocolitica*
- Yeast associated with development of struvite calculi include *Candida humicola, Cryptococcus* species, *Rhodotorula* species, *Sporobolomyces* species, and *Trichosporon cutaneum*

Presence of Uric Acid Calculi (5%–8%)

- Increased levels of uric acid or increased urinary excretion of uric acid
- Anemias (pernicious, lead poisoning) *(related to cellular destruction and turnover)*
- Chemotherapy and radiation therapy *(related to high cell turnover)*
- Gout *(usually related to excess dietary intake)*
- Glycogen storage disease type I (von Gierke disease) *(related to a genetic deficiency of the enzyme G-6-P-D, ultimately resulting in hyperuricemia, increased production of uric acid via the pentose phosphate pathway, and increased purine catabolism)*
- Hemoglobinopathies (sickle cell anemia, thalassemias) *(related to cellular destruction and turnover)*
- Ileostomy *(related to imbalances in mineral salts)*
- Lesch-Nyhan syndrome *(related to a disorder of uric acid metabolism)*
- Metabolic syndrome *(elevated uric acid levels are associated with metabolic syndrome; there is evidence that uric acidemia is a risk factor for cardiovascular and renal disease)*
- Polycythemia *(related to increased cellular destruction)*
- Psoriasis *(related to increased skin cell turnover)*
- Tumors *(related to high cell turnover)*

Presence of Cystine Calculi (Approximately 1%)

- Fanconi syndrome (hereditary hypercistinuria) *(related to increased excretion of cystine)*

Negative findings in: N/A

K

NURSING IMPLICATIONS

POTENTIAL NURSING PROBLEMS: ASSESSMENT & NURSING DIAGNOSIS

Problems	Signs and Symptoms
Pain *(related to obstruction of urinary flow by stone, presence of stone, movement of stone)*	Report of pain, restlessness, grimace, moan, sleeplessness, diaphoresis, nausea, vomiting, elevated blood pressure
Fever *(related to infection secondary to stone formation)*	Elevated temperature, flushed, warm skin, diaphoresis
Infection *(related to stasis, interrupted urinary flow, gravel, urinary tract instrumentation)*	Elevated temperature, elevated white blood cell (WBC) count, cloudy urine, sediment in urine, blood in urine.

Teaching the Patient What to Expect

▶ Inform the patient this test can assist in identification of the presence of kidney stones.
▶ The patient presenting with symptoms indicating the presence of kidney stones may be provided with a device to strain the urine. The patient should be informed to transfer any particulate matter remaining in the strainer into the specimen collection container provided. Stones removed by the health-care provider (HCP) should be placed in the appropriate collection container.

Potential Nursing Actions

▶ Promptly transport any strained specimen to the laboratory for processing and analysis.

Avoiding Complications

▶ Inform the patient with kidney stones that the likelihood of recurrence is high. Educate the patient regarding risk factors that contribute to the likelihood of kidney stone formation, including family history, osteoporosis, UTIs, gout, magnesium deficiency, Crohn disease with prior resection, age, gender (males are two to three times more likely than females to develop stones), ethnicity (Caucasians are three to four times more likely than people of African descent to develop stones), and climate.

Treatment Considerations

▶ Pain: Administer prescribed medication for pain and assesses effectiveness of pain medication. Assess characteristics of pain (location, duration, intensity). Consider nonpharmacological pain interventions that have worked for the patient in the past.
▶ Fever: Assess the patient's temperature frequently. Encourage the use of light bedding and lightweight clothing to prevent overheating. Increase fluid intake to offset insensible fluid loss and dehydration. Encourage bathing with tepid water for comfort and promotion of cooling. Administer prescribed medication for elevated temperature.
▶ Infection: Monitor urinary output. Assess urine color, odor, and for presence of blood. Monitor and trend temperature and WBC count. Obtain urine for culture and sensitivity as required, encourage fluid intake in excess of 3,000 mL/day, and administer prescribed antibiotics.

Nutritional Considerations

▶ Nutritional therapy is indicated for individuals identified as being at high risk for developing kidney stones. Educate the patient that diets rich in protein, salt, and oxalates increase the risk of stone formation. Adequate fluid intake should be encouraged (more than 3,000 mL/day). Cranberry juice and cranberry supplements have been used for years as a home remedy for UTIs; cranberries contain A-type proanthocyanidins, which are believed to prevent bacteria from adhering to the bladder wall and causing a UTI. Clinical studies continue to provide conflicting results regarding the efficacy of cranberry products, and patients should rely on the advice of their HCP.

Follow-Up, Evaluation, and Desired Outcomes

▶ Successfully demonstrates how to strain urine to check for stones and accurately self-administer prescribed medication that may decrease stone formation (cholestyramine, thiazide, allopurinol).
▶ Recognizes the importance of reporting worsening symptoms of infection such as fever, chills, and pain; discusses the importance in reporting changes in the characteristics of the urine in relation to infection risk.
▶ Understands that follow-up testing of urine may be requested, but usually not for 1 mo after the stones have passed or been removed.

K

Kidney, Ureter, and Bladder Study

SYNONYM/ACRONYM: Flat plate of the abdomen; kidney, urine, and bladder (KUB); plain film of the abdomen.

RATIONALE: To visualize and assess the abdominal organs for obstruction or abnormality related to mass, trauma, bleeding, stones, or congenital anomaly.

PATIENT PREPARATION: There are no food, fluid, activity, or medication restrictions unless by medical direction.

NORMAL FINDINGS
- Normal size and shape of kidneys
- Normal bladder, absence of masses and renal calculi, and no abnormal accumulation of air or fluid.

CRITICAL FINDINGS AND POTENTIAL INTERVENTIONS
- Bowel obstruction
- Ischemic bowel
- Visceral injury

Timely notification to the requesting health-care provider (HCP) of any critical findings and related symptoms is a role expectation of the professional nurse. A listing of these findings varies among facilities.

K

OVERVIEW: (Study type: X-ray, plain; related body system: Digestive and Urinary systems.) A KUB x-ray examination provides information regarding the structure, size, and position of the abdominal organs; it also indicates whether there is any obstruction or abnormality of the abdomen caused by disease or congenital malformation. Calcifications of the renal calyces, renal pelvis, and any radiopaque calculi present in the urinary tract or surrounding organs may be visualized in addition to normal air and gas patterns within the intestinal tract. Perforation of the intestinal tract or an intestinal obstruction can be visualized on erect KUB images. KUB x-rays are among the first examinations done to diagnose intra-abdominal diseases such as intestinal obstruction, masses, tumors, ruptured organs, abnormal gas accumulation, and ascites.

INDICATIONS
- Determine the cause of acute abdominal pain or palpable mass.
- Evaluate the effects of lower abdominal trauma, such as internal hemorrhage.
- Evaluate known or suspected intestinal obstructions.
- Evaluate the presence of renal, ureter, or other organ calculi.
- Evaluate the size, shape, and position of the liver, kidneys, and spleen.
- Evaluate suspected abnormal fluid, air, or metallic objects in the abdomen.

INTERFERING FACTORS
Contraindications

 Patients who are pregnant or suspected of being pregnant, unless the potential benefits of a procedure using radiation far outweigh the risk of radiation exposure to the fetus and mother.

Factors that may alter the results of the study
- Retained barium from a previous radiological procedure.
- Metallic objects (e.g., jewelry, body rings) within the examination field, which may inhibit organ visualization and cause unclear images.
- Inability of the patient to cooperate or remain still during the procedure, because movement can produce blurred or otherwise unclear images.

POTENTIAL MEDICAL DIAGNOSIS: CLINICAL SIGNIFICANCE OF RESULTS
Abnormal findings related to
- Abnormal accumulation of bowel gas
- Ascites
- Bladder distention
- Congenital renal anomaly
- Foreign body
- Hydronephrosis
- Intestinal obstruction
- Organomegaly
- Renal calculi
- Renal hematomas
- Ruptured viscus
- Soft tissue masses
- Trauma to liver, spleen, kidneys, and bladder
- Vascular calcification

NURSING IMPLICATIONS

BEFORE THE STUDY: PLANNING AND IMPLEMENTATION

Teaching the Patient What to Expect
- Inform the patient this procedure can assist in assessing the status of the abdomen.
- Pregnancy is a general contraindication to procedures involving radiation. Explain to the female patient that she will be asked the date of her last menstrual period. Pregnancy testing may be performed to determine the possibility of pregnancy before exposure to radiation.
- Review the procedure with the patient. Address concerns about pain and explain that little to no pain is expected during the test, but there may be moments of discomfort.
- Explain that the procedure is performed in the radiology department or at the bedside by a registered radiologic technologist and takes approximately 5 to 15 min to complete.
- Advise removal of all metallic objects from the area to be examined. Instruct the patient to remain still throughout the procedure because movement produces unreliable results.
- Positioning for this procedure is on the table in a supine position with hands relaxed at the side.
- Explain that the patient will be asked to inhale deeply and hold his or her breath while the x-ray images are taken, and then to exhale after the images are taken.

AFTER THE STUDY: POTENTIAL NURSING ACTIONS

Treatment Considerations
- Assess pain character, location, duration, intensity; use an easily understood pain rating scale; place in a position of comfort; administer ordered analgesics; consider alternative measures for pain management (imagery, relaxation, music, etc.); administer ordered parenteral fluids; monitor and trend laboratory results (hemoglobin, hematocrit, electrolytes); maintain NPO status as appropriate; evaluate response and readjust pain management strategies.
- Insufficient fluid volume can be a concern in relation to the disease processes associated with the need for a KUB. Some interventions that can be used to address these concerns are to monitor and trend vital signs, urine output, urine color, and intake and

output. Administer ordered parenteral fluids and encourage the intake of oral fluids. Administer ordered antiemetics and monitor and trend laboratory studies (uric acid, BUN, Cr, electrolytes).

Follow-Up, Evaluation, and Desired Outcomes
⬥ Understands that additional testing may be necessary to monitor disease progression and determine the need for a change in therapy.

Kleihauer-Betke Test

SYNONYM/ACRONYM: Fetal hemoglobin, hemoglobin F, acid elution slide test.

RATIONALE: To assist in assessing occurrence and extent of fetal maternal hemorrhage and calculate the amount of Rh immune globulin to be administered.

PATIENT PREPARATION: There are no food, fluid, activity, or medication restrictions unless by medical direction.

NORMAL FINDINGS: (Method: Microscopic examination of treated and stained peripheral blood smear) Less than 1% fetal cells present.

CRITICAL FINDINGS AND POTENTIAL INTERVENTIONS: N/A

OVERVIEW: (**Study type:** Blood collected in a lavender-top [EDTA] tube; **related body system:** Circulatory/Hematopoietic, Immune, and Reproductive systems. Freshly prepared blood smears are also acceptable. Cord blood may be requested for use as a positive control.) The Kleihauer-Betke test is used to determine the degree of fetal-maternal hemorrhage (FMH) and to help calculate the dosage of Rh(D) immune globulin RhoGAM intramuscular (IM) or Rhophylac IM or IV—to be given in some cases of Rh-negative mothers. Administration of Rh immune globulin (RhIG) inhibits formation of Rh antibodies in the mother to prevent Rh disease in future pregnancies with Rh-positive children. The test is also used to resolve the question of whether FMH was the cause of fetal death in the case of stillbirth. A sample of maternal blood should be collected within 1 hr of delivery. A blood film of maternal red blood cells (RBCs) is prepared, treated with an acid buffer, and stained. The acid solution causes hemoglobin to be leached from the maternal cells, giving them a ghostlike appearance. Fetal cells containing hemoglobin F retain their hemoglobin and are stained bright red. Approximately 2,000 cells are examined microscopically and counted. A percentage of fetal cells is reported. Enumeration of a total of 2,000 cells is important to achieve the accuracy and precision to detect an FMH of 15 mL of fetal RBCs or 30 mL of fetal whole blood, which is the amount of FMH that corresponds to a 300-mcg dose of RhIG. Recommendations for initial RhIG doses range from 100 to 300 mcg to cover 10 to 30 mL of fetal blood volumes. Many manufacturers recommend additional 50 mcg doses for each 2.5 mL of fetal blood. Calculation of RhIG dosage is based on the

K

calculated size of FMH and should be done only after reviewing the information in the manufacturer's package insert. The formula to calculate quantity of fetal bleed in milliliters of fetal blood is to multiply the percentage of fetal cells in maternal circulation by 50, based on the assumption that maternal blood volume is 5 liters. Conversion of absolute cells counted to percent cells counted changes the factor representing maternal blood volume from 5000 to 50. For example, if 12 fetal cells were counted out of a total of 2,000 total RBCs, then 0.006 cells were counted/2000 cells which when converted to percentage is 0.6% fetal cells. Then FMH = 0.6 × 50 = 30 mL (this is the same as multiplying the number of cells 0.006 by 5000 mL = 30 mL). The formula to calculate FMH in relation to fetal blood cell volume is to multiply the percentage of fetal cells in maternal circulation by 2, based on the assumption that the hematocrit of fetal whole blood is 50%. For example, if the quantity of fetal bleed is 30 mL of fetal whole blood, then FMH = (30/2) = 15 mL fetal RBCs. Postpartum RhIG should be given within 72 hr of delivery. The test can also be used to distinguish some forms of thalassemia from the hereditary persistence of fetal hemoglobin, but hemoglobin electrophoresis and flow cytometry methods are more commonly used for this purpose.

INDICATIONS
- Assist in the diagnosis of certain types of anemia.
- Calculate dosage of RhoGAM.
- Determine whether FMH was a potential cause of death in stillborn delivery.

- Screening postpartum maternal blood for the presence of FMH.

INTERFERING FACTORS
Factors that may alter the results of the study
Specimens must be obtained before transfusion.

POTENTIAL MEDICAL DIAGNOSIS: CLINICAL SIGNIFICANCE OF RESULTS
Positive findings in
- Fetal-maternal hemorrhage *(related to leakage of fetal RBCs into maternal circulation)*
- Hereditary persistence of fetal hemoglobin *(the test does not differentiate fetal hemoglobin from neonate and adult)*

Negative findings in: N/A

NURSING IMPLICATIONS

BEFORE THE STUDY: PLANNING AND IMPLEMENTATION

Teaching the Patient What to Expect
▶ Inform the patient this test can assist in identifying how much Rh(D) immune globulin should be given to Rh negative mother after delivery of an Rh positive neonate.
▶ Explain that a blood sample is needed for the test.

Potential Nursing Actions
▶ Verify Rh status of mother and baby prior to RhD administration.

AFTER THE STUDY: POTENTIAL NURSING ACTIONS

Treatment Considerations
▶ Explain the benefit of testing and medication administration in relation to mother's health and as a preventative measure against Rh disease in future pregnancies.

Follow-Up, Evaluation, and Desired Outcomes
▶ Understands the importance of knowing and communicating her Rh status as it relates to future pregnancies.

Lactate Dehydrogenase and Isoenzymes

SYNONYM/ACRONYM: LDH and isos, LD, and isos.

RATIONALE: To assess myocardial or skeletal muscle damage toward diagnosing disorders such as myocardial infarction or damage to brain, liver, kidneys, and skeletal muscle.

PATIENT PREPARATION: There are no food, fluid, activity, or medication restrictions unless by medical direction.

NORMAL FINDINGS: (Method: Enzymatic [L to P] for lactate dehydrogenase, electrophoretic analysis for isoenzymes) Reference ranges are method dependent and may vary among laboratories.

Lactate Dehydrogenase

Age	Conventional and SI Units
0–2 yr	125–275 units/L
2–3 yr	166–232 units/L
4–6 yr	104–206 units/L
7–12 yr	90–203 units/L
13–14 yr	90–199 units/L
15–43 yr	90–156 units/L
Greater than 43 yr	90–176 units/L

LDH Fraction	% of Total	Fraction of Total
LDH_1	14–26	0.14–0.26
LDH_2	29–39	0.29–0.39
LDH_3	20–26	0.2–0.26
LDH_4	8–16	0.08–0.16
LDH_5	6–16	0.06–0.16

CRITICAL FINDINGS AND POTENTIAL INTERVENTIONS: N/A

OVERVIEW: (**Study type:** Blood collected in a gold-, red-, or red/gray-top tube; **related body system:** Circulatory, Circulatory/Hematopoietic, Digestive, Musculoskeletal, and Urinary systems.) Lactate dehydrogenase (LDH) is an enzyme that catalyzes the reversible conversion of lactate to pyruvate within numerous tissues in the body, making it a nonspecific indicator of cellular damage. Determining tissue origin can be accomplished by electrophoretic analysis of the five isoenzymes found in certain tissues. The heart and erythrocytes are rich sources of LDH_1, LDH_2, and LDH_3; the kidneys contain large amounts of LDH_3 and LDH_4; and the liver and skeletal muscles are high in LDH_4 and LDH_5. Certain glands (e.g., thyroid, adrenal, thymus), the pancreas, spleen, lungs, lymph nodes, and white blood cells contain LDH_3, whereas the ileum is an additional source of

LDH_5. Documented reports identify a sixth isoenzyme of LDH. It is seen in patients with severe liver disease and is an indicator of an extremely poor prognosis. Testing for the presence of LDH and isoenzymes is rarely used anymore to confirm acute myocardial infarction (MI), having been replaced by more sensitive and specific creatine kinase (CK-MB) and troponin assays. Acute MI releases LDH into the serum within the first 12 hr, causing a "flip" isoenzyme pattern within 48 hr of MI, and levels remain elevated for 1 to 2 wk after CK and aspartate aminotransferase have returned to normal levels. For additional information regarding screening guidelines for *atherosclerotic cardiovascular disease* (ASCVD), refer to the study titled "Cholesterol, Total and Fractions."

INDICATIONS

- Differentiate acute MI from pulmonary infarction and liver problems *(acute MI elevates LDH_1 and LDH_2 levels; pulmonary infarction and liver problems elevate LDH_4 and LDH_5)*.
- Evaluate the degree of muscle wasting in muscular dystrophy *(LDH levels rise early in this disorder and approach normal as muscle mass is reduced by atrophy)*.
- Evaluate red cell hemolysis or renal infarction, especially as indicated by reversal of the LDH_1:LDH_2 ratio.
- Investigate acute MI or extension thereof *(indicated by elevation [usually] of total LDH, elevation of LDH_1 and LDH_2, and reversal of the LDH_1:LDH_2 ratio within 48 hr of the infarction)*.

- Investigate chronicity of liver, lung, and kidney disorders *(evidenced by LDH levels that remain persistently high)*.

INTERFERING FACTORS
Factors that may alter the results of the study

- Drugs and other substances that may increase total LDH levels include amiodarone, etretinate, oxacillin, plicamycin, and streptokinase.
- Drugs and other substances that may decrease total LDH levels include ascorbic acid, cefotaxime, enalapril, fluorides, naltrexone, and oxylate.
- Hemolysis will cause significant false elevations in total LDH and a false flip pattern of the isoenzymes because LDH_1 fraction is of red blood cell origin.
- Some isoenzymes are temperature sensitive; therefore, prolonged storage at refrigerated temperatures may cause false decreases.

POTENTIAL MEDICAL DIAGNOSIS: CLINICAL SIGNIFICANCE OF RESULTS

Total LDH Increased In
LDH is released from any damaged cell in which it is stored so conditions that affect the heart, liver, kidneys, red blood cells, skeletal muscle, or other tissue source and cause cellular destruction demonstrate elevated LDH levels.

- Alcohol misuse
- Cancer of the liver
- Cirrhosis
- Heart failure
- HELLP (hemolysis, elevated liver enzymes, low platelet count) syndrome of pregnancy
- Hemolytic anemias
- Hypoxia
- Kidney disease (severe)
- Leukemias
- Megaloblastic and pernicious anemia
- MI or pulmonary infarction

L

- Musculoskeletal disease
- Obstructive jaundice
- Pancreatitis
- Shock
- Viral hepatitis

Total LDH Decreased In: N/A

LDH Isoenzymes
- LDH_1 fraction increased over LDH_2 can be seen in acute MI, anemias (pernicious, hemolytic, acute sickle cell, megaloblastic, hemolytic), and acute kidney injury due to any cause. The LDH_1 fraction in particular is elevated in cases of germ cell tumors.
- Increases in the middle fractions are associated with conditions in which massive platelet destruction has occurred (e.g., pulmonary embolism, posttransfusion period) and in lymphatic system disorders (e.g., infectious mononucleosis, lymphomas, lymphocytic leukemias).
- An increase in LDH_5 occurs with musculoskeletal damage and many types of liver damage (e.g., cirrhosis, cancer, hepatitis).

NURSING IMPLICATIONS

BEFORE THE STUDY: PLANNING AND IMPLEMENTATION

Teaching the Patient What to Expect
- Inform the patient this test can assist in evaluating skeletomuscular and organ damage (brain, heart, kidneys, liver, and some blood cells).
- Explain that a blood sample is needed for the test.

AFTER THE STUDY: POTENTIAL NURSING ACTIONS

Treatment Considerations
- Explain the study results will provide valuable information to assist in addressing health concerns related to

coronary artery disease, type 1 and type 2 diabetes, insulin resistance, and metabolic syndrome.

Nutritional Considerations
- Discuss ideal body weight and the purpose of and relationship between ideal weight and caloric intake to support cardiac health. Review ways to decrease intake of saturated fats and increase intake of polyunsaturated fats. Discuss limiting intake of refined processed sugar and sodium; discuss limiting cholesterol intake to less than 300 mg per day. Encourage the intake of fresh fruits and vegetables, unprocessed carbohydrates, poultry, and grains.
- Nutritional therapy is recommended for those with identified coronary artery disease risk, especially for those with elevated low-density lipoprotein cholesterol levels, other lipid disorders, diabetes, insulin resistance, or metabolic syndrome. Always consider cultural influences with dietary choices to ensure better adherence to a change in lifestyle. A variety of dietary patterns are beneficial for people with ASCVD. For additional information regarding nutritional guidelines, refer to the study titled "Cholesterol, Total and Fractions."
- Other changeable risk factors warranting education include strategies to encourage regular participation of moderate aerobic physical activity three to four times per week, eliminate tobacco use, and adhere to a heart-healthy diet.
- Those with elevated triglycerides should be advised to eliminate or reduce alcohol.

Follow-Up, Evaluation, and Desired Outcomes
- Acknowledges contact information provided for the American Heart Association (www.heart.org/HEARTORG), National Heart, Lung, and Blood Institute (www.nhlbi.nih.gov), and U.S. Department of Agriculture's resource for nutrition (www.choosemyplate.gov).

L

Lactic Acid

SYNONYM/ACRONYM: Lactate.

RATIONALE: To assess for lactic acid acidosis related to poor organ perfusion and liver failure. May also be used to differentiate between lactic acid acidosis and ketoacidosis by evaluating blood glucose levels.

PATIENT PREPARATION: There are no activity or medication restrictions unless by medical direction. Instruct the patient to fast and to restrict fluids overnight. Instruct the patient not to ingest alcohol for 12 hr before the test. Protocols may vary among facilities.

NORMAL FINDINGS: Method: Spectrophotometry/enzymatic analysis.

	Conventional Units	SI Units (Conventional Units × 0.111)
0–90 d	3–32 mg/dL	0.3–3.6 mmol/L
3–24 mo	3–30 mg/dL	0.3–3.3 mmol/L
2 yr–adult	3–23 mg/dL	0.3–2.6 mmol/L

CRITICAL FINDINGS AND POTENTIAL INTERVENTIONS

Adults
• Greater than 31 mg/dL (SI: Greater than 3.4 mmol/L).

Children
• Greater than 37 mg/dL (SI: Greater than 4.1 mmol/L).

Timely notification to the requesting health-care provider (HCP) of any critical findings and related symptoms is a role expectation of the professional nurse. A listing of these findings varies among facilities.

Consideration may be given to verification of critical findings before action is taken. Policies vary among facilities and may include requesting immediate recollection and retesting by the laboratory or retesting using a rapid point-of-care testing instrument at the bedside, if available.

Observe the patient for signs and symptoms of elevated levels of lactate, such as Kussmaul breathing and increased pulse rate. In general, there is an inverse relationship between critically elevated lactate levels and survival.

OVERVIEW: (**Study type:** Blood collected in a gray-top [sodium fluoride] or a green-top [lithium heparin] tube; **related body system:** Circulatory and Digestive systems. The patient should be instructed *not* to clench and unclench fist immediately before or during specimen collection; a tourniquet should not be used prior to or during venipuncture. The tightly capped sample should be placed in an ice slurry immediately after collection. Information on the specimen label should be protected from water in the ice slurry by first placing the specimen in a protective plastic bag.)

Lactic acid, also known as *lactate,* is a by-product of anaerobic carbohydrate metabolism. Pyruvate, the normal end product of glucose metabolism, is converted to lactate in situations when energy is needed but there is insufficient oxygen in the system to favor the aerobic and customary energy cycle. Lactic acid levels increase with strenuous exercise, heart failure, severe infection, sepsis, or shock. Lactic acid levels can also increase from liver disease or damage, because lactate is normally metabolized by the liver. Lactic acidosis can be differentiated from ketoacidosis by the absence of ketosis and grossly elevated glucose levels.

INDICATIONS
• Assess tissue oxygenation.
• Evaluate acidosis.

INTERFERING FACTORS
Factors that may alter the results of the study
• Drugs and other substances that may increase lactate levels include albuterol, aspirin, anticonvulsants (long-term use), isoniazid, metformin (Glucophage), oral contraceptives, sodium bicarbonate, and sorbitol.
• Falsely low lactate levels are obtained in samples with elevated levels of the enzyme lactate dehydrogenase because this enzyme reacts with the available lactate substrate.
• Using a tourniquet or instructing the patient to clench his or her fist during a venipuncture can cause elevated levels.
• Engaging in strenuous physical activity (i.e., activity in which blood flow and oxygen distribution cannot keep pace with increased

energy needs) before specimen collection can cause an elevated result.

Other considerations
• Delay in transport of the specimen to the laboratory must be avoided. Specimens not processed by centrifugation in a tightly stoppered collection container within 15 min of collection should be rejected for analysis. It is preferable to transport specimens to the laboratory in an ice slurry to further retard cellular metabolism that might shift lactate levels in the sample before analysis.

POTENTIAL MEDICAL DIAGNOSIS: CLINICAL SIGNIFICANCE OF RESULTS
Increased in
The liver is the major organ responsible for the breakdown of lactic acid. Any condition affecting normal liver function may also reflect increased blood levels of lactic acid.

• Cardiac failure *(decreased blood flow and insufficient oxygen in tissues result in accumulation of lactic acid from anaerobic glycolysis)*
• Diabetes *(inefficient aerobic glycolysis and decreased blood flow caused by diabetes result in accumulation of lactic acid from anaerobic glycolysis)*
• Hemorrhage *(decreased blood circulation and insufficient oxygen in tissues result in accumulation of lactic acid from anaerobic glycolysis)*
• Hepatic coma *(related to liver damage and decreased tissue oxygenation)*
• Ingestion of large doses of alcohol or acetaminophen *(related to liver damage)*
• Lactic acidosis *(related to strenuous exercise that results in accumulations in metabolic by-products of anaerobic breakdown of sugars for energy)*

L

- Pulmonary embolism *(decreased blood flow and insufficient oxygen in tissues result in accumulation of lactic acid from anaerobic glycolysis)*
- Pulmonary failure *(decreased blood flow and insufficient oxygen in tissues result in accumulation of lactic acid from anaerobic glycolysis)*

- Reye syndrome *(related to liver damage)*
- Shock *(decreased blood flow and insufficient oxygen in tissues result in accumulation of lactic acid from anaerobic glycolysis)*
- Strenuous exercise *(related to lactic acidosis)*

Decreased in: N/A

NURSING IMPLICATIONS

POTENTIAL NURSING PROBLEMS: ASSESSMENT & NURSING DIAGNOSIS

Problems	Signs and Symptoms
Confusion *(related to hepatic dysfunction, decreased tissue oxygenation)*	Disorganized thinking, restlessness, irritability, altered concentration and attention span, changeable mental function over the day, hallucinations
Electrolyte imbalance *(related to altered metabolic process, decreased oxygenation, hepatic dysfunction, shock, sepsis, excessive alcohol intake)*	Altered EKG, decreased serum bicarbonate, elevated lactic acid, symptoms of shock (cool, clammy skin; decreased mental status; decreased urinary output; hypotension), diagnosis of liver failure, elevated WBCs (sepsis, HIV infection), elevated blood glucose (diabetic ketoacidosis [DKA])
Fever *(related to liver disease, infection)*	Continuous low-grade temperature that is unaltered by treatment with antibiotics; temperature variances secondary to cirrhosis and liver damage; WBCs; positive sepsis screen
Gas exchange *(related to obstruction secondary to embolism, shock)*	Decreased activity tolerance, increased shortness of breath with activity, weakness, orthopnea, cyanosis, cough, increased heart rate, weight gain, edema in the lower extremities, weakness, increased respiratory rate, use of respiratory accessory muscles

BEFORE THE STUDY: PLANNING AND IMPLEMENTATION

Teaching the Patient What to Expect
- Inform the patient this test can assist with assessing organ function.
- Explain that a blood sample is needed for the test.

AFTER THE STUDY: POTENTIAL NURSING ACTIONS

Treatment Considerations
- Confusion: Correlate and treat the medical condition associated with the laboratory results. Consider electrolyte alterations that could contribute to the confusion and

reversal measures. Evaluate medications that could contribute to the confusion.
- Electrolyte Imbalance: Correlate lactic acid imbalance with disease process; liver function, shock, and DKA. Collaborate with the pharmacist and HCP for appropriate pharmacologic interventions. Monitor and trend serum lactic acid, arterial blood gas bicarbonate, glucose, and sodium results. Monitor EKG and assess for alcohol misuse, which could cause hepatic dysfunction.
- Fever: Take temperature every 4 hr and trend for continuous low-grade fever. Administer prescribed antipyretics and antibiotics. Provide clean linens to keep cool and comfortable (diaphoresis) and cooling measures (light clothing).
- Gas Exchange: Auscultate and trend breath sounds, administer ordered oxygen and use pulse oximetry to monitor oxygenation. Place the head of the bed in high Fowler position to promote ease of chest expansion and improve oxygenation, administer

ordered diuretics and vasodilators, and prepare for intubation. Monitor potassium level.

Safety Considerations
- Prevent falls and injury by appropriate use of fall precautions and consider postural support, bed alarm, or restraints as needed.

Follow-Up, Evaluation, and Desired Outcomes
- Understands that adequate hydration is necessary to prevent dehydration.
- Acknowledges the importance of monitoring self for dehydration. Symptoms for early dehydration are dry mouth, thirst, and concentrated dark yellow urine; for moderate dehydration are extreme thirst, dry oral mucus membranes, inability to produce tears, decreased urinary output, and lightheadedness; and for severe dehydration are confusion, lethargy, vertigo, tachycardia, anuria, diaphoresis, and loss of consciousness.

Lactose Tolerance Test

SYNONYM/ACRONYM: LTT.

RATIONALE: To assess for lactose intolerance or other metabolic disorders.

PATIENT PREPARATION: For the breath test or the glucose challenge test, there are no fluid restrictions unless by medical direction. Inform the patient that antibiotics, laxatives, antacids and stool softeners should not be taken within 2 wk prior to the test. Fasting for at least 12 hr before the test is required, and strenuous activity should also be avoided for at least 12 hr before the test. The patient should be instructed not to smoke cigarettes or chew gum during the test. Instructions for the breath test may also include brushing the teeth and/ or rinsing the mouth with water prior to and during the breath test. Obtain the pediatric patient's weight to calculate dose of lactose to be administered. Protocols may vary among facilities.

NORMAL FINDINGS: Method: Spectrophotometry.

Change in Glucose Value*	Conventional Units	SI Units (Conventional Units × 0.0555)
Normal	Greater than 30 mg/dL	Greater than 1.7 mmol/L
Inconclusive	20–30 mg/dL	1.1–1.7 mmol/L
Abnormal	Less than 20 mg/dL	Less than 1.1 mmol/L

*Compared to fasting sample for infants, children, adults, and older adults.

CRITICAL FINDINGS AND POTENTIAL INTERVENTIONS

Glucose
Adults and Children
- Less than 40 mg/dL (SI: Less than 2.22 mmol/L)
- Greater than 400 mg/dL (SI: Greater than 22.2 mmol/L).

Timely notification to the requesting health-care provider (HCP) of any critical findings and related symptoms is a role expectation of the professional nurse. A listing of these findings varies among facilities.

Consideration may be given to verification of critical findings before action is taken. Policies vary among facilities and may include requesting immediate recollection and retesting by the laboratory or retesting using a rapid point-of-care testing instrument at the bedside, if available.

Symptoms of decreased glucose levels include headache, confusion, polyphagia, irritability, nervousness, restlessness, diaphoresis, and weakness. Possible interventions include oral or IV administration of glucose, IV or intramuscular injection of glucagon, and continuous glucose monitoring.

Symptoms of elevated glucose levels include abdominal pain, fatigue, muscle cramps, nausea, vomiting, polyuria, polyphagia, and polydipsia. Possible interventions include fluid replacement in addition to subcutaneous or IV injection of insulin with continuous glucose monitoring.

OVERVIEW: (**Study type:** Plasma collected in a gray-top [fluoride/oxalate] tube; **related body system:** Digestive system.) Lactose is a disaccharide found in dairy products. When ingested, lactose is broken down in the intestine by the sugar-splitting enzyme lactase into glucose and galactose. When sufficient lactase is not available, intestinal bacteria metabolize the lactose, resulting in abdominal bloating, pain, flatus, and diarrhea. The most commonly used method to determine lactose intolerance is accomplished using the noninvasive hydrogen breath test. The breakdown of lactose by intestinal bacteria produces hydrogen gas. Before the administration of lactose, the patient breathes into a balloon. The concentration of hydrogen is measured from a sample of the gas in the balloon. After the administration of lactose, the patient breathes into a balloon at 15-min intervals over a period of 2 to 3 hr, and subsequent samples are measured for levels of hydrogen gas. The breath test is considered abnormal if the hydrogen measurements increase over the fasting or pretest level. The blood tolerance test screens for lactose intolerance by monitoring glucose levels after ingestion of a dose of lactose. There is also a stool acidity test used for pediatric patients who may not be able to be tested by the breath or glucose blood methods. After administration of a lactose solution, a stool sample is collected and tested for acidity. Normally, stool has a neutral or slightly alkaline pH. If the patient is unable to metabolize the lactose into glucose and galactose, lactic acid (and other acids) will be excreted in the stool and the stool pH will be acidic.

INDICATIONS
• Evaluate patients for suspected lactose intolerance.

INTERFERING FACTORS
Contraindications: N/A

Factors that may alter the results of the study
• Numerous medications may alter glucose levels (see study titled "Glucose").
• Delayed gastric emptying may decrease glucose levels.
• Smoking may falsely increase glucose levels.

POTENTIAL MEDICAL DIAGNOSIS: CLINICAL SIGNIFICANCE OF RESULTS

Glucose Levels Increased In
• Normal response

Glucose Levels Decreased In
• Lactose intolerance (lactase is insufficient to break down ingested lactose into glucose)

NURSING IMPLICATIONS

POTENTIAL NURSING PROBLEMS: ASSESSMENT & NURSING DIAGNOSIS

Problems	Signs and Symptoms
Diarrhea *(related to gastric irritation secondary to bowel irritation from undigested lactose)*	Frequent diarrhea after ingesting dairy products with lower abdominal cramping, gas, bloating
Nutrition *(related to the inability to digest dairy products secondary to lactase deficiency)*	Intolerance to dairy products; a history of lower abdominal cramping, gas, bloating, and diarrhea with the ingestion of dairy products
Pain *(related to altered gastrointestinal [GI] motility secondary to lactase deficiency)*	Lower abdominal cramping, gas, bloating, diarrhea

BEFORE THE STUDY: PLANNING AND IMPLEMENTATION

Teaching the Patient What to Expect
▶ Inform the patient this test can assist with evaluating tolerance to dairy products which contain lactose.
▶ Review the procedure with the patient. Obtain the pediatric patient's weight to calculate dose of lactose to be administered.

▶ For the glucose blood test, hydrogen breath test, or stool acidity test, lactose will be dissolved in a small amount of room temperature water (250 mL) and administered over a 5- to 10-min period. Dosage is 2 g/kg body weight to a maximum of 50 g for patients of all ages. The requesting HCP may specify a lower challenge dose if severe lactose intolerance is suspected. One pound is equal to 0.45 kg; therefore, a weight of 50 lb is equal to 22.7 kg. The appropriate dosage of lactose in this example would be 45.4 g. Record body weight, dose administered, and time of ingestion.

▶ Encourage the patient to drink one to two glasses of water during the test. Record any symptoms the patient reports throughout the course of the test.

▶ Explain that the test may produce symptoms such as cramps and diarrhea.

▶ *Glucose Blood Sample:* A baseline specimen will be collected with additional samples collected every 15 min over a 120 min interval. Subsequent specimens will be collected at 15, 30, 60, 90, and 120 min.

▶ *Hydrogen Breath Test:* A baseline specimen will be collected with additional samples collected every 15 min over an interval of 2 to 3 hr. Breath samples are collected by blowing into a collection device that resembles a balloon.

AFTER THE STUDY: POTENTIAL NURSING ACTIONS

Avoiding Complications

▶ Ensure the patient understands that the preparation designed for this test may cause cramping and diarrhea ranging in intensity from mild to severe.

Treatment Considerations

▶ Diarrhea: There are some interventions that can help when the patient has diarrhea. One approach is to eliminate or reduce the consumption of dairy products and to self-administer an oral enzyme medication to manage lactose when ingested.

▶ Nutrition: An accurate history of GI upset with the ingestion of dairy products can be helpful in identifying causal factors. Consider a trial lactose-free diet to see if the symptoms of GI upset resolve. Ensure the patient understands the importance of self-administering the oral enzyme medication that manages ingested lactalose. Explain how limiting or eliminating the consumption of obvious sources of dairy, such as milk, ice cream, and cheese, can be a valuable preventative measure. Encourage evaluation of foods for hidden dairy ingredients, such as found in sherbet, sauces, gravy, and desserts.

▶ Pain: Reducing or eliminating the consumption of dairy products can do a great deal to prevent the pain experienced with lactose ingestion.

Nutritional Considerations

▶ Advise those with lactose intolerance to avoid milk products and to carefully read labels on prepared products. Yogurt, which contains inactive lactase enzyme, may be ingested. The lactase in yogurt is activated by the temperature and pH of the duodenum and substitutes for the lack of endogenous lactase. Advise the patient that products such as Lactaid tablets or drops may allow ingestion of milk products without sequelae. Many lactose-free food products are now available in grocery stores.

Follow-Up, Evaluation, and Desired Outcomes

▶ Understands that dietary choices will need to be altered if lactose intolerance is identified.

▶ Considers collaboration with a registered dietitian to ensure proper diet selections and nutritional balance.

Laparoscopy, Abdominal

SYNONYM/ACRONYM: Abdominal peritoneoscopy.

RATIONALE: To visualize and assess the liver, gallbladder, and spleen to assist with surgical interventions, staging tumor, and performing diagnostic biopsies.

PATIENT PREPARATION: Inform the patient that a laxative and cleansing enema may be needed the day before the procedure, with cleansing enemas on the morning of the procedure. There are no activity or medication restrictions unless by medical direction. Instruct the patient that to reduce the risk of aspiration related to nausea and vomiting, solid food and milk or milk products are restricted for at least 6 hr and clear liquids are restricted for at least 2 hr prior to general anesthesia, regional anesthesia, or sedation/analgesia (monitored anesthesia). The patient may be asked to be NPO after midnight. The American Society of Anesthesiologists has fasting guidelines for risk levels according to patient status. More information can be located at www.asahq.org.

Regarding the patient's risk for bleeding, the patient should be instructed to avoid taking natural products and medications with known anticoagulant, antiplatelet, or thrombolytic properties or to reduce dosage, as ordered, prior to the procedure. Number of days to withhold medication is dependent on the type of anticoagulant. Note the last time and dose of medication taken. Protocols may vary among facilities.

Patients on beta blockers before the surgical procedure should be instructed to take their medication as ordered during the perioperative period.

NORMAL FINDINGS
- Normal appearance of the liver, spleen, gallbladder, pancreas, and other abdominal contents.

CRITICAL FINDINGS AND POTENTIAL INTERVENTIONS
- Appendicitis

Timely notification to the requesting health-care provider (HCP) of any critical findings and related symptoms is a role expectation of the professional nurse. A listing of these findings varies among facilities.

OVERVIEW: (Study type: Endoscopy; related body system: Digestive system.) Abdominal or gastrointestinal (GI) laparoscopy provides direct visualization of the liver, gallbladder, spleen, and stomach after insufflation of carbon dioxide (CO_2). In this procedure, a rigid laparoscope is introduced into the body cavity through a 1- to 2-cm abdominal incision. The endoscope has a microscope to allow visualization of the organs, and it can be used to insert instruments for performing certain procedures, such as biopsy and tumor resection. Under general anesthesia, the peritoneal cavity is inflated with 2 to 3 L of CO_2. The gas distends the abdominal wall so that the instruments can be inserted safely. Advantages of this procedure compared to an open laparotomy include reduced pain, reduced length of stay at the hospital or surgical center, and reduced time off from work.

INDICATIONS
- Assist in performing surgical procedures such as cholecystectomy, appendectomy, hernia repair, hiatal hernia repair, and bowel resection.
- Detect cirrhosis of the liver.
- Detect pancreatic disorders.
- Evaluate abdominal pain or abdominal mass of unknown origin.
- Evaluate abdominal trauma in an emergency.
- Evaluate and treat appendicitis.
- Evaluate the extent of splenomegaly as a result of portal hypertension.

- Evaluate jaundice of unknown origin.
- Obtain biopsy specimens of benign or cancerous tumors.
- Stage neoplastic disorders such as lymphomas, Hodgkin disease, and hepatic cancer.

INTERFERING FACTORS
Contraindications

⬥ Patients who are pregnant or suspected of being pregnant, unless the potential benefits of a procedure using radiation far outweigh the risk of radiation exposure to the fetus and mother.

⬥ Patients with bleeding disorders, especially those associated with uremia and cytotoxic chemotherapy.

⬥ Patients with cardiac conditions or dysrhythmias.

⬥ Patients with advanced respiratory or cardiovascular disease.

⬥ Patients with intestinal obstruction, abdominal mass, abdominal hernia, or suspected intra-abdominal hemorrhage.

⬥ Patients with a history of peritonitis or multiple abdominal operations causing dense adhesions.

Factors that may alter the results of the study

- Gas or feces in the GI tract resulting from inadequate cleansing or failure to restrict food intake before the study.
- Retained barium from a previous radiological procedure.
- Metallic objects (e.g., jewelry, body rings) within the examination field, which may inhibit organ visualization and cause unclear images.

Other considerations

- Patients who are in a hypoxemic or hypercapnic state will require continuous oxygen administration.

POTENTIAL MEDICAL DIAGNOSIS: CLINICAL SIGNIFICANCE OF RESULTS
Abnormal findings related to

- Abdominal adhesions
- Appendicitis
- Ascites
- Cancer of any of the organs
- Cirrhosis of the liver
- Gangrenous gallbladder
- Intra-abdominal bleeding
- Portal hypertension
- Splenomegaly

NURSING IMPLICATIONS

POTENTIAL NURSING PROBLEMS: ASSESSMENT & NURSING DIAGNOSIS

Problems	Signs and Symptoms
Breathing (related to postoperative pain, abdominal distention)	Adventitious breath sounds, shallow respirations
Insufficient fluid volume (related to postoperative vomiting, nausea, pre- and postoperative NPO status)	Dry mucous membranes, low blood pressure, increased heart rate, slow capillary refill, diminished skin turgor, diminished urine output
Skin (related to surgical incision)	Postoperative incision or staples; drains; elevated white blood cell (WBC) count; elevated C-reactive protein (CRP); redness, swelling, or drainage at incision site; fever

Teaching the Patient What to Expect

▶ Inform the patient this procedure can assist in assessing the abdominal organs.

▶ Explain to the female patient that she will be asked the date of her last menstrual period and pregnancy testing may be performed to determine the possibility of pregnancy before she undergoes the procedure in order to prevent any harm in the event of an unsuspected pregnancy.

▶ Review the procedure with the patient. Address concerns about pain and explain that there may be moments of discomfort or pain experienced when the IV line or catheter is inserted to allow infusion of fluids such as saline, anesthetics, sedatives, medications used in the procedure, or emergency medications.

▶ Explain that the procedure is performed in a surgery department by an HCP, with support staff, and takes approximately 30 to 60 min.

▶ Baseline vital signs are recorded and monitored throughout the procedure. Protocols may vary among facilities.

▶ The patient is placed in a modified lithotomy position with the head tilted downward on the laparoscopy table. If general anesthesia is to be used, it is administered at this time. The abdomen is cleansed with an antiseptic solution. The patient is draped and catheterized.

▶ The HCP identifies the site for the scope insertion and administers local anesthesia if that is to be used. After deeper layers are anesthetized, a pneumoperitoneum needle is placed between the visceral and parietal peritoneum.

▶ CO_2 is insufflated through the pneumoperitoneum needle to separate the abdominal wall from the viscera and to aid in visualization of the abdominal structures. The pneumoperitoneum needle is removed, and the trocar and laparoscope are inserted through the incision.

▶ After the examination, collection of tissue samples, and performance of therapeutic procedures, the scope is withdrawn. All possible CO_2 is evacuated via the trocar, which is then removed. The skin incision is closed with sutures, clips, or sterile strips, and a small dressing or adhesive strip is applied.

Potential Nursing Actions

✸ *Make sure a written and informed consent has been signed prior to the procedure and before administering any medications.*

Safety Considerations

▶ Anticoagulants, aspirin, and other salicylates should be discontinued by medical direction for the appropriate number of days prior to a procedure in which bleeding is a potential complication.

Avoiding Complications

▶ Complications of the procedure may include bleeding and cardiac dysrhythmias. Those with acute infection or advanced malignancy involving the abdominal wall are at increased risk for infection because organisms may be introduced into the normally sterile peritoneal cavity. Postprocedure, observe the incision site for bleeding, inflammation, or hematoma formation. Instruct the patient that persistent shoulder pain, abdominal pain, vaginal bleeding, fever, redness, or swelling of the incisional area must be reported to the HCP immediately.

Treatment Considerations

▶ After the procedure instruct the patient to resume usual diet, fluids, and medication, as directed by the HCP.

▶ Monitor vital signs and neurological status every 15 min for 1 hr, then every 2 hr for 4 hr, and as ordered. Take temperature every 4 hr for 24 hr. Monitor intake and output at least every 8 hr. Compare with baseline values. Notify the HCP if temperature is elevated. Protocols may vary among facilities.

L

▶ Instruct the patient to restrict activity for 2 to 7 days after the procedure.

▶ Inform the patient that shoulder discomfort may be experienced for 1 or 2 days after the procedure as a result of abdominal distention caused by insufflation of CO_2 into the abdomen and that mild analgesics and cold compresses, as ordered, can be used to relieve the discomfort.

▶ Breathing: Assess for changes in respiratory status and rate, work of breathing, and breath sounds. Elevate the head of the bed to facilitate breathing, facilitate mobility, and administer ordered pain medications.

▶ Insufficient Fluid Volume: Administer ordered parenteral and oral fluids. Perform strict intake and output, monitor color of urine, administer ordered antiemetics, and monitor and trend laboratory studies (uric acid, BUN, creatinine, electrolytes), and trend vital signs.

▶ Pain management is an important aspect of postprocedural care. Assess pain character, location, duration, and intensity. Use an easily understood pain rating scale, place in a position of comfort, and administer ordered analgesics. Consider alternative measures for pain management (imagery, relaxation, music), as appropriate.

▶ Skin: Monitor the surgical site and any drains for redness, drainage, swelling or warmth. Monitor and trend temperature, and WBC (immature WBCs and bands), and CRP as indicators of infection. Observe for abdominal distention or rigidity, and administer ordered antibiotics and antipyretics. Send ordered culture and sensitivity in the presence of drainage.

▶ Instruct the patient in the care and assessment of the incision site.

▶ If indicated, inform the patient of a follow-up appointment for the removal of sutures.

Follow-Up, Evaluation, and Desired Outcomes

▶ Recognizes reportable signs and symptoms of infection.

▶ Acknowledges the value of good nutrition in wound healing (iron, protein, vitamin C, zinc).

Laparoscopy, Gynecologic

SYNONYM/ACRONYM: Gynecologic pelviscopy, gynecologic laparoscopy, pelvic endoscopy, peritoneoscopy.

RATIONALE: To visualize and assess the ovaries, fallopian tubes, and uterus toward diagnosing inflammation, malformations, cysts, and fibroids and to evaluate causes of infertility.

PATIENT PREPARATION: Inform the patient that a laxative and cleansing enema may be needed the day before the procedure, with cleansing enemas on the morning of the procedure. There are no activity or medication restrictions unless by medical direction. Instruct the patient that to reduce the risk of aspiration related to nausea and vomiting, solid food and milk or milk products are restricted for at least 6 hr and clear liquids are restricted for at least 2 hr prior to general anesthesia, regional anesthesia, or sedation/analgesia (monitored anesthesia). The patient may be asked to be NPO after midnight. The American Society of Anesthesiologists has fasting guidelines for risk levels according to patient status. More information can be located at www.asahq.org.

Regarding the patient's risk for bleeding, the patient should be instructed to avoid taking natural products and medications with known anticoagulant, antiplatelet, or thrombolytic properties or to reduce dosage, as ordered, prior to the procedure. Number of days to withhold medication is dependent on the type of anticoagulant. Note the last time and dose of medication taken. Protocols may vary among facilities.

Patients on beta blockers before the surgical procedure should be instructed to take their medication as ordered during the perioperative period.

NORMAL FINDINGS
• Normal appearance of uterus, ovaries, fallopian tubes, and other pelvic contents.

CRITICAL FINDINGS AND POTENTIAL INTERVENTIONS
• Ectopic pregnancy
• Foreign body
• Tumor with significant mass effect.

Timely notification to the requesting health-care provider (HCP) of any critical findings and related symptoms is a role expectation of the professional nurse. A listing of these findings varies among facilities.

OVERVIEW: (Study type: Endoscopy; **related body system:** Reproductive system.) Gynecologic laparoscopy provides direct visualization of the internal pelvic contents, including the ovaries, fallopian tubes, and uterus, after insufflation of carbon dioxide (CO_2). It is done to diagnose and treat pelvic organ disorders as well as to perform surgical procedures on the organs. In this procedure, a rigid laparoscope is introduced into the body cavity through a 1- to 2-cm periumbilical incision. The endoscope has a microscope to allow visualization of the organs, and it can be used to insert instruments for performing procedures such as biopsy (e.g., biopsy of suspected endometrial lesions) and tumor resection. Under general or local anesthesia, the peritoneal cavity is inflated with 2 to 3 L of CO_2. The gas distends the abdominal wall so that the instruments can be inserted safely. Advantages of this procedure compared to an open laparotomy include reduced pain, reduced length of stay at the hospital or surgical center, and reduced time off from work.

INDICATIONS
• Detect ectopic pregnancy and determine the need for surgery.
• Detect pelvic inflammatory disease or abscess.
• Detect uterine fibroids, ovarian cysts, and uterine malformations (ovarian cysts may be aspirated during the procedure).
• Evaluate amenorrhea and infertility.
• Evaluate fallopian tubes and anatomic defects to determine the cause of infertility.
• Evaluate known or suspected endometriosis, salpingitis, and hydrosalpinx.
• Evaluate pelvic pain or masses of unknown cause.
• Evaluate reproductive organs after therapy for infertility.
• Obtain biopsy specimens to confirm suspected pelvic malignancies or metastasis.

L

- Perform tubal sterilization and ovarian biopsy.
- Perform vaginal hysterectomy.
- Remove adhesions or foreign bodies such as intrauterine devices.
- Treat endometriosis through electrocautery or laser vaporization.

INTERFERING FACTORS

Contraindications

⚜️ Patients who are pregnant or suspected of being pregnant, unless the potential benefits of a procedure using radiation far outweigh the risk of radiation exposure to the fetus and mother.

⚜️ Patients with bleeding disorders, especially those associated with uremia and cytotoxic chemotherapy.

⚜️ Patients with cardiac conditions or dysrhythmias.

⚜️ Patients with advanced respiratory or cardiovascular disease.

⚜️ Patients with intestinal obstruction, abdominal mass, abdominal hernia, or suspected intra-abdominal hemorrhage.

Factors that may alter the results of the study

- Gas or feces in the gastrointestinal (GI) tract resulting from inadequate cleansing or failure to restrict food intake before the study.
- Retained barium from a previous radiological procedure.
- Metallic objects (e.g., jewelry, body rings) within the examination field, which may inhibit organ visualization and cause unclear images.

Other considerations

- Patients who are in a hypoxemic or hypercapnic state will require continuous oxygen administration.

POTENTIAL MEDICAL DIAGNOSIS: CLINICAL SIGNIFICANCE OF RESULTS

Abnormal findings related to

- Abscesses
- Adhesions or scar tissue

- Ascites
- Cancer staging
- Ectopic pregnancy
- Endometriosis
- Enlarged fallopian tubes
- Infection
- Ovarian cyst
- Ovarian tumor
- Pelvic adhesions
- Pelvic inflammatory disease
- Pelvic tumor
- Salpingitis
- Uterine fibroids

NURSING IMPLICATIONS

BEFORE THE STUDY: PLANNING AND IMPLEMENTATION

Teaching the Patient What to Expect

▶ Inform the patient this procedure can assist in assessing the abdominal and pelvic organs.

▶ Explain to the female patient that she will be asked the date of her last menstrual period and pregnancy testing may be performed to determine the possibility of pregnancy before she undergoes the procedure in order to prevent any harm in the event of an unsuspected pregnancy.

▶ Review the procedure with the patient. Address concerns about pain and explain that there may be moments of discomfort or pain experienced when the IV line or catheter is inserted to allow infusion of fluids such as saline, anesthetics, sedatives, medications used in the procedure, or emergency medications.

▶ Inform the patient that the procedure is performed in a surgery department, by an HCP, with support staff, and takes approximately 30 to 60 min.

▶ Baseline vital signs are recorded and monitored throughout the procedure. Protocols may vary among facilities.

▶ The patient is placed in a modified lithotomy position with the head tilted downward on the laparoscopy table. If general anesthesia is to be used, it is administered at this time.

The abdomen is cleansed with an antiseptic solution. The patient is draped and catheterized.

♦ The HCP identifies the site for the scope insertion and administers local anesthesia if that is to be used. After deeper layers are anesthetized, a pneumoperitoneum needle is placed between the visceral and parietal peritoneum.

♦ CO_2 is insufflated through the pneumoperitoneum needle to separate the abdominal wall from the viscera and to aid in visualization of the abdominal structures. The pneumoperitoneum needle is removed, and the trocar and laparoscope are inserted through the incision.

♦ The HCP inserts a uterine manipulator through the vagina and cervix and into the uterus so that the uterus, fallopian tubes, and ovaries can be moved to permit better visualization.

♦ After the examination, collection of tissue samples, and performance of therapeutic procedures (e.g., tubal ligation), the scope is withdrawn. All possible CO_2 is evacuated via the trocar, which is then removed. The skin incision is closed with sutures, clips, or sterile strips and a small dressing or adhesive strip is applied. After the perineum is cleansed, the uterine manipulator is removed and a sterile pad applied.

Potential Nursing Actions

◆ *Make sure a written and informed consent has been signed prior to the procedure and before administering any medications.*

Safety Considerations

♦ Anticoagulants, aspirin, and other salicylates should be discontinued by medical direction for the appropriate number of days prior to a procedure in which bleeding is a potential complication.

AFTER THE STUDY: POTENTIAL NURSING ACTIONS

Avoiding Complications

♦ Complications of the procedure may include bleeding and cardiac

dysrhythmias. Those with acute infection or advanced malignancy involving the abdominal wall are at increased risk for infection because organisms may be introduced into the normally sterile peritoneal cavity. Postprocedure, observe the incision site for bleeding, inflammation, or hematoma formation. Instruct the patient that persistent shoulder pain, abdominal pain, vaginal bleeding, fever, redness, or swelling of the incisional area must be reported to the HCP immediately.

Treatment Considerations

♦ After the procedure instruct the patient to resume usual diet, fluids, and medication, as directed by the HCP.

♦ Monitor vital signs and neurological status every 15 min for 1 hr, then every 2 hr for 4 hr, and as ordered. Take temperature every 4 hr for 24 hr. Monitor intake and output at least every 8 hr. Compare with baseline values. Notify the HCP if temperature is elevated. Protocols may vary among facilities.

♦ Instruct the patient to restrict activity for 2 to 7 days after the procedure.

♦ Inform the patient that shoulder discomfort may be experienced for 1 or 2 days after the procedure as a result of abdominal distention caused by insufflation of CO_2 into the abdomen and that mild analgesics and cold compresses, as ordered, can be used to relieve the discomfort.

♦ Pain management is an important aspect of postprocedural care. Assess pain character, location, duration, and intensity. Use an easily understood pain rating scale, place in a position of comfort, and administer ordered analgesics. Consider alternative measures for pain management (e.g., imagery, relaxation, music), as appropriate.

♦ Teach the patient the signs and symptoms of pelvic inflammatory disease and to seek medical attention as soon as possible if they occur.

♦ Infection is always a risk with any invasion procedure. Advise the patient to complete ordered antibiotics for infection. Monitor and trend WBC and C-reactive protein and compare culture

L

and sensitivity results to prescribed antibiotics.

▶ This procedure can be emotionally difficult for the patient in relation to reproductive failure or success. Assess the level of anxiety and possible coping mechanisms to mitigate that anxiety. Allow verbalization of fears, concerns related to potential to fetal viability, and provide clear and easy-to-understand information related to reproductive challenges and treatment options.

▶ Instruct the patient in the care and assessment of the incision site.

▶ If indicated, inform the patient of a follow-up appointment for the removal of sutures.

Follow-Up, Evaluation, and Desired Outcomes

▶ Understands the necessity of refraining from sexual activity and tampon use until an infection is resolved.

▶ States the importance of good personal hygiene and perineal care after bowel movement to minimize bacteria.

Lead

SYNONYM/ACRONYM: Pb.

RATIONALE: To assess for lead toxicity and monitor exposure to lead to assist in diagnosing lead poisoning.

PATIENT PREPARATION: There are no food, fluid, activity, or medication restrictions unless by medical direction.

NORMAL FINDINGS: Method: Atomic absorption spectrophotometry.

	Conventional Units	SI Units (Conventional Units × 0.0483)
Children and adults (CDC)	Less than 5 mcg/dL	Less than 0.24 micromol/L

CDC = Centers for Disease Control and Prevention.

CRITICAL FINDINGS AND POTENTIAL INTERVENTIONS

• Levels equal to or greater than 5 mcg/dL (SI: Greater than 0.24 micromol/L) indicate exposure above the reference level.

• Levels equal to or greater than 45 mcg/dL (SI: Greater than 2.2 micromol/L) require chelation therapy.

• Levels greater than 70 mcg/dL (SI: Greater than 3.3 micromol/L) may cause severe brain damage and result in death.

Timely notification to the requesting health-care provider (HCP) of any critical findings and related symptoms is a role expectation of the professional nurse. A listing of these findings varies among facilities.

Observe the patient for signs and symptoms of elevated lead levels to include headache, impaired hearing, weight loss, disturbances of the nervous system, severe stomach cramps, and anemia. The pediatric patient may also demonstrate delayed learning and delayed growth.

OVERVIEW: (Study type: Blood collected in a special lead-free royal blue or tan-top tube; a lavender-top [EDTA] tube is also acceptable; related body system: Circulatory/Hematopoietic, Digestive, Musculoskeletal, Nervous, and Urinary systems.) Lead is a heavy metal and trace element found in the environment. It is absorbed through the respiratory and gastrointestinal systems. It can also be transported from mother to fetus through the placenta. When there is frequent exposure to lead-containing items (e.g., paint, batteries, gasoline, pottery, bullets, printing materials) or occupations (mining, automobile, printing, and welding industries), lead poisoning can cause severe behavioral and neurological effects. The blood test is considered the best indicator of lead poisoning.

INDICATIONS
Assist in the diagnosis and treatment of lead poisoning.

INTERFERING FACTORS
Other considerations
Contamination of the collection site and/or specimen with lead in dust can be avoided by taking special care to have the surfaces surrounding the collection location cleaned. Extra care should also be used to avoid contamination during the actual venipuncture.

POTENTIAL MEDICAL DIAGNOSIS: CLINICAL SIGNIFICANCE OF RESULTS
Increased in
Heme synthesis involves the conversion of D-amino levulinic acid to porphobilinogen. Lead interferes with the enzyme that is responsible for this critical step in heme synthesis, amino levulinic acid dehydrase.

- Anemia of lead intoxication
- Lead encephalopathy
- Metal poisoning

Decreased in: N/A

NURSING IMPLICATIONS

BEFORE THE STUDY: PLANNING AND IMPLEMENTATION

Teaching the Patient What to Expect
- Inform the patient this test can assist in detecting lead exposure.
- Explain that a blood sample is needed for the test.

AFTER THE STUDY: POTENTIAL NURSING ACTIONS

Avoiding Complications
- Avoid herbal or traditional folk remedies that contain lead.

Treatment Considerations
- Assess the environment for lead exposure, which can cause pediatric developmental delay; old leaded paint; contaminated soil of older homes; lead pipes; leaded ceramics or pottery used for food preparation and dining; old toys with lead.
- Assess for lead exposure related to adult hobbies, which may disrupt mental acuity; the use of products containing lead; restoration that includes sanding or removal of old leaded paint; work-related lead exposure (mining, battery manufacturing, construction).
- Modify diet and food purchasing habits to ensure absence of lead-contaminated kitchen cookware (ceramics), utensils, and foods; decrease environmental exposure by removing all decorative ceramics, toys, loose paint that contain lead.

Safety Considerations
- Slow exposure to lead-based environment or products can cause irreversible damage over time to brain, kidneys, and nervous system and can lead to death.

L

Nutritional Considerations
▶ Some canned goods and candies imported from other countries may have been produced using lead-contaminated ingredients (e.g., tamarind products packed in lead-glazed pots, minimally refined chili powder), lead-contaminated ink used to label candy packaging, or by poor manufacturing and storage processes. As appropriate, health-care providers should provide culturally sensitive education and discuss the safety issues related to consuming imported canned foods and candies.

Follow-Up, Evaluation, and Desired Outcomes
▶ Understands that further testing may be necessary to evaluate or monitor progression of the disease process and determine the need for a change in therapy.
▶ Agrees to institute environmental and dietary changes to prevent further lead exposure.

Leukocyte Alkaline Phosphatase

SYNONYM/ACRONYM: LAP, LAP score, LAP smear.

RATIONALE: To monitor response to therapy in Hodgkin disease and diagnose other disorders of the hematological system such as aplastic anemia.

PATIENT PREPARATION: There are no food, fluid, activity, or medication restrictions unless by medical direction.

NORMAL FINDINGS: (Method: Microscopic evaluation of specially stained blood smears) 25 to 130 (score based on 0 to 4+ rating of 100 neutrophils).

CRITICAL FINDINGS AND POTENTIAL INTERVENTIONS: N/A

OVERVIEW: (Study type: Blood collected in a lavender-top [EDTA] tube; related body system: Circulatory/Hematopoietic and Immune systems.) Alkaline phosphatase is present in the cytoplasm of neutrophilic granulocytes from the metamyelocyte to the segmented stage of development. The study involves counting 100 neutrophils from a stained smear. Segmented and band forms are counted; eosinophils, basophils, and other immature neutrophil forms are excluded. The reaction is subjectively scored from 0 to 4 based on the number of stained granules observed in the counted cells as well as the intensity of the staining. The number of cells counted is then multiplied by the score to arrive at the result. Leukocyte alkaline phosphatase (LAP) concentrations may be altered by the presence of infection, stress, chronic inflammatory diseases, Hodgkin disease, and hematological disorders. Low levels are associated with the presence of leukemic leukocytes, and high levels are present in normal white blood cells (WBCs). The test has been used for many years as a supportive test in the differential diagnosis of leukemia.

As time from its inception has passed and other technologies such as polymerase chain reaction (PCR) and fluoresence in-situ hybridization (FISH) have emerged, the LAP assay is used less often. The current World Health Organization classification of chronic myeloproliferative tumors does not use the LAP score; rather, by consensus, experts have developed international criteria such as morphology, immunophenotype, genetics, and clinical features. PCR and FISH technologies are used to evaluate blood or bone marrow specimens collected in a sodium heparin collection tube. The testing can be used to identify BCR/ABL-1 or JAK2 gene rearrangements that assist in the classification and treatment of hematologic conditions such as chronic myelogenous leukemia (CML), polcythemia vera, and other myeloproliferative tumors.

INDICATIONS
- Differentiate chronic myelocytic leukemia from other disorders that increase the WBC count.
- Monitor response of Hodgkin disease to therapy.

INTERFERING FACTORS
Factors that may alter the results of the study
Drugs that may increase the LAP score include steroids.

POTENTIAL MEDICAL DIAGNOSIS: CLINICAL SIGNIFICANCE OF RESULTS
Increased in
Conditions that result in an increase in leukocytes in all stages of maturity will reflect a corresponding increase in LAP.

- Aplastic leukemia
- Chronic inflammation
- Down syndrome
- Hairy cell leukemia
- Hodgkin disease

- Leukemia (acute and chronic lymphoblastic)
- Myelofibrosis with myeloid metaplasia
- Multiple myeloma
- Polycythemia vera *(increase in all blood cell lines, including leukocytes)*
- Pregnancy
- Stress
- Thrombocytopenia

Decreased in
- Chronic myelogenous leukemia
- Hereditary hypophosphatemia *(insufficient phosphorus levels)*
- Idiopathic thrombocytopenia purpura
- Nephrotic syndrome *(excessive loss of phosphorus)*
- Paroxysmal nocturnal hemoglobinuria *(possibly related to the absence of LAP and other proteins anchored to the red blood cell wall, resulting in complement-mediated hemolysis)*
- Sickle cell anemia
- Sideroblastic anemia

L

NURSING IMPLICATIONS

BEFORE THE STUDY: PLANNING AND IMPLEMENTATION

Teaching the Patient What to Expect
- Inform the patient this test can assist in evaluating for blood disorders.
- Explain that a blood sample is needed for the test.

AFTER THE STUDY: POTENTIAL NURSING ACTIONS

Treatment Considerations
- Instruct the patient to avoid exposure to infection if WBC count is decreased.

Follow-Up, Evaluation, and Desired Outcomes
- Recognizes the value of this study in relation to disease management and monitoring.

Lipase

SYNONYM/ACRONYM: Triacylglycerol acylhydrolase.

RATIONALE: To assess for pancreatic disease related to inflammation, tumor, or cyst, specific to the diagnosis of pancreatitis.

PATIENT PREPARATION: There are no food, fluid, activity, or medication restrictions unless by medical direction. Ensure specimen collection takes place prior to endoscopic retrograde cholangiopancreatography (ECRP).

NORMAL FINDINGS: Method: Enzymatic spectrophotometry.

	Conventional and SI Units
Newborn–older adult	0–60 units/L

CRITICAL FINDINGS AND POTENTIAL INTERVENTIONS: N/A

OVERVIEW: (**Study type:** Blood collected in a gold-, red-, red/gray-, or green-top [heparin] tube; related body system: Digestive system.) Lipases are digestive enzymes secreted mainly by the pancreas into the duodenum. There are different lipolytic enzymes with specific substrates, but they are collectively described as lipase. Other lipases produced by the body include sources such as the salivary glands, tongue, liver, intestines, and stomach. Lipase participates in fat digestion by breaking down triglycerides into fatty acids and glycerol so the fatty acids can be absorbed and either used for energy or stored for later use. Lipase is released into the bloodstream when damage occurs to the pancreatic acinar cells.

INDICATIONS

- Assist in the diagnosis of acute and chronic pancreatitis.
- Assist in the diagnosis of pancreatic cancer.

INTERFERING FACTORS

Factors that may alter the results of the study

- Drugs and other substances that may increase lipase levels include acetaminophen, asparaginase, azathioprine, calcitriol, cholinergics, codeine, diazoxide, didanosine, felbamate, glycocholate, hydrocortisone, indomethacin, meperidine, methacholine, methylprednisolone, metolazone, morphine, narcotics, nitrofurantoin, pancreozymin, pentazocine, and taurocholate.
- Drugs and other substances that may decrease lipase levels include protamine and saline IV infusions.

Other considerations

- ERCP may increase lipase levels; specimens should be collected prior to ERCP.
- Serum lipase levels increase with hemodialysis. Therefore, predialysis specimens should be collected for lipase analysis.

POTENTIAL MEDICAL DIAGNOSIS: CLINICAL SIGNIFICANCE OF RESULTS

Increased in

Lipase is contained in pancreatic tissue and is released into the serum when cell damage or necrosis occurs.

- Acute cholecystitis
- Bowel obstruction
- Cystic fibrosis
- Chronic diseases of the pancreas that cause permanent damage to acinar cells
- Chronic kidney disease *(related to decreased urinary excretion)*
- Obstruction of the pancreatic duct
- Pancreatic cancer (early)
- Pancreatic cyst or pseudocyst
- Pancreatic inflammation
- Pancreatitis (acute and chronic)

Decreased in: N/A

NURSING IMPLICATIONS

POTENTIAL NURSING PROBLEMS: ASSESSMENT & NURSING DIAGNOSIS

Problems	Signs and Symptoms
Breathing *(related to abdominal distention, ascites, pleural effusion, respiratory failure)*	Dyspnea, shortness of breath, increased work of breathing, nasal flare, respiratory rate greater than 24 breaths/min, tachypnea, use of accessory muscles for breathing, anxiety
Fluid volume *(related to vomiting, decreased oral intake, diaphoresis, nothing by mouth with a nasogastric tube, overly aggressive fluid resuscitation, compromised renal function, overly aggressive diuresis)*	**Deficit:** Decreased urinary output, fatigue, sunken eyes, dark urine, decreased blood pressure, increased heart rate, altered mental status **Excess:** Edema, shortness of breath, increased weight, ascites, rales, rhonchi, diluted laboratory values
Nutrition *(related to altered pancreatic function, excess alcohol intake, insufficient eating habits, altered pancreatic and liver function)*	Known inadequate caloric intake, weight loss, muscle wasting in arms and legs, stool that is pale or gray colored, skin that is flaky with loss of elasticity
Pain *(related to organ inflammation and surrounding tissues, excessive alcohol intake, infection)*	Emotional symptoms of distress, crying, agitation, facial grimace, moaning, verbalization of pain, rocking motions, irritability, disturbed sleep, diaphoresis, altered blood pressure and heart rate, nausea, vomiting, self-report of pain, upper abdominal and gastric pain after eating fatty foods or alcohol intake with acute pancreatic disease; pain may be decreased or absent in chronic pancreatic disease

L

BEFORE THE STUDY: PLANNING AND IMPLEMENTATION

Teaching the Patient What to Expect
⏵ Inform the patient this test can assist in diagnosing pancreatitis.
⏵ Explain that a blood sample is needed for the test.

AFTER THE STUDY: POTENTIAL NURSING ACTIONS

Treatment Considerations
⏵ Breathing: Monitor for cyanosis, pallor, snoring, adventitious breath sounds, and respiratory rate and effort. Evaluate the effect of administered medication on respiratory effort. Consider the need for intubation or mechanical ventilation. Monitor and trend vital signs. Teach the patient and the patient's family that they should report any difficulty of breathing or shortness of breath to the nurse for immediate intervention.
⏵ Fluid Volume: Perform accurate intake and output, perform and record daily weight. Collaborate with health-care provider (HCP) regarding IV fluid administration to support hydration. Trend laboratory values that reflect alterations in fluid status: potassium, BUN, creatinine, calcium, Hgb, and Hct. Manage the underlying cause of fluid alteration while assessing urine characteristics and respiratory status.

⏵ Nutrition: Consider barriers to eating, use of a food diary, and assessment of cultural food selections. Explain that continued alcohol use is a barrier to adequate protein intake. Monitor glucose levels.
⏵ Pain: Collaborate with the patient and HCP to identify the best pain management modality to provide relief. Refrain from activities that aggravate the pain. Consider appropriate use of heat or cold to manage pain. Identify pain location, intensity, and severity.

Nutritional Considerations
⏵ Administer vitamin B_{12}, as ordered, to the patient with decreased lipase levels, especially if his or her disease prevents adequate absorption of the vitamin.
⏵ Instruct patients with gastrointestinal disorders to eat small, frequent meals.
⏵ As compromised bowels improve and acute symptoms subside with the return of bowel sounds, patients are usually prescribed a clear liquid diet, progressing to a low-fat, high-carbohydrate diet.

Follow-Up, Evaluation, and Desired Outcomes
⏵ Patients with issues pertaining to alcohol misuse agree to avoid alcohol and to seek appropriate counseling for substance misuse.

Liver and Spleen Scan

SYNONYM/ACRONYM: Liver and spleen scintigraphy, radionuclide liver scan, spleen scan.

RATIONALE: To visualize and assess the liver and spleen related to tumors, inflammation, cysts, abscess, trauma, and portal hypertension.

PATIENT PREPARATION: There are no food, fluid, activity, or medication restrictions unless by medical direction. No other radionuclide tests should be scheduled within 24 to 48 hr before this procedure. Protocols may vary among facilities.

NORMAL FINDINGS
• Normal size, contour, position, and function of the liver and spleen.

CRITICAL FINDINGS AND POTENTIAL INTERVENTIONS
• Visceral injury

Timely notification to the requesting health-care provider (HCP) of any critical findings and related symptoms is a role expectation of the professional nurse. A listing of these findings varies among facilities.

OVERVIEW: (Study type: Nuclear scan; related body system: Digestive system.) The liver and spleen scan is performed to help diagnose abnormalities in the function and structure of the liver and spleen. It is often performed in combination with lung scanning to help diagnose masses or inflammation in the diaphragmatic area. This procedure is useful for evaluating right-upper-quadrant pain, metastatic disease, jaundice, cirrhosis, ascites, traumatic infarction, and radiation-induced organ cellular necrosis. Technetium-99m (Tc-99m) sulfur colloid is injected by IV access and rapidly taken up through phagocytosis by the reticuloendothelial cells, which normally function to remove particulate matter, including radioactive colloids in the liver and spleen. Radionuclide uptake in the spleen should always be less than uptake in the liver. False-negative results may occur in patients with space-occupying lesions that prevent normal hepatic filling (e.g., tumors, cysts, abscesses) smaller than 2 cm. For evaluation of a suspected hemangioma, the most common benign cause of a hepatic filling defect, the patient's red blood cells are combined with Tc-99m and images are recorded of the liver. This scan can detect portal hypertension, demonstrated by a greater uptake of the radionuclide in the spleen than in the liver. Liver and spleen scans are generally being ordered with less frequency and are in some cases being replaced by more advanced technology, including computed tomography (CT), magnetic resonance imaging (MRI), ultrasonography (US), and single-photon emission computed tomography (SPECT) scans. SPECT has significantly improved the resolution and accuracy of liver scanning. SPECT enables images to be recorded from multiple angles around the body and reconstructed by a computer to produce images, or *slices,* representing the organ at different levels. Diagnostic test results are interpreted in light of the results of liver function tests (alanine aminotransferase, albumin, alkaline phosphatase, aspartate aminotransferase, bilirubin, total protein). Liver scans are also used to assist with tumor staging, monitor disease progress, and follow response to therapeutic interventions.

INDICATIONS
• Assess the condition of the liver and spleen after abdominal trauma.
• Detect a bacterial or amebic abscess.
• Detect and differentiate between primary and metastatic tumor focal disease.
• Detect benign tumors, such as adenoma and cavernous hemangioma.
• Detect cystic focal disease.
• Detect diffuse hepatocellular disease, such as hepatitis and cirrhosis.

- Detect infiltrative processes that affect the liver, such as sarcoidosis and amyloidosis.
- Determine superior vena cava obstruction or Budd-Chiari syndrome.
- Differentiate between splenomegaly and hepatomegaly.
- Evaluate the effects of lower abdominal trauma, such as internal hemorrhage.
- Evaluate jaundice.
- Evaluate liver and spleen damage caused by radiation therapy or toxic drug therapy.
- Evaluate palpable abdominal masses.
- Evaluate post–liver transplantation for indications of organ rejection.

INTERFERING FACTORS
Contraindications

Patients who are pregnant or suspected of being pregnant, unless the potential benefits of a procedure using radiation far outweigh the risk of radiation exposure to the fetus and mother.

Factors that may alter the results of the study
- The scan may fail to detect focal lesions smaller than 2 cm in diameter.
- Metallic objects (e.g., jewelry, body rings) within the examination field, other nuclear scans done within the previous 24 to 48 hr, or retained barium from a previous radiological procedure, which may inhibit organ visualization and cause unclear images.
- Improper injection of the radionuclide that allows the tracer to seep deep into the muscle tissue can produce erroneous hot spots.

- Inability of the patient to cooperate or remain still during the procedure because movement can produce blurred or otherwise unclear images.

POTENTIAL MEDICAL DIAGNOSIS: CLINICAL SIGNIFICANCE OF RESULTS
Abnormal findings related to
The radioactive tracer accumulates in abnormal tissue, and "hot spots" identify specific areas of concern. "Cold spots," or the absence of tracer in areas where uptake is expected, also can identify specific areas of concern. Images can identify abnormalities in anatomical structures with regard to size, shape, and function (e.g., unexpected cold spots may inform with regard to dysfunctional tissue, filling defects).

- Abscesses
- Cirrhosis
- Cysts
- Hemangiomas *(evidenced by immediate uptake of the radionuclide by the filling defect)*
- Hematomas
- Hepatitis
- Hodgkin disease
- Infarction
- Infection
- Infiltrative process (amyloidosis and sarcoidosis)
- Inflammation of the diaphragmatic area
- Metastatic tumors
- Nodular hyperplasia
- Portal hypertension *(related to a reversal in the radionuclide uptake ratio [liver to spleen], which indicates a reversal in blood flow as a result of portal hypertension)*
- Primary benign or malignant tumors
- Traumatic lesions

NURSING IMPLICATIONS

POTENTIAL NURSING PROBLEMS: ASSESSMENT & NURSING DIAGNOSIS

Problems	Signs and Symptoms
Excess fluid volume (water) *(related to changes in portal pressure, low albumin, imbalanced aldosterone)*	Visual notation of increased abdominal girth, edema, shortness of breath, tachycardia, hypertension, positive jugular vein distention, electrolyte imbalance (potassium, sodium)
Inadequate nutrition *(related to pain, nausea, vomiting, inadequate metabolic function)*	Self-report of pain, nausea, vomiting
Pain *(related to inflammation, distention, obstruction, infection, infarction, tumor, trauma)*	Self-report of pain, facial grimace, crying, moaning, elevated heart rate, elevated blood pressure

BEFORE THE STUDY: PLANNING AND IMPLEMENTATION

Teaching the Patient What to Expect

▶ Inform the patient this procedure can assist in evaluating liver and spleen function.
▶ Pregnancy is a general contraindication to procedures involving radiation. Explain to the female patient that she will be asked the date of her last menstrual period. Pregnancy testing may be performed to determine the possibility of pregnancy before exposure to radiation.
▶ Review the procedure with the patient. Address concerns about pain and explain that there may be moments of discomfort or pain experienced when the IV line is inserted to allow infusion of fluids such as saline, anesthetics, sedatives, radionuclides, medications used in the procedure, or emergency medications.
▶ Explain that the procedure is performed in a nuclear medicine department by a health-care provider (HCP) specializing in this procedure, with support staff, and takes approximately 30 to 60 min.

▶ Reassure the patient that the radionuclide poses no radioactive hazard and rarely produces adverse effects.
▶ Instruct the patient to remove jewelry and other metallic objects from the area to be examined prior to the procedure.
▶ Baseline vital signs and neurological status are recorded. Protocols may vary among facilities.
▶ Positioning for the procedure is in a supine position on a flat table with foam wedges to help maintain position and immobilization.
▶ Once the IV radionuclide is administered, the abdomen is scanned immediately to screen for vascular lesions with images taken in various positions.
▶ Explain that once the study is completed, the needle or catheter will be removed and a pressure dressing applied over the puncture site.
▶ The patient may be imaged by SPECT techniques to further clarify areas of suspicious radionuclide localization.

Potential Nursing Actions
 Make sure a written and informed consent has been signed prior to

the procedure and before administering any medications.

AFTER THE STUDY: POTENTIAL NURSING ACTIONS

Avoiding Complications

▶ Establishing an IV site and injection of radionuclides are invasive procedures. Complications are rare but include risk for allergic reaction *(related to contrast reaction)*, hematoma *(related to blood leakage into the tissue following needle insertion)*, bleeding from the puncture site *(related to a bleeding disorder or the effects of natural products and medications with known anticoagulant, antiplatelet, or thrombolytic properties)*, or infection *(which might occur if bacteria from the skin surface is introduced at the puncture site)*. Monitor the patient for complications related to the procedure (e.g., allergic reaction, anaphylaxis, bronchospasm). Immediately report symptoms such as fast heart rate, difficulty breathing, skin rash, itching, or chest pain to the appropriate HCP. Observe/assess the needle/catheter insertion site for bleeding, inflammation, or hematoma formation.

Treatment Considerations

▶ Explain that the radionuclide is eliminated from the body within 6 to 24 hr. Advise the patient to drink increased amounts of fluids for 24 to 48 hr to eliminate the radionuclide from the body, unless contraindicated.
▶ Instruct the patient to resume usual medication and activity, as directed by the HCP.
▶ Excess Fluid Volume: Monitor fluid and electrolytes, heart rate, blood pressure, and perform a daily weight. Consider a low sodium diet, and administer ordered antihypertensives, diuretics, and spironolactone. Consider the use of an abdominal binder for support.
▶ Inadequate Nutrition: Complete a culturally appropriate nutritional assessment and trend specific laboratory studies: lipase, amylase, albumin, total protein, electrolytes, glucose, calcium, iron, and folic acid. Administer ordered IV fluids with supplements such as electrolytes as well as ordered antiemetics and antacids. Facilitate a dietary consult and administer ordered dietary supplements. Small, frequent meals may be beneficial.
▶ Pain: Assess pain character, location, duration, and intensity using an easily understood pain rating scale. Place the patient in a position of comfort and administer ordered medications: analgesics, narcotics, and anti-inflammatory. Consider alternative measures for pain management (imagery, relaxation, music, etc.).
▶ Instruct the patient in the care and assessment of the injection site.
▶ Explain that application of cold compresses to the puncture site may reduce discomfort or edema.

Safety Considerations

▶ The patient who is breastfeeding should consult with the requesting HCP regarding alternate testing that does not involve radiation. In general, if a woman who is breastfeeding must have a nuclear scan, she should not breastfeed the infant for 72 hr after the scan, until the radionuclide has been eliminated. She should be instructed to express the milk in order to prevent cessation of milk production; the milk can be stored and used after the 3-day period.
▶ Refer to organizational policy for additional precautions that may include instructions on handwashing, toilet flushing, limited contact with others, and other aspects of nuclear medicine safety.

Nutritional Considerations

▶ A low-fat, low-cholesterol, and low-sodium diet should be consumed to reduce current disease processes. High fat consumption increases the amount of bile acids in the colon and should be avoided.

Follow-Up, Evaluation, and Desired Outcomes

▶ Recognizes the importance of adequate caloric intake for positive health as well as the value of taking dietary supplements.

Lung Scans
(Perfusion and Ventilation studies)

SYNONYM/ACRONYM: Lung Perfusion Scan: Lung perfusion scintigraphy, lung scintiscan, pulmonary scan, radioactive perfusion scan, radionuclide lung scan, ventilation-perfusion scan, V/Q scan. Lung Ventilation Scan: Aerosol lung scan, radioactive ventilation scan, ventilation scan, VQ lung scan, xenon lung scan.

RATIONALE: To assess pulmonary blood flow and ventilation to assist in diagnosis of pulmonary embolism.

PATIENT PREPARATION: There are no food, fluid, activity, or medication restrictions unless by medical direction. No other radionuclide tests should be scheduled within 24 to 48 hr before this procedure. Protocols may vary among facilities.

NORMAL FINDINGS

Lung Perfusion Scan
• Diffuse and homogeneous uptake of the radioactive material by the lungs

Lung Ventilation Scan
• Equal distribution of radioactive gas throughout both lungs and a normal wash-out phase.

CRITICAL FINDINGS AND POTENTIAL INTERVENTIONS
• PE

Timely notification to the requesting health-care provider (HCP) of any critical findings and related symptoms is a role expectation of the professional nurse. A listing of these findings varies among facilities.

OVERVIEW: (**Study type:** Nuclear scan; **related body system:** Respiratory system.) The lung perfusion scan is a nuclear medicine study performed to evaluate a patient for pulmonary embolus (PE) or other pulmonary disorders. Technetium (Tc-99m) is injected by IV access and distributed throughout the pulmonary vasculature. The scan, which produces a visual image of pulmonary blood flow, is useful in diagnosing or confirming pulmonary vascular obstruction. The diameter of the IV-injected macroaggregated albumin (MAA) is larger than that of the pulmonary capillaries; therefore, the MAA becomes temporarily lodged in the pulmonary vasculature. A gamma camera detects the radiation emitted from the injected radioactive material, and a representative image of the lung is obtained. This procedure is often done in conjunction with the lung ventilation scan to obtain clinical information that assists in differentiating among the many possible pathological conditions revealed by the procedure; the combined study is a V/Q scan. The results are correlated with other diagnostic studies, such as thoracic computed tomography, pulmonary function, chest x-ray, pulmonary angiography, ECG, and arterial blood gases. A recent chest x-ray is essential for accurate interpretation of the lung perfusion scan. An area of nonperfusion seen in the same area as a pulmonary parenchymal abnormality on the chest x-ray indicates that a

L

PE is not present; the defect may represent some other pathological condition, such as pneumonia.

The lung ventilation scan is used to evaluate respiratory function (i.e., demonstrating areas of the lung that are patent and capable of ventilation) and dysfunction (e.g., parenchymal abnormalities affecting ventilation, such as pneumonia). The procedure is performed after the patient inhales air mixed with a radioactive gas (xenon gas or technetium-DTPA) through a face mask and mouthpiece. The radioactive gas delineates areas of the lung during ventilation. The distribution of the gas throughout the lung is measured in three phases:

- *Wash-in Phase:* Phase during buildup of the radioactive gas
- *Equilibrium Phase:* Phase after the patient rebreathes from a closed delivery system
- *Wash-out Phase:* Phase after the radioactive gas has been removed

When PE is present, ventilation scans display a normal wash-in and wash-out of radioactivity from the lung areas. Parenchymal disease responsible for perfusion abnormalities will produce abnormal wash-in and wash-out phases. This test can be used to quantify regional ventilation in patients with pulmonary disease.

INDICATIONS

General
- Aid in the diagnosis of PE in a patient with a normal chest x-ray.

Lung Perfusion Scan
- Detect malignant tumor.
- Differentiate between PE and other pulmonary diseases, such as

pneumonia, pulmonary effusion, atelectasis, asthma, bronchitis, and tumors.
- Evaluate perfusion changes associated with heart failure and pulmonary hypertension.
- Evaluate pulmonary function preoperatively in a patient with pulmonary disease.

Lung Ventilation Scan
- Evaluate regional respiratory function.
- Identify areas of the lung that are capable of ventilation.
- Locate hypoventilation (regional), which can result from chronic obstructive pulmonary disease (COPD) or excessive smoking.

INTERFERING FACTORS
Contraindications

General
Patients who are pregnant or suspected of being pregnant, unless the potential benefits of a procedure using radiation far outweigh the risk of radiation exposure to the fetus and mother.

Lung Perfusion Scan
Patients with atrial and ventricular septal defects, *because the MAA particles will not reach the lungs.*
Patients with pulmonary hypertension.

Factors that may alter the results of the study
- The presence of conditions that affect perfusion or ventilation (e.g., tumors that obstruct the pulmonary artery, vasculitis, pulmonary edema, sickle cell disease, parasitic disease, COPD, effusion, infection) can simulate a perfusion defect similar to PE.
- Metallic objects (e.g., jewelry, body rings) within the examination field or other nuclear scans done within the previous 24 to 48 hr which

may inhibit organ visualization and cause unclear images.

- Improper injection of the radionuclide that allows the tracer to seep deep into the muscle tissue can produce erroneous hot spots.
- Inability of the patient to cooperate or remain still during the procedure because movement can produce blurred or otherwise unclear images.

POTENTIAL MEDICAL DIAGNOSIS: CLINICAL SIGNIFICANCE OF RESULTS

Abnormal findings related to

The radioactive tracer accumulates in abnormal tissue, and "hot spots" in areas that would otherwise be expected to demonstrate a diffusely uniform distribution of radionuclide identify specific areas of concern.

General

- Atelectasis
- Bronchitis
- COPD
- PE
- Pneumonia
- Tuberculosis

Lung Perfusion Scan

- Asthma
- Left atrial or pulmonary hypertension
- Lung displacement by fluid or chest masses
- Pneumonitis
- Tuberculosis

Lung Ventilation Scan

- AIDS-related respiratory conditions
- Airway obstruction
- Bronchogenic cancer
- Cyanosis
- Cystic fibrosis
- Regional hypoventilation
- Sarcoidosis
- Tumor

NURSING IMPLICATIONS

BEFORE THE STUDY: PLANNING AND IMPLEMENTATION

Teaching the Patient What to Expect

- Inform the patient this procedure can assist in assessing blood flow to the lungs.
- Pregnancy is a general contraindication to procedures involving radiation. Explain to the female patient that she will be asked the date of her last menstrual period. Pregnancy testing may be performed to determine the possibility of pregnancy before exposure to radiation.
- Review the procedure with the patient. Address concerns about pain and explain that there may be moments of discomfort or pain experienced when the IV line is inserted to allow infusion of fluids such as saline, anesthetics, sedatives, radionuclides, medications used in the procedure, or emergency medications.
- Explain that the procedure is performed in a nuclear medicine department, by a health-care provider (HCP) specializing in this procedure, with support staff, and takes approximately 30 to 60 min.
- Reassure the patient that the radionuclide poses no radioactive hazard and rarely produces adverse effects.
- Instruct the patient to remove jewelry and other metallic objects from the area to be examined prior to the procedure.
- Baseline vital signs and neurological status are recorded. Protocols may vary among facilities.
- Positioning for the study is in the supine position on a flat table with foam wedges to help maintain position and immobilization.

Lung Perfusion Scan

- Once IV radionuclide is administered, a camera rotates around the patient, taking pictures in various positions and in multiple views (anterior, posterior, lateral, and oblique).

▶ Explain that once the study is completed, the needle or catheter will be removed and a pressure dressing applied over the puncture site.

Lung Ventilation Scan
▶ The radionuclide is administered through a mask placed over the nose and mouth, and the patient is asked to hold his or her breath for a short period of time while the scan is taken.

Potential Nursing Actions
✧ *Make sure a written and informed consent has been signed prior to the procedure and before administering any medications.*

AFTER THE STUDY: POTENTIAL NURSING ACTIONS

Avoiding Complications
▶ Establishing an IV site and injection of radionuclides are invasive procedures. Complications are rare but include risk for allergic reaction *(related to contrast reaction)*, hematoma *(related to blood leakage into the tissue following needle insertion)*, bleeding from the puncture site *(related to a bleeding disorder or the effects of natural products and medications with known anticoagulant, antiplatelet, or thrombolytic properties)*, or infection *(which might occur if bacteria from the skin surface is introduced at the puncture site)*. Monitor the patient for complications related to the procedure (e.g., allergic reaction, anaphylaxis, bronchospasm). Immediately report symptoms such as fast heart rate, difficulty breathing, skin rash, itching, or chest pain to the appropriate HCP. Observe/assess the needle/catheter insertion site for bleeding, inflammation, or hematoma formation.

Treatment Considerations
▶ Explain that the radionuclide is eliminated from the body within 6 to 24 hr. Advise the patient to drink increased amounts of fluids for 24 to 48 hr to eliminate the radionuclide from the body, unless contraindicated.
▶ Instruct the patient to resume usual medication and activity, as directed by the HCP.
▶ Monitor vital signs and neurological status every 15 min for 1 hr, then every

2 hr for 4 hr, and then as ordered by the HCP. Compare with baseline values. Protocols may vary among facilities.
▶ Alterations in gas exchange are a concern with lung perfusion and ventilation issues. Applicable interventions include establishing a respiratory status baseline regarding rate, rhythm, and depth. Pulse oximetry is a good tool to evaluate the effectiveness of ordered oxygen. Other interventions include elevating the head of the bed to facilitate breathing, monitoring and trending ABG results, and assessing for cyanosis and work of breathing. Thrombolytics may be ordered when occlusion is a concern.
▶ Ineffective breathing can also be a problem related to lung perfusion and ventilation in combination with gas exchange. Similar interventions are applicable. Assess and trend breath sounds, work of breathing, ABGs, and respiratory rate. The use of coping mechanisms to decrease anxiety can be beneficial, as can elevating the head of the bed. Administer ordered analgesics, instruct patient to cough and deep breathe as appropriate, and prepare for intubation.
▶ Poor pain management can contribute to altered respiratory patterns. It is advisable to complete a good pain assessment related to character, location, duration, and intensity with an easily understood pain rating scale and administer the ordered analgesic. Other interventions may include repositioning, imagery, relaxation, music, and head elevation.
▶ Instruct the patient in the care and assessment of the injection site.
▶ Explain that application of cold compresses to the puncture site may reduce discomfort or edema.

Safety Considerations
▶ The patient who is breastfeeding should consult with the requesting HCP regarding alternate testing that does not involve radiation. In general, if a woman who is breastfeeding must have a nuclear scan, she should not breastfeed the infant for 72 hr after the scan, until the radionuclide has been eliminated. She should be instructed

to express the milk in order to prevent cessation of milk production; the milk can be stored and used after the 3-day period.

▶ Refer to organizational policy for additional precautions that may include instructions on handwashing, toilet flushing, limited contact with others, and other aspects of nuclear medicine safety.

Follow-Up, Evaluation, and Desired Outcomes

▶ Is aware of reportable signs of bleeding: bleeding gums, black tarry stools, blood in urine, and hematoma when taking thrombolytics.

▶ Acknowledges the importance of remaining on bed rest to prevent movement of the embolus if present.

Lupus Anticoagulant Antibodies

SYNONYM/ACRONYM: Lupus inhibitor phospholipid type, lupus antiphospholipid antibodies, LA.

RATIONALE: To assess for systemic dysfunction related to anticoagulation and assist in diagnosing conditions such as lupus erythematosus and fetal loss.

PATIENT PREPARATION: There are no food, fluid, or activity restrictions unless by medical direction. Heparin therapy should be discontinued 2 days before specimen collection, with medical direction. Warfarin (Coumadin) therapy should be discontinued 2 wk before specimen collection, with medical direction.

NORMAL FINDINGS: (Method: Dilute Russell viper venom test time) Negative.

CRITICAL FINDINGS AND POTENTIAL INTERVENTIONS: N/A

OVERVIEW: (Study type: Blood collected in a completely filled blue-top [3.2% sodium citrate] tube; **related body system:** Circulatory/Hematopoietic, Immune, and Reproductive systems. If the patient's hematocrit exceeds 55%, the volume of citrate in the collection tube must be adjusted. Fill tube completely. *Important note:* When multiple specimens are drawn, the blue-top tube should be collected after sterile [i.e., blood culture] tubes. Otherwise, when using a standard vacutainer system, the blue-top tube is the first tube collected. When a butterfly is used, due to the added tubing, an extra red-top tube should be collected before the blue-top tube to ensure complete

filling of the blue-top tube. Promptly transport the specimen to the laboratory for processing and analysis. The recommendation for processed and unprocessed samples stored in unopened tubes is that testing should be completed within 1 to 4 hr of collection.) Lupus anticoagulant (LA) antibodies are immunoglobulins, usually of the immunoglobulin G class. They are also called *lupus antiphospholipid antibodies* because they interfere with phospholipid-dependent coagulation tests such as activated partial thromboplastin time (aPTT) by reacting with the phospholipids in the test system. They are not associated with a bleeding disorder unless thrombocytopenia or antiprothrombin antibodies are already present. They are associated with an increased risk of thrombosis. The combination of noninflammatory thrombosis of blood vessels, low platelet count, and history of miscarriage is termed *antiphospholipid antibody syndrome* and is confirmed by the presence of at least one of the clinical criteria (vascular thrombosis confirmed by histopathology or imaging studies; pregnancy morbidity defined as either one or more unexplained deaths of a morphologically normal fetus at or beyond the 10th week of gestation, one or more premature births of a morphologically normal neonate before the 34th week of gestation due to eclampsia or severe pre-eclampsia, or three or more unexplained consecutive spontaneous abortions before the 10th week of gestation) and one of the laboratory criteria (Anticardiolipin antibody, IgG, or IgM, detectable at greater than 40 units on two or more occasions at least 12 wk apart; or LA detectable on two or more occasions at least 12 wk apart; or anti-β_2 glycoprotein 1 antibody, IgG, or IgM, detectable on two or more occasions at least 12 wk apart, all measured by a standardized ELISA, according to recommended procedures).

INDICATIONS
• Evaluate prolonged aPTT.
• Investigate reasons for fetal death.

INTERFERING FACTORS
Factors that may alter the results of the study
• Drugs and other substances that may cause a positive LA test result include calcium channel blockers, chlorpromazine, heparin, hydralazine, hydantoins, isoniazid, methyldopa, phenytoin, phenothiazines, procainamide, quinine, and quinidine.
• Placement of a tourniquet for longer than 1 min can result in venous stasis and changes in the concentration of plasma proteins to be measured. Platelet activation may also occur under these conditions, causing erroneous results.
• Vascular injury during phlebotomy can activate platelets and coagulation factors, causing erroneous results.
• Hemolyzed specimens must be rejected because hemolysis is an indication of platelet and coagulation factor activation.
• Icteric or lipemic specimens interfere with optical testing methods, producing erroneous results.
• Hematocrit greater than 55% may cause falsely prolonged results because of anticoagulant excess relative to plasma volume.
• Incompletely filled collection tubes, specimens contaminated with heparin, clotted specimens, or unprocessed specimens not delivered to the laboratory within 1 to 2 hr of collection should be rejected.

POTENTIAL MEDICAL DIAGNOSIS: CLINICAL SIGNIFICANCE OF RESULTS
Positive findings in
• Antiphospholipid antibody syndrome *(LA are nonspecific antibodies associated with this syndrome)*
• Fetal loss *(thrombosis associated with LA can form clots that lodge in the placenta and disrupt nutrition to the fetus)*
• Raynaud disease *(LA can be detected with this condition and can cause vascular inflammation)*
• Rheumatoid arthritis *(LA can be detected with this condition and can cause vascular inflammation)*
• Systemic lupus erythematosus *(related to formation of thrombi as*

a result of LA binding to phospholipids on cell walls)

• **Thromboembolism** *(related to formation of thrombi as a result of LA binding to phospholipids on cell walls)*

Negative findings in: N/A

NURSING IMPLICATIONS

BEFORE THE STUDY: PLANNING AND IMPLEMENTATION

Teaching the Patient What to Expect

▸ Inform the patient that this test can assist in evaluation of clotting disorders.

▸ Explain that a blood sample is needed for the test.

AFTER THE STUDY: POTENTIAL NURSING ACTIONS

Treatment Considerations

▸ Pain management is an important aspect of care. Careful assessment to identify the best pain management modality to provide relief is a good place to start. Discuss with patient what has worked to relieve joint pain in the past; the effect of pain on personal, social, and professional obligations; and what activities that may aggravate pain. Some interventions are to apply heat or cold to the best effect and administer ordered medications such as opioids or anti-inflammatory medication. Collaborate with physical therapy to splint joints and avoid prolonged periods of inactivity that could exacerbate joint pain and stiffness.

▸ Fatigue can occur from multiple causes. Some of these are loss of sleep, anemia, or depression. Simple interventions include pacing activities to preserve energy stores, identify what aggravates and decreases fatigue, and assess for related emotional factors.

Follow-Up, Evaluation, and Desired Outcomes

▸ Acknowledges contact information provided for the American College of Rheumatology (www.rheumatology.org/I-Am-A/Patient-Caregiver/Diseases-Conditions/Antiphospholipid-Syndrome).

L

Luteinizing Hormone

SYNONYM/ACRONYM: LH, luteotropin, interstitial cell–stimulating hormone (ICSH).

RATIONALE: To assess gonadal function related to fertility issues and response to therapy.

PATIENT PREPARATION: There are no food, fluid, activity, or medication restrictions unless by medical direction.

NORMAL FINDINGS: Method: Immunoassay.

Concentration by Gender and by Phase (in Females)	Conventional and SI Units
Male	
Less than 2 yr	0.5–1.9 international units/mL
2–10 yr	Less than 0.5 international units/mL
11–20 yr	0.5–5.3 international units/mL
Adult	1.2–7.8 international units/mL

(table continues on page 794)

Concentration by Gender and by Phase (in Females)	Conventional and SI Units
Female	
Less than 2–10 yr	Less than 0.5 international units/mL
11–20 yr	0.5–9 international units/mL
Phase in Females	
Follicular	1.7–15 international units/mL
Ovulatory	21.9–80 international units/mL
Luteal	0.6–16.3 international units/mL
Postmenopausal	14.2–52.3 international units/mL

CRITICAL FINDINGS AND POTENTIAL INTERVENTIONS: N/A

OVERVIEW: (Study type: Blood collected in a gold-, red-, red/gray, or green-top [heparin] tube; related body system: Endocrine and Reproductive systems.) The secretion and inhibition of human reproductive hormones is maintained by a fine balance of feedback mechanisms involving the hypothalmus, pituitary gland, ovaries, and testes. Gonadotropin-releasing hormone (Gn-RH), a peptide neurohormone produced and released by the hypothalamus, signals the anterior pituitary gland to release luteinizing hormone and follicle-stimulating hormone. Gn-RH is secreted during the neonatal period, and gonadotropins are detectable in the blood at an early age. A negative feedback mechanism initiated by follicle-stimulating hormone and luteinizing hormone (LH) levels inhibits further secretion by suppressing the release of Gn-RH until puberty. During the prepubital period and following into adulthood, nocturnal pulses of Gn-RH induce nocturnal, pulsatile secretions of LH. The mechanism by which increased release of Gn-RH permits increased secretion of gonadotropins is not well understood. LH affects gonadal function in both men and women. In women, a surge of LH normally occurs at the midpoint of the menstrual cycle (ovulatory phase) due to initiation of a positive feedback loop involving estrogen and which results in ovulation. As the corpus luteum develops, progesterone levels rise, signaling the pituitary to stop secreting LH. In males, LH stimulates the interstitial cells of Leydig, located in the testes, to produce testosterone. For this reason, in reference to males, LH is sometimes called *interstitial cell–stimulating hormone.* Serial specimens may be required to accurately demonstrate blood levels.

INDICATIONS
- Distinguish between primary and secondary causes of gonadal failure.
- Evaluate children with precocious puberty.
- Evaluate male and female infertility, as indicated by decreased LH levels.
- Evaluate response to therapy to induce ovulation.

- Support diagnosis of infertility caused by anovulation, as evidenced by lack of LH surge at the midpoint of the menstrual cycle.

INTERFERING FACTORS
Factors that may alter the results of the study
- Drugs and other substances that may increase LH levels include clomiphene, gonadotropin-releasing hormone, goserelin, ketoconazole, leuprolide, mestranol, nafarelin, naloxone, nilutamide, spironolactone, and tamoxifen.
- Drugs and other substances that may decrease LH levels include anabolic steroids, anticonvulsants, conjugated estrogens, cyproterone, danazol, digoxin, D-Trp-6-LHRH, estradiol valerate, estrogen/progestin therapy, finasteride, ganirelix, goserelin, ketoconazole, leuprolide, desogestrel/ethinylestradiol (Marvelon), medroxyprogesterone, megestrol, metformin, octreotide, oral contraceptives, phenothiazine, pimozide, pravastatin, progesterone, and tamoxifen.

Other considerations
- In menstruating women, values vary in relation to the phase of the menstrual cycle.
- LH secretion follows a circadian rhythm, with higher levels occurring during sleep.

POTENTIAL MEDICAL DIAGNOSIS: CLINICAL SIGNIFICANCE OF RESULTS
Increased in
Conditions of decreased gonadal function cause a feedback response that stimulates LH secretion.

- Anorchia
- Gonadal failure
- Menopause
- Primary gonadal dysfunction

Decreased in
- Anorexia nervosa *(pathophysiology is unclear)*
- Kallmann syndrome *(pathophysiology is unclear)*
- Malnutrition *(pathophysiology is unclear)*
- Pituitary or hypothalamic dysfunction *(these organs control production of LH; failure of the pituitary to produce LH or of the hypothalamus to produce gonadotropin-releasing hormone results in decreased LH levels)*
- Severe stress *(pathophysiology is unclear)*

NURSING IMPLICATIONS

BEFORE THE STUDY: PLANNING AND IMPLEMENTATION
Teaching the Patient What to Expect
- Inform the patient this test can assist in assessing hormone and fertility disorders.
- Explain that a blood sample is needed for the test.
- Review the procedure with the patient. If the test is being performed to detect ovulation, inform the patient that it may be necessary to obtain a series of samples over a period of several days to detect peak LH levels.

AFTER THE STUDY: POTENTIAL NURSING ACTIONS
Treatment Considerations
- Record the date of the last menstrual period and determine the possibility of pregnancy in women who are perimenopausal.
- Fertility issues can be an emotional land mine for many people. Failure to conceive can cause great anxiety and engender feelings of hopelessness, depression, and a sense of powerlessness that affect the patient's

L

sense of self. Encourage verbalization of feelings and discuss therapeutic options offered by the health-care provider (HCP).
▶ Explain the purpose of repeating laboratory studies is to monitor and trend hormone levels.

Follow-Up, Evaluation, and Desired Outcomes
▶ States the proper use of home ovulation test kits approved by the U.S. Food and Drug Administration.
▶ Understands the alternative methods to achieve pregnancy, as described by HCP.

Lyme Disease Testing

SYNONYM/ACRONYM: N/A

RATIONALE: To detect antibodies to the organism that causes Lyme disease.

PATIENT PREPARATION: There are no food, fluid, activity, or medication restrictions unless by medical direction.

NORMAL FINDINGS: (Method: Enzyme immunoassay [EIA]) Less than 0.91 index; positives are confirmed by blot analysis (immunoblot). The criterion for interpretation of a positive immunoblot test requires the identification of at least five specific bands.

CRITICAL FINDINGS AND POTENTIAL INTERVENTIONS: N/A

OVERVIEW: (Study type: Blood collected in a gold-, red-, or red/gray-top tube; **related body system:** Immune system.) *Borrelia burgdorferi,* a deer tick–borne spirochete, is the organism that causes Lyme disease. Lyme disease affects multiple systems and is characterized by fever, arthralgia, and arthritis. The circular, red rash characterizing erythema migrans can appear 3 to 30 days after the tick bite. About one-half of patients in the early stage of Lyme disease (stage 1) and generally all of those in the advanced stage (stage 2, with cardiac, neurological, and rheumatoid manifestations) will have a positive test result. Patients in remission will also have a positive test response. The presence of immunoglobulin M (IgM) antibodies indicates acute infection. The presence of

IgG antibodies indicates current or past infection. However, other diseases such as anaplasmosis (formerly granulocytic ehrlichiosis), autoimmune disorders (e.g., lupus erythematosus, rheumatoid arthritis), endocarditis (bacterial), Epstein-Barr virus infection, *Helicobacter pylori* infection, leptospirosis, syphilis, tick-borne relapsing fever, or *Treponema denticola* infection can produce a positive EIA test, when the patient does not have Lyme disease. It is for this reason the Centers for Disease Control and Prevention (CDC) recommends a two-step testing process that begins with an immunofluorescence or enzyme-linked immunosorbent assay (ELISA) and is confirmed by using a Western blot or other FDA-approved immunoblot test. Immunoblot tests for Lyme disease testing can also detect IgM and IgG antibodies. It is desirable to perform confirmatory immunoblot testing for IgM antibodies because they are produced early in the disease process, but the incidence of false-positive results is higher than it is for IgG immunoblot testing, and a positive IgM immunoblot is meaningful only during the first 4 weeks of illness. Development of IgG antibodies can lag by 4 to 6 weeks after infection before being produced at detectable levels. Illness for longer than 4 to 6 weeks with a negative IgG immunoblot test and a positive IgM immunoblot most likely indicates the patient does not have Lyme disease.

INDICATIONS
Assist in establishing a diagnosis of Lyme disease.

INTERFERING FACTORS
• High rheumatoid-factor titers as well as cross-reactivity with Epstein-Barr virus and other spirochetes (e.g., *Rickettsia, Treponema*) may cause false-positive results.
• Positive test results should be confirmed by an FDA-approved immunoblot method (e.g., Western blot).

POTENTIAL MEDICAL DIAGNOSIS: CLINICAL SIGNIFICANCE OF RESULTS
Positive findings in
Lyme disease

Negative findings in: N/A

NURSING IMPLICATIONS

POTENTIAL NURSING PROBLEMS: ASSESSMENT & NURSING DIAGNOSIS

Problems	Signs and Symptoms
Infection (related to Borrelia burgdorferi bacteria, transmission of B. burgdorferi bacteria in utero from infected mother to baby)	Macular flush, flu-like symptoms, headache, extreme fatigue, neck pain, joint pain, joint swelling, bone pain, classic bull's-eye rash, unexplained fever, difficulty swallowing, chest pain, shortness of breath, heart palpitations, nausea, vomiting, pain in feet, twitching, numbness, irritability, visual disturbance, mood swings, depression, paranoia

BEFORE THE STUDY: PLANNING AND IMPLEMENTATION
Teaching the Patient What to Expect
▶ Inform the patient this test can assist in diagnosing Lyme disease.
▶ Explain that a blood sample is needed for the test. Warn the patient that false-positive and false-negative test results can occur.

Potential Nursing Actions
▶ Discuss history of exposure; ask the patient if he or she lives in or visits wooded areas, wears long pants and long-sleeved shirts when in wooded areas or when doing yard work, or has ever been bitten by a tick.

AFTER THE STUDY: POTENTIAL NURSING ACTIONS
Treatment Considerations
▶ Infection: Administer prescribed antibiotics and other medications to treat symptoms. Minimize future exposure to ticks by staying out of the woods in spring and summer

and staying toward the center of the hiking trail when hiking. Do not sit on the ground in leafy/grassy wooded areas. Complete frequent self-checks for ticks, wear long-sleeved shirts, tuck pants into socks, tuck shirt into pants, wear light-colored clothing to make attached ticks more visible, and use bug repellant with DEET. Do a full body check after being outdoors in endemic areas, and check pets for ticks.

Follow-Up, Evaluation, and Desired Outcomes
▶ Recognizes the importance of wearing light-colored clothing that covers extremities when in areas infested by ticks.
▶ Understands the importance of reporting continued signs and symptoms of the infection.
▶ Understands the importance of taking the prescribed antibiotic to treat infection, including that repeated antibiotic treatments that may be necessary.

Lymphangiography

SYNONYM/ACRONYM: Lymphangiogram.

RATIONALE: To visualize and assess the lymphatic system related to diagnosis of lymphomas such as Hodgkin disease.

PATIENT PREPARATION: There are no food, fluid, or activity restrictions unless by medical direction.

Note: If iodinated contrast medium is scheduled to be used in patients receiving metformin or drugs containing metformin for type 2 diabetes, the drug may be discontinued on the day of the test and continue to be withheld for 48 hr after the test.

Regarding the patient's risk for bleeding, the patient should be instructed to avoid taking natural products and medications with known anticoagulant, antiplatelet, or thrombolytic properties or to reduce dosage, as ordered, prior to the procedure. Number of days to withhold medication is dependent on the type of anticoagulant. Note the last time and dose of medication taken. Protocols may vary among facilities.

Ensure that barium studies were performed more than 4 days before lymphangiography.

NORMAL FINDINGS
• Normal lymphatic vessels and nodes that fill completely with contrast medium on the initial films. On 24-hr images, the lymph nodes are fully opacified and well circumscribed. The lymphatic channels are emptied a few hours after injection of the contrast medium.

CRITICAL FINDINGS AND POTENTIAL INTERVENTIONS: N/A

OVERVIEW: (Study type: X-ray, contrast/special; related body system: Immune system.) Lymphangiography involves visualization of the lymphatic system after the injection of an iodinated oil–based contrast medium into a lymphatic vessel in the hand or foot. The lymphatic system collects and filters lymph fluid, moving the fluid in one direction from the surrounding tissues to the neck where it reenters the circulatory system. The lymphatic system consists of lymph vessels, lymph ducts, lymph nodes, tonsils, adenoids, spleen, and thymus. Lymph is a colorless to white fluid composed of lymphocytes (white blood cells produced by the bone marrow and thymus), excess plasma proteins, and chyle (emulsified fats) from the intestines. The filtration units of the lymphatic system are the lymph nodes and organs located in different parts of the body, such as the neck, armpit, groin, chest, and abdomen. The main function of the lymphatic system is to provide immunological defense for the body against injury from disease or toxic chemicals. Assessment of this system is important because cancer (e.g., lymphoma and Hodgkin disease) often spreads via the lymphatic system. Painful edema of the extremities usually occurs when the flow of lymphatic fluid becomes obstructed by infection, injury, or cancer. Lymphangiography is performed for evaluating edema of unknown cause in an extremity; identifying lymph node involvement, which may indicate metastases from a primary tumor; staging cancer in patients with an established diagnosis of lymphoma or metastatic tumor to assist in monitoring progression of the disease; planning surgical intervention; and monitoring the effectiveness of therapeutic modalities such as chemotherapy or radiation treatment. Injection into the hand allows visualization of the axillary and supraclavicular nodes. Injection into the foot allows visualization of the lymphatics of the leg, inguinal and iliac regions, and retroperitoneum up to the thoracic duct. Less commonly, injection into the foot can be used to visualize the cervical region (retroauricular area).

INDICATIONS

- Determine the extent of adenopathy.
- Determine lymphatic cancer staging.
- Distinguish primary from secondary lymphedema.
- Evaluate edema of an extremity without known cause.
- Evaluate effects of chemotherapy or radiation therapy.
- Plan surgical treatment or evaluate effectiveness of chemotherapy or radiation therapy in controlling malignant tumors.

INTERFERING FACTORS

Contraindications

Patients who are pregnant or suspected of being pregnant, unless the potential benefits of a procedure using radiation far outweigh the risk of radiation exposure to the fetus and mother.

Patients with conditions associated with adverse reactions to contrast medium (e.g., asthma, food allergies, or allergy to contrast medium). Although patients are asked specifically if they have a known allergy to iodine or shellfish (shellfish contain high levels of iodine), it has been well established that the reaction is not to iodine; an actual iodine allergy would be problematic because iodine is required for the production of thyroid hormones. In the case of shellfish, the reaction is to a muscle protein called *tropomyosin*; in the case of iodinated contrast medium, the reaction is to the noniodinated part of the contrast molecule. Patients with a known hypersensitivity to the medium may benefit from premedication with corticosteroids and diphenhydramine; the use of nonionic contrast or an alternative noncontrast imaging study,

L

if available, may be considered for patients who have severe asthma or who have experienced moderate to severe reactions to ionic contrast medium.

✹ Patients with conditions associated with preexisting renal insufficiency (e.g., chronic kidney disease, single kidney transplant, nephrectomy, diabetes, multiple myeloma, treatment with aminoglycosides and NSAIDs), *because iodinated contrast is nephrotoxic.*

✹ Patients who are chronically dehydrated before the test, especially older adults and patients whose health is already compromised, *because of their risk of contrast-induced acute kidney injury.*

✹ Patients with bleeding disorders or receiving anticoagulant therapy, *because the puncture site may not stop bleeding.*

✹ Patients with severe chronic lung disease, cardiac disease, or advanced liver disease.

Factors that may alter the results of the study
- Gas or feces in the gastrointestinal tract resulting from inadequate cleansing or failure to restrict food intake before the study.
- Retained barium from a previous radiological procedure.
- Inability to cannulate the lymphatic vessels.
- Metallic objects (e.g., jewelry, body rings) within the examination field, which may inhibit organ visualization and cause unclear images.
- Inability of the patient to cooperate or remain still during the procedure, because movement can produce blurred or otherwise unclear images.

POTENTIAL MEDICAL DIAGNOSIS: CLINICAL SIGNIFICANCE OF RESULTS
Abnormal findings related to
- Abnormal lymphatic vessels
- Hodgkin disease

- Metastatic tumor involving the lymph glands
- Nodal lymphoma
- Retroperitoneal lymphomas associated with Hodgkin disease

NURSING IMPLICATIONS

BEFORE THE STUDY: PLANNING AND IMPLEMENTATION

Teaching the Patient What to Expect
◗ Inform the patient this procedure can assist in assessing the lymphatic system.
◗ Explain that prior to the procedure, laboratory testing may be required to assess for impaired kidney function (creatinine level and estimated glomerular filtration rate) if use of iodinated contrast medium is anticipated.
◗ Pregnancy is a general contraindication to procedures involving radiation. Explain to the female patient that she will be asked the date of her last menstrual period. Pregnancy testing may be performed to determine the possibility of pregnancy before exposure to radiation.
◗ Review the procedure with the patient. Address concerns about pain and explain that there may be moments of discomfort or pain experienced when the IV line or catheter is inserted to allow infusion of fluids such as saline, anesthetics, sedatives, contrast medium, medications used in the procedure, or emergency medications.
◗ Explain that contrast medium will be injected, by catheter, at a separate site from the IV line.
◗ Inform the patient that the procedure is performed by a health-care provider (HCP), with support staff, and takes approximately 1 to 2 hr.
◗ Advise that it will be necessary to return the next day for an additional set of images that will take about 30 min.
◗ Instruct the patient to remove jewelry and other metallic objects from the area of examination.
◗ Baseline vital signs and neurological status are assessed.
◗ Positioning for this study is in a supine position on an x-ray table.

▶ The selected area is cleansed and covered with a sterile drape.

▶ A local anesthetic is injected at the site, and a small incision is made or a needle inserted. A blue dye is injected intradermally into the area between the toes or fingers. The lymphatic vessels are identified as the dye moves. A local anesthetic is then injected into the dorsum of each foot or hand, and a small incision is made and cannulated for injection of the contrast medium.

▶ The contrast medium is then injected, and the flow of the contrast medium is followed by fluoroscopy or images. When the contrast medium reaches the upper lumbar level, the infusion of contrast medium is discontinued. X-ray images are taken of the chest, abdomen, and pelvis to determine the extent of filling of the lymphatic vessels. To examine the lymphatic nodes and to monitor the progress of delayed flow, 24-hr delayed images are taken.

▶ Explain to the patient that he or she will be monitored for complications related to the procedure (e.g., allergic reaction, anaphylaxis, bronchospasm).

▶ Explain that once the study is completed, the needle or catheter is removed, and a pressure dressing is applied over the puncture site.

▶ Once the cannula is removed, the incision is sutured and bandaged.

Potential Nursing Actions

✦ *Make sure a written and informed consent has been signed prior to the procedure and before administering any medications.*

Safety Considerations

▶ If iodinated contrast medium is scheduled to be used in patients receiving metformin or drugs containing metformin for type 2 diabetes, the drug may be discontinued on the day of the test and continue to be withheld for 48 hr after the test. Protocols may vary among facilities

▶ Anticoagulants, aspirin and other salicylates should be discontinued by medical direction for the appropriate number of days prior to a procedure in which bleeding is a potential complication.

Avoiding Complications

▶ Establishing an IV site and injection of contrast medium are invasive procedures. Complications are rare but include risk for allergic reaction *(related to contrast reaction);* bleeding from the puncture site *(related to a bleeding disorder or the effects of natural products and medications with known anticoagulant, antiplatelet, or thrombolytic properties);* dyspnea, pain, or hypotension *(caused by micropulmonary emboli);* hematoma *(related to blood leakage into the tissue following needle insertion);* infection *(which might occur if bacteria from the skin surface is introduced at the puncture site);* lipoid pneumonia *(caused by contrast dye entering the thoracic duct);* tissue damage *(related to extravasation or leaking of contrast into the tissues during injection);* nerve injury *(which might occur if the needle strikes a nerve);* or nephrotoxicity *(a deterioration of renal function associated with contrast administration).* Monitor the patient for complications related to the procedure (e.g., allergic reaction, anaphylaxis, bronchospasm, infection, injury, lipid pneumonia, pulmonary embolus). Immediately report symptoms such as difficulty breathing, chest pain, fever, hyperpnea, hypertension, nausea, palpitations, pruritus, rash, tachycardia, urticaria, or vomiting to the appropriate HCP. Observe/assess the needle/catheter insertion site for bleeding, inflammation, or hematoma formation. Administer ordered antihistamines or prophylactic steroids if the patient has an allergic reaction.

Treatment Considerations

▶ The usual diet, fluids, medications, or activity can be resumed, as directed by the HCP. Kidney function should be assessed before metformin is resumed.

▶ Monitor vital signs and neurological status every 15 min for 30 min. Take temperature every 4 hr for 24 hr. Monitor intake and output at least every 8 hr. Compare with baseline values. Notify the HCP if temperature is elevated. Protocols may vary among facilities.

L

▶ Instruct the patient to maintain bedrest up to 24 hr to reduce extremity swelling after the procedure or as ordered.

▶ Explain the care and assessment of the site and how to apply cold compresses to the puncture site as needed to reduce discomfort or edema.

▶ Explain that the skin, urine, and stool may retain a bluish hue from the dye for 2 to 3 days after the procedure until the dye clears from the body.

Safety Considerations

▶ Advise patients with diabetes to avoid all medications containing metformin for 48 hr following a procedure with iodinated contrast. Iodinated contrast can temporarily impair kidney function, and failure to withhold metformin may indirectly result in drug-induced lactic acidosis, a dangerous and sometimes fatal adverse effect of metformin (related to renal impairment that does not support sufficient excretion of metformin).

Follow-Up, Evaluation, and Desired Outcomes

▶ Acknowledges additional testing may be needed to monitor disease progression and evaluate the need for change in therapy.

L

Magnesium, Blood

RATIONALE: To assess electrolyte balance related to magnesium levels to assist in diagnosis, monitoring diseases, and therapeutic interventions such as hemodialysis, preeclampsia, and eclampsia.

PATIENT PREPARATION: There are no food, fluid, activity, or medication restrictions unless by medical direction.

NORMAL FINDINGS: Method: Spectrophotometry.

Age	Conventional Units	SI Units (Conventional Units × 0.4114)
Newborn	1.7–2.5 mg/dL	0.7–1 mmol/L
Child	1.7–2.3 mg/dL	0.7–0.95 mmol/L
Adult	1.6–2.2 mg/dL	0.66–0.91 mmol/L
Pregnant female		
First and second trimester	1.5–2.2 mg/dL	0.63–0.91 mmol/L
Third trimester	1.1–2.2 mg/dL	0.46–0.91 mmol/L

CRITICAL FINDINGS AND POTENTIAL INTERVENTIONS

Adults
- Less than 1.2 mg/dL (SI: Less than 0.5 mmol/L)
- Greater than 4.9 mg/dL (SI: Greater than 2 mmol/L)

Children
- Less than 1.2 mg/dL (SI: Less than 0.5 mmol/L)
- Greater than 4.3 mg/dL (SI: Greater than 1.8 mmol/L)

Timely notification to the requesting health-care provider (HCP) of any critical findings and related symptoms is a role expectation of the professional nurse. A listing of these findings varies among facilities.

Consideration may be given to verification of critical findings before action is taken. Policies vary among facilities and may include requesting immediate recollection and retesting by the laboratory or retesting using a rapid point-of-care testing instrument at the bedside, if available.

Symptoms such as tetany, weakness, dizziness, tremors, hyperactivity, nausea, vomiting, and convulsions occur at decreased (less than 1.2 mg/dL [SI: less than 0.5 mmol/L]) concentrations. Electrocardiographic (ECG) changes (prolonged P-R and Q-T intervals; broad, flat T waves; and ventricular tachycardia) may also occur. Treatment may include IV or oral administration of magnesium salts, monitoring for respiratory depression and areflexia (IV administration of magnesium salts), and monitoring for diarrhea and metabolic alkalosis (oral administration to replace magnesium).

Respiratory paralysis, decreased reflexes, and cardiac arrest occur at grossly elevated (greater than 15 mg/dL [SI: greater than 6.2 mmol/L]) levels. ECG changes, such as prolonged P-R and Q-T intervals, and bradycardia may be seen. Toxic levels of magnesium may be reversed with the administration of calcium, dialysis treatments, and removal of the source of excessive intake.

M

OVERVIEW: (Study type: Blood collected in a gold-, red-, or red/gray-top tube; **related body system:** Circulatory, Digestive, Endocrine, Reproductive, and Urinary systems.) Magnesium is required as a cofactor in numerous crucial enzymatic processes, such as protein synthesis, nucleic acid synthesis, and muscle contraction. Magnesium is also required for the use of adenosine diphosphate as a source of energy. It is the fourth-most abundant cation and the second-most abundant intracellular ion. Magnesium is needed for the transmission of nerve impulses and muscle relaxation. It controls absorption of sodium, potassium, calcium, and phosphorus; utilization of carbohydrate, lipid, and protein; and activation of enzyme systems that enable the B vitamins to function. Magnesium is also essential for oxidative phosphorylation, nucleic acid synthesis, and blood clotting. Urine magnesium levels reflect magnesium deficiency before serum levels. Magnesium deficiency severe enough to cause hypocalcemia and cardiac dysrhythmias can exist despite normal serum magnesium levels. The increased nutritional demands of a developing fetus during pregnancy are often associated with corresponding maternal deficiencies, including a lower than normal magnesium level. Magnesium supplementation during pregnancy may be ordered in the form of oral prenatal vitamins, intermittent intromuscular injections, or by IV administration depending on the degree of deficiency. Magnesium can be used to inhibit preterm labor by lowering calcium in uterine cells, causing the uterine muscles to relax.

Magnesium is also used to help prevent and treat pre-eclampsia and eclampsia.

INDICATIONS

- Determine electrolyte balance in chronic kidney disease and alcohol misuse.
- Evaluate cardiac dysrhythmias (decreased magnesium levels can lead to excessive ventricular irritability).
- Evaluate known or suspected disorders associated with altered magnesium levels.
- Monitor the effects of various drugs on magnesium levels.

INTERFERING FACTORS
Factors that may alter the results of the study

- Drugs and other substances that may increase magnesium levels include acetylsalicylic acid and progesterone.
- Drugs and other substances that may decrease magnesium levels include albuterol, aminoglycosides, amphotericin B, bendroflumethiazide, chlorthalidone, cisplatin, citrates, cyclosporine, digoxin, glucagon, and oral contraceptives.
- Magnesium is present in higher intracellular concentrations; therefore, hemolysis will result in a false elevation in values, and such specimens should be rejected for analysis.
- Specimens should never be collected above an IV line because of the potential for dilution when the specimen and the IV solution combine in the collection container, falsely decreasing the result. There is also the potential of contaminating the sample with the substance of interest if it is present in the IV solution, falsely increasing the result.

POTENTIAL MEDICAL DIAGNOSIS: CLINICAL SIGNIFICANCE OF RESULTS

Increased in

- Addison disease *(related to insufficient production of aldosterone, decreased renal excretion)*
- Adrenocortical insufficiency *(related to decreased renal excretion)*
- Dehydration *(related to hemoconcentration)*
- Diabetic acidosis (severe) *(related to acid-base imbalance)*
- Hypothyroidism *(pathophysiology is unclear)*
- Massive hemolysis *(related to release of intracellular magnesium; intracellular concentration is three times higher than normal plasma levels)*
- Overuse of antacids *(related to excessive intake of magnesium-containing antacids)*
- Renal insufficiency *(related to decreased urinary excretion)*
- Tissue trauma

Decreased in

- Alcohol misuse *(related to increased renal excretion and possible insufficient dietary intake)*
- Diabetic acidosis *(insulin treatment lowers blood glucose and appears to increase intracellular transport of magnesium)*
- Glomerulonephritis (chronic) *(related to diminished renal function; magnesium is reabsorbed in the renal tubules)*
- Hemodialysis *(related to loss of magnesium due to dialysis treatment)*
- Hyperaldosteronism *(related to increased excretion)*
- Hypocalcemia *(decreased magnesium is associated with decreased calcium and vitamin D levels)*
- Hypoparathyroidism *(related to decreased calcium)*
- Inadequate intake
- Inappropriate secretion of antidiuretic hormone *(related to fluid overload)*
- Long-term hyperalimentation
- Malabsorption *(related to impaired absorption of calcium and vitamin D)*
- Pancreatitis *(secondary to alcohol misuse)*
- Pregnancy
- Severe loss of body fluids *(diarrhea, lactation, sweating, laxative abuse)*

M

NURSING IMPLICATIONS

POTENTIAL NURSING PROBLEMS: ASSESSMENT & NURSING DIAGNOSIS

Problems	Signs and Symptoms
Cardiac output *(related to increased preload, increased afterload, impaired cardiac contractility, cardiac muscle disease, altered cardiac conduction)*	Decreased peripheral pulses; decreased urinary output; cool, clammy skin; tachypnea; dyspnea; edema; altered level of consciousness; abnormal heart sounds; crackles in lungs; decreased activity tolerance; weight gain; fatigue; hypoxia
Electrolyte imbalance *(related to metabolic imbalance)*	**Excess:** Nausea, vomiting, diarrhea, diaphoresis, flushing, sensation of heat, decreased mental functioning, weakness, drowsiness, hypotension, bradycardia, respiratory depression, coma

(table continues on page 806)

Problems	Signs and Symptoms
Fluid volume (water) *(related to metabolic imbalances associated with disease process)*	**Deficit:** Nystagmus, fatigue, convulsions, weakness, numbness **Deficit:** Decreased urinary output, fatigue, sunken eyes, dark urine, decreased blood pressure, increased heart rate, and altered mental status **Excess:** Edema, shortness of breath, increased weight, ascites, rales, rhonchi, and diluted laboratory values
Nutrition *(related to excess caloric intake with large amounts of dietary sodium and fat; cultural lifestyle; overeating associated with anxiety, depression, compulsive disorder; genetics; inadequate or unhealthy food resources)*	Observable obesity, high-fat or sodium food selections, high body mass index, high consumption of ethnic foods, sedentary lifestyle, dietary religious beliefs and food selections, binge eating, diet high in refined sugar, repetitive dieting and failure

BEFORE THE STUDY: PLANNING AND IMPLEMENTATION

Teaching the Patient What to Expect
▸ Inform the patient this test can assist in the evaluation of electrolyte balance.
▸ Explain that a blood sample is needed for the test.

AFTER THE STUDY: POTENTIAL NURSING ACTIONS

Treatment Considerations
▸ Cardiac Output: Assess peripheral pulses, capillary refill, respiratory rate, breath sounds, skin color and temperature, and level of consciousness. Monitor urinary output, oxygenation with pulse oximetry, and blood pressure, including orthostatic changes. Monitor sodium, potassium, and B-type natriuretic peptide levels. Administer ordered angiotensin-converting enzyme inhibitors, beta-blockers, diuretics, aldosterone antagonists, and vasodilators.
▸ Fluid Volume and Electrolyte Balance: Complete a daily weight and intake and output. Monitor laboratory values that reflect alterations in fluid status (potassium, BUN, creatinine, calcium, magnesium, Hgb, Hct). Manage the underlying cause of fluid alterations, monitor urine characteristics and respiratory status. Establish baseline assessment data and collaborate with HCP to adjust oral and IV fluids to provide optimal hydration, including replacement of electrolytes.

Nutritional Considerations
▸ Review the concept of an ideal body weight. Explain the purpose of and relationship between ideal weight and caloric intake to support cardiac health. Review ways to decrease the intake of saturated fats and increase the intake of polyunsaturated fats. Discuss limiting the intake of cholesterol, sodium, and refined processed sugar. Encourage the intake of fresh fruits and vegetables, unprocessed carbohydrates, poultry, and grains. Educate the magnesium-deficient patient regarding good dietary sources of magnesium, such as green vegetables, seeds, legumes, shrimp, and some bran cereals. Advise the patient that high intake of substances such as phosphorus, calcium, fat, and protein interferes with the absorption of magnesium.

M

Follow-Up, Evaluation, and Desired Outcomes

▶ Understands the importance of reporting any signs or symptoms of electrolyte imbalance, such as dehydration, diarrhea, vomiting, or prolonged anorexia.

▶ Recognizes the value of nutritional counseling services with a registered dietitian.

▶ Acknowledges provided contact information for the U.S. Department of Agriculture's resource for nutrition (www.choosemyplate.gov).

Magnesium, Urine

SYNONYM/ACRONYM: Urine Mg^{2+}.

RATIONALE: To assess magnesium levels related to renal function.

PATIENT PREPARATION: There are no food, fluid, activity, or medication restrictions unless by medical direction. Either a random or a 24-hr urine collection may be ordered. As appropriate, provide the required urine collection container and specimen collection instructions.

NORMAL FINDINGS: Method: Spectrophotometry.

Conventional Units	SI Units (Conventional Units × 0.4114)
20–200 mg/24 hr	8.2–82.3 mmol/24 hr

CRITICAL FINDINGS AND POTENTIAL INTERVENTIONS: N/A

OVERVIEW: (**Study type:** Urine from a random or timed specimen collected in a clean plastic collection container with 6N hydrochloride as a preservative; **related body system:** Digestive and Urinary systems.) Magnesium is required as a cofactor in numerous crucial enzymatic processes, such as protein synthesis, nucleic acid synthesis, and muscle contraction. Magnesium is also required for the use of adenosine diphosphate as a source of energy. It is the fourth-most abundant cation and the second-most abundant intracellular ion. Magnesium is needed for the transmission of nerve impulses and muscle relaxation. It controls absorption of sodium, potassium, calcium, and phosphorus; utilization of carbohydrate, lipid, and protein; and activation of enzyme systems that enable the B vitamins to function. Magnesium is also essential for oxidative phosphorylation, nucleic acid synthesis, and blood clotting. Urine magnesium levels reflect magnesium deficiency before serum levels. Magnesium deficiency severe enough to cause hypocalcemia and cardiac dysrhythmias can exist despite normal serum magnesium levels.

Regulating electrolyte balance is one of the major functions of the kidneys. In normally

M

functioning kidneys, urine levels increase when serum levels are high and decrease when serum levels are low to maintain homeostasis. Analyzing these urinary levels can provide important clues as to the functioning of the kidneys and other major organs. Tests for electrolytes, such as magnesium, in urine usually involve timed urine collections over a 12- or 24-hr period. Measurement of random specimens may also be requested.

INDICATIONS
- Determine the potential cause of renal calculi.
- Evaluate known or suspected endocrine disorder.
- Evaluate known or suspected kidney disease.
- Evaluate magnesium imbalance.
- Evaluate a malabsorption problem.

INTERFERING FACTORS
Factors that may alter the results of the study
- Drugs and other factors that may increase urine magnesium levels include cisplatin, cyclosporine, ethacrynic acid, furosemide, mercaptomerin, mercurial diuretics, thiazides, torsemide, and triamterene.
- Drugs and other substances that may decrease urine magnesium levels include amiloride, angiotensin, oral contraceptives, parathyroid extract, and phosphates.

Other considerations
- Magnesium levels follow a circadian rhythm, and for this reason 24-hr collections are recommended.
- All urine voided for the timed collection period must be included in the collection, or else falsely decreased values may be obtained. Compare output records with volume collected to verify that all voids were included in the collection.

POTENTIAL MEDICAL DIAGNOSIS: CLINICAL SIGNIFICANCE OF RESULTS
Increased in
- Alcohol misuse *(related to impaired absorption and increased urinary excretion)*
- Bartter syndrome *(inherited defect in renal tubules that results in urinary wasting of potassium and magnesium)*
- Transplant recipients on cyclosporine and prednisone *(related to increased excretion by the kidney)*
- Use of corticosteroids *(related to increased excretion by the kidney)*
- Use of diuretics *(related to increased urinary excretion)*

Decreased in
- Abnormal kidney function *(related to diminished ability of renal tubules to reabsorb magnesium)*
- Crohn disease *(related to inadequate intestinal absorption)*
- Inappropriate secretion of antidiuretic hormone *(related to diminished renal absorption)*
- Salt-losing conditions *(related to diminished renal absorption)*

NURSING IMPLICATIONS

BEFORE THE STUDY: PLANNING AND IMPLEMENTATION

Teaching the Patient What to Expect
- Inform the patient this test can assist in evaluating magnesium balance.
- Explain that a urine sample is needed for the test. Information regarding specimen collection is presented with other general guidelines in Appendix A: Patient Preparation and Specimen Collection.

Potential Nursing Actions
- Include on the collection container's label urine total volume, test start and

stop times/dates, and any medications that may interfere with test results.

Avoiding Complications
▶ Instruct the patient to report any signs or symptoms of electrolyte imbalance, such as dehydration, diarrhea, vomiting, or prolonged anorexia.

Nutritional Considerations
▶ Educate the magnesium-deficient patient regarding good dietary sources of magnesium, such as green vegetables, seeds, legumes, shrimp, and some bran cereals. Advise the patient that high intake of substances such as phosphorus, calcium, fat, and protein interferes with the absorption of magnesium.

Follow-Up, Evaluation, and Desired Outcomes
▶ Understands that additional testing may be necessary to evaluate or monitor disease progression and determine the need for a change in therapy.

Magnetic Resonance Imaging, Various Sites
(Abdomen, Blood Vessels, Brain, Breast, Chest, Musculoskeletal, Pancreas, Pelvis, Pituitary)

SYNONYM/ACRONYM: Magnetic resonance angiography: MRA; magnetic resonance imaging: MRI.

RATIONALE: To visualize and assess internal organs/structures and blood vessels for abnormal or absent anatomical features, abscess, aneurysm, cancer or other masses, infection, or presence of disease. Used as an evaluation tool for surgical, radiation, and medical therapeutic interventions.

PATIENT PREPARATION: *General:* There are no food, fluid, activity, or medication restrictions unless by medical direction. *MRA:* Some protocols may require the patient to restrict prescribed oral iron supplements prior to the study because the iron may interfere with the study results. Restriction of food, fluids, alcohol, nicotine, and caffeine for 1 to 2 hr before the procedure may also be required in order to avoid vasoconstriction or vasodilation as well as nausea and vomiting related to anxiety while in the MRI scanner.

NORMAL FINDINGS
• MRA: Normal blood flow/rate in the area being examined.
• MRI: Normal anatomic structures, function, soft tissue density, and biochemical constituents of body tissues, including blood flow/rate.

CRITICAL FINDINGS AND POTENTIAL INTERVENTIONS
• Abscess
• Acute gastrointestinal (GI) bleed
• Aortic aneurysm
• Aortic dissection
• Cerebral aneurysm
• Cerebral emboli
• Cerebral infarct

M

- Hydrocephalus
- Infection
- Occlusion
- Pulmonary emboli
- Skull fracture or contusion
- Tumor with significant mass effect
- Vertebral artery dissection

Timely notification to the requesting health-care provider (HCP) of any critical findings and related symptoms is a role expectation of the professional nurse. A listing of these findings varies among facilities.

OVERVIEW

MRI

(Study type: MRI; related body system: Circulatory, Digestive, Endocrine, Musculoskeletal, Nervous, Reproductive, and Respiratory systems.) MRI is useful when the area of interest is soft tissue. The study can be performed with or without the contrast medium gadopentetate dimeglumine (Magnevist), which is administered IV to enhance contrast differences between normal and abnormal tissues. The technology does not involve radiation exposure and is considered safer than other imaging methods, such as radiographs and computed tomography (CT). MRI uses a magnet and radio waves to produce an energy field that can be displayed as an image of the anatomic area of interest based on the water content of the tissue. The magnetic field causes the hydrogen atoms in tissue to line up, and when radio waves are directed toward the magnetic field, the hydrogen atoms absorb the radio waves and change their position. This change in the energy field is detected by the equipment, and an image is generated by the equipment's computer system using assigned values that correspond to the strength of the signal produced; the anatomical images are represented in various shades of gray. MRI produces cross-sectional images of the vessels in multiple planes without the use of ionizing radiation or the interference of bone or surrounding tissue. Images can be obtained in two-dimensional (series of slices) or three-dimensional sequences. Standard or closed MRI equipment has the appearance of an open tube or tunnel; open MRI equipment has no sides and provides an alternative for people who suffer from claustrophobia, pediatric patients, and patients who are obese. Some open MRI units are designed to allow the patient to stand or sit while images are taken in various body positions. IV gadolinium-based contrast media may be used to better visualize the vessels and tissues in the area of interest. Clear, high-quality images of abnormalities and disease processes significantly improve the diagnostic value of the study.

MRA

MRA is an application of MRI that provides images of blood flow and diseased and normal blood vessels. In patients who are allergic to iodinated contrast medium, MRA is used in place of angiography. MRA is particularly useful for visualizing vascular abnormalities, dissections, and other pathology.

M

Special imaging sequences allow the visualization of moving blood within the vascular system, and two common techniques are used to obtain images of flowing blood: time-of-flight and phase-contrast MRA. In time-of-flight imaging, incoming blood makes the vessels appear bright and surrounding tissue is suppressed. Phase-contrast images are produced by subtracting the stationary tissue surrounding the vessels where the blood is moving through vessels during the imaging, producing high-contrast images. MRA is the most accurate technique for imaging blood flowing in veins and small arteries (*laminar flow*), but it does not accurately depict blood flow in tortuous sections of vessels and distal to bifurcations and stenosis. Swirling blood may cause a signal loss and result in inadequate images, and the degree of vessel stenosis may be overestimated.

MRI Abdomen

Abdominal MRI is performed to assist in diagnosing abnormalities of abdominal and hepatic structures. Contrast-enhanced imaging is effective for distinguishing peritoneal metastases from primary tumors of the GI tract. Primary tumors of the stomach, pancreas, colon, and appendix often spread by intraperitoneal tumor shedding and subsequent peritoneal carcinosis (condition in which cancer advances throughout large areas of the body).

Magnetic resonance cholangiopancreatography (MRCP) is an imaging technique used specifically to evaluate the hepatobiliary system that is comprised of the liver, gallbladder, bile ducts, pancreas, and pancreatic ducts. MRCP is a less invasive way than endoscopic retrograde cholangiopancreatography (ERCP) to investigate abdominal pain, suspected malignancy, gall stones, or pancreatitis.

MRI Brain

Standard brain MRI can distinguish solid, cystic, and hemorrhagic components of lesions. This procedure is done to aid in the diagnosis of intracranial abnormalities, including tumors, ischemia, infection, and multiple sclerosis, and in assessment of brain maturation in pediatric patients. Rapidly flowing blood on spin-echo MRI appears as an absence of signal or a void in the vessel's lumen. Blood flow can be evaluated in the cavernous and carotid arteries. Contrast-enhanced imaging is effective for enhancing differences between normal and abnormal tissues. Aneurysms may be diagnosed without traditional iodine-based contrast angiography, and old clotted blood in the walls of the aneurysm appears white.

Functional MRI (fMRI) is a neuroimaging application of MRI used to study how the brain is working. It identifies changes in blood flow, reflected by changes in the level of blood oxygenation, in response to activity. fMRI can identify metabolic changes in normal, diseased, or injured brain tissue. It is also used in research to study which parts of the brain are responsible for speech, physical movement, thought, and sensations; this type of research is also called *brain mapping* and has significant implications in understanding and managing the effects of stroke, brain tumors, and diseases such as Alzheimer disease. fMRI is based on the blood oxygen level–dependent contrast mechanism that takes advantage

M

of the inherent paramagnetic quality of deoxyhemoglobin. In a properly performed study, the patient is asked to perform a task; the MRI scanner detects changes in the signal strength of brain water protons produced as blood oxygen levels change, and the corresponding strength of the natural paramagnetic signal of deoxyhemoglobin changes.

Magnetic resonance spectroscopy (MRS) is an application of MRI based on the same principles as MRI, but instead of as an anatomical image, the data is displayed graphically as a series of peaks. The peaks represent specific elements and compounds that provide physiological data regarding the tissue of interest. MRS can be performed using MRI equipment with software adapted for the collection and interpretation of spectral data. MRS may be used alone or in conjunction with MRI whereby anatomical images are first collected by MRI followed by focused MRS images that reflect specific active metabolic processes. The frequency information used in MRS identifies specific chemical compounds, such as amino acids, lipids, and lactate, that are commonly involved in or produced by cellular activity. The presence or absence of different metabolites in the spectral analysis can be used to identify metabolic activity associated with a suspected tumor, differentiate between tumor types, provide information about brain lesions (brain tumors, Alzheimer disease), and monitor response to therapeutic interventions.

MRI Breast
MRI imaging of the breast is not a replacement for traditional mammography, ultrasound, or biopsy. This examination is extremely helpful in evaluating mammogram abnormalities and identifying early breast cancer in women at high risk. Women at high risk include those who have had breast cancer, have an abnormal mutated breast cancer gene (BRCA1 or BRCA2), or have a mother or sister who has been diagnosed with breast cancer. Breast MRI is used most commonly in women at high risk when findings of a mammogram or ultrasound are inconclusive because of dense breast tissue or there is a suspected abnormality that requires further evaluation. MRI is also an excellent examination in the augmented breast, including both the breast implant and the breast tissue surrounding the implant. This same examination is also useful for staging breast cancer and determining the most appropriate treatment.

MRI Chest
Chest MRI scanning is performed to assist in diagnosing abnormalities of cardiovascular and pulmonary structures. Two special techniques are available for evaluation of cardiovascular structures. One is the electrocardiograph (ECG)–gated multislice spin-echo sequence, used to diagnose anatomic abnormalities of the heart and aorta, and the other is the ECG-referenced gradient refocused sequence used to diagnose heart function and analyze blood flow patterns.

MRI Musculoskeletal
Musculoskeletal MRI is performed to assist in diagnosing abnormalities of bones and joints and surrounding soft tissue structures, including cartilage, synovium,

ligaments, and tendons. MRI eliminates the risks associated with exposure to x-rays and causes no harm to cells. Contrast-enhanced imaging is effective for evaluating scarring from previous surgery, vascular abnormalities, and differentiation of metastases from primary tumors.

As with brain studies, MRS applications can also be used to provide information about the spine (e.g., demyelinating diseases) or conditions involving skeletal muscle disease (muscular dystrophies), and monitor response to therapeutic interventions.

MRI Pancreas

MRI of the pancreas is employed to evaluate small pancreatic adenocarcinomas, islet cell tumors, ductal abnormalities and calculi, or parenchymal abnormalities. A T1-weighted, fat-saturation series of images is probably best for evaluating the pancreatic parenchyma. This sequence is ideal for showing fat planes between the pancreas and peripancreatic structures and for identifying abnormalities such as fatty infiltration of the pancreas, hemorrhage, adenopathy, and cancers. T2-weighted images are most useful for depicting intrapancreatic or peripancreatic fluid collections, pancreatic tumors, and calculi. Imaging sequences can be adjusted to display fluid in the biliary tree and pancreatic ducts.

MRI Pelvis

Pelvic MRI is performed to assist in diagnosing abnormalities of the pelvis and associated structures. Contrast-enhanced MRI is effective for evaluating metastases from primary tumors. MRI is highly effective for depicting small-volume peritoneal tumors,

carcinosis, and peritonitis and for determining the response to surgical and chemical therapies. Oral and rectal contrast administration may be used to isolate the bowel from adjacent pelvic organs and improve organ visualization.

MRI Pituitary

Pituitary MRI shows the relationship of pituitary lesions to the optic chiasm and cavernous sinuses. MRI has the capability of distinguishing the solid, cystic, and hemorrhagic components of lesions. Rapidly flowing blood on spin-echo MRI appears as an absence of signal or a void in the vessel's lumen. Blood flow can be evaluated in the cavernous and carotid arteries. Suprasellar aneurysms may be diagnosed without angiography, and old clotted blood in the walls of the aneurysms appears white.

MRI Venography

Magnetic resonance venography (MRV) is an accurate, noninvasive technique used to detect deep vein thrombosis (DVT). This application of MRI provides images of blood flow in diseased and normal veins. In patients who are allergic to iodinated contrast medium, MRV is used in place of venography or CT venography. MRV is particularly useful for visualizing vascular abnormalities, thrombosis, and other pathology. MRV can be accomplished with a contrast-enhanced (CE) or non–contrast-enhanced method. Special imaging sequences allow the visualization of moving blood within the venous system. Two common techniques to obtain images of flowing blood are time-of-flight (TOF) and steady-state free precession (SSFP). In TOF imaging, incoming blood makes

M

the vessels appear bright, and surrounding tissue is suppressed. SSFP is generally used for assessment of veins in the chest, abdomen, and pelvis. Although the initial evaluation of the iliac and lower extremity veins is usually accomplished with sonography, MRV is more efficient in detecting venous thrombus in the pelvic and calf veins, especially in obese patients and those with chronic asymptomatic thrombus.

INDICATIONS

General
• Detect and locate tumors.
• Differentiate tumors from tissue abnormalities, such as cysts, cavernous hemangiomas, and abscesses.
• Monitor and evaluate the effectiveness of medical or surgical treatment.

MRA
• Detect pericardial abnormalities.
• Detect peripheral arterial disease (PAD).
• Detect thoracic and abdominal vascular diseases.
• Determine renal artery stenosis.
• Differentiate aortic aneurysms from tumors near the aorta.
• Evaluate cardiac chambers and pulmonary vessels.
• Evaluate postoperative angioplasty sites and bypass grafts.
• Identify congenital vascular diseases.

Abdomen
• Detect abdominal aortic diseases.
• Detect and stage cancer (primary or metastatic tumors of liver, pancreas, prostate, uterus, and bladder).
• Detect chronic pancreatitis.
• Detect renal vein thrombosis.
• Detect soft tissue abnormalities.
• Determine and monitor tissue damage in renal transplant patients.

• Determine the presence of blood clots, cysts, fluid or fat accumulation in tissues, hemorrhage, and infarctions.
• Determine vascular complications of pancreatitis, venous thrombosis, or pseudoaneurysm.
• Differentiate aortic aneurysms from tumors near the aorta.
• Evaluate postoperative angioplasty sites and bypass grafts.

Brain
• Detect cause of cerebrovascular accident, cerebral infarct, or hemorrhage.
• Detect cranial bone, face, throat, and neck soft tissue lesions.
• Evaluate the cause of seizures, such as intracranial infection, edema, or increased intracranial pressure.
• Evaluate cerebral changes associated with dementia.
• Evaluate demyelinating disorders.
• Evaluate intracranial infections.
• Evaluate optic and auditory nerves.
• Evaluate the potential causes of headache, visual loss, and vomiting.
• Evaluate shunt placement and function in patients with hydrocephalus.
• Evaluate the solid, cystic, and hemorrhagic components of lesions.
• Evaluate vascularity of the brain and vascular integrity.

Breast
• Evaluate breast implants.
• Evaluate dense breasts.
• Evaluate for residual cancer after lumpectomy.
• Evaluate inverted nipples.
• Evaluate tissue after lumpectomy or mastectomy.
• Evaluate women at high risk for breast cancer.

Chest
• Confirm diagnosis of cardiac and pericardiac masses.
• Detect aortic aneurysms.

- Detect myocardial infarction and cardiac muscle ischemia.
- Detect pericardial abnormalities.
- Detect pleural effusion.
- Detect thoracic aortic diseases.
- Determine blood, fluid, or fat accumulation in tissues, pleuritic space, or vessels.
- Determine cardiac ventricular function.
- Differentiate aortic aneurysms from tumors near the aorta.
- Evaluate cardiac chambers and pulmonary vessels.
- Evaluate postoperative angioplasty sites and bypass grafts.
- Identify congenital heart diseases.

Musculoskeletal
- Confirm diagnosis of osteomyelitis.
- Detect avascular necrosis of the femoral head or knee.
- Detect benign and cancerous tumors and cysts of the bone or soft tissue.
- Detect bone infarcts in the epiphyseal or diaphyseal sites.
- Detect changes in bone marrow.
- Detect tears or degeneration of ligaments, tendons, and menisci resulting from trauma or pathology.
- Determine cause of low back pain, including herniated disk and spinal degenerative disease.
- Differentiate between primary and secondary malignant processes of the bone marrow.
- Differentiate between a stress fracture and a tumor.
- Evaluate meniscal detachment of the temporomandibular joint.

Pancreas
- Detect pancreatic fatty infiltration, hemorrhage, and adenopathy.
- Detect a pancreatic mass.
- Detect pancreatitis.
- Detect primary or metastatic tumors of the pancreas and provide cancer staging.
- Detect soft tissue abnormalities.

- Determine vascular complications of pancreatitis, venous thrombosis, or pseudoaneurysm.

Pelvis
- Detect cancer (primary or metastatic tumors of ovary, prostate, uterus, and bladder) and provide cancer staging.
- Detect pelvic vascular diseases.
- Detect peritonitis.
- Detect soft tissue abnormalities.
- Determine blood clots, cysts, fluid or fat accumulation in tissues, hemorrhage, and infarctions.

Pituitary
- Detect microadenoma or macroadenoma of the pituitary.
- Detect parasellar abnormalities.
- Detect tumors of the pituitary.
- Evaluate potential cause of headache, visual loss, and vomiting.
- Evaluate the solid, cystic, and hemorrhagic components of lesions.
- Evaluate vascularity of the pituitary.

Venography
- Detect peripheral vascular disease (PVD).
- Detect axillary subclavian DVT.
- Detect cerebral vein disease.
- Detect pulmonary vein disease.
- Evaluate iliac and lower-extremity vein disease.
- Evaluate postoperative venous sites and bypass grafts.
- Identify deep vein thrombus in postsurgical patients.

INTERFERING FACTORS
Contraindications

⬥ Patients who are pregnant or suspected of being pregnant, unless the potential benefits of MRI far outweigh the risks to the fetus and mother. *In pregnancy, gadolinium-based contrast medium (GBCAs) cross the placental barrier, enter the fetal circulation, and pass via the kidneys into the amniotic fluid. Although no definite adverse effects of GBCA administration*

M

on the human fetus have been documented, the potential bioeffects of fetal GBCA exposure are not well understood. GBCA administration should therefore be avoided during pregnancy unless no suitable alternative imaging is possible and the benefits of contrast administration outweigh the potential risk to the fetus.

✹ Conditions associated with adverse reactions to contrast medium (e.g., asthma, food allergies, or allergy to contrast medium). Although patients are asked specifically if they have a known allergy to iodine or shellfish (shellfish contain high levels of iodine), it has been well established that the reaction is not to iodine; an actual iodine allergy would be problematic because iodine is required for the production of thyroid hormones. In the case of shellfish, the reaction is to a muscle protein called *tropomyosin*; in the case of iodinated contrast medium, the reaction is to the noniodinated part of the contrast molecule. Patients with a known hypersensitivity to the medium may benefit from premedication with corticosteroids and diphenhydramine; the use of nonionic contrast or an alternative noncontrast imaging study, if available, may be considered for patients who have severe asthma or who have experienced moderate to severe reactions to ionic contrast medium.

✹ Patients with moderate to marked renal impairment (glomerular filtration rate less than 30 mL/min/ 1.73 m²). Patients should be screened for kidney dysfunction prior to administration. The use of GBCAs should be avoided in these patients unless the benefits of the studies outweigh the risks and essential diagnostic information is not available using non–contrast-enhanced diagnostic studies.

✹ Patients with cardiac pacemakers that can be deactivated by MRI.

✹ Patients with metal in their body, such as dental amalgams, metallic body piercing items, tattoo inks containing iron (including tattooed eyeliners), shrapnel, bullet, ferrous metal in the eye, certain ferrous metal prosthetics, valves, aneurysm clips, intrauterine device, inner ear prostheses, or other metallic objects; these items can impair image quality. Metallic objects are also a significant safety issue for patients and health-care staff in the examination room during performance of an MRI. The MRI equipment consists of an extremely powerful magnet that can inactivate, move, or shift metallic objects inside a patient. Many metallic objects currently used in health-care procedures are made of materials that do not interfere with MRI studies; it is important for patients to provide specific information regarding medical procedures they have undergone in order to identify whether their device is safe to undergo MRI. Required information includes the date of the procedure and identification of the device. Metallic objects are not allowed inside the room with the MRI equipment because items such as watches, credit cards, and car keys can become dangerous projectiles.

✹ Patients with transdermal patches containing metallic components. The patch's liner contains a metal that controls absorption of the substance from the patch (e.g., drugs, nicotine, steroids, hormones). The patch may cause burns to the skin *related to energy conducted through the metal which is converted to heat during the MRI.* Other metallic objects on the skin may also cause burns.

✹ Patients who are claustrophobic.

Factors that may alter the results of the study
• Metallic objects (e.g., jewelry, body rings, dental amalgams) within

the examination field, which may inhibit organ visualization and cause unclear images.

- Patients with extreme cases of claustrophobia, unless sedation is given before the study.
- Patients who are extremely obese may require more radiation to obtain a clear image.

Other considerations

General

- If contrast medium is allowed to seep deep into the muscle tissue, vascular visualization will be impossible.

Breast

- The procedure can be nonspecific; the examination is unable to image calcifications that can indicate breast cancer, and there may be difficulty distinguishing between cancerous and noncancerous tumors.

POTENTIAL MEDICAL DIAGNOSIS: CLINICAL SIGNIFICANCE OF RESULTS
Abnormal findings related to

General

- Abscess
- Aneurysm
- Hematoma
- Hemorrhage
- Infarct
- Masses, lesions, infections, or inflammations
- Metastasis
- Tumor
- Vascular abnormalities

MRA

- Coarctations
- Dissections
- PAD
- Thrombosis within a vessel
- Vascular abnormalities
- Vessel occlusion
- Vessel stenosis

MRI Abdomen

- Acute tubular necrosis
- Cholangitis
- Glomerulonephritis
- Hydronephrosis
- Renal vein thrombosis
- Vena cava obstruction

MRI Brain

- Acoustic neuroma
- Alzheimer disease
- Arteriovenous malformation
- Benign meningioma
- Cerebral infarction
- Craniopharyngioma or meningioma
- Granuloma
- Intraparenchymal hematoma or hemorrhage
- Lipoma
- Multiple sclerosis
- Optic nerve tumor
- Parkinson disease
- Pituitary microadenoma
- Subdural empyema
- Ventriculitis

MRI Breast

- Breast cancer
- Breast implant rupture

MRI Chest

- Aortic dissection
- Congenital heart diseases, including pulmonary atresia, aortic coarctation, agenesis of the pulmonary artery, and transposition of the great vessels
- Constrictive pericarditis
- Intramural and periaortic hematoma
- Myocardial infarction
- Pericardial hematoma or effusion
- Pleural effusion

MRI Musculoskeletal

- Avascular necrosis of femoral head or knee, as found in Legg-Calvé-Perthes disease
- Bone marrow disease, such as Gaucher disease, aplastic anemia, sickle cell disease, or polycythemia

M

- Degenerative spinal disease, such as spondylosis or arthritis
- Fibrosarcoma
- Hemangioma (muscular or osseous)
- Herniated disk
- Meniscal tears or degeneration
- Osteochondroma
- Osteogenic sarcoma
- Osteomyelitis
- Rotator cuff tears
- Spinal stenosis
- Stress fracture
- Synovitis

MRI Pancreas
- Islet cell tumor
- Pancreatic duct obstruction or calculi
- Pancreatic fatty infiltration, hemorrhage
- Pancreatitis

MRI Pelvis
- Adenomyosis
- Ascites
- Fibroids
- Peritonitis
- Pseudomyxoma peritonei

MRI Pituitary
- Choristoma
- Craniopharyngioma or meningioma
- Empty sella
- Granuloma
- Macroadenoma or microadenoma

MRI Venography
- Cerebral vein thrombosis
- DVT
- Pulmonary emboli
- PVD
- Vascular abnormalities
- Vein occlusion
- Vein stenosis

NURSING IMPLICATIONS

POTENTIAL NURSING PROBLEMS: ASSESSMENT & NURSING DIAGNOSIS

Problems	Signs and Symptoms
Angiography: Tissue perfusion *(related to dissection, rupture, hypertension)*	Elevated blood pressure, pulsing abdominal mass, elevated heart rate
Angiography: Pain *(related to diminished perfusion, rupture, dissection)*	Self-report of pain that is severe in nature, located in the abdomen, and radiates to the flank; pain may be located in the back and groin areas
Angiography: Cardiac output (diminished) *(related to dissection, rupture)*	Altered level of consciousness, hypotension, increased pulse that may be thready, delayed capillary refill, diminished peripheral pulses, cool skin, restlessness, anxiety
MRI Abdomen: Nutrition *(related to pain, nausea, vomiting, anorexia)*	Weight loss, emaciation, malabsorption, poor intake
MRI Brain: Inadequate cerebral tissue perfusion *(related to infarct, hemorrhage, mass, edema, infection, plaque, atrophy)*	Diminished or altered level of consciousness, aphasia that can be expressive or receptive, loss of sensory functionality, slurred speech, difficulty swallowing, difficulty in completing a learned activity or in recognizing familiar objects (apraxia, agnosia), motor function deficits, spatial neglect, facial droop and/or varying degrees of flaccid extremities

M

Problems	Signs and Symptoms
MRI Brain: Mobility *(related to altered muscular function secondary to cerebral injury)*	Loss of sensation, weakness on one side, uncoordinated movement, difficulty understanding and following instructions, spatial neglect
MRI Brain: Inadequate self-care *(related to loss of cognitive or motor function)*	Unable to complete the activities of daily living without assistance (eating, bathing, dressing, toileting)
MRI Chest: Inadequate tissue perfusion *(related to blood flow obstruction, oxygen supply/demand mismatch)*	Chest pain, chest pressure, shortness of breath, increased heart rate, cool skin, decreased capillary refill, diminished peripheral pulses, altered cardiac enzymes, confusion, restlessness
MRI Chest: Pain *(related to myocardial ischemia, inadequate oxygenation)*	Self-report of chest pain, pressure; radiating pain to the neck, jaw, arm
MRI Chest: Activity *(related to myocardial ischemia, increased oxygen demands)*	Weakness, fatigue, chest pain with exertion, anxiety
MRI Pancreas: Pain *(related to necrosis or inflammation)*	Self-report of pain located in the left upper quadrant of the abdomen, which may radiate to the left flank area; complaint of epigastric pain and discomfort after consuming fatty foods; moaning; crying; restlessness; anxiety; increased heart rate; increased blood pressure
MRI Pancreas: Nutrition (insufficient) *(related to decreased oral intake associated with pain)*	Self-report of pain with eating, presence of nausea and vomiting, NPO order, inflammation
MRI Pancreas: Insufficient fluid volume *(related to nausea, vomiting, pain)*	Elevated heart rate; low blood pressure; cool, clammy skin; poor urine output (less than 30 mL/hr); confusion; restlessness; agitation; capillary refill delay; hemoconcentration; dehydration
MRI Venography: Tissue perfusion, ineffective *(related to obstruction secondary to thrombus, tumor, stenosis, anatomical abnormalities)*	Pain, tenderness, warmth, edema, palpable vein
MRI Venography: Bleeding *(related to anticoagulant use secondary to venous obstruction)*	Easy bruising, bleeding gums, blood in urine or stool, bleeding from invasive procedure sites such as IV access (central or peripheral)
MRI Venography: Pain *(related to vascular occlusion, diminished circulatory blood flow, inflammation, obstruction)*	Self-report of pain, facial grimace, crying, restlessness, anxiety, elevated blood pressure and heart rate

M

BEFORE THE STUDY: PLANNING AND IMPLEMENTATION

Teaching the Patient What to Expect

▶ Inform the patient this procedure can assist in assessing internal organs and other anatomical areas of interest.

▶ Obtain a history of the patient's kidney dysfunction if the use of GBCA is anticipated.

▶ Those with a hypersensitivity to contrast medium may benefit from premedication with corticosteroids and diphenhydramine.

▶ Explain to the female patient that she will be asked the date of her last menstrual period. Generally, MRI during pregnancy is not specifically contraindicated in the first trimester, as there is no association with fetal harm. However, if contrast (e.g., gadolinium) is being used for the MRI during pregnancy, there is an increased risk of fetal harm, including stillbirth and fetal death. In all cases, the benefits versus the risks should be discussed with the HCP on a case-by-case basis before proceeding with the MRI.

▶ Review the procedure with the patient. Address concerns about pain and explain that there may be moments of discomfort or pain experienced when the IV line or catheter is inserted to allow infusion of fluids such as saline, anesthetics, sedatives, contrast medium, medications used in the procedure, or emergency medications.

▶ Reassure the patient that if contrast is used, it poses no radioactive hazard and rarely produces adverse effects.

▶ Explain that the procedure is performed in an MRI department by an HCP who specializes in this procedure, with support staff, and takes approximately 30 to 60 min.

▶ Explain that there will be a loud banging from the scanner and possibly some visual magnetophosphenes (flickering lights in the visual field), which will stop once the procedure is over. Earplugs will be provided to block the sound.

▶ During the procedure, communication with the technologist will occur by way of the microphone located inside the scanner.

▶ Explain the need to remain still during the procedure, as movement produces unreliable results. ECG or respiratory gating may be performed in conjunction with the scan to reduce artifacts due to respiratory or cardiac movement during data collection.

▶ MRI-safe electrodes will be applied to the appropriate sites if an ECG or respiratory gating is to be performed in conjunction with the scan.

▶ Upon arrival for scanning, the patient will be assisted onto the examination table and positioned for imaging to begin.

▶ Positioning for this study is in a supine position on a flat table in a large cylindrical scanner.

▶ Imaging can begin shortly after the injection, if contrast is used.

▶ The patient will be asked to inhale deeply and hold his or her breath while the images are taken, and then to exhale after the images are taken.

▶ The patient will be instructed to take slow, deep breaths if nausea occurs during the procedure.

▶ The patient will be monitored for complications related to the procedure (e.g., allergic reaction, anaphylaxis, bronchospasm).

▶ Once the procedure is completed, the needle or catheter will be removed and a pressure dressing applied.

Potential Nursing Actions

◆ *Make sure a written and informed consent has been signed prior to the procedure and before administering any medications.*

▶ Verify the MRI screening form has been completed if required by the organization.

Safety Considerations

▶ Determine if the patient has ever had any device implanted into his or her body, including copper intrauterine devices, pacemakers, ear implants, and heart valves.

▶ Obtain occupational history to determine the presence of metal in the body, such as shrapnel or flecks of ferrous metal in the eye (which can cause retinal hemorrhage).

Avoiding Complications

▶ Injection of the contrast is an invasive procedure. Complications are rare but include risk for allergic reaction *(related to contrast reaction);* cardiac dysrhythmias; hematoma *(related to blood leakage into the tissue following needle insertion);* bleeding from the puncture site *(related to a bleeding disorder or the effects of natural products and medications with known anticoagulant, antiplatelet, or thrombolytic properties);* vascular or nerve injury *(which might occur if the needle strikes a nerve or nearby blood vessel);* or infection *(which might occur if bacteria from the skin surface are introduced at the puncture site).* Monitor the patient for complications related to the procedure (e.g., allergic reaction, anaphylaxis, bronchospasm, infection, injury). Immediately report symptoms such as difficulty breathing, chest pain, fever, hyperpnea, hypertension, nausea, palpitations, pruritus, rash, tachycardia, urticaria, or vomiting to the appropriate HCP. Observe/assess the needle/catheter insertion site for bleeding, inflammation, or hematoma formation. Administer ordered antihistamines or prophylactic steroids if the patient has an allergic reaction.

▶ Some patients are at risk for developing nephrogenic systemic fibrosis as a result of the use of gadolinium-based contrast medium *(related to ineffective renal clearance in patients with impaired kidney function).*

Treatment Considerations
General

▶ Pain: Pain can occur with any disease process. Accurate pain assessment in all cases involves an evaluation of pain characteristics, which include location, duration, and intensity. The pain rating scale used for this assessment should be reflective of individualized needs. Types of interventions selected will be dependent on assessment findings and may include analgesics, narcotics, anti-inflammatory medications, heat and cold application, or repositioning. Evaluate the effectiveness of the chosen pain management strategy and make any necessary adjustments to provide relief. Consider alternative interventions such as imagery, relaxation, and music.

▶ Instruct the patient in the care and assessment of the injection site.

▶ Instruct the patient to apply cold compresses to the puncture site as needed to reduce discomfort or edema.

Angiography

▶ Cardiac Output: Administer ordered IV fluid to support blood pressure or blood transfusion. Monitor and trend vital signs and ECG. Assess for changes in sensorium and monitor renal status.

▶ Pain: Assess for pain that is located in the abdomen, back, groin, or flank. Administer ordered pain and blood pressure medications; morphine or nitroglycerine.

▶ Tissue Perfusion: Assess abdominal mass without palpation, trend heart rate and blood pressure. Assess pulses at femoral arteries, for cool or clammy extremities, and for altered level of consciousness or confusion. Administer ordered vasodilator to decrease blood pressure, or beta blockers. Monitor results of complementary ordered diagnostic studies: x-ray, ultrasound, complete blood count, prothrombin time, international normalized ratio, and activated partial thromboplastin time.

MRI Abdomen

▶ Nutrition: Obtain a nutritional history, perform a daily weight, calorie count, dietary consult, and monitor and trend albumin.

MRI Brain

▶ Cerebral Tissue Perfusion: Complete a baseline neurological assessment for ongoing comparison to evaluate improvement or deterioration. Facilitate complementary diagnostic studies: MRI, positron emission tomography, ultrasound, and subtraction

M

angiography. Elevate the head of the bed, and administer ordered antiplatelet, anticoagulant, thrombolytics, antihypertensives, steroids, diuretics, calcium channel blockers, or antiseizure medications.

▶ Mobility: Assess current functional level. Facilitate physical therapy evaluation and treatment, use of assistive devices (walker, cane), and active or passive range of motion to maintain muscle strength. Provide assistance with activities to decrease fall risk (gait belt), assess the skin for pressure ulcers, and teach proper turning and assisting techniques.

▶ Self-Care: Assess self-care deficits, identify areas where the patient can provide own care and encourage them, and assess the family's ability to assist with self-care needs. Facilitate use of assistive devices to assist with self-care such as a commode or special utensils. Alter the diet to match swallowing ability with the use of thick liquids, puree, or small bites and remind the patient to chew and swallow slowly.

MRI Chest

▶ Activity: Identify the patient's normal activity patterns; maintain bedrest as required to rest the heart and conserve oxygen; administer ordered oxygen, and have patient wear oxygen with activity; pace activity and increase as tolerated; monitor and trend vital signs; discuss the effects of altered cardiac health on sexual activity

▶ Pain: Assess for pain in chest, back, or shoulders by evaluating pain character, location, duration, and intensity. Administer ordered medications: morphine, nitroglycerine, calcium channel blockers, beta blockers.

▶ Tissue Perfusion: Assess for characteristics of pain: quality, intensity, duration, and location. Monitor and trend heart rate, respiratory rate, and blood pressure. Facilitate continuous cardiac monitoring, administer oxygen and monitor with pulse oximetry. Assess skin color and temperature, breath sounds (rate, rhythm), capillary refill, peripheral pulses, and cyanosis. Monitor laboratory studies: ABGs, creatine phosphokinase, CK-MB, troponin, C-reactive protein, and lactate dehydrogenase. Observe for confusion and restlessness. Administer ordered thrombolytics, morphine, amiodarone, nitroglycerine, and beta blockers.

MRI Pancreas

▶ Fluid Volume: Monitor and trend laboratory studies; BUN, creatinine, Hgb, Hct, and electrolytes. Monitor skin turgor; daily weight, heart rate, temperature; capillary refill; and intake and output. Administer parenteral fluids, encourage oral fluids, discourage caffeine and advise the patient that alcohol use should be eliminated or reduced.

▶ Nutrition: Maintain NPO status with nasogastric tube to low suction, as ordered. Complete a culturally appropriate nutritional assessment, daily weight, and intake and output. Administer ordered IV fluids with supplements such as electrolytes. Monitor and trend specific laboratory studies: lipase, amylase, albumin, total protein, electrolytes, glucose, calcium, iron, and folic acid.

▶ Pain: Assess abdominal, back, or flank pain. Place in a side-lying position with knees to chest. Administer ordered anticholinergics. Maintain ordered NPO status.

MRI Venography

▶ Bleeding: Administer ordered anticoagulants: heparin, enoxaparin, or warfarin. Institute bleeding precautions and monitor for bleeding gums, easy bruising, blood in the urine or stool, or bleeding from invasive procedure sites. Monitor appropriate laboratory studies: activated partial thromboplastin time, prothrombin time, international normalized ratio, Hgb, and Hct. Be aware of the possibility of aggressive thrombolytic interventions: streptokinase, urokinase, or tissue plasma activator.

▶ Pain: Administer ordered anticoagulants.

▶ Tissue Perfusion: Assess and trend the DVT site for degree of warmth, redness, and edema. Review diagnostic study results: impedance plethysmography and ultrasound. Enforce bedrest, elevate affected limb, apply ordered moist heat packs to the affected limb, and encourage oral fluids to decrease blood viscosity.

Follow-Up, Evaluation, and Desired Outcomes

▶ *MRA:* Acknowledges contact information provided for the American Heart Association (www.heart.org/ HEARTORG), National Heart, Lung, and Blood Institute (www.nhlbi.nih .gov), Legs for Life (www.legsforlife .org), American College of Rheumatology (www.rheumatology.org), or Arthritis Foundation (www.arthritis .org).

▶ *MRI, Breast:* Understands that decisions regarding the need for and frequency of breast self-examination, mammography, MRI or ultrasound of the breast, or other cancer screening procedures, should be made after consultation between the patient and HCP. Acknowledges that the most current guidelines for breast cancer screening of the general population as well as of individuals with increased

risk are available from the American Cancer Society (www.cancer.org), American College of Obstetricians and Gynecologists (www.acog.org), and American College of Radiology (www.acr.org). Screening guidelines vary depending on the age and health history of those at average risk and those at high risk for breast cancer. Guidelines may not always agree between organizations; therefore, it is important for patients to participate in their health care, be informed, ask questions, and follow their HCP's recommendations regarding frequency and type of screening. For additional information regarding screening guidelines, refer to the study titled "Mammography."

▶ *MRI, Pancreas:* Understands the link between alcohol use and disease process and that increased amylase levels may be associated with gastrointestinal disease and/or alcohol misuse.

▶ *MRI, Pancreas:* Agrees to avoid alcohol and to seek appropriate counseling.

Mammography

M

SYNONYM/ACRONYM: Breast x-ray, mammogram.

RATIONALE: To visualize and assess breast tissue and surrounding lymph nodes for cancer, inflammation, abscess, tumor, and cysts.

PATIENT PREPARATION: There are no food, fluid, activity, or medication restrictions unless by medical direction. Inform the patient that the best time to schedule the examination is 1 wk after menses, when breast tenderness is decreased. Inform the patient not to apply deodorant, body creams, or powders on the day of the procedure, as these products may contain aluminum, which can be misinterpreted as calcifications in the breast tissue.

NORMAL FINDINGS

• Normal breast tissue, with no cysts, tumors, or calcifications.

CRITICAL FINDINGS AND POTENTIAL INTERVENTIONS: N/A

OVERVIEW: (Study type: X-ray; related body system: Immune and Reproductive systems.) Mammography, an x-ray examination

of the breast, is most commonly used to detect breast cancer; however, it can also be used to detect and evaluate symptomatic changes associated with other breast diseases, including mastitis, abscess, cystic changes, cysts, benign tumors, masses, and lymph nodes. In addition, mammography can be used to locate a nonpalpable lesion for breast biopsy studies. Although mammography cannot detect breast cancer with 100% accuracy, only about 10% to 15% of breast cancer cases are not detected. Recent advances in mammography technologies include full-field digital mammography (FFDM), computer-aided detection (CAD) systems, and three-dimensional breast imaging or breast tomosynthesis. FFDM is performed in the same manner as conventional screen film mammography (SFM). The difference is that FFDM images are created by digitized signals rather than from x-ray film as with SFM. The FFDM detectors convert x-rays into electrical signals that are digitalized. The digital images can be visualized on a computer screen or printed on special paper. CAD systems use software to search images from SFM or FFDM for abnormal areas of breast tissue evidenced by denseness, abnormal size, or calcifications that may indicate the presence of cancer. Abnormal areas are "marked" for further review by a radiologist. Three-dimensional breast imaging is performed in the same manner as conventional two-dimensional SFM. However, three-dimensional imaging uses equipment that rotates in an arc over the breast instead of the stationary system used in conventional SFM. Three-dimensional equipment generates a series of thin slices believed to produce clearer images, especially of dense breast tissue. The new technologies are becoming more frequently used in screening mammography programs across the United States. Preliminary studies have demonstrated some improvement in detection rates, especially for some types of invasive cancer, and a reduction in recalls for additional imaging.

When a mass is detected, additional studies are performed to help differentiate the nature of the mass, as follows:

- Magnification views of the area in question
- Focal or "spot" views of the area in question, done with a specialized paddle-style compression device
- Ultrasound images of the area in question, which help differentiate between a fluid-filled cystic lesion and a solid lesion indicative of cancer or fibroadenomas

INDICATIONS
- Differentiate between benign and neoplastic breast disease.
- Evaluate breast pain, skin retraction, nipple erosion, or nipple discharge.
- Evaluate known or suspected breast cancer.
- Evaluate nonpalpable breast masses.
- Evaluate opposite breast after mastectomy.
- Monitor postoperative and post-radiation treatment status of the breast.
- Evaluate size, shape, and position of breast masses.

INTERFERING FACTORS
Contraindications

Patients who are pregnant or suspected of being pregnant, unless the potential benefits of a procedure using radiation far outweigh the risks to the fetus and mother.

❖ Patients younger than age 25 or patients with very dense breast tissue, *because the density of the breast tissue is such that diagnostic x-rays are of limited value.*

Factors that may alter the results of the study
- Application of substances such as talcum powder, deodorant, or creams to the skin of breasts or underarms, which may alter test results.
- Previous breast surgery, breast augmentation, or the presence of breast implants, which may decrease the readability of the examination.
- Metallic objects (e.g., jewelry, body rings) within the examination field, which may inhibit organ visualization and cause unclear images.
- Inability of the patient to cooperate or remain still during the procedure, because movement can produce blurred or otherwise unclear images.

POTENTIAL MEDICAL DIAGNOSIS: CLINICAL SIGNIFICANCE OF RESULTS
Abnormal findings related to
- Breast calcifications
- Breast cysts or abscesses
- Breast tumors
- Hematoma resulting from trauma
- Mastitis
- Soft tissue masses
- Vascular calcification

NURSING IMPLICATIONS

POTENTIAL NURSING PROBLEMS: ASSESSMENT & NURSING DIAGNOSIS

Problems	Signs and Symptoms
Altered self-image *(related to self-depreciation secondary to breast removal)*	Stated loss or fear of intimacy, stated dissatisfaction with appearance, refusal to view postoperative site, crying, anger, grief, anxiety
Sexuality *(related to loss of breast and perceived change in desirability)*	Stated loss or fear of loss of attractiveness, sexual intimacy, desirability; fear of rejection by or repulsion of their sexual partner; stated loss of sexual partner secondary to breast removal

M

BEFORE THE STUDY: PLANNING AND IMPLEMENTATION

Teaching the Patient What to Expect
▶ Inform the patient this procedure can assist in assessing breast status.
▶ Pregnancy is a general contraindication to procedures involving radiation. Explain to the female patient that she will be asked the date of her last menstrual period. Pregnancy testing may be performed to determine the possibility of pregnancy before exposure to radiation.
▶ Review the procedure with the patient. Address concerns about pain related to the procedure. Explain that there may be discomfort while the breast is being compressed, but the compression allows for better visualization of the breast tissue.
▶ Explain that the procedure is performed in the mammography department by a registered mammographer and takes approximately 15 min to complete.
▶ The patient will be instructed to remove jewelry and other metallic objects from the area of examination.
▶ Assistance will be provided to help the patient into a standing or sitting position in front of the x-ray machine, which

is adjusted to the level of the breasts. The arms are positioned out of the range of the area to be imaged.
- Breasts will be placed one at a time between the compression apparatus.
- Two images or exposures are taken of each breast during which the patient will be asked to hold her breath during each exposure.
- Additional images may be taken as requested by the radiologist before the patient leaves the mammography room.

Potential Nursing Actions

- Obtain a history of the patient's known or suspected breast disease and family history of breast disease. Knowledge of genetics assists in identifying those who may benefit from additional education, risk assessment, and counseling. Genetics is the study and identification of genes, genetic mutations, and inheritance. For example, genetics provides some insight into the likelihood of inheriting a condition associated with a type of cancer such as breast cancer. Genomic studies evaluate the interaction of groups of genes. The combined activity or combined expression of groups of genes allows assumptions or predictions to be made. As an example, genomic studies measure the levels of activity in multiple genes to predict how they influence the development and growth of a tumor. Further information regarding inheritance of genes can be found in the study titled "Genetic Testing."

AFTER THE STUDY: POTENTIAL NURSING ACTIONS

Treatment Considerations

- Self Image: When a body part is removed by a surgical procedure, negative self-image thoughts may occur. Assure the patient that feelings of distress are normal, and facilitate the grieving process for the lost breast. Provide privacy to explore personal grief, listen to concerns, and support positive coping strategies. Encourage viewing the surgical site, as sometimes the imagined is worse than the real.

Consider the cultural aspects of body image and incorporate them into the plan of care.
- Sexuality: A negative change in self-image can have an impact on feelings of sexuality. Allow for verbalization of concerns related to sense of unattractiveness and feared loss of desirability with breast removal. Encourage open communication with sexual partner and provide information on prosthetic appliances.

Follow-Up, Evaluation, and Desired Outcomes

- Understands that decisions regarding the need for and frequency of breast self-examination, mammography, magnetic resonance imaging (MRI) or ultrasound of the breast, or other cancer screening procedures should be made after consultation between the patient and health-care provider (HCP).
- Acknowledges that the most current guidelines for breast cancer screening of the general population as well as of individuals with increased risk are available from the American Cancer Society (ACS) (www.cancer.org), the American College of Obstetricians and Gynecologists (ACOG) (www.acog.org), and the American College of Radiology (www.acr.org). Screening guidelines vary depending on the age and health history of those at average risk and those at high risk for breast cancer. Guidelines may not always agree between organizations; therefore, it is important for patients to participate in their health care, be informed, ask questions, and follow their HCP's recommendations regarding frequency and type of screening.

American Cancer Society

- The ACS defines women at average risk for breast cancer as those who have no personal or family history of breast cancer, genetic mutation (BRCA1 or BRCA2 gene), or exposure to chest radiation therapy before the age of 30 yr. Screening recommendations for women at average risk are as follows: Women ages 40 to 44 yr can begin screenings by this age if they choose to do so. Annual screenings should begin by age 45 yr. Women age 55 yr can choose to have screenings annually or every 2 yr and continue to do so as long as they maintain good health (ages 55+). The ACS recommends those at high risk for breast cancer have annual screening coupled with MRI evaluation. *High risk* is defined as those with known or a first-degree relative with a BRCA1 or BRCA2 gene, breast cancer, an at-risk syndrome (Li-Fraumeni syndrome, Cowden syndrome, or Bannayan-Riley-Ruvalcaba syndrome), or exposure to chest radiation between the ages 10 and 30 yr. High-risk patients should begin screening at age 30 yr and continue screening for as long as their health remains good.

American College of Obstetricians and Gynecologists
▶ In 2017, the ACOG updated its guidelines and recommends that for women with average risk, breast cancer screening by mammography be performed every 1 to 3 yr starting between the ages of 25 and 39 yr, annually or biennially for women ages 40 to 49 yr after consultation between patient and HCP, and annually or biennially for women 50 yr or older if screening has not yet been initiated. It recommends that consideration be given to discontinue screenings after age 75 yr based on a shared decision-making process between patient and HCP. Genetic testing for inherited mutations (BRCA1 and BRCA2) associated with increased risk of developing breast cancer may be ordered for women at risk.

Maternal Markers

SYNONYM/ACRONYM: α_1-Fetoprotein, cell-free DNA screening, maternal serum screening tests, prenatal screening tests, quad testing (AFP, HCG, estriol, inhibin-A), triple markers (AFP, HCG, estriol).

RATIONALE: To assist in the evaluation of fetal health related to chromosomal (e.g., trisomy 18, trisomy 21) or neural tube defects (e.g., spina bifida, anencephaly).

PATIENT PREPARATION: There are no food, fluid, activity, or medication restrictions unless by medical direction or as required by the specific collection procedure.

NORMAL FINDINGS: Each testing laboratory must establish its own reference ranges for quantitative measurements and its own cutoffs for negative and positive findings. Findings are then issued by laboratory report. Serum values for the tests evaluated vary with maternal race, weight, weeks of gestation, diabetic status, and number of fetuses. Variations exist between test methods; therefore, serial testing should be determined using the same test method. The calculated risk of a trisomy is based on the multiples of the median (MoM) of multiple markers, where the MoM is calculated for each marker and applied to an algorithm that includes other information known to influence the incidence of trisomy.

CRITICAL FINDINGS AND POTENTIAL INTERVENTIONS: N/A

OVERVIEW: (Study type: Maternal blood collected in a gold-, red-, or red/gray-top tube; related body system: Reproductive system. For maternal triple- or quad-marker testing, include α₁-fetoprotein [AFP], human chorionic gonadotropin [HCG], pregnancy-associated plasma protein A, and free estriol measurement. A blood sample from the fetus may be collected directly from the cord by percutaneous umbilical blood sampling [S] or cordocentesis and transferred to a red-top tube.) *Maternal genetic screening* is intended to assess a mother's risk for carrying a fetus with (specific) birth defects. Maternal genetic screening is a tiered and potentially complex paradigm that can begin prior to pregnancy, such as with carrier screening of the potential parents, or with carrier and/or prenatal screening after a diagnosis of pregnancy is made. Although the American College of Obstetricians and Gynecologists (ACOG) recommends maternal screening be offered to all expectant mothers, a discussion that covers the risks, benefits, and other choices (including the option to decline screening) should take place before any testing occurs and again after test results are available. Estimated risk stratification is based on algorithms that include blood test results, ultrasound measurements, and factors such as date of last menstrual period, maternal age, race, weight, diabetic status, and number of fetuses. Screening tests produce a number of false positives, and all positive screening test results should be confirmed using an approved diagnostic genetic test in combination with an offer of further genetic counseling by the requesting obstetric health care provider or by a specially trained genetic counselor. Factors that increase the risk of fetal abnormalities include the following:

- Maternal age of 35 years or older
- History of trisomy
- One or both parents are known carriers (having balanced chromosome translocations associated with trisomies 13, 18, and 21)
- Positive maternal screen results in the current pregnancy (first or second trimester)
- Ultrasound findings in the current pregnancy indicative of a fetal abnormality.

Genetic Testing for Carrier Status Before Pregnancy or in the Prenatal Period
A genetic carrier has the mutation for a disease, does not demonstrate symptoms of the disease, and can pass the mutation on to offspring. Depending on the carrier status of the parents, the offspring may inherit the disease or become carriers themselves. For more information on how genes are inherited, refer to the study titled "Genetic Testing." Carrier screening entails collection of a blood, saliva, or buccal sample (swab from inside the cheek). Conditions screened include cystic fibrosis, fragile X syndrome, sickle cell disease, spinal muscular atrophy, Tay-Sachs disease, and thalassemia.

Prenatal Genetic Screening Tests
First trimester screening is optimally performed between 11 and 14 wk; second trimester screening is optimally performed between 15 and 20 wk. A number of conventional screening tests for serum and amniotic fluid markers can be used in collaboration to screen for Down syndrome, neural

tube defects, and trisomy 18. These markers include AFP, HCG, unconjugated estriol, dimeric inhibin-A (DIA), pregnancy-associated plasma protein A, and nuchal translucency (NT) measurements.

Cell-free fetal DNA (cffDNA) analysis is a newer, noninvasive cytogenetic screening option for women with an increased risk for fetal aneuploidy (an abnormal number of fetal chromosomes). CffDNA is released by the placenta as early as the 10th week of pregnancy and is detectable in circulating maternal blood. Analysis of a maternal blood sample can be performed to identify trisomy 13 (Patau syndrome), trisomy 18 (Edwards syndrome), trisomy 21 (Down syndrome), and Klinefelter syndrome (XXY). It should be noted that there are a number of limitations with cffDNA testing that would not be encountered with conventional maternal screening and diagnostic testing strategies. Discussion regarding the limitations and benefits should occur between every patient who chooses this testing and the appropriate health-care provider (HCP). The most current ACOG screening recommendations for aneuploidy include a requirement that all cffDNA screens be confirmed by a diagnostic test such as amniocentesis or chorionic villus sampling, regardless of whether the screening test results were positive or negative.

First Trimester Screening
First trimester screening includes two blood tests (HCG and pregnancy-associated plasma protein-A [PAPP-A]) and an ultrasound marker called the *NT measurement*. It is performed between 10 or 11 and 13 wk/6 days.

HCG, a hormone secreted by the placenta, stimulates secretion of progesterone by the corpus luteum. (The use of HCG as a pregnancy test is also discussed in the study titled "Human Chorionic Gonadotropin.")

PAPP-A is a protein produced by first trimester trophoblasts, the earliest cells of a blastocyst that eventually forms a large portion of the placenta and also develops into fetal membranes; its function is to nourish the developing embryo. PAPP-A levels in maternal serum are related to fetal growth, are detectable at the start of the first trimester, and correspondingly increase throughout a normal pregnancy. Decreased levels are associated with an increased risk for Down syndrome and trisomy 18.

NT is obtained by measuring a saggital image of the fluid-filled space at the back of the fetus's neck (the nuchal region). NT measurements are evaluated in consideration of approximate gestational age, which is estimated by the corresponding crown rump length (CRL) during the first trimester. CRL is the length of the fetus from the top of its head (crown) to the bottom of its torso (rump). Normal NT at 11 weeks is up to 2 mm and at 13 weeks and 6 days is 2.8 mm; larger than normal NT measurements are found in trisomies, including Down syndrome.

Second Trimester Screening
Second trimester screening can be performed between 15 and 22 weeks and 6 days; optimal screening window is between 16 and 18 weeks. There are a number of different screening panels available.

M

Triple Marker Screen	Quad Screen	Penta Screen	Screening Results That Indicate Increased Risk for Down Syndrome (Trisomy 21)	Screening Results That Indicate Increased Risk for Edwards Syndrome (Trisomy 18)	Screening Results That Indicate Increased Risk for Open Spina Bifida (Myelomeningocele)
AFP	AFP	AFP	Low	Low	High
HCG	HCG	HCG	High	Low	Normal
Unconjugated estriol	Unconjugated estriol	Unconjugated estriol	Low	Low	Normal
	DIA	DIA	High	NA	NA

The incidence of Down syndrome in the United States is 1 in 750 live births. The triple screen detection rate for Down syndrome is 67% to 72%. The Down syndrome detection rate increases to 76% to 79% and maintains a false-positive rate of 5% when DIA is included. Some laboratories offer a Penta screen, which increases the detection rate for Down syndrome to 83%. The Penta screen includes the tests in a quad screen plus measurement of a carbohydrate isoform of HCG called *hyperglycosylated hCG* (h-HCG). h-HCG is produced during embryonic implantation by invasive trophoblast cells and was initially known as *invasive trophoblast antigen*. Increased levels of h-HCG are associated with Down syndrome. The incidence of trisomy 18 is 1 in 4,100 live births; most die within the first year after birth. The incidence of neural tube defects is 1 in 1,300 pregnancies.

AFP is a glycoprotein produced in the fetal liver, gastrointestinal tract, and yolk sac. AFP is the major serum protein produced for 10 wk in early fetal life. (See "Amniotic Fluid Analysis and L/S Ratio" study for measurement of AFP levels in amniotic fluid.) After 10 wk of gestation, levels of fetal AFP can be detected in maternal blood, with peak levels occurring at 16 to 18 wk. Elevated maternal levels of AFP on two tests taken 1 wk apart suggest further investigation into fetal well-being by ultrasound or amniocentesis.

During intrauterine development, the normal fetus and placenta produce estriol, a form of estrogen, some of which passes into maternal circulation. Decreased estriol levels are an independent indicator of neural tube defects.

DIA is the fourth biochemical marker used in prenatal quad screening. DIA is a glycoprotein secreted by the placenta. Maternal blood levels of DIA normally remain fairly stable during the 15th to 18th weeks of pregnancy. Blood levels are twice as high in the second trimester of pregnancies affected by Down syndrome.

Integrated Screening and Sequential Screening

Integrated and sequential screening are combinations of the first and second trimester screening tests. Integrated screening has the highest detection rate, but results of the first trimester screening are not reported until the second trimester testing has been completed. Sequential screening has a higher detection rate than any individual screening test, results of first trimester screening are reported when they become available, and the results are used to determine whether second trimester screening should be considered.

Prenatal Genetic Diagnostic Tests

Prenatal *genetic diagnostic tests* are used to identify, with a high level of confidence, the presence of an inherited fetal disease or genetic disorder. Diagnostic tests are those performed on amniotic fluid (performed between 15 and 20 wk) or chorionic villus sampling (CVS) (performed between 10 and 13 wk) to include AFP, acetylcholinesterase, chromosome analysis, chromosomal microarray analysis, and fetal hemoglobin. They are discussed in the studies "Amniotic Fluid Analysis and L/S Ratio" and "Biopsy, Chorionic Villus."

Cordocentesis or Percutaneous Umbilical Cord Blood Sampling

PUBS is a less frequently used option, performed after the 18th week of pregnancy, to obtain a sample of fetal blood when diagnostic information cannot be obtained through amniocentesis, CVS, or ultrasound. During the procedure, ultrasound is used to guide a needle through the abdominal and uterine walls into the umbilical cord at the point where the umbilical cord attaches to the placenta. A sample of fetal blood is withdrawn and submitted for genetic testing. PUBS is associated with a number of significant risks to the health of the fetus, including fetal bleeding, hematoma of the cord, and fetal death. More often, PUBS is used therapeutically to treat fetal blood conditions such as types of anemia requiring transfusion.

M

INDICATIONS
- Genetic screening and diagnostic testing either before pregnancy or during specific weeks of pregnancy for fetal neural tube defects and other disorders, as indicated by elevated levels in maternal serum and amniotic fluid.

INTERFERING FACTORS
Factors that may alter the results of the study

AFP
- Drugs and other substances that may decrease AFP levels in pregnant women include acetaminophen and acetylsalicylic acid.
- Multiple fetuses can cause increased levels.

Other considerations
- Inaccurate estimation of gestational age is the most common cause of an abnormal MoM (where gestational age is defined as weeks from the first day of the last menstrual period).
- Maternal AFP levels vary by ethnicity.

POTENTIAL MEDICAL DIAGNOSIS: CLINICAL SIGNIFICANCE OF RESULTS
Maternal serum screening test results report actual values and MoM by gestational age (in weeks). MoM are calculated by dividing each of the patient's test values by the midpoint (or median) of values expected for a large population of unaffected women at the same gestational age in weeks. MoM should be corrected for maternal weight as well as for maternal insulin requirement, ethnicity, and multiple fetuses.

Calculated Screen Risks for Down Syndrome (Trisomy 21)
Negative findings in
- First trimester screening— Calculated screen risk less than 1/230

- Second trimester screening— Calculated screen risk less than 1/270

Positive findings in
- First trimester screening— Calculated screen risk equal to or greater than 1/230
- Second trimester screening— Calculated screen risk equal to or greater than 1/270

Calculated Screen Risks for Edwards Syndrome (Trisomy 18)
Negative findings in
- First trimester screening— Calculated screen risk less than 1/100
- Second trimester screening— Calculated screen risk less than 1/100

Positive findings in
- First trimester screening— Calculated screen risk less than 1/100
- Second trimester screening— Calculated screen risk equal to or greater than 1/100

AFP (Note: Neural tube defect risk is based mainly on AFP MoM)
Increased in
- Pregnant women:
  Congenital nephrosis *(related to defective renal reabsorption)*
  Fetal abdominal wall defects *(related to release of AFP from open body wall defect)*
  Fetal distress
  Fetal neural tube defects (e.g., anencephaly, spina bifida, myelomeningocele) *(related to release of AFP from open body wall defect)*
  Low birth weight *(related to inaccurate estimation of gestational age)*
  Multiple pregnancy *(related to larger quantities from multiple fetuses)*
  Polycystic kidneys *(related to defective renal reabsorption)*
  Underestimation of gestational age *(related to the expectation of a lower value based on incorrect prediction of gestational age, i.e., AFP increases with*

age; therefore, if the age is believed to be less than it is actually, the expectation of the corresponding AFP value will be lower than it is actually, and the result appears to be elevated)

Decreased in
* Pregnant women:
  Down syndrome (trisomy 21)
  Edwards syndrome (trisomy 18)
  Fetal demise (undetected over a lengthy period of time) *(related to cessation of AFP production)*
  Hydatidiform moles *(partial mole may secrete some AFP)*
  Overestimation of gestational age *(related to the expectation of a higher value based on incorrect prediction of gestational age; i.e., AFP increases with age; therefore, if the age is believed to be greater than it actually is, the expectation of the corresponding AFP value will be greater than it actually is, and the result appears to be decreased)*
  Pseudopregnancy *(there is no fetus to produce AFP)*
  Spontaneous abortion *(there is no fetus to produce AFP)*

NURSING IMPLICATIONS

BEFORE THE STUDY: PLANNING AND IMPLEMENTATION

Teaching the Patient What to Expect
* Inform the patient that this test can assist in evaluating fetal health.
* Explain that a blood sample is needed for the test. The sample may be collected from the mother by venipuncture or from the baby, directly from the cord using a syringe, and transferred to a red-top tube.
* Explain that required information will need to be provided to the laboratory for triple-marker testing, including maternal birth date, weight, age, race, calculated gestational age, gestational age by ultrasound, gestational date by physical examination, first day of last menstrual period, estimated date of delivery, and whether the patient has type 1 diabetes.

Potential Nursing Actions
* Consent may be required for this type of testing. As appropriate, make sure a written and informed consent has been signed prior to the venipuncture procedure.

AFTER THE STUDY: POTENTIAL NURSING ACTIONS

Treatment Considerations
* Provide education related to the clinical implications of the test results.
* Discuss the implications of abnormal test results on lifestyle choices.
* Provide a nonjudgmental, nonthreatening atmosphere for discussing the risks and difficulties of delivering and raising a developmentally challenged infant as well as for exploring other options (termination of pregnancy or adoption). It is also important to discuss feelings the mother and father may experience (e.g., guilt, depression, anger) if fetal abnormalities are detected.

Nutritional Considerations
* Hyperhomocysteinemia resulting from folate deficiency in pregnant women is believed to increase the risk of neural tube defects. Elevated levels of homocysteine are thought to chemically damage the exposed neural tissue of the developing fetus. As appropriate, instruct pregnant patients to eat foods rich in folate, such as liver, salmon, eggs, asparagus, green leafy vegetables, broccoli, sweet potatoes, beans, and whole wheat.

Follow-Up, Evaluation, and Desired Outcomes
* Understands that an ultrasound may be performed and AFP levels in amniotic fluid may be analyzed if maternal blood levels are elevated in two samples obtained 1 wk apart.
* Acknowledges anxiety related to test results and accepts information provided regarding counseling if concerned with pregnancy termination or for genetic counseling if a chromosomal abnormality is determined. Decisions regarding elective abortion should take place in the presence of both parents.

M

Meckel Diverticulum Scan

SYNONYM/ACRONYM: Ectopic gastric mucosa scan, Meckel scan, Meckel scintigraphy.

RATIONALE: To assess, evaluate, and diagnose the cause of abdominal pain and gastrointestinal bleeding.

PATIENT PREPARATION: There are no activity or medication restrictions unless by medical direction. Instruct the patient to fast and refrain from fluids for 8 hr prior to the procedure. Instruct the patient to take a histamine blocker, as ordered, 2 days before the study to block gastrointestinal (GI) secretion.

Regarding the patient's risk for bleeding, the patient should be instructed to avoid taking natural products and medications with known anticoagulant, antiplatelet, or thrombolytic properties or to reduce dosage, as ordered, prior to the procedure. Number of days to withhold medication is dependent on the type of anticoagulant. Note the last time and dose of medication taken. Protocols may vary among facilities.

No other radionuclide scans or procedures using barium contrast medium should be scheduled within 24 to 48 hr before this procedure.

NORMAL FINDINGS
• Normal distribution of radionuclide by gastric mucosa at normal sites.

CRITICAL FINDINGS AND POTENTIAL INTERVENTIONS: N/A

OVERVIEW: (**Study type:** Nuclear scan; **related body system:** Digestive system.) Meckel diverticulum scan is a nuclear medicine study performed to assist in diagnosing the cause of abdominal pain or occult GI bleeding and to assess the presence and size of a congenital anomaly of the GI tract (especially in pediatric or young adult patients). After IV injection of technetium-99m pertechnetate, immediate and delayed imaging is performed, with various views of the abdomen obtained. The radionuclide is taken up and concentrated by parietal cells of the gastric mucosa, whether located in the stomach or in a Meckel diverticulum. Up to 25% of Meckel diverticulum is lined internally with ectopic gastric mucosal tissue. This tissue is usually located in the ileum and right lower quadrant of the abdomen; it secretes acid that causes ulceration of intestinal tissue, which results in abdominal pain and occult blood in stools.

INDICATIONS
• Aid in the diagnosis of unexplained abdominal pain and GI bleeding caused by hydrochloric acid and pepsin secreted by ectopic gastric mucosa, which ulcerates nearby mucosa.
• Detect sites of ectopic gastric mucosa.

INTERFERING FACTORS
Contraindications

Patients who are pregnant or suspected of being pregnant, unless the potential benefits of a procedure using radiation far outweigh the risk of radiation exposure to the fetus and mother.

Factors that may alter the results of the study
- False-positive results may occur from nondiverticular bleeding, intussusception, duplication cysts, inflammatory bowel disease, hemangioma of the bowel, and other organ infections.
- Inadequate amount of gastric mucosa within Meckel diverticulum can affect the ability to visualize abnormalities.
- Inaccurate timing for imaging after the radionuclide injection can affect the results.
- Metallic objects (e.g., jewelry, body rings) within the examination field, other nuclear scans done within the previous 24 to 48 hr, or retained barium from a previous radiological procedure, which may inhibit organ visualization and cause unclear images.
- Improper injection of the radionuclide that allows the tracer to seep deep into the muscle tissue can produce erroneous hot spots.
- Inability of the patient to cooperate or remain still during the procedure, because movement can produce blurred or otherwise unclear images.

POTENTIAL MEDICAL DIAGNOSIS: CLINICAL SIGNIFICANCE OF RESULTS
Abnormal findings related to
- Meckel diverticulum, as evidenced by focally increased radioactive uptake in areas other than normal structures

NURSING IMPLICATIONS

BEFORE THE STUDY: PLANNING AND IMPLEMENTATION

Teaching the Patient What to Expect
- Inform the patient this procedure can assist in assessing GI bleeding.

- Pregnancy is a general contraindication to procedures involving radiation. Explain to the female patient that she will be asked the date of her last menstrual period. Pregnancy testing may be performed to determine the possibility of pregnancy before exposure to radiation.
- Review the procedure with the patient. Address concerns about pain and explain that there may be moments of discomfort or pain experienced when the IV line is inserted to allow infusion of fluids such as saline, anesthetics, sedatives, radionuclides, medications used in the procedure, or emergency medications.
- Explain that the procedure is performed in a nuclear medicine department by a health-care provider (HCP) specializing in this procedure, with support staff, and takes approximately 60 min.
- Reassure the patient that the radionuclide poses no radioactive hazard and rarely produces adverse effects.
- **Pediatric Considerations:** Preparing children for a Meckel diverticulum scan depends on the age of the child. Encourage parents to be truthful about what the child may experience during the procedure (e.g., he or she may feel a pinch or minor discomfort when the IV needle is inserted) and to use words that they know their child will understand. Toddlers and preschool-age children have a very short attention span, so the best time to talk about the test is right before the procedure. The child should be assured that he or she will be allowed to bring a favorite comfort item into the examination room, and if appropriate, that a parent will be with the child during the procedure. Explain the importance of remaining still while the images are taken.
- Instruct the patient to remove jewelry and other metallic objects from the area to be examined.
- Baseline vital signs and neurological status will be recorded. Protocols may vary among facilities.
- Positioning for this study is in a supine position on a flat table with foam wedges to help maintain position and immobilization.

M

▸ Once the IV radionuclide is administered, the abdomen is scanned immediately to screen for vascular lesions. Images are taken in various positions every 5 min for the next hour.

▸ Once the study is completed, the needle or catheter will be removed and a pressure dressing applied over the puncture site.

Potential Nursing Actions

◈ *Make sure a written and informed consent has been signed prior to the procedure and before administering any medications.*

Safety Considerations

▸ Anticoagulants, aspirin, and other salicylates should be discontinued by medical direction for the appropriate number of days prior to a procedure in which bleeding is a potential complication.

AFTER THE STUDY: POTENTIAL NURSING ACTIONS

Avoiding Complications

▸ Establishing an IV site and injection of radionuclides are invasive procedures. Complications are rare but include risk for allergic reaction *(related to contrast reaction)*, hematoma *(related to blood leakage into the tissue following needle insertion)*, bleeding from the puncture site *(related to a bleeding disorder or the effects of natural products and medications with known anticoagulant, antiplatelet, or thrombolytic properties)*, or infection *(which might occur if bacteria from the skin surface are introduced at the puncture site)*. Monitor the patient for complications related to the procedure (e.g., allergic reaction, anaphylaxis, bronchospasm). Immediately report symptoms such as fast heart rate, difficulty breathing, skin rash, itching, or chest pain to the appropriate HCP. Observe/assess the needle/catheter insertion site for bleeding, inflammation, or hematoma formation.

Treatment Considerations

▸ Explain that the radionuclide is eliminated from the body within 6 to 24 hr. Advise the patient to drink increased

amounts of fluids for 24 to 48 hr to eliminate the radionuclide from the body, unless contraindicated.

▸ Instruct the patient to resume usual diet, fluids, and medications, as directed by the HCP.

▸ Monitor vital signs and neurological status every 15 min for 1 hr, then every 2 hr for 4 hr and compare with baseline values. Take temperature every 4 hr for 24 hr and notify the HCP if the temperature becomes elevated. Monitor intake and output at least every 8 hr. Protocols may vary among facilities.

▸ Instruct the patient in the care and assessment of the injection site.

▸ Explain that application of cold compresses to the puncture site may reduce discomfort or edema.

Safety Considerations

▸ The patient who is breastfeeding should consult with the requesting HCP regarding alternate testing that does not involve radiation. In general, if a woman who is breastfeeding must have a nuclear scan, she should not breastfeed the infant for 72 hr after the scan, until the radionuclide has been eliminated. She should be instructed to express the milk in order to prevent cessation of milk production; the milk can be stored and used after the 3-day period.

▸ Refer to organizational policy for additional precautions that may include instructions on handwashing, toilet flushing, limited contact with others, and other aspects of nuclear medicine safety.

Nutritional Considerations

▸ A low-fat, low-cholesterol, and low-sodium diet should be consumed to reduce current disease processes.

▸ High fat consumption increases the amount of bile acids in the colon and should be avoided.

Follow-Up, Evaluation, and Desired Outcomes

▸ Acknowledges further testing may be required to better manage treatment and evaluate disease progression.

Mediastinoscopy

SYNONYM/ACRONYM: N/A

RATIONALE: To visualize and assess structures under the mediastinum to assist in obtaining biopsies for diagnosing and staging cancer and to evaluate the effectiveness of therapeutic interventions.

PATIENT PREPARATION: There are no activity restrictions unless by medical direction. Instruct the patient to fast and restrict fluids for at least 8 hr prior to general anesthesia. The American Society of Anesthesiologists has fasting guidelines for risk levels according to patient status. More information can be located at www.asahq.org.

Regarding the patient's risk for bleeding, the patient should be instructed to avoid taking natural products and medications with known anticoagulant, anti-platelet, or thrombolytic properties or to reduce dosage, as ordered, prior to the procedure. Number of days to withhold medication is dependent on the type of anticoagulant. Note the last time and dose of medication taken. Protocols may vary among facilities.

Ensure that this procedure is performed before an upper gastrointestinal study or barium swallow.

NORMAL FINDINGS
- Normal appearance of mediastinal structures
- No abnormal lymph node tissue.

CRITICAL FINDINGS AND POTENTIAL INTERVENTIONS: N/A

OVERVIEW: (Study type: Endoscopy; **related body system:** Immune and Respiratory systems.) Mediastinoscopy provides direct visualization of the structures that lie beneath the mediastinum, which is the area behind the sternum and between the lungs. The test is performed under general anesthesia by means of a mediastinoscope inserted through a surgical incision at the suprasternal notch. Structures that can be viewed include the trachea, the esophagus, the heart and its major vessels, the thymus gland, and the lymph nodes that receive drainage from the lungs. The procedure is performed primarily to visualize and obtain biopsy specimens of the mediastinal lymph nodes and to determine the extent of metastasis into the mediastinum for the determination of treatment planning in cancer patients.

INDICATIONS
- Confirm radiological evidence of a thoracic infectious process of an indeterminate nature, coccidioidomycosis, or histoplasmosis.
- Confirm radiological or cytological evidence of cancer or sarcoidosis.
- Detect Hodgkin disease.
- Detect metastasis into the anterior mediastinum or extrapleurally into the chest.
- Determine stage of known bronchogenic cancer, as indicated by the extent of mediastinal lymph node involvement.
- Evaluate a patient with signs and symptoms of obstruction of

M

mediastinal lymph flow and a history of head or neck cancer to determine recurrence or spread.

INTERFERING FACTORS
Contraindications

✺ Patients who are pregnant or suspected of being pregnant, unless the potential benefits of a procedure using anesthesia outweigh the risk to the fetus and mother.

✺ Patients who have had a previous mediastinoscopy, *because scarring can make insertion of the scope and biopsy of lymph nodes difficult.*

✺ Patients who have superior vena cava obstruction, *because this condition causes increased venous collateral circulation in the mediastinum.*

POTENTIAL MEDICAL DIAGNOSIS: CLINICAL SIGNIFICANCE OF RESULTS
Abnormal findings related to

• Bronchogenic cancer
• Coccidioidomycosis
• Granulomatous infections
• Histoplasmosis
• Hodgkin disease
• *Pneumocystis jiroveci*
• Sarcoidosis
• Tuberculosis

NURSING IMPLICATIONS

BEFORE THE STUDY: PLANNING AND IMPLEMENTATION

Teaching the Patient What to Expect

▶ Inform the patient this procedure can assist in assessing structure in the middle of the chest.
▶ Review the procedure with the patient. Address concerns about pain and explain that there may be moments of discomfort or pain experienced when the IV line or catheter is inserted to allow infusion of fluids such as saline, anesthetics, sedatives, medications used in the procedure, or emergency medications.
▶ Explain that prophylactic antibiotics may be administered prior to the procedure.

▶ Inform the patient that the procedure is performed in the operating room by a health care provider (HCP) specializing in this procedure, with support staff, and usually takes 30 to 60 min to complete. Explain that general anesthesia will be administered to promote relaxation and reduce discomfort prior to the mediastinoscopy but that some pain may be experienced after the test.
▶ The patient will be asked to remove jewelry and external metallic objects from the area to be examined prior to the procedure.
▶ Baseline vital signs and neurological status will be recorded. Protocols may vary among facilities.
▶ Electrocardiographic electrodes are placed on the patient for cardiac monitoring. A baseline rhythm is established to determine if the patient has ventricular dysrhythmias.
▶ Positioning for this study is in the supine position.
▶ Lymph node biopsy specimens are obtained by incision that allows access to specific tissue.
▶ Tissue samples are placed in properly labelled specimen containers, and promptly transport the specimen to the laboratory for processing and analysis.
▶ Once the procedure is completed, the scope is removed and the incision closed.
▶ The incision site is observed for bleeding, inflammation, or hematoma formation.
▶ The patient is extubated once deemed stable and no further surgery is immediately indicated.

Potential Nursing Actions

✺ *Make sure a written and informed consent has been signed prior to the procedure and before administering any medications.*
▶ Ensure that the results of blood typing and crossmatching are obtained and recorded before the procedure in the event that an emergency thoracotomy is required. Check to verify that ordered blood is available.

Safety Considerations
▶ Avoid using morphine sulfate in patients with asthma or other pulmonary disease. This drug can further exacerbate bronchospasms and respiratory impairment.

AFTER THE STUDY: POTENTIAL NURSING ACTIONS

Avoiding Complications

♦ Complications of the procedure may include bleeding, pneumothorax, infection, and cardiac arrhythmias. Emphasize that any excessive bleeding, fast heart rate, difficulty breathing, skin rash, itching, chest pain, abdominal pain, excessive coughing, fever, redness, swelling, or pain of the incisional area must be reported to the HCP immediately.

Treatment Considerations

♦ Do not allow the patient to eat or drink for 12 to 24 hr.

♦ Instruct the patient to resume normal activity, medication, and diet in 24 hr or as tolerated after the examination, unless otherwise indicated.

♦ Patient may be placed in a semi-Fowler position, which prevents compression of the chest from gravity, relaxes abdominal muscles and promotes improved breathing, until vital signs revert to baseline.

♦ A chest x-ray will be performed to check for presence of pneumothorax.

♦ Monitor vital signs and neurological status every 15 min for 1 hr, then every 2 hr for 4 hr, and then as ordered by the HCP. Compare with baseline values. Take temperature every 4 hr for 24 hr and notify the HCP if the temperature changes. Monitor intake and output at least every 8 hr. Protocols may vary among facilities.

♦ Instruct the patient in the care and assessment of the site.

Safety Considerations

♦ Assess the patient's ability to swallow before allowing the patient to attempt liquids or solid foods.

Follow-Up, Evaluation, and Desired Outcomes

♦ Understands that a follow up appointment for the removal of stitches is required, as ordered.

♦ Understands that additional testing may be needed to monitor disease progression.

Metanephrines

M

SYNONYM/ACRONYM: N/A

RATIONALE: To assist in the diagnosis of cancer of the adrenal medulla or to assess for the cause of hypertension.

PATIENT PREPARATION: There are no food, fluid, or medication restrictions unless by medical direction. Instruct the patient to avoid excessive exercise and stress during the 24-hr collection of urine. Usually a 24-hr urine collection may be ordered. As appropriate, provide the required urine collection container and specimen collection instructions.

NORMAL FINDINGS: Method: High-pressure liquid chromatography.

Age	Conventional Units	SI Units
Normetanephrines		*(Conventional Units × 5.07)*
3 mo–4 yr	54–249 mcg/24 hr	274–1,262 micromol/day
5–9 yr	31–398 mcg/24 hr	157–2,018 micromol/day
10–17 yr	67–531 mcg/24 hr	340–2,692 micromol/day
18–39 yr	35–482 mcg/24 hr	177–2,444 micromol/day
Greater than 40 yr	88–676 mcg/24 hr	446–3,427 micromol/day

(table continues on page 840)

Age	Conventional Units	SI Units
Metanephrines, Total		*(Conventional Units × 5.07)*
3 mo–4 yr	79–345 mcg/24 hr	401–1,749 micromol/day
5–9 yr	49–409 mcg/24 hr	248–2,074 micromol/day
10–17 yr	107–741 mcg/24 hr	543–3,757 micromol/day
18–39 yr	94–695 mcg/24 hr	477–3,524 micromol/day
40–49 yr	182–739 mcg/24 hr	923–3,747 micromol/day
Greater than 50 yr	224–832 mcg/24 hr	1,136–4,218 micromol/day

CRITICAL FINDINGS AND POTENTIAL INTERVENTIONS: N/A

OVERVIEW: (Study type: Urine from a timed specimen collected in a clean amber plastic collection container with 6N hydrochloride as a preservative; related body system: Endocrine system.) Metanephrines are the inactive metabolites of epinephrine and norepinephrine. Metanephrines are either excreted or further metabolized into vanillylmandelic acid. Release of metanephrines in the urine is indicative of disorders associated with excessive catecholamine production, particularly pheochromocytoma. Vanillylmandelic acid and catecholamines are normally measured with urinary metanephrines. Creatinine is usually measured simultaneously to ensure adequate collection and to calculate an excretion ratio of metabolite to creatinine.

INDICATIONS
- Assist in the diagnosis of suspected pheochromocytoma.
- Assist in identifying the cause of hypertension.
- Verify suspected tumors associated with excessive catecholamine secretion.

INTERFERING FACTORS
Factors that may alter the results of the study
- Drugs and other substances that may increase metanephrine levels include monoamine oxidase inhibitors and prochlorperazine.
- Methylglucamine in x-ray contrast medium may cause false-negative results.

Other considerations
- All urine voided for the timed collection period must be included in the collection, or else falsely decreased values may be obtained. Compare output records with volume collected to verify that all voids were included in the collection.

POTENTIAL MEDICAL DIAGNOSIS: CLINICAL SIGNIFICANCE OF RESULTS
Increased in
- Ganglioneuroma
- Neuroblastoma
- Pheochromocytoma
- Severe stress

Decreased in: N/A

NURSING IMPLICATIONS

BEFORE THE STUDY: PLANNING AND IMPLEMENTATION
Teaching the Patient What to Expect
- Inform the patient this test can assist in diagnosing adrenal gland health and hypertension.
- Explain that a urine sample is needed for the test. Information regarding specimen collection is presented with

M

other general guidelines in Appendix A: Patient Preparation and Specimen Collection.

Potential Nursing Actions
♦ Include on the collection container's label urine total volume, test start and stop times/dates, and any medications that may interfere with test results.

AFTER THE STUDY: POTENTIAL NURSING ACTIONS

Treatment Considerations
♦ Grief is an emotional response associated with a diagnosis of cancer that places one at risk for death. Monitor for observable symptoms of this response, which are crying, withdrawal, anxiety, fear, anger, denial, and disrupted sleep.
♦ Maintain clear communication with the patient that keeps the patient informed of his or her health status, and consider facilitating participation in a support group or connection with spiritual support.
♦ Facilitate open discussions on treatment options and outcomes, including consideration of hospice care.

Follow-Up, Evaluation, and Desired Outcomes
♦ Understands that additional testing may be necessary to evaluate or monitor disease progression and determine the need for a change in therapy.

Microalbumin

SYNONYM/ACRONYM: Albumin, urine.

RATIONALE: To assist in the identification and management of early diabetes in order to avoid or delay onset of diabetic associated kidney disease.

PATIENT PREPARATION: There are no food, fluid, activity, or medication restrictions unless by medical direction. Either a random or a 24-hr urine collection may be ordered. As appropriate, provide the required urine collection container and specimen collection instructions.

NORMAL FINDINGS: Method: Immunoassay.

Test	Conventional and SI Units
24-hr microalbumin to creatinine ratio	Less than 30 mg/g creatinine/24 hr
24-hr microalbumin	
Normal	Less than 30 mg/24 hr
Microalbuminuria	30–299 mg/24 hr
Clinical albuminuria	300 mg or greater/24 hr

The American Diabetes Association (ADA) recommends annual measurement of microalbumin (spot or 24-hr, as requested by the health-care provider [HCP]) with serum creatinine (Cr) and estimated glomerular filtration rate (eGFR). Numerous factors, such as hydration status, the presence of an infection, or significant hyperglycemia, can produce falsely increased or decreased microalbumin levels. The National Kidney Foundation defines microalbuminuria as equal to or greater than 30 mg/g Cr/24 hr based on eGFR measurements.

CRITICAL FINDINGS AND POTENTIAL INTERVENTIONS: N/A

OVERVIEW: (Study type: Urine from a random or timed specimen collected in a clean plastic collection container; related body system: Endocrine and Urinary systems.) The term *microalbumin* describes concentrations of albumin in urine that are greater than normal but undetectable by dipstick or traditional spectrophotometry methods. Microalbuminuria precedes the nephropathy associated with diabetes and is often elevated years before Cr clearance shows abnormal values. Studies have shown that the median duration from onset of microalbuminuria to development of nephropathy is 5 to 7 yr. For additional information regarding screening guidelines and management of diabetes, refer to the study titled "Glucose."

INDICATIONS
- Evaluate kidney disease.
- Screen patients with diabetes for early signs of nephropathy.

INTERFERING FACTORS
Factors that may alter the results of the study
- Drugs and other substances that may decrease microalbumin levels include captopril, dipyridamole, enalapril, furosemide, indapamide, perindopril, quinapril, ramipril, tolrestat, and simvastatin.

Other considerations
- All urine voided for the timed collection period must be included in the collection, or else falsely decreased values may be obtained. Compare output records with volume collected to verify that all voids were included in the collection.

POTENTIAL MEDICAL DIAGNOSIS: CLINICAL SIGNIFICANCE OF RESULTS
Increased in
Conditions resulting in increased renal excretion or loss of protein.

- Cardiomyopathy
- Diabetic nephropathy
- Exercise
- Hypertension (uncontrolled)
- Kidney disease
- Pre-eclampsia
- Urinary tract infections

Decreased in: N/A

M

NURSING IMPLICATIONS

POTENTIAL NURSING PROBLEMS: ASSESSMENT & NURSING DIAGNOSIS

Problems	Signs and Symptoms
Blood glucose *(related to sedentary lifestyle, circulating insulin deficiency secondary to pancreatic insufficiency, excessive dietary intake, insulin resistance, pregnancy)*	**Excess:** Fatigue, mild dehydration, elevated blood glucose, weight loss, weakness, polyuria, polydipsia, polyphagia, blurred vision, headache, paresthesia, poor skin turgor, dry mouth, nausea, vomiting, abdominal pain, Kussmaul respirations **Deficit:** Tremor, diaphoresis, decreased concentration, elevated blood pressure, palpitations, headache,

Problems	Signs and Symptoms
	polyphagia, restlessness, lethargy, altered mental status, combativeness, altered speech, altered coordination
Nutrition *(related to excessive dietary intake more than body requirements, insulin deficiency, stress, anxiety, depression, cultural lifestyle, unhealthy food sources, financial restrictions)*	Increased thirst, increased urination, **weight loss, fatigue, elevated blood glucose levels, inadequate glucose management, increased hunger**
Renal impairment *(related to elevated blood glucose levels over time, decreased renal perfusion, prolonged hypotension, heart disease with altered cardiac output)*	Altered fluid, electrolyte, and acid base balance; decreasing urinary output; elevated blood glucose

BEFORE THE STUDY: PLANNING AND IMPLEMENTATION

Teaching the Patient What to Expect

▶ Inform the patient this test can assist in evaluating for early kidney disease associated with diabetes.

▶ Emphasize that good glycemic management delays the onset and slows the progression of diabetic retinopathy, nephropathy, and neuropathy.

▶ Explain that a urine sample is needed for the test. Information regarding specimen collection is presented with other general guidelines in Appendix A: Patient Preparation and Specimen Collection.

Potential Nursing Actions

▶ Include on the timed collection container's label urine total volume, test start and stop times/dates, and any medications that may interfere with test results.

AFTER THE STUDY: POTENTIAL NURSING ACTIONS

Avoiding Complications

▶ Emphasize, as appropriate, that good management of glucose levels delays the onset and slows the progression of diabetic retinopathy, nephropathy, and neuropathy.

▶ Explain that unmanaged diabetes can cause multiple health issues, including diabetic kidney disease, amputation of limbs, and ultimately in death.

Treatment Considerations

▶ Emphasize the importance of adhering to the HCP-recommended therapeutic regime to manage diabetes.

▶ Discuss the advantages that attendance in support group meetings has to learn how to manage the disease process from other people with diabetes.

▶ Blood Glucose: Instruct the patient and caregiver to report signs and symptoms of hypoglycemia or hyperglycemia. Glucose should be checked before meals and at bedtime and prescribed insulin or oral drugs should be administered. Make sure the patient understands how to perform glucose self-checks and provide education for deficits in learning. Collaborate with the HCP and registered dietitian to support medical nutritional therapy. Encourage activity commensurate with the patient's physical abilities. Discuss the lifestyle alterations necessary to support positive health management secondary to disease process. Monitor and trend results: hemoglobin (Hgb) A_{1c}, BUN, Cr, electrolytes, arterial pH, magnesium, urine ketones and microalbumin, WBC count, amylase, Hgb/Hct, C-reactive protein, liver enzymes, and serum insulin levels.

▶ Renal Impairment: Review and trend diagnostic tests: BUN, Cr, urine osmolality, Cr clearance, microalbumin, GFR, and blood glucose. Ensure adherence

M

to recommended dietary and exercise regimes.

Nutritional Considerations

◗ Abnormal findings may be associated with diabetes. There is no "diabetic diet"; however, many meal-planning approaches with nutritional goals are endorsed by the ADA. Patients who adhere to dietary recommendations report a better general feeling of health, better weight management, better management of glucose and lipid values, and improved use of insulin. Instruct the patient, as appropriate, in nutritional management of diabetes. A variety of dietary patterns are beneficial for people with diabetes. Encourage consultation with a registered dietitian who is a certified diabetes educator.

Follow-Up, Evaluation, and Desired Outcomes

◗ Acknowledges contact information provided for the ADA (www.diabetes.org), American Heart Association (www.heart.org/HEARTORG), the National Heart, Lung, and Blood Institute (www.nhlbi.nih.gov), National Institute of Diabetes and Digestive and Kidney Disease (www.niddk.nih.gov), and U.S. Department of Agriculture's resource for nutrition (www.choosemyplate.gov).

Mononucleosis Testing

SYNONYM/ACRONYM: Monospot, Epstein-Barr test, heterophil antibody test, IM serology.

RATIONALE: To assess for Epstein-Barr virus (EBV) and assist with diagnosis of infectious mononucleosis.

PATIENT PREPARATION: There are no food, fluid, activity, or medication restrictions unless by medical direction.

NORMAL FINDINGS: (Method: Heterophile antibody test by agglutination; serological tests for EBV early antigen D antibody IgG, EBV nuclear antigen antibody IgG, EBV viral capsid antigen antibody IgG, EBV viral capsid antigen antibody IgM by immunoassay) Negative.

CRITICAL FINDINGS AND POTENTIAL INTERVENTIONS: N/A

OVERVIEW: (**Study type:** Blood collected in a gold-, red-, or red/gray-top tube; **related body system:** Immune system.) Infectious mononucleosis is caused by the human herpesvirus 4, more commonly known as the *Epstein-Barr virus.* The incubation period is 10 to 50 days, and the symptoms last 1 to 4 wk after the infection has fully developed. The hallmark of EBV infection is the presence of heterophil antibodies, also called *Paul-Bunnell-Davidsohn antibodies,* which are immunoglobulin M (IgM) antibodies that agglutinate sheep or horse red blood cells. The disease induces formation of abnormal lymphocytes in the lymph nodes; stimulates increased formation of heterophil antibodies; and is characterized by fever, cervical lymphadenopathy, tonsillopharyngitis, and hepatosplenomegaly. EBV is also thought to play a role in Burkitt lymphoma, nasopharyngeal cancer, and chronic fatigue syndrome. If the results of the heterophil antibody screening test are negative and infectious mononucleosis is highly suspected, EBV-specific serology should be requested (EBV early antigen D antibody IgG, EBV nuclear antigen antibody IgG, EBV viral capsid antigen antibody IgG, EBV viral capsid antigen antibody IgM). Molecular testing methods (e.g., polymerase chain reaction) are available to identify the presence of EBV viral DNA and to monitor viral load in patients being treated for other EBV-related diseases.

INDICATIONS

• Assist in confirming infectious mononucleosis.

INTERFERING FACTORS

Factors that may alter the results of the study

• False-positive results may occur in the presence of narcotic addiction, serum sickness, lymphomas, hepatitis, leukemia, cancer of the pancreas, and phenytoin therapy.
• A false-negative result may occur if treatment was begun before antibodies developed or if the test was done less than 6 days after exposure to the virus.

POTENTIAL MEDICAL DIAGNOSIS: CLINICAL SIGNIFICANCE OF RESULTS

Positive findings in

• Infectious mononucleosis

Negative findings in: N/A

NURSING IMPLICATIONS

POTENTIAL NURSING PROBLEMS: ASSESSMENT & NURSING DIAGNOSIS

Problems	Signs and Symptoms
Fatigue *(related to EBV infection secondary to exposure through kissing, cough, sneeze, sharing food utensils of an infected person)*	Decreased concentration, increased physical health concerns, unable to restore energy with sleep, reports being tired, unable to maintain normal routine
Infection *(related to EBV infection secondary to exposure through kissing, cough, sneeze, sharing food utensils of an infected person)*	Fatigue, malaise, sore throat, fever, enlarged lymph nodes in the neck and armpits, swollen tonsils, headache, rash, swollen spleen

BEFORE THE STUDY: PLANNING AND IMPLEMENTATION

Teaching the Patient What to Expect

▶ Inform the patient this test can assist with diagnosing a mononucleosis infection.
▶ Explain that a blood sample is needed for the test. Inform the patient that approximately 10% of all results are false-negative or false-positive.

AFTER THE STUDY: POTENTIAL NURSING ACTIONS

Treatment Considerations

▶ Fatigue: Monitor and trend mononucleosis screening results. Trend the degree of fatigue over time and pace activities to preserve energy stores. Identify what aggravates and decreases fatigue. Consider related emotional factors such as depression, current medications in relation to

M

fatigue, and physiologic factors such as anemia.

▶ Infection: Review signs and symptoms of infection: fever, chills, sore throat, enlarged lymph nodes, and fatigue. Encourage rest and ingestion of plenty of fluids (water and fruit juice). Administer ordered antibiotics to treat strep throat and steroids to treat swollen throat or tonsils. Discuss gargling with warm saltwater to decrease sore throat pain and the use of over-the-counter ibuprofen or acetaminophen. Discuss the importance of avoiding at-risk activities that may cause trauma and spleen rupture.

▶ Advise the patient to refrain from direct contact with others because the disease is transmitted through saliva.

Follow-Up, Evaluation, and Desired Outcomes

▶ Acknowledges the importance of fluids and rest for recovery, avoiding vigorous activities, heavy lifting, roughhousing, and contact sports for at least 1 mo or as recommended by the health-care provider.

Mumps Testing

SYNONYM/ACRONYM: N/A

RATIONALE: To assist in diagnosing a present or past mumps infection.

PATIENT PREPARATION: There are no food, fluid, activity, or medication restrictions unless by medical direction.

NORMAL FINDINGS: Method: Indirect immunofluorescence.

	IgM	Interpretation	IgG	Interpretation
Negative	0.89 index or less	No significant level of detectable antibody	Less than 5 IU/mL	No significant level of detectable antibody; indicative of nonimmunity
Indeterminate	0.9–1 index	Equivocal results; retest in 10–14 days	6–9 IU/mL	Equivocal results; retest in 10–14 days
Positive	1.1 index or greater	Antibody detected; indicative of recent immunization, current or recent infection	10 IU/mL or greater	Antibody detected; indicative of immunization, current or past infection

CRITICAL FINDINGS AND POTENTIAL INTERVENTIONS: N/A

OVERVIEW: (Study type: Blood collected in a gold-, red-, or red/gray-top tube; related body system: Immune system.) Mumps serology is done to determine the presence of mumps antibody, indicating exposure to or active presence of mumps. Mumps, also known as *parotitis,* is an infectious viral disease of the parotid glands caused by a myxovirus that is transmitted by direct contact with or droplets spread from the saliva of an infected person. The incubation period averages 3 wk. Virus can be shed in saliva for 2 wk after infection and in urine for 2 wk after the onset of symptoms. Complications of infection include aseptic meningitis; encephalitis; and inflammation of the testes, ovaries, and pancreas. The presence of immunoglobulin M (IgM) antibodies indicates acute infection. The presence of immunoglobulin G (IgG) antibodies indicates current or past infection.

INDICATIONS

- Determine resistance to or protection against the mumps virus by a positive reaction or susceptibility to mumps by a negative reaction.
- Document immunity.
- Evaluate mumps-like diseases and differentiate between these and actual mumps.

INTERFERING FACTORS: N/A

POTENTIAL MEDICAL DIAGNOSIS: CLINICAL SIGNIFICANCE OF RESULTS
Past or current mumps infection.

NURSING IMPLICATIONS

BEFORE THE STUDY: PLANNING AND IMPLEMENTATION

Teaching the Patient What to Expect
- Inform the patient this test can assist in diagnosing a mumps infection.
- Explain that a blood sample is needed for the test and that several tests may be necessary to confirm diagnosis.
- Any individual positive result should be repeated in 7 to 14 days to monitor a change in detectable levels of antibodies.

AFTER THE STUDY: POTENTIAL NURSING ACTIONS

Treatment Considerations
- Instruct the patient in isolation precautions during the time of communicability or contagion.
- Emphasize that the patient must return to have a convalescent blood sample taken in 7 to 14 days.
- Inform the patient that the presence of mumps antibodies ensures lifelong immunity.

Follow-Up, Evaluation, and Desired Outcomes
- Acknowledges contact information provided regarding vaccine-preventable diseases (e.g., mumps), as indicated, for the Centers for Disease Control and Prevention (www.cdc.gov/vaccines/vpd/vaccines-diseases.html).

M

Myocardial Infarct Scan

SYNONYM/ACRONYM: PYP cardiac scan, infarct scan, pyrophosphate cardiac scan, acute myocardial infarction scan.

RATIONALE: To identify myocardial infarcts and evaluate myocardial perfusion.

PATIENT PREPARATION

• Instruct the patient to fast, restrict fluids, and refrain from smoking for 4 hr prior to the procedure. Instruct the patient to withhold medications for 24 hr before the procedure. No other radionuclide scans should be scheduled within 24 to 48 hr before this procedure. Protocols may vary among facilities.

NORMAL FINDINGS

• Normal coronary blood flow and tissue perfusion, with no pyrophosphate (PYP) localization in the myocardium
• No uptake above background activity in the myocardium (*Note:* When PYP uptake is present, it is graded in relation to adjacent rib activity.)

CRITICAL FINDINGS AND POTENTIAL INTERVENTIONS: N/A

OVERVIEW: (Study type: Nuclear medicine; related body system: Circulatory system.) Technetium-99m stannous PYP scanning, also known as *myocardial infarct imaging,* can identify areas of infarct or necrosis due to insufficient myocardial perfusion and provide information about the extent of myocardial infarction (MI). This procedure can distinguish new from old infarcts when a patient has had abnormal electrocardiograms (ECGs) and cardiac enzymes have returned to normal.

PYP uptake by acutely infarcted tissue may be related to the influx of calcium through damaged cell membranes, which accompanies myocardial necrosis; that is, the radionuclide may be binding to calcium phosphate crystals (hydroxyapatite). The PYP in these damaged cells can be viewed as spots of increased radionuclide uptake that appear in 12 hr at the earliest. PYP uptake usually takes place 24 to 72 hr after MI, and the radionuclide remains detectable for approximately 10 to 14 days after the MI. PYP uptake is proportional to the blood flow to the affected area; with large areas of necrosis, PYP uptake may be maximal around the periphery of a necrotic area, with little uptake being detectable in the poorly perfused center. Most of the PYP is concentrated in regions that have 20% to 40% of the normal blood flow. Single-photon emission computed tomography (SPECT) can be used to visualize the heart from multiple angles and planes, enabling areas of MI to be viewed with greater accuracy and resolution. This technique removes overlying structures that may confuse interpretation of the results. multigated acquisition (MUGA) scan, also known as *blood pool imaging scan and radionuclide ventriculogram,* may also be performed in conjunction with a PYP scan. MUGA provides information about cardiac function such as ejection fraction, ventricular wall motion, ventricular dilation, stroke volume, and cardiac output. With the availability of newer biomarkers such as troponin, myocardial infarct imaging has become less important in the diagnosis of acute MI. For additional information regarding screening guidelines for *atherosclerotic cardiovascular disease* (ASCVD), refer to the study titled "Cholesterol, Total and Fractions."

Comparison of Cardiac Nuclear Scans

	Common Use	Radionuclide/ Radiopharmaceutical/ Action	Alternate Names
Myocardial Infarct Scan	Evaluate extent of myocardial damage after acute MI; the PYP adheres to calcium deposits in irreversibly damaged myocardium	Tc-99m (PYP)	PYP cardiac scan, infarct scan, pyrophosphate cardiac scan, acute myocardial infarction scan
Related Study			
Myocardial Perfusion Scan With or Without SPECT	Visualizes areas of reversible ischemia and irreversibly infarcted cardiac tissue; heart movement visualized in three-dimensional images with SPECT; used to evaluate the pharmacological stress test	Tc-99m (sestamibi) or Cardiolite, Tc-99m (tetrofosmin) or Myoview, thallium-201 chloride	Sestamibi scan, cardiac stress scan (because it is often performed with the pharmacological cardiac stress test)

Further information regarding the evaluation of cardiac blood flow can be found in the study titled "Stress Testing: Exercise and Pharmacological."

INDICATIONS

- Aid in the diagnosis of (or confirm and locate) acute MI when ECG and enzyme testing do not provide a diagnosis.
- Aid in the diagnosis of perioperative MI.
- Differentiate between a new and old infarction.
- Evaluate possible reinfarction or extension of the infarct.
- Obtain baseline information about infarction before cardiac surgery.

INTERFERING FACTORS

Contraindications

- Patients who are pregnant or suspected of being pregnant, unless the potential benefits of a procedure using radiation far outweigh the risk of radiation exposure to the fetus and mother.

Factors that may alter the results of the study

- Conditions such as chest wall trauma, cardiac trauma, or recent cardioversion procedure.

- Other conditions that may interfere include:
  - Aneurysms
  - Cardiac tumors
  - Left ventricular aneurysm
  - Metastasis
  - Myocarditis
  - Pericarditis
  - Valvular and coronary artery calcifications
- Metallic objects (e.g., jewelry, body rings) within the examination field or other nuclear scans done within the previous 24 to 48 hr, which may inhibit organ visualization and cause unclear images.

- Improper injection of the radionuclide may allow the tracer to seep deep into the muscle tissue, producing erroneous hot spots.
- Inability of the patient to cooperate or remain still during the procedure, because movement can produce blurred or otherwise unclear images.

POTENTIAL MEDICAL DIAGNOSIS: CLINICAL SIGNIFICANCE OF RESULTS
Abnormal findings related to
- MI, indicated by increased PYP uptake in the myocardium.

NURSING IMPLICATIONS

POTENTIAL NURSING PROBLEMS: ASSESSMENT & NURSING DIAGNOSIS

Problems	Signs and Symptoms
Activity *(related to myocardial ischemia, increased oxygen demands)*	Weakness, fatigue, chest pain with exertion, anxiety
Inadequate cardiac tissue perfusion *(related to blood flow obstruction, oxygen supply/demand mismatch)*	Chest pain, chest pressure, shortness of breath, increased heart rate, cool skin, decreased capillary refill, diminished peripheral pulses, altered cardiac enzymes, confusion, restlessness
Pain *(related to myocardial ischemia, inadequate oxygenation)*	Self-report of chest pain, pressure; radiating pain to the neck, jaw, arm

BEFORE THE STUDY: PLANNING AND IMPLEMENTATION

Teaching the Patient What to Expect
- Inform the patient this procedure can assess blood flow to the heart.
- Pregnancy is a general contraindication to procedures involving radiation. Explain to the female patient that she will be asked the date of her last menstrual period. Pregnancy testing may be performed to determine the possibility of pregnancy before exposure to radiation.
- Review the procedure with the patient. Address concerns about pain and explain that there may be moments of

discomfort or pain experienced when the IV line is inserted to allow infusion of fluids such as saline, anesthetics, sedatives, radionuclides, medications used in the procedure, or emergency medications.
- Explain that the procedure is performed in a nuclear medicine department by a health-care provider (HCP), and staff, specializing in this procedure and takes approximately 30 and 60 min.
- Reassure the patient that the radionuclide poses no radioactive hazard and rarely produces adverse effects.
- Explain that a technologist will administer an IV injection of the radionuclide

and that it will be necessary to return 2 to 4 hr later for the scan.

▶ Instruct the patient to remove jewelry and other metallic objects from the area to be examined.

▶ Positioning for the procedure is in the supine position. Foam wedges may be used to help maintain position and immobilization.

▶ The chest is exposed, and the ECG leads are attached. Baseline readings are recorded immediately prior to administration of the IV radionuclide, and the heart is then scanned.

▶ Scanning of the heart begins after injection and is performed from various positions. In most circumstances, however, SPECT is done so that the heart can be viewed from multiple angles and planes.

▶ Vital signs to monitor oxygen level (pulse oximetry) and blood pressure (sphygmomanometer) are measured before, during (peak), and after the study.

▶ Reassure the patient that he or she will be closely monitored for any complications related to the procedure (e.g., allergic reaction, anaphylaxis, bronchospasm).

▶ Explain that once the study is completed, the needle or catheter is removed and a pressure dressing is applied over the puncture site.

Potential Nursing Actions

✦ *Make sure a written and informed consent has been signed prior to the procedure and before administering any medications.*

▶ Investigate the presence of other risk factors, such as family history of heart disease, smoking, obesity, diet, lack of physical activity, hypertension, diabetes, previous myocardial infarction, and previous vascular disease. Knowledge of genetics assists in identifying those who may benefit from additional education, risk assessment, and counseling. Genetics is the study and identification of genes, genetic mutations, and inheritance. For example, genetics provides some insight into the likelihood of inheriting a medical condition such as coronary

artery disease (CAD). Genomic studies evaluate the interaction of groups of genes. The combined activity or combined expression of groups of genes allows assumptions or predictions to be made. As an example, genomic studies measure the levels of activity in multiple genes to predict how they, along with environmental and lifestyle decisions, influence the development of type 2 diabetes, CAD, MI, or ischemic stroke. Further information regarding inheritance of genes can be found in the study titled "Genetic Testing."

AFTER THE STUDY: POTENTIAL NURSING ACTIONS

Avoiding Complications

▶ Establishing an IV site and injection of radionuclides are invasive procedures. Complications are rare but include risk for allergic reaction *(related to contrast reaction)*, hematoma *(related to blood leakage into the tissue following needle insertion)*, bleeding from the puncture site *(related to a bleeding disorder or the effects of natural products and medications with known anticoagulant, antiplatelet, or thrombolytic properties)*, or infection *(which might occur if bacteria from the skin surface are introduced at the puncture site)*. Monitor the patient for complications related to the procedure (e.g., allergic reaction, anaphylaxis, bronchospasm). Immediately report symptoms such as fast heart rate, difficulty breathing, skin rash, itching, or chest pain to the appropriate HCP. Observe/assess the needle/catheter insertion site for bleeding, inflammation, or hematoma formation.

Treatment Considerations

▶ Explain that the radionuclide is eliminated from the body within 6 to 24 hr. Advise the patient to drink increased amounts of fluids for 24 to 48 hr to eliminate the radionuclide from the body, unless contraindicated.

▶ Instruct the patient to resume usual dietary, medication, and activity, as directed by the HCP.

▶ Monitor vital signs, and neurological status every 15 min for 1 hr, then every

M

2 hr for 4 hr, and compare with baseline values. Monitor intake and output at least every 8 hr and ECG tracings until stable. Protocols may vary among facilities.
▶ Activity: Identify the patient's normal activity patterns. Maintain bedrest as required to rest the heart and conserve oxygen. Administer ordered oxygen, and have patient wear it with activity. Pace activity and increase as tolerated. Monitor and trend vital signs. Discuss the effects of altered cardiac health on sexual activity.
▶ Explain the link between activity and cardiac health and how oxygen administration supports cardiac function.
▶ Inadequate Cardiac Tissue Perfusion: Assess for characteristics of pain: quality, intensity, duration, and location. Monitor and trend vital signs: heart rate, respiratory rate, and blood pressure. Administer ordered oxygen with continuous pulse oximetry and cardiac monitoring. Assess skin color, temperature, and cyanosis. Assess breath sounds rate and rhythm, capillary refill, peripheral pulses, confusion, and restlessness. Monitor and trend laboratory studies: ABGs, creatine phosphokinase, CK-MB, C-reactive protein, and troponin. Administer ordered thrombolytics, morphine, amiodarone, nitroglycerin, beta-blockers.
▶ Discuss the recommended treatment and expected outcomes in relation to the patient's cardiac status.
▶ Discuss the importance of rest periods during the day to conserve oxygen.
▶ Teach the pathophysiology of MI and the purpose of ordered medications (morphine, nitroglycerin, calcium channel blockers, beta blockers).
▶ Describe the lifestyle changes that will need to be made to support positive cardiac health.
▶ Provide access to a registered dietitian to make heart-healthy changes that are culturally congruent.
▶ Encourage the patient and family to meet with a support group to decrease risk of depression.

▶ Assist with recognition and acceptance of the importance of cardiac rehabilitation.
▶ Pain: Administer ordered oxygen. Assess pain character, location, duration, and intensity. Administer ordered medications: morphine, nitroglycerin, calcium channel blockers, beta blockers. Consider alternative measures for pain management (imagery, relaxation, music).

Safety Considerations
▶ The patient who is breastfeeding should consult with the requesting HCP regarding alternate testing that does not involve radiation. In general, if a woman who is breastfeeding must have a nuclear scan, she should not breastfeed the infant for 72 hr after the scan, until the radionuclide has been eliminated. She should be instructed to express the milk in order to prevent cessation of milk production; the milk can be stored and used after the 3-day period.
▶ Refer to organizational policy for additional precautions that may include instructions on handwashing, toilet flushing, limited contact with others, and other aspects of nuclear medicine safety.

Nutritional Considerations
▶ Discuss ideal body weight and the purpose of and relationship between ideal weight and caloric intake to support cardiac health. Review ways to decrease intake of saturated fats and increase intake of polyunsaturated fats. Discuss limiting intake of refined processed sugar and sodium; discuss limiting cholesterol intake to less than 300 mg per day. Encourage the intake of fresh fruits and vegetables, unprocessed carbohydrates, poultry, and grains.
▶ Nutritional therapy is recommended for those with identified CAD risk, especially for those with elevated low-density lipoprotein cholesterol levels, other lipid disorders, diabetes, insulin resistance, or metabolic syndrome. Always consider cultural influences with dietary choices to ensure better

M

adherence to a change in lifestyle. A variety of dietary patterns are beneficial for people with ASCVD. For additional information regarding nutritional guidelines, refer to the study titled "Cholesterol, Total and Fractions."
▶ Other changeable risk factors warranting education include strategies to encourage regular participation of moderate aerobic physical activity three to four times per week, eliminating tobacco use, and adhering to a heart-healthy diet.

▶ Those with elevated triglycerides should be advised to eliminate or reduce alcohol.

Follow-Up, Evaluation, and Desired Outcomes
▶ Acknowledges contact information provided for the American Heart Association (www.heart.org/HEARTORG), National Heart, Lung, and Blood Institute (www.nhlbi.nih.gov), and U.S. Department of Agriculture's resource for nutrition (www.choosemyplate.gov).

Myocardial Perfusion Heart Scan

SYNONYM/ACRONYM: Cardiac stress scan, nuclear stress test, sestamibi scan, stress thallium, thallium scan.

RATIONALE: To assess cardiac blood flow to evaluate for and assist in diagnosing coronary artery disease and myocardial infarction.

PATIENT PREPARATION
• Instruct the patient to fast and refrain from consuming caffeinated beverages for 4 hr, refrain from smoking for 4 to 6 hr, and withhold medications for 24 hr before the test. Instruct the patient to avoid taking anticoagulant medication or to reduce dosage as ordered prior to the procedure. No other radionuclide scans should be scheduled within 24 to 48 hr before this procedure. Protocols may vary among facilities.

NORMAL FINDINGS
• Normal wall motion, ejection fraction (55%–70%), coronary blood flow, tissue perfusion, and ventricular size and function. Mitochondria are responsible for generating the energy required for all cellular function; the amount of radionuclide visualization should reflect normal, active cardiac tissue.

CRITICAL FINDINGS AND POTENTIAL INTERVENTIONS: N/A

OVERVIEW: (Study type: Nuclear scan; related body system: Circulatory system.) Cardiac scanning is a nuclear medicine study that reveals clinical information about coronary blood flow, ventricular size, and cardiac function. Thallium or technetium rest and stress studies are used to evaluate myocardial blood flow to assist in diagnosing or determining the risk for ischemic cardiac disease, coronary artery disease (CAD), and myocardial infarction (MI). This procedure is an alternative to angiography or cardiac catheterization in cases in which these procedures may pose a risk to the patient. Thallium-201 is a potassium analog and is taken up

M

by myocardial cells proportional to blood flow to the cell and cell viability. Technetium-99m radionuclides such as sestamibi (2-methoxyisobutylisonitrile) and tetrofosmin are delivered similarly to thallium-201 (chloride) during myocardial perfusion imaging, but they are extracted to a lesser degree on the first pass through the heart and are taken up by the mitochondria in heart tissue cells. Over a short period, the Tc-99m analogs concentrate in the heart. The advantage of Tc-99m is that immediate imaging is unnecessary because it remains fixed to the heart muscle for several hours. The examination may require two separate injections, one for the rest portion and one for the stress portion of the procedure. These injections can take place on the same day or preferably over a 2-day period. Examination quality is improved if the patient is given a light, fatty meal after the radionuclide is injected to facilitate hepatobiliary clearance of the radioactivity.

Single-photon emission computed tomography (SPECT) can be used to visualize the heart from multiple angles and planes, providing three-dimensional functional images in color that enable areas of ischemia to be viewed with greater accuracy and resolution. This technique removes overlying structures that may confuse interpretation of the results. SPECT also provides accurate, quantitative information regarding the degree of cardiac damage. Myocardial perfusion SPECT is being successfully used as a predictor of the likelihood of future cardiac events in patients with known CAD. Based on the study findings, multigated acquisition (MUGA) scan, also known as *blood pool imaging scan and radionuclide ventriculogram,* may be performed in conjunction with a myocardial perfusion scan. MUGA provides information about cardiac function such as ejection fraction, ventricular wall motion, ventricular dilation, stroke volume, and cardiac output.

For additional information regarding screening guidelines for *atherosclerotic cardiovascular disease* (ASCVD), refer to the study titled "Cholesterol, Total and Fractions."

Comparison of Cardiac Nuclear Scans

	Common Use	Radionuclide/ Radiopharmaceutical/ Action	Alternate Names
Myocardial Perfusion Scan With or Without SPECT	Visualizes areas of reversible ischemia and irreversibly infarcted cardiac tissue; heart movement visualized in three-dimensional images with SPECT; used to evaluate the pharmacological stress test	Tc-99m (sestamibi), Tc-99m (tetrofosmin), thallium-201 chloride	Sestamibi scan, cardiac stress scan (because myocardial perfusion testing is often performed with the exercise or pharmacological cardiac stress test)
Related Studies			
Blood Pool (MUGA): Gated Equilibrium Studies	These studies collect images of heart function and blood flow over numerous cardiac cycles to evaluate the direction of blood flow, wall motion, and most frequently to determine cardiac ejection fraction	Tc-99m (pertechnetate) for in vitro procedure; pyrophosphate (PYP) injection followed by a second injection of Tc-99m (pertechnetate) for in vivo procedure	Blood pool imaging, cardiac flow studies, cardiac equilibrium studies, cardiac nuclear scan, multigated acquisition scan, radionuclide ventriculogram, wall motion study
Blood Pool Scan: First Pass Studies	Determination of direction of blood flow, wall movement, and ejection fraction based on data collected from the initial movement of the radiopharmaceutical as it passes through the heart	Tc-99m (pertechnetate), Tc-99m (pentetate)	Blood pool imaging, cardiac flow studies, cardiac nuclear scan, radionuclide ventriculogram, wall motion study
Myocardial Infarct Scan	Evaluate extent of myocardial damage after acute MI; PYP adheres to calcium deposits in irreversibly damaged myocardium	Tc-99m (PYP)	PYP cardiac scan, infarct scan, pyrophosphate cardiac scan, acute myocardial infarction scan

Further information regarding the evaluation of cardiac blood flow can be found in the study titled "Stress Testing: Exercise and Pharmacological."

INDICATIONS

Adult

- Aid in the diagnosis of CAD or risk for CAD.
- Determine rest defects and reperfusion with delayed imaging in unstable angina.
- Evaluate the extent of CAD and determine cardiac function.
- Assess the function of collateral coronary arteries.
- Evaluate bypass graft patency and general cardiac status after surgery.
- Evaluate the site of an old MI to determine obstruction to cardiac muscle perfusion.
- Evaluate the effectiveness of medication regimen and balloon angioplasty procedure on narrow coronary arteries.

Pediatric

- Assess athletic potential.
- Establish baseline prior to physical rehabilitation therapy.
- Evaluate for cardiac dysfunction related to diagnosed or undiagnosed congenital heart defects or other cardiac issues that manifest symptoms when individual engages in physical activity or exertion.

INTERFERING FACTORS

Contraindications

�֍ Patients who are pregnant or suspected of being pregnant, unless the potential benefits of a procedure using radiation far outweigh the risk of radiation exposure to the fetus and mother.

✖ Patients who have taken sildenafil (Viagra) within the previous 48 hr, *because this test may require the use of nitrates (nitroglycerin) that can precipitate life-threatening low blood pressure.*

✖ Patients with bleeding disorders.

✖ Patients with left ventricular hypertrophy, right and left bundle branch block, and hypokalemia, and patients receiving cardiotonic therapy.

✖ Patients with anginal pain at rest or patients with severe atherosclerotic coronary vessels *in whom dipyridamole testing cannot be performed.*

✖ Patients with asthma, *because chemical stress with vasodilators can cause bronchospasms.*

Factors that may alter the results of the study

- Medications such as digoxin and quinidine, *related to altered cardiac contractility* and nitrates, *related to altered cardiac performance.*
- Single-vessel disease, which can produce false-negative thallium-201 scanning results.
- Excessive eating or exercising between initial and redistribution imaging 4 hr later, which produces false-positive results.
- Conditions such as chest wall trauma, cardiac trauma, angina that is difficult to control, significant cardiac dysrhythmias, or a recent cardioversion procedure may affect test results.
- Metallic objects (e.g., jewelry, body rings) within the examination field or other nuclear scans done within the previous 24 to 48 hr, which may inhibit organ visualization and cause unclear images.
- Improper injection of the radionuclide that allows the tracer to seep deep into the muscle tissue can produce erroneous hot spots.
- Inability of the patient to cooperate or remain still during the procedure, because movement can produce blurred or otherwise unclear images.

POTENTIAL MEDICAL DIAGNOSIS: CLINICAL SIGNIFICANCE OF RESULTS

Abnormal findings related to

Poor visualization or "cold spots" are seen in areas of poor perfusion and diminished cardiac muscle activity.

- Abnormal stress and resting images, indicating previous MI
- Abnormal stress images with normal resting images, indicating transient ischemia
- Cardiac hypertrophy, indicated by increased radionuclide uptake in the myocardium
- Enlarged left ventricle
- Heart chamber disorder
- Heart failure
- Ventricular septal defects

NURSING IMPLICATIONS

BEFORE THE STUDY: PLANNING AND IMPLEMENTATION

Teaching the Patient What to Expect

▶ Inform the patient this procedure can assist in assessing blood flow to the heart.

▶ Pregnancy is a general contraindication to procedures involving radiation. Explain to the female patient that she will be asked the date of her last menstrual period. Pregnancy testing may be performed to determine the possibility of pregnancy before exposure to radiation.

▶ Review the procedure with the patient. Address concerns about pain and explain that there may be moments of discomfort or pain experienced when the IV line is inserted to allow infusion of fluids such as saline, anesthetics, sedatives, radionuclides, medications used in the procedure, or emergency medications.

▶ Explain that the procedure is performed in a nuclear medicine department by a health-care provider (HCP), and staff, specializing in this procedure and takes approximately 30 to 60 min.

▶ Reassure the patient that the radionuclide poses no radioactive hazard and rarely produces adverse effects.

▶ **Pediatric Considerations:** Preparing children for a perfusion heart scan depends on the age of the child. Encourage parents to be truthful about what the child may experience during the procedure and to use words that they know their child will understand. Toddlers and preschool-aged children have a short attention span, so the best time to talk about the test is right before the procedure. The child should be assured that he or she will be allowed to bring a favorite comfort item into the examination room, and if appropriate, that a parent will be with the child during the procedure. Provide older children with information about the test, and allow them to participate in as many decisions as possible (e.g., choice of clothes to wear to the appointment) in order to reduce anxiety and encourage cooperation. If the child will be asked to perform specific movements or exercises for the test, encourage the child to practice the required activities, provide a CD that demonstrates the procedure, and teach strategies to remain calm, such as deep breathing, humming, or counting to himself or herself.

▶ Instruct the patient to remove jewelry and other metallic objects from the area to be examined.

▶ Positioning for the procedure is in the supine position. Foam wedges may be used to help maintain position and immobilization.

▶ The chest is exposed, and the ECG leads are attached. Baseline readings are recorded immediately prior to administration of the IV radionuclide, and the heart is scanned with images taken in various positions over the entire cardiac cycle.

▶ Vital signs to monitor oxygen level (pulse oximetry) and blood pressure (sphygmomanometer) are measured before, during (peak), and after the study.

▶ Depending on results of the resting test, an exercise or pharmacological stress test may also be performed.

▶ Reassure the patient that he or she will be closely monitored for any for

M

complications related to the procedure (e.g., allergic reaction, anaphylaxis, bronchospasm).

◆ Once the scan is completed, the needle or catheter is removed and a pressure dressing is applied over the puncture site.

Potential Nursing Actions

✻ *Make sure a written and informed consent has been signed prior to the procedure and before administering any medications.*

◆ Investigate the presence of other risk factors, such as family history of heart disease, smoking, obesity, diet, lack of physical activity, hypertension, diabetes, previous myocardial infarction, and previous vascular disease. Knowledge of genetics assists in identifying those who may benefit from additional education, risk assessment, and counseling. Genetics is the study and identification of genes, genetic mutations, and inheritance. For example, genetics provides some insight into the likelihood of inheriting a medical condition such as CAD. Genomic studies evaluate the interaction of groups of genes. The combined activity or combined expression of groups of genes allows assumptions or predictions to be made. As an example, genomic studies measure the levels of activity in multiple genes to predict how they, along with environmental and lifestyle decisions, influence the development of type 2 diabetes, CAD, MI, or ischemic stroke. Further information regarding inheritance of genes can be found in the study titled "Genetic Testing."

AFTER THE STUDY: POTENTIAL NURSING ACTIONS

Avoiding Complications

◆ Establishing an IV site and injection of radionuclides are invasive procedures. Complications are rare but include risk for allergic reaction *(related to contrast reaction),* hematoma *(related to blood leakage into the tissue following needle insertion),* bleeding from the puncture site *(related to a bleeding disorder or the effects of natural products and medications with known anticoagulant, antiplatelet, or thrombolytic properties),* or infection *(which might occur if bacteria from the skin surface are introduced at the puncture site).* Monitor the patient for complications related to the procedure (e.g., allergic reaction, anaphylaxis, bronchospasm). Immediately report symptoms such as fast heart rate, difficulty breathing, skin rash, itching, or chest pain to the appropriate HCP. Observe/assess the needle/catheter insertion site for bleeding, inflammation, or hematoma formation.

Treatment Considerations

◆ Explain that the radionuclide is eliminated from the body within 6 to 24 hr. Advise the patient to drink increased amounts of fluids for 24 to 48 hr to eliminate the radionuclide from the body, unless contraindicated.

◆ Instruct the patient to resume usual dietary, medication, and activity, as directed by the HCP.

◆ Monitor vital signs, and neurological status every 15 min for 1 hr, then every 2 hr for 4 hr, and compare with baseline values. Monitor intake and output at least every 8 hr and ECG tracings until stable. Protocols may vary among facilities.

◆ Poor cardiac perfusion can be seen in physical assessment results. Alterations will be seen in skin color (cyanosis), temperature, breath sounds (rate, rhythm), confusion, capillary refill, and peripheral pulses. Appropriate interventions could include administration of ordered medications: thrombolytics, amiodarone, nitroglycerin. Monitor laboratory studies: arterial blood gases, creatine phosphokinase, CK-MB, C-reactive protein, and troponin.

◆ Evaluate the patient's ability to perform activities. Decreasing tolerance can be an indicator of diminishing cardiac health. Identify the patient's normal

M

activity patterns and encourage pacing activities to rest the heart.

◗ Discuss the importance of rest periods during the day to conserve oxygen.

◗ Explain the link between activity and cardiac health and how oxygen administration supports cardiac function.

◗ Discuss the recommended treatment and expected outcomes in relation to their cardiac status.

◗ Pain is a common concern with poor cardiac health. Assess pain character, location, duration, and intensity using an easily understood pain rating scale. Place in a position of comfort, administer ordered medications, and consider alternative measures for pain management (imagery, relaxation, music).

◗ Teach the pathophysiology of MI and the purpose of ordered medications (morphine, nitroglycerin, calcium channel blockers, beta blockers).

◗ Describe the lifestyle changes that will need to be made to support positive cardiac health.

◗ Provide access to a registered dietician to make heart-healthy changes that are culturally congruent.

◗ Encourage the patient and family to meet with a support group to decrease risk of depression.

◗ Assist with recognition and acceptance of the importance of cardiac rehabilitation.

Safety Considerations

◗ The patient who is breastfeeding should consult with the requesting HCP regarding alternate testing that does not involve radiation. In general, if a woman who is breastfeeding must have a nuclear scan, she should not breastfeed the infant for 72 hr after the scan, until the radionuclide has been eliminated. She should be instructed to express the milk in order to prevent cessation of milk production; the milk can be stored and used after the 3-day period.

◗ Refer to organizational policy that may include additional precautions that may include instructions on handwashing, toilet flushing, limited contact with others, and other aspects of nuclear medicine safety.

Nutritional Considerations

◗ Discuss ideal body weight and the purpose of and relationship between ideal weight and caloric intake to support cardiac health. Review ways to decrease intake of saturated fats and increase intake of polyunsaturated fats. Discuss limiting intake of refined processed sugar and sodium; discuss limiting cholesterol intake to less than 300 mg per day. Encourage the intake of fresh fruits and vegetables, unprocessed carbohydrates, poultry, and grains.

◗ Nutritional therapy is recommended for those with identified CAD risk, especially for those with elevated low-density lipoprotein cholesterol levels, other lipid disorders, diabetes, insulin resistance, or metabolic syndrome. Always consider cultural influences with dietary choices to ensure better adherence to a change in lifestyle. A variety of dietary patterns are beneficial for people with ASCVD. For additional information regarding nutritional guidelines, refer to the study titled "Cholesterol, Total and Fractions."

◗ Other changeable risk factors warranting education include strategies to encourage regular participation of moderate aerobic physical activity three to four times per week, eliminating tobacco use, and adhering to a heart-healthy diet.

◗ Those with elevated triglycerides should be advised to eliminate or reduce alcohol.

Follow-Up, Evaluation, and Desired Outcomes

◗ Acknowledges contact information provided for the American Heart Association (www.heart.org/HEARTORG), National Heart, Lung, and Blood Institute (www.nhlbi.nih.gov), and U.S. Department of Agriculture's resource for nutrition (www.choosemyplate.gov).

M

Myoglobin

SYNONYM/ACRONYM: MB.

RATIONALE: A general assessment of damage to skeletal or cardiac muscle from trauma or inflammation.

PATIENT PREPARATION: There are no food, fluid, activity, or medication restrictions unless by medical direction.

NORMAL FINDINGS: Method: Electrochemiluminescent immunoassay.

	Conventional Units	SI Units (Conventional Units × 0.0571)
Male	28–72 ng/mL	1.6–4.1 nmol/L
Female	25–58 ng/mL	1.4–3.3 nmol/L

Values are higher in males, *related to higher muscle mass,* and lower in older adults, *related to decreased muscle mass.*

CRITICAL FINDINGS AND POTENTIAL INTERVENTIONS: N/A

OVERVIEW: (Study type: Blood collected in a red- or red/gray-top tube; **related body system:** Circulatory and Musculoskeletal systems.) Myoglobin is an oxygen-binding muscle protein normally found in skeletal and cardiac muscle. It is released into the bloodstream after muscle damage from ischemia, trauma, or inflammation.

Although myoglobin testing is more sensitive than creatinine kinase and isoenzymes, it does not indicate the specific site involved. For additional information regarding screening guidelines for *atherosclerotic cardiovascular disease* (ASCVD), refer to the study titled "Cholesterol, Total and Fractions."

Timing for Appearance and Resolution of Serum/Plasma Cardiac Markers in Acute Myocardial Infarction

Cardiac Marker	Appearance (Hr)	Peak (Hr)	Resolution (Days)
CK (total)	4–6	24	2–3
CK-MB	4–6	15–20	2–3
LDH	12	24–48	10–14
Myoglobin	1–3	4–12	1
Troponin I	2–6	15–20	5–7

CK = creatine kinase; CK-MB = creatine kinase myocardial band; LDH = lactate dehydrogenase.

INDICATIONS
• Assist in predicting a flare-up of polymyositis.
• Estimate damage from skeletal muscle injury or myocardial infarction (MI).

INTERFERING FACTORS: N/A

POTENTIAL MEDICAL DIAGNOSIS: CLINICAL SIGNIFICANCE OF RESULTS

Increased in

Conditions that cause muscle damage; damaged muscle cells release myoglobin into circulation.

- Cardiac surgery
- Chronic kidney disease
- Cocaine use *(rhabdomyolysis is a complication of cocaine use or overdose)*
- Exercise
- Malignant hyperthermia
- MI
- Progressive muscular dystrophy
- Rhabdomyolysis
- Shock
- Thrombolytic therapy

Decreased in
- Myasthenia gravis
- Presence of antibodies to myoglobin, as seen in patients with polymyositis
- Rheumatoid arthritis

NURSING IMPLICATIONS

BEFORE THE STUDY: PLANNING AND IMPLEMENTATION

Teaching the Patient What to Expect
- Inform the patient this test can assist in diagnosing cardiac or skeletal muscle damage.
- Explain that a blood sample is needed for the test.

AFTER THE STUDY: POTENTIAL NURSING ACTIONS

Treatment Considerations
- Cardiac output may be decreased. This can be seen through assessment results that show dizziness, altered level of consciousness, peripheral edema, cool skin, cyanosis, and weak peripheral pulses. Some interventions that can be used to address this concern are the administration of oxygen and ordered medications such as diuretics, procainamide, beta blockers, antidysrhythmics, atropine, calcium channel blockers, and amiodarone. Electrocardiogram results and vital signs should be trended, and it may be necessary to prepare for cardioversion or pacemaker placement.
- Mobility can be a concern for those with cardiac disease. To facilitate mobility, encourage the use of appropriate assistive devices, including braces and wheelchairs. Encourage active and passive range-of-motion exercises, promote independence, and facilitate physical therapy as prescribed by the health-care provider (HCP).

Nutritional Considerations
- Discuss ideal body weight and the purpose of and relationship between ideal weight and caloric intake to support cardiac health. Review ways to decrease intake of saturated fats and increase intake of polyunsaturated fats. Discuss limiting intake of refined processed sugar and sodium; discuss limiting cholesterol intake to less than 300 mg per day. Encourage the intake of fresh fruits and vegetables, unprocessed carbohydrates, poultry, and grains.
- Nutritional therapy is recommended for those with identified coronary artery disease risk, especially for those with elevated low-density lipoprotein cholesterol levels, other lipid disorders, diabetes, insulin resistance, or metabolic syndrome. Always consider cultural influences with dietary choices to ensure better adherence to a change in lifestyle. A variety of dietary patterns are beneficial for people with ASCVD. For additional information regarding nutritional guidelines, refer to the study titled "Cholesterol, Total and Fractions."
- Other changeable risk factors warranting education include strategies to encourage regular participation of moderate aerobic physical activity three to four times per week, eliminating tobacco use, and adhering to a heart-healthy diet.

M

▶ Those with elevated triglycerides should be advised to eliminate or reduce alcohol.

Follow-Up, Evaluation, and Desired Outcomes

▶ Acknowledges provided contact information the American Heart Association (www.heart.org/HEARTORG),

National Heart, Lung, and Blood Institute (www.nhlbi.nih.gov), and U.S. Department of Agriculture's resource for nutrition (www.choosemyplate .gov).

▶ Recognizes that further testing, treatment, or referral to another HCP may be necessary to treat and manage the disease.

M

Nerve Fiber Analysis

SYNONYM/ACRONYM: NFA.

RATIONALE: To assist in measuring the thickness of the retinal nerve fiber layer, to assist in diagnosing diseases of the eye such as glaucoma.

PATIENT PREPARATION: There are no food, fluid, activity, or medication restrictions unless by medical direction.

NORMAL FINDINGS
• Normal nerve fiber layer thickness.

CRITICAL FINDINGS AND POTENTIAL INTERVENTIONS: N/A

OVERVIEW: (Study type: Sensory (ocular); related body system: Nervous system.) There are over 1 million ganglion nerve cells in the retina of each eye. Each nerve cell has a long fiber that travels through the nerve fiber layer of the retina and exits the eye through the optic nerve. The optic nerve is made up of all the ganglion nerve fibers and connects the eye to the brain for vision to occur. As the ganglion cells die, the nerve fiber layer becomes thinner and an empty space in the optic nerve, called the *cup*, becomes larger. The thinning of the nerve fiber layer and the enlargement of the nerve fiber cup are measurements used to gauge the extent of damage to the retina. Significant damage to the nerve fiber layer occurs before loss of vision is noticed by the patient. Damage can be caused by glaucoma, aging, or occlusion of the vessels in the retina. Ganglion cell loss due to glaucoma begins in the periphery of the retina, thereby first affecting peripheral vision. This change in vision can also be detected by visual field testing. There are several different techniques for measuring nerve fiber layer thickness. The equipment used to perform the test determines whether dilation of the pupils is required (by optical coherence tomography [OCT]) or avoided (by GDx scanning laser polarimetry). One of the most common is scanning laser polarimetry. The amount of change in polarization correlates to the thickness of the retinal nerve fiber layer.

INDICATIONS
• Assist in the diagnosis of eye diseases.
• Determine retinal nerve fiber layer thickness.
• Monitor the effects of various therapies or the progression of conditions resulting in loss of vision.

INTERFERING FACTORS
Factors that may alter the results of the study
• Inability of the patient to fixate on focal point.
• Corneal disorder that prevents proper alignment of the retinal nerve fibers.
• Dense cataract that prevents visualization of a clear nerve fiber image.

POTENTIAL MEDICAL DIAGNOSIS: CLINICAL SIGNIFICANCE OF RESULTS
Abnormal findings related to
• Glaucoma or suspicion of glaucoma
• Ocular hypertension
• Optic nerve disease

N

NURSING IMPLICATIONS

BEFORE THE STUDY: PLANNING AND IMPLEMENTATION

Teaching the Patient What to Expect

▶ Inform the patient this procedure can assist in diagnosing eye disease.

▶ Review the procedure with the patient and explain that no pain will be experienced during the test, but there may be moments of discomfort after the test when the numbness wears off from anesthetic drops administered prior to the test.

▶ Explain that a health-care provider (HCP) performs the test and that to evaluate both eyes, the test can take 10 to 15 min.

▶ The patient will be seated during the test and instructed to look straight ahead, keeping the eyes open and unblinking.

▶ Topical anesthetic drops will be instilled in each eye and allowed time to take effect.

▶ The equipment used to perform the test determines whether dilation of the pupils is required (OCT) or avoided (GDx).

▶ The patient will be asked to look straight ahead at a fixation light with the chin in the chin rest and forehead against the support bar.

▶ There should be no movement of the eyes or blinking as the measurement is taken.

▶ Baseline data is stored, and the mean image from current and previous data can be retrieved as the computer makes a comparison against previous images.

Potential Nursing Actions

▶ Investigate history of the patient's known or suspected vision loss, including type and cause; eye conditions with treatment regimens; eye surgery; and other tests and procedures to assess and diagnose visual deficit.

▶ Investigate history of narrow-angle glaucoma, known or suspected visual impairment, changes in visual acuity, and use of glasses or contact lenses.

▶ Advise the patient to remove contact lenses or glasses, as appropriate.

AFTER THE STUDY: POTENTIAL NURSING ACTIONS

Treatment Considerations

▶ Instruct the patient in the use of any ordered medications, usually eye drops.

▶ Explain the ocular adverse effects associated with the prescribed medication and encourage a review of corresponding literature provided by a pharmacist.

▶ Explain the importance of adhering to the therapy regimen, especially because glaucoma does not present symptoms.

▶ Be supportive of impaired activity related to vision loss or anticipated loss of driving privileges.

Follow-Up, Evaluation, and Desired Outcomes

▶ Acknowledges contact information provided for the Glaucoma Research Foundation (www.glaucoma.org).

Newborn Screening

SYNONYM/ACRONYM: NBS, newborn metabolic screening, tests for inborn errors of metabolism, early hearing loss detection and intervention for newborns.

RATIONALE: To evaluate newborns for congenital abnormalities, which may include hearing loss; identification of hemoglobin variants such as thalassemias and sickle cell anemia; presence of antibodies that would indicate an HIV infection; or metabolic disorders such as homocystinuria, maple syrup urine disease (MSUD), phenylketonuria (PKU), tyrosinuria, and unexplained physical or intellectual disabilities.

PATIENT PREPARATION: There are no food, fluid, activity, or medication restrictions unless by medical direction.

NORMAL FINDINGS: Method: Thyroxine, TSH, and HIV—immunoassay; amino acids—tandem mass spectrometry; hemoglobin variants—electrophoresis.

Hearing Test

Age	Normal Findings
Neonates–3 days	Normal pure tone average of −10 to 15 dB

Thyroid-Stimulating Hormone (TSH)

Age	Conventional Units	SI Units (Conventional Units × 1)
Neonates–3 days	Less than 40 micro-international units/mL	Less than 40 milli-international units/L

Thyroxine, Total

Age	Conventional Units	SI Units (Conventional Units × 12.9)
Neonates–30 days	5.4–22.6 mcg/dL	69.7–291.5 nmol/L

Hemoglobinopathies	Normal Hemoglobin Pattern
Blood spot amino acid analysis	Normal findings. Numerous amino acids are evaluated by blood spot testing, and values vary by method and laboratory. The testing laboratory should be consulted for corresponding reference ranges.

Infectious disease	Normal Findings
HIV antibodies	Negative

CRITICAL FINDINGS AND POTENTIAL INTERVENTIONS: N/A

OVERVIEW: (Study type: Blood [see individual studies for specimen requirements]; related body system: Circulatory/Hematopoietic, Endocrine, Digestive, Immune, Nervous, and Reproductive systems.) Newborn screening is a process used to evaluate infants for disorders that are treatable but difficult to identify by direct observation of diagnosable symptoms. The testing is conducted shortly after birth through a collaborative effort between government agencies, local public health departments, hospitals, and parents. Knowledge of genetics assists in identifying those who may benefit from additional education, risk assessment, and counseling. Genetics is the study and identification of genes, genetic mutations, and inheritance. For example, genetics provides some insight into the likelihood of inheriting a medical condition such as cystic fibrosis (CF), an aminoacidopathy, or a hemoglobinopathy. Some conditions are the result of mutations involving a single gene, whereas other conditions may involve multiple genes and/or multiple chromosomes. Sickle cell disease is an example of an autosomal recessive disorder in which the offspring inherits a copy of the defective gene from each parent. Further information regarding inheritance of genes can be found in the study titled "Genetic Testing."

Every state and territory in the United States has a newborn screening program that includes early hearing loss detection and intervention (EHDI). The goal of EHDI is to assure that permanent hearing loss is identified before 3 mo of age, appropriate and timely intervention services are provided before 6 mo of age, families of infants with hearing loss receive culturally competent support, and tracking and data management systems for newborn hearing screens are linked with other relevant public health information systems. For more detailed information, refer to the study titled "Audiometry, Hearing Loss." Testing of interest that is not included in the mandatory list can be requested by a health-care provider (HCP), as appropriate. Confirmatory testing is performed if abnormal findings are produced by screening methods. Properly collected blood spot cards contain sufficient sample to perform both screening and confirmatory testing. Confirmatory testing varies depending on the initial screen and can include fatty acid oxidation probe tests on skin samples, enzyme uptake testing of skin or muscle tissue samples, enzyme assays of blood samples, DNA testing, gas chromatography/mass spectrometry, and tandem mass spectrometry. Testing for common genetically transferred conditions can be performed on either or both prospective parents by blood tests, skin tests, or DNA testing. DNA testing can also be performed on the fetus, in utero, through the collection of fetal cells by amniocentesis or chorionic villus sampling. Counseling and written, informed consent are recommended and sometimes required before genetic testing.

The adrenal glands are responsible for production of the hormones cortisol, aldosterone, and male sex androgens. Most infants born with congenital adrenal hyperplasia (CAH) make too much of the androgen hormones and not enough cortisol or aldosterone. The complex feedback loops in the body call for the adrenal glands to increase production of cortisol and aldosterone, and as the adrenal glands work harder to increase production, they increase in size, resulting in hyperplasia. CAH is a group of conditions.

Most frequently, lack of or dysfunction of an enzyme called *21-hydroxylase* results in one of two types of CAH. The first is a salt-wasting condition in which insufficient levels of aldosterone causes too much salt and water to be lost in the urine. Newborns with this condition are poor feeders and appear lethargic or sleepy. Other symptoms include vomiting, diarrhea, and dehydration, which can lead to weight loss, low blood pressure, and decreased electrolytes. If untreated, these symptoms can result in metabolic acidosis and shock, which in CAH infants is called an *adrenal crisis.* Signs of an adrenal crisis include confusion, irritability, tachycardia, and coma. The second-most common type of CAH is a condition in which having too much of the androgen hormones in the blood causes female babies to develop masculinized or virilized genitals. High levels of androgens leads to precocious sexual development, well before the normal age of puberty, in both boys and girls.

Inadequate production of the thyroid hormone thyroxine can result in congenital hypothyroidism, which when untreated manifests in severely delayed physical and intellectual development. Inadequate production may be due to a defect such as a missing, misplaced, or malfunctioning thyroid gland. Inadequate production may also be due to the mother's thyroid condition or treatment during pregnancy or, less commonly encountered in developed nations, a maternal deficiency of iodine. Most newborns do not exhibit signs and symptoms of thyroxine deficiency during the first few weeks of life while they function on the hormone provided by their mother. As the maternal thyroxine is metabolized, some of the symptoms that ensue include coarse, swollen facial features; wide, short hands; respiratory problems; a hoarse-sounding cry; poor weight gain and small stature; delayed occurrence of developmental milestones such as sitting up, crawling, walking, and talking; goiter; anemia; bradycardia; myxedema (accumulation of fluid under the skin); and hearing loss. Children who remain untreated usually demonstrate physical and intellectual disabilities. They may have an unsteady gait and lack coordination. Most demonstrate delays in development of speech, and some have behavioral problems.

Hemoglobin (Hgb) A is the main form of Hgb in the healthy adult. Hgb F is the main form of Hgb in the fetus, the remainder being composed of Hgb A_1 and A_2. Hgb S and C result from abnormal amino acid substitutions during the formation of Hgb and are inherited hemoglobinopathies. Hgb S results from an amino acid substitution during Hgb synthesis whereby valine replaces glutamic acid. Hgb C Harlem results from the substitution of lysine for glutamic acid. Hgb electrophoresis is a separation process used to identify normal and abnormal forms of Hgb. Electrophoresis and high-performance liquid chromatography as well as molecular genetics testing for mutations can also be used to identify abnormal forms of Hgb. Individuals with sickle cell disease have chronic anemia because the abnormal Hgb is unable to carry oxygen. The red blood cells of affected

N

individuals are also abnormal in shape, resembling a crescent or sickle rather than the normal disk shape. This abnormality, combined with cell-wall rigidity, prevents the cells from passing through smaller blood vessels. Blockages in blood vessels result in hypoxia, damage, and pain. Individuals with the sickle cell trait do not have the clinical manifestations of the disease but may pass the disease on to children if the other parent has the trait (or the disease) as well.

Amino acids are required for the production of proteins, enzymes, coenzymes, hormones, nucleic acids used to form DNA, pigments such as Hgb, and neurotransmitters. Testing for specific aminoacidopathies is generally performed on infants after an initial screening test with abnormal results. Certain congenital enzyme deficiencies interfere with normal amino acid metabolism and cause excessive accumulation of or deficiencies in amino acid levels. The major genetic disorders include PKU, MSUD, and tyrosinuria. Enzyme disorders can also result in conditions of dysfunctional fatty acid or organic acid metabolism in which toxic substances accumulate in the body and, if untreated, can result in death. Infants with these conditions often appear normal and healthy at birth. Symptoms can appear soon after feeding begins or not until the first months of life, depending on the specific condition. Most of the signs and symptoms of amino acid disorders in infants include poor feeding, lethargy, vomiting,

and irritability. Newborns with MSUD produce urine that smells like maple syrup or burned sugar. Accumulation of ammonia, a by-product of protein metabolism, and the corresponding amino acids results in progressive liver damage, hepatomegaly, jaundice, and tendency to bruise and bleed. If untreated, there may be delays in growth, lack of coordination, and permanent learning and intellectual disabilities. Early diagnosis and treatment of certain aminoacidopathies can prevent intellectual disabilities, reduced growth rates, and various unexplained symptoms.

CF is a genetic disease that affects normal functioning of the exocrine glands, causing them to excrete large amounts of electrolytes. CF is characterized by abnormal exocrine secretions within the lungs, pancreas, small intestine, bile ducts, and skin. Some of the signs and symptoms that may be demonstrated by the newborn with CF include failure to thrive, salty sweat, chronic respiratory problems (constant coughing or wheezing, thick mucus, recurrent lung and sinus infections, nasal polyps), and chronic gastrointestinal problems (diarrhea, constipation, pain, gas, and greasy, malodorous stools that are bulky and pale colored). Patients with CF have sweat electrolyte levels two to five times normal. Sweat test values, with family history and signs and symptoms, are required to establish a diagnosis of CF. Clinical presentation may include chronic problems of the gastrointestinal and/or respiratory system. CF is more common in Caucasians than in other populations. Testing of stool samples for decreased trypsin activity has been used as a screen for CF in infants and children, but this is a much less reliable method than the sweat test. Sweat conductivity is a screening method that estimates chloride levels. Sweat conductivity values greater than or equal to 50 mEq/L should be referred for quantitative analysis of sweat chloride. The sweat electrolyte test is still considered the gold standard diagnostic for CF.

Biotin is an important water-soluble vitamin/cofactor that aids in the metabolism of fats, carbohydrates, and proteins. A congenital enzyme deficiency of biotinidase prevents biotin released during normal cellular turnover or via digested dietary proteins from being properly recycled and absorbed, resulting in biotin deficiency. Signs and symptoms of biotin deficiency appear within the first few months and can result in hypotonia, poor coordination, respiratory problems, delays in development, seizures, behavioral disorders, and learning disabilities. Untreated, the deficiency can lead to loss of vision and hearing, ataxia, skin rashes, and hair loss.

Lactose, the main sugar in milk and milk products, is composed of galactose and glucose. Galactosemia occurs when there is a deficiency of the enzyme galactose-1-phosphate uridyl transferase, which is responsible for the conversion of galactose into glucose. The inability of dietary galactose and lactose to be metabolized results in the accumulation of galactose-1-phosphate,

which causes damage to the liver, central nervous system, and other body systems. Newborns with galactosemia usually have diarrhea and vomiting within a few days of drinking milk or formula containing lactose. Other early symptoms include poor suckling and feeding, failure to gain weight or grow in length, lethargy, and irritability. The accumulation of galactose-1-phosphate and ammonia is damaging to the liver, and symptoms likely to follow if untreated include hypoglycemia, seizures, coma, hepatomegaly, jaundice, bleeding, shock, and life-threatening bacteremia or septicemia. Early cataracts can occur in about 10% of children with galactosemia. Most untreated children eventually die of liver failure.

HIV is the cause of AIDS and is transmitted through bodily secretions, especially by blood or sexual contact. The virus preferentially binds to the T4 helper lymphocytes and replicates within the cells. Current assays detect several viral proteins. Positive results should be confirmed by Western blot assay. This test is routinely recommended as part of a prenatal work-up and is required for evaluating donated blood units before release for transfusion. The Centers for Disease Control and Prevention (CDC) has structured its recommendations to increase identification of HIV-infected patients as early as possible; early identification increases treatment options, increases frequency of successful treatment, and can decrease further spread of disease.

(text continues on page 878)

N

Core Conditions Evaluated

Condition	Affected Component	Marker for Disease	Incidence	Potential Therapeutic Interventions	Outcomes of Therapeutic Interventions
Hearing loss	Damage to or malformations of the inner ear	Abnormal audiogram	1 in 3,000 births	Surgery, medications for infections, removal of substances blocking the ear canal, hearing aids	A shorter period of auditory deprivation has a positive impact on normal development.
CAH (classical)	Multiple types of CAH; majority have a deficiency of or nonfunctioning enzyme: 21-hydroxylase	17-Hydroxyprogesterone (17-OHP)	1 in 15,000 births (75% have salt-wasting type; 25% have virilization type)	Oral cortisone administration, surgery for females with virilization	Patients who begin treatment soon after birth usually have normal growth and development.
Congenital hypothyroidism	Missing, misplaced, or malfunctioning thyroid gland resulting in insufficient thyroxine; insufficient thyroxine due to maternal thyroid condition or treatment with antithyroid medications during pregnancy	Thyroxine (total), thyroid-stimulating hormone	1 in 3,000–4,000 births	Administration of L-thyroxine	Patients who begin treatment soon after birth usually have normal growth and development.

Sickle cell disease (SCD) and thalassemia	Variant hemoglobin	Hgb S: amino acid substitution of valine for glutamic acid in the beta-globin chain; Hgb C: amino acid substitution of lysine for glutamic acid in the beta-globin chain; thalassemia: loss of two amino acids in the alpha-globin chain or decreased production of the beta-globin chain	Hgb S: 1 in 3,700 births; Hgb S/C: 1 in 7,400 births; Hgb S/beta-thalassemia 1 in 50,000 births (found more often in people of African, Mediterranean, Middle Eastern, and Asian descent and in parts of the world where malaria is endemic)	Care of patients with Hgb S is complex, and the main goal is to prevent complications from infection, blindness from damaged blood vessels in the eye, anemia, dehydration, and fatigue; some thalassemias may require iron supplementation	The goal with treatment is to lessen symptoms. Treatment cannot cure the condition. Symptoms may occur in spite of good treatment.

Inborn Errors of Amino Acid Metabolism

Argininosuccinic aciduria (ASA)	Deficiency of or nonfunctioning enzyme: argininosuccinic acid lyase	Argininosuccinic acid lyase	1 in 70,000 births	Consultation with a dietitian; low-protein diet supplemented by special medical foods and formula	Patients who begin treatment soon after birth and continue treatment throughout life usually have normal growth and development. Early treatment can help prevent high ammonia levels.

(table continues on page 872)

Core Conditions Evaluated

Condition	Affected Component	Marker for Disease	Incidence	Potential Therapeutic Interventions	Outcomes of Therapeutic Interventions
					Accumulation of ammonia can cause brain damage, resulting in lifelong learning problems, intellectual disabilities, or lack of coordination.
Citrullinemia type I	Deficiency of or nonfunctioning enzyme: argininosuccinate synthetase	Citrulline	1 in 57,000 births	Consultation with a dietitian; low-protein diet supplemented by special medical foods and formula	Patients who begin treatment soon after birth and continue treatment throughout life usually have normal growth and development. Early treatment can help prevent high ammonia levels. Accumulation of ammonia can cause brain damage, resulting in lifelong learning problems, intellectual disabilities, or lack of coordination.

Disease	Deficiency of or nonfunctioning enzyme	Amino acid	Incidence	Treatment	Outcome
Homocystinuria	Deficiency of or nonfunctioning enzyme: cystathionine beta-synthase	Methionine	Less than 1 in 50,000 births (found more often in white people from the New England region of the United States and in people of Irish ancestry)	Consultation with dietitian; diet low in methionine supplemented by special medical foods; administration of vitamin B_6, vitamin B_{12}, folic acid, betaine, and L-cystine	Patients who begin treatment soon after birth and continue treatment throughout life usually have normal growth and development. Treatment may lower the chance of blood clots, heart disease, and stroke. Treatment also lessens the chance of eye problems such as cataract or lens dislocation, which can often be corrected by surgery.
MSUD	Deficiency of or nonfunctioning enzyme group: branched-chain ketoacid dehydrogenase	Leucine and isoleucine	Less than 1 in 100,000 births (found more often in Mennonite people: about 1 in 380 babies of Mennonite background are born with MSUD; also	Consultation with a dietitian; diet low in branched-chain amino acids supplemented by special medical foods and formula; administration of thiamine; liver transplant	Patients who begin treatment soon after birth and continue treatment throughout life usually have normal growth and development. Untreated or delayed treatment results in brain damage and intellectual disabilities.

(table continues on page 874)

Core Conditions Evaluated

Condition	Affected Component	Marker for Disease	Incidence	Potential Therapeutic Interventions	Outcomes of Therapeutic Interventions
Phenylketonuria	Deficiency of or nonfunctioning enzyme: phenylalanine hydroxylase (PAH)	Phenylalanine	1 in 10,000 births (found more often in people of Irish, Northern European, Turkish, or Native American ancestry; found more often in people of French-Canadian ancestry)	Consultation with a dietitian; diet low in phenylalanine supplemented by special medical foods and formula; administration of BH4 (tetrahydrobiopterin), which helps the PAH enzyme convert phenylalanine to tyrosine; patients with this condition should avoid foods and vitamins containing the sugar substitute aspartame, which increases blood levels of phenylalanine	Patients who begin treatment soon after birth and continue treatment throughout life usually have normal growth and development. Some patients may experience delays in learning even after treatment, but without treatment or if treatment is delayed until after 6 mo of age, intellectual disabilities usually result.

N

Inborn Errors of Fatty Acid Metabolism

Medium-chain acyl-CoA dehydrogenase deficiency	Deficiency of or nonfunctioning enzyme: medium-chain acyl-CoA dehydrogenase	Octanoylcarnitine and acylcarnitine	1 in 15,000 births (found more often in white people from Northern Europe and the United States)	Consultation with a dietitian; low-fat, high-carbohydrate diet supplemented by special medical foods and formula consumed in small, frequent meals to avoid hypoglycemia; infants may need to be woken up to eat if they do not wake up on their own; administration of medium-chain triglycerides (MCT) oil and L-carnitine	Patients who begin treatment soon after birth and continue treatment throughout life usually have normal growth and development. Continued episodes of hypoglycemia can lead to lack of coordination, chronic muscle weakness, learning or intellectual disabilities.

Inborn Errors of Organic Acid Metabolism

Glutaric acidemia type 1	Deficiency of or nonfunctioning enzyme: glutaryl-CoA dehydrogenase	Glutarylcarnitine	1 in 40,000 births (found more often in people of Amish background in the United States, the Ojibway Indian population	Consultation with a dietitian; diet high in carbohydrates, low in protein, especially lysine and tryptophan, supplemented by special medical foods and formula consumed in small,	Patients who begin treatment soon after birth and continue treatment throughout life usually have normal growth and development.

(table continues on page 876)

Core Conditions Evaluated

Condition	Affected Component	Marker for Disease	Incidence	Potential Therapeutic Interventions	Outcomes of Therapeutic Interventions
			in Canada, and people of Swedish ancestry)	frequent meals; administration of riboflavin, carnitine	Patients who begin treatment soon after birth and continue treatment throughout life usually have normal growth and development. Some patients may experience delays in learning even after treatment, but without treatment or if treatment is delayed until after 10 days of age, developmental delays and learning disabilities usually result.
Inborn Errors of Carbohydrate Metabolism					
Galactosemia (classical)	Deficiency of or nonfunctioning enzyme: galactose-1-phosphate uridyl transferase	Galactose-1-phosphate	Greater than 1 in 50,000 births	Consultation with a dietitian; diet free of lactose and galactose supplemented by special medical foods and formula; administration of calcium, vitamin D, and vitamin K	

2

Other Multisystem Diseases

Disease	Deficiency of Enzyme or Function	Screening Test	Incidence	Treatment	Prognosis
CF	Deficiency of or nonfunctioning protein: CF transmembrane conductance regulator protein	CF mutation analysis or immunoreactive trypsinogen	1 in 3,600 to 3,700 births	Consultation with a dietitian; higher calorie diet supplemented by special medical foods and formula, additional hydration, administration of pancreatic enzymes and vitamins; bronchodilators, antibiotics, mucus thinners; percussive therapy, airway clearance vest; gene therapy, lung transplant	Patients who begin treatment soon after birth and continue treatment throughout life usually have normal growth and development. The goal of treatment is to lessen symptoms. Treatment cannot cure the condition. Symptoms may occur in spite of good treatment.

Rare Conditions

Inborn Errors of Amino Acid Metabolism
- Tyrosinemia type 1

Inborn Errors of Fatty Acid Metabolism
- Carnitine uptake disorder
- Long-chain L-3-hydroxyacyl-CoA dehydrogenase deficiency
- Trifunctional protein (TFP) deficiency
- Very-long-chain acyl-CoA dehydrogenase deficiency

Inborn Errors of Organic Acid Metabolism
- 3-Hydroxy, 3-methylglutaric aciduria
- Beta ketothiolase
- Isovaleric acidemia
- Methyl malonic acidemias (vitamin B_{12} disorders)
- Multiple carboxylase (holocarboxylase)
- Propionic acidemia

Other Multisystem Diseases
- Biotinidase deficiency

INDICATIONS

Hearing Tests
- Screen for hearing loss in infants to determine the need for a referral to an audiologist.

Blood Spot Testing
- Assist in the diagnosis of CAH.
- Assist in the diagnosis of congenital hypothyroidism.
- Assist in the diagnosis of abnormal hemoglobins as with Hgb C disease, sickle cell trait or sickle cell disease, and thalassemias, especially in patients with a family history positive for any of the disorders.
- Assist in identifying the cause of hemolytic anemia resulting from glucose-6-phosphate dehydrogenase (G6PD) enzyme deficiency.

- Detect congenital errors of amino acid, fatty acid, or organic acid metabolism.
- Detect congenital errors responsible for urea cycle disorders.
- Screen for multisystem disorders such as CF, biotinidase deficiency, or galactosemia.
- Test for HIV antibodies in infants who have documented and significant exposure to other infected individuals.

INTERFERING FACTORS

Factors that may alter the results of the study
- Specimens for newborn screening that are collected earlier than 24 hr after the first feeding *(false-negative results related to insufficient time after feeding for the abnormal metabolites to accumulate)* or from neonates receiving total parenteral nutrition *(false-negative results if circulating levels of the amino acids are increased above the detectable limit of the test)* may produce invalid results.
- Specimens for newborn screening that are improperly applied to the filter paper circles may produce invalid results.
- Touching blood spots after collection on the filter paper card may contaminate the sample and produce invalid results.
- Failure to let the filter paper sample dry may affect test results.
- Specimens for newborn screening collected after transfusion may produce invalid results.
- Nonreactive HIV test results occur during the acute stage of the disease, when the virus is present but antibodies have not developed sufficiently to be detected. It may take up to 6 mo for the test to become positive. During this stage, the test for HIV antigen may not confirm an HIV infection.

POTENTIAL MEDICAL DIAGNOSIS: CLINICAL SIGNIFICANCE OF RESULTS
Abnormal findings related to

Hearing Test
- Abnormal audiogram *(related to congenital damage or malformations of the inner ear, infections, residual amniotic fluid or vernix in the ear canal)*

Endocrine Disorders
Increased in
- Congenital hypothyroidism (TSH) *(related to decrease in total thyroxine hormone levels, which activates the feedback loop to increase production of TSH)*
- CAH (adrenocorticotropic hormone [ACTH] and androgens) *(related to an autosomal recessive inherited disorder that results in missing or malfunctioning enzymes responsible for the production of cortisol and which may result in a salt-wasting condition or virilization of female genitalia)*

Decreased in
- Congenital hypothyroidism (total T4) *(related to missing or malfunctioning thyroid gland resulting in absence or decrease in total thyroxine hormone levels)*
- CAH (21-hydroxylase) *(related to an autosomal recessive inherited disorder that results in missing or malfunctioning enzymes responsible for the production of cortisol and which may result in one of several conditions, including a salt-wasting condition or virilization of female genitalia)*
- CAH (cortisol) *(related to an autosomal recessive inherited disorder that results in missing or malfunctioning enzymes responsible for the production of cortisol and which may result in a salt-wasting condition or virilization of female genitalia)*

- CAH (aldosterone) *(related to an autosomal recessive inherited disorder that results in missing or malfunctioning enzymes responsible for the production of cortisol and which may result in a salt-wasting condition)*

Abnormal findings related to

Hemoglobinopathies
- Hgb S: Sickle cell trait or sickle cell anemia *(related to an autosomal recessive inherited disorder that results in a genetic variation in the beta-chain of Hgb, causing a conformational change in the hemoglobin molecule and affecting the oxygen-binding properties of hemoglobin, which results in sickle-shaped red blood cells)*
- Hgb SC disease *(related to an autosomal recessive inherited disorder that results in the presence of an abnormal combination of Hgb S with Hgb C and presents a milder form of sickle cell anemia)*
- Hgb S/β-thalassemias *(related to an autosomal recessive inherited disorder that results in the presence of abnormal Hbg S/β-thalassemia, which combines the effects of thalassemia, a genetic disorder that results in decreased production of hemoglobin and sickle cell anemia, where sickled red blood cells lack the ability to combine effectively with oxygen)*

RBC Enzyme Defect
Decreased in
- G6PD deficiency *(usually related to an X-linked recessive inherited disorder that results in a deficiency of G6PD, which causes a hemolytic anemia)*

Inborn Errors of Amino Acid Metabolism/Disorders of the Urea Cycle
- Aminoacidopathies *(usually related to an autosomal recessive inherited*

disorder that results in insufficient or nonfunctional enzyme levels; specific amino acids are implicated)

- Disorders of the urea cycle; specifically argininemia, argininosuccinic acidemia, citrullinemia, and hyperammonemia/hyperornithinemia/homocitrullinemia *(usually related to an autosomal recessive inherited disorder that results in insufficient or nonfunctional enzyme levels; specific amino acids are implicated)*

Inborn Errors of Organic Acid Metabolism

- Organic acid disorders *(usually related to an autosomal recessive inherited disorder that results in insufficient or nonfunctional enzyme levels; specific organic acids are implicated)*

Inborn Errors of Fatty Acid Metabolism

- Fatty acid oxidation disorders *(usually related to an autosomal recessive inherited disorder that results in insufficient or nonfunctional enzyme levels; specific fatty acids are implicated)*

Other Multisystem Diseases

- Biotinidase deficiency *(related to an autosomal recessive inherited disorder that results in deficiency of the enzyme biotinidase, which prevents absorption or recycling of the essential vitamin biotin)*
- CF *(related to an autosomal recessive inherited disorder that results in insufficient or nonfunctional CF transmembrane conductance regulator protein, which results in poor transport of salts, especially sodium and chloride, and significantly impairs pulmonary and gastrointestinal function)*
- Galactosemia (classical) *(usually related to an autosomal recessive inherited disorder that results in insufficient or nonfunctional*

galactose-1-phosphate uridyl transferase enzyme levels

Infectious Diseases
Positive findings in
- HIV-1 or HIV-2 infection

NURSING IMPLICATIONS

BEFORE THE STUDY: PLANNING AND IMPLEMENTATION

Teaching the Patient What to Expect

▶ Newborn screening education should start during the prenatal period and be reinforced during preadmission testing. Many facilities provide educational brochures to the parents.

▶ A physician or delegate is responsible to inform parents of the newborn screening process before discharge.

▶ These procedures can assist in evaluating a number of congenital conditions, including hearing loss, thyroid function, adrenal gland function, and other metabolic enzyme disorders.

▶ Evaluation may also include HIV antibody testing if not performed prenatally or if otherwise clinically indicated.

▶ Explain that a blood sample is needed for some of the tests.

Blood Tests (Filter Paper Tests)

▶ Review the procedure with the parents or caregiver. Explain that blood specimens from neonates are collected by heelstick and applied to filter paper spots on the birth state's specific screening program card.

▶ Most regulations require screening specimens to be collected between 24 and 48 hr after birth to allow sufficient time after protein intake for abnormal metabolites to be detected and preferably before blood product transfusion or physical transfer to another facility.

▶ Prior to the heelstick, the site is cleansed with an antiseptic.

▶ When the heelstick is performed, the infant's heel is gently squeezed and the filter paper touched to the puncture site.

N

- When collecting samples for newborn screening, it is important to apply each blood drop to the correct side of the filter paper card and fill each circle with a single application of blood.
- Overfilling or underfilling the circles causes the specimen card to be rejected by the testing facility. Additional information is required on newborn screening cards and may vary by testing location.
- Newborn screening cards should be allowed to air dry for several hours on a level, nonabsorbent, unenclosed area. If multiple patients are tested, cards should not be stacked.
- The puncture site should be assessed for bleeding or hematoma formation, and secured with gauze and an adhesive bandage.

Hearing Test
- Review the procedure with the parents or caregiver. Address concerns about pain and explain that no discomfort will be experienced during the test. For further information, refer to the study titled "Otoscopy."

AFTER THE STUDY: POTENTIAL NURSING ACTIONS

Treatment Considerations
- Receiving a diagnosis for any of these conditions can be very fearful for a parent. Provide access to social services, including culturally appropriate education. Facilitate a safe environment to discuss fear and explore cultural influences that may enhance fear.
- Identify concerns about the child's diagnosed disease or disability and provide information related to genetic counseling and support group information on caring for a disabled child. Disease- or disability-specific education and treatment options should be discussed.
- Be supportive of the perceived loss of impaired activity or independence related to hearing loss or physical limitations and parents' fear of shortened life expectancy for the newborn.
- Offer support to victims of sexual assault in a nonjudgmental, nonthreatening atmosphere for a discussion

where the risks of sexually transmitted infections to the newborn are explained.
- Provide information related to access to genetic or other support counseling services.

Nutritional Considerations
- Provide education in special dietary modifications to treat deficiencies and references to the appropriate resource for dietary consultation.
- Amino acids are classified as essential (i.e., must be present simultaneously in sufficient quantities), conditionally or acquired essential (i.e., under certain stressful conditions, they become essential), and nonessential (i.e., can be produced by the body, when needed, if diet does not provide them).
- Essential amino acids include lysine, threonine, histidine, isoleucine, methionine, phenylalanine, tryptophan, and valine.
- Conditionally essential amino acids include cysteine, tyrosine, arginine, citrulline, taurine, and carnitine.
- Nonessential amino acids include alanine, glutamic acid, aspartic acid, glycine, serine, proline, glutamine, and asparagine.
- A high intake of specific amino acids can cause other amino acids to become essential.

Follow-Up, Evaluation, and Desired Outcomes
- Acknowledges contact information provided regarding guidelines on sexually transmitted infections (www.cdc.gov/DiseasesConditions) and vaccine-preventable diseases (e.g., diphtheria, hepatitis B, measles, mumps, pertussis, polio, rotavirus, rubella, varicella), as indicated (www.cdc.gov/vaccines/vpd/vaccines-diseases.html).
- Acknowledges contact information provided for the March of Dimes (www.marchofdimes.com), National Library of Medicine (https://medlineplus.gov/newbornscreening.html), general information (http://newbornscreening.info/Parents/facts.html), and state department of health newborn screening program. There are numerous support groups and informational Web

sites for specific conditions, including the National Center for Hearing Assessment and Management (www.infanthearing.org), American Speech-Language-Hearing Association (www.asha.org), Sickle Cell Disease Association of America (www.sicklecelldisease.org), Fatty Oxidation Disorders (FOD) Family Support Group (www.fodsupport.org), Organic Acidemia Association (www.oaanews.org), United Mitochondrial Disease Foundation (www.umdf.org), Cystic Fibrosis Foundation (www.cff.org), and for AIDS information, the National Institutes of Health (https://.aidsinfo.nih.gov) and the CDC (www.cdc.gov).

❱ Accepts that positive neonatal HIV findings must be reported to local health department officials.

❱ Recognizes the importance of facilitating alternative language training (sign language) for an infant with hearing loss to enhance growth and development.

❱ Understands that failure to refrain from feeding the child prohibited foods can result in severe disability and death.

Osmolality, Blood and Urine

SYNONYM/ACRONYM: Osmo.

RATIONALE: To assess fluid and electrolyte balance related to hydration, acid-base balance, and screening for toxins.

PATIENT PREPARATION: There are no food, fluid, activity, or medication restrictions unless by medical direction. As appropriate, provide the required urine collection container and specimen collection instructions.

NORMAL FINDINGS: Method: Freezing point depression.

	Conventional Units	SI Units (Conventional Units × 1)
Serum	275–295 mOsm/kg	275–295 mmol/kg
Urine (random)	50–1200 mOsm/kg	50–1200 mmol/kg
Urine (24-hr collection)		
Newborn	75–300 mOsm/kg	75–300 mmol/kg
Children and adults	250–900 mOsm/kg	250–900 mmol/kg

CRITICAL FINDINGS AND POTENTIAL INTERVENTIONS

Serum

- Less than 265 mOsm/kg (SI: Less than 265 mmol/kg)
- Greater than 320 mOsm/kg (SI: Greater than 320 mmol/kg)

Timely notification to the requesting health-care provider (HCP) of any critical findings and related symptoms is a role expectation of the professional nurse. A listing of these findings varies among facilities.

Serious clinical conditions may be associated with elevated or decreased serum osmolality. The following conditions are associated with elevated serum osmolality:

- *Respiratory arrest:* 360 mOsm/kg (SI: 360 mmol/kg)
- *Stupor of hyperglycemia:* 385 mOsm/kg (SI: 385 mmol/kg)
- *Grand mal seizures:* 420 mOsm/kg (SI: 420 mmol/kg)
- *Death:* Greater than 420 mOsm/kg (SI: Greater than 420 mmol/kg)

Symptoms of critically high levels include poor skin turgor, listlessness, acidosis (decreased pH), shock, seizures, coma, and cardiopulmonary arrest. Intervention may include close monitoring of electrolytes, administering intravenous fluids with the appropriate composition to shift water either into or out of the intravascular space as needed, monitoring cardiac signs, continuing neurological checks, and taking seizure precautions.

OVERVIEW: (**Study type:** Blood collected in a gold-, red-, or red/gray-top tube; urine from an unpreserved random specimen collected in a clean plastic collection container; related body system: Endocrine and Urinary systems.) Osmolality is a measure of the number of particles in a solution; it is independent of particle size, shape, and charge. Measurement of osmotic

O

concentration in serum provides clinically useful information about water and dissolved-particle transport across fluid compartment membranes. Urine osmolality provides information about the ability of the kidneys to concentrate urine. Urine osmolality, like serum osmolality, can be used to evaluate, monitor, and treat imbalances in fluid and electrolyte concentrations. Osmolality is used to assist in the diagnosis of metabolic, renal, and endocrine disorders. The simultaneous determination of serum and urine osmolality provides the opportunity to compare values between the two fluids. A normal urine-to-serum ratio is approximately 0.2 to 4.7 for random samples and greater than 3 for first-morning samples (dehydration normally occurs overnight). The major dissolved particles that contribute to osmolality are sodium, chloride, bicarbonate, urea, and glucose. Some of these substances are used in the following calculated estimate:

$$\text{Serum osmolality} = (2 \times Na^+) + (\text{glucose}/18) + (BUN/2.8)$$

Measured osmolality in serum or urine is higher than the estimated value because of other unmeasured organic particles in solution contributing to the osmotic concentration. The osmal gap is the difference between the measured and calculated values and is normally 5 to 10 mOsm/kg. If the difference is greater than 15 mOsm/kg, consider ethylene glycol, isopropanol, methanol, or ethanol toxicity. These substances behave like antifreeze, lowering the freezing point in the blood, and provide misleadingly high results.

INDICATIONS

Serum
- Assist in the evaluation of antidiuretic hormone (ADH) function.
- Assist in rapid screening for toxic substances, such as ethylene glycol, ethanol, isopropanol, and methanol.
- Evaluate electrolyte and acid-base balance.
- Evaluate state of hydration.

Urine
- Evaluate concentrating ability of the kidneys.
- Evaluate diabetes insipidus, *a condition related to a dysfunction of the kidneys (nephrogenic diabetes insipidus) or pituitary gland (central diabetes insipidus); unrelated to type 1 or type 2 diabetes.*
- Evaluate neonatal patients with protein or glucose in the urine.
- Perform work-up for kidney disease.

INTERFERING FACTORS
Factors that may alter the results of the study
- Drugs and other substances that may increase serum osmolality include corticosteroids, glycerin, inulin, ioxitalamic acid, and mannitol.
- Drugs and other substances that may decrease serum osmolality include bendroflumethiazide, carbamazepine, chlorpromazine, chlorthalidone, cyclophosphamide, cyclothiazide, doxepin, hydrochlorothiazide, lorcainide, methyclothiazide, and polythiazide.
- Drugs and other substances that may increase urine osmolality include anesthetic drugs, chlorpropamide, cyclophosphamide, furosemide, mannitol, metolazone, octreotide, and vincristine.
- Drugs and other substances that may decrease urine osmolality

include captopril, demeclocycline, glyburide, lithium, octreotide, tolazamide, and verapamil.

POTENTIAL MEDICAL DIAGNOSIS: CLINICAL SIGNIFICANCE OF RESULTS

Increased in

- **Serum**

  Azotemia *(related to accumulation of nitrogen-containing waste products that contribute to osmolality)*

  Dehydration *(related to hemoconcentration)*

  Diabetes insipidus *(related to excessive loss of water through urination that results in hemoconcentration)*

  Diabetic ketoacidosis *(related to excessive loss of water through urination that results in hemoconcentration)*

  Hypercalcemia *(related to electrolyte imbalance that results in water loss and hemoconcentration)*

  Hypernatremia *(related to insufficient intake of water or excessive loss of water; sodium is a major cation in the determination of osmolality)*

- **Urine**

  Amyloidosis

  Azotemia *(related to decrease in renal blood flow; decrease in water excreted by the kidneys results in a more concentrated urine)*

  Heart failure *(decrease in renal blood flow related to diminished cardiac output; decrease in water excreted by the kidneys results in a more concentrated urine)*

  Dehydration *(related to decrease in water excreted by the kidneys that results in a more concentrated urine)*

  Hyponatremia

  Syndrome of inappropriate antidiuretic hormone production (SIADH) *(related to decrease in water excreted by the kidneys that results in a more concentrated urine)*

Decreased in

- **Serum**

  Adrenocorticoid insufficiency

  Hyponatremia *(sodium is a major influence on osmolality; decreased sodium contributes to decreased osmolality)*

SIADH *(related to increase in water reabsorbed by the kidneys that results in a more dilute serum)*

Water intoxication *(related to excessive water intake, which has a dilutional effect)*

- **Urine**

  Diabetes insipidus *(related to decreased ability of the kidneys to concentrate urine)*

  Hypernatremia *(related to increased water excreted by the kidneys that results in a more dilute urine)*

  Hypokalemia *(related to increased water excreted by the kidneys that results in a more dilute urine)*

  Primary polydipsia *(related to increase in water intake that results in dilute urine)*

NURSING IMPLICATIONS

BEFORE THE STUDY: PLANNING AND IMPLEMENTATION

Teaching the Patient What to Expect

- Inform the patient that the test is used to evaluate electrolyte and water balance.
- Explain that a blood or urine sample is needed for the test.
- Either a random or a timed urine collection may be requested. Information regarding specimen collection is presented with other general guidelines in Appendix A: Patient Preparation and Specimen Collection.

Potential Nursing Actions

- Include on the timed collection container's label urine total volume, test start and stop times/dates, and any medications that may interfere with test results.

AFTER THE STUDY: POTENTIAL NURSING ACTIONS

Treatment Considerations

- Increased osmolality may be associated with dehydration. Evaluate the patient for signs and symptoms of dehydration.
- Dehydration is a significant and common finding in older adults and other patients in whom renal function has deteriorated.

O

Nutritional Considerations
▶ Decreased osmolality may be associated with overhydration. Observe for signs and symptoms of fluid-volume excess related to excess electrolyte intake, fluid-volume deficit related to active body fluid loss, or risk of injury related to an alteration in body chemistry. (For electrolyte-specific dietary references, see blood studies titled "Chloride," "Potassium," and "Sodium.")

Follow-Up, Evaluation, and Desired Outcomes
▶ Acknowledges contact information provided for the National Kidney Foundation (www.kidney.org).

Osmotic Fragility

SYNONYM/ACRONYM: Red blood cell osmotic fragility, OF.

RATIONALE: To assess the fragility of erythrocytes related to red blood cell (RBC) lysis toward diagnosing diseases such as hemolytic anemia.

PATIENT PREPARATION: There are no food, fluid, activity, or medication restrictions unless by medical direction.

NORMAL FINDINGS: (Method: Spectrophotometry) Hemolysis (unincubated) begins at 0.5% sodium chloride (NaCl) solution and is complete at 0.3% NaCl solution. Results are compared to a normal curve.

CRITICAL FINDINGS AND POTENTIAL INTERVENTIONS: N/A

OVERVIEW: (Study type: Blood collected in a green-top [heparin] tube and two peripheral blood smears; related body system: Circulatory/Hematopoietic system.) Osmotic fragility (OF) is an indication of the ability of RBCs to experience osmotic stress and take on water without lysing. Normal RBC membranes must be flexible to changes in plasma concentrations of electrolytes and other substances. In this test, RBCs are placed in graded dilutions of NaCl. Swelling of the cells occurs at lower concentrations of NaCl as they take on water in the hypotonic solution; that is, the concentration of electrolyte is higher inside the RBC, and in order to establish equilibrium with the surrounding fluid, the RBC must take on water by osmosis. Normal RBCs can absorb an increased volume; because of their bicocave shape, they have more surface area and can swell. Thicker cells, such as spherocytes, have an increased OF because they are already spherical, already have weak membranes, and cannot take on more volume without lysing; thinner cells have a decreased OF.

INDICATIONS
Evaluate hemolytic anemia.

INTERFERING FACTORS
Factors that may alter the results of the study
• Drugs and other substances that may increase osmotic fragility include dapsone.

- Parasitic infestations, such as malaria, may independently cause cell hemolysis.

Other considerations
- Specimens should be submitted for analysis immediately after collection.

POTENTIAL MEDICAL DIAGNOSIS: CLINICAL SIGNIFICANCE OF RESULTS
Increased in
Conditions that produce RBCs with a small surface-to-volume ratio or RBCs that are rounder than normal will have increased osmotic fragility.

- Acquired immune hemolytic anemias *(abnormal RBCs in size and shape; spherocytes)*
- Hemolytic disease of the newborn *(abnormal RBCs in size and shape; spherocytes)*
- Hereditary spherocytosis *(abnormal RBCs in size and shape; spherocytes)*
- Malaria *(related to effect of parasite on RBC membrane integrity)*
- Pyruvate kinase deficiency *(abnormal RBCs in size and shape; spherocytes)*

Decreased in
Conditions that produce RBCs with a large surface-to-volume ratio or RBCs that are flatter than normal will have decreased osmotic fragility.

- Asplenia *(abnormal cells are not removed from circulation due to absence of spleen; target cells)*
- Hemoglobinopathies *(abnormal RBCs in size and shape; target cells, drepanocytes)*
- Iron-deficiency anemia *(abnormal RBCs in size and shape; target cells)*
- Liver disease *(abnormal RBCs in size and shape; target cells)*
- Thalassemias *(abnormal RBCs in size and shape; target cells)*

NURSING IMPLICATIONS

BEFORE THE STUDY: PLANNING AND IMPLEMENTATION
Teaching the Patient What to Expect
- Inform the patient this test can assist in assessing for anemia.
- Explain that a blood sample is needed for the test.

AFTER THE STUDY: POTENTIAL NURSING ACTIONS
Follow-Up, Evaluation, and Desired Outcomes
- Acknowledges that additional testing may be necessary to monitor disease progression or evaluate the need for a change in therapy.

Osteocalcin

SYNONYM/ACRONYM: Bone GLA protein, BGP.

RATIONALE: To assist in assessment of risk for osteoporosis and to evaluate effectiveness of therapeutic interventions.

PATIENT PREPARATION: There are no food, fluid, activity, or medication restrictions unless by medical direction.

NORMAL FINDINGS: Method: Electrochemiluminescence.

Age and Sex	Conventional Units	SI Units (Conventional Units × 1)
6 mo–6 yr		
Male	39–121 ng/mL	39–121 mcg/L
Female	44–130 ng/mL	44–130 mcg/L
7–9 yr		
Male	66–182 ng/mL	66–182 mcg/L
Female	73–206 ng/mL	73–206 mcg/L
10–12 yr		
Male	85–232 ng/mL	85–232 mcg/L
Female	77–262 ng/mL	77–262 mcg/L
13–15 yr		
Male	70–336 ng/mL	70–336 mcg/L
Female	33–222 ng/mL	33–222 mcg/L
16–17 yr		
Male	43–237 ng/mL	43–237 mcg/L
Female	24–99 ng/mL	24–99 mcg/L
Adult		
Male	3–40 ng/mL	3–40 mcg/L
Female		
Premenopausal	5–30 ng/mL	5–30 mcg/L
Postmenopausal	9–50 ng/mL	9–50 mcg/L

CRITICAL FINDINGS AND POTENTIAL INTERVENTIONS: N/A

OVERVIEW: (**Study type:** Blood collected in a gold-, red/gray, red-, lavender [EDTA]-pink [K2EDTA], or green [sodium or lithium heparin]-top tube; **related body system:** Musculoskeletal system.) Osteocalcin is an important bone cell matrix protein and a sensitive marker in bone metabolism. It is produced by osteoblasts during the matrix mineralization phase of bone formation and is the most abundant noncollagenous bone cell protein. Synthesis of osteocalcin is dependent on vitamin K and vitamin D. Osteocalcin levels parallel alkaline phosphatase levels. Osteocalcin levels are affected by a number of factors, including estrogen levels. Assessment of osteocalcin levels permits indirect measurement of osteoblast activity and bone formation. Because it is released into the bloodstream during bone resorption, there is some speculation as to whether osteocalcin might also be considered a marker for bone matrix degradation and turnover.

INDICATIONS
- Assist in the diagnosis of bone cancer.
- Evaluate bone disease.
- Evaluate bone metabolism.
- Monitor effectiveness of estrogen replacement therapy.

INTERFERING FACTORS
Factors that may alter the results of the study
- Drugs and other substances that may increase osteocalcin levels

include anabolic steroids, calcitonin, calcitriol, danazol, nafarelin, pamidronate, and parathyroid hormone.

- Drugs and other substances that may decrease osteocalcin levels include alendronate, antithyroid therapy, corticosteroids, cyproterone, estradiol valerate, estrogen/progesterone therapy, glucocorticoids, hormone replacement therapy, methylprednisolone, oral contraceptives, pamidronate, parathyroid hormone, prednisolone, prednisone, raloxifene, tamoxifen, and vitamin D.

POTENTIAL MEDICAL DIAGNOSIS: CLINICAL SIGNIFICANCE OF RESULTS

Increased in

- Adolescents undergoing a growth spurt *(levels in the blood increase as the rate of bone formation increases)*
- Chronic kidney disease *(related to accumulation in circulation due to decreased renal excretion)*
- Hyperthyroidism (primary and secondary) *(related to increased bone turnover)*
- Metastatic skeletal disease *(levels in the blood increase as bone destruction releases it into circulation)*
- Paget disease *(levels in the blood increase as bone destruction releases it into circulation)*
- Renal osteodystrophy *(related to bone degeneration secondary to hyperparathyroidism of chronic kidney disease)*
- Some patients with osteoporosis *(levels in the blood increase as bone destruction releases it into circulation)*

Decreased in

- Growth hormone deficiency *(bone mineralization is stimulated by growth hormone)*

- Pregnancy *(increased demand by developing fetus results in an increase in maternal bone resorption)*
- Primary biliary cholangitis *(related to increased bone loss)*

NURSING IMPLICATIONS

BEFORE THE STUDY: PLANNING AND IMPLEMENTATION

Teaching the Patient What to Expect

- Inform the patient this test can assist in evaluating for bone disease.
- Explain that a blood sample is needed for the test.

AFTER THE STUDY: POTENTIAL NURSING ACTIONS

Treatment Considerations

- Explain that the test may need to be repeated to evaluate disease progression and therapy effectiveness.

Nutritional Considerations
Osteocalcin Levels

- Increased osteocalcin levels may be associated with skeletal disease. Nutritional therapy is indicated for those at high risk for developing osteoporosis.
- Educate the patient regarding the National Osteoporosis Foundation's guidelines (www.nof.org), which include a regular regimen of weight-bearing exercises, limited alcohol intake, avoidance of tobacco products, and adequate dietary intake of vitamin D and calcium.

Abnormal Calcium Values

- Patients with abnormal calcium values should be informed that daily intake of calcium is important even though body stores in the bones can be called on to supplement circulating levels.
- Dietary calcium can be obtained from animal or plant sources.
- Milk and milk products, sardines, clams, oysters, salmon, rhubarb, spinach, beet greens, broccoli, kale, tofu, legumes, and fortified orange juice are

O

high in calcium. Milk and milk products also contain vitamin D and lactose, which assist calcium absorption.

▸ Cooked vegetables provide more absorbable calcium than raw vegetables.

▸ Explain that there are substances that can inhibit calcium absorption by irreversibly binding to some of the calcium, making it unavailable for absorption. Examples include oxalates, which naturally occur in some vegetables (e.g., beet greens, collards, leeks, okra, parsley, quinoa, spinach, Swiss chard) and are found in tea; phytic acid, found in some cereals (e.g., wheat bran, wheat germ); phosphoric acid, found in dark cola; and insoluble dietary fiber (in excessive amounts).

▸ Excessive protein intake can negatively affect calcium absorption, especially when combined with foods high in phosphorus and in the presence of a reduced dietary calcium intake.

Vitamin D Deficiency
▸ Educate that the main dietary sources of vitamin D are fortified dairy foods and cod liver oil. Explain that vitamin D is also synthesized by the body, in the skin, and is activated by sunlight.

Vitamin K Deficiency
▸ Explain that the main dietary sources of vitamin K are broccoli, cabbage, cauliflower, kale, spinach, leaf lettuce, watercress, parsley, and other raw green leafy vegetables, pork, liver, soybeans, mayonnaise, and vegetable oils.

Follow-Up, Evaluation, and Desired Outcomes
▸ Acknowledges contact information provided for the U.S. Department of Agriculture's resource for nutrition (www.choosemyplate.gov).

Otoscopy

SYNONYM/ACRONYM: Ear examination.

RATIONALE: To visualize and assess internal and external structures of the ear to evaluate for pain or hearing loss.

PATIENT PREPARATION: There are no food, fluid, activity, or medication restrictions unless by medical direction.

NORMAL FINDINGS
• Normal structure and appearance of the external ear, auditory canal, and tympanic membrane.
  Pinna: Funnel-shaped cartilaginous structure; no evidence of infection, pain, dermatitis with swelling, redness, or itching
  External Auditory Canal: S-shaped canal lined with fine hairs, sebaceous and ceruminous glands; no evidence of redness, lesions, edema, scaliness, pain, accumulation of cerumen, drainage, or presence of foreign bodies
  Tympanic Membrane: Shallow, circular cone that is shiny and pearl gray in color, semi-transparent whitish cord crossing from front to back just under the upper edge, cone of light on the right side at the 4 o'clock position; no evidence of bulging, retraction, lusterless membrane, or obliteration of the cone of light

CRITICAL FINDINGS AND POTENTIAL INTERVENTIONS: N/A

OVERVIEW: (Study type: Sensory, auditory; related body system: Nervous system.) This noninvasive procedure is used to inspect the external ear, auditory canal, and tympanic membrane. Otoscopy is an essential part of any general physical examination but is also done before any other audiological studies when symptoms of ear pain or hearing loss are present.

INDICATIONS

- Detect causes of deafness, obstruction, stenosis, or swelling of the pinna or canal causing a narrowing or closure that prevents sound from entering.
- Detect ear abnormalities during routine physical examination.
- Diagnose cause of ear pain.
- Remove impacted cerumen (with a dull ring curette) or foreign bodies (with a forceps) that are obstructing the entrance of sound waves into the ear.
- Evaluate acute or chronic otitis media and effectiveness of therapy in controlling infections.

INTERFERING FACTORS

Factors that may alter the results of the study

- Obstruction of the auditory canal with cerumen, dried drainage, or foreign bodies that prevent introduction of the otoscope.

POTENTIAL MEDICAL DIAGNOSIS: CLINICAL SIGNIFICANCE OF RESULTS

Abnormal findings related to

- Cerumen accumulation
- Ear trauma
- Foreign bodies
- Otitis externa
- Otitis media
- Tympanic membrane perforation or rupture

NURSING IMPLICATIONS

BEFORE THE STUDY: PLANNING AND IMPLEMENTATION

Teaching the Patient What to Expect

- Inform the patient this procedure can assist in investigating suspected ear disorders.
- Review the procedure with the patient or family. Address concerns about pain and explain that no discomfort will be experienced during the test.
- Explain that a health-care provider (HCP) performs the test and that it may take 5 to 10 minutes to evaluate both ears.
- If the auditory canal is not clear, administer ordered ear drops or irrigation to prepare for cerumen removal.
- Positioning for testing is in the sitting position for an adult and supine position on the caregiver's lap for a child.
- An otoscope with the correct-size speculum to fit the size of the patient's ear will be selected for use.
- Both adults and children will be assisted to position their heads appropriately for gentle speculum insertion and examination.
- Any effusion will be cultured with a sterile swab and culture tube (see "Culture, Bacterial Various Sites (Anal/Genital, Ear, Eye, Skin, Wound, Blood, Sputum, Stool, Throat/Nasopharyngeal, Urine)" study); alternatively, an HCP will perform a needle aspiration from the middle ear through the tympanic membrane during the examination. Other procedures such as cerumen and foreign body removal can also be performed.
- Pneumatic otoscopy can be done to determine tympanic membrane flexibility. This test permits the introduction of

air into the canal that reveals a reduction in movement of the membrane in otitis media and absence of movement in chronic otitis media.

Potential Nursing Actions
▶ Obtain a list of the patient's current medications (especially antibiotic regimen), including over-the-counter medications and dietary supplements.
▶ Investigate history of the patient's known or suspected hearing loss, including type and cause; ear conditions with treatment regimens; ear surgery; and other tests and procedures to assess and diagnose auditory deficit; presence of tympanotomy tube, symptoms (especially pain, itching, drainage).
▶ Explain that it may be necessary to assist in restraining a child in order to

prevent damage to the ear if the child cannot remain still.
▶ Ensure that the external auditory canal is clear of impacted cerumen.

AFTER THE STUDY: POTENTIAL NURSING ACTIONS

Treatment Considerations
▶ Administer ear drops of a soothing oil, as ordered, if the canal is irritated by removal of cerumen or foreign bodies.

Follow-Up, Evaluation, and Desired Outcomes
▶ Recognize anxiety related to test results, and be supportive of impaired activity related to hearing loss.
▶ Discuss the implications of abnormal test results on the patient's lifestyle.

Oxalate, Urine

SYNONYM/ACRONYM: N/A

RATIONALE: To identify patients who are at risk for renal calculus formation or hyperoxaluria related to malabsorption.

PATIENT PREPARATION: There are no fluid, activity, or medication restrictions unless by medical direction. Instruct the patient to abstain from calcium supplements, gelatin, rhubarb, spinach, strawberries, tomatoes, and vitamin C for at least 24 hr before the test. High-protein meals should also be avoided for 24 hr before specimen collection. Protocols may vary among facilities. Usually, a 24-hr urine collection is ordered. As appropriate, provide the required urine collection container and specimen collection instructions.

NORMAL FINDINGS: Method: Spectrophotometry.

	Conventional Units	SI Units (Conventional Units × 11.1)
Children and adults	Less than 40 mg/24 hr	Less than 444 micromol/24 hr

CRITICAL FINDINGS AND POTENTIAL INTERVENTIONS: N/A

OVERVIEW: (Study type: Urine from a timed specimen collected in a clean plastic collection container with hydrogen chloride [HCl] as a preservative; related body system: Digestive and Urinary systems.) Oxalate is derived from the metabolism of oxalic acid, glycine, and ascorbic acid. Some individuals with malabsorption disorders absorb and excrete abnormally high amounts of oxalate, resulting in hyperoxaluria. Hyperoxaluria may be seen in patients who consume large amounts of animal protein, certain fruits and vegetables, or megadoses of vitamin C (ascorbic acid). Hyperoxaluria is also associated with ethylene glycol poisoning (oxalic acid is used in cleaning and bleaching agents). Patients who absorb and excrete large amounts of oxalate may form calcium oxalate kidney stones. Simultaneous measurement of serum and urine calcium is often requested.

INDICATIONS

• Assist in the evaluation of patients with ethylene glycol poisoning.
• Assist in the evaluation of patients with a history of kidney stones.
• Assist in the evaluation of patients with malabsorption syndromes or patients who have had jejunoileal bypass surgery.

INTERFERING FACTORS

Factors that may alter the results of the study
• Drugs and other substances that may increase oxalate levels include ascorbic acid and calcium.

• Drugs and other substances that may decrease oxalate levels include nifedipine and pyridoxine.

Other considerations
• Failure to collect sample in proper preservative may cause the procedure to be repeated. HCl helps keep oxalate dissolved in the urine. If the pH rises above 3, oxalate may precipitate from the sample, causing falsely decreased values. The acid also prevents oxidation of vitamin C to oxalate in the sample, causing falsely increased values.
• All urine voided for the timed collection period must be included in the collection or else falsely decreased values may be obtained. Compare output records with volume collected to verify that all voids were included in the collection.

POTENTIAL MEDICAL DIAGNOSIS: CLINICAL SIGNIFICANCE OF RESULTS

Increased in
Conditions that result in malabsorption for any reason can lead to increased levels. Chronic diarrhea results in excessive loss of calcium to bind oxalate. Increased oxalate is absorbed by the intestine and excreted by the kidneys.

• Bacterial overgrowth
• Biliary tract disease
• Bowel disease
• Celiac disease
• Cirrhosis
• Crohn disease
• Diabetes
• Ethylene glycol poisoning *(ethylene glycol is metabolized to oxalate and excreted by the kidneys; crystals are present in urine)*
• Ileal resection

O

- Jejunal shunt
- Pancreatic disease
- Primary hereditary hyperoxaluria (rare)
- Pyridoxine (vitamin B$_6$) deficiency *(pyridoxine is a cofactor in an enzyme reaction that converts glyoxylic acid to glycine; deficiency results in an increase in oxalate)*
- Sarcoidosis

Decreased in

- Hypercalciuria *(related to formation of calcium oxalate crystals)*
- Kidney disease *(related to oxalate kidney stone disease)*

NURSING IMPLICATIONS

BEFORE THE STUDY: PLANNING AND IMPLEMENTATION

Teaching the Patient What to Expect
▶ Inform the patient this test can assist in evaluating risk for kidney stones.
▶ Explain that a urine sample is needed for the test. Information regarding specimen collection is presented with

other general guidelines in Appendix A: Patient Preparation and Specimen Collection.

Potential Nursing Actions
▶ Include on the collection container's label urine total volume, test start and stop times/dates, and any medications that may interfere with test results.

AFTER THE STUDY: POTENTIAL NURSING ACTIONS

Treatment Considerations
▶ Instruct the patient to resume usual diet, as directed by the health-care provider.

Nutritional Considerations
▶ Consideration may be given to lessening dietary intake of oxalate if urine levels are increased.
▶ Facilitate those with abnormal results to seek advice regarding dietary modifications from a registered dietitian.
▶ Discuss the use of magnesium supplementation for those with gastrointestinal disease to prevent the development of calcium oxalate kidney stones.

Follow-Up, Evaluation, and Desired Outcomes
▶ Accepts that dietary changes are necessary to better manage health.

O

Pachymetry

SYNONYM/ACRONYM: N/A

RATIONALE: To assess the thickness of the cornea prior to LASIK surgery and evaluate glaucoma risk.

PATIENT PREPARATION: There are no food, fluid, activity, or medication restrictions unless by medical direction.

NORMAL FINDINGS
• Normal corneal thickness of 535 to 555 micron.

CRITICAL FINDINGS AND POTENTIAL INTERVENTIONS: N/A

OVERVIEW: (Study type: Sensory, ocular; related body system: Nervous system.) Pachymetry is the measurement of the thickness of the cornea using an ultrasound device called a *pachymeter.* Refractive surgery procedures such as LASIK (laser-assisted in situ keratomileusis) remove tissue from the cornea. Pachymetry is used to ensure that enough central corneal tissue remains after surgery to prevent ectasia, or abnormal bowing, of thin corneas. Also, studies point to a correlation between increased risk of glaucoma and decreased corneal thickness. This correlation has influenced some health-care providers (HCPs) to include pachymetry as part of a regular eye health examination for patients who have a family history of glaucoma, have high blood pressure, or are part of a high-risk population. People of African descent have a higher incidence of glaucoma than any other ethnic group.

INDICATIONS
• Assist in the diagnosis of glaucoma (*Note:* The intraocular pressure in glaucoma patients with a thin cornea, 530 micron or less, may be higher than in patients whose corneal thickness is within normal limits).

• Determine corneal thickness in potential refractive surgery candidates.
• Monitor the effects of various therapies using eyedrops, laser, or filtering surgery.

INTERFERING FACTORS
Factors that may alter the results of the study
• Improper technique during application of the probe tip to the cornea.

POTENTIAL MEDICAL DIAGNOSIS: CLINICAL SIGNIFICANCE OF RESULTS
Abnormal findings related to
• Bullous keratopathy
• Corneal rejection after penetrating keratoplasty
• Fuchs endothelial dystrophy
• Glaucoma

NURSING IMPLICATIONS

BEFORE THE STUDY: PLANNING AND IMPLEMENTATION

Teaching the Patient What to Expect
◗ Inform the patient this procedure can assist in measuring the thickness of the cornea in the eye.
◗ Review the procedure and address concerns about pain. Explain that some discomfort may be experienced after the test when the numbness wears off from anesthetic drops administered prior to the test, or discomfort may occur if too much pressure is used during the test.

P

▶ Explain that an HCP performs the test and that it can take 3 to 5 min to evaluate both eyes.

▶ During the procedure, the patient will be comfortably seated and instructed to look straight ahead, keeping the eyes open and unblinking.

▶ Topical anesthetic drops will be instilled in each eye and allowed time to work.

▶ Advise the patient that he or she will be asked to look straight ahead while the probe of the pachymeter is applied directly on the cornea of the eye.

▶ An average of three readings are taken for each eye. Individual readings should be within 10 microns. Results on both eyes should be similar.

Potential Nursing Actions

▶ Obtain a history of known or suspected visual impairment, including type and cause (e.g., dry eye, narrow-angle glaucoma); eye conditions with treatment regimens; eye surgery; changes in visual acuity; and use of glasses or contact lenses.

▶ Instruct the patient to remove contact lenses or glasses, as appropriate.

AFTER THE STUDY: POTENTIAL NURSING ACTIONS

Treatment Considerations

▶ Anticipate anxiety related to test results and provide teaching related to the clinical implications of the test results.

▶ Encourage the family to recognize and be supportive of impaired activity related to vision loss, anticipated loss of driving privileges, or the possibility of requiring corrective lenses (self-image).

▶ Discuss the implications of test results on lifestyle choices.

▶ Provide reassurance regarding concerns related to impending corneal surgery.

Follow-Up, Evaluation, and Desired Outcomes

▶ Acknowledges contact information provided for patient education on the topic of eye care, such as the American Academy of Ophthalmologists (www.aao.org), American Optometric Association (www.aoa.org), or All About Vision (www.allaboutvision.com).

▶ Acknowledges contact information provided for the Glaucoma Research Foundation (www.glaucoma.org).

Papanicolaou Smear

SYNONYM/ACRONYM: Pap smear, cervical smear.

RATIONALE: To establish a cytological diagnosis of cervical and vaginal disease and identify the presence of genital infections, such as human papillomavirus, herpes, and cytomegalovirus.

PATIENT PREPARATION: There are no food, fluid, activity, or medication restrictions unless by medical direction. Instruct the patient to avoid douching or sexual intercourse for 24 hr before specimen collection. Verify that the patient is not menstruating.

NORMAL FINDINGS: Method: (Microscopic examination of fixed and stained smear) Reporting of Pap smear findings may follow one of several formats and may vary by laboratory. Simplified content of the two most common formats for interpretation are listed in the table.

Manual Review (Bethesda System)

Specimen type: Smear, liquid-based, or other.

Specimen adequacy:

- *Satisfactory* for evaluation—endocervical transformation zone component is described as present or absent, along with other quality indicators (e.g., partially obscuring blood, inflammation).
- *Unsatisfactory* for evaluation—either the specimen is rejected and the reason given or the specimen is processed and examined but not evaluated for epithelial abnormalities and the reason is given.

General categorization:

- *Negative for intraepithelial lesion or malignancy.*
- *Epithelial cell abnormality* (abnormality is specified in the interpretation section of the report).
- *Other comments*

Interpretation/result:

1. Negative for intraepithelial lesion or malignancy
   A. *List organisms causing infection:*
      - *Trichomonas vaginalis;* fungal organisms consistent with *Candida* spp.; shift in flora suggestive of bacterial vaginosis; bacteria morphologically consistent with *Actinomyces* spp.; cellular changes consistent with herpes simplex virus
   B. Other nonneoplastic findings:
      - Reactive cellular changes associated with inflammation, radiation, intrauterine device; glandular cell status post-hysterectomy; atrophy
2. Epithelial cell abnormalities
   A. *Squamous cell abnormalities*
      - ASC of undetermined significance (ASC-US) cannot exclude HSIL (ASC-H)
      - LSIL encompassing HPV, mild dysplasia, CIN 1
      - HSIL encompassing moderate and severe dysplasia, CIS/CIN 2 and CIN 3 with features suspicious for invasion (if invasion is suspected)
      - Squamous cell cancer
   B. *Glandular cell*
      - Atypical glandular cells (NOS or specify otherwise)
      - Atypical glandular cells, favor neoplastic (NOS or specify otherwise)
      - Endocervical adenocarcinoma in situ
      - Adenocarcinoma
3. Other
   A. Endometrial cells (in a woman of 40 yr or greater)

Automated review (any system):

Indicates the case was examined by an automated device and the results are listed along with the name of the device.

Ancillary testing:

Describes the test method and result.

Educational notes and suggestions:

Should be consistent with clinical follow-up guidelines published by professional organizations with references included.

P

ASC = atypical squamous cells; ASC-H = high-grade atypical squamous cells; ASC-US = atypical squamous cells undetermined significance; CIN = cervical intraepithelial neoplasia; CIS = cancer in situ; HSIL = high-grade squamous intraepithelial lesion; LSIL = low-grade squamous intraepithelial lesion.

CRITICAL FINDINGS AND POTENTIAL INTERVENTIONS: N/A

OVERVIEW: (Study type: Tissue and cell microscopy, cervical cells; related body system: Immune and Reproductive systems.)
The Papanicolaou (Pap) smear is primarily used for the early detection of cervical cancer. The interpretation of Pap smears is as heavily dependent on the collection and fixation technique as it is on the completeness and accuracy of the clinical information provided with the specimen. The patient's age, date of last menstrual period, parity, surgical status, postmenopausal status, use of hormone therapy (including use of oral contraceptives), history of radiation or chemotherapy, history of abnormal vaginal bleeding, and history of previous Pap smears are essential for proper interpretation. Human papillomavirus (HPV) is the most common sexually transmitted virus and primary causal factor in the development of cervical cancer. Therefore, specimens for HPV are often collected simultaneously with the PAP smear. The laboratory should be consulted about the availability of this option prior to specimen collection because specific test kits are required to allow for simultaneous sample collection. HPV infection can be successfully treated once it has been identified. There are three HPV vaccines (Cervarix, Gardasil, and Gardasil 9), usually given as a series of three injections, at 2 and 6 mo after the initial injection. Vaccination is recommended in the preteen years because the vaccine's protection is most effective if the immune response to HPV develops prior to sexual activity. All three vaccines protect against the HPV strains that carry the highest infection risk (strains 16 and 18), which are associated with approximately 65% to 70% of cervical cancers and the majority of other HPV-related anal/genital cancers. Cervarix is a 2-valent vaccine that targets HPV types 16 and 18; Gardasil is a 4-valent vaccine that targets HPV types 6, 11, 16, and 18; and Gardasil 9 is a 9-valent vaccine that targets HPV types 6, 11, 16, 18, 31, 33, 45, 52, and 58. Gardasil and Gardasil 9 are effective against HPV types that account for another 15% to 20% of cervical cancers; they are also effective against HPV types 6 and 11, the types that cause genital warts. The Centers for Disease Control and Prevention (CDC) recommends vaccination for males (4-v HPV or 9-v HPV) aged 11 or 12 yr through 21 yr who are not already vaccinated or who have not completed the entire three-dose series; vaccination of males through age 26 yr (4-v HPV or 9-v HPV) for immunocompromised men or men who have oral or anal intercourse with other men; and for females (2-v HPV, 4-v HPV, or 9-v HPV) aged 11 or 12 yr through 26 yr who are not already vaccinated or who have not completed the entire three-dose series.

Vaccination can begin at age 9 yr for both males and females. FDA approval was recently received for administration of Gardasil 9 for females aged 9 to 25 yr and males aged 9 to 15 yr. Additional FDA approval has been requested for males aged 16 to 26 yr. The Advisory Committee on Immunization Practices has reviewed the preliminary data and recommended off-label use for males aged 16 to 26 yr.

P

A wet prep can be prepared simultaneously from a cervical or vaginal sample. The swab is touched to a microscope slide, and a small amount of saline is dropped on the slide. The slide is examined by microscope to determine the presence of harmful bacteria or *Trichomonas*.

A Schiller test entails applying an iodine solution to the cervix. Normal cells pick up the iodine and stain brown. Abnormal cells do not pick up any color.

Improvements in specimen preparation have added to the increased quality of screening procedures. Liquid-based Pap tests have largely replaced the traditional Pap smear. Cervical cells collected in the liquid media are applied in a very thin layer onto slides, using a method that clears away contaminants such as blood or vaginal discharge. Samples can be "split" so that questionable findings by cytological screening can be followed up with more specific molecular methods such as nucleic acid hybridization probes, polymerase chain reaction, intracellular microRNA quantification, or immunocytochemistry to detect the presence of high-risk HPV, *Chlamydia trachomatis,* and *Neisseria gonorrhoeae.* Computerized scanning systems are also being used to reduce the number of smears that require manual review by a cytotechnologist or pathologist.

There are now some alternatives to cone biopsy and cryosurgery for the treatment of cervical dysplasia. Patients with abnormal Pap smear results may have a cervical loop electrosurgical excision procedure (LEEP) performed to remove or destroy abnormal cervical tissue. In the LEEP procedure, a speculum is inserted into the vagina, the cervix is numbed, and a special electrically charged wire loop is used to painlessly remove the suspicious area. Postprocedure cramping and bleeding can occur. Laser ablation is another technique that can be employed for the precise removal of abnormal cervical tissue.

INDICATIONS
- Assist in the diagnosis of cervical dysplasia.
- Assist in the diagnosis of endometriosis, condyloma, and vaginal adenosis.
- Assist in the diagnosis of genital infections (herpes, *Candida* spp., *Trichomonas vaginalis,* cytomegalovirus, *Chlamydia,* lymphogranuloma venereum, HPV, and *Actinomyces* spp.).
- Assist in the diagnosis of primary and metastatic tumors.
- Evaluate hormonal function.

INTERFERING FACTORS
Factors that may alter the results of the study
- The smear should not be allowed to air dry before fixation.
- Lubricating jelly should not be used on the speculum *because the viability of some organisms is adversely affected by gels and disinfectants.*
- Improper collection site may result in specimen rejection. Samples for cancer screening are obtained from the posterior vaginal fornix and from the cervix. Samples for hormonal evaluation are obtained from the vagina.
- Douching, sexual intercourse, using tampons, or using vaginal medication within 24 hr prior to specimen collection can interfere with the specimen's results.
- Collection of other specimens prior to the collection of the Pap smear may be cause for specimen rejection.

P

• Contamination with blood from samples collected during the patient's menstrual period may be cause for specimen rejection.

POTENTIAL MEDICAL DIAGNOSIS: CLINICAL SIGNIFICANCE OF RESULTS

Abnormal findings related to (See table [Manual review, Bethesda system or Automated review, any system])

NURSING IMPLICATIONS

BEFORE THE STUDY: PLANNING AND IMPLEMENTATION

Teaching the Patient What to Expect

‣ Inform the patient this procedure can assist in diagnosing infection or disease of the reproductive system.

‣ Explain that a swab of cells from the cervical or vaginal area is needed for the test.

‣ Review the procedure with the patient. Address concerns about pain and explain that there may be some discomfort during the procedure.

‣ Explain that specimen collection is performed by a health-care provider (HCP) specializing in this procedure and takes approximately 5 to 10 min.

‣ Explain that it will be necessary to remove all clothes below the waist.

‣ Positioning for this procedure is in the lithotomy position on a gynecological examination table (with feet in stirrups). The legs are draped.

‣ Once the patient is positioned correctly, a plastic or metal speculum is inserted into the vagina and opened to gently spread apart the vagina for inspection of the cervix. The speculum may be dipped in warm water to aid in comfortable insertion.

‣ After the speculum is properly positioned, the cervical and vaginal specimens are obtained by inserting a synthetic fiber brush deep enough into the cervix to reach the endocervical canal. The brush is then rotated one turn and removed. A plastic or wooden spatula is used to lightly scrape the cervix and vaginal wall.

Conventional Collection

‣ Specimens from both the brush and the spatula are plated on the glass slide.

‣ The brush specimen is plated using a gentle rolling motion, whereas the spatula specimen is plated using a light gliding motion across the slide.

‣ The specimens are immediately fixed to the slide with a liquid or spray containing 95% ethanol.

‣ The speculum is removed from the vagina.

‣ A pelvic and/or rectal examination is usually performed after specimen collection is completed.

ThinPrep Collection

‣ The ThinPrep bottle lid is opened and removed, exposing the solution.

‣ The brush and spatula specimens are then gently swished in the ThinPrep solution to remove the adhering cells, and then the bottle lid is replaced and secured.

General

‣ Samples are placed in a properly labelled specimen container and promptly transported to the laboratory for processing and analysis.

Potential Nursing Actions

   Make sure a written and informed consent has been signed prior to the procedure and before administering any medications.

‣ Ask if the patient is taking vaginal antibiotic medication, as testing should be delayed for 1 mo after the treatment has been completed.

‣ Verify adherence to the request to avoid douching or sexual intercourse for 24 hr before specimen collection.

‣ Verify that the patient is not menstruating.

AFTER THE STUDY: POTENTIAL NURSING ACTIONS

Treatment Considerations

‣ Assist in cleansing secretions or excess lubricant (if a pelvic and/or rectal examination is also performed) from the perineal area. Provide a sanitary pad if cervical bleeding occurs. Provide instructions if the patient wishes to complete this task herself.

▶ There may be concerns related to changes to sexual intimacy associated with sexually transmitted infection. Provide a relaxed atmosphere in which to discuss sexuality concerns and support group contact information.

▶ Provide information regarding vaccine-preventable diseases when indicated (e.g., cervical cancer and sexually transmitted infections such as hepatitis B and human papillomavirus).

Follow-Up, Evaluation, and Desired Outcomes

▶ Acknowledges provided contact information for the CDC (www.cdc.gov/vaccines/vpd/vaccines-diseases.html) for guidelines on vaccine preventable diseases.

▶ Understands that decisions regarding the need for and frequency of conventional or liquid-based Pap tests or other cancer screening procedures should be made after consultation between the patient and HCP. The American Cancer Society's (ACS) guidelines for preventing cervical cancer no longer recommend annual cytological screening because of the extended period of time (10–20 years) it takes for cervical cancer to develop; more frequent screening in low-risk women is believed to result in unnecessary procedures. ACS recommends cytological screening every 3 yr for women aged 21 to 29 yr and co-testing for HPV with cytological screening every 5 yr for women aged 30 to 65 yr; no screening is recommended for women over age 65 years who have had regular screening with normal findings; no screening is recommended for women who have had a total hysterectomy (removal of uterus and cervix). The most current guidelines for cervical cancer screening of the general population as well as of individuals with increased risk are available from the ACS (www.cancer.org) and the American College of Obstetricians and Gynecologists (www.acog.org).

Parathyroid Hormone

SYNONYM/ACRONYM: Parathormone, PTH, intact PTH, whole molecule PTH.

RATIONALE: To assist in the diagnosis of parathyroid disease and disorders of calcium balance. Also used to monitor patients receiving renal dialysis.

PATIENT PREPARATION: There are no food, fluid, activity, or medication restrictions unless by medical direction.

NORMAL FINDINGS: Method: Immunoassay.

Age	Conventional Units	SI Units (Conventional Units × 1)
Cord blood	Less than 3 pg/mL	Less than 3 ng/L
2–20 yr	9–52 pg/mL	9–52 ng/L
Adult	10–65 pg/mL	10–65 ng/L

CRITICAL FINDINGS AND POTENTIAL INTERVENTIONS: N/A

OVERVIEW: (Study type: Blood collected in a gold-, red-, or red/gray-top tube; related body system: Endocrine system. The specimen should be promptly transported to the laboratory for processing and analysis. The sample should be placed in an ice slurry immediately after collection. Information on the specimen label should be protected from water in the ice slurry by first placing the specimen in a protective plastic bag.) Parathyroid hormone (PTH) is secreted by the parathyroid glands in response to decreased levels of circulating calcium. PTH assists in raising serum calcium levels by

- Stimulating the release of calcium from bone into the bloodstream.
- Promoting renal tubular reabsorption of calcium and decreased reabsorption of phosphate.
- Enhancing renal production of active vitamin D metabolites, which increases calcium absorption in the small intestine.

C-terminal and N-terminal assays were used prior to the development of reliable intact or whole molecule PTH assays. A rapid PTH assay has been developed specifically for intraoperative monitoring of PTH in the surgical treatment of primary hyperparathyroidism. Rapid PTH assays have proved valuable because the decision whether the hyperparathyroidism involves one or multiple glands depends on measurement of circulating PTH levels. Surgical outcomes indicate that a 50% decrease or more in intraoperative PTH from baseline measurements can predict successful treatment with up to 97% accuracy. An intraoperative decrease of less than 50% indicates the need to identify and remove additional malfunctioning parathyroid tissue. In healthy individuals, intact PTH has a circulating half-life of about 5 min. N-terminal PTH has a circulating half-life of about 2 min and is found in minute quantities. Intact and N-terminal PTH are the only biologically active forms of the hormone. Ninety percent of circulating PTH is composed of inactive C-terminal and midregion fragments. PTH is cleared from the body by the kidneys.

INDICATIONS

- Assist in the diagnosis of hyperparathyroidism.
- Assist in the diagnosis of suspected secondary hyperparathyroidism due to chronic kidney disease, malignant tumors that produce ectopic PTH, and malabsorption syndromes.
- Detect incidental damage or inadvertent removal of the parathyroid glands during thyroid or neck surgery.
- Differentiate parathyroid and nonparathyroid causes of hypercalcemia.
- Evaluate autoimmune destruction of the parathyroid glands.
- Evaluate parathyroid response to altered serum calcium levels, especially those that result from malignant processes, leading to decreased PTH production.
- Evaluate source of altered calcium metabolism.

INTERFERING FACTORS
Factors that may alter the results of the study
- Drugs and other substances that may increase PTH levels include anticonvulsants, clodronate, estrogen/progestin therapy, foscarnet,

furosemide, hydrocortisone, isoniazid, lithium, nifedipine, octreotide,
pamidronate, phosphates, prednisone, rifampin, steroids, tamoxifen,
and verapamil.
• Drugs and other substances that
may decrease PTH levels include
alfacalcidol, aluminum hydroxide,
calcitriol, cimetidine, diltiazem,
magnesium sulfate, parathyroid
hormone, pindolol, prednisone,
propranolol, and vitamin D.

Other considerations
• PTH levels are subject to diurnal
variation, with highest levels occurring in the morning.
• PTH levels should always be measured in conjunction with calcium
for proper interpretation.

POTENTIAL MEDICAL DIAGNOSIS: CLINICAL SIGNIFICANCE OF RESULTS
Increased in
• Fluorosis *(skeletal fluorosis can
cause a condition resembling
secondary hyperparathyroidism,
disruption in calcium homeostasis,
and excessive PTH production)*
• Hyperparathyroidism: primary,
secondary, or tertiary *(all result in
excess PTH production)*
• Hypocalcemia *(compensatory
increase in PTH in response to low
calcium levels)*
• Pseudogout *(calcium is lost due to
deposits in the joint; decrease in calcium stimulates PTH production)*
• Pseudohypoparathyroidism
*(related to a congenital defect of
the kidney that prevents a normal
response to PTH in the presence of
low calcium levels, signaling the
parathyroid glands to secrete additional PTH)*
• Zollinger-Ellison syndrome
*(related to poor intestinal absorp-
tion of calcium and vitamin D;
decreased calcium stimulates PTH
production)*

Decreased in
• Autoimmune destruction of the
parathyroids *(related to decreased
parathyroid function)*
• DiGeorge syndrome *(related to
hypoparathyroidism)*
• Hypercalcemia for any reason (e.g.,
tumors of the bone, breast, lung,
kidney, pancreas, ovary) *(compensatory response to high calcium levels)*
• Hyperthyroidism *(related to
increased calcium from bone loss;
increased calcium levels inhibit PTH
production)*
• Hypomagnesemia *(magnesium is a
calcium channel blocker; low magnesium levels allow for increased
calcium, which inhibits PTH
production)*
• Nonparathyroid hypercalcemia
(in the absence of kidney disease)
*(increased calcium levels inhibit
PTH production)*
• Sarcoidosis *(related to increased
calcium levels)*
• Secondary hypoparathyroidism due
to surgery

NURSING IMPLICATIONS

BEFORE THE STUDY: PLANNING AND IMPLEMENTATION

**Teaching the Patient What
to Expect**
▸ Inform the patient this test can assist in
diagnosing parathyroid disease.
▸ Explain that a blood sample is needed
for the test.
▸ For most patients with primary hyperparathyroidism, it is usually a single
gland, rather than multiple of the four
glands present, that is abnormal.
▸ Surgical removal of abnormal glands
combined with intraoperative PTH
monitoring has become the treatment
of choice.
▸ Inform the surgical patient that a baseline
PTH level will be collected prior to resection of the abnormal parathyroid glands.

P

▶ Explain that additional specimens will be collected during the procedure to indicate that all abnormal parathyroid tissue has been removed and the procedure can be concluded.

▶ The protocol may vary among healthcare providers (HCPs) regarding when the baseline level should be drawn (i.e., prior to anesthesia or prior to incision).

▶ The amount of change between the baseline and intraoperative values considered adequate for determining successful, complete resection of the abnormal tissue may also vary by HCP; a decrease of 50% is typically used as a cutoff.

▶ Early-morning specimen collection is recommended because of the diurnal variation in PTH levels.

AFTER THE STUDY: POTENTIAL NURSING ACTIONS

Treatment Considerations

▶ A deficit or excess of parathyroid hormone can result in observable symptoms. Deficits in hormone levels can result in pain and altered sensory perception. Observable symptoms of pain include muscle and carpopedal spasms, abdominal cramping, and tetany. Observable symptoms of altered sensory perception are paresthesia of the lips, hands, and feet and hyperactive reflexes. Excess in hormone levels can result in abdominal pain, peptic ulcer formation, and constipation. Some interventions to manage this excess are to monitor and trend serum calcium and phosphorus levels and collaborate with the pharmacist and HCP to pharmacologically manage calcium levels and monitor and trend serum parathyroid hormone levels.

Nutritional Considerations

▶ Patients with abnormal parathyroid levels are also likely to experience the effects of calcium-level imbalances. Instruct the patient to report signs and symptoms of hypocalcemia and hypercalcemia to the HCP. (For critical findings, signs, and symptoms of calcium imbalance and for nutritional information, see study titled "Calcium, Blood, Total and Ionized.")

Follow-Up, Evaluation, and Desired Outcomes

▶ Correctly states reportable symptoms of parathyroid disease that should be reported to the HCP.

▶ Agrees to institute recommended dietary changes and follow-up laboratory studies.

Parathyroid Scan

P

SYNONYM/ACRONYM: Parathyroid scintiscan.

RATIONALE: To assess the parathyroid gland toward diagnosing cancer and to perform postoperative evaluation of the parathyroid gland.

PATIENT PREPARATION: There are no food, fluid, activity, or medication restrictions unless by medical direction. No other radionuclide scans or procedures using iodinated contrast medium should be scheduled within 24 to 48 hr before this procedure. Protocols may vary among facilities.

NORMAL FINDINGS
• No areas of increased perfusion or uptake in the thyroid or parathyroid.

CRITICAL FINDINGS AND POTENTIAL INTERVENTIONS: N/A

OVERVIEW: (Study type: Nuclear scan; related body system: Endocrine system.) Parathyroid scanning is performed to assist in the preoperative identification and localization of the parathyroid glands. Parathyroid hyperplasia has the effect of enlarging all four glands; parathyroid adenoma results in enlargement of a single gland while suppressing growth of the unaffected glands. The scan is also performed after surgery to verify the presence of the parathyroid gland in children and adults after thyroidectomy.

The radionuclide (iodine-123, technetium-99m [Tc-99m] pertechnetate, Tc-99m sestamibi, or a combination of the three radionuclides) is administered either orally or by IV 10 to 20 min before the imaging is performed. There are two types of parathyroid scan: single-tracer double-phase (STDP) scan and double-tracer subtraction test (DTST). In STDP, images are taken at 15 min and 3 hr after the Tc-99m sestamibi is injected. The tracer is observed in both the thyroid and parathyroid tissue at 15 min but is only retained and observed in abnormal parathyroid tissue after 3 hr. In DTST, images are taken about 15 min after administration of either iodine-123 or Tc-99m pertechnetate where it can be observed that the thyroid gland has taken up the radionuclide; Tc-99m sestamibi is then injected and is taken up by both the thyroid and the parathyroid tissue. A second set of images is taken, and the first image is "subtracted" from the second so that the image of the thyroid is removed and images of the parathyroid glands remain.

Fine-needle aspiration biopsy guided by ultrasound is occasionally necessary to differentiate thyroid pathology, as well as pathology of other tissues, from parathyroid neoplasia.

INDICATIONS
- Aid in the diagnosis of hyperparathyroidism.
- Differentiate between extrinsic and intrinsic parathyroid adenoma but not between benign and malignant conditions.
- Evaluate the parathyroid in patients with severe hypercalcemia or in patients before parathyroidectomy.

INTERFERING FACTORS
Contraindications
　　Patients who are pregnant or suspected of being pregnant, unless the potential benefits of a procedure using radiation far outweigh the risk of radiation exposure to the fetus and mother.

Factors that may alter the results of the study
- Ingestion of foods containing iodine (e.g., iodized salt) and medications containing iodine (e.g., cough syrup, potassium iodide, vitamins, Lugol solution, thyroid replacement medications), which can decrease uptake of the radionuclide.
- Metallic objects (e.g., jewelry, body rings) within the examination field, other nuclear scans or radiographic procedures using iodinated contrast medium done within the previous 24 to 48 hr, or retained barium from a previous radiological procedure, which may inhibit organ visualization and cause unclear images.
- Improper injection of the radionuclide that allows the tracer to seep

P

deep into the muscle tissue can produce erroneous hot spots.
- Inability of the patient to cooperate or remain still during the procedure, because movement can produce blurred or otherwise unclear images.

POTENTIAL MEDICAL DIAGNOSIS: CLINICAL SIGNIFICANCE OF RESULTS

Abnormal findings related to
- Intrinsic and extrinsic parathyroid adenomas

NURSING IMPLICATIONS

BEFORE THE STUDY: PLANNING AND IMPLEMENTATION

Teaching the Patient What to Expect
- Inform the patient this procedure can assist in diagnosing parathyroid disease.
- Pregnancy is a general contraindication to procedures involving radiation. Explain to the female patient that she will be asked the date of her last menstrual period and pregnancy testing may be performed to determine the possibility of pregnancy before she is exposed to radiation.
- Review the procedure with the patient. Address concerns about pain and explain that there may be moments of discomfort or pain experienced when the IV line is inserted to allow infusion of fluids such as saline, anesthetics, sedatives, radionuclides, medications used in the procedure, or emergency medications.
- Explain that the procedure is performed in a nuclear medicine department by a health-care provider (HCP) specializing in this procedure, with support staff, and takes approximately 30 to 60 min.
- Tc-99m pertechnetate is injected by IV; iodine-123 may be administered orally in place of Tc-99m pertechnetate.
- Tc-99m sestamibi is injected, and a second image is obtained after 10 min.
- Reassure the patient that the radionuclide poses no radioactive hazard and rarely produces adverse effects.

- Instruct the patient to remove jewelry and other metallic objects from the area to be examined prior to the procedure.
- Prior to the procedure, baseline vital signs and neurological status are recorded. Protocols may vary among facilities.
- Positioning for the procedure is in a supine position under a radionuclide gamma camera. Images are performed 15 min after the injection.
- Once the scan is completed, the needle or catheter is removed and a pressure dressing is applied over the puncture site.

Potential Nursing Actions
- ✦ *Make sure a written and informed consent has been signed prior to the procedure and before administering any medications.*

AFTER THE STUDY: POTENTIAL NURSING ACTIONS

Avoiding Complications
- Establishing an IV site and injection of radionuclides are invasive procedures. Complications are rare but include risk for allergic reaction *(related to contrast reaction),* hematoma *(related to blood leakage into the tissue following needle insertion),* bleeding from the puncture site *(related to a bleeding disorder or the effects of natural products and medications with known anticoagulant, antiplatelet, or thrombolytic properties),* or infection *(which might occur if bacteria from the skin surface is introduced at the puncture site).* Monitor the patient for complications related to the procedure (e.g., allergic reaction, anaphylaxis, bronchospasm). Immediately report symptoms such as fast heart rate, difficulty breathing, skin rash, itching, or chest pain to the appropriate HCP. Observe/assess the needle/catheter insertion site for bleeding, inflammation, or hematoma formation.

Treatment Considerations
- Explain that the radionuclide is eliminated from the body within 6 to 24 hr. Advise the patient to drink increased amounts of fluids for 24 to 48 hr to eliminate the radionuclide from the body, unless contraindicated.

- Administer ordered antiemetics as needed.
- Evaluate pain and facilitate pain management with administration of ordered narcotics, anticholinergics, and alternative methods of pain management (relaxation, imagery, music, etc.)
- Instruct in the care and assessment of the injection site.
- Explain that application of cold compresses to the puncture site may reduce discomfort or edema.

Safety Considerations
- The patient who is breastfeeding should consult with the requesting HCP regarding alternate testing that does not involve radiation. In general, if a woman who is breastfeeding must have a nuclear scan, she should not breastfeed the infant for 72 hr after the scan, until the radionuclide has been eliminated. She should be instructed to express the milk in order to prevent cessation of milk production; the milk can be stored and used after the 3-day period.
- Refer to organizational policy for additional precautions that may include instructions on handwashing, toilet flushing, limited contact with others, and other aspects of nuclear medicine safety.

Follow-Up, Evaluation, and Desired Outcomes
- Understands that depending on the results of this procedure, additional testing may be needed to evaluate or monitor progression of the disease process and determine the need for a change in therapy.

Partial Thromboplastin Time, Activated

SYNONYM/ACRONYM: aPTT, APTT.

RATIONALE: To assist in assessing coagulation disorders and monitor the effectiveness of therapeutic interventions.

PATIENT PREPARATION: There are no food, fluid, activity, or medication restrictions unless by medical direction.

NORMAL FINDINGS: (Method: Clot detection) 25 to 35 sec. The activated partial thromboplastin time (aPTT) is slightly prolonged in infants and children and is slightly shortened in older adults. Reference ranges vary with respect to the equipment and reagents used to perform the assay. For the patient on anticoagulants, therapeutic levels of heparin are achieved by adjusting the dosage so the aPTT value is 1.5 to 2.5 times the normal.

P

CRITICAL FINDINGS AND POTENTIAL INTERVENTIONS
- *Adults and Children:* Greater than 70 sec

Timely notification to the requesting health-care provider (HCP) of any critical findings and related symptoms is a role expectation of the professional nurse. A listing of these findings varies among facilities.

Consideration may be given to verification of critical findings before action is taken. Policies vary among facilities and may include requesting immediate recollection and retesting by the laboratory or retesting using a rapid point-of-care testing instrument at the bedside, if available.

Important signs to note are prolonged bleeding from cuts or gums, hematoma at a puncture site, bruising easily, blood in the stool, persistent epistaxis, heavy or prolonged menstrual flow, and shock. Monitor vital signs, aPTT levels, unusual ecchymosis, occult blood, severe headache, unusual dizziness, and neurological changes until aPTT is within normal range.

OVERVIEW: (Study type: Blood collected in a completely filled blue-top [3.2% sodium citrate] tube; related body system: Circulatory/Hematopoietic system. If the patient's hematocrit [Hct] exceeds 55%, the volume of citrate in the collection tube must be adjusted. *Important Note:* The collection tube should be completely filled. When multiple specimens are drawn, the blue-top tube should be collected after sterile [i.e., blood culture] tubes. Otherwise, when using a standard vacutainer system, the blue top is the first tube collected. When a butterfly is used, due to the added tubing, an extra red-top tube should be collected before the blue-top tube to ensure complete filling of the blue-top tube.) The aPTT test evaluates the function of the contact activation pathway, formerly known as intrinsic pathway (factors XII, XI, IX, VIII, prekallikrein, and high molecular weight kininogen) and the common pathway (factors V, X, II, and I) of the coagulation sequence. The aPTT time represents the time required for formation of a firm fibrin clot after tissue thromboplastin reagents and calcium are added to a plasma specimen. The aPTT is abnormal in 90% of patients with coagulation disorders and is useful in monitoring effective inactivation of factor II (thrombin) by heparin therapy. The test is prolonged when there is a 30% to 40% deficiency in one of the factors required or when factor inhibitors (e.g., antithrombin III, protein C, or protein S)

are present. The aPTT and prothrombin time (PT) tests assist in identifying the cause of or tendency for bleeding as related to coagulation defects. A comparison between the results of aPTT and PT tests can allow some inferences to be made that a factor deficiency exists. A normal aPTT with a prolonged PT can occur only with factor VII deficiency. A prolonged aPTT with a normal PT could indicate a deficiency in factors XII, XI, IX, VIII, and VIII:C (von Willebrand factor). Factor deficiencies can also be identified by correction or substitution studies using normal serum. These studies are easy to perform and are accomplished by adding plasma from a healthy patient to a sample from a patient suspected to be factor deficient. When the aPTT is repeated and is corrected, or is within the reference range, it can be assumed that the prolonged aPTT is caused by a factor deficiency. If the result remains uncorrected, the prolonged aPTT is most likely due to a circulating anticoagulant. (For more information on factor deficiencies, see the "Coagulation Factors" study.)

INDICATIONS
- Detect congenital deficiencies in clotting factors, as seen in diseases such as hemophilia A (factor VIII) and hemophilia B (factor IX).
- Evaluate response to anticoagulant therapy with heparin or warfarin derivatives.
- Identify individuals who may be prone to bleeding during surgical,

obstetric, dental, or invasive diagnostic procedures.
- Identify the possible cause of abnormal bleeding, such as epistaxis, hematoma, gingival bleeding, hematuria, and menorrhagia.
- Monitor the hemostatic effects of conditions such as liver disease, protein deficiency, and fat malabsorption.

INTERFERING FACTORS
Factors that may alter the results of the study
- Drugs and other substances such as anistreplase, antihistamines, chlorpromazine, salicylates, and ascorbic acid may cause prolonged aPTT.
- Anticoagulant therapy with heparin will prolong the aPTT.
- Copper is a component of factor V, and severe copper deficiencies may result in prolonged aPTT values.
- Traumatic venipunctures can activate the coagulation sequence by contamination of the sample with tissue thromboplastin and can produce falsely shortened results.
- Excessive agitation that causes sample hemolysis can falsely shorten the aPTT because the hemolyzed cells activate plasma-clotting factors.
- High platelet count or inadequate centrifugation will result in decreased values.
- Hct greater than 55% may cause falsely prolonged results because of anticoagulant excess relative to plasma volume.

Other considerations
- Inadequate mixing of the tube can produce erroneous results.
- Incompletely filled collection tubes, specimens contaminated with heparin, or clotted specimens. If delays in specimen transport and processing occur, it is important to consult with the testing laboratory. Whole blood specimens are stable at room temperature for up to 24 hr. Specimen stability requirements may also vary if the patient is receiving heparin therapy. Some laboratories require frozen plasma if testing will not be performed within 1 hr of collection. Criteria for rejection of specimens based on collection time may vary among facilities.

POTENTIAL MEDICAL DIAGNOSIS: CLINICAL SIGNIFICANCE OF RESULTS
Prolonged in
- Afibrinogenemia, dysfibrinogenemia, or hypofibrinogenemia *(related to insufficient levels of fibrinogen, which is required for clotting)*
- Circulating anticoagulants *(related to the presence of coagulation factor inhibitors, e.g., developed from long-term factor VIII therapy, or circulating anticoagulants associated with conditions like tuberculosis, systemic lupus erythematosus, rheumatoid arthritis, and chronic glomerulonephritis)*
- Circulating products of fibrin and fibrinogen degradation *(related to the presence of circulating breakdown products of fibrin)*
- Disseminated intravascular coagulation *(related to increased consumption of clotting factors)*
- Factor deficiencies *(related to insufficient levels of coagulation factors)*
- Patients on hemodialysis *(related to the anticoagulant effect of heparin)*
- Severe liver disease *(insufficient production of clotting factors related to liver damage)*
- Vitamin K deficiency *(related to insufficient vitamin K levels required for clotting)*
- Von Willebrand disease *(related to a congenital deficiency of clotting factors)*

P

NURSING IMPLICATIONS

POTENTIAL NURSING PROBLEMS: ASSESSMENT & NURSING DIAGNOSIS

Problems	Signs and Symptoms
Bleeding *(related to alerted clotting factors secondary to heparin use or depleted clotting factors)*	Altered level of consciousness; hypotension; increased heart rate; decreased Hgb and Hct; capillary refill greater than 3 sec; cool extremities; blood in urine, stool, sputum; bleeding gums; nosebleed; bruises easily; elevated PTT
Gas exchange *(related to deficient oxygen capacity of the blood secondary to blood loss)*	Irregular breathing pattern, use of accessory muscles, altered chest excursion, adventitious breath sounds (crackles, rhonchi, wheezes, diminished breath sounds), copious secretions, signs of hypoxia, altered blood gas results, confusion, lethargy, cyanosis
Tissue perfusion *(related to decreased hemoglobin secondary to bleeding, altered clotting factors)*	Hypotension, dizziness, cool extremities, pallor, capillary refill greater than 3 sec in fingers and toes, weak pedal pulses, altered level of consciousness, altered sensation

BEFORE THE STUDY: PLANNING AND IMPLEMENTATION

Teaching the Patient What to Expect
- Inform the patient this test can assist in evaluating the effectiveness of blood clotting.
- Explain that a blood sample is needed for the test.

Potential Nursing Actions
- Observe for symptoms of altered coagulation such as bruising, bleeding gums, or blood in urine, sputum, or stool.

Safety Considerations
- Bleeding precautions may be necessary if there is a known or suspected coagulation problem.

AFTER THE STUDY: POTENTIAL NURSING ACTIONS

Treatment Considerations
- Bleeding: Increase the frequency of vital sign assessment with variances and trends in results. Monitor and trend Hgb/Hct results. Administer ordered blood or blood products, vitamin K, and stool softener. Assess skin for petechiae, purpura, or hematoma. Monitor for blood in emesis, sputum, urine, or stool. Institute bleeding precautions, which include avoiding unnecessary venipuncture, avoiding intramuscular (IM) injections, preventing trauma, being gentle with oral care and suctioning, and avoiding the use of a sharp razor.
- Gas Exchange: Monitor respiratory rate and effort based on assessment of patient condition. Assess lung sounds

P

frequently, monitor for secretions and bloody sputum, and suction as necessary. Use pulse oximetry to monitor oxygen saturation and collaborate with HCP to administer oxygen as needed. Elevate the head of the bed 30 degrees or higher. Monitor IV fluids and avoid aggressive fluid resuscitation. Assess level of consciousness and anticipate the need for possible intubation.

♦ Tissue Perfusion: Monitor blood pressure; assess extremities for skin temperature, color, and warmth; assess capillary refill and pedal pulses. Monitor for dizziness, numbness, tingling, hyperesthesia, or hypoesthesia. Monitor and trend PT and INR. Administer ordered IV fluids, fluid bolus, and medication to support blood pressure. Monitor and trend aPTT results.

Safety Considerations
♦ Instruct the patient to report severe bruising or bleeding from any areas of the skin or mucous membranes.

♦ Teach the patient at risk for bleeding to use a soft-bristle toothbrush, an electric razor, and to avoid constipation, acetylsalicylic acid and similar products, and IM injections.

Nutritional Considerations
♦ Discuss the importance of including foods high in vitamin K; the main dietary sources of vitamin K are broccoli, brussels sprouts, cabbage, cauliflower, greens (beet, collards, dandelion, mustard, and turnip), kale, spinach, leaf lettuce, watercress, parsley, and other raw green leafy vegetables, pork, liver, soybeans, mayonnaise, and vegetable oils.

Follow-Up, Evaluation, and Desired Outcomes
♦ Agrees to periodic laboratory testing while taking an anticoagulant.
♦ Complies with the request to refrain from at-risk behavior that would cause bleeding.

Parvovirus B19 Testing

SYNONYM/ACRONYM: N/A

RATIONALE: To assist in confirming a diagnosis of a present or past parvovirus infection.

PATIENT PREPARATION: There are no food, fluid, activity, or medication restrictions unless by medical direction.

NORMAL FINDINGS: Method: Immunoassay.

Negative	Less than 0.9 index
Equivocal	0.9–1 index
Positive	Greater than 1 index

CRITICAL FINDINGS AND POTENTIAL INTERVENTIONS: N/A

OVERVIEW: (Study type: Blood collected in a gold-, red-, or red/gray-top tube; related body system: Immune system.) Parvovirus B19, a single-stranded DNA virus transmitted by respiratory secretions, is the only parvovirus known to infect humans. Parvovirus B19 can also be transmitted in infected blood products and

P

across the placental barrier to the fetus. Its primary site of replication is in red blood cell precursors in the bone marrow. It is capable of causing disease along a wide spectrum ranging from a self-limited erythema (fifth disease) to bone marrow failure or aplastic crisis in patients with sickle cell anemia, spherocytosis, or thalassemia. Fetal hydrops and spontaneous abortion may also occur as a result of infection during pregnancy. The incubation period is approximately 1 wk after exposure. The infection is more common in children than adults. B19-specific antibodies appear in the serum approximately 3 days after the onset of symptoms. The presence of immunoglobulin M (IgM) antibodies indicates acute infection. The presence of immunoglobulin G (IgG) antibodies indicates past infection and is believed to confer lifelong immunity. Parvovirus B19 can also be detected by DNA hybridization using a polymerase chain reaction method.

INDICATIONS
• Assist in establishing a diagnosis of parvovirus B19 infection.

INTERFERING FACTORS
Factors that may alter the results of the study
• Patients who are immunocompromised may not develop sufficient antibody to be detected.

POTENTIAL MEDICAL DIAGNOSIS: CLINICAL SIGNIFICANCE OF RESULTS
Positive findings in
Parvovirus infection can be evidenced in a variety of conditions.

• Arthritis
• Erythema infectiosum (fifth disease)
• Erythrocyte aplasia
• Hydrops fetalis

Negative findings in: N/A

NURSING IMPLICATIONS

BEFORE THE STUDY: PLANNING AND IMPLEMENTATION

Teaching the Patient What to Expect
▶ Inform the patient this test can assist in diagnosing a viral infection.
▶ Explain that a blood sample is needed for the test.

AFTER THE STUDY: POTENTIAL NURSING ACTIONS

Treatment Considerations
▶ Be supportive of anxiety related to test results, and impaired activity related to lack of neuromuscular control, perceived loss of independence, and fear of shortened life expectancy.
▶ Provide teaching related to the clinical implications of the test results and access to counseling services.

Follow-Up, Evaluation, and Desired Outcomes
▶ Understands the necessity of returning to have a convalescent blood sample taken in 7 to 14 days.

Pericardial Fluid Analysis

SYNONYM/ACRONYM: N/A

RATIONALE: To evaluate and classify the type of fluid between the pericardium membranes to assist with diagnosis of infection or fluid balance disorder.

PATIENT PREPARATION: There are no activity restrictions unless by medical direction. Note that food and fluids should be restricted for 6 to 8 hr before the procedure, as directed by the health-care provider (HCP), unless the procedure is performed in an emergency situation to correct pericarditis.

Regarding the patient's risk for bleeding, the patient should be instructed to avoid taking natural products and medications with known anticoagulant, antiplatelet, or thrombolytic properties or to reduce dosage, as ordered, prior to the procedure. Number of days to withhold medication is dependent on the type of anticoagulant. Note the last time and dose of medication taken. Protocols may vary among facilities.

NORMAL FINDINGS: Method: Spectrophotometry for glucose; automated or manual cell count, macroscopic examination of cultured organisms, and microscopic examination of specimen for microbiology and cytology; microscopic examination of cultured microorganisms.

Pericardial Fluid	Reference Value
Appearance	Clear
Color	Pale yellow
Glucose	Parallels serum values
Red blood cell (RBC) count	None seen
White blood cell (WBC) count	Less than 300 cells/microL
Culture	No growth
Gram stain	No organisms seen
Cytology	No abnormal cells seen

CRITICAL FINDINGS AND POTENTIAL INTERVENTIONS
• Positive culture findings in any sterile body fluid.

Timely notification to the requesting HCP of any critical findings and related symptoms is a role expectation of the professional nurse. A listing of these findings varies among facilities.

OVERVIEW: (Study type: Body fluid [pericardial fluid] collected in a red- or green-top [heparin] tube for glucose, a lavender-top [EDTA] tube for cell count, and sterile containers for microbiology specimens; fluid in a clear container for cytology; related body system: Circulatory and Immune systems. Ensure that there is an equal amount of fixative and fluid in the container for cytology.) The heart is located within a protective membrane called the *pericardium*. The fluid between the pericardial membranes is called *serous fluid*.

Normally, only a small amount of fluid is present because the rates of fluid production and absorption are about the same. Many abnormal conditions can result in the buildup of fluid within the pericardium. Specific tests are usually ordered in addition to a common battery of tests used to distinguish a transudate from an exudate. *Transudates* are effusions that form as a result of a systemic disorder that disrupts the regulation of fluid balance, such as a suspected perforation. *Exudates* are caused by conditions involving the tissue of

P

the membrane itself, such as an infection or malignancy. Fluid is withdrawn from the pericardium by needle aspiration and tested as listed in the previous and following tables.

Characteristic	Transudate	Exudate
Appearance	Clear to pale yellow	Cloudy, bloody, or turbid
Specific gravity	Less than 1.015	Greater than 1.015
Total protein	Less than 2.5 g/dL	Greater than 3 g/dL
Fluid protein–to–serum protein ratio	Less than 0.5	Greater than 0.5
Lactate dehydrogenase (LDH)	Less than 2/3 the upper limit of normal serum LDH	Greater than 2/3 the upper limit of normal serum LDH
Fluid LDH–to–serum LDH ratio	Less than 0.6	Greater than 0.6
Fluid cholesterol	Less than 55 mg/dL	Greater than 55 mg/dL
WBC count	Less than 100 cells/microL	Greater than 1,000 cells/microL

INDICATIONS
- Evaluate effusion of unknown etiology.
- Investigate suspected hemorrhage, immune disease, malignancy, or infection.

INTERFERING FACTORS
Factors that may alter the results of the study
- Bloody fluid may be the result of a traumatic tap.

Other considerations
- Unknown hyperglycemia or hypoglycemia may be misleading in the comparison of fluid and serum glucose levels. Therefore, it is advisable to collect comparative serum samples a few hours before performing pericardiocentesis.

POTENTIAL MEDICAL DIAGNOSIS: CLINICAL SIGNIFICANCE OF RESULTS
Increased in
Condition/Test Showing Increased Result
- Bacterial pericarditis (RBC count, WBC count with a predominance of neutrophils)
- Hemorrhagic pericarditis (RBC count, WBC count)
- Malignancy (RBC count, abnormal cytology)
- Post-myocardial infarction syndrome, also called *Dressler syndrome* (RBC count, WBC count with a predominance of neutrophils)
- Rheumatoid disease or systemic lupus erythematosus (SLE) (RBC count, WBC count)
- Tuberculous or fungal pericarditis (RBC count, WBC count with a predominance of lymphocytes)
- Viral pericarditis (RBC count, WBC count with a predominance of neutrophils)

Decreased in
Condition/Test Showing Decreased Result
- Bacterial pericarditis (glucose)
- Malignancy (glucose)
- Rheumatoid disease or SLE (glucose)

P

NURSING IMPLICATIONS

BEFORE THE STUDY: PLANNING AND IMPLEMENTATION

Teaching the Patient What to Expect
▶ Inform the patient this procedure can assist with evaluating fluid around the heart.
▶ Explain that a pericardial fluid sample is needed for the test.
▶ Explain that prior to the procedure, laboratory testing may be required to determine the possibility of bleeding risk (coagulation testing).
▶ Explain that reducing health-care-associated infections is an important patient safety goal and a number of different safety practices will be implemented during their procedure. Advise the patient that hair in the area near the catheter insertion site may be clipped or shaved and the area cleaned with an antiseptic solution to cleanse bacteria from the skin in order to reduce the risk for infection. *Note:* The World Health Organization, Centers for Disease Control and Prevention, and Association of periOperative Registered Nurses recommend that hair not be removed at all unless it interferes with the incision site or other aspects of the procedure because hair removal by any means is associated with increased infection rates. When hair removal is necessary, facilities must use a protocol that is based on scientific literature or the endorsement of a professional organization. Clipping immediately before the procedure and in a location outside the procedure area is preferred to shaving with a razor. Shaving creates a break in skin integrity and provides a way for bacteria on the skin to enter the incision site.
▶ Explain that a pericardial fluid sample is needed for the test.
▶ Review the procedure with the patient. Address concerns about pain and explain that there may be moments of discomfort or pain experienced when the IV line is inserted to allow infusion of fluids such as saline, anesthetics, sedatives, antibiotics, medications used in the procedure, or emergency medications; a sedative and/or analgesia will be administered to promote relaxation and reduce discomfort prior to needle insertion through the chest wall into the pericardium.
▶ Explain that any discomfort with the needle insertion will be minimized with local anesthetics and systemic analgesics.
▶ Advise that the anesthetic injection may cause a stinging sensation and that after the skin has been anesthetized, a large needle will be inserted through the chest to obtain the fluid.
▶ The specimen collection is performed by an HCP specializing in this procedure and usually takes approximately 30 min to complete.
▶ Baseline vital signs are recorded and continuously monitored throughout the procedure. Protocols may vary among facilities.
▶ Positioning for this procedure is in a comfortable supine position with the head elevated 45 to 60 degrees.
▶ The area is draped, and then the skin at the injection site is anesthetized. Explain that the cardiac needle is inserted just below and to the left of the breastbone, and fluid is removed.
▶ Vital signs are monitored every 15 min for signs of hypovolemia or shock.
▶ The electrocardiogram is monitored for needle-tip positioning to indicate accidental puncture of the right atrium.
▶ Once the procedure is completed, the needle is withdrawn, and slight pressure is applied to the site along with a sterile dressing.
▶ Samples are placed in properly labelled specimen containers and promptly transported to the laboratory for processing and analysis.

Potential Nursing Actions
❖ *Make sure a written and informed consent has been signed prior to the procedure and before administering any medications.*

Safety Considerations
▶ Anticoagulants, aspirin, and other salicylates should be discontinued by medical direction for the appropriate number of days prior to a procedure in which bleeding is a potential complication.

P

AFTER THE STUDY: POTENTIAL NURSING ACTIONS

Avoiding Complications

❯ Establishing an IV site and performing a pericardiocentesis are invasive procedures. Complications are rare but include risk for bleeding *(related to a bleeding disorder, or the effects of natural products and medications with known anticoagulant, antiplatelet, or thrombolytic properties)*, infection, or injury *(related to puncture of surrounding vessels or organs)*. Monitor the patient for complications related to the procedure (e.g., bleeding, infection, injury). Immediately report the appropriate elevated WBC count, fever, malaise, or tachycardia (indications of infection). Observe/assess the needle insertion site for bleeding, drainage, inflammation, or hematoma formation.

Treatment Considerations

❯ Instruct the patient to resume usual diet and medications, as directed by the HCP.
❯ Inform the patient that 1 hr or more of bedrest is required after the procedure.
❯ Monitor vital signs and cardiac status every 15 min for the first hour, every 30 min for the next 2 hr, every hr for the next 4 hr, and every 4 hr for the next 24 hr. Take the patient's temperature every 4 hr for 24 hr. Monitor intake and output for 24 hr. Notify the HCP if temperature is elevated. Protocols may vary among facilities.
❯ Observe for signs of respiratory and cardiac distress, such as shortness of breath, cyanosis, or rapid pulse.
❯ Continue IV fluids until vital signs are stable and the patient can resume fluid intake independently.
❯ Observe for nausea and pain. Administer antiemetic and analgesic medications as needed and as directed by the HCP.
❯ Administer ordered antibiotics and explain the importance of completing the entire course of antibiotic therapy even if no symptoms are present.

Follow-Up, Evaluation, and Desired Outcomes

❯ Understands that further testing, along with a referral to another HCP, may be necessary to manage the disease process and monitor the effectiveness of therapeutic interventions.

Peritoneal Fluid Analysis

SYNONYM/ACRONYM: Ascites fluid analysis.

RATIONALE: To evaluate and classify the type of fluid within the peritoneal cavity to assist with diagnosis of cancer, infection, necrosis, and perforation.

PATIENT PREPARATION: There are no food, fluid, or activity restrictions unless by medical direction. Regarding the patient's risk for bleeding, the patient should be instructed to avoid taking natural products and medications with known anticoagulant, antiplatelet, or thrombolytic properties or to reduce dosage, as ordered, prior to the procedure. Number of days to withhold medication is dependent on the type of anticoagulant. Note the last time and dose of medication taken.

NORMAL FINDINGS: Method: Spectrophotometry for glucose, amylase, and alkaline phosphatase; automated or manual cell count, macroscopic examination of cultured organisms, and microscopic examination of specimen for microbiology and cytology; microscopic examination of cultured microorganisms.

Peritoneal Fluid	Reference Value
Appearance	Clear
Color	Pale yellow
Amylase	Parallels serum values
Alkaline phosphatase	Parallels serum values
CEA	Parallels serum values
Glucose	Parallels serum values
Red blood cell (RBC) count	None seen
White blood cell (WBC) count	Less than 300 cells/microL
Culture	No growth
Acid-fast stain	No organisms seen
Gram stain	No organisms seen
Cytology	No abnormal cells seen

CRITICAL FINDINGS AND POTENTIAL INTERVENTIONS
• Positive culture findings in any sterile body fluid.

Timely notification to the requesting health-care provider (HCP) of any critical findings and related symptoms is a role expectation of the professional nurse. A listing of these findings varies among facilities.

OVERVIEW: (Study type: Body fluid [peritoneal fluid] collected in a red- or green-top [heparin = tube for amylase, glucose, and alkaline phosphatase; lavender-top [EDTA] tube for cell count; sterile containers for microbiology specimens; fluid in a clear container with anticoagulant for cytology; related body system: Digestive and Immune systems. Ensure that there is an equal amount of fixative and fluid in the container for cytology.) The peritoneal cavity and organs within it are lined with a protective membrane. The fluid between the membranes is called *serous fluid.* Normally, only a small amount of fluid is present because the rates of fluid production and absorption are about the same. Many abnormal conditions can result in the buildup of fluid within the peritoneal cavity. Specific tests are usually ordered in addition to a common battery of tests used to distinguish a transudate from an exudate. *Transudates* are effusions that form as a result of a systemic disorder that disrupts the regulation of fluid balance, such as a suspected perforation. *Exudates* are caused by conditions involving the tissue of the membrane itself, such as an infection or malignancy. Fluid (ascites) is withdrawn from the peritoneal cavity by needle aspiration (paracentesis) and tested as listed in the previous and following tables.

INDICATIONS
• Evaluate ascites of unknown cause.
• Investigate suspected peritoneal rupture, perforation, malignancy, or infection.

P

Characteristic	Transudate	Exudate
Appearance	Clear to pale yellow	Cloudy, bloody, or turbid
Specific gravity	Less than 1.015	Greater than 1.015
Total protein	Less than 2.5 g/dL	Greater than 3 g/dL
Fluid protein–to–serum protein ratio	Less than 0.5	Greater than 0.5
Lactate dehydrogenase (LDH)	Less than 2/3 the upper limit of normal serum LDH	Greater than 2/3 the upper limit of normal serum LDH
Fluid LDH–to–serum LDH ratio	Less than 0.6	Greater than 0.6
Fluid cholesterol	Less than 55 mg/dL	Greater than 55 mg/dL
WBC count	Less than 100 cells/ microL	Greater than 1,000 cells/ microL

INTERFERING FACTORS

Factors that may alter the results of the study
- Bloody fluids may result from a traumatic tap.

Other considerations
- Unknown hyperglycemia or hypoglycemia may be misleading in the comparison of fluid and serum glucose levels. Therefore, it is advisable to collect comparative serum samples a few hours before performing paracentesis.

POTENTIAL MEDICAL DIAGNOSIS: CLINICAL SIGNIFICANCE OF RESULTS

Increased in
Condition/Test Showing Increased Result
- Abdominal malignancy (RBC count, carcinoembryonic antigen, abnormal cytology)
- Abdominal trauma (RBC count)
- Ascites caused by cirrhosis (WBC count, neutrophils greater than 25% but less than 50%)
- Bacterial peritonitis (WBC count, neutrophils greater than 50%)
- Peritoneal effusion due to gastric strangulation, perforation, or necrosis (amylase, ammonia, alkaline phosphatase)
- Peritoneal effusion due to pancreatitis, pancreatic trauma, or pancreatic pseudocyst (amylase)
- Rupture or perforation of urinary bladder (ammonia, creatinine, urea)
- Tuberculous effusion (elevated lymphocyte count, positive acid-fast bacillus smear and culture [25% to 50% of cases])

Decreased in
Condition/Test Showing Decreased Result
- Abdominal malignancy (glucose)
- Tuberculous effusion (glucose)

NURSING IMPLICATIONS

BEFORE THE STUDY: PLANNING AND IMPLEMENTATION

Teaching the Patient What to Expect
- Inform the patient this procedure can assist with evaluation of fluid surrounding the abdominal organs.
- Explain that prior to the procedure, laboratory testing may be required to determine the possibility of bleeding risk (coagulation testing).

P

◗ Explain that reducing health-care-associated infections is an important patient safety goal and a number of different safety practices will be implemented during their procedure. Advise the patient that hair in the area near the catheter insertion site may be clipped or shaved and the area cleaned with an antiseptic solution to cleanse bacteria from the skin in order to reduce the risk for infection. *Note:* The World Health Organization, Centers for Disease Control and Prevention, and Association of periOperative Registered Nurses recommend that hair not be removed at all unless it interferes with the incision site or other aspects of the procedure because hair removal by any means is associated with increased infection rates. When hair removal is necessary, facilities must use a protocol that is based on scientific literature or the endorsement of a professional organization. Clipping immediately before the procedure and in a location outside the procedure area is preferred to shaving with a razor. Shaving creates a break in skin integrity and provides a way for bacteria on the skin to enter the incision site.

◗ Explain that a peritoneal fluid sample is needed for the test.

◗ Review the procedure with the patient. Address concerns about pain and explain that there may be moments of discomfort or pain experienced when the IV line is inserted to allow infusion of fluids such as saline, anesthetics, sedatives, antibiotics, medications used in the procedure, or emergency medications; a sedative and/or analgesia will be administered to promote relaxation and reduce discomfort prior to needle insertion through the abdomen wall. Explain that any discomfort with the needle insertion will be minimized with local anesthetics and systemic analgesics. The anesthetic injection may cause an initial stinging sensation.

◗ Explain that after the skin has been anesthetized, a large needle will be inserted through the abdominal wall and a "popping" sensation may be experienced as the needle penetrates the peritoneum.

◗ The patient's weight and abdominal girth measurements will be taken for those with ascites.

◗ Inform the patient that specimen collection is performed under sterile conditions by an HCP specializing in this procedure and usually takes approximately 30 min to complete.

◗ Baseline vital signs are recorded and continuously monitored throughout the procedure. Protocols may vary among facilities.

◗ Positioning for this procedure is in a seated comfortable position with feet and back supported or in high Fowler position.

◗ Explain that hair is clipped from the site as needed, and the site is cleansed with an antiseptic solution and draped with sterile towels prior to the administration of local anesthesia. The skin at the injection site is then anesthetized.

◗ Explain the process for fluid removal is to insert a paracentesis needle 1 to 2 in. below the umbilicus, allowing fluid to be removed.

◗ If lavage fluid is required (helpful if malignancy is suspected), saline or Ringer lactate can be infused via the needle over a 15- to 20-min period before the lavage fluid is removed.

◗ The patient's vital signs are monitored every 15 min for signs of hypovolemia or shock.

◗ Explain that the amount of fluid removed at a time will be no more than 1,500 to 2,000 mL of fluid, even in the case of a therapeutic paracentesis, due to the risk of hypovolemia and shock.

◗ Once the needle is withdrawn, slight pressure is applied to the site, and the site is covered with a sterile dressing.

Potential Nursing Actions

✦ *Make sure a written and informed consent has been signed prior to the procedure and before administering any medications.*

Safety Considerations

◗ Anticoagulants, aspirin, and other salicylates should be discontinued by medical direction for the appropriate number of days prior to a procedure where bleeding is a potential complication.

AFTER THE STUDY: POTENTIAL NURSING ACTIONS

Avoiding Complications
▶ Establishing an IV site and performing a paracentesis are invasive procedures. Complications are rare but include risk for bleeding (related to a bleeding disorder, or the effects of natural products and medications with known anticoagulant, antiplatelet, or thrombolytic properties), infection, or injury (related to puncture of surrounding vessels or organs). Monitor the patient for complications related to the procedure (e.g., bleeding, infection, injury). Immediately report to the appropriate elevated WBC count, fever, malaise, or tachycardia (indications of infection). Instruct the patient to immediately report severe abdominal pain. (Note: Rigidity of abdominal muscles indicates developing peritonitis.) Report to HCP if abdominal rigidity or pain is present. Observe/assess the needle insertion site for bleeding, drainage, inflammation, or hematoma formation.

Treatment Considerations
▶ Instruct the patient to resume usual medications, as directed by the HCP.

▶ Inform the patient that 1 hr or more of bedrest is required after the procedure.
▶ Monitor vital signs every 15 min for the first hr, every 30 min for the next 2 hr, every hour for the next 4 hr, and every 4 hr for the next 24 hr. Take the patient's temperature every 4 hr for 24 hr. Monitor intake and output for 24 hr. Protocols may vary among facilities.
▶ Observe the puncture site each time vital signs are taken and daily thereafter for several days. Report to the HCP if bleeding is present.
▶ Obtain weight and measure abdominal girth if a large amount of fluid was removed.
▶ Observe for nausea and pain. Administer antiemetic and analgesic medications as needed and as directed by the HCP.
▶ Administer ordered antibiotics and instruct in the importance of completing the entire course of antibiotic therapy even if no symptoms are present.

Follow-Up, Evaluation, and Desired Outcomes
▶ Understands that further testing, along with a referral to another HCP, may be necessary to manage the disease process, and monitor the effectiveness of therapeutic interventions.

Phosphorus, Blood

SYNONYM/ACRONYM: Inorganic phosphorus, phosphate, PO_4.

RATIONALE: To assist in evaluating multiple body system functions by monitoring phosphorus levels in relation to other electrolytes. Used specifically to evaluate renal function in at-risk patients.

PATIENT PREPARATION: There are no food, fluid, activity, or medication restrictions unless by medical direction.

NORMAL FINDINGS: Method: Spectrophotometry.

Age	Conventional Units	SI Units (Conventional Units × 0.323)
0–5 days	4.6–8 mg/dL	1.5–2.6 mmol/L
1–3 yr	3.9–6.5 mg/dL	1.3–2.1 mmol/L
4–6 yr	4–5.4 mg/dL	1.3–1.7 mmol/L
7–11 yr	3.7–5.6 mg/dL	1.2–1.8 mmol/L
12–13 yr	3.3–5.4 mg/dL	1.1–1.7 mmol/L
14–15 yr	2.9–5.4 mg/dL	0.9–1.7 mmol/L
16–19 yr	2.8–4.6 mg/dL	0.9–1.5 mmol/L
Adult	2.5–4.5 mg/dL	0.8–1.4 mmol/L

Values may be slightly decreased in older adults due to dietary insufficiency or the effects of medications and the presence of multiple chronic or acute diseases with or without muted symptoms.

CRITICAL FINDINGS AND POTENTIAL INTERVENTIONS

Adults
- Less than 1 mg/dL (SI: Less than 0.3 mmol/L)
- Greater than 8.9 mg/dL (SI: Greater than 2.9 mmol/L)

Children
- Less than 1.3 mg/dL (SI: Less than 0.4 mmol/L)
- Greater than 8.9 mg/dL (SI: Greater than 2.9 mmol/L)

Timely notification to the requesting health-care provider (HCP) of any critical findings and related symptoms is a role expectation of the professional nurse. A listing of these findings varies among facilities.

Interventions including IV replacement therapy with sodium or potassium phosphate may be necessary. Close monitoring of both phosphorus and calcium is important during replacement therapy.

OVERVIEW: (Study type: Blood collected in a gold-, red-, red/gray, or green-top [heparin] tube; related body system: Digestive, Endocrine, Musculoskeletal, and Urinary systems.) Phosphorus, in the form of phosphate, is distributed throughout the body. Approximately 85% of the body's phosphorus is stored in bones; the remainder is found in cells and body fluids. It is the major intracellular anion and plays a crucial role in cellular metabolism, maintenance of cellular membranes, and formation of bones and teeth. Phosphorus also indirectly affects the release of oxygen from hemoglobin by affecting the formation of 2,3-bisphosphoglycerate. The reabsorption and excretion of phosphorus is largely regulated by the parathyroid glands and the kidneys. Levels of phosphorus are also affected by dietary intake and are dependent on the presence of activated vitamin D for absorption by the intestines. Calcium and phosphorus are interrelated with respect to absorption and metabolic function. They

P

have an inverse relationship with respect to concentration; serum phosphorus is increased when serum calcium is decreased.

An infant fed only cow's milk during the first few weeks of life can develop hyperphosphatemia because of the combination of a high phosphorus content in cow's milk and the inability of infants' kidneys to clear the excess phosphorus.

INDICATIONS
• Assist in establishing a diagnosis of hyperparathyroidism.
• Assist in the evaluation of chronic kidney disease.

INTERFERING FACTORS
Factors that may alter the results of the study
• Drugs and other substances that may increase phosphorus levels include anabolic steroids, β-adrenergic blockers, ergocalciferol, furosemide, hydrochlorothiazide, methicillin (occurs with nephrotoxicity), oral contraceptives, parathyroid extract, phosphates, sodium etidronate, tetracycline (occurs with nephrotoxicity), and vitamin D.
• Drugs and other substances that may decrease phosphorus levels include acetazolamide, albuterol, aluminum salts, amino acids (via IV hyperalimentation), anesthetic drugs, anticonvulsants, calcitonin, epinephrine, fibrin hydrolysate, fructose, glucocorticoids, glucose, insulin, mannitol, oral contraceptives, pamidronate, phenothiazine, phytate, and plicamycin.
• Hemolysis will falsely increase phosphorus values.
• Specimens should never be collected above an IV line because of the potential for dilution when the specimen and the IV solution combine in the collection container, thereby falsely decreasing the result. There is also the potential of contaminating the sample with the substance of interest if it is present in the IV solution, thereby falsely increasing the result.

Other considerations
• Serum phosphorus levels are subject to diurnal variation: They are highest in late morning and lowest in the evening; therefore, serial samples should be collected at the same time of day for consistency in interpretation.

POTENTIAL MEDICAL DIAGNOSIS: CLINICAL SIGNIFICANCE OF RESULTS
Increased in
• **Acromegaly** *(related to increased renal absorption)*
• **Bone metastases** *(related to release from bone stores)*
• **Chronic kidney disease** *(related to decreased renal excretion)*
• **Diabetic ketoacidosis** *(acid-base imbalance causes intracellular phosphorus to move into the extracellular fluid)*
• **Excessive levels of vitamin D** *(vitamin D promotes intestinal absorption of phosphorus; excessive levels promote phosphorus release from bone stores)*
• **Hyperthermia** *(tissue damage causes intracellular phosphorus to be released into circulation)*
• **Hypocalcemia** *(calcium and phosphorus have an inverse relationship)*
• **Hypoparathyroidism** *(related to increased renal absorption)*
• **Lactic acidosis** *(acid-base imbalance causes intracellular*

P

phosphorus to move into the extra-cellular fluid)
- Milk alkali syndrome *(increased dietary intake)*
- Pseudohypoparathyroidism *(related to increased renal absorption)*
- Pulmonary embolism *(related to respiratory acid-base imbalance and compensatory mechanisms)*
- Respiratory acidosis *(acid-base imbalance causes intracellular phosphorus to move into the extracellular fluid)*

Decreased in
- Acute gout *(related to decreased circulating calcium in calcium crystal–induced gout; calcium and phosphorus have an inverse relationship)*
- Alcohol withdrawal *(related to malnutrition)*
- Gram-negative bacterial septicemia
- Growth hormone deficiency
- Hyperalimentation therapy
- Hypercalcemia *(calcium and phosphorus have an inverse relationship)*
- Hyperinsulinism *(insulin increases intracellular movement of phosphorus)*
- Hyperparathyroidism *(parathyroid hormone [PTH] increases renal excretion)*
- Hypokalemia
- Impaired renal absorption *(decreases return of phosphorus to general circulation)*
- Malabsorption syndromes *(related to insufficient intestinal absorption of phosphorus)*
- Malnutrition *(related to deficient intake)*
- Osteomalacia *(evidenced by hypophosphatemia)*
- PTH-producing tumors *(PTH increases renal excretion)*
- Primary hyperparathyroidism *(PTH increases renal excretion)*

- Renal tubular acidosis
- Renal tubular defects *(related to decreased renal absorption)*
- Respiratory alkalosis
- Respiratory infections
- Rickets *(related to vitamin D deficiency)*
- Salicylate poisoning
- Severe burns
- Severe vomiting and diarrhea *(related to excessive loss)*
- Vitamin D deficiency *(related to vitamin D deficiency, which reduces intestinal and renal tubular absorption of phosphorus)*

NURSING IMPLICATIONS

BEFORE THE STUDY: PLANNING AND IMPLEMENTATION

Teaching the Patient What to Expect
- Inform the patient this test can assist in a general evaluation of body systems.
- Explain that a blood sample is needed for the test.

AFTER THE STUDY: POTENTIAL NURSING ACTIONS

Treatment Considerations
- Discuss dietary changes that need to be made to support positive health.

Nutritional Considerations
- Severe hypophosphatemia is common in older adult patients or patients who have been hospitalized for long periods of time. Good dietary sources of phosphorus include meat, dairy products, nuts, and legumes. To decrease phosphorus levels to normal in the patient with hyperphosphatemia, dietary restriction may be recommended. Other interventions may include the administration of phosphate binders or calcitriol (the activated form of vitamin D).
- Vitamin D is necessary for the body to absorb phosphorus. Educate the patient with vitamin D deficiency, as appropriate, that the main dietary

P

sources of vitamin D are cod liver oil and fortified dairy foods such as milk, cheese, and orange juice. Explain to the patient that vitamin D is also synthesized by the body, in the skin, and is activated by sunlight.

Follow-Up, Evaluation, and Desired Outcomes

◗ Acknowledges contact information provided for the U.S. Department of Agriculture's resource for nutrition (www.choosemyplate.gov/).

Phosphorus, Urine

SYNONYM/ACRONYM: Urine phosphate.

RATIONALE: To assist in evaluating calcium and phosphorus levels related to use of diuretics in progression of kidney disease.

PATIENT PREPARATION: There are no food, fluid, activity, or medication restrictions unless by medical direction. Usually, a 24-hr urine collection is ordered. As appropriate, provide the required urine collection container and specimen collection instructions.

NORMAL FINDINGS: (Method: Spectrophotometry) Reference values are dependent on phosphorus and calcium intake. Phosphate excretion exhibits diurnal variation and is significantly higher at night.

Conventional Units	SI Units (Conventional Units × 0.0323)
400–1,300 mg/24 hr	12.9–42 mmol/24 hr

CRITICAL FINDINGS AND POTENTIAL INTERVENTIONS: N/A

OVERVIEW: (**Study type:** Urine from an unpreserved random or timed specimen collected in a clean plastic collection container; **related body system:** Endocrine and Urinary systems.) Phosphorus, in the form of phosphate, is distributed throughout the body. Approximately 85% of the body's phosphorus is stored in bones; the remainder is found in cells and body fluids. It is the major intracellular anion and plays a crucial role in cellular metabolism, maintenance of cellular membranes, and formation of bones and teeth. Phosphorus also indirectly affects the release of oxygen from hemoglobin by affecting the formation of 2,3-bisphosphoglycerate. Levels of phosphorus are dependent on dietary intake.

Analyzing urinary phosphorus levels can provide important clues to the functioning of the kidneys and other major organs. Tests for phosphorus in urine usually involve timed urine collections over a 12- or 24-hr period. Measurement of random specimens may also be requested. Children with thalassemia may have normal phosphorus absorption but increased excretion, which may result in a phosphorus deficiency.

P

INDICATIONS

- Assist in the diagnosis of hyperparathyroidism.
- Assist in the evaluation of calcium and phosphorus balance.
- Assist in the evaluation of nephrolithiasis.
- Assist in the evaluation of renal tubular disease.

INTERFERING FACTORS

Factors that may alter the results of the study

- Drugs and other substances that can cause an increase in urine phosphorus levels include acetazolamide, acetylsalicylic acid, bismuth salts, calcitonin, corticosteroids, dihydrotachysterol, glucocorticoids, hydrochlorothiazide, mestranol, metolazone, parathyroid extract, and parathyroid hormone.
- Drugs and other substances that can cause a decrease in urine phosphorus levels include aluminum-containing antacids and diltiazem.

Other considerations

- Urine phosphorus levels are subject to diurnal variation: Output is highest in the afternoon, which is why 24-hr urine collections are recommended.
- All urine voided for the timed collection period must be included in the collection or else falsely decreased values may be obtained. Compare output records with volume collected to verify that all voids were included in the collection.

POTENTIAL MEDICAL DIAGNOSIS: CLINICAL SIGNIFICANCE OF RESULTS

Increased in

- Misuse of diuretics *(related to increased renal excretion)*
- Primary hyperparathyroidism *(parathyroid hormone [PTH] increases renal excretion)*

- Renal tubular acidosis
- Vitamin D deficiency *(related to decreased renal reabsorption)*

Decreased in

- Hypoparathyroidism *(PTH enhances renal excretion; therefore, a lack of PTH will decrease urine phosphorus levels)*
- Pseudohypoparathyroidism *(PTH enhances renal reabsorption; therefore, a lack of response to PTH, as in pseudohypoparathyroidism, will decrease urine phosphorus levels)*
- Vitamin D intoxication *(vitamin D promotes renal excretion of phosphorus)*

NURSING IMPLICATIONS

BEFORE THE STUDY: PLANNING AND IMPLEMENTATION

Teaching the Patient What to Expect

▸ Inform the patient this test can assist in evaluating calcium and phosphorus balance.
▸ Explain that a urine sample is needed for the test. Information regarding specimen collection is presented with other general guidelines in Appendix A: Patient Preparation and Specimen Collection.

Potential Nursing Actions

▸ Include on the collection container's label the amount of urine, test start and stop times, and ingestion of any foods or medications that can affect test results.

AFTER THE STUDY: POTENTIAL NURSING ACTIONS

Treatment Considerations

▸ Explain that increased urine phosphorus levels may be associated with the formation of kidney stones.
▸ Advise the patient on the importance of drinking a sufficient amount of water when kidney stones are suspected.

P

Nutritional Considerations
▶ Vitamin D is necessary for the body to absorb phosphorus.
▶ Educate the patient with vitamin D deficiency that the main dietary sources of vitamin D are cod liver oil and fortified dairy foods such as milk, cheese, and orange juice.
▶ Explain that vitamin D is also synthesized by the body, in the skin, and is activated by sunlight.

Plasminogen

SYNONYM/ACRONYM: Profibrinolysin, PMG.

RATIONALE: To assess thrombolytic disorders such as disseminated intravascular coagulation (DIC) and monitor thrombolytic therapy.

PATIENT PREPARATION: There are no food, fluid, activity, or medication restrictions unless by medical direction.

NORMAL FINDINGS: Method: Chromogenic substrate for plasminogen activity and nephelometric for plasminogen antigen.

Plasminogen activity	70%–150% of normal
Plasminogen antigen	7.5–15.5 mg/dL

Plasminogen activity in newborns is half of adult ranges.

CRITICAL FINDINGS AND POTENTIAL INTERVENTIONS: N/A

OVERVIEW: (**Study type:** Blood collected in a completely filled blue-top [3.2% sodium citrate] tube; **related body system:** Circulatory/Hematopoietic system. If the patient's hematocrit [Hct] exceeds 55%, the volume of citrate in the collection tube must be adjusted. *Important Note:* The collection tube should be completely filled. When multiple specimens are drawn, the blue-top tube should be collected after sterile [i.e., blood culture] tubes. Otherwise, when using a standard vacutainer system, the blue top is the first tube collected. When a butterfly is used, due to the added tubing, an extra red-top tube should be collected before the blue-top tube to ensure complete filling of the blue-top tube. The specimen should be promptly transported to the specimen to the laboratory for processing and analysis. The recommendation for processed and unprocessed samples stored in unopened tubes is that testing should be completed within 1 to 4 hr of collection.) Plasminogen is a plasma glycoprotein produced by the liver. It is the circulating, inactive precursor to plasmin. Damaged tissues release a substance called *plasminogen activator* that initiates the conversion of plasminogen to plasmin. Plasmin participates in fibrinolysis and is capable of degrading fibrin, factor I (fibrinogen), factor V, and factor VIII. (For more information on fibrin degradation, see studies titled "Fibrinogen" and "Fibrinogen Degradation Products.")

INDICATIONS

Evaluate the level of circulating plasminogen in patients with thrombosis or disseminated intravascular coagulation (DIC).

INTERFERING FACTORS

Factors that may alter the results of the study
- Drugs and other substances that may decrease plasminogen levels include streptokinase and urokinase.
- Hct greater than 55% may cause falsely prolonged results because of anticoagulant excess relative to plasma volume.

Other considerations
- Incompletely filled collection tubes, specimens contaminated with heparin, clotted specimens, or unprocessed specimens not delivered to the laboratory within 1 to 2 hr of collection should be rejected.

POTENTIAL MEDICAL DIAGNOSIS: CLINICAL SIGNIFICANCE OF RESULTS

Increased in
- Pregnancy (late) *(pathophysiology is unclear)*

Decreased in
- DIC *(related to increased consumption during the hyperfibrinolytic state by conversion to plasmin)*
- Fibrinolytic therapy with tissue plasminogen activators such as streptokinase or urokinase *(related to increased consumption by conversion to plasmin)*

- Hereditary deficiency
- Liver disease *(related to decreased production by damaged liver cells)*
- Neonatal hyaline membrane disease *(possibly related to deficiency of plasminogen)*
- Postsurgical period *(possibly related to trauma of surgery)*

NURSING IMPLICATIONS

BEFORE THE STUDY: PLANNING AND IMPLEMENTATION

Teaching the Patient What to Expect
- Inform the patient that this test can assist in evaluating the effectiveness of blood clotting.
- Explain that a blood sample is needed for the test.

Potential Nursing Actions
- Observe for symptoms of altered coagulation such as bruising, bleeding gums, or blood in urine, sputum, or stool.

AFTER THE STUDY: POTENTIAL NURSING ACTIONS

Treatment Considerations
- Explain to those who have a bleeding disorder the importance of taking precautions against bruising and bleeding.
- Provide education for bleeding precautions, including the use of a soft-bristle toothbrush, electric razor; and avoidance of constipation, intramuscular injections, and acetylsalicylic acid (and similar products).

Follow-Up, Evaluation, and Desired Outcomes
- Acknowledges that depending on the results of this procedure, additional testing may be performed to evaluate or monitor progression of the disease process and determine the need for a change in therapy, including referral to another health-care provider.

P

Platelet Antibodies

SYNONYM/ACRONYM: Antiplatelet antibody; platelet-bound IgG/IgM, direct and indirect.

RATIONALE: To assess for the presence of platelet antibodies to assist in diagnosing thrombocytopenia related to autoimmune conditions and platelet transfusion compatibility issues.

PATIENT PREPARATION: There are no food, fluid, activity, or medication restrictions unless by medical direction.

NORMAL FINDINGS: (Method: Solid-phase enzyme-linked immunoassay) Negative.

CRITICAL FINDINGS AND POTENTIAL INTERVENTIONS: N/A

OVERVIEW: (Study type: Blood collected in a red-top tube for indirect immunoglobulin G [IgG] antibody. Whole blood collected in a lavender- [EDTA], yellow- [ACD], or pink- [K2EDTA]-top tube for direct antibody; related body system: Circulatory/Hematopoietic and Immune systems.) Platelet antibodies can be formed by autoimmune response, or they can be acquired in reaction to transfusion products or medications. Platelet autoantibodies are immunoglobulins of autoimmune origin (i.e., immunoglobulin G [IgG]), and they are present in various autoimmune disorders, including thrombocytopenias. Platelet alloantibodies develop in patients who become sensitized to platelet antigens of transfused blood. As a result, destruction of both donor and native platelets occurs along with a shortened survival time of platelets in the transfusion recipient. The platelet antibody detection test is also used for platelet typing, which allows compatible platelets to be transfused to patients with

disorders such as aplastic anemia and cancer. Platelet typing decreases the alloimmunization risk resulting from repeated transfusions from random donors. Platelet typing may also provide additional support for a diagnosis of post-transfusional purpura.

INDICATIONS
- Assist in the detection of platelet alloimmune disorders.
- Determine platelet type for refractory patients.

INTERFERING FACTORS
Factors that may alter the results of the study
- There are many drugs and other substances that may induce immune thrombocytopenia (production of antibodies that destroy platelets in response to the drugs). The most common include acetaminophen, gold salts, heparin (type II HIT), oral diabetic medications, penicillin, quinidine, quinine, salicylates, sulfonamides, and sulfonylurea.
- There are many drugs and other substances that may induce nonimmune thrombocytopenia (effect

P

of the drug includes bone marrow suppression or nonimmune platelet destruction). The most common include anticancer medications (e.g., bleomycin), ethanol, heparin (type I HIT), procarbazine, protamine, ristocetin, thiazide, and valproic acid.

Other considerations
• Hemolyzed or clotted specimens will affect results.

POTENTIAL MEDICAL DIAGNOSIS: CLINICAL SIGNIFICANCE OF RESULTS
Increased in
Development of platelet antibodies is associated with autoimmune conditions and medications.

• AIDS *(related to medications used therapeutically)*
• Acute myeloid leukemia *(related to medications used therapeutically)*
• Idiopathic thrombocytopenic purpura *(related to development of platelet-associated IgG antibodies)*
• Immune complex diseases
• Multiple blood transfusions *(related in most cases to sensitization to PLA1 antigens on donor red blood cells that will stimulate formation of antiplatelet antibodies)*
• Multiple myeloma *(related to medications used therapeutically)*
• Neonatal immune thrombocytopenia *(related to maternal platelet–associated antibodies directed against fetal platelets)*
• Paroxysmal hemoglobinuria
• Rheumatoid arthritis *(related to medications used therapeutically)*
• Systemic lupus erythematosus *(related to medications used therapeutically)*
• Thrombocytopenias provoked by drugs

Decreased in: N/A

BEFORE THE STUDY: PLANNING AND IMPLEMENTATION
Teaching the Patient What to Expect
▶ Inform the patient this test can assist in evaluating for issues related to platelet compatibility.
▶ Explain that a blood sample is needed for the test.

Potential Nursing Actions
▶ Observe for symptoms of altered coagulation such as bruising, bleeding gums, or blood in urine, sputum, or stool.

Safety Considerations
▶ Bleeding precautions may be necessary if there is a known or suspected coagulation problem.

AFTER THE STUDY: POTENTIAL NURSING ACTIONS
Treatment Considerations
▶ Note the patient's response to ordered platelet transfusions.
▶ Explain to those with a bleeding disorder the importance of taking precautions against bruising and bleeding.
▶ Instruct the patient to report severe bruising or bleeding from any areas of the skin or mucous membranes.
▶ Provide education for bleeding precautions, including the use of a soft-bristle toothbrush, electric razor; and avoidance of constipation, intramuscular injections, and acetylsalicylic acid (and similar products).

Follow-Up, Evaluation, and Desired Outcomes
▶ Acknowledges that depending on the results of this procedure, additional testing may be performed to evaluate or monitor progression of the disease process and determine the need for a change in therapy including referral to another health-care provider.

P

Platelet Count

SYNONYM/ACRONYM: Thrombocytes.

RATIONALE: To assist in diagnosing and evaluating treatment for blood disorders such as thrombocytosis and thrombocytopenia and to evaluate preprocedure or preoperative coagulation status.

PATIENT PREPARATION: There are no food, fluid, activity, or medication restrictions unless by medical direction.

NORMAL FINDINGS: Method: Automated, computerized, multichannel analyzers.

Age	Platelet Count*	SI Units (Conventional Units × 1)	MPV (fL)	IPF (%)
Birth	150–450 × 10³/microL	150–450 × 10⁹/L	7.1–10.2	1.1–7.1
Child, adult, older adult	140–400 × 10³/microL	140–400 × 10⁹/L	7.1–10.2	1.1–7.1

Note: Platelet counts may decrease slightly with age.
*Conventional units.
MPV = mean platelet volume.

CRITICAL FINDINGS AND POTENTIAL INTERVENTIONS
- Less than 30 × 10³/microL (SI: Less than 30 × 10⁹/L)
- Greater than 1,000 × 10³/microL (SI: Greater than 1,000 × 10⁹/L)

Timely notification to the requesting health-care provider (HCP) of any critical findings and related symptoms is a role expectation of the professional nurse. A listing of these findings varies among facilities.

Consideration may be given to verifying the critical findings before action is taken. Policies vary among facilities and may include requesting immediate recollection and retesting by the laboratory.

Critically low platelet counts can lead to brain bleeds or gastrointestinal hemorrhage, which can be fatal. Some signs and symptoms of decreased platelet count include spontaneous nosebleeds or bleeding from the gums, bruising easily, prolonged bleeding from minor cuts and scrapes, and bloody stool. Possible interventions for decreased platelet count may include transfusion of platelets or changes in anticoagulant therapy.

OVERVIEW: (**Study type:** Blood collected in a lavender-top [EDTA] tube; **related body system:** Circulatory/Hematopoietic and Immune systems. The specimen should be mixed gently by inverting the tube 10 times. The specimen should be analyzed within 24 hr when stored at room temperature or within 48 hr if stored at refrigerated temperature. If it is anticipated the specimen will not be analyzed within 24 hr, two blood smears should be made immediately after the venipuncture and submitted with the blood sample.) *Platelets* are nonnucleated, cytoplasmic, round or oval disks formed by budding off of large, multinucleated cells (megakaryocytes). Platelets have an essential function in coagulation, hemostasis, and blood thrombus formation. Activated platelets release a number of procoagulant factors, including thromboxane, a very potent platelet activator, from storage granules. These factors enter the circulation and activate other platelets, and the cycle continues. The activated platelets aggregate at the site of vessel injury, and at this stage of hemostasis the glycoprotein IIb/IIIa receptors on the activated platelets bind fibrinogen, causing the platelets to stick together and form a plug. Coagulation must be localized to the site of vessel wall injury, or the growing platelet plug would eventually occlude the affected vessel. The fibrinolytic system, under normal circumstances, begins to work, once fibrin begins to form, to ensure coagulation is limited to the appropriate site. *Thrombocytosis* is an increase in platelet count. In reactive thrombocytosis, the increase is transient and short-lived, and it usually does not pose a health risk. One exception may be reactive thrombocytosis occurring after coronary bypass surgery. This circumstance has been identified as an important risk factor for postoperative infarction and thrombosis. The term *thrombocythemia* describes platelet increases associated with chronic myeloproliferative disorders; *thrombocytopenia* describes platelet counts of less than 140 × 10^3/microL Decreased platelet

counts occur whenever the body's need for platelets exceeds the rate of platelet production; this circumstance will arise if production rate decreases or platelet loss increases. The severity of bleeding is related to platelet count as well as platelet function. Platelet counts can be within normal limits, but the patient may exhibit signs of internal bleeding; this circumstance usually indicates an anomaly in platelet function. Abnormal findings by automated cell counters may indicate the need to review a smear of peripheral blood for platelet estimate. Abnormally large or giant platelets may result in underestimation of automated counts by 30% to 50%. A large discrepancy between the automated count and the estimate requires that a manual count be performed. Platelet clumping may result in the underestimation of the platelet count. Clumping may be detected by the automated cell counter or upon microscopic review of a blood smear. A citrated platelet count, performed on a specimen collected in a blue-top tube, can be performed to obtain an accurate platelet count from patients who demonstrate platelet clumping in EDTA-preserved samples.

Thrombopoiesis or platelet production is reflected by the measurement of the immature platelet fraction (IPF). This parameter can be correlated to the total platelet count in the investigation of platelet disorders. A low platelet count with a low IPF can indicate a disorder of platelet production (e.g., drug toxicity, aplastic anemia or bone marrow failure of another cause), whereas a low platelet count with an increased IPF might indicate platelet destruction or abnormally high platelet consumption (e.g., mechanical destruction, disseminated intravascular coagulation, idiopathic thrombocytopenic purpura [ITP], thrombotic thrombocytopenic purpura).

Platelet size, reflected by mean platelet volume (MPV), and cellular age are inversely related; that is, younger platelets tend to be larger. An increase in MPV indicates an increase in platelet turnover. Therefore, in a healthy patient, the platelet count and MPV have an inverse relationship. Abnormal platelet size may also indicate the presence of a disorder. MPV and platelet distribution width are both increased in ITP. MPV is also increased in May-Hegglin anomaly, Bernard-Soulier syndrome, myeloproliferative disorders, hyperthyroidism, and pre-eclampsia. MPV is decreased in Wiskott-Aldrich syndrome, septic thrombocytopenia, and hypersplenism.

Platelets have receptor sites that are essential for normal platelet function and activation. Drugs such as clopidogrel (Plavix), abciximab (ReoPro), eptifibatide (Integrilin), and tirofiban block these receptor sites and inhibit platelet function. Aspirin also can affect platelet function by the irreversible inactivation of a crucial cyclooxygenase enzyme. Medications such as clopidogrel and aspirin are prescribed to prevent heart attack, stroke, and blockage of coronary stents. Studies have confirmed that up to 30% of patients receiving these medications may be nonresponsive. There are several commercial test systems that can assess aspects

of platelet function in addition to platelet count and size. Platelet adhesion, platelet aggregation, or bleeding time studies provide measurable responses that represent the time it might take for platelet closure to occur after a vascular injury. Platelet function testing helps ensure alternative or additional platelet therapy is instituted, if necessary. The test results can also be used preoperatively to determine whether antiplatelet medications have been sufficiently cleared from the patient's circulation such that surgery can safely be performed without risk of excessive bleeding. Thromboxane A2 is a potent stimulator of platelet activation. Activated platelets release 11-dehydrothromboxane B2 (11-D B2), the stable, inactive product of thromboxane A2 metabolism. Urine levels of 11-D B2 can be used to monitor response to aspirin therapy.

The metabolism of many commonly prescribed medications is driven by the cytochrome P450 (CYP450) family of enzymes. Genetic variants can alter enzymatic activity that results in a spectrum of effects ranging from the total absence of drug metabolism to ultrafast metabolism. Impaired drug metabolism can prevent the intended therapeutic effect or even lead to serious adverse drug reactions. Poor metabolizers are at increased risk for drug-induced adverse effects due to accumulation of drug in the blood, while ultra-rapid metabolizers require a higher than normal dosage because the drug is metabolized over a shorter duration than intended. Other genetic phenotypes used to report CYP450 results are intermediate metabolizer and extensive metabolizer. CYP2C19 is a gene in the CYP450 family that metabolizes drugs such as clopidogrel. Genetic testing can be performed on blood samples submitted to a laboratory. Testing for the most common genetic variants of CYP2C19 is used to predict altered enzyme activity and anticipate the most effective therapeutic plan. The test method commonly used is polymerase chain reaction. Counseling and informed written consent are generally required for genetic testing.

Knowledge of genetics assists in identifying those who may benefit from additional education, risk assessment, and counseling. Genetics is the study and identification of genes, genetic mutations, and inheritance. For example, genetics provides some insight into the likelihood of inheriting a tendency to abnormally metabolize drugs. Some conditions are the result of mutations involving a single gene, whereas other conditions may involve multiple genes and/or multiple chromosomes. Further information regarding inheritance of genes can be found in the study titled "Genetic Testing."

INDICATIONS

- Confirm an elevated platelet count (thrombocytosis), which can cause increased clotting.
- Confirm a low platelet count (thrombocytopenia), which can be associated with bleeding.
- Identify the possible cause of abnormal bleeding, such as epistaxis, hematoma, gingival bleeding, hematuria, and menorrhagia.
- Provide screening as part of a complete blood count (CBC) in a general physical examination, especially upon admission to a healthcare facility or before surgery.

INTERFERING FACTORS

Factors that may alter the results of the study

- Drugs and other substances that may decrease platelet counts include acetophenazine, amphotericin B, antazoline, anticonvulsants, antimony compounds, arsenicals, azathioprine, barbiturates, benzene, busulfan, butaperazine, chlordane, chlorophenothane, dactinomycin, dextromethorphan, diethylstilbestrol, ethoxzolamide, floxuridine, hydantoin derivatives, hydroxychloroquine, iproniazid, mechlorethamine, mefenamic acid, miconazole, mitomycin, nitrofurantoin, novobiocin, nystatin, phenolphthalein, phenothiazine, pipamazine, plicamycin, procarbazine, pyrazolones, streptomycin, sulfonamides, tetracycline, thiabendazole, thiouracil, tolazamide, tolazoline, tolbutamide, trifluoperazine, and urethane.
- Drugs and other substances that may increase platelet counts include glucocorticoids.
- X-ray therapy may also decrease platelet counts.
- The results of blood counts may vary depending on the patient's position. Platelet counts can decrease when the patient is recumbent, as a result of hemodilution, and can increase when the patient rises, as a result of hemoconcentration.
- Platelet counts normally increase under a variety of stressors, such as high altitudes or strenuous exercise.

P

- Platelet counts are normally decreased before menstruation and during pregnancy.

Other considerations
- Leaving the tourniquet in place for longer than 60 sec can affect the results.
- Traumatic venipunctures may lead to erroneous results as a result of activation of the coagulation sequence.
- Failure to fill the tube sufficiently (i.e., tube less than three-quarters full) may yield inadequate sample volume for automated analyzers and may be a reason for specimen rejection.
- Hemolysis or clotted specimens are reasons for rejection.
- CBC should be carefully evaluated after transfusion or acute blood loss because the value may appear to be normal.

POTENTIAL MEDICAL DIAGNOSIS: CLINICAL SIGNIFICANCE OF RESULTS
Increased in
Conditions that involve inflammation activate and increase the number of circulating platelets:

- Acute infections
- After exercise (transient)
- Anemias (posthemorrhagic, hemolytic, iron deficiency) *(bone marrow response to anemia; platelet formation is unaffected by iron deficiency)*
- Cirrhosis
- Essential thrombocythemia
- Leukemias (chronic)
- Malignancies (cancer, Hodgkin's, lymphomas)
- Pancreatitis (chronic)
- Polycythemia vera *(hyperplastic bone marrow response in all cell lines)*
- Rebound recovery from thrombocytopenia *(initial response)*

- Rheumatic fever (acute)
- Rheumatoid arthritis
- Splenectomy (2 mo postprocedure) *(normal function of the spleen is to cull aging cells from the blood; without the spleen, the count increases)*
- Surgery (2 wk postprocedure)
- Trauma
- Tuberculosis
- Ulcerative colitis

Decreased in
Conditions that are a result of megakaryocytic hypoproliferation:
- Alcohol toxicity
- Aplastic anemia
- Congenital abnormalities (Fanconi syndrome, May-Hegglin anomaly, Bernard-Soulier syndrome, Wiskott-Aldrich syndrome, Gaucher disease, Chédiak-Higashi syndrome)
- Drug toxicity
- Prolonged hypoxia

Conditions that are a result of ineffective thrombopoiesis:
- Alcohol misuse without malnutrition
- Iron-deficiency anemia
- Megaloblastic anemia (B_{12}/folate deficiency)
- Paroxysmal nocturnal hemoglobinuria
- Thrombopoietin deficiency
- Viral infection

Conditions that are a result of bone marrow replacement:
- Lymphoma
- Granulomatous infections
- Metastatic cancer
- Myelofibrosis

Conditions that are a result of increased destruction, loss, or consumption:
- Contact with foreign surfaces (dialysis membranes, artificial organs, grafts, prosthetic devices)

- Disseminated intravascular coagulation
- Extensive transfusion
- HELLP syndrome of pregnancy (hemolysis, elevated liver enzymes, low platelet count)
- Severe hemorrhage
- Thrombotic thrombocytopenic purpura
- Uremia

Conditions that are a result of increased destruction as a result of an immune reaction:
- Antibody/human leukocyte antigen reactions
- Hemolytic disease of the newborn *(target is platelets instead of RBCs)*
- Idiopathic thrombocytopenic purpura

- Refractory reaction to platelet transfusion

Conditions that are a result of increased destruction as a result of an immune reaction secondary to infection:
- Bacterial infections
- Burns
- Congenital infections (cytomegalovirus, herpes, syphilis, toxoplasmosis)
- Histoplasmosis
- Malaria
- Rocky Mountain spotted fever

Conditions that are a result of increased destruction as a result of other causes:
- Radiation
- Splenomegaly caused by liver disease

NURSING IMPLICATIONS

POTENTIAL NURSING PROBLEMS: ASSESSMENT AND NURSING DIAGNOSIS

Problems	Signs and Symptoms
Confusion *(related to decreased tissue perfusion secondary to platelet clumping and altered blood flow)*	Disorganized thinking; restlessness; irritability; altered concentration and attention span; changeable mental function over the day; hallucinations; inability to follow directions; disoriented to person, place, time, and purpose; inappropriate affect
Pain *(related to joint disturbances associated with bleeding, bleeding into the tissues)*	Expression of pain, facial grimace, moaning, crying, report of pain
Protection *(related to decreased platelet count, bleeding risk)*	Ease of bruising; blood in urine, stool, sputum; nosebleed; bleeding gums; presence of hematoma or petechiae; headache; vision changes
Tissue perfusion (cerebral, peripheral, renal) *(related to altered blood flow associated with platelet clumping)*	Confusion, altered mental status, headaches, dizziness, visual disturbances, hypotension, cool extremities, capillary refill greater than 3 sec, weak pedal pulses, altered level of consciousness, decreased urine output

P

BEFORE THE STUDY: PLANNING AND IMPLEMENTATION

Teaching the Patient What to Expect
- Inform the patient this test can assist in diagnosing, evaluating, and monitoring bleeding disorders.
- Explain that a blood sample is needed for the test.

AFTER THE STUDY: POTENTIAL NURSING ACTIONS

Treatment Considerations
- Confusion: Treat the medical condition that may be responsible for the confusion. Monitor and trend platelet count. Evaluate medications as a causative factor. Prevent falls and injury through appropriate use of postural support, bed alarm, or appropriate restraints. Administer prescribed medications (IV immunoglobulin, recombinant interleukin).
- Pain: Assess level of pain and identify pain characteristics, what makes it better or worse. Administer prescribed analgesics, assess effectiveness, and collaborate with HCP to provide adequate pain management.
- Tissue Perfusion: Monitor blood pressure, and dizziness. Check skin temperature for warmth, assess capillary refill, assess pedal pulses, and monitor level of consciousness. Verify urine output to be in excess of 30 mL/hr and ensure adequate fluid intake or administer IV fluids as ordered.
- The results of a CBC should be carefully evaluated during transfusion or acute blood loss because the body is not in a state of homeostasis and values may be misleading. Considerations for draw times after transfusion include the type of product, the amount of product transfused, and the patient's clinical situation. Generally, specimens collected an hour after transfusion will provide an acceptable reflection of the effects of the transfused product. Measurements taken during a massive transfusion are an exception, providing essential guidance for therapeutic decisions during critical care.

Safety Considerations
- Protection: Assess for bruising, petechiae, or hematoma. Monitor and trend platelet count. Administer platelets, blood, or other blood products. Administer ordered stool softeners or corticosteroids. Monitor and trend vital signs and report significant variances. Monitor stool, urine, sputum, gums, and nose for blood. Coordinate laboratory draws to decrease frequency of venipuncture. Institute bleeding precautions, avoid intramuscular (IM) injections, prevent trauma, be gentle with oral care and suctioning, and avoid use of a sharp razor. Administer prescribed medications.

Nutritional Considerations
- Instruct patients to consume a variety of foods within the basic food groups, maintain a healthy weight, be physically active, limit salt intake, limit alcohol intake, and avoid the use of tobacco.

Follow-Up, Evaluation, and Desired Outcomes
- Acknowledges the importance of taking precautions against bruising and bleeding, including the use of a soft bristle toothbrush, use of an electric razor, avoidance of constipation to prevent straining while having a bowel movement, avoidance of acetylsalicylic acid and similar products, and avoidance of IM injections.
- Recognizes the importance of periodic laboratory testing if taking an anticoagulant.
- Adheres to the request to refrain from participating in at-risk activities that could cause trauma and bleeding.

P

Plethysmography

SYNONYM/ACRONYM: Impedance plethysmography, PVR.

RATIONALE: To measure changes in blood vessel size or changes in gas volume in the lungs to assist in diagnosing diseases such as deep vein thrombosis (DVT), chronic obstructive pulmonary disease (COPD), and some peripheral vascular disorders.

PATIENT PREPARATION: There are no food, fluid, or medication restrictions unless by medical direction. Instruct the patient to refrain from smoking for 2 hr prior to the procedure.

NORMAL FINDINGS
- Arterial plethysmography:

  Normal arterial pulse waves: Steep upslope, more gradual downslope with narrow pointed peaks

  Normal pressure: Less than 20 mm Hg systolic difference between the lower and upper extremities; toe pressure greater than or equal to 80% of ankle pressure and finger pressure greater than or equal to 80% of wrist pressure
- Venous plethysmography:

  Normal venous blood flow in the extremities

  Venous filling times greater than 20 sec
- Body plethysmography:

  Thoracic gas volume: 2,400 mL

  Compliance: 0.2 L/cm H_2O

  Airway resistance: 0.6 to 2.5 cm H_2O/L per sec
- Impedance plethysmography:

  Sharp rise in volume with temporary occlusion

  Rapid venous outflow with release of the occlusion

CRITICAL FINDINGS AND POTENTIAL INTERVENTIONS
- DVT

Timely notification to the requesting health-care provider (HCP) of any critical findings and related symptoms is a role expectation of the professional nurse. A listing of these findings varies among facilities.

P

OVERVIEW: (Study type: Manometry; related body system: Circulatory and Respiratory systems.) Plethysmography is a noninvasive diagnostic manometric study used to measure changes in the size of blood vessels by determining volume changes in the blood vessels of the eye, extremities, and neck or to measure gas volume changes in the lungs.

Arterial plethysmography assesses arterial circulation in an upper or lower limb; it is used to diagnose extremity arteriosclerotic disease and to rule out occlusive disease. The test requires a normal extremity for comparison of results. The test is performed by applying a series of three blood pressure cuffs to the extremity. The amplitude of each pulse wave is then recorded.

Venous plethysmography, done with a series of cuffs, measures changes in venous capacity and outflow (volume and rate of outflow); it is used to diagnose a thrombotic condition that causes obstruction of the major veins of the extremity. When the cuffs are applied to an extremity in patients with venous obstruction, no initial increase in leg volume is recorded because the venous volume of the leg cannot dissipate quickly.

Body plethysmography measures the total amount (volume) of air within the thorax, whether or not the air is in ventilatory communication with the lung; the elasticity (compliance) of the lungs; and the resistance to airflow in the respiratory tree. It is used in conjunction with pulmonary stress testing and pulmonary function testing.

Impedance plethysmography is widely used to detect acute DVT of the leg, but it can also be used in the arm, abdomen, neck, or thorax. Doppler flow studies now are used to identify DVT, but ultrasound studies are less accurate in examinations below the knee.

INDICATIONS

Arterial Plethysmography
- Confirm suspected acute arterial embolization.
- Detect vascular changes associated with Raynaud phenomenon and disease.
- Determine changes in toe or finger pressures when ankle pressures are elevated as a result of arterial calcifications.
- Determine the effect of trauma on the arteries in an extremity.
- Determine peripheral small-artery changes (ischemia) caused by diabetes, and differentiate these changes from neuropathy.
- Evaluate suspected arterial occlusive disease.
- Locate and determine the degree of arterial atherosclerotic obstruction and vessel patency in peripheral

atherosclerotic disease, as well as inflammatory changes causing obliteration in the vessels in thromboangiitis obliterans.

Venous Plethysmography
- Detect partial or total venous thrombotic obstruction.
- Determine valve competency in conjunction with Doppler ultrasonography in the diagnosis of varicose veins.

Body Plethysmography
- Detect acute pulmonary disorders, such as atelectasis.
- Detect or determine the status of COPD, such as asthma or chronic bronchitis.
- Detect or determine the status of restrictive pulmonary disease, such as fibrosis.
- Detect infectious pulmonary diseases, such as pneumonia.
- Determine baseline pulmonary status before pulmonary rehabilitation to determine potential therapeutic benefit.
- Differentiate between obstructive and restrictive pulmonary pathology.

Impedance Plethysmography
- Act as a diagnostic screen for patients at risk for DVT.
- Detect and evaluate DVT.
- Evaluate degree of resolution of DVT after treatment.
- Evaluate patients with suspected pulmonary embolism (most pulmonary emboli are complications of DVT in the leg).

INTERFERING FACTORS
Arterial Plethysmography
Factors that may alter the results of the study
- Cigarette smoking 2 hr before the study, which causes inaccurate results because the nicotine constricts the arteries
- Alcohol consumption
- Low cardiac output
- Shock

- Compression of pelvic veins (tumors or external compression by dressings)
- Environmental temperatures (hot or cold)
- Arterial occlusion proximal to the extremity to be examined, which can prevent blood flow to the limb

Venous Plethysmography
Factors that may alter the results of the study
- Low environmental temperature or cold extremity, which constricts the vessels
- High anxiety level or muscle tenseness
- Venous thrombotic occlusion proximal to the extremity to be examined, which can affect blood flow to the limb

Body Plethysmography
Factors that may alter the results of the study
- Inability of the patient to follow breathing instructions during the procedure

Impedance Plethysmography
Factors that may alter the results of the study
- Movement of the extremity during electrical impedance recording, poor electrode contact, or nonlinear electrical output, which can cause false-positive results
- Constricting clothing or bandages

POTENTIAL MEDICAL DIAGNOSIS: CLINICAL SIGNIFICANCE OF RESULTS
Abnormal findings related to
- COPD, restrictive lung disease, lung infection, or atelectasis (body plethysmography)
- DVT (arterial, venous, or impedance plethysmography)
- Incompetent valves, thrombosis, or thrombotic obstruction in a major vein in an extremity
- Small-vessel diabetic changes
- Vascular disease (Raynaud phenomenon)
- Vascular trauma

NURSING IMPLICATIONS

POTENTIAL NURSING PROBLEMS: ASSESSMENT & NURSING DIAGNOSIS

Problems	Signs and Symptoms
Breathing *(related to fear, anxiety, lack of oxygen, inflammation, infection, obstruction, trauma)*	Shortness of breath; skin that is cool, clammy, and cyanotic; anxiety; pain; decreased oxygenation; abnormal blood gas; increased work of breathing (use of accessory muscles); increased respiratory rate
Gas exchange *(related to obstruction, trauma, infection, thrombus, tumor inflammation)*	Difficulty breathing, shortness of breath (dyspnea), chest pain (pleuritic), diminished oxygenation, cyanosis, increased heart rate, increased respiratory rate, restlessness, anxiety, fear, adventitious breath sounds (rales, crackles), sense of impending death and doom, hemoptysis, abnormal arterial blood gas
Pain *(related to obstruction, trauma, infection, inflammation, tumor, ischemic tissue)*	Self-report of chest, extremity pain; increased respiratory rate; increased heart rate; fear; anxiety

P

BEFORE THE STUDY: PLANNING AND IMPLEMENTATION

Teaching the Patient What to Expect

♦ Inform the patient this procedure can assist in evaluating blood vessel size and lung ventilation.
♦ Review the procedure with the patient.
♦ Address concerns about pain related to the procedure and explain that no discomfort will be experienced during the test. However, there may be some discomfort during insertion of the nasoesophageal catheter if compliance testing is done.
♦ Explain that the procedure is generally performed in a specialized area or at the bedside by a health-care provider (HCP) who specializes in this procedure and usually takes 30 to 60 min.
♦ For body plethysmography, the patient's weight, height, and gender are recorded.
♦ Explain to the patient that he or she will be placed in a body box, and determine whether the patient is claustrophobic; if so, notify the HCP.
♦ Baseline vital signs are taken and recorded.
♦ Explain to the patient that cuffs are applied to the extremity to measure and compare blood flow.
♦ Positioning for this procedure is in a semi-Fowler position on an examination table or in bed.
♦ Explain that any unexpected symptoms that occur during the test should be reported.

Arterial Plethysmography

♦ Explain to the patient that cuffs are applied to the extremity to measure and compare blood flow.
♦ Explain that three blood pressure cuffs are applied to the extremity, and a pulse volume recorder (plethysmograph) is attached. This device records the amplitude of each pulse wave.
♦ Explain that the cuffs will be inflated to 65 mm Hg to measure the pulse waves of each cuff. When compared with a normal limb, these measurements determine the presence of arterial occlusive disease.

Venous Plethysmography

♦ Explain that two blood pressure cuffs are applied to the extremity, one on the proximal part of the extremity (occlusion cuff) and the other on the distal part of the extremity (recorder cuff). A third cuff is attached to the pulse volume recorder.
♦ The recorder cuff is inflated to 10 mm Hg, the effects of respiration on venous volume are evaluated. Absence of changes during respirations indicates venous thrombotic occlusion.
♦ The occlusion cuff is inflated to 50 mm Hg, and venous volume is recorded on the pulse monitor. The occlusion cuff is deflated after the highest volume is recorded in the recorder cuff. A delay in the return to preocclusion volume indicates venous thrombotic occlusion.

Body Plethysmography

♦ Positioning for this procedure is in a sitting position on a chair in the body box. Explain to the patient that the cuffs are applied to the extremities to measure and compare blood flow.
♦ A nose clip is positioned to prevent breathing through the nose, and a mouthpiece is connected to a measuring instrument.
♦ Explain to the patient that he or she will be asked to breathe through the mouthpiece.
♦ Explain that when the door to the box is closed, the start time of the procedure is recorded. Advise the patient he or she will be asked to pant rapidly and shallowly, without allowing the glottis to close.
♦ For compliance testing, a double-lumen nasoesophageal catheter is inserted, and the bag is inflated with air. Intraesophageal pressure is recorded during normal breathing.

Impedance Plethysmography

♦ Explain to the patient that cuffs are applied to the extremity to measure and compare blood flow.
♦ Positioning for this procedure is on the back with the leg being tested above heart level.
♦ Explain that the knee will be slightly flexed and the hips will be slightly

rotated by shifting weight to the same side as the leg being tested.
- Conductive gel and electrodes are applied to the legs, near the cuffs.
- Explain that a blood pressure cuff will be applied to the thigh.
- The pressure cuff attached to the thigh is temporarily inflated to occlude venous return without interfering with arterial blood flow. Expect the blood volume in the other calf to increase.
- A tracing of changes in electrical impedance occurring during inflation and for 15 sec after cuff deflation is recorded.
- With DVT, blood volume increases less than expected because the veins are already at capacity.
- The conductive gel and electrodes are removed at the end of the procedure.

AFTER THE STUDY: POTENTIAL NURSING ACTIONS

Treatment Considerations
- Instruct the patient to resume usual activity, as directed by the HCP.
- Monitor vital signs every 15 min until they return to baseline levels.
- Monitor for severe ischemia, ulcers, and pain of the extremity after arterial, venous, or impedance plethysmography, and handle the extremity gently.
- Breathing: Assess and trend breath sounds and work of breathing. Monitor and trend respiratory rate and arterial blood gases. Elevate the head of the bed to promote breathing (semi-Fowler to high Fowler based on the level of comfort that best facilitates breathing),

and recommend bedrest as appropriate. Administer ordered analgesics, encourage cough and deep breathe as appropriate, and prepare for intubation.
- Monitor respiratory pattern after body plethysmography, and allow the patient time to resume a normal breathing pattern.
- Gas Exchange: Assess respiratory status to establish a baseline rate, rhythm, and depth. Assess for cyanosis and work of breathing. Apply pulse oximetry, administer ordered oxygen, and elevate the head of the bed. Administer ordered thrombolytic and anticoagulants. Institute bleeding precautions and bedrest as appropriate. Monitor and trend arterial blood gas results, D-dimer test, prothrombin time, international normalized ratio, and activated partial thromboplastin time.
- Pain: Assess pain character, location, duration, and intensity. Use an easily understood pain rating scale and place in a position of comfort. Administer ordered analgesics and consider alternative measures for pain management such as imagery, relaxation, music, etc.).

Follow-Up, Evaluation, and Desired Outcomes
- Understands the value of ordered medications.
- Acknowledges the importance of completing all follow-up diagnostic and laboratory studies needed to monitor health status and the effectiveness of treatment modalities.

P

Pleural Fluid Analysis

SYNONYM/ACRONYM: Thoracentesis fluid analysis.

RATIONALE: To assess and categorize fluid obtained from within the pleural space for infection, cancer, and blood as well as identify the cause of its accumulation.

PATIENT PREPARATION: There are no food, fluid, or activity restrictions unless by medical direction. Regarding the patient's risk for bleeding, the patient should be instructed to avoid taking natural products and medications with known anticoagulant, antiplatelet, or thrombolytic properties or to reduce dosage, as ordered, prior to the procedure. Number of days to withhold medication is dependent on the type of anticoagulant. Note the last time and dose of medication taken.

NORMAL FINDINGS: Method: Spectrophotometry for amylase, cholesterol, glucose, lactate dehydrogenase (LDH), protein, and triglycerides; ion-selective electrode for pH; automated or manual cell count; macroscopic and microscopic examination of cultured microorganisms; microscopic examination of specimen for microbiology and cytology.

Appearance	Clear
Color	Pale yellow
Amylase	Parallels serum values
Cholesterol	Parallels serum values
CEA	Parallels serum values
Glucose	Parallels serum values
LDH	Less than 2/3 the upper limit of normal serum LDH
Fluid LDH–to–serum LDH ratio	0.6 or less
Protein	3 g/dL
Fluid protein–to–serum protein ratio	0.5 or less
Triglycerides	Parallel serum values
pH	7.37–7.43
RBC count	None seen
WBC count	Less than 1,000 cells/microL
Culture	No growth
Gram stain	No organisms seen
Cytology	No abnormal cells seen

CEA = carcinoembryonic antigen; LDH = lactate dehydrogenase; RBC = red blood cell; WBC = white blood cell.

CRITICAL FINDINGS AND POTENTIAL INTERVENTIONS
• Positive culture findings in any sterile body fluid.

Timely notification to the requesting health-care provider (HCP) of any critical findings and related symptoms is a role expectation of the professional nurse. A listing of these findings varies among facilities.

P

OVERVIEW: (Study type: Pleural fluid collected in a green-top [heparin] tube for amylase, cholesterol, glucose, LDH, pH, protein, and triglycerides; lavender-top [EDTA] tube for cell count; sterile containers for microbiology specimens; 200–500 mL of fluid in a clear container with anticoagulant for cytology. Ensure that there is an equal amount of fixative and fluid in the container for cytology; **related body system:** Immune and Respiratory systems.) The pleural cavity and organs within it are lined with a protective membrane. The fluid between the membranes is called *serous fluid.* Normally, only a small amount of fluid is present because the rates of fluid production and absorption are about the same. Many abnormal conditions can result in the buildup of fluid within the pleural cavity. Specific tests are usually ordered in addition to a common battery of tests used to distinguish a transudate from an exudate. *Transudates* are effusions that form as a result of a systemic disorder that disrupts the regulation of fluid balance, such as a suspected perforation. *Exudates* are caused by conditions involving the tissue of the membrane itself, such as an infection or malignancy. Fluid is withdrawn from the pleural cavity by needle aspiration (thoracentesis) and tested as listed in the previous and following tables. A significant number of pleural effusion cases remain undiagnosed after pleural fluid analysis.

Further investigation, by pleural biopsy, is indicated in circumstances such as undiagnosed recurrent pleural effusion, identification or exclusion of conditions such as tuberculosis or tumor (e.g., malignant mesothelioma), or pleural thickening in the absence of abnormal accumulations of pleural fluid. Various biopsy techniques include closed needle biopsy, image guided biopsy, and thoracoscopic biopsy. Closed needle biopsy carries increased risk for pneumothorax, is mainly used in the presence of large effusions, requires multiple samples to provide sufficient specimen yield, and has largely been replaced by ultrasound or CT image guided and thoracoscopic biopsy in combination with immunohistochemistry. The newer techniques provide a higher quality specimen yield with more sensitive and accurate findings. Pleuroscopy or thoracoscopic biopsy is a technique that allows direct, minimally invasive visualization of the pleural space. It is usually performed by a pulmonologist in an endoscopy suite or operating room under conscious sedation with local anesthesia.

Characteristic	Transudate	Exudate
Appearance	Clear to pale yellow	Cloudy, bloody, or turbid
Specific gravity	Less than 1.015	Greater than 1.015
Total protein	Less than 2.5 g/dL	Greater than 3 g/dL
Fluid protein–to–serum protein ratio	Less than 0.5	Greater than 0.5
LDH	Less than 2/3 the upper limit of normal serum LDH	Greater than 2/3 the upper limit of normal serum LDH
Fluid LDH–to–serum LDH ratio	Less than 0.6	Greater than 0.6
Fluid cholesterol	Less than 55 mg/dL	Greater than 55 mg/dL
WBC count	Less than 100 cells/microL	Greater than 1,000 cells/microL

P

INDICATIONS
- Differentiate transudates from exudates.
- Evaluate effusion of unknown cause.
- Investigate suspected rupture, immune disease, malignancy, or infection.

INTERFERING FACTORS
Contraindications

⬥ Abnormal bleeding tendencies or diagnosed bleeding conditions.

Factors that may alter the results of the study
- Bloody fluids may be the result of a traumatic tap.
- Unknown hyperglycemia or hypoglycemia may be misleading in the comparison of fluid and serum glucose levels. Therefore, it is advisable to collect comparative serum samples a few hours before performing thoracentesis.

POTENTIAL MEDICAL DIAGNOSIS: CLINICAL SIGNIFICANCE OF RESULTS
- *Bacterial or Tuberculous Empyema:* Elevated WBC count with a predominance of neutrophils, increased fluid protein-to-serum protein ratio, increased fluid LDH-to-serum LDH ratio, decreased glucose, pH less than 7.3
- *Chylous Pleural Effusion:* Marked increase in both triglycerides (two to three times serum level) and chylomicrons
- *Effusion Caused by Pneumonia:* Elevated WBC count with a predominance of neutrophils and some eosinophils, increased fluid protein-to-serum protein ratio, increased fluid LDH-to-serum LDH ratio, pH less than 7.4 (and decreased glucose if bacterial pneumonia)
- *Esophageal Rupture:* Significantly decreased pH (6) and elevated amylase
- *Hemothorax:* Bloody appearance, increased RBC count, elevated hematocrit

- *Malignancy:* Elevated WBC count with a predominance of lymphocytes, possible elevated RBC count, abnormal cytology, increased fluid protein-to-serum protein ratio, increased fluid LDH-to-serum LDH ratio, decreased glucose, pH less than 7.3
- *Pancreatitis:* Elevated WBC count with a predominance of neutrophils, elevated RBC count, pH greater than 7.3, increased fluid protein-to-serum protein ratio, increased fluid LDH-to-serum LDH ratio, increased amylase
- *Pulmonary Infarction:* Elevated RBC count, elevated WBC count with a predominance of neutrophils, pH greater than 7.3, normal glucose, increased fluid protein-to-serum protein ratio, and increased fluid LDH-to-serum LDH ratio
- *Pulmonary Tuberculosis:* Elevated WBC count with a predominance of lymphocytes, positive acid-fast bacillus stain and culture, increased protein, decreased glucose, pH less than 7.3
- *Rheumatoid Disease:* Elevated WBC count with a predominance of either lymphocytes or neutrophils, pH less than 7.3, decreased glucose, increased fluid protein-to-serum protein ratio, increased fluid LDH-to-serum LDH ratio, increased immunoglobulins
- *Systemic Lupus Erythematosus:* Similar findings as with rheumatoid disease, except that glucose is usually not decreased

NURSING IMPLICATIONS

BEFORE THE STUDY: PLANNING AND IMPLEMENTATION

Teaching the Patient What to Expect
▶ Inform the patient this test can assist in identifying the type of fluid being produced within the body cavity.

P

▶ Explain that prior to the procedure, laboratory testing may be required to determine the possibility of bleeding risk (coagulation testing).

▶ Pregnancy is a general contraindication to procedures involving radiation. Explain to the female patient that she will be asked the date of her last menstrual period. Pregnancy testing may be performed to determine the possibility of pregnancy before exposure to radiation if a chest x-ray is expected to be ordered.

▶ Explain that reducing health-care-associated infections is an important patient safety goal and a number of different safety practices will be implemented during their procedure. Advise the patient that hair in the area near the catheter insertion site may be clipped or shaved and the area cleaned with an antiseptic solution to cleanse bacteria from the skin in order to reduce the risk for infection. Note: The World Health Organization, Centers for Disease Control and Prevention, and Association of periOperative Registered Nurses recommend that hair not be removed at all unless it interferes with the incision site or other aspects of the procedure because hair removal by any means is associated with increased infection rates. When hair removal is necessary, facilities must use a protocol that is based on scientific literature or the endorsement of a professional organization. Clipping immediately before the procedure and in a location outside the procedure area is preferred to shaving with a razor. Shaving creates a break in skin integrity and provides a way for bacteria on the skin to enter the incision site.

▶ Explain that a pleural fluid sample is needed for the test and that chest x-ray is recommended immediately after a pleural biopsy in order to identify postprocedural complications.

▶ Review the procedure with the patient. Address concerns about pain and explain that there may be moments of discomfort or pain experienced when the IV line is inserted to allow infusion of fluids such as saline, anesthetics, sedatives, antibiotics, medications used in the procedure, or emergency medications; a sedative and/or analgesia will be administered to promote relaxation and reduce discomfort prior to needle insertion through the chest wall into the pleural space.

▶ Explain that the HCP may request that a cough suppressant be given before the thoracentesis.

▶ Explain that the needle insertion is performed under sterile conditions by an HCP specializing in this procedure and that the procedure usually takes about 20 min to complete.

▶ Baseline vital signs are recorded and monitored throughout the procedure. Protocols may vary among facilities.

▶ Advise the patient that he or she will be assisted into a comfortable sitting or side-lying position.

▶ Hair is clipped prior to the administration of local anesthesia, and the site is cleansed with an antiseptic solution and draped with sterile towels. The skin at the injection site is then anesthetized.

▶ The thoracentesis needle is inserted, and fluid is removed.

▶ The needle is withdrawn, and pressure is applied to the site with a petroleum jelly gauze. A pressure dressing is applied over the petroleum jelly gauze.

▶ Samples are placed in a properly labelled specimen container and promptly transported to the laboratory for processing and analysis.

Potential Nursing Actions

Make sure a written and informed consent has been signed prior to the procedure and before administering any medications.

Safety Considerations

▶ Avoid using morphine sulfate in those with asthma or other pulmonary disease. This drug can further exacerbate bronchospasms and respiratory impairment.

▶ Anticoagulants, aspirin, and other salicylates should be discontinued by medical direction for the appropriate number of days prior to a procedure where bleeding is a potential complication.

P

AFTER THE STUDY: POTENTIAL NURSING ACTIONS

Avoiding Complications

▶ Establishing an IV site and performing a thoracentesis are invasive procedures. Complications are rare but include risk for bleeding *(related to a bleeding disorder, or the effects of natural products and medications with known anticoagulant, antiplatelet, or thrombolytic properties)*, bronchospasm, hemoptysis, hypoxemia, infection, pneumothorax, or pulmonary edema. Observe/assess the patient for signs of respiratory distress or skin color changes. Monitor the patient for complications related to the procedure (e.g., bleeding, infection, pneumothorax). Immediately report to the appropriate HCP symptoms such as absent breathing sounds, air hunger, excessive coughing, or dyspnea (indications of hemoptysis); elevated WBC count, fever, malaise, or tachycardia (indications of infection); dyspnea, tachypnea, anxiety, decreased breathing sounds, or restlessness (symptoms of developing pneumothorax). A chest x-ray may be ordered to check for the presence of pneumothorax. Observe/assess the needle insertion site for bleeding, inflammation, or hematoma formation. The use of morphine sulfate in those with asthma or other pulmonary disease should be avoided. This drug can further exacerbate bronchospasms and respiratory impairment.

Emergency resuscitation equipment should be readily available in the case of respiratory impairment or laryngospasm after the procedure.

Treatment Considerations

▶ Instruct the patient to resume usual medications, as directed by the HCP.
▶ Monitor vital signs every 15 min for the first hr, every 30 min for the next 2 hr, every hour for the next 4 hr, and every 4 hr for the next 24 hr. Take the patient's temperature every 4 hr for 24 hr. Monitor intake and output for 24 hr. Notify the HCP if temperature is elevated. Protocols may vary among facilities.
▶ Inform the patient that 1 hr or more of bedrest (lying on the unaffected side) is required after the procedure. Elevate the patient's head for comfort.
▶ Observe/assess for nausea and pain. Administer antiemetic and analgesic medications as needed and as directed by the HCP.
▶ Administer antibiotics, as ordered, and instruct the patient in the importance of completing the entire course of antibiotic therapy even if no symptoms are present.

Follow-Up, Evaluation, and Desired Outcomes

▶ Acknowledges that depending procedure results, additional testing may be necessary to evaluate or monitor disease progression or the need for a change in therapy.

Porphyrins, Urine

SYNONYM/ACRONYM: Coproporphyrin, porphobilinogen, urobilinogen, and other porphyrins.

RATIONALE: To assess for porphyrins in the urine to assist with diagnosis of genetic disorders associated with porphyrin synthesis as well as heavy metal toxicity.

PATIENT PREPARATION: There are no food, fluid, activity, or medication restrictions unless by medical direction. Usually, a 24-hr urine collection is ordered. As appropriate, provide the required urine collection container and specimen collection instructions.

NORMAL FINDINGS: Method: High-performance liquid chromatography for porphyrins; spectrophotometry for δ-aminolevulinic acid and porphobilinogen.

Test	Conventional Units	SI Units
		(Conventional units × 1.53)
Coproporphyrin I	0–24 mcg/24 h	0–36.7 nmol/24 hr
Coproporphyrin III	0–74 mcg/24 hr	0–113.2 nmol/24 hr
		(Conventional units × 1.43)
Uroporphyrins	0–24 mcg/24 hr	0–34.3 nmol/24 hr
		(Conventional units × 1.34)
Hexacarboxylporphyrin	Less than 10 mcg/24 hr	Less than 10.34 nmol/24 hr
		(Conventional units × 1.27)
Heptacarboxylporphyrin	Less than 4 mcg/24 hr	Less than 5.1 nmol/24 hr
		(Conventional units × 4.42)
Porphobilinogen	Less than 2 mg/24 hr	Less than 8.8 micromol/24 hr
		(Conventional units × 7.626)
δ-Aminolevulinic acid	1.5–7.5 mg/24 hr	11.4–57.2 micromol/24 hr

CRITICAL FINDINGS AND POTENTIAL INTERVENTIONS: N/A

OVERVIEW: (Study type: Urine from a random or timed specimen collected in a clean, amber-colored plastic collection container with sodium carbonate as a preservative; related body system: Circulatory/Hematopoietic system.) Porphyrins are produced during the synthesis of heme. If heme synthesis is disturbed, these precursors accumulate and are excreted in the urine in excessive amounts. Conditions producing increased levels of heme precursors are called *porphyrias*. The two main categories of genetically determined porphyrias are erythropoietic porphyrias, in which major abnormalities occur in red blood cell (RBC) chemistry, and hepatic porphyrias, in which heme precursors are found in urine and feces.

Erythropoietic and hepatic porphyrias are rare. Acquired porphyrias are characterized by greater accumulation of precursors in urine and feces than in RBCs. Lead poisoning is the most common cause of acquired porphyrias. Porphyrins are reddish fluorescent compounds. Depending on the type of porphyrin present, the urine may be reddish, resembling port wine. Porphobilinogen is excreted as a colorless compound. A color change may occur in an acidic sample containing porphobilinogen if the sample is exposed to air for several hours.

INDICATIONS
- Assist in the diagnosis of congenital or acquired porphyrias characterized by abdominal pain, tachycardia,

P

emesis, fever, leukocytosis, and neurological abnormalities.
- Detect suspected lead poisoning, as indicated by elevated porphyrins.

INTERFERING FACTORS

Factors that may alter the results of the study
- Drugs and other substances that may increase urine porphyrin levels include acriflavine, ethoxazene, griseofulvin, hexachlorobenzene, oxytetracycline, and sulfonmethane
- Exposure of the specimen to light can falsely decrease values.
- Screening methods are not well standardized and can produce false-negative results.

Other considerations
- Numerous drugs and other substances are suspected as potential initiators of acute attacks, but drugs classified as unsafe for high-risk individuals include antipyrine, barbiturates, *N*-butylscopolammonium bromide, carbamazepine, carbromal, chlorpropamide, danazol, dapsone, diclofenac, diphenylhydantoin, ergot preparations, ethchlorvynol, ethinamate, glutethimide, griseofulvin, *N*-isopropyl meprobamate, meprobamate, methyprylon, novobiocin, phenylbutazone, primidone, pyrazolone preparations, succinimides, sulfonamide antibiotics, sulfonethylmethane, sulfonmethane, synthetic estrogens and progestins, tolazamide, tolbutamide, trimethadione, and valproic acid.
- Failure to collect all urine and store specimen properly during the 24-hour test period will interfere with results.

POTENTIAL MEDICAL DIAGNOSIS: CLINICAL SIGNIFICANCE OF RESULTS
Increased in
Accumulation of porphyrins or porphyrin precursors in the body is common to the various types of porphyrias.

Excessive amounts of circulating porphyrins and precursors are excreted in the urine.

- Acute intermittent porphyria *(related to an autosomal dominant disorder resulting in a deficiency of the enzyme porphobilinogen deaminase and increased excretion of porphobilinogen and delta-aminolevulinic acid [δ-ALA] in the urine)*
- Acquired or chemical porphyrias (heavy metal, benzene, or carbon tetrachloride toxicity; drug induced) *(related to a disturbance in the heme biosynthetic pathway and increased excretion of delta-aminolevulinic acid in the urine)*
- ALAD deficiency porphyria *(related to an autosomal recessive disorder resulting in a deficiency of the enzyme delta-aminolevulinic acid dehydratase and increased excretion of δ-ALA in the urine)*
- Hepatoerythropoietic porphyria *(related to an autosomal recessive disorder resulting in a deficiency of the enzyme uroporphyrinogen decarboxylase and increased excretion of uroporphyrin and heptacarboxylporphyrin in the urine)*
- Hereditary coproporphyria *(related to an autosomal dominant disorder resulting in a deficiency of the enzyme coproporphyrinogen oxidase and increased excretion of porphobilinogen, δ-ALA, and coproporphyrin in the urine)*
- Porphyria cutanea tarda *(related to an acquired deficiency of the enzyme uroporphyrinogen decarboxylase activated by exposure to triggers such as iron, alcohol, hepatitis C virus, HIV, or estrogens and increased excretion of uroporphyrin, heptacarboxylporphyrin, and coproporphyrin in the urine)*
- Variegate porphyrias *(related to an autosomal dominant disorder*

resulting in a deficiency of the enzyme protoporphyrinogen oxidase and increased excretion of porphobilinogen, coproporphyrin, and δ-ALA in the urine during attacks; excretion of normal levels may be found between attacks)

Decreased in: N/A

NURSING IMPLICATIONS

BEFORE THE STUDY: PLANNING AND IMPLEMENTATION

Teaching the Patient What to Expect

◗ Inform the patient this test can assist in evaluating for conditions producing increased levels of heme precursors called porphyrias.
◗ Explain that a urine sample is needed for the test. Information regarding specimen collection is presented with other general guidelines in Appendix A: Patient Preparation and Specimen Collection.

Potential Nursing Actions

◗ Include on the collection container's label the amount of urine, test start and stop times, and ingestion of any foods or medications that can affect test results.

AFTER THE STUDY: POTENTIAL NURSING ACTIONS

Treatment Considerations

◗ Discuss the implications of abnormal test results on the patient's lifestyle.
◗ Provide education related to the clinical implications of the test results.

Nutritional Considerations

◗ Increased δ-ALA levels may be associated with an acute porphyria attack.
◗ Patients prone to attacks should eat a normal or high-carbohydrate diet.
◗ Indicated dietary recommendations may vary depending on the condition and its severity; however, restrictions of or wide variations in dietary carbohydrate content should be avoided, even for short periods of time.
◗ After recovering from an attack, daily intake of carbohydrates should be 300 grams or more per day.

Follow-Up, Evaluation, and Desired Outcomes

◗ Acknowledges contact information provided for the American Porphyria Foundation (www.porphyriafoundation .com).

Positron Emission Tomography, Various Sites (Brain, Heart, Pelvis)

P

SYNONYM/ACRONYM: PET scan.

RATIONALE: To assess blood flow and metabolic processes at the site of interest, to assist in diagnosis of disorders such as ischemic or hemorrhagic stroke, cancer, and to evaluate head trauma (head/brain); coronary artery disease, infarct, and aneurysm (chest/thorax, heart, vascular system); colorectal tumor, to assist in tumor staging, and monitor the effectiveness of therapeutic interventions (pelvis).

PATIENT PREPARATION: There are no activity restrictions unless by medical direction. Instruct the patient to restrict food for 4 hr; restrict alcohol, nicotine, or caffeine-containing drinks for 24 hr; and withhold medications for 24 hr before the test. Protocols may vary among facilities.

NORMAL FINDINGS
• Normal patterns of tissue metabolism, blood flow, and homogeneous radionuclide distribution.

CRITICAL FINDINGS AND POTENTIAL INTERVENTIONS

Brain
• Aneurysm
• Cerebrovascular accident
• Tumor with significant mass effect

Timely notification to the requesting health-care provider (HCP) of any critical findings and related symptoms is a role expectation of the professional nurse. A listing of these findings varies among facilities.

OVERVIEW: (Study type: Nuclear scan; related body system: Circulatory, Digestive, Nervous systems.) Positron emission tomography (PET) combines the biochemical properties of nuclear medicine with the anatomic accuracy of computed tomography (CT). PET uses positron emissions from specific radionuclides. The positron radiopharmaceuticals generally have short half-lives, ranging from a few seconds to a few hours, and therefore they must be produced in a cyclotron located near where the test is being done. A radionuclide is basically composed of a measurable radioactive isotope and a biologically active molecule. The isotopes are derived from elements that are either naturally present in organic molecules (oxygen, nitrogen, and carbon) or can be substituted for naturally occurring elements (fluorine can be substituted for hydrogen). Selected molecules become biologically active radiolabelled analogs of their naturally occurring forms to create radionuclides that produce detailed functional images of the target organ's structure. Radionuclides are used to evaluate many aspects of organ function, including oxygen consumption and glucose metabolism; most PET studies are conducted in the areas of cardiology, neurology, and oncology. The studies are used to diagnose and stage diseases as well as to monitor the efficacy of therapeutic interventions. During the PET scan, the radiotracer is injected into the body where it migrates to the intended target organ, becomes involved in the physiological process of interest, and accumulates to the degree that radioactive emissions are detected by the PET scanner. The PET scanner translates the emissions from the radioactivity as the positron combines with the negative electrons from the tissues and forms gamma rays that can be detected by the scanner. This information is transmitted to the computer, which determines the location and its distribution and translates the emissions as color-coded images for viewing, quantitative measurements, activity changes in relation to time, and three-dimensional computer-aided analysis.

Major organs such as the brain, heart, and cardiac muscles and anatomical areas with high concentrations of tissue such as the pelvis, use oxygen and glucose almost exclusively to meet their energy needs, and therefore their metabolism has been studied widely with PET. Each radionuclide tracer is designed to measure a specific body process, such as glucose metabolism, blood flow, and brain or cardiac tissue perfusion. Fluorine-18, in the form of fluorodeoxyglucose (FDG), is one of the most versatile and commonly used radionuclides in PET. FDG is a glucose analogue. All cells use glucose, but diseases that involve increased metabolic activity will show a high level of radionuclide visualization, whereas those that are hypometabolic will show little to no radionuclide visualization. There is little localization of FDG in normal tissue with minimal amounts being evenly distributed, allowing rapid detection of abnormal disease states. The radionuclide can be administered by IV injection or inhaled as a gas. After the radionuclide becomes concentrated in the brain, PET images of blood flow or metabolic processes at the cellular level can be obtained. Oxygen-15 is used in circumstances that warrant the evaluation of blood flow in the brain to predict or identify areas affected by a stroke. PET scan of the brain has had the greatest clinical impact in patients with epilepsy, dementia, neurodegenerative diseases, inflammation, cerebrovascular disease (indirectly), and brain tumors. At one point in time Alzheimer disease could be diagnosed only upon autopsy. Currently the disease can be diagnosed by PET imaging and by biochemical analysis of CSF. There is a substantial campaign to develop noninvasive markers of the disease as well as development of complimentary drugs to provide effective treatment—and potentially a means of prevention. In 2016 a research application (for amyloid PET scans) was used in the "Imaging Dementia—Evidence for Amyloid Scanning (IDEAS) Study" to evaluate whether brain PET scans, an invasive and expensive study, could have a positive impact on the identification and treatment of cognitive disorders. The study was conducted on 18,488 Medicare patients who were 65 years or older and who had been diagnosed with dementia or mild cognitive impairment (MCI). The patients had to meet other criteria which included a diagnosed cognitive impairment (CI) of unknown cause, confirmed by objective evaluation. Interim results presented in 2017 showed that PET scans from a significant sample of patients being treated for dementia and MCI showed the presence of beta-amyloid plaque; the study results also showed that a significant sampling of study patients where Alzheimer was suspected, presented with scans that were negative for the presence of beta-amyloid plaque. The report stated that 66% of providers caring for the latter group of participants changed their plan of treatment based on the amyloid negative PET scans. The IDEAS study findings are currently pending but researchers are hopeful the final results will provide the basis for using amyloid PET scans in those with CI of unknown cause resulting in better treatment and more positive patient outcomes. Cardiac PET scans are used to diagnose coronary artery disease, identify areas of heart tissue that are dead or scarred as a

P

result of an MI, and identify areas of impaired or diminished blood flow that may be corrected with coronary angioplasty/stent or coronary artery bypass surgery. For additional information regarding screening guidelines for *atherosclerotic cardiovascular disease* (ASCVD), refer to the study titled "Cholesterol, Total and Fractions." Colorectal tumor detection, tumor staging, evaluation of the effects of therapy, detection of recurrent disease, and detection of metastases are the main reasons to do a pelvic PET scan.

The expense of the study and the limited availability of radiopharmaceuticals tend to restrict the use of PET even though it is more sensitive than traditional nuclear scanning and single-photon emission computed tomography (SPECT). PET/CT and SPECT/CT are imaging applications that superimpose PET or SPECT and CT findings. The images are collected and produced by a single gantry system. The coregistered or image fusion of PET/CT or SPECT/CT findings can provide a detailed combination of anatomical and functional images. PET images can also be superimposed on MRI images.

INDICATIONS

General
- Assess tissue permeability.
- Determine the effectiveness of therapy, as evidenced by biochemical activity of normal and abnormal tissues.
- Determine the effects of therapeutic drugs on malfunctioning or diseased tissue.
- Identify the site for biopsy.

Brain
- Detect Parkinson disease and Huntington disease, as evidenced by decreased metabolism.
- Determine physiological changes in psychosis and schizophrenia.
- Differentiate between tumor recurrence and radiation necrosis.
- Evaluate Alzheimer disease and differentiate it from other causes of dementia, as evidenced by decreased cerebral flow and metabolism.
- Evaluate cranial tumors pre- and postoperatively and determine stage and appropriate treatment or procedure.
- Identify cerebrovascular accident or aneurysm, as evidenced by decreased blood flow and oxygen use.
- Identify focal seizures, as evidenced by decreased metabolism between seizures.

Heart
- Determine localization of areas of heart metabolism.
- Determine the presence of coronary artery disease (CAD), as evidenced by metabolic state during ischemia and after angina.
- Determine the size of heart infarcts.
- Identify cerebrovascular accident or aneurysm, as evidenced by decreasing blood flow and oxygen use.

Pelvis
- Determine the presence of colorectal cancer.
- Determine the presence of metastases of a cancerous tumor.
- Determine the recurrence of tumor or cancer.

INTERFERING FACTORS
Contraindications
Patients who are pregnant or suspected of being pregnant, unless

the potential benefits of a procedure using radiation far outweigh the risk of radiation exposure to the fetus and mother.

Factors that may alter the results of the study
- Drugs that alter glucose metabolism, such as tranquilizers or insulin, because hypoglycemia can alter PET results.
- The use of alcohol, tobacco, or caffeine-containing drinks at least 24 hr before the study, because the effects of these substances would make it difficult to evaluate the patient's true physiological state (e.g., alcohol is a vasoconstrictor and would decrease blood flow to the target organ).
- False-positive findings may occur as a result of normal gastrointestinal tract uptake and uptake in areas of infection or inflammation.
- Metallic objects (e.g., jewelry, body rings) within the examination field, which may inhibit organ visualization and cause unclear images.
- Improper injection of the radionuclide that allows the tracer to seep deep into the muscle tissue produces erroneous hot spots.
- Inability of the patient to cooperate or remain still during the procedure because movement can produce blurred or otherwise unclear images.

POTENTIAL MEDICAL DIAGNOSIS: CLINICAL SIGNIFICANCE OF RESULTS
Abnormal findings related to
Brain
- Alzheimer disease *(evidenced in later stages by areas lacking radionuclide visualization related to decreased cellular activity; cellular activity decreases as the disease progresses)*

- Aneurysm *(evidenced by areas lacking radionuclide visualization related to decreased cellular activity; cellular activity decreases as the disease progresses)*
- Cerebral metastases *(evidenced by areas of intense radionuclide visualization related to abnormally increased cellular activity)*
- Cerebrovascular accident *(evidenced by areas lacking radionuclide visualization related to decreased cellular activity)*
- Creutzfeldt-Jakob disease
- Dementia *(evidenced by areas lacking radionuclide visualization related to decreased cellular activity; cellular activity decreases as the disease progresses)*
- Head trauma *(evidenced by areas lacking radionuclide visualization related to decreased cellular activity)*
- Huntington disease *(evidenced by focal areas of intense radionuclide visualization related to hyperactivity of the affected nerves and increased cellular metabolism; cellular activity decreases as the disease progresses)*
- Migraine
- Parkinson disease *(evidenced by focal areas of intense radionuclide visualization related to hyperactivity of the affected nerves and increased cellular metabolism; cellular activity decreases as the disease progresses)*
- Schizophrenia
- Seizure disorders *(evidenced by focal areas of intense radionuclide visualization related to hyperactivity of the affected nerves and increased cellular metabolism)*
- Tumors *(evidenced by areas of intense radionuclide visualization related to abnormally increased cellular activity)*

P

Heart
- Chronic obstructive pulmonary disease
- Areas of tissue necrosis and scar tissue *(indicated by the lack of radionuclide visualization in areas of decreased blood flow and decreased glucose concentration)*
- Enlarged left ventricle
- Heart chamber disorder
- Ischemia and myocardial infarction *(indicated by the lack of radionuclide visualization in areas of decreased blood flow and decreased glucose concentration)*
- Pulmonary edema

Pelvis
- Focal uptake of the radionuclide in pelvis
- Focal uptake in abnormal lymph nodes
- Focal uptake in tumor
- Focal uptake in metastases

NURSING IMPLICATIONS

POTENTIAL NURSING PROBLEMS: ASSESSMENT & NURSING DIAGNOSIS

Problems	Signs and Symptoms
Brain: Tissue perfusion, cerebral *(related to infarct, altered cerebral blood flow, tumor, mass, dementia, hemorrhage, seizure)*	Diminished or altered level of consciousness, aphasia that can be expressive or receptive, loss of sensory functionality, slurred speech, difficulty swallowing, difficulty in completing a learned activity or in recognizing familiar objects (apraxia, agnosia), motor function deficits, spatial neglect, facial droop and/or varying degrees of flaccid extremities
Brain: Self-care deficit *(related to loss of cognitive or motor function)*	Unable to complete the activities of daily living without assistance (eating, bathing, dressing, toileting), psychological deficits
Heart: Inadequate tissue perfusion *(related to blood flow obstruction, oxygen supply/demand mismatch)*	Chest pain, chest pressure, shortness of breath, increase heart rate, cool skin, decreased capillary refill, diminished peripheral pulses, altered cardiac enzymes, confusion, restlessness
Heart: Activity *(related to myocardial ischemia, increased oxygen demands)*	Weakness, fatigue, chest pain with exertion, anxiety
Pelvis: Infection *(related to bacterial growth secondary to postoperative status)*	Chills, fever, elevated white blood cell (WBC) count, elevated C-reactive protein (CRP), purulent drainage, foul odor, positive culture for bacterial infection, fatigue

P

Teaching the Patient What to Expect

General

▶ Inform the patient that this procedure can assist in assessing blood flow and tissue metabolism in the site of interest.

▶ Pregnancy is a general contraindication to procedures involving radiation. Explain to the female patient that she will be asked the date of her last menstrual period and pregnancy testing may be performed to determine the possibility of pregnancy before she is exposed to radiation.

▶ Review the procedure with the patient. Address concerns about pain and explain that there may be moments of discomfort or pain experienced when the IV line is inserted to allow infusion of fluids such as saline, anesthetics, sedatives, radionuclides, medications used in the procedure, or emergency medications.

▶ Sometimes FDG examinations are done after blood has been drawn to determine circulating blood glucose levels. If blood glucose levels are high, insulin may be given.

▶ Explain that the procedure is performed in a special department, usually in a radiology suite, by an HCP specializing in this procedure, with support staff, and takes approximately 60 to 120 min for PET of the brain or heart and 30 to 60 min for PET of the pelvis.

▶ Reassure the patient that the radionuclide poses no radioactive hazard and rarely produces adverse effects.

▶ Instruct the patient to remove jewelry and other metallic objects from the area to be examined prior to the procedure.

▶ Explain that baseline vital signs and neurological status will be recorded and monitored throughout the procedure. Protocols may vary among facilities.

▶ Positioning for the study will be in the supine position on a flat table with foam wedges to help maintain position and immobilization.

Brain

▶ The radionuclide is injected, and imaging is started after a 30-min delay. If comparative studies are indicated, additional injections may be needed.

▶ Explain to the patient that he or she may be asked to perform different cognitive activities (e.g., reading) to measure changes in brain activity during reasoning or remembering.

▶ Advise that it may be necessary to be blindfolded or asked to use earplugs to decrease auditory and visual stimuli.

Heart

▶ The radionuclide is injected and imaging is done at periodic intervals, with continuous scanning done for 1 hr. If comparative studies are indicated, additional injections may be needed.

Pelvis

▶ The radionuclide is injected, and imaging is started after a 45-min delay. Continuous scanning may be done for 1 hr. If comparative studies are indicated, additional injections of radionuclide may be needed.

▶ Explain that it may be necessary to lavage the bladder via a urinary catheter with 2 L of 0.9% saline solution to remove concentrated radionuclide.

General

▶ Explain that once the study is completed, the needle or catheter will be removed and a pressure dressing applied over the puncture site.

Potential Nursing Actions

✷ *Make sure a written and informed consent has been signed prior to the procedure and before administering any medications.*

Avoiding Complications

▶ Establishing an IV site and injection of radionuclides are invasive procedures. Complications are rare but include risk for allergic reaction *(related to contrast reaction)*, hematoma *(related to blood leakage into the tissue following needle insertion)*, bleeding from the puncture site *(related to a bleeding disorder*

P

or the effects of natural products and medications with known anticoagulant, antiplatelet, or thrombolytic properties), or infection *(which might occur if bacteria from the skin surface is introduced at the puncture site).* Monitor the patient for complications related to the procedure (e.g., allergic reaction, anaphylaxis, bronchospasm). Immediately report symptoms such as fast heart rate, difficulty breathing, skin rash, itching, or chest pain to the appropriate HCP. Observe/assess the needle/catheter insertion site for bleeding, inflammation, or hematoma formation.

Treatment Considerations
◗ Explain that the radionuclide is eliminated from the body within 6 to 24 hr. Advise the patient to drink increased amounts of fluids for 24 to 48 hr to eliminate the radionuclide from the body, unless contraindicated.
◗ Instruct the patient to resume usual diet, fluids, medications, and activity as directed by the HCP.
◗ Instruct in the care and assessment of the injection site.
◗ Explain that application of cold compresses to the puncture site may reduce discomfort or edema.

Brain
◗ Cerebral Tissue Perfusion: When there is inadequate tissue perfusion to the brain, it is important to assess for psychological changes such as Alzheimer, psychosis, or dementia. A baseline neurological assessment is necessary for ongoing comparison to evaluate improvement or deterioration. Prepare for potential complementary diagnostic studies such as magnetic resonance imaging, ultrasound, or subtraction angiography. Interventions may include elevating the head of the bed and administering ordered antiplatelet, anticoagulant, thrombolytic medication, antihypertensive steroids, diuretics, calcium channel blockers, or antiseizure medications.
◗ Self-Care Deficit: Changes in cognitive function will be noted by changes in the patient's ability to perform self-care. Assess self-care deficits and identify areas where the patient can provide own care and where he or she needs assistance. Evaluate the family's ability to assist with self-care needs and consider a home health evaluation for home care. Provide assistive devices to help with self-care: commode, special utensils, walker, or cane. Alter the diet to match the patient's swallowing ability: thick liquids, puree, small bites, and so on, and remind the patient to chew and swallow slowly. Evaluate swallowing as appropriate before oral feeding.

Heart
◗ Cardiac Tissue Perfusion: Pain can be a common complaint when there is poor cardiac tissue perfusion. Assess for characteristics of pain: quality, intensity, duration, and location. Monitor and trend vital signs, pulse oximetry, and institute continuous cardiac monitoring. Assess skin color and temperature, cyanosis, breath sounds rate and rhythm, capillary refill, peripheral pulses, and for confusion and restlessness. Monitor and trend arterial blood gases, creatine phosphokinase, CK-MB, troponin, CRP, and lactate dehydrogenase. Administer ordered thrombolytics, morphine, amiodarone, nitroglycerine beta blockers. Ensure patient understands risk factors for CAD, necessary lifestyle changes (diet, smoking, alcohol use), the importance of weight management, and reportable signs and symptoms of heart attack.
◗ Activity: Identify the patient's normal activity patterns, maintain bedrest as required to rest the heart and conserve oxygen. Administer ordered oxygen, and remind the patient to wear oxygen with all activity. Other interventions include pacing activity with increases as tolerated. Monitor and trend vital signs including oxygen saturation and cardiac rhythm.

Pelvis
◗ Infection: When there is a confirmed infection, administer ordered antibiotics and prescribed antipyretics for fever. Monitor and trend WBC and CRP and compare culture and sensitivity results to prescribed antibiotics. Some interventions are to use appropriate cooling

P

measures, increase oral intake, apply a cooling blanket, light clothing, or a cooling tepid bath. Administer ordered IV fluids. Monitor and trend temperature, and screen for sepsis.

Safety Considerations

▶ The patient who is breastfeeding should consult with the requesting HCP regarding alternate testing that does not involve radiation. In general, if a woman who is breastfeeding must have a nuclear scan, she should not breastfeed the infant for 72 hr after the scan, until the radionuclide has been eliminated. She should be instructed to express the milk in order to prevent cessation of milk production; the milk can be stored and used after the 3-day period.

▶ Refer to organizational policy for additional precautions that may include instructions on handwashing, toilet flushing, limited contact with others, and other aspects of nuclear medicine safety.

Nutritional Considerations

Heart

▶ Discuss ideal body weight and the purpose of and relationship between ideal weight and caloric intake to support cardiac health. Review ways to decrease intake of saturated fats and increase intake of polyunsaturated fats. Discuss limiting intake of refined processed sugar and sodium; discuss limiting cholesterol intake to less than 300 mg per day. Encourage the intake of fresh fruits and vegetables, unprocessed carbohydrates, poultry, and grains.

▶ Nutritional therapy is recommended for those with identified CAD risk, especially for those with elevated low-density lipoprotein cholesterol levels, other lipid disorders, diabetes, insulin resistance, or metabolic syndrome. Always consider cultural influences with dietary choices to ensure better adherence to a change in lifestyle. A variety of dietary patterns are beneficial for people with ASCVD. For additional information regarding nutritional guidelines, refer to the study titled "Cholesterol, Total and Fractions."

▶ Other changeable risk factors warranting education include strategies to encourage regular participation in moderate aerobic physical activity three to four times per week, eliminate tobacco use, and adhere to a heart-healthy diet.

▶ Those with elevated triglycerides should be advised to eliminate or reduce alcohol.

Follow-Up, Evaluation, and Desired Outcomes

▶ Acknowledges the potential implications of abnormal test results on current lifestyle and the overall clinical implications of the test results.

▶ Individuals with cardiac disease acknowledge contact information provided for the American Heart Association (www.heart.org/HEARTORG), National Heart, Lung, and Blood Institute (www.nhlbi.nih.gov), and U.S. Department of Agriculture's resource for nutrition (www.choosemyplate.gov).

▶ Patients with pelvic disease acknowledge cancer screening options and understand that decisions regarding the need for and frequency of occult blood testing, colonoscopy, or other cancer screening procedures may be made after consultation between the patient and HCP. The American Cancer Society (ACS) recommends that regular screening for colon cancer begin at age 50 yr for individuals with average risk and sooner for those with increased or high risk for developing colon cancer. Its recommendations for frequency of screening are to use one of the following: (1) annual for occult blood testing (fecal occult blood testing or fecal immunochemical testing); (2) every 5 yr for flexible sigmoidoscopy, double-contrast barium enema, or CT colonography; (3) every 10 yr for colonoscopy; or (4) every 3 yr for stool DNA testing. Abnormal findings should be followed up by colonoscopy. There are both advantages and disadvantages to the screening tests that are available today. The stool DNA test is designed to identify abnormal changes in DNA from the cells in the lining of the colon that are normally shed and excreted in stool. Unlike some of the current screening methods, the DNA tests would be able to detect precancerous polyps. The most current guidelines for colon cancer screening of the general population as well as of individuals with increased risk are available from the ACS (www.cancer.org), U.S. Preventive Services Task Force (www.uspreventiveservices-taskforce.org), and American College of Gastroenterology (http://gi.org).

Potassium, Blood

SYNONYM/ACRONYM: Serum K⁺.

RATIONALE: To evaluate fluid and electrolyte balance related to potassium levels toward diagnosing disorders such as acidosis, acute kidney injury, chronic kidney disease, and dehydration and to monitor the effectiveness of therapeutic interventions.

PATIENT PREPARATION: There are no food, fluid, activity, or medication restrictions unless by medical direction. Instruct the patient not to clench and unclench the fist immediately before or during specimen collection.

NORMAL FINDINGS: Method: Ion-selective electrode.

Serum Potassium	Conventional and SI Units
Newborn	3.2–5.5 mEq/L or mmol/L
7–29 days	3.4–6 mEq/L or mmol/L
1–5 mo	3.5–5.6 mEq/L or mmol/L
6–12 mo	3.5–6.1 mEq/L or mmol/L
Child–18 yr	3.8–5.1 mEq/L or mmol/L
Adult–older adult	3.5–5.3 mEq/L or mmol/L
Anion Gap	**Conventional and SI Units**
Child or adult	8–16 mmol/L

Note: Value ranges may vary depending on the laboratory. Serum values are 0.1 mmol/L higher than plasma values, and reference ranges should be adjusted accordingly. It is important that serial measurements be collected using the same type of collection container to reduce variability of results from collection to collection.

Older adults are at risk for hyperkalemia due to the decline in aldosterone levels, decline in kidney function, and effects of commonly prescribed medications that inhibit the renin-angiotensin-aldosterone system.

CRITICAL FINDINGS AND POTENTIAL INTERVENTIONS

Adults and Children
- Less than 2.5 mEq/L or mmol/L (SI: Less than 2.5 mmol/L)
- Greater than 6.2 mEq/L or mmol/L (SI: Greater than 6.2 or mmol/L)

Newborns
- Less than 2.8 mEq/L or mmol/L (SI: Less than 2.8 mmol/L)
- Greater than 7.6 mEq/L or mmol/L (SI: Greater than 7.6 mmol/L)

Timely notification to the requesting health-care provider (HCP) of any critical findings and related symptoms is a role expectation of the professional nurse. A listing of these findings varies among facilities.

Consideration may be given to verification of critical findings before action is taken. Policies vary among facilities and may include requesting immediate recollection and retesting by the laboratory or retesting using a rapid point-of-care testing instrument at the bedside, if available.

Symptoms of hyperkalemia include irritability, diarrhea, cramps, oliguria, difficulty speaking, and cardiac dysrhythmias (peaked T waves and ventricular fibrillation). Continuous cardiac monitoring is indicated. Administration of sodium bicarbonate or calcium chloride may be requested. If the patient is receiving an IV supplement, verify that the patient is voiding.

Symptoms of hypokalemia include malaise, thirst, polyuria, anorexia, weak pulse, low blood pressure, vomiting, decreased reflexes, and electrocardiographic changes (depressed T waves and ventricular ectopy). Replacement therapy is indicated.

OVERVIEW: (**Study type:** Blood collected in a gold-, red-, red/gray-, or green-top [heparin] tube; **related body system:** Circulatory, Circulatory/Hematopoietic, Digestive, Endocrine, Respiratory, and Urinary systems.) Electrolytes dissociate into electrically charged ions when dissolved. Cations, including potassium, carry a positive charge. Body fluids contain approximately equal numbers of anions and cations, although the nature of the ions and their mobility differs between the intracellular and extracellular compartments. Both types of ions affect the electrical and osmolar functions of the body. Electrolyte quantities and the balance among them are controlled by oxygen and carbon dioxide exchange in the lungs; absorption, secretion, and excretion of many substances by the kidneys; and secretion of regulatory hormones by the endocrine glands. Potassium is the most abundant intracellular cation with a number of essential functions to include transmission of electrical impulses in cardiac and skeletal muscle and participation in enzyme reactions that transform glucose into energy and amino acids into proteins. Potassium also helps maintain acid-base equilibrium, and it has a significant and inverse relationship to pH: A decrease in pH of 0.1 increases the potassium level by 0.6 mmol/L.

Abnormal potassium levels can be caused by a number of contributing factors, which can be categorized as follows:

Altered Renal Excretion: Normally, 80% to 90% of the body's potassium is filtered out through the kidneys each day (the remainder is excreted in sweat and stool); kidney disease can result in abnormally high potassium levels.

Altered Dietary Intake: A severe potassium deficiency can be caused by an inadequate intake of dietary potassium.

Altered Cellular Metabolism: Damaged red blood cells (RBCs) release potassium into the circulating fluid, resulting in increased potassium levels.

The anion gap is a calculated value often reported from a set of electrolytes (sodium, potassium, chloride, and carbon dioxide) and is used most frequently as a clinical indicator of metabolic acidosis. The most common causes of an increased gap are lactic acidosis and ketoacidosis. The concept of estimating electrolyte disturbances in the extracellular fluid is based on the principle of electrical neutrality. The formula includes the major cation (sodium) and anions (chloride and bicarbonate) found in extracellular fluid. The anion gap is calculated as follows: anion gap = sodium − (chloride + HCO_3^-). Some laboratories may include potassium in the calculation of the anion gap. Calculations including potassium can be invalidated because minor amounts of hemolysis can contribute significant levels of potassium leaked into the serum as a result of cell rupture.

Because bicarbonate (HCO_3^-) is not directly measured on most chemistry analyzers, it is estimated by substitution of the total carbon dioxide (Tco_2) value in the calculation. The anion gap is also widely used as a laboratory quality-control measure because low gaps usually indicate a reagent, calibration, or instrument error.

INDICATIONS

- Assess a known or suspected disorder associated with kidney disease, glucose metabolism, trauma, or burns.
- Assist in the evaluation of electrolyte imbalances; this test is especially indicated in older adult patients, patients receiving hyperalimentation supplements, patients on hemodialysis, and patients with hypertension.
- Evaluate cardiac dysrhythmia to determine whether altered

potassium levels are contributing to the problem, especially during digoxin therapy, which leads to ventricular irritability.
- Evaluate the effects of drug therapy, especially diuretics.
- Evaluate the response to treatment for abnormal potassium levels.
- Monitor known or suspected acidosis, because potassium moves from RBCs into the extracellular fluid in acidotic states.
- Routine screen of electrolytes in acute and chronic illness.

INTERFERING FACTORS
Factors that may alter the results of the study

- Drugs and other substances that can cause an increase in potassium levels include ACE inhibitors, atenolol, basiliximab, captopril, clofibrate in association with kidney disease, cyclosporine, dexamethasone, enalapril, etretinate, lisinopril in association with heart failure or hypertension, NSAIDs, some drugs with potassium salts (e.g., antibiotics such as penicillin), spironolactone, succinylcholine, and tacrolimus.
- Drugs and other substances that can cause a decrease in potassium levels include acetazolamide, acetylsalicylic acid, aldosterone, ammonium chloride, amphotericin B, bendroflumethiazide, benzthiazide, bicarbonate, captopril, cathartics, chlorothiazide, chlorthalidone, cisplatin, clorexolone, corticosteroids, cyclothiazide, dichlorphenamide, digoxin, diuretics, enalapril, foscarnet, fosphenytoin, furosemide, insulin, laxatives, metolazone, moxalactam (common when coadministered with amikacin), large doses of any IV penicillin, phenolphthalein

(with chronic laxative misuse), polythiazide, quinethazone, sodium bicarbonate, tacrolimus, IV theophylline, thiazides, triamterene, and trichlormethiazide. A number of these medications initially increase the serum potassium level, but they also have a diuretic effect, which promotes potassium loss in the urine except in cases of renal insufficiency.

• Leukocytosis, as seen in leukemia, causes elevated potassium levels.

• False elevations can occur with vigorous pumping of the hand immediately before or during venipuncture.

• Hemolysis of the sample and high platelet counts also increase potassium levels, as follows: (1) Because potassium is an intracellular ion and concentrations are approximately 150 times extracellular concentrations, even a slight amount of hemolysis can cause a significant increase in levels. (2) Platelets release potassium during the clotting process, and therefore serum samples collected from patients with elevated platelet counts may produce spuriously high potassium levels. Plasma is the specimen of choice in patients known to have elevated platelet counts.

• False increases are seen in unprocessed samples left at room temperature because a significant amount of potassium leaks out of the cells within a few hours. Plasma or serum should be separated from cells within 4 hr of collection.

• Specimens should never be collected above an IV line because of the potential for dilution when the specimen and the IV solution combine in the collection container, falsely decreasing the result. There is also the potential of contaminating the sample with the substance of interest, if it is present in the IV solution, falsely increasing the result.

POTENTIAL MEDICAL DIAGNOSIS: CLINICAL SIGNIFICANCE OF RESULTS

Increased in

• Acidosis *(intracellular potassium ions are expelled in exchange for hydrogen ions in order to achieve electrical neutrality)*

• Acute kidney injury *(potassium excretion is diminished, and it accumulates in the blood)*

• Addison disease *(due to lack of aldosterone, potassium excretion is diminished, and it accumulates in the blood)*

• Asthma *(related to chronic inflammation and damage to lung tissue)*

• Burns *(related to tissue damage and release by damaged cells)*

• Chronic interstitial nephritis *(potassium excretion is diminished, and it accumulates in the blood)*

• Dehydration *(related to hemoconcentration)*

• Dialysis *(dialysis treatments simulate kidney function, but potassium builds up between treatments)*

• Diet *(related to excessive intake of salt substitutes or of potassium salts in medications)*

• Exercise *(related to tissue damage and release by damaged cells)*

• Hemolysis (massive) *(potassium is the major intracellular cation)*

• Hyperventilation *(in response to respiratory alkalosis, blood levels of potassium are increased in order to achieve electrical neutrality)*

• Hypoaldosteronism *(due to lack of aldosterone, potassium excretion is diminished, and it accumulates in the blood)*

• Insulin deficiency *(insulin deficiency results in movement of*

P

potassium from the cell into the extracellular fluid)
- Ketoacidosis *(insulin deficiency results in movement of potassium from the cell into the extracellular fluid)*
- Leukocytosis
- Muscle necrosis *(related to tissue damage and release by damaged cells)*
- Near drowning
- Pregnancy
- Prolonged periods of standing
- Tissue trauma *(related to release by damaged cells)*
- Transfusion of old banked blood *(aged cells hemolyze and release intracellular potassium)*
- Tubular unresponsiveness to aldosterone
- Uremia

Decreased in
- Alcohol misuse *(related to insufficient dietary intake)*
- Alkalosis *(potassium uptake by cells is increased in response to release of hydrogen ions from cells)*
- Anorexia nervosa *(related to significant changes in renal function that result in hypokalemia)*
- Bradycardia *(hypokalemia can cause bradycardia)*
- Chronic, excessive licorice ingestion *(from licorice root. Licorice inhibits short-chain dehydrogenase/reductase enzymes. These enzymes normally prevent cortisol from binding to aldosterone receptor sites in the kidney. In the absence of these enzymes, cortisol acts on the kidney and triggers the same effects as aldosterone, which include increased potassium excretion, sodium retention, and water retention.)*

- Crohn's disease *(insufficient intestinal absorption)*
- Cushing's syndrome *(aldosterone facilitates the excretion of potassium by the kidneys)*
- Diet deficient in meat and vegetables *(insufficient dietary intake)*
- Excess insulin *(insulin causes glucose and potassium to move into cells)*
- Familial periodic paralysis *(related to fluid retention)*
- Gastrointestinal (GI) loss due to vomiting, diarrhea, nasogastric suction, or intestinal fistula
- Heart failure *(related to fluid retention and hemodilution)*
- Hyperaldosteronism *(aldosterone facilitates the excretion of potassium by the kidneys)*
- Hypertension *(medications used to treat hypertension may result in loss of potassium; hypertension is often related to diabetes and kidney disease, which affect cellular retention and renal excretion of potassium, respectively)*
- Hypomagnesemia *(magnesium levels tend to parallel potassium levels)*
- IV therapy with inadequate potassium supplementation
- Laxative misuse *(related to medications that cause potassium wasting)*
- Malabsorption *(related to insufficient intestinal absorption)*
- Pica (eating substances of no nutritional value, e.g., clay)
- Renal tubular acidosis *(condition results in excessive loss of potassium)*
- Sweating *(related to increased loss)*
- Theophylline administration, excessive *(theophylline drives potassium into cells, reducing circulating levels)*
- Thyrotoxicosis *(related to changes in kidney function)*

P

NURSING IMPLICATIONS

POTENTIAL NURSING PROBLEMS: ASSESSMENT & NURSING DIAGNOSIS

Problems	Signs and Symptoms
Activity *(related to compromised cardiac status, compromised renal status, weakness, lack of motivation, oxygen supply and demand imbalance)*	Verbal report of weakness; inability to tolerate activity; shortness of breath with activity; altered heart rate, blood pressure, and respiratory rate with activity
Electrolyte imbalance *(related to metabolic imbalance associated with disease process)*	**Excess:** Nausea, weak or irregular pulse, sudden collapse, cardiac arrest
Deficit: Thirst, tetany, weakness, constipation, arrhythmias, hypotension, nausea, vomiting, anorexia, polyuria, mental depression, cardiac arrest
Fluid volume (water) *(related to metabolic imbalances associated with disease process)*	**Deficit:** Decreased urinary output, fatigue, sunken eyes, dark urine, decreased blood pressure, increased heart rate, altered mental status
Excess: Edema, shortness of breath, increased weight, ascites, rales, rhonchi, diluted laboratory values
Health management *(related to complexity of health-care system, complexity of therapeutic management, altered metabolic process resulting in increased or decreased potassium, knowledge deficit, conflicted decision making, cultural family health patterns, barriers to healthy decisions, mistrust of HCP)*	Health choices are ineffective in making a difference on outcomes; increasing symptoms of illness; verbalizes that therapeutic regime is too difficult; patient and family do not support HCP's suggestions for health improvement; refuses to follow recommended therapeutic regime

P

BEFORE THE STUDY: PLANNING AND IMPLEMENTATION

Teaching the Patient What to Expect
▶ Inform the patient this test can assist in evaluating electrolyte balance.
▶ Explain that a blood sample is needed for the test.

AFTER THE STUDY: POTENTIAL NURSING ACTIONS

Avoiding Complications
▶ Observe the patient for signs and symptoms of fluid volume excess related to excess potassium intake (hyperkalemia), fluid volume deficit related to active loss (hypokalemia), or risk of injury related to an alteration in body chemistry.

Treatment Considerations

▶ Activity: Assess current level of physical activity, monitor and trend vital signs in response to activity, monitor blood pressure for orthostatic changes. Monitor for oxygen desaturation with activity and administer ordered oxygen to maintain prescribed saturation level. Collaborate with physical therapy and the patient to facilitate activity and establish activity goals and guidelines. Remember to pace activities to match energy stores.

▶ Electrolyte Balance: Correlate potassium imbalance with disease process, nutritional intake, renal function, and medications. Monitor electrocardiogram status, and respiratory changes. Collaborate with the pharmacist and HCP for appropriate pharmacologic interventions and adjust medication dosage to compensate for renal impairment. Collaborate with dietitian for dietary modifications and begin hemodialysis or peritoneal dialysis treatments if necessary. Reduce the intake of high-potassium foods and dietary supplements.

▶ Fluid Volume: Monitor and trend daily weight, intake and output, urine characteristics, respiratory status and laboratory values that reflect alterations in fluid status: potassium, BUN, Cr, calcium, Hgb, and Hct. Collaborate with the HCP to manage the underlying cause of fluid alteration; administer and adjust oral or IV fluids to support hydration and replacement of electrolytes. Increased potassium levels may be associated with dehydration. Evaluate the patient for signs and symptoms of dehydration. Dehydration is a significant and common finding in older adult patients and other patients in whom kidney function has deteriorated.

▶ Health Management: Assess the effort to follow the recommended therapeutic regime. Evaluate for any family or cultural factors that may impact the success of the therapeutic plan. Consider the patient's assessment of his or her own health in tailoring the plan of care to the patient's lifestyle. Include the patient and family in designing the plan of care and work toward a system of self-management that works within the context of their lives. Focus on behaviors that will make the biggest positive impact on improved health. Decreased potassium levels may occur in patients receiving digoxin or potassium-wasting diuretics. Potassium levels should be monitored carefully because cardiac dysrhythmias can occur. Instruct the patient in electrolyte replacement therapy and changes in dietary intake that affect electrolyte levels, as ordered.

Nutritional Considerations

▶ Potassium is present in all plant and animal cells, making dietary replacement simple to achieve in the potassium-deficient patient. Fruits and vegetables (artichokes, avocados, bananas, cantaloupe, dried fruits, kiwi, mango, dried beans, nuts, oranges, peaches, pears, pomegranates, potatoes, prunes, pumpkin, spinach, sunflower seeds, swiss chard, tomatoes, and winter squash), dairy products (especially milk and milk products such as ice cream, yogurt, cream, buttermilk, half & half), and meats are rich in potassium.

Follow-Up, Evaluation, and Desired Outcomes

▶ Acknowledges contact information provided for the U.S. Department of Agriculture's resource for nutrition (www.choosemyplate.gov).

P

Potassium, Urine

SYNONYM/ACRONYM: Urine K+.

RATIONALE: To evaluate electrolyte balance, acid-base balance, and hypokalemia.

PATIENT PREPARATION: There are no food, fluid, activity, or medication restrictions unless by medical direction. Usually, a 24-hr urine collection is ordered. As appropriate, provide the required urine collection container and specimen collection instructions.

NORMAL FINDINGS: Method: Ion-selective electrode.

Age	Conventional Units	SI Units (Conventional Units × 1)
6–10 yr		
Male	17–54 mEq/24 hr or mmol/24 hr	17–54 mmol/24 hr
Female	8–37 mEq/24 hr or mmol/24 hr	8–37 mmol/24 hr
10–14 yr	18–58 mEq/24 hr or mmol/24 hr	18–58 mmol/24 hr
Adult–older adult	26–123 mEq/24 hr or mmol/24 hr	26–123 mmol/24 hr

Note: Reference values depend on potassium intake and diurnal variation. Excretion is significantly higher at night.

Potassium excretion declines in older adults due to the decline in aldosterone levels, decline in kidney function, and effects of commonly prescribed medications that inhibit the renin-angiotensin-aldosterone system.

CRITICAL FINDINGS AND POTENTIAL INTERVENTIONS: N/A

OVERVIEW: (Study type: Urine from an unpreserved random or timed specimen collected in a clean plastic collection container; related body system: Circulatory, Digestive, Endocrine, and Urinary systems.) Electrolytes dissociate into electrically charged ions when dissolved. Cations, including potassium, carry a positive charge. Body fluids contain approximately equal numbers of anions and cations, although the nature of the ions and their mobility differs between the intracellular and extracellular compartments. Both types of ions affect the electrical and osmolar functions of the body. Electrolyte quantities and the balance among them are controlled by oxygen and carbon dioxide exchange in the lungs; absorption, secretion, and excretion of many substances by the kidneys; and secretion of regulatory hormones by the endocrine glands. Potassium is the most abundant intracellular cation. It is essential for the transmission of electrical impulses in cardiac and skeletal muscle. It also functions in enzyme reactions

P

that transform glucose into energy and amino acids into proteins. Potassium helps maintain acid-base equilibrium, and it has a significant and inverse relationship to pH: A decrease in pH of 0.1 increases the potassium level by 0.6 mEq/L.

Abnormal potassium levels can be caused by a number of contributing factors, which can be categorized as follows:

Altered Renal Excretion: Normally, 80% to 90% of the body's potassium is filtered out through the kidneys each day (the remainder is excreted in sweat and stool); renal disease can result in abnormally high potassium levels.

Altered Dietary Intake: A severe potassium deficiency can be caused by an inadequate intake of dietary potassium.

Altered Cellular Metabolism: Damaged red blood cells (RBCs) release potassium into the circulating fluid, resulting in increased potassium levels.

Regulating electrolyte balance is one of the major functions of the kidneys. In normally functioning kidneys, urine potassium levels increase when serum levels are high and decrease when serum levels are low to maintain homeostasis. The kidneys respond to alkalosis by excreting potassium to retain hydrogen ions and increase acidity. In acidosis, the body excretes hydrogen ions and retains potassium. Analyzing these urinary levels can provide important clues to the functioning of the kidneys and other major organs. Urine potassium tests usually involve timed urine collections over a 12- or 24-hr period. Measurement of random specimens also may be requested.

INDICATIONS
- Determine the potential cause of renal calculi.
- Evaluate known or suspected endocrine disorder.
- Evaluate known or suspected kidney disease.
- Evaluate malabsorption disorders.

INTERFERING FACTORS
Factors that may alter the results of the study
- Drugs and other substances that can cause an increase in urine potassium levels include acetazolamide, acetylsalicylic acid, ammonium chloride, bendroflumethiazide, chlorthalidone, clopamide, corticosteroids, cortisone, diapamide, dichlorphenamide, diuretics, ethacrynic acid, fludrocortisone, furosemide, hydrochlorothiazide, hydrocortisone, intra-amniotic saline, mefruside, niacinamide, some oral contraceptives, thiazides, torsemide, triflocin, and viomycin.
- Drugs and other substances that can cause a decrease in urine potassium levels include anesthetic drugs, felodipine, and levarterenol.
- Diuretic therapy with excessive loss of electrolytes into the urine may falsely elevate results.

Other considerations
- A dietary deficiency or excess of potassium can lead to spurious results.
- Potassium levels are subject to diurnal variation (output being highest at night), which is why 24-hr collections are recommended.
- All urine voided for the timed collection period must be included in the collection, or else falsely decreased values may be obtained. Compare output records with volume collected to verify that all voids were included in the collection.

POTENTIAL MEDICAL DIAGNOSIS: CLINICAL SIGNIFICANCE OF RESULTS

Increased in

- Albright-type kidney disease *(related to excessive production of cortisol)*
- Cushing syndrome *(excessive corticosteroids, especially aldosterone levels, will increase urinary excretion of potassium)*
- Diabetic ketoacidosis *(insulin deficiency forces potassium into the extracellular fluid; excess potassium is excreted in the urine)*
- Diuretic therapy *(related to potassium-wasting effects of the medications)*
- Hyperaldosteronism *(excessive aldosterone levels will increase urinary excretion of potassium)*
- Starvation (onset) *(cells involved in providing energy through tissue breakdown release potassium into circulation)*
- Vomiting *(elevated urine potassium is a hallmark of bulimia)*

Decreased in

- Addison disease *(reduced aldosterone levels will diminish excretion of potassium by the kidneys)*
- Chronic kidney disease with decreased urine flow
- Potassium deficiency (chronic)

NURSING IMPLICATIONS

BEFORE THE STUDY: PLANNING AND IMPLEMENTATION

Teaching the Patient What to Expect

▶ Inform the patient this test can assist in evaluating electrolyte balance.
▶ Explain that a urine sample is needed for the test. Information regarding specimen collection is presented with other general guidelines in Appendix A: Patient Preparation and Specimen Collection.

Potential Nursing Actions

▶ Patients receiving digoxin or diuretics should have potassium levels monitored carefully because cardiac dysrhythmias can occur.
▶ Include on the collection container's label the amount of urine, test start and stop times, and ingestion of any foods or medications that can affect test results.

AFTER THE STUDY: POTENTIAL NURSING ACTIONS

Avoiding Complications

▶ Increased urine potassium levels may be associated with the formation of kidney stones.
▶ Explain the importance of drinking a sufficient amount of water when kidney stones are suspected.

Treatment Considerations

▶ Observe for signs and symptoms of fluid volume excess related to excess potassium intake, fluid volume deficit related to active loss, or risk of injury related to an alteration in body chemistry. Symptoms include dehydration, diarrhea, vomiting, or prolonged anorexia. Dehydration is a significant and common finding in older adult patients and other patients in whom renal function has deteriorated.

Nutritional Considerations

▶ Potassium is present in all plant and animal cells, making dietary replacement simple to achieve in the potassium-deficient patient. Fruits and vegetables (artichokes, avocados, bananas, cantaloupe, dried fruits, kiwi, mango, dried beans, nuts, oranges, peaches, pears, pomegranates, potatoes, prunes, pumpkin, spinach, sunflower seeds, swiss chard, tomatoes, and winter squash), dairy products (especially milk and milk products such as ice cream, yogurt, cream, buttermilk, half & half), and meats are rich in potassium.
▶ Instruct the patient in electrolyte replacement therapy and changes in dietary intake that affect electrolyte levels, as ordered.

P

Prealbumin

SYNONYM/ACRONYM: Transthyretin.

RATIONALE: To assess nutritional status and evaluate liver function toward diagnosing disorders such as malnutrition and chronic kidney disease.

PATIENT PREPARATION: There are no fluid, activity, or medication restrictions unless by medical direction. The patient may be instructed to fast prior to the test; protocols vary among facilities.

NORMAL FINDINGS: Method: Nephelometry.

Age	Conventional Units	SI Units (Conventional Units × 10)
Newborn–1 mo	7–39 mg/dL	70–390 mg/L
1–6 mo	8–34 mg/dL	80–340 mg/L
6 mo–4 yr	11–23 mg/dL	110–230 mg/L
5–15 yr	14–35 mg/dL	140–350 mg/L
16–17 yr	20–43 mg/dL	20–43 mg/L
Adult/older adult	20–42 mg/dL	200–420 mg/L

CRITICAL FINDINGS AND POTENTIAL INTERVENTIONS: N/A

OVERVIEW: (Study type: Blood collected in a gold-, red-, or red/gray-top tube; **related body system:** Digestive, Endocrine, and Immune systems.) Prealbumin is a protein primarily produced by the liver. It is the major transport protein for triiodothyronine and thyroxine. It is also important in the metabolism of retinol-binding protein, which is needed for transporting vitamin A (retinol). Prealbumin has a short biological half-life of 2 days. It is used as an indicator of protein status and a marker for malnutrition. Prealbumin is often measured simultaneously with transferrin and albumin. The role of prealbumin in nutritional management has come into question by some

health care providers (HCPs) because it is a negative acute-phase protein. Prealbumin levels decrease during the acute phase of an inflammatory process such as in burns, infection, tumors, strenuous exercise, surgery, tissue infarction, and trauma, making the use of prealbumin less reliable as a predictor of malnutrition in certain clinical situations. Prealbumin may also be measured with C-reactive protein to assess for the coexistence of an inflammatory process and provide a more complete interpretation of the results.

INDICATIONS
Evaluate nutritional status.

INTERFERING FACTORS
Factors that may alter the results of the study
- Drugs and other substances that may increase prealbumin levels include anabolic steroids, anticonvulsants, danazol, oral contraceptives, prednisolone, prednisone, and propranolol.
- Drugs and other substances that may decrease prealbumin levels include amiodarone and diethylstilbestrol.

Other considerations
- Reference ranges are often based on fasting populations to provide some level of standardization for comparison. The presence of lipids in the blood may also interfere with the test method; fasting eliminates this potential source of error, especially if the patient has elevated lipid levels.

POTENTIAL MEDICAL DIAGNOSIS: CLINICAL SIGNIFICANCE OF RESULTS
Increased in
- Alcohol misuse *(related to leakage of prealbumin from damaged hepatocytes and/or poor nutrition)*
- Chronic kidney disease *(related to rapid turnover of prealbumin, which reflects a perceived elevation in the presence of overall loss of other proteins that take longer to produce)*
- Patients receiving steroids *(these drugs stimulate production of prealbumin)*

Decreased in
- Acute-phase inflammatory response *(prealbumin is a negative acute-phase reactant protein; levels decrease in the presence of inflammation)*
- Diseases of the liver *(related to decreased ability of the damaged liver to synthesize protein)*

- Hepatic damage *(related to decreased ability of the damaged liver to synthesize protein)*
- Malnutrition *(synthesis is decreased due to lack of proper diet)*
- Tissue necrosis *(prealbumin is a negative acute-phase reactant protein; levels decrease in the presence of inflammation)*

NURSING IMPLICATIONS

BEFORE THE STUDY: PLANNING AND IMPLEMENTATION

Teaching the Patient What to Expect
- Inform the patient this test can assist in assessing nutritional status.
- Explain that a blood sample is needed for the test.

AFTER THE STUDY: POTENTIAL NURSING ACTIONS

Treatment Considerations
- Instruct the patient to resume usual diet if fasting was required and as directed by the HCP.

Nutritional Considerations
- Nutritional therapy may be indicated for patients with decreased prealbumin levels. Educate the patient, as appropriate, that good dietary sources of complete protein (containing all eight essential amino acids) include meat, fish, eggs, and dairy products and that good sources of incomplete protein (lacking one or more of the eight essential amino acids) include grains, nuts, legumes, vegetables, and seeds.

Follow-Up, Evaluation, and Desired Outcomes
- Understands that depending on the results of this procedure, additional testing may be performed to evaluate or monitor disease progression and determine the need for a change in therapy.

P

Prion Disease Testing

SYNONYM/ACRONYM: Transmissible spongiform encephalopathies, TSEs.

RATIONALE: Testing for prion diseases may be considered for patients with undiagnosed, rapidly progressive dementia.

PATIENT PREPARATION: There are no activity restrictions unless by medical direction. Follow the food, fluid, or medication instructions indicated in the individual studies.

NORMAL FINDINGS: Negative biopsy, normal cerebrospinal fluid (CSF) protein levels, normal electroencephalogram (EEG), normal magnetic resonance imaging (MRI), normal neurologic examination.

- No evidence of prion disease
- Negative tonsillar biopsy (if variant Creutzfeldt-Jakob disease [vCJD] is being considered), *as vCJD is the only type known to involve the lymph nodes, spleen, tonsil, and appendix. Note:* A negative biopsy does not rule out vCJD.

CRITICAL FINDINGS AND POTENTIAL INTERVENTIONS: N/A

OVERVIEW: (Study type: Information is collected from a variety of sources that may include brain or tonsillar biopsy, CSF. Analysis for the presence of 14-3-3 type protein, EEG, brain MRI, neurologic examinations, and patient history; **related body system:** Musculoskeletal and Nervous systems.) Prion diseases have been identified in humans and animals throughout the world. They are classified in a general category of brain diseases called *proteinopathies.* Prion diseases are rare, fatal (no known cure), and very difficult to diagnose. Prion diseases are caused by abnormal protein molecules called *scrapie prion proteins* (PrPSc) that cause irreversible damage to brain tissue. The protein molecules themselves appear to be capable of initiating the disease process, do not stimulate an immune response, and are extraordinarily resistant to destruction. Records describing the first prion disease date back to the 1700s, and the pathophysiology of transmissible spongiform encephalopathy (TSE) continues to elude scientists, as there is no known test that can reliably detect either the disease or its cause by conventional methods. The term *prion* is derived from a combination of the words *protein* and *infectious* and was given to the protein in the 1980s by its Nobel Prize–winning discoverer, Stanley Prusiner. Cellular prion protein (PrPC) exists normally in humans and all other mammals; the highest concentration of PrPC is found in brain tissue, but it is also present in other tissue types (e.g., tonsil, appendix, spleen, intestinal, lymphatic). The trigger that leads to the aberrant conformational changes in the PrPC remains unknown, but the aberrant PrPSc protein will serve as a template to produce more abnormal protein once it has been transmitted into its host. There is significant

P

scientific evidence that as the structurally abnormal PrPSc protein molecules develop, they gather in clusters and accumulate in affected tissue, especially brain tissue. The resulting damage leaves spongelike holes in the tissue that are evident upon microscopic examination of brain tissue; hence, the condition is termed *spongiform encephalopathy.* Difficulty in diagnosis is due to a number of factors that include latency (the infection can be developing for years before signs and symptoms appear) and the lack of specific, minimally invasive, rapid disease markers. Brain biopsy and neuropathologic examination at autopsy are the only methods that can positively confirm a diagnosis of prion disease. It is hoped that a growing understanding of molecular science will open doors that have thus far prevented our discovery of the cause, treatment, and cure for prion diseases. Current research projects are investigating the possibility of a connection between prion disease and the progressive loss of neuromuscular abilities associated with Alzheimer disease, another familiar proteinopathy. Some research studies have reported positive correlations between abnormal brain FDG-PET scans (i.e., those showing lower than normal metabolic activity) and prion disease diagnosed upon autopsy. The rare occurrence of patients with prion disease or who have died from it presents a significant obstacle for researchers who are trying to identify the cause of prion disease in humans. Other diseases classified as proteinopathies include Parkinson disease and amyotrophic lateral sclerosis.

Specific prion diseases are known to affect humans and animals. Scrapie, the first prion disease identified, affects sheep and goats. The scrapie-infected animals "scrape" off their wool or hair and exhibit signs and symptoms of a central nervous system disorder.

Prion Diseases Associated With Animals

- Bovine spongiform encephalopathy (BSE)—affects cattle; also known as *mad cow disease*
- Chronic wasting disease—affects deer, elk, and moose
- Feline spongiform encephalopathy
- Scrapie—affects sheep and goats
- Transmissible mink encephalopathy
- Ungulate spongiform encephalopathy—affects exotic animals such as kudu, nyala, and oryx

Human prion diseases can be acquired or inherited, or they can occur sporadically, unassociated with any cause. Even though the diseases are rare, there is cause for public health concern because transmission of tiny amounts of prion-contaminated material can initiate the conversion of normal to abnormal protein production in a healthy individual, and the disease that develops is always fatal. Some infections occur strictly within an animal species (e.g., sheep-to-sheep transmission), and some occur across animal species (e.g., animal-to-human transmission). Infection of animals is believed to occur as a result of direct transmission from animal to animal or by consumption of feed processed with infected animal parts; infection of humans is believed to occur

P

as a result of the consumption of infected flesh (human or animal), blood transfusion, administration of human-derived pituitary growth hormones (production of genetically engineered hormones began in the 1980s), implantation of infected tissue (corneas and skin) or infected grafts (during spinal cord or brain surgery), and exposure to contaminated objects (e.g., surgical instruments used in neurosurgery). Blood product services have developed strict deferral policies regarding Creutzfeldt-Jakob disease (CJD), a human prion disease.

Three Types of Human Prion Disease

1. Acquired and iatrogenic prion diseases are very rare, accounting for less than 1% of reported cases. Kuru and vCJD are types of acquired prion diseases caused by exposure to exogenous sources of PrPSc. Kuru is a disease that was originally identified in a New Guinea tribe that practiced cannibalism as part of the funeral ritual. Kuru is rarely encountered today because education regarding the mechanism of its transmission has resulted in its virtual eradication. vCJD is linked to exposure to BSE through consumption of contaminated beef, although there have been some cases of vCJD linked to blood transfusion. Unlike classic CJD, vCJD appears to affect younger patients (average age of 28 yr) and has a longer duration of illness (average of 12 to 14 mo). Iatrogenic prion disease occurs accidentally during a medical procedure (e.g., as a result of receiving prion-contaminated tissue implants or grafts, by injections of human derived hormones, or through exposure during a surgical procedure using contaminated instruments).

2. Inherited or familial prion diseases have a low incidence, accounting for 10% to 15% of reported cases. Familial prion diseases are defined by the presence of a mutation in the PrPC gene as determined by genetic testing. There are three distinct types of familial prion disease: familial Creutzfeldt-Jakob disease (fCJD), fatal familial insomnia (FFI), and Gerstmann-Sträussler-Scheinker disease (GSS).

3. Sporadic prion diseases are the most common, have no known cause, and comprise 85% to 90% of reported cases. There are also three types of sporadic diseases: sporadic Creutzfeldt-Jakob disease (sCJD), sporadic fatal insomnia (sFI), and variably protease-sensitive prionopathy (VPSPr). sCJD, or classical CJD, is the most common of all prion diseases. The average age of onset ranges between 45 and 75 yr and has a relatively short duration of illness; 70% of patients diagnosed with sCJD die in 6 mo or less. The period between production of the abnormal PrPSc protein and the onset of symptoms (latency period) can be anywhere between 1 and 30 yr. Once the abnormal protein begins accumulating, symptoms appear suddenly. Cognitive changes include memory lapses, moodiness, lack of interest in normal activities, and withdrawal from social contacts. Motor changes include unsteady gait, slurred speech, and difficulty swallowing. Blurred vision and hallucinations sometimes occur in the later phase of the disease. Mental and physical deterioration rapidly

progress until, eventually, movement and speech are lost. Death is usually a complication of heart failure or respiratory failure.

INDICATIONS
- Identify family history of prion disease.
- Identify undiagnosed, rapidly progressive dementia.

INTERFERING FACTORS: N/A

POTENTIAL MEDICAL DIAGNOSIS: CLINICAL SIGNIFICANCE OF RESULTS
Abnormal findings related to
Testing for sCJD, the most common type of prion disease, may include noninvasive testing such as brain MRI and EEG. Two types of MRI studies may be used to identify abnormalities in the cerebral cortex, striatum, and/or thalamus of the brain: fluid attenuated inversion recovery and diffusion weighted imaging. EEG studies of people with sCJD show the characteristic abnormal findings associated with CJD (periodic, sharp brain waves) at some stage of the disease in 65% of cases. The problem is that the abnormal patterns may be only intermittently manifested or they may not be demonstrated at all until the later stages of the disease. CSF analysis is a more invasive procedure and is used to identify an increase in CSF protein levels. Protein 14-3-3, brain-specific enolase, and tau protein have been associated with proteinopathies but are not specific for CJD. Two newer methods to detect prion proteins have been developed with good promise for detecting tiny amounts of PrPSc in human specimens. The real-time quaking-induced conversion (RT-QUIC) method utilizes a CSF specimen to detect CJD-associated prions. The protein misfolding cyclic amplification (PMCA) urine test detects evidence of vCJD-associated prions. More studies need to be done to determine whether these assays can be used diagnostically, but the hope is that reliable antemortem testing for TSEs, prior to the development of symptoms, may become a possibility.

- CJD *(evidenced by abnormal brain biopsy and neuropathologic findings at autopsy)*

NURSING IMPLICATIONS

BEFORE THE STUDY: PLANNING AND IMPLEMENTATION

Teaching the Patient What to Expect
- Inform the patient that the testing ordered by the health-care provider (HCP) can assist in the differential diagnosis of types of conditions that affect the brain and nervous system.
- Explain that specimen type varies by study; blood, CSF, or tissue samples may be needed for the test.
- Review the procedure with the patient.
- Explain that several tests may be necessary to establish a presumptive diagnosis.
- Advise that CSF specimens are collected by lumbar puncture, as described in the "Cerebrospinal Fluid Analysis" study.
- Address concerns about pain, and explain that there may be some discomfort during CSF specimen collection.

Safety Considerations
- CJD-specific infection-control guidelines have been developed to assist those involved in the care of CJD patients and disposal or cleaning of contaminated materials and equipment. Methods include steam autoclaving materials or immersing them in sodium hydroxide solution. Additional information can be obtained from the Centers for Disease Control and Prevention (CDC) (www.cdc.gov/prions/cjd/infection-control.html) and the World Health Organization

(www.who.int/csr/resources/publications/bse/whocdscsraph2003.pdf?ua=1).

▶ CJD-specific infection control guidelines have been developed to assist funeral directors and their employees who are involved in funeral preparations. Information can be accessed at the Web sites provided for health-care workers.

AFTER THE STUDY: POTENTIAL NURSING ACTIONS

Treatment Considerations

▶ Teach the patient and family about the disease progression. Explain that fear, anxiety, and grief are normal reactions. The patient may experience visual hallucinations, myoclonus, and dysesthesia, which can be very distressing for patients and their caregivers.

▶ Explain that with disease progression there is a loss of awareness of surroundings, of the disease, and of the symptoms.

▶ Explain that there are drugs available that can help alleviate the discomfort associated with some of the symptoms.

▶ Provide emotional support for anxiety related to test results that may be indicative of CJD.

▶ Encourage the family to seek counseling if concerned with providing care to the patient at home or for assistance to address fears about disease transmission during home care, especially regarding considerations for end-of-life preparations, including special funeral arrangements and the possibility of a postmortem autopsy.

Follow-Up, Evaluation, and Desired Outcomes

▶ Understands that prion diseases are reportable in some state health departments; state health departments should be notified by HCPs as required by law.

▶ Acknowledges contact information provided for the Creutzfeldt-Jacob Disease Foundation (https://cjdfoundation.org) and CDC (www.cdc.gov/DiseasesConditions).

▶ Teach the pathophysiology associated with the disease process, including mode of transmission if known.

▶ Provide advance directive options to the patient and family with a discussion on end-of-life care.

Procalcitonin

SYNONYM/ACRONYM: PCT.

RATIONALE: To assist in diagnosing bacterial infection and risk for developing sepsis.

PATIENT PREPARATION: There are no food, fluid, activity, or medication restrictions unless by medical direction.

NORMAL FINDINGS: Method: Fluorescence immunoassay.

Age	Conventional Units	SI Units (Conventional Units × 1)
Newborn	Less than 2 ng/mL	Less than 2 mcg/L
18–20 hr	Less than 20 ng/mL	Less than 20 mcg/L
48 hr	Less than 5 ng/mL	Less than 5 mcg/L
3 d–adult	Less than 0.1 ng/mL	Less than 0.1 mcg/L

Interpretive Guidelines

Interpretation	Conventional Units	SI Units
Bacterial infection absent or highly unlikely	Less than 0.1 ng/mL	Less than 0.1 mcg/L
Bacterial infection possible, low risk for development of sepsis	Less than 0.5 ng/mL	Less than 0.5 mcg/L
Bacterial infection likely, development of sepsis is possible	0.5–2 ng/mL	0.5–2 mcg/L
Bacterial infection highly likely, high risk for development of sepsis	2.1–9.9 ng/mL or greater	2.1–9.9 mcg/L or greater
Bacterial infection severe, septic shock is probable	10 ng/mL or greater	10 mcg/L or greater

The value of individual levels or absolute cutoffs varies between facilities; many have adopted multivariate criteria for the evaluation and management of sepsis that may or may not include procalcitonin measurements.

CRITICAL FINDINGS AND POTENTIAL INTERVENTIONS: N/A

OVERVIEW: (Study type: Blood collected in a gold-, red-, red/gray-, lavender- [EDTA], or green- [lithium or sodium heparin] top tube; related body system: Immune system.) Procalcitonin, blood cultures, C-reactive protein (CRP), and lactate levels are all used as indicators of infection, inflammation—and as sepsis markers. Normally, procalcitonin, the precursor of the hormone calcitonin, is produced by the C cells of the thyroid. In sepsis and septic shock, microbial toxins and inflammatory mediator proteins, including cytokines, tumor necrosis factor α, interleukin 1, prostaglandins, and platelet activating factor, are thought to trigger the production of large amounts of procalcitonin (bacterial sources are believed to stimulate production of procalcitonin to a greater degree than viral sources) by nonthyroidal, non-neuroendocrine cells throughout the body. Procalcitonin is detectable within 2 to 4 hr after a sepsis initiating event, peaks within 12 to 24 hr, and remains detectable for up to 7 days. Serial measurements are useful to monitor patients at risk of developing sepsis or to monitor response to therapy.

Sepsis is a very serious, potentially life-threatening systemic inflammatory response to infection with a significantly high mortality rate. Sepsis involves a systemic inflammatory response to infectious organisms that suppresses the immune system, activates the coagulation process (reflected by prolonged prothrombin time and activated partial thromboplastin time, elevated D-dimer, and deficiency of protein C), and results in

P

cardiovascular insufficiency, and multiple organ failure. The incidence of sepsis in hospitals is especially high in noncardiac intensive care units.

Another patient population with a high risk of developing sepsis includes neonates in cases of early- and late-onset. Early-onset neonatal sepsis is also a significant concern. It occurs in the first 72 hr of life with 85% of cases presenting in the first 24 hr. Early-onset neonatal sepsis is the result of colonization of the neonate from the mother as it moves through the birth canal before delivery. The Centers for Disease Control and Prevention recommends universal screening for group B *Streptococcus* for all pregnant women at 35 to 37 weeks' gestation. Other organisms associated with early-onset neonatal sepsis include coagulase-negative *Staphylococcus, Escherichia coli, Haemophilus influenzae,* and *Listeria monocytogenes.*

Late-onset neonatal sepsis, during days 4 to 90, is acquired from the environment and has been associated with infection by *Acinetobacter, Candida,* coagulase-negative *Staphylococci, Enterobacter, E. coli,* group B *Streptococcus, Klebsiella, Pseudomonas, Serratia,* and *Staphylococcus aureus,* as well as some anaerobes.

Surviving sepsis depends on rapid, accurate identification, intervention, and management. The host inflammatory reaction was termed *systemic inflammatory response syndrome* (SIRS) by the American College of Chest Physicians and the Society of Critical Care Medicine in 1992. SIRS is defined by documented clinical evidence of bacterial infection (e.g., culture results) in the presence of two of four other criteria: temperature greater than 100.4°F or less than 96.8°F, heart rate greater than 90 beats/min, hyperventilation (greater than 20 breaths/minute or $Paco_2$ less than 32 mm Hg), or white blood cell (WBC) count greater than 12×10^3/microL or less than 4×10^3/microL. The SIRS criteria is sensitive in identifying people who show signs of infection or inflammation and who may be at risk for developing sepsis, but retrospective studies show the criteria lacks specificity. Lower specificity resulted in overidentification of patients "at risk for developing sepsis" and overconsumption of interventional resources. The criteria was reevaluated, and in 2001 diagnostic criteria for sepsis was developed to include the following:

- Evidence or diagnosis of infection in the presence of other factors
- General metabolic factors associated with sepsis (fever, hypothermia, increased heart rate, altered mental status, positive fluid imbalance, hyperglycemia not associated with diabetes)
- Inflammatory factors (elevated WBC count, bandemia, elevated CRP, elevated procalcitonin)
- Hemodynamic factors (arterial hypotension, elevated mixed venous oxygen saturation, elevated cardiac output/index)
- Organ/system dysfunction indicators (arterial hypoxemia, significant oliguria, elevated serum creatinine, abnormally elevated coagulation test levels, thrombocytopenia, elevated total bilirubin)
- Tissue perfusion factors (elevated lactate, hypotension *evidenced by decreased capillary refilling, e.g., skin mottling*)

In 2016, a revised description, with newer recommendations, was proposed for sepsis and septic shock. The criteria also include clinical guidelines to facilitate more rapid identification of patients at risk. As with any transition of paradigms, it is important to consider the established guidelines as long as the information remains applicable, accurate, and relevant, which is to say that the SIRS and 2001 criteria should not be eliminated from consideration while the new tools are used to collect additional data. The latest recommendations define sepsis as life-threatening organ dysfunction brought about when the body's normal regulatory response to infection is impaired. Septic shock is defined as a subset of sepsis in which the associated abnormalities place the patient at greater risk of death than from sepsis alone. The newest sepsis assessment tools include objective *measurements of parameters widely available* in health-care facilities and laboratories. Although blood cultures, lactate, and procalcitonin are valued studies, they have the liabilities of turnaround times that exceed the urgent timeframe needed for effective intervention. Also, these established markers are not available in all laboratories and point-of-care testing options are available in even fewer facilities. Research continues for more sensitive and specific biomarkers for sepsis and include assays for pancreatic stone protein, soluble CD14 (presepsin), the midregion precursor fragment of adrenomedullin (MR-pro-ADM), and heparin binding protein (HBP).

The Sequential (Sepsis-Related) Organ Failure Assessment (SOFA) score is a point system developed to provide an objective tool to assess organ failure. Points (0–4) are assigned for each measurement, representing an organ system. Organ dysfunction is determined by an increase in the SOFA score of 2 points or more when evaluated over a fairly limited period of time, that is, less than 24 hrs, using the worst values collected over time in comparison to the baseline values. A number of SOFA calculators are available on the Internet; some scoring methods use additional qualifiers such as vasopressor specific criteria, but the basic assessment covers multiple organs/systems using objective measurements to include the following:

- Respiratory system: Partial pressure of oxygen in arterial blood (P_{AO_2})
- Coagulation process: Platelet count
- Liver function: Total bilirubin
- Cardiovascular system: Mean arterial pressure
- Central nervous system/altered mental status: Glasgow Coma Scale score
- Kidney function: Creatinine (serum) or urine output

The bedside companion to SOFA is called the *Quick Sepsis-Related Organ Failure Assessment* (qSOFA). The qSOFA algorithm utilizes yes/no responses as well as numeric data to calculate a score based on the following:

- Patient location (ICU or outside ICU, e.g., emergency department or noncritical in-patient location; Y or N)
- Evidence of altered mentation (Y or N)

- Respiration rate in BPM (numeric value)
- Systolic blood pressure (numeric value)

INDICATIONS

- Assist in the diagnosis of bacteremia and septicemia.
- Assist in the differential diagnosis of bacterial versus viral meningitis.
- Assist in the differential diagnosis of community-acquired bacterial versus viral pneumonia.
- Monitor response to antibacterial therapy.

INTERFERING FACTORS: N/A

POTENTIAL MEDICAL DIAGNOSIS: CLINICAL SIGNIFICANCE OF RESULTS

Increased in

- Bacteremia or septicemia *(related to SIRS induced overproduction of procalcitonin)*
- Major surgery *(related to inflammation in the absence of sepsis)*
- Multiorgan failure *(related to inflammation in the absence of sepsis)*
- Neuroendocrine tumors (medullary thyroid cancer, small-cell lung cancer, and carcinoid tumors) *(related to procalcitonin-secreting tumor cells)*
- Severe burns *(related to inflammation in the absence of sepsis)*
- Severe trauma *(related to inflammation in the absence of sepsis)*

- Treatment with OKT3 antibodies (antibody used to protect a transplanted organ or graft from attack by T cells and subsequent rejection) and other drugs that stimulate the release of cytokines *(related to inflammatory response in the absence of sepsis)*

Decreased in: N/A

NURSING IMPLICATIONS

BEFORE THE STUDY: PLANNING AND IMPLEMENTATION

Teaching the Patient What to Expect
◗ Inform the patient this test can assist in assessing for infection and response to antibiotic treatment.
◗ Explain that a blood sample is needed for the test.

AFTER THE STUDY: POTENTIAL NURSING ACTIONS

Treatment Considerations
◗ Answer any questions or address any concerns voiced by the patient or family.

Follow-Up, Evaluation, and Desired Outcomes
◗ Understands that depending on the results of this procedure, additional testing may be performed to evaluate or monitor disease progression and determine the need for a change in therapy.

P

Progesterone

SYNONYM/ACRONYM: N/A

RATIONALE: To assess ovarian function, assist in fertility work-ups, and monitor placental function during pregnancy related to disorders such as tumor, cysts, and threatened abortion.

PATIENT PREPARATION: There are no food, fluid, activity, or medication restrictions unless by medical direction.

NORMAL FINDINGS: Method: Immunochemiluminometric assay (ICMA).

Hormonal State	Conventional Units	SI Units (Conventional Units × 3.18)
Prepubertal	Less than 1 ng/mL	Less than 3 nmol/L
Adult male	Less than 1 ng/mL	Less than 3 nmol/L
Adult female		
Follicular phase	Less than 1 ng/mL	Less than 3 nmol/L
Luteal phase	2–25 ng/mL	6.4–79.5 nmol/L
Pregnancy, first trimester	10–44 ng/mL	31.8–140 nmol/L
Pregnancy, second trimester	19.5–82.5 ng/mL	62–262.4 nmol/L
Pregnancy, third trimester	65–229 ng/mL	206.7–728.2 nmol/L
Postmenopausal period	Less than 1 ng/mL	Less than 3 nmol/L

CRITICAL FINDINGS AND POTENTIAL INTERVENTIONS: N/A

OVERVIEW: (Study type: Blood collected in a gold-, red-, or red/gray-top tube; related body system: Endocrine and Reproductive systems.) Progesterone is a female sex hormone. Its function is to prepare the uterus for pregnancy and the breasts for lactation. Progesterone testing can be used to confirm that ovulation has occurred and to assess the functioning of the corpus luteum. Serial measurements can be performed to help determine the day of ovulation.

INDICATIONS
- Assist in the diagnosis of luteal-phase defects (performed in conjunction with endometrial biopsy).
- Evaluate patients at risk for early or spontaneous abortion.
- Identify patients at risk for ectopic pregnancy and assessment of corpus luteum function.

- Monitor patients ovulating during the induction of human chorionic gonadotropin (HCG), human menopausal gonadotropin, follicle stimulating hormone/luteinizing hormone–releasing hormone, or clomiphene (serial measurements can assist in pinpointing the day of ovulation).
- Monitor patients receiving progesterone replacement therapy.

INTERFERING FACTORS
Factors that may alter the results of the study
- Drugs and other substances that may increase progesterone levels include clomiphene, corticotropin, hydroxyprogesterone, ketoconazole, mifepristone, progesterone, tamoxifen, and valproic acid.
- Drugs and other substances that may decrease progesterone levels include ampicillin, danazol, epostane, goserelin, and leuprolide.

P

POTENTIAL MEDICAL DIAGNOSIS: CLINICAL SIGNIFICANCE OF RESULTS

Increased in

- Chorioepithelioma of the ovary *(related to progesterone-secreting tumor)*
- Congenital adrenal hyperplasia *(related to excessive production of progesterone precursors)*
- Hydatidiform mole *(related to progesterone-secreting tumor)*
- Lipoid ovarian tumor *(related to progesterone-secreting tumor)*
- Ovulation *(related to normal production of progesterone)*
- Pregnancy *(related to normal production of progesterone)*
- Theca lutein cyst *(related to progesterone-secreting cyst)*

Decreased in

- Galactorrhea-amenorrhea syndrome *(progesterone is not produced in the absence of ovulation)*
- Primary or secondary hypogonadism *(related to diminished production of progesterone)*
- Short luteal-phase syndrome *(related to diminished time frame for production and secretion)*
- Threatened abortion, fetal demise, toxemia of pregnancy, pre-eclampsia, placental failure

(related to decreased production by threatened placenta)

NURSING IMPLICATIONS

BEFORE THE STUDY: PLANNING AND IMPLEMENTATION

Teaching the Patient What to Expect

- Inform the patient this test can assist in evaluating hormone level during pregnancy.
- Explain that a blood sample is needed for the test.

AFTER THE STUDY: POTENTIAL NURSING ACTIONS

Treatment Considerations

- Reinforce information given by the patient's health-care provider (HCP) regarding further testing, treatment, or referral to another HCP.
- Instruct the patient in the use of home pregnancy test kits approved by the U.S. Food and Drug Administration.
- Provide a nonjudgmental, nonthreatening atmosphere for exploring other options (e.g., adoption).
- Provide contact information for access to counseling services, as appropriate.

Follow-Up, Evaluation, and Desired Outcomes

- Understands the clinical implications of the study results and corresponding therapeutic interventions.

Prolactin

SYNONYM/ACRONYM: Luteotropic hormone, lactogenic hormone, lactogen, HPRL, PRL.

RATIONALE: To assess for lactation disorders and identify the presence of prolactin-secreting tumors to assist in diagnosing disorders such as lactation failure.

PATIENT PREPARATION: There are no fluid, activity, or medication restrictions unless by medical direction. Instruct the patient to fast for 12 hr before specimen collection because hyperglycemia can cause a short-term increase in prolactin levels. Specimen collection should occur between 0800 and 1000.

NORMAL FINDINGS: Method: Immunoassay.

Age	Conventional Units	SI Units (Conventional Units × 1)
Prepubertal males and females	3.2–20 ng/mL	3.2–20 mcg/L
Adult males	4–23 ng/mL	4–23 mcg/L
Adult females	4–30 ng/mL	4–30 mcg/L
Pregnant	5.3–215.3 ng/mL	5.3–215.3 mcg/L
Postmenopausal	2.4–24 ng/mL	2.4–24 mcg/L

CRITICAL FINDINGS AND POTENTIAL INTERVENTIONS: N/A

OVERVIEW: (**Study type:** Blood collected in a gold-, red-, or red/gray-top tube; **related body system:** Endocrine and Reproductive systems. Specimen should be tightly capped and transported in an ice slurry.) Prolactin is a hormone secreted by the pituitary gland. It is normally elevated in pregnant and lactating females. The main function of prolactin is to induce and sustain milk production in lactating females. Prolactin levels rise late in pregnancy, peak with the initiation of lactation, and surge each time a woman breastfeeds. Prolactin levels are highest at night during sleep and shortly after awakening. Levels are known to increase during periods of physical and emotional stress. Elevated prolactin levels are also known to affect fertility by inhibiting secretion of gonadotropin-releasing hormone from the hypothalamus, thereby also inhibiting secretion of luteinizing hormone and follicle-stimulating hormone from the pituitary gland and suppressing ovulation. Reduced fertility during lactation offers some natural protection against pregnancy. The function of prolactin in males and nonpregnant females is unknown, but there is an association between high levels and infertility.

INDICATIONS
- Assist in the diagnosis of primary hypothyroidism, as indicated by elevated levels.
- Assist in the diagnosis of suspected tumor involving the lungs or kidneys (elevated levels indicating ectopic prolactin production).
- Evaluate failure of lactation in the postpartum period.
- Evaluate sexual dysfunction of unknown cause in men and women.
- Evaluate suspected postpartum hypophyseal infarction (Sheehan syndrome), as indicated by decreased levels.

INTERFERING FACTORS
Factors that may alter the results of the study
- Drugs and other substances that may increase prolactin levels include amitriptyline, amoxapine, azosemide, benserazide,

P

butaperazine, butorphanol, carbidopa, chlorpromazine, cimetidine, clomipramine, desipramine, diethylstilbestrol, enalapril, enflurane, fenoldopam, flunarizine, fluphenazine, fluvoxamine, furosemide, growth hormone–releasing hormone, haloperidol, hexarelin, imipramine, insulin, interferon, labetalol, loxapine, megestrol, mestranol, methyldopa, metoclopramide, molindone, morphine, nitrous oxide, oral contraceptives, oxcarbazepine, parathyroid hormone, pentagastrin, perphenazine, phenytoin, pimozide, prochlorperazine, ranitidine, remoxipride, reserpine, sulpiride, sultopride, thiethylperazine, thioridazine, thiothixene, thyrotropin-releasing hormone, trifluoperazine, trimipramine, tumor necrosis factor, veralipride, verapamil, and zometapine.

- Drugs and other substances that may decrease prolactin levels include anticonvulsants, apomorphine, bromocriptine, cabergoline, calcitonin, cyclosporine, dexamethasone, D-Trp-6-LHRH, levodopa, metoclopramide, morphine, nifedipine, octreotide, pergolide, ranitidine, rifampin, ritanserin, ropinirole, secretin, and tamoxifen.
- Prolactin secretion is subject to diurnal variation with highest levels occurring in the morning.
- Episodic elevations can occur in response to sleep, stress, exercise, hypoglycemia, and breastfeeding.

POTENTIAL MEDICAL DIAGNOSIS: CLINICAL SIGNIFICANCE OF RESULTS

Increased in
- Adrenal insufficiency *(secondary to hypopituitarism)*
- Amenorrhea *(pathophysiology is unclear)*
- Anorexia nervosa *(pathophysiology is unclear)*
- Breastfeeding *(stimulates secretion of prolactin)*
- Chiari-Frommel and Argonz–Del Castillo syndromes *(endocrine disorders in which pituitary or hypothalamic tumors secrete excessive amounts of prolactin)*
- Chest wall injury *(trauma in this location can stimulate production of prolactin)*
- Chronic kidney disease *(related to decreased renal excretion)*
- Ectopic prolactin-secreting tumors (e.g., lung, kidney)
- Galactorrhea *(production of breast milk related to prolactin-secreting tumor)*
- Hypothalamic and pituitary disorders
- Hypothyroidism (primary) *(related to pituitary gland dysfunction)*
- Pituitary tumor
- Polycystic ovary (Stein-Leventhal) syndrome
- Pregnancy
- Shingles
- Stress *(stimulates secretion of prolactin)*
- Surgery (pituitary stalk section)

Decreased in
- Sheehan syndrome *(severe hemorrhage after obstetric delivery that causes pituitary infarct; secretion of all pituitary hormones is diminished)*

NURSING IMPLICATIONS

BEFORE THE STUDY: PLANNING AND IMPLEMENTATION

Teaching the Patient What to Expect
▶ Inform the patient that test can assist in evaluating breast feeding hormone level.

P

▶ Explain that a blood sample is needed for the test.

AFTER THE STUDY: POTENTIAL NURSING ACTIONS

Treatment Considerations
▶ Answer any questions or address any concerns voiced by the patient or family.

Follow-Up, Evaluation, and Desired Outcomes
▶ Understands that depending on the results of this procedure, additional testing may be performed to evaluate or monitor disease progression and determine the need for a change in therapy.

Prostate-Specific Antigen

SYNONYM/ACRONYM: PSA.

RATIONALE: To assess prostate health and assist in diagnosis of disorders such as prostate cancer, inflammation, and benign tumor and to evaluate effectiveness of medical and surgical therapeutic interventions.

PATIENT PREPARATION: There are no food, fluid, activity, or medication restrictions unless by medical direction.

NORMAL FINDINGS: Method: Immunoassay.

Conventional Units	SI Units (Conventional Units × 1)
Total PSA	
0–4 ng/mL	0–4 mcg/L

Some guidelines recommend a lower range: 0–2.5 ng/mL.

CRITICAL FINDINGS AND POTENTIAL INTERVENTIONS: N/A

OVERVIEW: (Study type: Blood collected in a gold-, red-, or red/gray-top tube; related body system: Immune, Reproductive, and Urinary systems.) Prostate-specific antigen (PSA) is produced exclusively by the epithelial cells of the prostate, periurethral, and perirectal glands. PSA testing may be used in conjunction with the digital rectal examination (DRE) and ultrasound for detection and monitoring cancer of the prostate. Risk of diagnosis is higher in men of African descent, who are 61% more likely than Caucasian men to develop prostate cancer. Family history and age at diagnosis are other strong correlating factors. PSA circulates in both free and bound (complexed) forms. A low ratio of free to complexed PSA (i.e., less than 10%) is suggestive of prostate cancer; a ratio of greater than 30% is rarely associated with prostate cancer. PSA velocity (PSAV), the rate of PSA increase over time, is being used to indicate the potential

P

aggressiveness of the cancer in order to identify the appropriate interventions and to monitor the effectiveness of treatment; at least three serial samples are required.

Prostate Cancer in Men With a Slightly Elevated Total PSA (Between 4 and 10 ng/mL)

Free PSA (%)	Probability of Developing Prostate Cancer
Greater than 30%	8%–20%
21%–30%	16%–19%
11%–20%	20%–25%
1%–10%	40%–50%
PSA velocity ng/mL	
Change of less than 0.75/yr	Low
Change of greater than 0.75/yr	Suspicious

Approximately 15% to 40% of patients who have had their prostate removed will encounter an increase in PSA. Patients treated for prostate cancer and who have had a PSA recurrence can still develop a metastasis for as long as 8 years after the postsurgical PSA level increased. The majority of prostate tumors develop slowly and require minimal intervention, but patients with an increase in PSA greater than 2 ng/mL in a year are more likely to have an aggressive form of prostate cancer with a greater risk of death.

The Prostate Health Index (PHI) is another multimarker strategy being used to improve the positive prediction rate of prostate cancer, especially when PSA levels are considered to be moderately increased (between 4–10 ng/mL). The PHI applies information provided by the results of prostate marker blood tests to a mathematical formula and offers additional information for clinical decision making. The three tests used in the formula are the total PSA, free PSA, and p2PSA (an isoform of PSA) where:

$$PHI = p2PSA/(free\ PSA \times total\ PSA)$$

PHI less than 27% have a relatively low probability for prostate cancer, PHI between 27% and 55% predict a moderate probability for prostate cancer, and PHI greater than 55% have an increased risk for prostate cancer.

The prostate cancer antigen 3 gene (PCA3) is a nucleic acid amplification test performed on a urine sample. The sample is collected after DRE because stimulation of the prostate releases a greater number of prostate cancer cells containing PCA3 into the urinary tract, where they can be collected and measured in the first-catch urine. PCA3 is overexpressed in prostate cancer but not in benign hypertrophy, which assists in determining the need for repeat biopsy in men 50 years of age or older who have had positive screening tests with one or more negative prostate biopsies.

Precision medicine provides a technology to predict the progression of prostate cancer, likelihood of recurrence, or development of related metastatic disease. New technology makes it possible to combine data such as analysis of molecular biomarkers and cellular structure specific to the individual's biopsy tissue, standard tissue biopsy results, Gleason score, number of positive tumor cores, tumor stage, presurgical and postsurgical PSA levels, and postsurgical margin status with computerized mathematical programs to create a personalized report that predicts the likelihood of post-prostatectomy disease progression. Serial measurements of PSA in the blood are often performed before and after surgery.

PSA is also produced in females, most notably in breast tissue. There is some evidence that elevated PSA levels in breast cancer patients are associated with positive estrogen and progesterone status.

Important Note: When following patients using serial testing, the same method of measurement should be consistently used.

INDICATIONS
• Evaluate the effectiveness of treatment for prostate cancer (prostatectomy): Levels decrease if treatment is effective; rising levels are associated with recurrence and a poor prognosis.
• Investigate or evaluate an enlarged prostate gland, especially if prostate cancer is suspected.
• Stage prostate cancer.

INTERFERING FACTORS
Factors that may alter the results of the study
• Drugs and other substances that decrease PSA levels include buserelin, dutasteride, finasteride, and flutamide.
• Increases may occur if ejaculation occurs within 24 hr prior to specimen collection. Increases can occur due to prostatic needle biopsy, cystoscopy, or prostatic infarction either by undergoing catheterization or the presence of an indwelling catheter; therefore, specimens should be collected prior to or

6 wk after the procedure. There is conflicting information regarding the effect of DRE on PSA values, and some health-care providers (HCPs) may specifically request specimen collection prior to DRE.

POTENTIAL MEDICAL DIAGNOSIS: CLINICAL SIGNIFICANCE OF RESULTS
Increased in
A breach in the protective barrier between the prostatic lumen and the bloodstream due to significant disease will allow measurable levels of circulating PSA.

• Benign prostatic hyperplasia
• Prostate cancer
• Prostatic infarct
• Prostatitis
• Urinary retention

Decreased in: N/A

NURSING IMPLICATIONS

BEFORE THE STUDY: PLANNING AND IMPLEMENTATION
Teaching the Patient What to Expect
▶ Inform the patient this test can assist in assessing prostate health.
▶ Explain that a blood sample is needed for the test.

AFTER THE STUDY: POTENTIAL NURSING ACTIONS
Treatment Considerations
▶ A diagnosis of cancer can be devastating and scary. Assess understanding of treatment options including radiation therapy, chemotherapy, and surgery.
▶ When the surgical option is chosen discuss postoperative infection risk, associated signs and symptoms, the possibility of postoperative incontinence and erectile dysfunction within the context of the clinical situation.
▶ A sense of powerlessness can be experienced by patients with a serious illness. Assess for feelings of hopelessness, depression, and apathy.

Encourage verbalization of feelings and assist in identifying strengths and development of coping strategies.

Nutritional Considerations

▶ There is growing evidence that inflammation and oxidation play key roles in the development of numerous diseases, including prostate cancer. Research also indicates that diets containing dried beans, fresh fruits and vegetables, nuts, spices, whole grains, and smaller amounts of red meats can increase the amount of protective antioxidants.

▶ Regular exercise in combination with a healthy diet can bring about changes in the body's metabolism that decrease inflammation and oxidation.

Follow-Up, Evaluation, and Desired Outcomes

General

▶ Understands that decisions regarding the need for and frequency of routine PSA testing or other cancer screening procedures should be made after consultation between the patient and HCP. Recommendations made by various medical associations and national health organizations regarding prostate cancer screening are moving away from routine PSA screening and toward informed decision making. Men who want to be screened should be tested with the PSA test in conjunction with DRE. Counsel the patient, as appropriate, that sexual dysfunction related to altered body function, drugs, or radiation may occur. Answer any questions or address any concerns voiced by the patient or family.

American Cancer Society (ACS) (www.cancer.org)

▶ The ACS's guidelines recommend that discussions about screening should begin at age 50 yr for men at average risk and whose life expectancy is 10 or more years, 45 yr for men at high risk (men of African descent and men with a first-degree relative who was diagnosed with prostate cancer at age 65 years or younger), and 40 yr for men at the highest risk of developing prostate cancer (men with multiple first-degree relatives who were

diagnosed with prostate cancer at age 65 yr or younger; first-degree relative is a father, brother, or son). The decision should be based on information about the limitations, risks, and potential benefits of PSA screening. If screening results do not indicate the presence of prostate cancer, future screenings may be recommended annually for men whose PSA is greater than 2.5 ng/mL and every 2 yr for men whose PSA is less than 2.5 ng/mL. Overall health status, age, ethnicity, and life expectancy are important variables when making decisions about screening and re-testing.

U.S. Preventive Services Task Force (USPSTF) (www.uspreventiveservicestaskforce.org)

▶ The USPSTF recommends against routine screening for healthy men in any age group. Their position is that the frequency of overdiagnosis and overtreatment outweighs the potential benefits. The USPSTF recommends that HCPs inform men between the ages of 55 and 69 yr about the potential limitations, risks, and potential benefits of PSA screening. The decision should be arrived at on a case-by-case basis that allows each patient to consider the information while incorporating his values and personal preferences. The USPSTF recommends against PSA screening for men age 70 yr and older.

American Urological Association (AUA) (www.auanet.org)

▶ The AUA recommends against screening for men under the age of 40 yr and does not recommend screening for men between 40 and 54 yr of age who have average risk.

▶ The AUA recommends that HCPs inform men between the ages of 55 and 69 yr about the potential limitations, risks, and potential benefits of PSA screening. The decision should be arrived at on an individualized basis, and rescreening be offered at a 2-yr interval instead of on an annual basis. The AUA recommends against routine screening after age 70 yr.

P

Protein, Blood, Total and Fractions

SYNONYM/ACRONYM: TP, SPEP (fractions include albumin, α_1-globulin, α_2-globulin, β-globulin, and γ-globulin).

RATIONALE: To assess nutritional status related to various disease and conditions such as dehydration, burns, and malabsorption.

PATIENT PREPARATION: There are no food, fluid, activity, or medication restrictions unless by medical direction.

NORMAL FINDINGS: Method: Spectrophotometry for total protein, electrophoresis for protein fractions.

Total Protein

Age	Conventional Units	SI Units (Conventional Units × 10)
Newborn–5 days	3.8–6.2 g/dL	38–62 g/L
1–3 yr	5.9–7 g/dL	59–70 g/L
4–6 yr	5.9–7.8 g/dL	59–78 g/L
7–9 yr	6.2–8.1 g/dL	62–81 g/L
10–19 yr	6.3–8.6 g/dL	63–86 g/L
Adult	6–8 g/dL	60–80 g/L

Values may be slightly decreased in older adults due to insufficient intake or the effects of medications and the presence of multiple chronic or acute diseases with or without muted symptoms.

Protein Fractions

	Conventional Units	SI Units (Conventional Units × 10)
Albumin	3.4–4.8 g/dL	34–48 g/L
α_1-Globulin	0.2–0.4 g/dL	2–4 g/L
α_2-Globulin	0.4–0.8 g/dL	4–8 g/L
β-Globulin	0.5–1 g/dL	5–10 g/L
γ-Globulin	0.6–1.2 g/dL	6–12 g/L

Values may be slightly decreased in older adults due to insufficient intake or the effects of medications and the presence of multiple chronic or acute diseases with or without muted symptoms.

CRITICAL FINDINGS AND POTENTIAL INTERVENTIONS: N/A

OVERVIEW: (Study type: Blood collected in a gold-, red-, or red/gray-top tube; related body system: Digestive and Immune systems.) Protein is essential to all physiological functions. Proteins consist of amino acids, the building blocks of blood and body tissues. Protein is also required for the regulation of metabolic processes, immunity, and proper water balance. Total protein includes albumin and globulins. Albumin, the protein present in the highest concentrations, is the main transport protein in the

P

body. Albumin also significantly affects plasma oncotic pressure, which regulates the distribution of body fluid between blood vessels, tissues, and cells. α_1-Globulin includes α_1-antitrypsin, α_1-fetoprotein, α_1-acidglycoprotein, α_1-antichymotrypsin, inter-α_1-trypsin inhibitor, high-density lipoproteins, and group-specific component (vitamin D–binding protein). α_2-Globulin includes haptoglobin, ceruloplasmin, and α_2-macroglobulin. β-Globulin includes transferrin, hemopexin, very-low-density lipoproteins, low-density lipoproteins, β_2-microglobulin, fibrinogen, complement, and C-reactive protein. γ-Globulin includes immunoglobulin (Ig) G, IgA, IgM, IgD, and IgE. After an acute infection or trauma, levels of many of the liver-derived proteins increase, whereas albumin level decreases; these conditions may not reflect an abnormal total protein determination.

INDICATIONS
- Evaluation of edema, as seen in patients with low total protein and low albumin levels.
- Evaluation of nutritional status.

INTERFERING FACTORS
Factors that may alter the results of the study
- Drugs and other substances that may increase protein levels include amino acids (if given by IV), anabolic steroids, angiotensin, anticonvulsants, corticosteroids, corticotropin, furosemide, insulin, isotretinoin, levonorgestrel, oral contraceptives, progesterone, radiographic medium, and thyroid drugs.
- Drugs and other substances that may decrease protein levels include acetylsalicylic acid, arginine, benzene, carvedilol, citrates, floxuridine, laxatives, mercury compounds, oral contraceptives, pyrazinamide, rifampin, trimethadione, and valproic acid.
- Values are significantly lower (5% to 10%) in recumbent patients.
- Hemolysis can falsely elevate results.
- Venous stasis can falsely elevate results; the tourniquet should not be left on the arm for longer than 60 sec.

POTENTIAL MEDICAL DIAGNOSIS: CLINICAL SIGNIFICANCE OF RESULTS
Increased in
- α_1-Globulin proteins in acute and chronic inflammatory diseases
- α_2-Globulin proteins occasionally in diabetes, pancreatitis, and hemolysis
- β-Globulin proteins in hyperlipoproteinemias and monoclonal gammopathies
- γ-Globulin proteins in chronic liver diseases, chronic infections, autoimmune disorders, hepatitis, cirrhosis, and lymphoproliferative disorders
- Total protein:
  Dehydration *(related to hemoconcentration)*
  Monoclonal and polyclonal gammopathies *(related to excessive γ-globulin protein synthesis)*
  Myeloma *(related to excessive γ-globulin protein synthesis)*
  Sarcoidosis *(related to excessive γ-globulin protein synthesis)*
  Some types of chronic liver disease
  Tropical diseases (e.g., leprosy) *(related to inflammatory reaction)*
  Waldenström macroglobulinemia *(related to excessive γ-globulin protein synthesis)*

Decreased in
- α_1-Globulin proteins in hereditary deficiency
- α_2-Globulin proteins in nephrotic syndrome, malignancies, numerous subacute and chronic inflammatory disorders, and recovery stage of severe burns

- β-Globulin proteins in hypo-β-lipoproteinemias and IgA deficiency
- γ-Globulin proteins in immune deficiency or suppression
- Total protein:
  Administration of IV fluids *(related to hemodilution)*
  Burns *(related to fluid retention, loss of albumin from chronic open burns)*
  Chronic alcohol misuse *(related to insufficient dietary intake; diminished protein synthesis by damaged liver)*
  Chronic ulcerative colitis *(related to poor intestinal absorption)*
  Cirrhosis *(related to damaged liver, which cannot synthesize adequate amount of protein)*
  Crohn disease *(related to poor intestinal absorption)*
  Glomerulonephritis *(related to alteration in permeability that results in excessive loss by kidneys)*
  Heart failure *(related to fluid retention)*
  Hyperthyroidism *(possibly related to increased metabolism and corresponding protein synthesis)*
  Malabsorption *(related to insufficient intestinal absorption)*
  Malnutrition *(related to insufficient intake)*
  Tumors
  Nephrotic syndrome *(related to alteration in permeability that results in excessive loss by kidneys)*
  Pregnancy *(related to fluid retention, dietary insufficiency, increased demands of growing fetus)*
  Prolonged immobilization *(related to fluid retention)*

Protein-losing enteropathies *(related to excessive loss)*
Severe skin disease
Starvation *(related to insufficient intake)*

NURSING IMPLICATIONS

BEFORE THE STUDY: PLANNING AND IMPLEMENTATION

Teaching the Patient What to Expect
- Inform the patient this test can assist in assessing nutritional status related to disease process.
- Explain that a blood sample is needed for the test.

AFTER THE STUDY: POTENTIAL NURSING ACTIONS

Nutritional Considerations
- Provide education on good dietary sources of complete protein (containing all eight essential amino acids) include meat, fish, eggs, and dairy products and that good sources of incomplete protein (lacking one or more of the eight essential amino acids) include grains, nuts, legumes, vegetables, and seeds.

Follow-Up, Evaluation, and Desired Outcomes
- Understands that depending on the results of this procedure, additional testing may be performed to evaluate or monitor disease progress and determine the need for a change in therapy.

Protein C

SYNONYM/ACRONYM: Protein C activity or protein C functional; protein C antigen.

RATIONALE: To assess coagulation function and assist in diagnosis of disorders such as thrombosis related to protein C deficiency.

PATIENT PREPARATION: There are no food, fluid, or activity restrictions unless by medical direction. Patients should discontinue warfarin therapy for 2 wk prior to specimen collection, as ordered. Specimen collection should not be performed sooner than 10 days following a thrombotic or clotting event.

NORMAL FINDINGS:

Protein C Activity or Functional Protein C (Method: Clot Detection)	Protein C Antigen (Method: Enzyme Immunoassay)
70%–170%	70%–140%

Values are significantly reduced in children because of liver immaturity. Levels rise to approximately 50% to 70% of adult levels by age 5 yr and reach adult levels by age 16 yr.

CRITICAL FINDINGS AND POTENTIAL INTERVENTIONS: N/A

OVERVIEW: (Study type: Blood collected in a completely filled blue-top [3.2% sodium citrate] tube; related body system: Circulatory/Hematopoietic system. If the patient's hematocrit exceeds 55%, the volume of citrate in the collection tube must be adjusted. *Important Note:* The collection tube should be completely filled. When multiple specimens are drawn, the blue-top tube should be collected after sterile (i.e., blood culture) tubes. Otherwise, when using a standard vacutainer system, the blue top is the first tube collected. When a butterfly is used, due to the added tubing, an extra red-top tube should be collected before the blue-top tube to ensure complete filling of the blue-top tube. The recommendation for processed and unprocessed samples stored in unopened tubes is that testing should be completed within 1 to 4 hr of collection.) Protein C is a vitamin K–dependent protein that originates in the liver and circulates in plasma as an enzyme precursor or inactive zymogen. Activated protein C (aPC) has a significant role in the process of coagulation. Protein C activation occurs on thrombomodulin receptors on the endothelial cell surface. Thrombin bound to thrombomodulin receptors preferentially activates protein C. Freely circulating thrombin mainly converts fibrinogen to fibrin. Other steps in the activation process of protein C require calcium and protein S cofactor binding (see "Protein S" and "Fibrinogen" studies). It also plays a role in anti-inflammatory and cytoprotective reactions mediated by receptor sites that appear to function independently from those involved in the coagulation process. aPC exhibits potent anticoagulant effects by degrading activated factors V and VIII, which affects the activation of other coagulation factors and ultimately disrupts the generation of thrombin. A deficiency of aPC disturbs the equilibrium between proteins that act as procoagulants and those that act as anticoagulants, tipping the balance to favor the development of blood clots or thromboses. Protein C deficiency can be an acquired or congenital condition. Acquired protein C deficiency is identified more frequently than the congenital condition and includes acute phase (systemic) reactions, antithrombin deficiency, DVT, DIC, liver disease, protein S deficiency, PE, sickle cell disease, and use of vitamin K antagonists. Congenital protein C deficiency is caused by mutations in the PROC gene, is usually transmitted as an autosomal dominant, and is the more common cause of a group of inherited thrombophilias, which include antithrombin deficiency, dysfibrinogenemia, factor V Leiden mutation, protein S deficiency, and prothrombin gene mutation. Activated protein C factor V Leiden is a genetic variant of factor V and is resistant to inactivation by protein C. Factor V Leiden is the most common inherited hypercoagulability disorder identified among individuals of Eurasian descent.

There are two types of inherited protein C deficiency. Identification of the subtype begins by screening for functional protein C activity; a decreased protein C activity or functional level is required to make the diagnosis of protein C deficiency. Decreased protein C activity results should be confirmed by repeat testing, and if confirmed an immunoassay for protein C antigen is usually reflexed to distinguish between type I and type II.

Type I: Quantitative protein C deficiency, that is, deficiency in both the plasma protein C antigen concentration and protein C functional activity

Type II: Functional protein C deficiency (less common than type I disease), that is, associated with decreased functional activity and normal levels of protein C

INDICATIONS
- Differentiate inherited deficiency from acquired deficiency.
- Investigate protein C deficiency as a possible cause for multiple miscarriages.
- Investigate the mechanism of idiopathic venous thrombosis, especially in the case of patients with a family history of blood clots or patients less than age 50 yr (including newborns being evaluated for possible clotting disorders, e.g., DIC, purpura fulminans).
- Screen relatives of patients with a known protein C deficiency.

INTERFERING FACTORS
Factors that may alter the results of the study
- Drugs and other substances that may increase protein C levels include desmopressin and oral contraceptives.
- Drugs and other substances that may decrease protein C levels include warfarin.
- Hematocrit greater than 55% may cause falsely prolonged results because of anticoagulant excess relative to plasma volume.
- Incompletely filled collection tubes, specimens contaminated with heparin, clotted specimens, or unprocessed specimens not delivered to the laboratory within 1 to 2 hr of collection should be rejected.
- Placement of the tourniquet for longer than 1 min can result in venous stasis and changes in the

P

concentration of the plasma proteins to be measured. Platelet activation may also occur under these conditions, resulting in erroneous measurements.

- Vascular injury during phlebotomy can activate platelets and coagulation factors, causing erroneous results.
- Hemolyzed specimens must be rejected because hemolysis is an indication of platelet and coagulation factor activation.
- Icteric or lipemic specimens interfere with optical testing methods, producing erroneous results.

POTENTIAL MEDICAL DIAGNOSIS: CLINICAL SIGNIFICANCE OF RESULTS
Increased in: N/A

Decreased in
- Congenital deficiency
- Disseminated intravascular coagulation *(related to increased consumption)*
- Liver disease *(related to decreased synthesis by the liver)*
- Oral anticoagulant therapy *(patients deficient in protein C may be at risk of developing warfarin-induced skin necrosis unless an immediate-acting anticoagulant like heparin is administered until therapeutic warfarin levels are achieved)*
- Septic shock *(related to increased consumption and decreased synthesis due to hepatic impairment)*
- Vitamin K deficiency *(related to production of dysfunctional protein in the absence of vitamin K)*

NURSING IMPLICATIONS

BEFORE THE STUDY: PLANNING AND IMPLEMENTATION

Teaching the Patient What to Expect
- Inform the patient this test can assist in assessing anticoagulant function.
- Explain that a blood sample is needed for the test.

Potential Nursing Actions
- Observe for symptoms of altered coagulation such as bruising, bleeding gums, or blood in urine, sputum, or stool.

AFTER THE STUDY: POTENTIAL NURSING ACTIONS

Treatment Considerations
- Discuss the implications of abnormal test results on the patient's lifestyle.
- Help those with bleeding disorders to understand the importance of taking precautions against bruising and bleeding.
- Provide education for precautions to include the use of a soft-bristle toothbrush, use of an electric razor, and avoidance of constipation, intramuscular injections, and acetylsalicylic acid (and similar products).

Safety Considerations
- Consider implementation of bleeding precautions for patients with coagulation disorders.

Follow-Up, Evaluation, and Desired Outcomes
- Understands that depending on the results of this procedure, additional testing may be performed to evaluate or monitor disease progress and determine the need for a change in therapy.

P

Protein S

SYNONYM/ACRONYM: Protein S antigen, protein S functional.

RATIONALE: To assess coagulation function, assist in the diagnosis of disorders such as venous thromboembolus (VTE) or disseminated intravascular coagulation (DIC).

PATIENT PREPARATION: There are no food, fluid, or activity restrictions unless by medical direction. Patients should discontinue warfarin therapy for 2 weeks prior to specimen collection, as ordered. Specimen collection should not be performed sooner than 10 days following a thrombotic event.

NORMAL FINDINGS:

Protein S Activity or Functional Protein S (Method: Clot Detection)	Protein S Total Antigen (Method: Enzyme Immunoassay)	Protein S Free Antigen (Method: Enzyme Immunoassay)
Male 70%–140%	Male 80%–130%	Male 70%–150%
Female 60%–130%	Female 60%–130%	Female 50%–120%

Note: Values are significantly reduced in children because of liver immaturity. Levels rise to approximately 50% to 70% of adult levels by age 5 yr and reach adult levels by age 16 yr.

CRITICAL FINDINGS AND POTENTIAL INTERVENTIONS: N/A

OVERVIEW: (Study type: Blood collected in a completely filled blue-top [3.2% sodium citrate] tube; **related body system:** Circulatory/Hematopoietic system. If the patient's hematocrit exceeds 55%, the volume of citrate in the collection tube must be adjusted. *Important Note:* The collection tube should be completely filled. When multiple specimens are drawn, the blue-top tube should be collected after sterile [i.e., blood culture] tubes. Otherwise, when using a standard vacutainer system, the blue top is the first tube collected. When a butterfly is used, due to the added tubing, an extra red-top tube should be collected before the blue-top tube to ensure complete filling of the blue-top tube. The recommendation for processed and unprocessed samples stored in unopened tubes is that testing should be completed within 1 to 4 hr of collection.) Protein S is a vitamin K–dependent protein that circulates in the plasma and is made by the liver, megakaryocytes, and endothelial cells. It is a cofactor required for the activation of protein C (see studies titled "Protein C" and "Fibrinogen"). Protein S exists in two forms: free (biologically active) and bound. Approximately 40% of protein S circulates in the free form; the remainder is bound and is functionally inactive. Protein S deficiency can be an acquired or congenital condition. Acquired protein S deficiency is usually due to hepatic disease or a vitamin K deficiency. Hereditary protein S deficiency is transmitted as an autosomal dominant trait.

There are three types of inherited protein S deficiency. Identification of the subtype begins with quantitation of total and free protein S antigen concentration; there are a number of conditions that produce misleading functional protein S levels; therefore, the free antigen assay is recommended for detection of protein S deficiency.

Type I: Quantitative protein S deficiency, that is, decreased total and free protein S antigen concentrations

Type II: Normal quantitative free and total protein S, but with decreased functional protein S activity (rare)

P

Type III: quantitative protein S deficiency, that is, decreased free protein S antigen concentration and normal total protein S antigen concentration

INDICATIONS
- Differentiate inherited deficiency from acquired deficiency.
- Investigate the cause of hypercoagulable states, especially in the case of patients with a family history of blood clots or patients less than age 50 years (including newborns being evaluated for possible clotting disorders, e.g., DIC, purpura fulminans, VTE).
- Screen relatives of patients with a known protein S deficiency.

Investigate the cause of hypercoagulable states.

INTERFERING FACTORS
Factors that may alter the results of the study
- Drugs and other substances that may decrease protein S levels include estrogen and warfarin.
- Placement of tourniquet for longer than 60 sec can result in venous stasis and changes in the concentration of plasma proteins to be measured. Platelet activation may also occur under these conditions, causing erroneous results.
- Vascular injury during phlebotomy can activate platelets and coagulation factors, causing erroneous results.
- Hemolyzed specimens must be rejected because hemolysis is an indication of platelet and coagulation factor activation.
- Icteric or lipemic specimens interfere with optical testing methods, producing erroneous results.
- Hematocrit greater than 55% may cause falsely prolonged results because of anticoagulant excess relative to plasma volume.
- Incompletely filled collection tubes, specimens contaminated with heparin, clotted specimens, or unprocessed specimens not delivered to the laboratory within 1 to 2 hr of collection should be rejected.

POTENTIAL MEDICAL DIAGNOSIS: CLINICAL SIGNIFICANCE OF RESULTS
Increased in: N/A

Decreased in
- Acute phase inflammatory reactions *(related to increased levels of C4b-binding protein in response to inflammation, which decrease levels of available functional protein)*
- Congenital deficiency
- DIC *(related to increased consumption)*
- Estrogen (replacement therapy, oral contraceptives, and pregnancy) *(elevated estrogen levels are associated with decreased protein levels; estrogen does not stimulate hypercoagulable states)*
- Kidney disease *(related to the chronic inflammation of impaired endothelial cells due to vascular damage)*
- Liver disease *(related to decreased synthesis by the liver)*
- Oral anticoagulant therapy
- Severe infections
- Vitamin K deficiency *(related to production of dysfunctional protein in the absence of vitamin K)*

NURSING IMPLICATIONS

BEFORE THE STUDY: PLANNING AND IMPLEMENTATION

Teaching the Patient What to Expect
- Inform the patient this test can assist in assessing anticoagulant function.
- Explain that a blood sample is needed for the test.

P

Potential Nursing Actions
♦ Observe for symptoms of altered coagulation such as bruising, bleeding gums, or blood in urine, sputum, or stool.

Treatment Considerations
♦ Discuss the implications of abnormal test results on the patient's lifestyle.
♦ Help those with bleeding disorders to understand the importance of taking precautions against bruising and bleeding.
♦ Provide education for precautions to include the use of a soft-bristle toothbrush, use of an electric razor, and avoidance of constipation, intramuscular injections, and acetylsalicylic acid (and similar products).

Safety Considerations
♦ Consider implementation of bleeding precautions for patients with coagulation disorders.

Follow-Up, Evaluation, and Desired Outcomes
♦ Understands that depending on the results of this procedure, additional testing may be performed to evaluate or monitor disease progress and determine the need for a change in therapy.

Protein, Urine, Total and Fractions

SYNONYM/ACRONYM: N/A

RATIONALE: To assess for the presence of protein in the urine toward diagnosing disorders affecting the kidneys and urinary tract, such as cancer, infection, and pre-eclampsia.

PATIENT PREPARATION: There are no food, fluid, activity, or medication restrictions unless by medical direction. Usually, a 24-hr time frame for urine collection is ordered. As appropriate, provide the required urine collection container and specimen collection instructions.

NORMAL FINDINGS: Method: Spectrophotometry for total protein, electrophoresis for protein fractions.

Normal 24-Hour Urine Volume

The ranges are very general averages and were not calculated on the basis of normal average body weights. Literature shows that the expected urinary output can be estimated by formula where the expected output is as follows: Infants: 1–2 mL/kg/hr Children and adolescents: 0.5–1 mL/kg/hr Adults: 1 mL/kg/hr	
Newborns	15–60 mL
Infants	
3–10 days	100–300 mL
11–59 days	250–450 mL
2–12 mo	400–500 mL

P

Children and adolescents

13 mo–4 yr	500–700 mL
5–7 yr	650–1,000 mL
8–14 yr	800–1,400 mL
Adults and older adults	800–2,500 mL (average 1,200 mL)

Normally, more urine is produced during the day than at night. With advancing age, the reverse will often occur. The total expected outcome for adults appears to remain the same regardless of age.

	Conventional Units	SI Units (Conventional Units × 0.001)
Total protein	30–150 mg/24 hr	0.03–0.15 g/24 hr
Second and third trimesters of pregnancy	45–185 mg/24 hr	0.045–0.185 g/24 hr

The 24-hr urine volume is recorded and provided with the results of the protein measurement. Electrophoresis for fractionation is qualitative: No monoclonal gammopathy detected. (Urine protein electrophoresis should be ordered along with serum protein electrophoresis.)

CRITICAL FINDINGS AND POTENTIAL INTERVENTIONS: N/A

OVERVIEW: (Study type: Urine from an unpreserved random or timed specimen collected in a clean plastic collection container; related body system: Urinary system.) Most proteins, with the exception of the immunoglobulins, are synthesized and catabolized in the liver, where they are broken down into amino acids. The amino acids are converted to ammonia and ketoacids. Ammonia is converted to urea via the urea cycle. Urea is excreted in the urine. Normally, proteins do not pass from the blood through the kidneys' filtration process into the urine. The presence of protein in the urine is a significant indication of kidney disease. The predominant causes of proteinuria are (1) lack of filtration due to damaged glomeruli and (2) a breakdown in the kidneys' tubular reabsorption process. Chronic conditions such as diabetes, hypertension, and sickle cell anemia cause incremental and potentially irreversible kidney damage. Acute conditions such as urinary tract infections and kidney stones can also damage the kidneys. Proteinuria can also be the result of extremely elevated serum protein levels, as seen with immunoglobulin-secreting malignancies such as multiple myeloma. The kappa and lambda light chain portions of the immunoglobulins, also known as *Bence Jones proteins,* are detected using electrophoresis techniques and are classic findings in conditions such as myeloma, Waldenström macroglobulinemia, and lymphoma.

INDICATIONS
- Assist in the detection of Bence Jones proteins (light chains).
- Assist in the diagnosis of myeloma, Waldenström macroglobulinemia, lymphoma, and amyloidosis.
- Evaluate kidney function.

INTERFERING FACTORS

Factors that may alter the results of the study

- Drugs and other substances that may increase urine protein levels include acetaminophen, aminosalicylic acid, amphotericin B, ampicillin, antimony compounds, antipyrine, arsenicals, ascorbic acid, bacitracin, bismuth subsalicylate, bromate, capreomycin, captopril, carbamazepine, carbarsone, cephaloglycin, cephaloridine, chlorpromazine, chlorpropamide, chlorthalidone, chrysarobin, colistimethate, colistin, corticosteroids, cyclosporine, demeclocycline, diatrizoic acid, dihydrotachysterol, doxycycline, enalapril, gentamicin, gold, hydrogen sulfide, iodopyracet, iopanoic acid, iophenoxic acid, ipodate, kanamycin, corn oil (Lipomul), lithium, mefenamic acid, melarsoprol, mercury compounds, methicillin, methylbromide, mezlocillin, mitomycin, nafcillin, naphthalene, neomycin, NSAIDs, oxacillin, paraldehyde, penicillamine, penicillin, phenolphthalein, phenols, phensuximide, piperacillin, plicamycin, polymyxin, probenecid, pyrazolones, radiographic medium, rifampin, sodium bicarbonate, streptokinase, sulfisoxazole, suramin, tetracyclines, thallium, thiosemicarbazones, tolbutamide, tolmetin, triethylenemelamine, and vitamin D.
- Drugs and other substances that may decrease urine protein levels include benazepril, captopril, cyclosporine, diltiazem, enalapril, fosinopril, interferon, lisinopril, losartan, lovastatin, prednisolone, prednisone, and quinapril.
- All urine voided for the timed collection period must be included in the collection, or else falsely decreased values may be obtained.

Compare output records with volume collected to verify that all voids were included in the collection.

POTENTIAL MEDICAL DIAGNOSIS: CLINICAL SIGNIFICANCE OF RESULTS

Increased in

- Diabetic nephropathy *(related to disease involving renal glomeruli, which increases permeability of protein)*
- Fanconi's syndrome *(related to abnormal protein deposits in the kidney, which can cause Fanconi syndrome)*
- Heavy metal poisoning *(related to disease involving renal glomeruli, which increases permeability of protein)*
- Malignancies of the urinary tract *(tumors secrete protein into the urine)*
- Monoclonal gammopathies *(evidenced by large amounts of Bence Jones protein light chains excreted in the urine)*
- Multiple myeloma *(evidenced by large amounts of Bence Jones protein light chains excreted in the urine)*
- Nephrotic syndrome *(related to disease involving renal glomeruli, which increases permeability of protein)*
- Postexercise period *(related to muscle exertion)*
- Pre-eclampsia *(numerous factors contribute to increased permeability of the kidneys to protein)*
- Sickle cell disease *(related to increased destruction of red blood cells and excretion of hemoglobin protein)*
- Urinary tract infections *(related to disease involving renal glomeruli, which increases permeability of protein)*

Decreased in: N/A

P

NURSING IMPLICATIONS

BEFORE THE STUDY: PLANNING AND IMPLEMENTATION

Teaching the Patient What to Expect
▶ Inform the patient this test can assist in assessing the cause of protein in the urine.
▶ Explain that a urine sample is needed for the test. Information regarding specimen collection is presented with other general guidelines in Appendix A: Patient Preparation and Specimen Collection.

Potential Nursing Actions
▶ Include on the collection container's label urine total volume, test start and stop times/dates, and any medications that may interfere with test results.

AFTER THE STUDY: POTENTIAL NURSING ACTIONS

Treatment Considerations
▶ Provide education related to the clinical implications of the test results.

Follow-Up, Evaluation, and Desired Outcomes
▶ Understands that depending on the results of this procedure, additional testing may be performed to evaluate or monitor disease progress and determine the need for a change in therapy.

Prothrombin Time and International Normalized Ratio

SYNONYM/ACRONYM: Protime, PT, and INR.

RATIONALE: To assess and monitor coagulation status related to therapeutic interventions and disorders such as vitamin K deficiency.

PATIENT PREPARATION: There are no food, fluid, activity, or medication restrictions unless by medical direction.

NORMAL FINDINGS: (Method: Clot detection) 10 to 13 sec.

- International normalized ratio (INR) = 0.9 to 1.1 for patients not receiving anticoagulation therapy.
- INR = 2 to 3 for patients receiving conventional anticoagulation therapy with warfarin.
- INR = 2.5 to 3.5 for patients receiving intensive anticoagulation therapy with warfarin.

CRITICAL FINDINGS AND POTENTIAL INTERVENTIONS

INR
- Greater than 5

Prothrombin Time
- Greater than 27 sec

Timely notification to the requesting health-care provider (HCP) of any critical findings and related symptoms is a role expectation of the professional nurse. A listing of these findings varies among facilities.

Consideration may be given to verification of critical findings before action is taken. Policies vary among facilities and may include requesting immediate recollection and retesting by the laboratory or retesting using a rapid point-of-care testing instrument at the bedside, if available.

Important signs to note relate to bleeding in specific areas of the body and include prolonged bleeding from cuts or gums, hematoma at a puncture site, hemorrhage, blood in the stool, backache or flank pain, dark-colored urine, joint pain, persistent epistaxis, heavy or prolonged menstrual flow, and shock. Monitor vital signs, unusual ecchymosis, occult blood, severe headache, unusual dizziness, and neurological changes until PT is within normal range. Intramuscular (IM) administration of vitamin K, an anticoagulant reversal drug, may be requested by the HCP.

OVERVIEW: (**Study type:** Blood collected in a completely filled blue-top [3.2% sodium citrate] tube; **related body system:** Circulatory/Hematopoietic system. If the patient's hematocrit exceeds 55%, the volume of citrate in the collection tube must be adjusted. *Important Note:* The collection tube should be completely filled. When multiple specimens are drawn, the blue-top tube should be collected after sterile [i.e., blood culture] tubes. Otherwise, when using a standard vacutainer system, the blue top is the first tube collected. When a butterfly is used, due to the added tubing, an extra red-top tube should be collected before the blue-top tube to ensure complete filling of the blue-top tube. The recommendation for processed and unprocessed samples stored in unopened tubes is that testing should be completed within 1 to 4 hr of collection.) PT is a coagulation test performed to measure the time it takes for a firm fibrin clot to form after tissue thromboplastin (factor III) and calcium are added to a sample of plasma. Coagulation factors in the patient's sample, including prothrombin (factor II) react with the reagents and complete the process of coagulation in proportion to the amount of available coagulation factors. The PT is used to evaluate the tissue factor pathway, formerly called the extrinsic pathway, of the coagulation sequence in patients receiving oral warfarin anticoagulants. Prothrombin is a vitamin K–dependent protein produced by the liver; measurement is reported as time in seconds or percentage of normal activity.

The goal of long-term anticoagulation therapy is to achieve a balance between in vivo thrombus formation and hemorrhage. It is a delicate clinical balance, and because of differences in instruments and reagents, there is a wide variation in PT results among laboratories. Worldwide concern for the need to provide more consistency in monitoring patients receiving anticoagulant therapy led to the development of an international committee. In the early 1980s, manufacturers of instruments and reagents began comparing their measurement systems with a single reference material provided by the World Health Organization (WHO). The international effort successfully developed an algorithm to provide comparable PT values regardless of differences in laboratory methodology. Reagent and instrument manufacturers compare their results to the WHO

P

reference and derive a factor called an *international sensitivity index* (ISI) that is applied to a mathematical formula to standardize the results. Laboratories convert their PT values into an INR by using the following formula:

$$INR = (patient\ PT\ result/normal\ patient\ average)^{(ISI)}$$

PT evaluation can now be based on an INR using a standardized thromboplastin reagent to assist in making decisions regarding oral anticoagulation therapy.

The metabolism of many commonly prescribed medications is driven by the cytochrome P450 (CYP450) family of enzymes. Genetic variants can alter enzymatic activity that results in a spectrum of effects ranging from the total absence of drug metabolism to ultrafast metabolism. Impaired drug metabolism can prevent the intended therapeutic effect or even lead to serious adverse drug reactions. Poor metabolizers are at increased risk for drug-induced adverse effects due to accumulation of drug in the blood, whereas ultra-rapid metabolizers require a higher-than-normal dosage because the drug is metabolized over a shorter duration than intended. In the case of prodrugs that require activation before metabolism, the opposite occurs: Poor metabolizers may require a higher dose because the activated drug is becoming available more slowly than intended, and ultra-rapid metabolizers may require less because the activated drug is becoming available sooner than intended. Other genetic phenotypes used to report CYP450 results are intermediate metabolizer and extensive metabolizer. Genetic testing can be performed on blood samples submitted to a laboratory. Test method commonly used is polymerase chain reaction. Counseling and informed written consent are generally required for genetic testing. CYP2C9 is a gene in the CYP450 family that metabolizes prodrugs like the anticoagulant warfarin. Three major gene mutations, CYP2CP*2, CYP2C9*3, and VKORC1, are associated with warfarin response and are estimated to account for up to 45% of variations in warfarin dose response. CYP450 testing is available and should be used in conjunction with other factors, including all prescription and over-the-counter medications being used; mode of drug administration; use of tobacco products, foods, and supplements; age, weight, environment, activity level, and diseases with which the patient may be dealing.

Some inferences of factor deficiency can be made by comparison of results obtained from the activated partial thromboplastin time (aPTT) and PT tests. A normal aPTT with a prolonged PT can occur only with factor VII deficiency. A prolonged aPTT with a normal PT could indicate a deficiency in factors XII, XI, IX, and VIII as well as VIII:C (von Willebrand factor). Factor deficiencies can also be identified by correction or substitution studies using normal serum. These studies are easy to perform and are accomplished by adding plasma from a healthy patient to a sample from a suspected factor-deficient patient. When the PT is repeated and corrected, or within the reference range, it can be assumed that the prolonged PT is due to a factor deficiency (see study titled

"Coagulation Factors"). If the result remains uncorrected, the prolonged PT is most likely due to a circulating anticoagulant.

INDICATIONS

- Differentiate between deficiencies of clotting factors II, V, VII, and X, which prolong the PT, and congenital coagulation disorders such as hemophilia A (factor VIII) and hemophilia B (factor IX), which do not alter the PT.
- Evaluate the response to anticoagulant therapy with warfarin derivatives and determine dosage required to achieve therapeutic results.
- Identify individuals who may be prone to bleeding during surgical, obstetric, dental, or invasive diagnostic procedures.
- Identify the possible cause of abnormal bleeding, such as epistaxis, hematoma, gingival bleeding, hematuria, and menorrhagia.
- Monitor the effects of conditions such as liver disease, protein deficiency, and fat malabsorption on hemostasis.
- Screen for prothrombin deficiency.
- Screen for vitamin K deficiency.

INTERFERING FACTORS

Factors that may alter the results of the study

- Drugs and other substances that may increase the PT in patients receiving anticoagulation therapy include acetaminophen, acetylsalicylic acid, amiodarone, anabolic steroids, anisindione, anistreplase, antibiotics, antipyrine, carbenicillin, cathartics, chloral hydrate, chlorthalidone, cholestyramine, clofibrate, corticotropin, demeclocycline, diazoxide, diflunisal, disulfiram, diuretics, doxycycline, erythromycin, ethyl alcohol, hydroxyzine, laxatives, mercaptopurine, miconazole, nalidixic acid, neomycin, niacin,

oxyphenbutazone, phenytoin, quinidine, quinine, thyroxine, and tosylate bretylium.

- Drugs and other substances that may decrease the PT in patients receiving anticoagulation therapy include amobarbital, anabolic steroids, antacids, antihistamines, barbiturates, carbamazepine, chloral hydrate, chlordane, chlordiazepoxide, cholestyramine, clofibrate, colchicine, corticosteroids, diuretics, oral contraceptives, penicillin, primidone, raloxifene, rifabutin, rifampin, simethicone, spironolactone, tacrolimus, tolbutamide, and vitamin K.
- Placement of the tourniquet for longer than 1 min can result in venous stasis and changes in the concentration of the plasma proteins to be measured. Platelet activation may also occur under these conditions, resulting in erroneous measurements.
- Traumatic venipunctures can activate the coagulation sequence by contaminating the sample with tissue thromboplastin and producing falsely shortened PT.
- Hematocrit greater than 55% may cause falsely prolonged results because of anticoagulant excess relative to plasma volume.
- Incompletely filled collection tubes, specimens contaminated with heparin, clotted or hemolyzed specimens, or unprocessed specimens not delivered to the laboratory within 24 hr of collection should be rejected.
- Excessive agitation causing sample hemolysis can falsely shorten the PT because the hemolyzed cells activate plasma-clotting factors.
- Hemolyzed specimens must be rejected because hemolysis is an indication of platelet and coagulation factor activation.
- Icteric or lipemic specimens interfere with optical testing methods, producing erroneous results.

P

POTENTIAL MEDICAL DIAGNOSIS: CLINICAL SIGNIFICANCE OF RESULTS

Increased in

- Afibrinogenemia, dysfibrinogenemia, or hypofibrinogenemia *(related to insufficient levels of fibrinogen, which is required for clotting; its absence prolongs PT)*
- Alcohol use *(related to decreased liver function, which results in decreased production of clotting factors and prolonged PT)*
- Biliary obstruction *(related to poor absorption of fat-soluble vitamin K; vitamin K is required for clotting and its absence prolongs PT)*
- Disseminated intravascular coagulation *(related to increased consumption of clotting factors; PT is increased)*
- Hereditary deficiencies of factors II, V, VII, and X *(related to deficiency of factors required for clotting; their absence prolongs PT)*
- Liver disease (cirrhosis) *(related to decreased liver function, which results in decreased production of clotting factors and prolonged PT)*
- Massive transfusion of packed red blood cells (RBCs) *(related to dilutional effect of replacing a significant fraction of the total blood volume; there are insufficient clotting factors in plasma-poor, packed RBC products. Blood products contain anticoagulants, which compound the lack of adequate clotting factors in the case of massive transfusion)*
- Poor fat absorption *(tropical sprue, celiac disease, and chronic diarrhea are conditions that prevent absorption of fat-soluble vitamins, including vitamin K, which is required for clotting; its absence prolongs PT)*
- Presence of circulating anticoagulant *(related to the production of inhibitors of specific factors, e.g., developed from long-term factor VIII therapy or circulating anticoagulants associated with conditions like tuberculosis, systemic lupus erythematosus, rheumatoid arthritis, and chronic glomerulonephritis)*
- Salicylate intoxication *(related to decreased liver function)*
- Vitamin K deficiency *(related to dietary deficiency or disorders of malabsorption; vitamin K is required for clotting; its absence prolongs PT)*

Decreased in

- Increased absorption of vitamin K *(related to dietary increases in fat, which enhances absorption of vitamin K, or increases of green leafy vegetables that contain large amounts of vitamin K)*
- Ovarian hyperfunction
- Regional enteritis or ileitis

P

NURSING IMPLICATIONS

POTENTIAL NURSING PROBLEMS: ASSESSMENT & NURSING DIAGNOSIS

Problems	Signs and Symptoms
Bleeding *(related to altered clotting factors secondary to warfarin use or depleted clotting factors)*	Altered level of consciousness; hypotension; increased heart rate; decreased Hgb and Hct; capillary refill greater than 3 sec; cool extremities; blood in urine, stool, sputum; bleeding gums; nosebleed; bruises easily

Problems	Signs and Symptoms
Gas exchange *(related to deficient oxygen capacity of the blood secondary to blood loss)*	Irregular breathing pattern, use of accessory muscles, altered chest excursion, adventitious breath sounds (crackles, rhonchi, wheezes, diminished breath sounds), copious secretions, signs of hypoxia, altered blood gas results, confusion, lethargy, cyanosis
Tissue perfusion *(related to decreased Hgb secondary to bleeding, altered clotting factors)*	Hypotension, dizziness, cool extremities, pallor, capillary refill greater than 3 sec in fingers and toes, weak pedal pulses, altered level of consciousness, altered sensation

BEFORE THE STUDY: PLANNING AND IMPLEMENTATION

Teaching the Patient What to Expect
▶ Inform the patient this test can assist in evaluating coagulation and monitor therapy.
▶ Explain that a blood sample is needed for the test.

Potential Nursing Actions
▶ Observe for symptoms of altered coagulation such as bruising, bleeding gums, or blood in urine, sputum, or stool.
▶ Investigate and document the patient's use of any over-the-counter medications, dietary supplements, anticoagulants, aspirin, and other salicylates, in addition to prescribed medications.

AFTER THE STUDY: POTENTIAL NURSING ACTIONS

Treatment Considerations
▶ Frequent monitoring of the PT/INR is important. Concern with monitoring is mostly involved with elevated values. However, decreased PT results can indicate a risk for thrombosis. There are three factors, known as the *Virchow triad,,* that increase the risk of developing a venous thrombus:
  ▶ Hypercoagulability, or a tendency for blood to coagulate at an abnormally rapid rate
  ▶ Venous stasis, or an impaired rate of blood flow through a vessel
  ▶ Vessel wall trauma or injury

Possible nursing interventions to decrease risk of thrombus include education for the patient regarding leg exercises, avoidance of constrictive clothing (e.g., stockings or tight socks), and avoidance of behaviors that might constrict blood flow, such as crossing of the legs or maintaining a dependent position for long periods of time.
▶ Bleeding: Monitor, trend, and increase the frequency of vital sign assessment noting variances in results. Administer ordered blood or blood products, vitamin K, and stool softener. Monitor and trend Hgb/Hct and PT/INR in relation to warfarin dosage. Assess skin for petechiae, purpura, or hematoma. Monitor for blood in emesis, sputum, urine or stool. Instruct the patient to report bleeding from any areas of the skin or mucous membranes. Institute bleeding precautions, prevent unnecessary venipuncture, avoid IM injections, prevent trauma, be gentle with oral care and suctioning, and avoid use of a sharp razor.
▶ Gas Exchange: Monitor respiratory rate and effort based on assessment the clinical condition. Assess lung sounds, work of breathing and oxygen saturation frequently. Monitor for bloody sputum and suction as necessary to maintain airway clearance. Administer ordered oxygen and monitor oxygen saturation with continuous pulse oximetry. Elevate the head of the bed 30 degrees or higher. Assess level of consciousness; anticipate the need for possible intubation.

P

◆ Tissue Perfusion: Monitor and trend blood pressure. Assess for dizziness, skin temperature, color, warmth, capillary refill, pedal pulses, numbness, tingling, hyperesthesia, or hypoesthesia. Monitor and trend PT and INR. Administer ordered blood or blood products, vitamin K, and intravenous fluids. Administer medication to support blood pressure as ordered.

Safety Considerations

◆ Consider implementation of bleeding precautions for patients with coagulation disorders.

Nutritional Considerations

◆ Foods high in vitamin K may alter PT/INR findings for patients on anticoagulant therapy if consumed in quantities that differ significantly (either more or less) from the normal dietary intake. Foods that contain vitamin K include asparagus, beans, cabbage, cauliflower, chickpeas, egg yolks, green tea, pork, liver, milk, soybean products, tomatoes, mayonnaise, vegetable oils, and green leafy vegetables such as leaf lettuce, watercress, parsley, broccoli, brussels sprouts, kale, spinach, swiss chard, and collard, mustard, and turnip greens.

Follow-Up, Evaluation, and Desired Outcomes

◆ Understands the importance of taking precautions against bruising and bleeding, including the use of a soft bristle toothbrush, use of an electric razor, avoidance of constipation, avoidance of aspirin products, and avoidance of IM injections with a prolonged PT/INR.

◆ Understands the importance of periodic laboratory testing while taking an anticoagulant.

◆ Acknowledges the importance of refraining from alcohol use while on warfarin because the combination of the two increases the risk of gastrointestinal bleeding.

Pseudocholinesterase and Dibucaine Number

SYNONYM/ACRONYM: CHS, PCHE, AcCHS.

RATIONALE: To assess for pseudocholinesterase deficiency to assist in diagnosing a congenital deficiency. Special attention must be given to results for preoperative patients because positive results indicate risk for apnea with use of succinylcholine as an anesthetic drug.

PATIENT PREPARATION: There are no food, fluid, activity, or medication restrictions unless by medical direction.

NORMAL FINDINGS: Method: Spectrophotometry, kinetic.

Test	Conventional Units
Pseudocholinesterase	
Males	3,334–7,031 units/L
Females	2,504–6,297 inits/L

Dibucaine Number	Fraction (%) of Activity Inhibited
Normal homozygote	79%–84%
Heterozygote	55%–70%
Abnormal homozygote	16%–28%

P

CRITICAL FINDINGS AND POTENTIAL INTERVENTIONS

• A positive result indicates that the patient is at risk for prolonged or unre-coverable apnea related to the inability to metabolize succinylcholine. Notify the anesthesiologist if the test result is positive and surgery is scheduled.

Timely notification to the requesting health-care provider (HCP) of any critical findings and related symptoms is a role expectation of the professional nurse. A listing of these findings varies among facilities.

OVERVIEW: (Study type: Blood collected in a red-, or lavender-top [EDTA] tube; related body system: Digestive and Musculo-skeletal systems.) There are two types of cholinesterase: *acetylcho-linesterase* (AChE), or "true cholin-esterase," which is found in red blood cells, lung tissue, and brain (nerve) tissue (see study titled "Red Blood Cell Cholinesterase"); and *pseudocholinesterase,* which is found mainly in the plasma, liver, and heart. Pseudocholines-terase is a nonspecific enzyme that hydrolyzes acetylcholine and noncholine esters. Carbamate and organophosphate insecticides (e.g., parathion, malathion) inhibit its activity.

Patients with inherited pseudocholinesterase deficiency are at risk during administration of anesthesia if succinylcholine is administered as an anesthetic. Succinylcholine, a short-acting muscle relaxant, is a revers-ible inhibitor of acetylcholin-esterase and is hydrolyzed by cholinesterase. Succinylcholine-sensitive patients may be unable to metabolize the anesthetic quickly, resulting in prolonged or unrecoverable apnea. Abnormal genotypes of pseudocholines-terase are detected using the dibucaine and fluoride inhibition tests because, in normal indi-viduals, these chemicals inhibit pseudocholinesterase activity. The prevalence of succinylcho-line sensitivity is 1 in 2,000 to 4,000 homozygote and 1 in 500 heterozygote patients. There are more than 15 identified phe-notypes; A, AS, S1, S2, F, AF, and FS are associated with prolonged apnea following the use of succi-nylcholine. Widespread preop-erative screening is not routinely performed.

INDICATIONS

• Assist in the evaluation of liver function.
• Screen for abnormal genotypes of pseudocholinesterase in patients with a family history of succi-nylcholine sensitivity who are about to undergo anesthesia using succinylcholine.

INTERFERING FACTORS

Factors that may alter the results of the study

• Drugs and other substances that may decrease pseudocholinester-ase levels include ambenonium, bambuterol, barbiturates, chlor-promazine, cyclophosphamide, echothiophate, edrophonium, esmolol, estrogens, fluorides, glucocorticoids, hexafluorenium, ibuprofen, iodipamide (contrast medium), iopanoic acid (con-trast medium), isoflurophate, metoclopramide, monoamine oxidase inhibitors, neostigmine, pancuronium, parathion, phen-elzine, physostigmine, procain-amide, pyridostigmine, and oral contraceptives.
• Drugs and other substances that may increase pseudocholinesterase

P

levels include carbamazepine, phenytoin, and valproic acid.

- Plasmapheresis decreases pseudocholinesterase levels.
- Pregnancy decreases pseudocholinesterase levels by about 30%.
- Improper anticoagulant; fluoride interferes with the measurement and causes a falsely decreased value.

POTENTIAL MEDICAL DIAGNOSIS: CLINICAL SIGNIFICANCE OF RESULTS

Increased in

Increased levels are observed in a number of conditions without specific cause.

- Diabetes
- Hyperthyroidism
- Nephrotic syndrome
- Obesity

Decreased in

The enzyme is produced in the liver, and any condition affecting liver function may result in decreased production of circulating enzyme.

- Acute infection
- Anemia (severe)
- Carcinomatosis
- Cirrhosis
- Congenital deficiency
- Hepatic cancer
- Hepatocellular disease
- Infectious hepatitis
- Insecticide exposure *(organic phosphate exposure decreases enzyme activity)*
- Malnutrition *(possibly related to decreased availability of transport proteins; condition associated with decreased enzyme activity)*
- Muscular dystrophy
- Myocardial infarction
- Plasmapheresis *(iatrogenic cause)*
- Succinylcholine hypersensitivity *(this chemical is a trigger in susceptible individuals)*

- Tuberculosis *(chronic infection is known to decrease enzyme activity)*
- Uremia *(pathological condition known to decrease enzyme activity)*

NURSING IMPLICATIONS

BEFORE THE STUDY: PLANNING AND IMPLEMENTATION

Teaching the Patient What to Expect
- Inform the patient this test can assist in evaluating for enzyme deficiency.
- Explain that a blood sample is needed for the test.

Potential Nursing Actions
- Discuss health concerns related to pseudocholinesterase deficiency, especially exposure to pesticides causing symptoms including blurred vision, muscle weakness, nausea, vomiting, headaches, pulmonary edema, salivation, sweating, or convulsions.

AFTER THE STUDY: POTENTIAL NURSING ACTIONS

Treatment Considerations
- Provide support for concerns related to impaired activity secondary to weakness and fear of shortened life expectancy.
- Discuss the implications of abnormal test results on the patient's lifestyle.
- Provide education related to the clinical implications of the test results.

Follow-Up, Evaluation, and Desired Outcomes
- Acknowledges contact information provided regarding genetic counseling services and screening tests for other family members.
- Understands the value of using a medic alert bracelet to notify health-care workers of increased risk from exposure to medications that may lower pseudocholinesterase activity.

P

Pulmonary Function Studies

SYNONYM/ACRONYM: Pulmonary function tests (PFTs).

RATIONALE: To assess respiratory function to assist in evaluating obstructive versus restrictive lung disease and to monitor and assess the effectiveness of therapeutic interventions.

PATIENT PREPARATION: There are no fluid restrictions unless by medical direction. Instruct the patient to refrain from smoking tobacco or eating a heavy meal for 4 to 6 hr prior to the study. Protocols may vary among facilities. Instruct the patient to avoid bronchodilators (oral or inhalant) for at least 4 hr before the study, as directed by the health-care provider (HCP).

NORMAL FINDINGS
• Normal respiratory volume and capacities, gas diffusion, and distribution
• No evidence of chronic obstructive pulmonary disease (COPD) or restrictive pulmonary disease

CRITICAL FINDINGS AND POTENTIAL INTERVENTIONS
• Hypoxia occurs at oxygen saturation levels less than 90%. Significant hypoxia, levels less than 85%, require immediate evaluation and treatment.

Timely notification to the requesting HCP of any critical findings and related symptoms is a role expectation of the professional nurse. A listing of these findings varies among facilities.

OVERVIEW: (Study type: Pulmonary function tests; related body system: Respiratory system.) Pulmonary function studies provide information about the volume, pattern, and rates of airflow involved in respiratory function. These studies may also include tests involving the diffusing capabilities of the lungs (i.e., volume of gases diffusing across a membrane). A complete pulmonary function study includes the determination of all lung volumes, spirometry, diffusing capacity, maximum voluntary ventilation, flow-volume loop, and maximum expiratory and inspiratory pressures. (See Figure 1 showing lung volumes measured during PFT.) Other studies include assessment of small airway volumes.

The studies are conducted using a mechanical device called a *spirometer.* The amount of gas breathed in and out by the patient is measured and converted into a series of electrical signals that are displayed in a *spirogram.*

Pulmonary function studies are classified according to lung volumes and capacities, rates of flow, and gas exchange. The exception is the diffusion test, which records the movement of a gas during inspiration and expiration. Lung volumes and capacities constitute the amount of air inhaled or exhaled from the lungs; this value is compared to normal reference values specific for the patient's age, height, and gender. The following are volumes and capacities measured by spirometry that do not require timed testing.

P

Tidal volume (TV)	Total amount of air inhaled and exhaled with one breath
Residual volume (RV)	Amount of air remaining in the lungs after a maximum expiration effort; this indirect type of measurement can be done by body plethysmography (see study titled "Plethysmography")
Inspiratory reserve volume (IRV)	Maximum amount of air inhaled at the point of maximum expiration
Expiratory reserve volume (ERV)	Maximum amount of air exhaled after a resting expiration; can be calculated by the VC minus the IC
Vital capacity (VC)	Maximum amount of air exhaled after a maximum inspiration (can be calculated by adding the IC and the ERV)
Total lung capacity (TLC)	Total amount of air that the lungs can hold after maximum inspiration; can be calculated by adding the VC and the RV
Inspiratory capacity (IC)	Maximum amount of air inspired after normal expiration; can be calculated by adding the IRV and the TV
Functional residual capacity (FRC)	Volume of air that remains in the lungs after normal expiration can be calculated by adding the RV and ERV

The volumes, capacities, and rates of flow measured by spirometry that do require timed testing include the following:

Forced vital capacity (FVC)	Maximum amount of air that can be forcefully exhaled after a full inspiration
Forced expiratory volume (FEV1)	Amount of air that can be forcefully exhaled in the first second after a full inspiration (can also be determined at 2 or 3 sec)
Maximal midexpiratory flow (MMEF)	Also known as *forced expiratory flow rate* (FEF_{25-75}), or the maximal rate of airflow during a forced expiration
Forced inspiratory flow rate (FIF)	Volume inspired from the RV at a point of measurement (can be expressed as a percentage to identify the corresponding volume pressure and inspired volume)
Peak inspiratory flow rate (PIFR)	Maximum airflow during a forced maximal inspiration
Peak expiratory flow rate (PEFR)	Maximum airflow expired during FVC
Flow-volume loops (F-V)	Flows and volumes recorded during forced expiratory volume and forced inspiratory VC procedures
Maximal inspiratory-expiratory pressures	Strengths of the respiratory muscles in neuromuscular disorders
Maximal voluntary ventilation (MVV)	Maximal volume of air inspired and expired in 1 min (may be done for shorter periods and multiplied to equal 1 min)

P

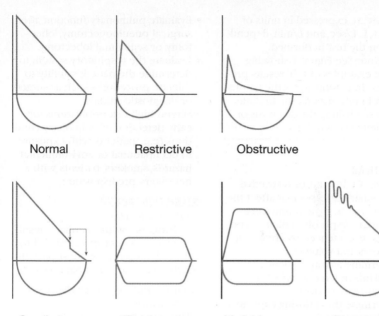

Figure 1 Examples of PFT results presented in graphic form.

Other studies for gas-exchange capacity, small airway abnormalities, and allergic responses in hyperactive airway disorders can be performed during the conventional pulmonary function study. These include the following:

Diffusing capacity of the lungs (DL)	Rate of transfer of carbon monoxide through the alveolar and capillary membrane in 1 min
Closing volume (CV)	Measure of the closure of small airways in the lower alveoli by monitoring volume and percentage of alveolar nitrogen after inhalation of 100% oxygen
Isoflow volume (isoV)	Flow-volume loop test followed by inhalation of a mixture of helium and oxygen to determine small airway disease
Body plethysmography	Measure of thoracic gas volume and airway resistance
Bronchial provocation	Quantification of airway response after inhalation of methacholine
Arterial blood gases (ABGs)	Measure of oxygen, pH, and carbon dioxide in arterial blood

P

Values are expressed in units of mL, %, L, L/sec, and L/min, depending on the test performed.

Note: See Figure 1 showing some examples of PFT results presented in graphic form; the graphs assist in interpreting the findings and establishing the diagnosis of respiratory conditions.

INDICATIONS

- Detect COPD and/or restrictive pulmonary diseases that affect the chest wall (e.g., neuromuscular disorders, kyphosis, scoliosis) and lungs, as evidenced by abnormal airflows and volumes.
- Determine airway response to inhalants in patients with an airway-reactive disorder.
- Determine the diffusing capacity of the lungs (DCOL).
- Determine the effectiveness of therapy regimens, such as bronchodilators, for pulmonary disorders.
- Determine the presence of lung disease when other studies, such as x-rays, do not provide a definitive diagnosis, or determine the progression and severity of known COPD and restrictive pulmonary disease.
- Evaluate the cause of dyspnea occurring with or without exercise.
- Evaluate lung compliance to determine changes in elasticity, as evidenced by changes in lung volumes (decreased in restrictive pulmonary disease, increased in COPD and in older adult patients).
- Evaluate pulmonary disability for legal or insurance claims.

- Evaluate pulmonary function after surgical pneumonectomy, lobectomy, or segmental lobectomy.
- Evaluate the respiratory system to determine the patient's ability to tolerate procedures such as surgery or diagnostic studies.
- Screen high-risk populations for early detection of pulmonary conditions (e.g., patients with exposure to occupational or environmental hazards, smokers, patients with a hereditary predisposition).

INTERFERING FACTORS

Contraindications

Patients with cardiac insufficiency, recent myocardial infarction, and presence of chest pain that affects inspiration or expiration ability.

Factors that may alter the results of the study

- The aging process can cause decreased values (FVC, DCOL) depending on the study done.
- Inability of the patient to put forth the necessary breathing effort affects the results.
- Medications such as bronchodilators can affect results.
- Improper placement of the nose clamp or mouthpiece that allows for leakage can affect volume results.

Other considerations

- Exercise caution with patients who have upper respiratory infections, such as a cold or acute bronchitis.

POTENTIAL MEDICAL DIAGNOSIS: CLINICAL SIGNIFICANCE OF RESULTS

Normal adult lung volumes, capacities, and flow rates are as follows:

TV	500 mL at rest
RV	1,200 mL (approximate)
IRV	3,000 mL (approximate)
ERV	1,100 mL (approximate)

P

VC	4,600 mL (approximate)
TLC	5,800 mL (approximate)
IC	3,500 mL (approximate)
FRC	2,300 mL (approximate)
FVC	3,000–5,000 mL (approximate)
FEV$_1$/FVC	81%–83%
MMEF	25%–75%
FIF	25%–75%
MVV	25%–35% or 170 L/min
PIFR	300 L/min
PEFR	450 L/min
F-V loop	Normal curve
DCOL	25 mL/min per mm Hg (approximate)
CV	10%–20% of VC
V$_{iso}$	Based on age formula
Bronchial provocation	No change, or less than 20% reduction in FEV$_1$

Note: Normal values listed are estimated values for adults. Actual pediatric and adult values are based on age, height, and gender. These normal values are included on the patient's pulmonary function laboratory report.

CV = closing volume; DCOL = diffusing capacity of the lungs; ERV = expiratory reserve volume; FEV$_1$ = forced expiratory volume in 1 sec; FIF = forced inspiratory flow rate; FRC = functional residual capacity; FVC = forced vital capacity; F-V loop = flow-volume loop; IC = inspiratory capacity; IRV = inspiratory reserve volume; MMEF = maximal midexpiratory flow (also known as FEF$_{25-75}$); MVV = maximal voluntary ventilation; PEFR = peak expiratory flow rate; PIFR = peak inspiratory flow rate; RV = residual volume; TLC = total lung capacity; TV = tidal volume; VC = vital capacity; V$_{iso}$ = isoflow volume. (See Figure 2.)

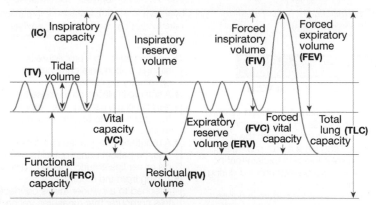

Figure 2 Showing lung volumes measured during PFT.

Abnormal findings related to
- Allergy
- Asbestosis
- Asthma

- Bronchiectasis
- Chest trauma
- COPD
- Curvature of the spine

- Myasthenia gravis
- Obesity
- Pulmonary fibrosis

- Pulmonary tumors
- Respiratory infections
- Sarcoidosis

NURSING IMPLICATIONS

POTENTIAL NURSING PROBLEMS: ASSESSMENT & NURSING DIAGNOSIS

Problems	Signs and Symptoms
Activity (related to ineffective oxygenation secondary to obstruction, infection, inflammation, ineffective cardiac function)	Weakness, fatigue, chest pain with exertion, anxiety, shortness of breath, cyanosis, decreasing oxygen saturation, increased heart rate
Breathing (related to obstruction, infection, inflammation, ineffective cardiac function, fear, anxiety, chest pain, lack of oxygen)	Shortness of breath; skin that is cool, clammy, and cyanotic; anxiety; pleuritic chest pain; decreased oxygenation; abnormal blood gas; increased work of breathing (use of accessory muscles); increased respiratory rate
Inadequate gas exchange (related to obstruction, e.g., obstructed pulmonary artery secondary to embolus; infection; inflammation; ineffective cardiac function)	Difficulty breathing, shortness of breath (dyspnea), chest pain (pleuritic), diminished oxygenation, cyanosis, increased heart rate, increased respiratory rate, restlessness, anxiety, fear, adventitious breath sounds (rales, crackles), sense of impending death and doom, hemoptysis, abnormal ABG
Pain (related to obstruction and ischemic tissue)	Chest pain (pleuritic), increased respiratory rate, increased heart rate, fear, anxiety

BEFORE THE STUDY: PLANNING AND IMPLEMENTATION

Teaching the Patient What to Expect

▶ Inform the patient this procedure can assist in assessing lung function.
▶ Review the procedure with the patient. Address concerns about pain related to the procedure and explain that no discomfort will be experienced during the test.
▶ Explain that the procedure is generally performed in a specially equipped room or in an office by a HCP specializing in this procedure and usually lasts 1 hr.
▶ An inhalant bronchodilator will be obtained to treat any bronchospasms that may occur with testing.

▶ Positioning for this procedure is in a sitting position on a chair near the spirometry equipment.
▶ A soft clip is placed on the nose to restrict nose breathing. The patient is then instructed to breathe through the mouth.
▶ A mouthpiece is placed in the mouth, and the patient is instructed to place his or her lips around it to form a seal.
▶ Tubing from the mouthpiece is attached to a cylinder that is connected to a computer that measures, records, and calculates the values for the tests done.
▶ Explain to the patient that he or she will be instructed to inhale deeply and then to quickly exhale as much air as possible into the mouthpiece.

P

▶ Additional breathing maneuvers are performed on inspiration and expiration (normal, forced, and breath-holding).

Safety Considerations

▶ Assess the patient for dizziness or weakness after the testing.

AFTER THE STUDY: POTENTIAL NURSING ACTIONS

Treatment Considerations

▶ Allow the patient to rest as long as needed to recover.

▶ Instruct the patient to resume usual diet and medications, as directed by the HCP.

▶ Activity: Activity becomes problematic when breathing is compromised. Identify normal activity patterns and enforce activity restrictions as necessary to rest the heart and conserve oxygen. Administer ordered oxygen and explain the importance of wearing oxygen with activity. Pacing activity can be useful in improving activity tolerance. Monitor and trend vital signs. Consider discussing the effects of altered cardiopulmonary status on sexual activity.

▶ Breathing: Assess and trend breath sounds, respiratory rate, and work of breathing. Elevate the head of the bed to improve ventilatory effort. Limit activity, administer ordered analgesics and oxygen, encourage cough and deep breathing, and prepare for intubation.

▶ Inadequate Gas Exchange: Assess respiratory status to establish baseline rate, rhythm, and depth. Assess for cyanosis and work of breathing. Monitor and trend ABG results; administer ordered oxygen and use pulse oximetry to monitor oxygenation. Administer ordered anticoagulants, antibiotics, bronchodilators, steroids, thrombolytic, and diuretics. Institute bleeding precautions; limit activity to support positive gas exchange. Monitor and trend for results of D-dimer test, international normalized ratio, and activated partial thromboplastin time.

▶ Pain: Assess pain character, location, duration, and intensity using an easily understood pain rating scale. Place in a position of comfort. Administer ordered oxygen, analgesics, anticoagulants or thrombolytics. Consider alternative measures for pain management (imagery, relaxation, music, etc.).

Follow-Up, Evaluation, and Desired Outcomes

▶ Understands that depending on the results of this procedure, additional testing may be performed to evaluate or monitor disease progression and determine the need for a change in therapy.

▶ Acknowledges information provided for smoking cessation, as appropriate.

Pulse Oximetry

P

SYNONYM/ACRONYM: Oximetry, pulse ox.

RATIONALE: To assess arterial blood oxygenation toward evaluating respiratory status during ventilation, acute illness, activity, and sleep and to evaluate the effectiveness of therapeutic interventions.

PATIENT PREPARATION: There are no food, fluid, or medication restrictions unless by medical direction.

NORMAL FINDINGS

• Greater than or equal to 95% (values may be at the lower end of the normal range in older adults).

CRITICAL FINDINGS AND POTENTIAL INTERVENTIONS

- Hypoxia occurs at oxygen saturation levels less than 90%. Significant hypoxia, levels less than 85%, require immediate evaluation and treatment.

Timely notification to the requesting health-care provider (HCP) of any critical findings and related symptoms is a role expectation of the professional nurse. A listing of these findings varies among facilities.

OVERVIEW: (Study type: Pulmonary function tests; related body system: Respiratory system.) Pulse oximetry is a noninvasive study that provides continuous readings of arterial blood oxygen saturation (SpO_2) using a sensor site (earlobe or fingertip). The SpO_2 equals the ratio of the amount of O_2 contained in the hemoglobin (Hgb) to the maximum amount of O_2 contained, with Hgb expressed as a percentage. The results obtained may compare favorably with O_2 saturation levels obtained by arterial blood gas analysis without the need to perform successive arterial punctures. The device used is a clip or probe that produces a light beam with two different wavelengths on one side. A sensor on the opposite side measures the absorption of each of the wavelengths of light to determine the O_2 saturation reading. The displayed result is a ratio, expressed as a percentage, between the actual O_2 content of the Hgb and the potential maximum O_2-carrying capacity of the Hgb.

INDICATIONS

- Determine the effectiveness of pulmonary gas exchange function.

- Evaluate suspected nocturnal hypoxemia in chronic obstructive pulmonary disease.
- Monitor oxygenation during testing for sleep apnea.
- Monitor oxygenation perioperatively and during acute illnesses.
- Monitor oxygenation status in patients on a ventilator, during surgery, and during bronchoscopy.
- Monitor O_2 saturation during activities such as pulmonary exercise stress testing or pulmonary rehabilitation exercises to determine optimal tolerance.
- Monitor response to pulmonary drug regimens, especially flow and O_2 content.

INTERFERING FACTORS

Factors that may alter the results of the study

- Patients who smoke or have experienced carbon monoxide inhalation, because O_2 levels may be falsely elevated.
- Patients with anemic conditions reflecting a reduction in hemoglobin, the O_2-carrying component in the blood.
- Excessive ambient light surrounding the patient, such as from surgical lights, interferes with accurate readings.
- Impaired cardiopulmonary function.
- Lipid emulsion therapy and presence of certain dyes.

P

- Movement of the finger or ear or improper placement of probe or clip.
- Nail polish, artificial fingernails, and skin pigmentation when a finger probe is used.
- Vasoconstriction from cool skin temperature, drugs, hypotension, or vessel obstruction causing a decrease in blood flow.

Other considerations
- Accuracy for most units is plus or minus 2% to 3%.

POTENTIAL MEDICAL DIAGNOSIS: CLINICAL SIGNIFICANCE OF RESULTS
Abnormal findings related to
- Abnormal gas exchange
- Hypoxemia with levels less than 95%
- Impaired cardiopulmonary function

NURSING IMPLICATIONS

BEFORE THE STUDY: PLANNING AND IMPLEMENTATION

Teaching the Patient What to Expect
- Inform the patient this procedure can assist in monitoring oxygen in the blood.
- Review the procedure with the patient. Address concerns about pain related to the procedure and explain that no pain is associated with the procedure.
- Explain that the procedure is generally performed at the bedside, in the operating room during a surgical procedure, or in the office of an HCP.
- Explain that the procedure lasts as long as the monitoring is needed and could be continuous.

- If a finger probe is used, instruct the patient to remove artificial fingernails and nail polish.
- The upper earlobe or finger can be massaged or have a warm towel applied to increase the blood flow.
- Normally, the index finger is used, but if the finger is too large for the probe, a smaller finger can be used.
- If the earlobe is used, make sure good contact is achieved.
- The big toe, top or bottom of the foot, or sides of the heel may be used in infants.
- A photodetector probe is placed over the finger in such a way that the light beams and sensors are opposite each other. The manufacturers' directions should be followed for the specific pulse oximeter being used. Typically, heart rate and peripheral capillary saturation are displayed.
- The clip used for monitoring is removed when the procedure is complete.

Safety Considerations
- When used in the presence of flammable gases, the equipment must be approved for that specific use.

AFTER THE STUDY: POTENTIAL NURSING ACTIONS

Avoiding Complications
- Closely observe SpO_2, and report to the HCP if it decreases to 90%.

Treatment Considerations
- Demonstrate how to use controlled breathing to improve breathing patterns.
- Explain how to pace and bundle activities to improve activity tolerance.

Follow-Up, Evaluation, and Desired Outcomes
- Understands that depending on the results of this procedure, additional testing may be performed to evaluate or monitor disease progress and determine the need for a change in therapy.

P

Pyruvate Kinase

SYNONYM/ACRONYM: PK.

RATIONALE: To assess for an enzyme deficiency to assist in diagnosis of hemolytic anemia.

PATIENT PREPARATION: There are no food, fluid, activity, or medication restrictions unless by medical direction.

NORMAL FINDINGS: (Method: Enzymatic) 4.6–11.2 units/g Hgb.

CRITICAL FINDINGS AND POTENTIAL INTERVENTIONS: N/A

OVERVIEW: (Study type: Blood collected in yellow-top [acid-citrate-dextrose (ACD)] tube. Specimens collected in a lavender-top [EDTA] or green-top [heparin] tube also may be acceptable in some laboratories; related body system: Circulatory/Hematopoietic system.) Pyruvate kinase (PK) is an enzyme that forms pyruvate and adenosine diphosphate during glycolysis. Isoenzymes of PK are present in specific tissue: M_1 type PK is mainly found in the heart, skeletal muscle, and brain; L type is found in the liver, kidney cortex, and intestine; M_2 is found in leukocytes and most other tissues; type R is specifically found in red blood cells (RBCs). Deficiency of this enzyme can be acquired by ingestion of a drug or as an effect of liver disease. There is also a hereditary form of pyruvate kinase deficiency that can be transmitted as an autosomal recessive trait, meaning both parents must have the affected gene for the enzyme deficiency to be passed on to their offspring. RBCs lacking this enzyme have a membrane defect resulting from low levels of adenosine triphosphate and are more susceptible to hemolysis.

INDICATIONS
Evaluate chronic hemolytic anemia.

INTERFERING FACTORS
Factors that may alter the results of the study
- Testing after blood transfusion may produce a falsely normal result.
- The enzyme is unstable. The specimen should be refrigerated immediately after collection.

POTENTIAL MEDICAL DIAGNOSIS: CLINICAL SIGNIFICANCE OF RESULTS
Increased in
Related to release of skeletal and cardiac specific isoenzymes of PK from damaged tissue cells.

- Carriers of Duchenne muscular dystrophy
- Muscle disease
- Myocardial infarction

Decreased in
- Hereditary pyruvate kinase deficiency (evidenced by autosomal recessive trait for PK enzyme deficiency): Congenital nonspherocytic hemolytic anemia
- Acquired pyruvate kinase deficiency (related to interaction of medications used for therapy; related to release of leukocyte specific isoenzymes from damaged leukocytes): Acute leukemia Aplasias Other anemias

P

NURSING IMPLICATIONS

Teaching the Patient What to Expect

▶ Inform the patient this test can assist in diagnosing anemia.
▶ Explain that a blood sample is needed for the test.

Treatment Considerations

▶ Address any concerns voiced by the patient or family.

Follow-Up, Evaluation, and Desired Outcomes

▶ Understands that depending on the results of this procedure, additional testing may be performed to evaluate or monitor disease progress determine the need for a change in therapy.

Radioactive Iodine Uptake

SYNONYM/ACRONYM: RAIU, thyroid uptake.

RATIONALE: To assess thyroid function toward diagnosing disorders such as hyperthyroidism and goiter.

PATIENT PREPARATION: There are no activity restrictions unless by medical direction. Instruct the patient to fast and restrict fluids for 8 to 12 hr before the procedure. The patient may be instructed, by medical direction, to restrict foods, medicines, or supplements containing iodine for one week before the study. Examples of restricted items include iodized salt, prepared or processed foods high in iodized salt, seaweed, kelp, shellfish; thyroid or anti-thyroid medications; vitamins and dietary supplements. The thyroid gland does not distinguish between radiolabeled and natural iodine; restricting dietary intake helps ensure optimal uptake of radiolabeled iodine for accurate study results. The patient may eat 4 hr after the injection unless otherwise indicated. Protocols may vary among facilities. Ensure that this procedure is performed before all radiographic procedures using iodinated contrast medium.

NORMAL FINDINGS

- Variations in normal ranges of iodine uptake can occur with differences in dietary intake, geographic location, and protocols among laboratories:

Iodine Uptake	Percentage of Radionuclide
2-hr absorption	1%–13%
6-hr absorption	2%–25%
24-hr absorption	15%–45%

CRITICAL FINDINGS AND POTENTIAL INTERVENTIONS: N/A

OVERVIEW: (**Study type:** Nuclear scan; **related body system:** Endocrine system.) Radioactive iodine uptake (RAIU) is a nuclear medicine study used for evaluating thyroid function. It directly measures the ability of the thyroid gland to concentrate and retain circulating iodide for the synthesis of thyroid hormone. RAIU assists in the diagnosis of both hyperthyroidism and hypothyroidism, but it is more useful in the diagnosis of hyperthyroidism.

A very small dose of radioactive iodine-123 (I-123) or I-131 is administered orally, and images are taken at specified intervals after the initial dose is administered. The radionuclide emits gamma radiation, which allows external measurement. The uptake of radionuclide in the thyroid gland is measured as the percentage of radionuclide absorbed in a specific amount of time. The iodine not used is excreted in the urine. The thyroid gland does not distinguish between radioactive and nonradioactive iodine. Uptake values are used in conjunction with measurements of circulating thyroid hormone levels to differentiate primary and secondary thyroid disease, and serial measurements are helpful in long-term management of thyroid disease and its treatment.

INDICATIONS
- Evaluate hyperthyroidism and/or hypothyroidism.
- Evaluate neck pain.

- Evaluate the patient as part of a complete thyroid evaluation for symptomatic patients (e.g., swollen neck, neck pain, extreme sensitivity to heat or cold, jitters, sluggishness).
- Evaluate thyroiditis, goiter, or pituitary failure.
- Monitor response to therapy for thyroid disease.

INTERFERING FACTORS
Contraindications

Patients who are pregnant or suspected of being pregnant, unless the potential benefits of a procedure using radiation far outweigh the risk of radiation exposure to the fetus and mother.

Factors that may alter the results of the study

- Recent use of iodinated contrast medium for radiographic studies (within the last 4 wk) or nuclear medicine procedures done within the previous 24 to 48 hr.
- Iodine deficiency (e.g., patients with inadequate dietary intake, patients on phenothiazine therapy), which can increase radionuclide uptake.
- Certain drugs and other external sources of excess iodine, which can decrease radionuclide uptake, as follows:
Foods containing iodine (e.g., iodized salt, shellfish)
Drugs and other substances such as aminosalicylic acid, antihistamines, antithyroid medications (e.g., propylthiouracil), corticosteroids, cough syrup, isoniazid, levothyroxine sodium/T_4, L-triiodothyronine, Lugol solution, nitrates, penicillins, potassium iodide, propylthiouracil, saturated solution of potassium iodide, sulfonamides, thyroid extract, tolbutamide, warfarin,
Multivitamins containing minerals
- Vomiting, severe diarrhea, and gastroenteritis, which can affect absorption of the oral radionuclide dose.
- Metallic objects (e.g., jewelry, body rings) within the examination field, which may inhibit organ visualization and cause unclear images.
- Inability of the patient to cooperate or remain still during the procedure, because movement can produce blurred or otherwise unclear images.

POTENTIAL MEDICAL DIAGNOSIS: CLINICAL SIGNIFICANCE OF RESULTS
Abnormal findings related to

- Decreased iodine intake or increased iodine excretion
- Graves disease
- Iodine-deficient goiter
- Hashimoto thyroiditis (early)
- Hyperthyroidism, increased uptake of radionuclide:
Rebound thyroid hormone withdrawal
Drugs and hormones such as barbiturates, diuretics, estrogens, lithium carbonate, phenothiazines, and thyroid-stimulating hormone
- Hypothyroidism, decreased uptake of 0% to 10% radionuclide over 24-hr period:
Chronic kidney disease
Hypoalbuminemia
Malabsorption
Subacute thyroiditis
Thyrotoxicosis as a result of ectopic thyroid metastasis

NURSING IMPLICATIONS

BEFORE THE STUDY: PLANNING AND IMPLEMENTATION

Teaching the Patient What to Expect

▶ Inform the patient this test can assist in assessing thyroid function.
▶ Pregnancy is a general contraindication to procedures involving radiation. Explain to the female patient that she will be asked the date of her last menstrual period and pregnancy testing

R

may be performed to determine the possibility of pregnancy before she is exposed to radiation.

▶ Review the procedure with the patient. Address concerns about pain and explain that there may be moments of discomfort or pain experienced if an IV line is inserted to allow infusion of fluids such as saline, anesthetics, sedatives, radionuclides, medications used in the procedure, or emergency medications.

▶ Explain that an I-123 will be administrated orally (pill form).

▶ Explain that the procedure is performed in a nuclear medicine department by a health-care provider (HCP) who specializes in this procedure, with support staff, and takes approximately 15 to 30 min.

▶ Explain that the radionuclide poses no radioactive hazard and rarely produces adverse effects.

▶ Advise that delayed images may be needed 2 to 24 hr later and that the patient may leave the department and return later to undergo delayed imaging.

▶ Reassure the patient that the radionuclide poses no radioactive hazard and rarely produces adverse effects.

▶ Instruct the patient to remove jewelry and other metallic objects from the area to be examined.

▶ Baseline vital signs and neurological status are recorded. Protocols may vary among facilities.

▶ Positioning for this procedure is in a sitting or supine position in front of a radionuclide detector.

▶ Explain that once the study is completed, the needle or catheter is removed and a pressure dressing applied over the puncture site.

Potential Nursing Actions

◈ *Make sure a written and informed consent has been signed prior to the procedure and before administering any medications.*

AFTER THE STUDY: POTENTIAL NURSING ACTIONS

Avoiding Complications

▶ Establishing an IV site and injection of radionuclides are invasive procedures. Complications are rare but include risk

for allergic reaction *(related to contrast reaction),* hematoma *(related to blood leakage into the tissue following needle insertion),* bleeding from the puncture site *(related to a bleeding disorder or the effects of natural products and medications with known anticoagulant, antiplatelet, or thrombolytic properties),* or infection *(which might occur if bacteria from the skin surface is introduced at the puncture site).* Monitor the patient for complications related to the procedure (e.g., allergic reaction, anaphylaxis, bronchospasm). Immediately report symptoms such as fast heart rate, difficulty breathing, skin rash, itching, or chest pain to the appropriate HCP. Observe/assess the needle/catheter insertion site for bleeding, inflammation, or hematoma formation.

Treatment Considerations

▶ Explain that the radionuclide is eliminated from the body within 6 to 24 hr. Advise the patient to drink increased amounts of fluids for 24 to 48 hr to eliminate the radionuclide from the body, unless contraindicated.

▶ Instruct the patient to resume usual diet, as directed by the HCP.

▶ Provide instruction in the care and assessment of the site.

▶ Explain that application of cold compresses to the puncture site may reduce discomfort or edema.

Safety Considerations

▶ The patient who is breastfeeding should consult with the requesting HCP regarding alternate testing that does not involve radiation. In general, if a woman who is breastfeeding must have a nuclear scan, she should not breastfeed the infant for 72 hr after the scan, until the radionuclide has been eliminated. She should be instructed to express the milk in order to prevent cessation of milk production; the milk can be stored and used after the 3-day period.

▶ Refer to organizational policy for additional precautions that may include instructions on handwashing, toilet flushing, limited contact with others, and other aspects of nuclear medicine safety.

Follow-Up, Evaluation, and Desired Outcomes

▶ Understands that depending on the results of this procedure, additional testing may be needed to evaluate or monitor disease progression and determine the need for a change in therapy.

Radiofrequency Ablation, Liver

SYNONYM/ACRONYM: RFA, RF ablation.

RATIONALE: To assist in treating tumors of the liver that are too small for surgery or have poor response to chemotherapy.

PATIENT PREPARATION: There are no activity restrictions unless by medical direction. Instruct the patient to fast and restrict fluids for 8 hr, or as ordered, prior to the procedure. Fasting may be ordered as a precaution against aspiration related to possible nausea and vomiting. The American Society of Anesthesiologists has fasting guidelines for risk levels according to patient status. More information can be located at www.asahq.org.

Note: If iodinated contrast medium is scheduled to be used in patients receiving metformin or drugs containing metformin for type 2 diabetes, the drug may be discontinued on the day of the test and continue to be withheld for 48 hr after the test.

Regarding the patient's risk for bleeding, the patient should be instructed to avoid taking natural products and medications with known anticoagulant, antiplatelet, or thrombolytic properties or to reduce dosage, as ordered, prior to the procedure. Number of days to withhold medication is dependent on the type of anticoagulant. Note the last time and dose of medication taken. Protocols may vary among facilities.

NORMAL FINDINGS
- Decrease in tumor size
- Normal size, position, contour, and texture of the liver.

CRITICAL FINDINGS AND POTENTIAL INTERVENTIONS: N/A

OVERVIEW: (Study type: Radiology, plain; related body system: Digestive system.) One minimally invasive therapy to eliminate tumors in organs such as the liver is called radiofrequency ablation (RFA). This technique works by passing electrical current in the range of radiofrequency waves between the needle electrode and the grounding pads placed on the patient's skin. A special needle electrode is placed in the tumor under the guidance of an imaging method such as ultrasound (US), computed tomography (CT) scanning (with or without iodinated contrast), or magnetic resonance imaging (MRI). A radiofrequency current is then passed through the electrode to heat the tumor tissue near the needle tip and to ablate, or eliminate, it. The current creates heat around the electrode inside the tumor, and this heat spreads out to destroy the entire tumor but little of the surrounding normal liver tissue. The heat

R

from radiofrequency energy also closes up small blood vessels, thereby minimizing the risk of bleeding. Because healthy liver tissue withstands more heat than a tumor, RFA is able to destroy a tumor and a small rim of normal tissue about its edges without affecting most of the normal liver. The dead tumor cells are gradually replaced by scar tissue that shrinks over time. This approach is used in destroying liver tumors that may have failed to respond to chemotherapy or have recurred after initial surgery. If there are multiple tumor nodules, they may be treated in one or more sessions. In general, RFA causes only minimal discomfort and may be done as an outpatient procedure without general anesthesia. The procedure can be performed percutaneously, laproscopically, or by open surgery. RFA is most effective if the tumor is less than 4 cm in diameter; results are not as good when RFA is used to treat larger tumors. Similar therapy is being used to treat tumors in the kidney, pancreas, bone, thyroid, breast, adrenal gland, and lung.

INDICATIONS
- Ablation of metastases to the liver.
- Ablation of primary liver tumors with hepatocellular cancer.
- Therapy for multiple small liver tumors that are too spread out to remove surgically.
- Therapy for recurrent liver tumors.
- Therapy for tumors that are less than 2 in. in diameter.
- Therapy for tumors that have failed to respond to chemotherapy.
- Therapy for tumors that have recurred after initial surgery.

INTERFERING FACTORS
Contraindications

❈ Patients who are pregnant or suspected of being pregnant, unless the potential benefits of a procedure using radiation (if CT is performed with or without contrast) far outweigh the risk of radiation exposure to the fetus.

❈ Patients with conditions associated with adverse reactions to contrast medium (e.g., asthma, food allergies, or allergy to contrast medium). Although patients are asked specifically if they have a known allergy to iodine or shellfish (shellfish contain high levels of iodine), it has been well established that the reaction is not to iodine; an actual iodine allergy would be problematic because iodine is required for the production of thyroid hormones. In the case of shellfish, the reaction is to a muscle protein called *tropomyosin;* in the case of iodinated contrast medium, the reaction is to the noniodinated part of the contrast molecule. Patients with a known hypersensitivity to the medium may benefit from premedication with corticosteroids and diphenhydramine; the use of nonionic contrast or an alternative noncontrast imaging study, if available, may be considered for patients who have severe asthma or who have experienced moderate to severe reactions to ionic contrast medium.

❈ Patients with conditions associated with preexisting renal insufficiency (e.g., chronic kidney disease, single kidney transplant, nephrectomy, diabetes, multiple myeloma, treatment with aminoglycosides and NSAIDs), *because iodinated contrast is nephrotoxic.*

❈ Patients who are chronically dehydrated before the test, especially older adults and patients whose health is already compromised, *because of their risk of contrast-induced acute kidney injury.*

❋ Patients with the presence of large or numerous tumors (studies show that RFA is most successful if fewer than three tumors are present and each lesion is not greater than 3 cm in size; ablation of tumors that occupy greater than 40% of the liver may not leave sufficient liver capacity to support normal function).

❋ Patients with metastasis to the bile duct or surrounding hepatic vessel.

❋ Patients with bile duct or major vessel invasion.

❋ Patients with significant extrahepatic disease.

❋ Patients with bleeding disorders who are receiving an arterial or venous puncture, because the site may not stop bleeding.

Factors that may alter the results of the study
• Metallic objects (e.g., jewelry, body rings) within the examination field, which may inhibit organ visualization and cause unclear images.
• Inability of the patient to cooperate or remain still during the procedure, because movement can produce blurred or otherwise unclear images.

POTENTIAL MEDICAL DIAGNOSIS: CLINICAL SIGNIFICANCE OF RESULTS:
Abnormal findings related to: N/A
This is a therapeutic procedure.

NURSING IMPLICATIONS

BEFORE THE STUDY: PLANNING AND IMPLEMENTATION

Teaching the Patient What to Expect
▸ Inform the patient this procedure can assist in removal of some types of liver tumors.
▸ Explain that prior to the procedure, laboratory testing may be required to determine the possibility of bleeding risk (coagulation testing) or to assess for impaired kidney function (creatinine level and estimated glomerular filtration rate) if use of iodinated contrast medium is anticipated.
▸ Pregnancy is a general contraindication to procedures involving radiation. Explain to the female patient that she will be asked the date of her last menstrual period. Pregnancy testing may be performed to determine the possibility of pregnancy before exposure to radiation.
▸ Review the procedure with the patient. Address concerns about pain and explain that there may be moments of discomfort or pain experienced when the IV line or catheter is inserted to allow infusion of fluids such as saline, anesthetics, sedatives, contrast medium, medications used in the procedure, or emergency medications.
▸ Explain that contrast medium will be injected, by catheter, at a separate site from the IV line.
▸ Advise that a burning and flushing sensation may be felt throughout the body during injection of the contrast medium, and the patient may experience an urge to cough, flushing, nausea, or a salty or metallic taste.
▸ Explain that a sedative and/or analgesia will be administered to promote relaxation and reduce discomfort prior to the needle electrode insertion.
▸ Explain that any discomfort with the needle electrode will be minimized with local anesthetics and systemic analgesics.
▸ Inform the patient that the procedure is performed in the radiology department by a health-care provider (HCP), with support staff, and takes approximately 30 to 90 min.
▸ Instruct the patient to remove jewelry and other metallic objects from the area to be examined prior to the procedure.
▸ Baseline vital signs are recorded and monitored throughout the procedure. Protocols may vary among facilities.
▸ Electrocardiographic electrodes are placed on the patient for cardiac

R

monitoring. A baseline rhythm is established and any ventricular dysrhythmias identified.

▶ Positioning for this procedure is in the supine position on an examination table.

▶ The selected area is cleansed and covered with a sterile drape.

▶ A local anesthetic is injected at the site and a needle electrode inserted under US, CT, or MRI guidance.

▶ A radiofrequency current is passed through the needle electrode, and the tumor is ablated.

▶ Advise taking slow, deep breaths if nausea occurs during the procedure. An ordered antiemetic drug can be administered as needed. An emesis basin can be ready for use.

▶ Explain that once the study is completed, the needle or catheter is removed, and a pressure dressing is applied over the puncture site.

Potential Nursing Actions

✦ *Make sure a written and informed consent has been signed prior to the procedure and before administering any medications.*

▶ If iodinated contrast medium is scheduled to be used in patients receiving metformin or drugs containing metformin for type 2 diabetes, the drug may be discontinued on the day of the test and continue to be withheld for 48 hr after the test. Protocols may vary among facilities.

Safety Considerations

▶ Anticoagulants, aspirin, and other salicylates should be discontinued by medical direction for the appropriate number of days prior to a procedure where bleeding is a potential complication.

AFTER THE STUDY: POTENTIAL NURSING ACTIONS

Avoiding Complications

▶ Establishing an IV site and injection of contrast medium are invasive procedures. Complications are rare but include risk for allergic reaction *(related to contrast reaction)*, bleeding from the puncture site *(related to a bleeding disorder or the effects of*

natural products and medications with known anticoagulant, antiplatelet, or thrombolytic properties) hematoma *(related to blood leakage into the tissue following needle insertion)*, infection *(which might occur if bacteria from the skin surface is introduced at the puncture site)*, nerve injury *(which might occur if the needle strikes a nerve)*, or nephrotoxicity *(a deterioration of renal function associated with contrast administration)*. Monitor the patient for complications related to the procedure (e.g., allergic reaction, anaphylaxis, bronchospasm, infection, injury). Immediately report symptoms such as difficulty breathing, chest pain, fever, hyperpnea, hypertension, nausea, palpitations, pruritus, rash, tachycardia, urticaria, or vomiting to the appropriate HCP. Observe/assess the needle/catheter insertion site for bleeding, inflammation, or hematoma formation. Administer ordered antihistamines or prophylactic steroids if the patient has an allergic reaction.

▶ Complications related to the ablation are rare but may include brief or long-lasting shoulder pain, hepatic abscess, biloma, inflammation of the gallbladder, damage to the bile ducts with resulting biliary obstruction, thermal damage to the bowel, thermal damage to surrounding tissue resulting in cellulitis, hemorrhage, or flu-like symptoms that appear 3 to 5 days after the procedure and last for approximately 5 days.

Treatment Considerations

▶ Instruct the patient to resume usual diet, fluids, medications, or activity, as directed by the HCP. Kidney function should be assessed before metformin is resumed.

▶ Monitor vital signs and neurological status every 15 min for 1 hr, then every 2 hr for 4 hr, and as ordered. Take temperature every 6 hr for 24 hr. Compare with baseline values. Notify the HCP if temperature is elevated. Protocols may vary among facilities.

▶ Instruct the patient to maintain bedrest for 4 to 6 hr after the procedure or as ordered.

▶ Instruct the patient in the care and assessment of the site.

R

Safety Considerations

◗ Advise diabetic patients to avoid all medications containing metformin for 48 hr following a procedure with iodinated contrast. Iodinated contrast can temporarily impair kidney function, and failure to withhold metformin may indirectly result in drug-induced lactic acidosis, a dangerous and sometimes fatal adverse effect of metformin (related to renal impairment that does not support sufficient excretion of metformin).

Follow-Up, Evaluation, and Desired Outcomes

◗ Understands the implications of abnormal test results on lifestyle choices and the clinical implications of the test results.

RBC Count, Indices, Morphology, and Inclusions

SYNONYM/ACRONYM: RBC.

RATIONALE: *RBC Count:* To evaluate the number of circulating red cells in the blood toward diagnosing disease and monitoring therapeutic treatment. *RBC Indices:* To evaluate cell size, shape, weight, and hemoglobin (Hgb) concentration. Used to diagnose and monitor therapy for diagnoses such as iron-deficiency anemia. Variations in the number of cells is most often seen in anemias, cancer, and hemorrhage. *Morphology and Inclusions:* To make a visual evaluation of the red blood cell (RBC) shape and/or size as a confirmation in assisting to diagnose and monitor disease progression.

PATIENT PREPARATION: There are no food, fluid, activity, or medication restrictions unless by medical direction.

NORMAL FINDINGS: Method: Automated, computerized, multichannel analyzers; microscopic, manual review of stained blood smear.

RBC Count		
Age	**Conventional Units (10^6 cells/microL)**	**SI Units (10^{12} cells/L) (Conventional Units × 1)**
Cord blood	3.61–5.81	3.61–5.81
0–1 wk	4.51–6.01	4.51–6.01
2–3 wk	3.99–6.11	3.99–6.11
1–2 mo	3.71–6.11	3.71–6.11
3–6 mo	3.81–5.61	3.81–5.61
7 mo–15 yr	3.81–5.21	3.81–5.21
16–18 yr	4.21–5.41	4.21–5.41
Adult		
Male	4.21–5.81	4.21–5.81
Female	3.61–5.11	3.61–5.11

Values are decreased in pregnancy related to the dilutional effects of increased fluid volume and potential nutritional deficiency related to decreased intake, nausea, and/or vomiting. Values are slightly lower in older adults associated with potential nutritional deficiency.

R

RBC Indices

Age	MCV (fL)	MCH (pg/cell)	MCHC (g/dL)	RDWCV	RDWSD
Cord blood	107–119	35–39	31–35	14.9–18.7	51–66
0–1 wk	104–116	29–45	24–36	14.9–18.7	51–66
2–3 wk	95–117	26–38	26–34	14.9–18.7	51–66
1–2 mo	81–125	25–37	26–34	14.9–18.7	44–55
3–11 mo	78–110	22–34	26–34	14.9–18.7	35–46
1–15 yr	74–94	24–32	30–34	11.6–14.8	35–42
16 yr–adult					
Male	77–97	26–34	32–36	11.6–14.8	38–48
Female	78–98	26–34	32–36	11.6–14.8	38–48
Older adult					
Male	79–103	27–35	32–36	11.6–14.8	38–48
Female	78–102	27–35	32–36	11.6–14.8	38–48

MCV = mean corpuscular volume; MCH = mean corpuscular hemoglobin; MCHC = mean corpuscular hemoglobin concentration; RDWCV = coefficient of variation in red blood cell distribution width; RDWSD = standard deviation in RBC distribution width.

RBC Morphology and Inclusions

RBC Morphology	Within Normal Limits	1+	2+	3+	4+
Size					
Anisocytosis	0–5	5–10	10–20	20–50	Greater than 50
Macrocytes	0–5	5–10	10–20	20–50	Greater than 50
Microcytes	0–5	5–10	10–20	20–50	Greater than 50
Shape					
Poikilocytes	0–2	3–10	10–20	20–50	Greater than 50
Burr cells	0–2	3–10	10–20	20–50	Greater than 50
Acanthocytes	Less than 1	2–5	5–10	10–20	Greater than 20
Schistocytes	Less than 1	2–5	5–10	10–20	Greater than 20
Dacryocytes (teardrop cells)	0–2	2–5	5–10	10–20	Greater than 20
Codocytes (target cells)	0–2	2–10	10–20	20–50	Greater than 50
Spherocytes	0–2	2–10	10–20	20–50	Greater than 50
Ovalocytes	0–2	2–10	10–20	20–50	Greater than 50
Stomatocytes	0–2	2–10	10–20	20–50	Greater than 50
Drepanocytes (sickle cells)	Absent	Reported as present or absent			

R

RBC Morphology and Inclusions

RBC Morphology	Within Normal Limits	1+	2+	3+	4+
Helmet cells	Absent	Reported as present or absent			
Agglutination	Absent	Reported as present or absent			
Rouleaux	Absent	Reported as present or absent			
Hgb Content					
Hypochromia	0–2	3–10	10–50	50–75	Greater than 75
Polychromasia					
Adult	Less than 1	2–5	5–10	10–20	Greater than 20
Newborn	1–6	7–15	15–20	20–50	Greater than 50
Inclusions					
Cabot rings	Absent	Reported as present or absent			
Basophilic stippling	0–1	1–5	5–10	10–20	Greater than 20
Howell-Jolly bodies	Absent	1–2	3–5	5–10	Greater than 10
Heinz bodies	Absent	Reported as present or absent			
Hgb C crystals	Absent	Reported as present or absent			
Pappenheimer bodies	Absent	Reported as present or absent			
Intracellular parasites (e.g., *Plasmodium, Babesia, Trypanosoma*)	Absent	Reported as present or absent			

CRITICAL FINDINGS AND POTENTIAL INTERVENTIONS

The presence of abnormal cells, other morphological characteristics, or cellular inclusions may signify a potentially life-threatening or serious health condition and should be investigated. Examples are the presence of sickle cells, moderate numbers of spherocytes, marked schistocytosis, oval macrocytes, basophilic stippling, nucleated RBCs (if the patient is not an infant), or malarial or other parasitic organisms.

Timely notification to the requesting health-care provider (HCP) of any critical findings and related symptoms is a role expectation of the professional nurse. A listing of these findings varies among facilities.

Consideration may be given to verifying the critical findings before action is taken. Policies vary among facilities and may include requesting immediate recollection and retesting by the laboratory or retesting using a rapid point-of-care instrument at the bedside, if available.

Low RBC count leads to anemia. Anemia can be caused by blood loss, decreased blood cell production, increased blood cell destruction, or hemodilution. Causes of blood loss include menstrual excess or frequency, gastrointestinal bleeding, inflammatory bowel disease, or hematuria. Decreased blood cell production can be caused by folic acid deficiency, vitamin B_{12} deficiency, iron deficiency, or chronic disease. Increased blood cell destruction can be caused by a hemolytic reaction, chemical reaction, medication reaction, or sickle cell disease. Hemodilution can be caused by heart failure, chronic kidney disease, polydipsia, or overhydration. Symptoms of anemia (due to these causes) include anxiety, dyspnea, edema, hypertension, hypotension, hypoxia, jugular venous distention, fatigue, pallor, rales, restlessness, and weakness. Treatment of anemia depends on the cause.

High RBC count leads to polycythemia. Polycythemia can be caused by dehydration, decreased oxygen levels in the body, and an overproduction of RBCs by the bone marrow. Dehydration by diuretic use, vomiting, diarrhea, excessive sweating, severe burns, or decreased fluid intake decreases the plasma component of whole blood, thereby increasing the ratio of RBCs to plasma, and leads to a higher than normal hematocrit (Hct). Causes of decreased oxygen include smoking, exposure to carbon monoxide, high altitude, and chronic lung disease, which leads to a mild hemoconcentration of blood in the body to carry more oxygen to the body's tissues. An overproduction of RBCs by the bone marrow leads to polycythemia vera, which is a rare chronic myeloproliferative disorder that leads to a severe hemoconcentration of blood. Severe hemoconcentration can lead to thrombosis (spontaneous blood clotting). Symptoms of hemoconcentration include decreased pulse pressure and volume, loss of skin turgor, dry mucous membranes, headaches, hepatomegaly, low central venous pressure, orthostatic hypotension, pruritus (especially after a hot bath), splenomegaly, tachycardia, thirst, tinnitus, vertigo, and weakness. Treatment of polycythemia depends on the cause. Possible interventions for hemoconcentration due to dehydration include IV fluids and discontinuance of diuretics if they are believed to be contributing to critically elevated Hct. Polycythemia due to decreased oxygen states can be treated by removal of the offending substance, such as smoke or carbon monoxide. Treatment includes oxygen therapy in cases of smoke inhalation, carbon monoxide poisoning, and desaturating chronic lung disease. Symptoms of polycythemic overload crisis include signs of thrombosis, pain and redness in extremities, facial flushing, and irritability. Possible interventions for hemoconcentration due to polycythemia include therapeutic phlebotomy and IV fluids.

OVERVIEW: (**Study type:** Blood collected in a lavender-top [EDTA] tube or Wright-stained, thin-film peripheral blood smear; related body system: Circulatory/Hematopoietic system. The laboratory should be consulted as to the necessity of thick-film smears for the evaluation of malarial inclusions. The specimen should be mixed gently by inverting the tube 10 times. The specimen should be analyzed within 6 hr when stored at room temperature or within 24 hr if stored at refrigerated temperature. If it is anticipated the specimen will not be analyzed within 4 to 6 hr, two blood smears should be made immediately after the venipuncture and submitted with the blood sample. Smears made from specimens older than 6 hr will contain an unacceptable number of misleading artifactual abnormalities of the RBCs, such as echinocytes and spherocytes, as well as necrobiotic white blood cells.)

RBC Count

The RBC count is a component of the complete blood count (CBC). It determines the number of RBCs per cubic millimeter of whole blood. The main role of RBCs, which contain the pigmented protein Hgb, is the transport and exchange of oxygen to the tissues. Some carbon dioxide is returned from the tissues to the lungs by RBCs. RBC production in healthy adults takes place in the bone marrow of the vertebrae, pelvis, ribs, sternum, skull, and proximal ends of the femur and humerus. Production of RBCs is regulated by a hormone called *erythropoietin,* which is produced and secreted by the kidneys. Normal RBC development and function are dependent on adequate levels of vitamin B_{12}, folic acid, vitamin E, and iron. The average life span of normal RBCs is 120 days. Old or damaged RBCs are removed from circulation by the spleen. The liver is responsible for the breakdown of Hgb and other cellular contents released from destroyed RBCs. *Polycythemia* is a condition resulting from an abnormal increase in Hgb, Hct, and RBC count. *Anemia* is a condition resulting from an abnormal decrease in Hgb, Hct, and RBC count. Results of the Hgb, Hct, and RBC count should be evaluated simultaneously because the same underlying conditions affect this triad of tests similarly. The RBC count multiplied by 3 should approximate the Hgb concentration. The Hct should be within three times the Hgb if the RBC population is normal in size and shape. The Hct plus 6 should approximate the first two figures of the RBC count within 3 (e.g., Hct is 40%; therefore, 40 + 6 = 46, and the RBC count should be 4.6 or in the range 4.3 to 4.9). (See the study titled "Hemoglobin and Hematocrit.")

RBC Indices

RBC indices provide information about RBC size and Hgb content. The indices are derived from mathematical relationships between the RBC count, Hgb level, and Hct percentage. RBC indices are frequently used to assist in the classification of anemias. The MCV reflects the average size of circulating RBCs and classifies size as normocytic, microcytic (smaller than normal), and macrocytic (larger than

R

normal). MCV is determined by dividing the Hct by the total RBC. The RDW is a measurement of cell size distribution. Many of the commonly used automated cell counters report the more sophisticated statistical indices, the RDWCV and RDWSD, instead of the RDW. The RDWCV is an indication of variation in cell size over the circulating RBC population. The RDWSD is also an indicator of variation in RBC size, is not affected by the MCV as with the RDWCV index, and is a more accurate measurement of the degree of variation in cell size. Review of peripheral smears is used to corroborate findings from automated instruments. Excessive variations in cell size are graded from 1+ to 4+, with 4+ indicating the most severe degree of anisocytosis, or variation in cell size. MCH, or average amount of Hgb in RBCs, and MCHC, or average amount of Hgb per volume of RBCs, are used to measure Hgb content. Microscopic review of the peripheral smear can also be used to visually confirm automated values. Terms used to describe the Hgb content of RBCs are *normochromic, hypochromic,* and *hyperchromic.* The findings are also visually graded from 1+ to 4+. The MCH is determined by dividing the total Hgb by the RBC count. MCHC is determined by dividing total Hgb by Hct. (See the study titled "Hemoglobin and Hematocrit.")

RBC Morphology and Inclusions
The decision to manually review a peripheral blood smear for abnormalities in RBC shape or size is made on the basis of criteria established by the reporting laboratory. Cues in the results of the CBC will point to specific abnormalities that can be confirmed visually by microscopic review of the sample on a stained blood smear.

INDICATIONS
- Assist in the diagnosis of anemia.
- Detect a hematological disorder involving RBC destruction (e.g., hemolytic anemia).
- Detect a hematological disorder, tumor, or immunological abnormality.
- Determine the presence of hereditary hematological abnormality.
- Evaluate the possibility of erythropoietin (EPO) abuse by athletes.
- Monitor the effects of acute or chronic blood loss.
- Monitor the effects of physical or emotional stress on the patient.
- Monitor patients with disorders associated with elevated erythrocyte counts (e.g., polycythemia vera, chronic obstructive pulmonary disease [COPD]).
- Monitor the progression of nonhematological disorders associated with elevated erythrocyte counts, such as COPD, liver disease, hypothyroidism, adrenal dysfunction, bone marrow failure, malabsorption syndromes, cancer, and chronic kidney disease.
- Monitor the response to drugs or chemotherapy and evaluate undesired reactions to drugs that may cause blood dyscrasias.
- Provide screening as part of a CBC in a general physical examination, especially upon admission to a health-care facility or before surgery.

INTERFERING FACTORS
Factors that may alter the results of the study
- Drugs and other substances that may decrease RBC count by causing hemolysis resulting from drug

sensitivity or enzyme deficiency include acetaminophen, aminosalicylic acid, amphetamine, anticonvulsants, antipyrine, arsenicals, benzene, busulfan, carbenicillin, cephalothin, chemotherapy drugs, chlorate, chloroquine, chlorothiazide, chlorpromazine, colchicine, diphenhydramine, dipyrone, glucosulfone, gold, indomethacin, nalidixic acid, neomycin, nitrofurantoin, penicillin, phenacemide, phenazopyridine, and phenothiazine.

- Drugs and other substances that may decrease RBC count by causing anemia include miconazole, penicillamine, phenylhydrazine, primaquine, probenecid, pyrazolones, pyrimethamine, quinines, streptomycin, sulfamethizole, sulfamethoxypyridazine, sulfisoxazole, suramin, thioridazine, tolbutamide, trimethadione, and tripelennamine.
- Drugs that may decrease RBC count by causing bone marrow suppression include floxuridine and phenylbutazone.
- Drugs and other substances that may decrease the MCHC include styrene (occupational exposure).
- Drugs and other substances that may decrease the MCV include nitrofurantoin.
- Drugs and vitamins that may increase the RBC count include amphotericin B, erythropoietin, glucocorticosteroids, pilocarpine, and vitamin B_{12}.
- Drugs and other substances that may increase the MCV include colchicine, pentamidine, pyrimethamine, and triamterene.
- Drugs and other substances that may increase the MCH and MCHC include oral contraceptives (long-term use).
- Drugs and other substances that may increase Heinz body formation as an initial precursor to significant

hemolysis include acetanilid, acetylsalicylic acid, antimalarials, antipyretics, furazolidone, methylene blue, naphthalene, and nitrofurans.
- Hemodilution (e.g., excessive administration of IV fluids, normal pregnancy) in the presence of a normal number of RBCs may lead to false decreases in RBC count.
- Diseases that cause agglutination of RBCs will alter test results. For example, cold agglutinins may falsely increase the mean corpuscular volume and decrease the RBC count. This can be corrected by warming the blood or diluting the sample with warmed saline and repeating the analysis.
- Excessive exercise, anxiety, pain, and dehydration may cause false elevations in RBC count.
- RBC counts can vary depending on the patient's position, decreasing when the patient is recumbent as a result of hemodilution and increasing when the patient rises as a result of hemoconcentration.
- Venous stasis can falsely elevate RBC counts; therefore, the tourniquet should not be left on the arm for longer than 60 sec.
- Lipemia will falsely increase the hemoglobin measurement, also affecting the MCV and MCH.

Other considerations
- Use of the dietary supplement liver extract is strongly contraindicated in patients with iron-storage disorders such as hemochromatosis because it is rich in heme (the iron-containing pigment in Hgb).
- Failure to fill the tube sufficiently (i.e., tube less than three-quarters full) may yield inadequate sample volume for automated analyzers and may be a reason for specimen rejection.
- Hemolyzed or clotted specimens must be rejected for analysis.

R

POTENTIAL MEDICAL DIAGNOSIS: CLINICAL SIGNIFICANCE OF RESULTS
Increased in

RBC Count
- Anxiety or stress *(related to physiological response)*
- Bone marrow failure *(initial response is stimulation of RBC production)*
- COPD with hypoxia and secondary polycythemia *(related to chronic hypoxia that stimulates production of RBCs and a corresponding increase in RBCs)*
- Dehydration with hemoconcentration *(related to decrease in total blood volume relative to unchanged RBC count)*
- Erythremic erythrocytosis *(related to unchanged total blood volume relative to increase in RBC count)*
- High altitude *(related to hypoxia that stimulates production of RBCs)*
- Polycythemia vera *(related to abnormal bone marrow response resulting in overproduction of RBCs)*

RBC Size, MCV
- Alcohol misuse *(vitamin deficiency related to malnutrition)*
- Antimetabolite therapy *(the therapy inhibits vitamin B$_{12}$ and folate)*
- Aplastic anemia
- Chemotherapy
- Chronic hemolytic anemia
- Grossly elevated glucose (hyperosmotic)
- Hemolytic disease of the newborn
- Hypothyroidism
- Leukemia
- Liver disease *(complex effect on RBCs that includes malnutrition, alterations in RBC shape and size, effects of chronic disease)*
- Lymphoma
- Metastatic cancer
- Myelofibrosis
- Myeloma

- Refractory anemia
- Sideroblastic anemia
- Vitamin B$_{12}$ (pernicious anemia)/folate deficiency *(related to impaired DNA synthesis and delayed cell division, which permits the cells to grow for a longer period than normal)*

MCH
- Macrocytic anemias *(related to increased Hgb or cell size)*

MCHC
- Spherocytosis *(artifact in measurement caused by abnormal cell shape)*

RDW
- Anemias with heterogeneous cell size as a result of hemoglobinopathy, hemolytic anemia, anemia following acute blood loss, iron-deficiency anemia, vitamin- and folate-deficiency anemia *(related to a mixture of cell sizes as the bone marrow responds to the anemia and/or to a mixture of cell shapes due to cell fragmentation as a result of the disease)*

Decreased in

RBC Count
- Chemotherapy *(related to reduced RBC survival)*
- Chronic inflammatory diseases *(related to anemia of chronic disease)*
- Chronic kidney disease *(related to decreased production of erythropoietin)*
- Hemoglobinopathy *(related to reduced RBC survival)*
- Hemolytic anemia *(related to reduced RBC survival)*
- Hemorrhage *(related to overall decrease in RBC count)*
- Hodgkin disease *(evidenced by bone marrow failure that results in decreased RBC production)*

- Leukemia *(evidenced by bone marrow failure that results in decreased RBC production)*
- Multiple myeloma *(evidenced by bone marrow failure that results in decreased RBC production)*
- Nutritional deficit *(related to deficiency of iron or vitamins required for RBC production and/or maturation)*
- Overhydration *(related to increase in blood volume relative to unchanged RBC count)*
- Pregnancy *(related to anemia; normal dilutional effect)*
- Subacute endocarditis

RBC Size, MCV
- Hereditary spherocytosis
- Inflammation
- Iron-deficiency anemia *(related to low Hgb)*
- Thalassemias *(related to low Hgb)*

MCH
- Hypochromic anemias *(related to low Hgb)*
- Microcytic anemias *(related to low Hgb)*

MCHC
- Iron-deficiency anemia *(the amount of Hgb in the RBC is small relative to RBC size)*

RBC Shape
Variations in cell shape are the result of hereditary conditions such as elliptocytosis, sickle cell anemia, spherocytosis, thalassemias, or hemoglobinopathies (e.g., hemoglobin C disease). Irregularities in cell shape can also result from acquired conditions, such as physical/mechanical cellular trauma, exposure to chemicals, or reactions to medications.

- Acquired spherocytosis can result from Heinz body hemolytic anemia, microangiopathic hemolytic anemia, secondary isoimmunohemolytic anemia, and transfusion of old banked blood.
- Acanthocytes are associated with acquired conditions such as alcohol associated cirrhosis with hemolytic anemia, disorders of lipid metabolism, hepatitis of newborns, malabsorptive diseases, metastatic liver disease, the postsplenectomy period, and pyruvate kinase deficiency.
- Burr cells are commonly seen in acquired renal insufficiency, burns, cardiac valve disease, disseminated intravascular coagulation (DIC), hypertension, IV fibrin deposition, metastatic malignancy, normal neonatal period, and uremia.
- Codocytes are seen in hemoglobinopathies, iron-deficiency anemia, obstructive liver disease, and the postsplenectomy period.
- Dacryocytes are most commonly associated with metastases to the bone marrow, myelofibrosis, myeloid metaplasia, pernicious anemia, and tuberculosis.
- Schistocytes are seen in burns, cardiac valve disease, DIC, glomerulonephritis, hemolytic anemia, microangiopathic hemolytic anemia, renal graft rejection, thrombotic thrombocytopenic purpura, uremia, and vasculitis.

RBC Hemoglobin Content
- RBCs with a normal Hgb level have a clear central pallor and are referred to as *normochromic.*
- Cells with low Hgb and lacking in central pallor are referred to as *hypochromic.* Hypochromia is associated with iron-deficiency anemia, thalassemias, and sideroblastic anemia.
- Cells with excessive Hgb levels are referred to as *hyperchromic* even though they technically lack a central pallor. Hyperchromia is usually

R

associated with an elevated mean corpuscular Hgb concentration as well as hemolytic anemias.

• Cells referred to as *polychromic* are young erythrocytes that still contain ribonucleic acid (RNA). The RNA is picked up by the Wright stain. Polychromasia is indicative of premature release of RBCs from bone marrow secondary to increased erythropoietin stimulation.

RBC Inclusions

RBC inclusions can result from certain types of anemia, abnormal Hgb precipitation, or parasitic infection.

• Cabot rings may be seen in megaloblastic and other anemias, lead poisoning, and conditions in which RBCs are destroyed before they are released from bone marrow.
• Basophilic stippling is seen whenever there is altered Hgb synthesis, as in thalassemias, megaloblastic anemias, alcohol misuse, and lead or arsenic intoxication.
• Howell-Jolly bodies are seen in sickle cell anemia, other hemolytic anemias, megaloblastic anemia, congenital absence of the spleen, and the postsplenectomy period.
• Pappenheimer bodies may be seen in cases of sideroblastic anemia, thalassemias, refractory anemia, dyserythropoietic anemias, hemosiderosis, and hemochromatosis.
• Heinz bodies are most often seen in the blood of patients who have ingested drugs known to induce the formation of these inclusion bodies. They are also seen in patients with hereditary glucose-6-phosphate dehydrogenase (G6PD) deficiency.
• Hgb C crystals can often be identified in stained peripheral smears of patients with hereditary hemoglobin C disease.

• Parasites such as *Plasmodium* (transmitted by mosquitoes and causing malaria) and *Babesia* (transmitted by ticks), known to invade human RBCs, can be visualized with Wright stain and other special stains of the peripheral blood.

NURSING IMPLICATIONS

BEFORE THE STUDY: PLANNING AND IMPLEMENTATION

Teaching the Patient What to Expect
▶ Inform the patient this test can assist in assessing for anemia and disorders affecting the appearance, shape, size, and number of circulating RBCs.
▶ Explain that a blood sample is needed for the test.

AFTER THE STUDY: POTENTIAL NURSING ACTIONS

Treatment Considerations
▶ The results of a CBC should be carefully evaluated during transfusion or acute blood loss because the body is not in a state of homeostasis and values may be misleading. Considerations for draw times after transfusion include the type of product, the amount of product transfused, and the patient's clinical situation. Generally, specimens collected an hour after transfusion will provide an acceptable reflection of the effects of the transfused product. Measurements taken during a massive transfusion are an exception, providing essential guidance for therapeutic decisions during critical care.

Nutritional Considerations
▶ Instruct patients to consume a variety of foods within the basic food groups, maintain a healthy weight, be physically active, limit salt intake, limit alcohol intake, and avoid the use of tobacco.
▶ Nutritional therapy may be indicated for patients with decreased RBC count. Iron deficiency is the most common nutrient deficiency in the United States. Patients at risk (e.g., children, pregnant

women and women of childbearing age, low-income populations) should be instructed to include foods that are high in iron in their diet, such as meats (especially liver), eggs, grains, green leafy vegetables, and multivitamins with iron. Iron absorption is affected by numerous factors (see study titled "Iron Studies: Iron (Total), Iron-Binding Capacity (Total), Transferrin, and Iron Saturation").

♦ Patients at risk for vitamin B_{12} or folate deficiency include those with the following conditions: malnourishment (inadequate intake), pregnancy (increased need), infancy, malabsorption syndromes (inadequate absorption/increased metabolic rate), infections, cancer, hyperthyroidism, serious burns, excessive blood loss, and gastrointestinal damage. Instruct the patient with vitamin B_{12} deficiency, as appropriate, in the use of vitamin supplements. Inform the patient, as appropriate, that the best dietary sources of vitamin B_{12} are meats, milk, cheese, eggs, and fortified soy milk products. Instruct the folate-deficient patient (especially pregnant women), as appropriate, to eat foods rich in folate, such as meats (especially liver), salmon, eggs, beets, asparagus, green leafy vegetables such as spinach, cabbage, oranges, broccoli, sweet potatoes, kidney beans, and whole wheat.

♦ A diet deficient in vitamin E puts the patient at risk for increased RBC destruction, which could lead to anemia. Nutritional therapy may be indicated for these patients. Educate the patient with a vitamin E deficiency, if appropriate, that the main dietary sources of vitamin E are vegetable oils (including olive oil), whole grains, wheat germ, nuts, milk, eggs, meats, fish, and green leafy vegetables. Vitamin E is fairly stable at most cooking temperatures (except frying) and when exposed to acidic foods. Supplemental vitamin E may also be taken, but the danger of toxicity should be explained to the patient. Overuse of vitamin E is associated with unexplained bleeding *evidenced by bruising or bleeding gums*. Vitamin E is heat stable but is very negatively affected by light.

Follow-Up, Evaluation, and Desired Outcomes

♦ Acknowledges contact information provided for the U.S. Department of Agriculture's resource for nutrition (www.choosemyplate.gov).

Red Blood Cell Cholinesterase

SYNONYM/ACRONYM: Acetylcholinesterase (AChE), erythrocyte cholinesterase, true cholinesterase.

RATIONALE: To assess for pesticide toxicity and screen for cholinesterase deficiency, which may contribute to unrecoverable apnea after surgical induction with succinylcholine.

PATIENT PREPARATION: There are no food, fluid, activity, or medication restrictions unless by medical direction.

NORMAL FINDINGS: Method: Enzymatic.

Test	Conventional Units
RBC cholinesterase	9,500–15,000 units/L

CRITICAL FINDINGS AND POTENTIAL INTERVENTIONS: N/A

OVERVIEW: (Study type: Blood collected in a lavender-top [EDTA] tube; related body system: Circulatory/Hematopoietic system.) There are two types of cholinesterase: *acetylcholinesterase* (AChE), or "true cholinesterase," which is found in red blood cells (RBCs), lung, and brain (nerve) tissue; and *pseudocholinesterase,* which is mainly found in the plasma, liver, and heart. RBC AChE is highly specific for acetylcholine. RBC cholinesterase is used to assist in the diagnosis of chronic carbamate or organophosphate insecticide (e.g., parathion, malathion) toxicity. Organophosphate pesticides bind irreversibly with cholinesterase, inhibiting normal enzyme activity. Carbamate insecticides bind reversibly. Serum or plasma pseudocholinesterase is used more frequently to measure acute pesticide toxicity. Pseudocholinesterase is also the test used to indicate succinylcholine sensitivity (see study titled "Pseudocholinesterase and Dibucaine Number").

Patients with inherited cholinesterase deficiency are at risk during anesthesia if succinylcholine is administered as an anesthetic. Succinylcholine, a short-acting muscle relaxant, is a reversible inhibitor of acetylcholinesterase and is hydrolyzed by cholinesterase. Succinylcholine-sensitive patients may be unable to metabolize the anesthetic quickly, resulting in prolonged or unrecoverable apnea. This test, along with the pseudocholinesterase test, is also used to identify individuals with atypical forms of the enzyme cholinesterase. The prevalence of succinylcholine sensitivity is 1 in 2,000 to 4,000 homozygote and 1 in 500 heterozygote patients. There are more than 15 identified phenotypes; A, AS, S1, S2, F, AF, and FS are associated with prolonged apnea following the use of succinylcholine. Widespread preoperative screening is not routinely performed.

INDICATIONS
• Monitor cumulative exposure to organic phosphate insecticides.
• Verify suspected exposure to organic phosphate insecticides.

INTERFERING FACTORS
Factors that may alter the results of the study
• Drugs and other substances that may increase RBC cholinesterase levels include echothiophate, parathion, and antiepileptic drugs such as carbamazepine, phenobarbital, phenytoin, and valproic acid.
• Improper anticoagulant; fluoride interferes with the measurement and causes a falsely decreased value.

POTENTIAL MEDICAL DIAGNOSIS: CLINICAL SIGNIFICANCE OF RESULTS
Increased in
• Hemolytic anemias (e.g., sickle cell anemia, thalassemias, spherocytosis, and acquired hemolytic anemias) *(increased in hemolytic anemias as AChE is released from the hemolyzed RBCs)*

Decreased in
• Insecticide exposure *(organic phosphate insecticides inhibit AChE activity)*
• Late pregnancy *(related to anemia of pregnancy)*
• Paroxysmal nocturnal hemoglobinuria *(related to lack of RBC production by bone marrow)*
• Relapse of megaloblastic anemia *(related to underproduction of normal RBCs containing AChE)*

R

NURSING IMPLICATIONS

BEFORE THE STUDY: PLANNING AND IMPLEMENTATION

Teaching the Patient What to Expect
▶ Inform the patient this test can assist in identification of pesticide poisoning.
▶ Explain that a blood sample is needed for the test.

Potential Nursing Actions
▶ Discuss health concerns related to exposure to pesticides causing symptoms including blurred vision, muscle weakness, nausea, vomiting, headaches, pulmonary edema, salivation, sweating, or convulsions.

AFTER THE STUDY: POTENTIAL NURSING ACTIONS

Treatment Considerations
▶ The patient with decreased values should be observed for signs of fluid volume excess related to compromised regulatory mechanisms, decreased cardiac output related to decreased myocardial contractility or dysrhythmias, and pain related to inflammation or ischemia.
▶ Be supportive of anxiety related to impaired activity secondary to weakness and fear of shortened life expectancy.
▶ Provide education regarding access to genetic counseling services and screening tests for other family members.
▶ Explain the importance of using a medic alert bracelet to notify health-care workers of increased risk from exposure to medications that may lower cholinesterase activity.

Follow-Up, Evaluation, and Desired Outcomes
▶ Understands that depending on the results of this procedure, additional testing may be performed to evaluate or monitor disease progression and determine the need for a change in therapy.

Refraction

SYNONYM/ACRONYM: N/A

RATIONALE: To assess the visual acuity of the eyes in patients of all ages, to evaluate visual acuity as required by driver licensing laws, and to assist in evaluating the eyes prior to therapeutic interventions such as eyeglasses, contact lenses, low vision aids, cataract surgery, or laser-assisted in situ keratomileusis (LASIK) surgery.

PATIENT PREPARATION: There are no food or fluid restrictions unless by medical direction. Instruct the patient to withhold eye medications (particularly miotic eye drops which may constrict the pupil, preventing a clear view of the fundus, and mydriatic eyedrops in order to avoid instigation of an acute open-angle attack in patients with narrow-angle glaucoma) for at least 1 day prior to the test. Ensure that the patient understands that he or she must refrain from driving until the pupils return to normal (about 4 hr) after the test and has made arrangements to have someone else be responsible for transportation after the test.

R

NORMAL FINDINGS
• Normal visual acuity; 20/20 (with corrective lenses if appropriate).

CRITICAL FINDINGS AND POTENTIAL INTERVENTIONS: N/A

OVERVIEW: (Study type: Sensory, ocular; **related body system:** Nervous system.) This noninvasive procedure tests the visual acuity (VA) of the eyes and determines abnormalities or refractive errors that need correction. Refractions are performed using a combination of different pieces of equipment. Refractive error can be quickly and accurately measured using computerized automatic refractors or manually with a viewing system consisting of an entire set of trial lenses mounted on a circular wheel (phoropter). A projector may also be used to display test letters and characters from Snellen eye charts for use in assessing VA. If the VA is worse than 20/20, the pinhole test may be used to quickly assess the best corrected vision. Refractive errors of the peripheral cornea and lens can be reduced or eliminated by having the patient look through a pinhole at the vision test. Patients with cataracts or visual field defects will not show improved results using the pinhole test. The retinoscope is probably the most valuable instrument that can be used to objectively assess VA. It is also the only objective means of assessing refractive error in pediatric patients and patients who are unable to cooperate with other techniques of assessing refractive error due to illiteracy, senility, or inability to speak the same language as the examiner. Visual defects identified through refraction, such as hyperopia (farsightedness), in which the point of focus lies behind the retina; myopia (nearsightedness), in which the point of focus lies in front of the retina; and astigmatism, in which the refraction is unequal in different curvatures of the eyeball, can be corrected by glasses, contact lenses, or refractive surgery.

INDICATIONS
• Determine if an optical defect is present and if light rays entering the eye focus correctly on the retina.
• Determine the refractive error prior to refractive surgery such as radial keratotomy, photorefractive keratotomy, LASIK, intracorneal rings, limbal relaxing incisions, implantable contact lens (phakic intraocular lens), clear lens replacement.
• Determine the type of corrective lenses (e.g., biconvex or plus lenses for hyperopia, biconcave or minus lenses for myopia, compensatory lenses for astigmatism) needed for refractive errors.
• Diagnose refractive errors in vision.

INTERFERING FACTORS
Contraindications
�֍ Patients with narrow-angle glaucoma if pupil dilation is performed; dilation can initiate a severe and sight-threatening open-angle attack.
✦ Patients with allergies to mydriatics if pupil dilation using mydriatics is performed.

Factors that may alter the results of the study
• Improper pupil dilation may prevent adequate examination for refractive error.

POTENTIAL MEDICAL DIAGNOSIS: CLINICAL SIGNIFICANCE OF RESULTS

Visual Acuity Scale

Foot	Meter	Decimal
20/200	6/60	0.1
20/160	6/48	0.13
20/120	6/36	0.17
20/100	6/30	0.2
20/80	6/24	0.25
20/60	6/18	0.33
20/50	6/15	0.4
20/40	6/12	0.5
20/30	6/9	0.67
20/25	6/7.5	0.8
20/20	6/6	1
20/16	6/4.8	1.25
20/12	6/3.6	1.67
20/10	6/3	2

VA can be expressed fractionally in feet, fractionally in meters, or as a decimal where perfect vision of 20/20 feet or 6/6 meters is equal to 1. Comparing the fraction in feet or meters to the decimal helps demonstrate that acuity less than 20/20, or less than 1.0, is "worse" vision, and acuity greater than 20/20, or greater than 1.0, is "better." A patient who cannot achieve best corrected VA of 20/200 or above (greater than 0.1) in his or her better eye is considered legally blind in the United States.

Uncorrected Visual Acuity	Foot	Meter	Decimal
Mild vision loss	20/30–20/70	6/9–6/21	0.67–0.29
Moderate vision loss	20/80–20/160	6/24–6/48	0.25–0.13
Severe vision loss	20/200–20/400	6/60–6/120	0.1–0.05
Profound vision loss	20/500–20/1,000	6/150–6/300	0.04–0.02

Abnormal findings related to
- Refractive errors such as anisometropia, astigmatism, hyperopia, myopia, and presbyopia.

NURSING IMPLICATIONS

BEFORE THE STUDY: PLANNING AND IMPLEMENTATION

Teaching the Patient What to Expect
- Inform the patient this procedure can assist in assessing visual acuity.
- Explain the importance of withholding eye medications for at least 1 day prior to the test. Miotic eye drops may constrict the pupil preventing a clear view of the fundus and mydriatic eyedrops may cause an instigation of an acute open angle attack in patients with narrow angle glaucoma.
- Review the procedure with the patient. Address concerns about pain and explain that mydriatics, if used, may cause blurred vision and sensitivity to light. There may also be a brief stinging sensation when the drop is put in the eye.
- Explain that a health-care provider (HCP) performs the test, in a quiet, darkened room, and that to evaluate both eyes, the test can take up to 30 min

R

(including time for the pupils to dilate before the test is actually performed).

▶ If dilation is to be performed, an ordered mydriatic will be administered to each eye and repeated in 5 to 15 min.

▶ Positioning for this procedure is seated with placement of the chin in the chin rest with the forehead gently pressed against the support bar.

▶ An examiner will sit at eye level about 2 ft away from the patient.

▶ A retinoscope light is held in front of the eyes and directed through the pupil.

▶ Each eye is examined for the characteristics of the red reflex, the reflection of the light from the retinoscope, which normally moves in the same direction as the light.

▶ Explain that there will be a request to look straight ahead while the eyes are examined with the instrument and while different lenses are tried to provide the best corrective lenses to be prescribed.

▶ Once an optimal VA is obtained with the trial lenses in each eye, a prescription for corrective lenses is written.

Potential Nursing Actions

▶ Obtain a history of allergies or sensitivities to mydriatics, if dilation is to be performed.

▶ Obtain a history of known or suspected vision loss; changes in visual acuity, including type and cause; use of glasses or contact lenses; eye conditions with treatment regimens; eye surgery; and other tests and procedures to assess and diagnose visual deficit.

▶ Instruct the patient to remove contact lenses or glasses, as appropriate.

AFTER THE STUDY: POTENTIAL NURSING ACTIONS

Avoiding Complications

▶ Dilation can initiate a severe and sight-threatening open-angle attack in patients with narrow-angle glaucoma.

Treatment Considerations

▶ Instruct the patient to resume usual medications, as directed by the HCP.

▶ Explain that visual acuity and responses to light may change.

▶ Remind the patient to wear dark glasses after the test until the pupils return to normal size.

▶ Review the implications of abnormal test results on the patient's lifestyle.

▶ Be supportive of impaired activity related to vision loss, anticipated loss of driving privileges, or the possibility of requiring corrective lenses (self-image).

Follow-Up, Evaluation, and Desired Outcomes

▶ Acknowledges contact information provided for patient education on the topic of eye care, such as the American Academy of Ophthalmologists (www .aao.org) or American Optometric Association (www.aoa.org or www .allaboutvision.com).

Renin

SYNONYM/ACRONYM: Plasma renin activity (PRA), angiotensinogenase.

RATIONALE: To assist in evaluating for a possible cause of hypertension.

PATIENT PREPARATION: There are no fluid restrictions unless by medical direction. The patient should be on a normal sodium diet (1–2 g sodium per day) for 2 to 4 wk before the test. Inform the patient or family member that the position required (supine or upright) must be maintained for 2 hr before specimen collection. By medical direction, the patient should avoid diuretics, antihypertensive drugs, herbals, cyclic progestogens, and estrogens for 2 to 4 wk before the test. Protocols may vary among facilities.

NORMAL FINDINGS: Method: Enzyme linked immunoassay.

Age and Position	Conventional Units	SI Units (Conventional Units × 1)
Newborn–12 mo	2–35 ng/mL/hr	2–35 mcg/L/hr
Supine, normal sodium diet		
1–3 yr	1.7–11.2 ng/mL/hr	1.7–11.2 mcg/L/hr
4–5 yr	1–6.5 ng/mL/hr	1.0–6.5 mcg/L/hr
6–10 yr	0.5–5.9 ng/mL/hr	0.5–5.9 mcg/L/hr
11–15 yr	0.5–3.3 ng/mL/hr	0.5–3.3 mcg/L/hr
Adult	0.2–2.3 ng/mL/hr	0.2–2.3 mcg/L/hr
Upright, normal sodium diet		
Adult–older adult	0.5–4 ng/mL/hr	0.5–4 mcg/L/hr

Values vary according to the laboratory performing the test, as well as the patient's age, gender, dietary pattern, state of hydration, posture, and physical activity.

CRITICAL FINDINGS AND POTENTIAL INTERVENTIONS: N/A

OVERVIEW: (**Study type:** Blood collected in a lavender-top [EDTA] or pink-top [K2-EDTA] tube; **related body system:** Endocrine and Urinary systems. Specify patient position [upright or supine] and exact source of specimen [peripheral vs. arterial]. Venipuncture should be performed after the patient has been in the upright [sitting or standing] position for 2 hr. If a supine specimen is requested on an inpatient, the specimen should be collected early in the morning before the patient rises. The specimen should be immediately transported in an ice slurry to the laboratory.) Renin is an enzymatic peptide hormone secreted by the granular cells of the juxtaglomerular apparatus in the kidney in response to sodium depletion and hypovolemia. Renin activates the renin-angiotensin system through the conversion of angiotensinogen to angiotensin I. Angiotensin I is converted to the biologically active angiotensin II by angiotensin-converting enzyme primarily within the capillaries of the lungs. Angiotensin II is a powerful vasoconstrictor that ultimately maintains the appropriate perfusion pressure in the kidneys. Angiotensin II stimulates aldosterone production in the adrenal cortex, secretion of antidiuretic hormone from the pituitary, and stimulates the thirst reflex from the hypothalmus. The net effect is regulation of blood pressure by regulating arterial vasoconstriction and the movement of extracellular fluids such as plasma, lymphatic fluid, and interstitial fluid. Excessive amounts of angiotensin II cause renal hypertension. The random collection of specimens without prior dietary preparations does not provide clinically significant information. Values should also be evaluated along with simultaneously collected aldosterone levels (see studies titled "Aldosterone" and "Angiotensin-Converting Enzyme").

INDICATIONS

- Assist in the identification of primary hyperaldosteronism resulting from aldosterone-secreting adrenal adenoma.
- Assist in monitoring patients on mineralocorticoid therapy.

R

• Assist in the screening of the origin of essential, renal, or renovascular hypertension.

INTERFERING FACTORS
Factors that may alter the results of the study
• Drugs and other substances that may increase renin levels include albuterol, amiloride, azosemide, benazepril, bendroflumethiazide, captopril, chlorthalidone, cilazapril, desmopressin, diazoxide, dihydralazine, doxazosin, enalapril, endralazine, felodipine, fenoldopam, fosinopril, furosemide, hydralazine, hydrochlorothiazide, laxatives, lisinopril, lithium, methyclothiazide, metolazone, muzolimine, nicardipine, nifedipine, opiates, oral contraceptives, perindopril, ramipril, spironolactone, triamterene, and xipamide.
• Drugs and other substances that may decrease renin levels include acetylsalicylic acid, angiotensin, angiotensin II, atenolol, bopindolol, bucindolol, carbenoxolone, carvedilol, clonidine, cyclosporin A, glycyrrhiza, ibuprofen, indomethacin, levodopa, metoprolol, naproxen, nicardipine, NSAIDs, oral contraceptives, oxprenolol, propranolol, sulindac, and vasopressin.
• Upright body posture, stress, and strenuous exercise can increase renin levels.
• Diet can significantly affect results (e.g., low-sodium diets stimulate the release of renin).
• Hyperkalemia, acute increase in blood pressure, and increased blood volume may suppress renin secretion.

POTENTIAL MEDICAL DIAGNOSIS: CLINICAL SIGNIFICANCE OF RESULTS
Increased in
• Addison disease *(related to hyponatremia, which stimulates production of renin)*

• Bartter syndrome *(related to hereditary defect in loop of Henle that affects sodium resorption; hyponatremia stimulates renin production)*
• Cirrhosis *(related to fluid buildup, which dilutes sodium concentration; hyponatremia is a strong stimulus for production of renin)*
• Gastrointestinal disorders with electrolyte loss *(related to hyponatremia, which stimulates production of renin)*
• Heart failure *(related to fluid buildup, which dilutes sodium concentration; hyponatremia is a strong stimulus for production of renin)*
• Hepatitis *(related to fluid buildup, which dilutes sodium concentration; hyponatremia is a strong stimulus for production of renin)*
• Hypokalemia *(related to decreased potassium levels, which stimulate renin production)*
• Malignant hypertension *(related to secondary hyperaldosteronism that constricts the blood vessels and results in hypertension)*
• Nephritis *(the kidneys can produce renin in response to inflammation or disease)*
• Nephropathies with sodium or potassium wasting *(related to hyponatremia, which stimulates production of renin)*
• Pheochromocytoma *(related to renin production in response to hypertension)*
• Pregnancy *(related to retention of fluid and hyponatremia that stimulates renin production; normal pregnancy is associated with changes in the balance between renin and angiotensin)*
• Renin-producing kidney tumors
• Renovascular hypertension *(related to decreased renal blood flow, which stimulates release of renin)*

Decreased in
• Cushing syndrome *(related to excessive production of glucocorticoids,*

which increase sodium levels and decrease potassium levels, inhibiting renin production)

- Primary hyperaldosteronism *(related to aldosterone-secreting adrenal tumor; aldosterone inhibits renin production)*

NURSING IMPLICATIONS

BEFORE THE STUDY: PLANNING AND IMPLEMENTATION

Teaching the Patient What to Expect
- Inform the patient this test can assist in evaluating for high blood pressure.
- Explain that a blood sample is needed for the test. Inform the patient that multiple specimens may be required.

Potential Nursing Actions
- Verify adherence to ordered pretest instructions regarding diet and medications.

AFTER THE STUDY: POTENTIAL NURSING ACTIONS

Treatment Considerations
- Instruct the patient to resume usual medications, as directed by the HCP.
- Explain the importance of notifying the HCP of any signs and symptoms of dehydration or fluid overload related to abnormal renin levels or compromised sodium regulatory mechanisms. Fluid loss or dehydration is signaled by the thirst response. Decreased skin turgor, dry mouth, and multiple longitudinal furrows in the tongue are symptoms of dehydration. Fluid overload may be signaled by a loss of appetite and

nausea. Excessive fluid also causes pitting edema: When firm pressure is placed on the skin over a bone (e.g., the ankle), the indentation will remain after 5 sec.
- Provide education on the importance of proper water balance. *In the case of hard water, untreated tap water contains minerals such as calcium, magnesium, and iron. Water-softening systems replace these minerals with sodium, and therefore patients on a low-sodium diet should avoid drinking treated tap water and drink bottled water instead.*

Nutritional Considerations
- Explain to patients with low sodium levels that the major source of dietary sodium is found in table salt. Many foods, such as milk and other dairy products, are also good sources of dietary sodium. Most other dietary sodium is available through the consumption of processed foods.
- Explain to patients on low-sodium diets to avoid beverages such as colas, ginger ale, sports drinks, lemon-lime sodas, and root beer. Many over-the-counter medications, including antacids, laxatives, analgesics, sedatives, and antitussives, contain significant amounts of sodium. A registered dietitian should be consulted before using salt substitutes.
- Explain that potassium is present in all plant and animal cells, making dietary replacement fairly simple to achieve.

Follow-Up, Evaluation, and Desired Outcomes
- Recognizes the value of reading all food, beverage, and medicine labels to evaluate nutritional value.
- Understands that renin levels affect the regulation of fluid balance and electrolytes.

R

Renogram

SYNONYM/ACRONYM: MAG$_3$ scan, radioactive renogram, renocystography, renocystogram, renal scintigraphy.

RATIONALE: To assist in diagnosing kidney disorders such as embolism, obstruction, infection, inflammation, trauma, stones, and bleeding.

PATIENT PREPARATION: There are no food, fluid, activity, or medication restrictions unless by medical direction. No other radionuclide tests should be scheduled within 24 to 48 hr before this procedure.

NORMAL FINDINGS
- Normal shape, size, position, symmetry, vasculature, perfusion, and function of the kidneys
- Radionuclide material circulates bilaterally, symmetrically, and without interruption through the renal parenchyma, ureters, and urinary bladder, with 50% of the radionuclide excreted within the first 10 min.

CRITICAL FINDINGS AND POTENTIAL INTERVENTIONS: N/A

OVERVIEW: (Study type: Nuclear scan; related body system: Urinary system.) A renogram is a nuclear medicine study performed to assist in diagnosing renal disorders, such as abnormal blood flow, collecting-system defects, and excretion dysfunction. Because renography uses no iodinated contrast medium, it is safe to use in patients who have iodine allergies or compromised renal function.

After IV administration of the radioisotope, information about the structures of the kidneys is obtained. Commonly used tracers include Tc-99 or MAG$_3$ (mercaptoacetyltriglycine). The radioactive material is detected by a gamma camera, which can detect the gamma rays emitted by the radionuclide in the kidney. Renography simultaneously tracks the rate at which the radionuclide flows into *(vascular phase),* through *(tubular phase),* and out of *(excretory phase)* the kidneys. The times are plotted on a graph and compared to normal parameters of organ function. Differential estimates of left and right kidney contributions to glomerular filtration rate and effective renal plasma flow can be calculated. With the use of diuretic stimulation during the excretory phase, it is possible to differentiate between anatomic obstruction and nonobstructive residual dilation from previous hydronephrosis. All information obtained is stored in a computer to be used for further interpretation and computations. Kidney function can be monitored by serially repeating this test and comparing results.

INDICATIONS
- Aid in the diagnosis of renal artery embolism or renal infarction causing obstruction.
- Aid in the diagnosis of renal artery stenosis resulting from renal dysplasia or atherosclerosis and causing arterial hypertension and reduced glomerular filtration rate.
- Aid in the diagnosis of renal vein thrombosis resulting from dehydration in infants or obstruction of blood flow in the presence of renal tumors in adults.
- Detect infectious or inflammatory diseases of the kidney, such as acute or chronic pyelonephritis, abscess, or nephritis.
- Determine the presence and effects of kidney trauma, such as arterial injury, renal contusion, hematoma, rupture, arteriovenous fistula, or urinary extravasation.
- Determine the presence, location, and cause of obstructive uropathy, such as calculi, tumor, congenital disorders, scarring, or inflammation.

R

- Evaluate acute kidney injury and chronic kidney disease.
- Evaluate chronic urinary tract infections, especially in children.
- Evaluate kidney transplant for acute or chronic rejection.
- Evaluate obstruction caused by stones or tumor.

INTERFERING FACTORS
Contraindications
⬥ Patients who are pregnant or suspected of being pregnant, unless the potential benefits of a procedure using radiation far outweigh the risk of radiation exposure to the fetus and mother.

Factors that may alter the results of the study
- Serum creatinine levels greater than or equal to 3 mg/dL (depending on the radionuclide used), which can decrease renal perfusion.
- Medications such as antihypertensives, angiotensin-converting enzyme (ACE) inhibitors, and β-blockers taken within 24 hr of the test.
- Dehydration, which can accentuate abnormalities, or overhydration, which can mask abnormalities.
- Metallic objects (e.g., jewelry, body rings) within the examination field, other nuclear scans done within the previous 24 to 48 hr, or retained barium from a previous radiological procedure, which may inhibit organ visualization and cause unclear images.
- Improper injection of the radionuclide that allows the tracer to seep deep into the muscle tissue can produce erroneous hot spots.
- Inability of the patient to cooperate or remain still during the procedure, because movement can produce blurred or otherwise unclear images.

Other considerations
- Inaccurate timing of imaging after the radionuclide injection can affect the results.

POTENTIAL MEDICAL DIAGNOSIS: CLINICAL SIGNIFICANCE OF RESULTS
Abnormal findings related to
- Acute tubular necrosis
- Chronic kidney disease, infarction, cyst, or abscess
- Congenital anomalies (e.g., absence of a kidney)
- Decreased kidney function
- Diminished blood supply
- Infection or inflammation (pyelonephritis, glomerulonephritis)
- Masses
- Obstructive uropathy
- Renal vascular disease, including renal artery stenosis or renal vein thrombosis
- Trauma

NURSING IMPLICATIONS

BEFORE THE STUDY: PLANNING AND IMPLEMENTATION

Teaching the Patient What to Expect
▶ Inform the patient this procedure can assist in assessing the renal system.
▶ Pregnancy is a general contraindication to procedures involving radiation. Explain to the female patient that she will be asked the date of her last menstrual period and pregnancy testing may be performed to determine the possibility of pregnancy before she is exposed to radiation.
▶ Review the procedure with the patient. Address concerns about pain and explain that there may be moments of discomfort or pain experienced when the IV line is inserted to allow infusion of fluids such as saline, anesthetics, sedatives, radionuclides, medications used in the procedure, or emergency medications.
▶ Explain that the procedure is performed in a nuclear medicine department by a

R

health-care provider (HCP) and usually takes approximately 60 to 90 min.

▶ Advise that delayed images are needed 2 to 24 hr later and that the patient may leave the department and return later to undergo delayed imaging.

▶ Reassure the patient that the radionuclide poses no radioactive hazard and rarely produces adverse effects.

▶ Instruct the patient to remove jewelry and other metallic objects from the area to be examined prior to the procedure.

▶ Explain that it will be necessary to drink several glasses of fluid before the study for hydration, unless there are fluid restrictions for other reasons.

▶ Baseline vital signs and neurological status are recorded. Protocols may vary among facilities.

▶ Positioning for this study is in a supine position on a flat table with foam wedges to help maintain position and immobilization.

▶ The radionuclide is administered IV, and the kidney area is scanned immediately with images taken every minute for 30 min; delayed imaging is conducted at additional intervals as ordered.

▶ During the flow and static imaging, the diuretic furosemide or ACE inhibitor (captopril) can be administered IV and images obtained.

▶ Urine and blood laboratory studies are done after the renogram to correlate findings before diagnosis.

▶ Explain that if a study for vesicoureteral reflux is done, the patient is asked to void, and a catheter is inserted into the bladder. The radionuclide is instilled into the bladder, and multiple images are obtained during bladder filling. The request is then made to void with the catheter in place or after catheter removal, depending on department policy. Imaging is continued during and after voiding. Reflux is determined by calculating the urine volume and counts obtained by imaging.

▶ Explain that once the study is completed, the needle or catheter is removed and a pressure dressing applied over the puncture site.

Potential Nursing Actions

▶ *Make sure a written and informed consent has been signed prior to the procedure and before administering any medications.*

AFTER THE STUDY: POTENTIAL NURSING ACTIONS

Avoiding Complications

▶ Establishing an IV site and injection of radionuclides are invasive procedures. Complications are rare but include risk for allergic reaction *(related to contrast reaction)*, hematoma *(related to blood leakage into the tissue following needle insertion)*, bleeding from the puncture site *(related to a bleeding disorder or the effects of natural products and medications with known anticoagulant, antiplatelet, or thrombolytic properties)*, or infection *(which might occur if bacteria from the skin surface is introduced at the puncture site)*. Monitor the patient for complications related to the procedure (e.g., allergic reaction, anaphylaxis, bronchospasm). Immediately report symptoms such as fast heart rate, difficulty breathing, skin rash, itching, or chest pain to the appropriate HCP. Observe/assess the needle/catheter insertion site for bleeding, inflammation, or hematoma formation.

Treatment Considerations

▶ Explain that the radionuclide is eliminated from the body within 6 to 24 hr. Advise the patient to drink increased amounts of fluids for 24 to 48 hr to eliminate the radionuclide from the body, unless contraindicated.

▶ Verification of infection may be the purpose of this procedure. Infection can also occur as an unexpected outcome related to performance of a procedure. Monitor indicators of infection such as WBC, CRP, urine culture, and body temperature.

▶ Pain may be present related to the individual diagnosis secondary to the disease progression. Always assess pain character, location, duration, and intensity with the use of an easily understood pain rating scale. Implement interventions as appropriate to the clinical situation.

R

▶ Provide instruction in the care and assessment of the site.

▶ Explain that application of cold compresses to the puncture site may reduce discomfort or edema.

Safety Considerations

▶ The patient who is breastfeeding should consult with the requesting HCP regarding alternate testing that does not involve radiation. In general, if a woman who is breastfeeding must have a nuclear scan, she should not breastfeed the infant for 72 hr after the scan, until the radionuclide has been eliminated. She should be instructed to express the milk in order to prevent cessation of milk production; the milk can be stored and used after the 3-day period.

▶ Refer to organizational policy for additional precautions that may include instructions on handwashing, toilet flushing, limited contact with others, and other aspects of nuclear medicine safety.

Nutritional Considerations

▶ Teach the patient to avoid foods that facilitate stone formation (tea, beer, chocolate) when diagnosed with stones.

▶ Teach the patient foods that can discourage stone formation, such as milk and milk products.

Follow-Up, Evaluation, and Desired Outcomes

▶ Understands that further testing may be necessary to monitor disease progression and evaluate the effectiveness of treatment options.

▶ The patient and family acknowledge the importance of completing prescribed antibiotic regimen.

▶ The patient agrees to diet changes that will facilitate renal health.

Reticulocyte Count

SYNONYM/ACRONYM: Retic count.

RATIONALE: To assess reticulocyte count in relation to bone marrow activity toward diagnosing anemias such as pernicious iron deficiency, and hemolytic anemia; to monitor response of therapeutic interventions.

PATIENT PREPARATION: There are no food, fluid, activity, or medication restrictions unless by medical direction.

NORMAL FINDINGS: Method: Automated analyzer or microscopic examination of specially stained peripheral blood smear.

Age	Reticulocyte Count %
Newborn	3%–6%
Infant	0.4%–2.8%
Child	0.8%–2.1%
Adult–older adult	0.5%–1.5%
	Reticulocyte Count (Absolute Number)
Birth–older adult	0.02–0.10 (10^6 cells/microL)
	Immature Reticulocyte Fraction %
Birth	2.5%–6.5%
Newborn–older adult	2.5%–17%

R

(table continues on page 1048)

Age	Reticulocyte Count %
	Reticulocyte Hemoglobin
Birth	22–32 pg/cell
Newborn–18 yr	23–34 pg/cell
Adult–older adult	30–35 pg/cell

CRITICAL FINDINGS AND POTENTIAL INTERVENTIONS: N/A

OVERVIEW: (**Study type:** Blood collected in a lavender-top [EDTA] tube; **related body system:** Circulatory/Hematopoietic system.) Normally, as it matures, the red blood cell (RBC) loses its nucleus. The remaining ribonucleic acid (RNA) produces a characteristic color when special stains are used, making these cells easy to identify and enumerate. Some automated cell counters have the ability to provide a reticulocyte panel, which includes the enumeration of circulating reticulocytes as an absolute count and as a percentage of total RBCs; the immature reticulocyte fraction, which reflects the number of reticulocytes released into the circulation within the past 24 to 48 hr; and the reticulocyte hemoglobin content, which reflects the amount of iron incorporated into the maturing RBCs. The presence of reticulocytes is an indication of the level of erythropoietic activity in the bone marrow. The information provided by the reticulocyte panel is useful in the evaluation of anemias, bone marrow response to therapy, degree of bone marrow engraftment following transplant, and the effectiveness of altitude training in high-performance athletes. In abnormal conditions, reticulocytes are prematurely released into circulation. (See studies titled "RBC Count, Indices, Morphology, and Inclusions.")

INDICATIONS
• Evaluate erythropoietic activity.
• Monitor response to therapy for anemias.

INTERFERING FACTORS
Factors that may alter the results of the study
• Drugs and other substances that may increase reticulocyte counts include acetylsalicylic acid, amyl nitrate, antimalarials, antipyretics, antipyrine, arsenicals, corticotropin, dimercaprol, etretinate, furazolidone, levodopa, methyldopa, nitrofurans, penicillin, procainamide, and sulfones.
• Drugs and other substances that may decrease reticulocyte counts include azathioprine, dactinomycin, hydroxyurea, methotrexate, and zidovudine.
• Reticulocyte count may be falsely increased by the presence of RBC inclusions (Howell-Jolly bodies, Heinz bodies, and Pappenheimer bodies) that stain with methylene blue.
• Reticulocyte count may be falsely decreased as a result of the dilutional effect after a recent blood transfusion.

Other considerations
• Specimens that are clotted or hemolyzed should be rejected for analysis.

POTENTIAL MEDICAL DIAGNOSIS: CLINICAL SIGNIFICANCE OF RESULTS
The reticulocyte production index (RPI) is a good estimate of RBC production. The calculation corrects the count for anemia and for the premature

R

release of reticulocytes into the peripheral blood during periods of hemolysis or significant bleeding. The RPI also takes into consideration the maturation time of large polychromatophilic cells or nucleated RBCs seen on the peripheral smear:

RPI = % reticulocytes × [patient hematocrit (Hct)/normal Hct] × (1/maturation time)

As the formula shows, the RPI is inversely proportional to Hct, as follows:

Hematocrit (%)	Maturation Time (d)
45	1
35	1.5
25	2
15	2.5

Increased in
Conditions that result in excessive RBC loss or destruction stimulate a compensatory bone marrow response by increasing production of RBCs.

- Blood loss
- Hemolytic anemias
- Iron-deficiency anemia
- Malaria
- Megaloblastic anemia

Other

- Pregnancy
- Treatment for anemia

Decreased in
- Alcohol misuse *(decreased production related to nutritional deficit)*

- Anemia of chronic disease
- Aplastic anemia *(related to overall lack of RBC)*
- Bone marrow replacement *(new marrow fails to produce RBCs until it engrafts)*
- Endocrine disease *(hypometabolism related to hypothyroidism is reflected by decreased bone marrow activity)*
- Kidney disease *(diseased kidneys cannot produce erythropoietin, which stimulates the bone marrow to produce RBCs)*
- RBC aplasia *(related to overall lack of RBCs)*
- Sideroblastic anemia *(RBCs are produced but are abnormal in that they cannot incorporate iron into hemoglobin, resulting in anemia)*

NURSING IMPLICATIONS

BEFORE THE STUDY: PLANNING AND IMPLEMENTATION

Teaching the Patient What to Expect
- Inform the patient this test can assist in assessing for anemia.
- Explain that a blood sample is needed for the test.

AFTER THE STUDY: POTENTIAL NURSING ACTIONS

Follow-Up, Evaluation, and Desired Outcomes
- Understands that depending on the results of this procedure, additional testing may be performed to evaluate or monitor disease progress and determine the need for a change in therapy.

R

Retrograde Ureteropyelography

SYNONYM/ACRONYM: Retrograde pyelography.

RATIONALE: To assess the urinary tract for trauma, obstruction, stones, infection, and abscess that can interfere with genitourinary function.

PATIENT PREPARATION: There are no activity restrictions unless by medical direction. Instruct the patient to fast and restrict fluids for 8 hr, or as ordered, prior to the procedure. Fasting may be ordered as a precaution against aspiration related to possible nausea and vomiting. The American Society of Anesthesiologists has fasting guidelines for risk levels according to patient status. More information can be located at www.asahq.org.

Note: If iodinated contrast medium is scheduled to be used in patients receiving metformin or drugs containing metformin for type 2 diabetes, the drug may be discontinued on the day of the test and continue to be withheld for 48 hr after the test.

Regarding the patient's risk for bleeding, the patient should be instructed to avoid taking natural products and medications with known anticoagulant, antiplatelet, or thrombolytic properties or to reduce dosage, as ordered, prior to the procedure. Number of days to withhold medication is dependent on the type of anticoagulant. Note the last time and dose of medication taken. Protocols may vary among facilities.

NORMAL FINDINGS
- Normal outline and opacification of renal pelvis and calyces
- Normal size and uniform filling of the ureters
- Symmetrical and bilateral outline of structures.

CRITICAL FINDINGS AND POTENTIAL INTERVENTIONS: N/A

OVERVIEW: (Study type: X-ray, contrast/special; **related body system:** Urinary system.) Retrograde ureteropyelography uses a contrast medium introduced through a ureteral catheter during cystography and radiographic visualization to view the renal collecting system (calyces, renal pelvis, and urethra). During a cystoscopic examination, a catheter is advanced through the ureters and into the kidney and contrast medium is injected through the catheter into the kidney. This procedure is primarily used in patients who are known to be hypersensitive to IV injected iodine-based contrast medium and when excretory ureterography does not adequately reveal the renal collecting system. The incidence of allergic reaction to the contrast medium is reduced because there is less systemic absorption of the contrast medium when injected into the kidney than when injected IV. Retrograde ureteropyelography sometimes provides more information about the anatomy of the different parts of the collecting system than can be obtained by excretory ureteropyelography. Computed tomography (CT) and ultrasound studies are replacing retrograde pyelography because they are less invasive and the quality of the technology has significantly improved.

INDICATIONS
- Evaluate the effects of urinary system trauma.
- Evaluate known or suspected ureteral obstruction.
- Evaluate placement of a ureteral stent or catheter.
- Evaluate the presence of calculi in the kidneys, ureters, or bladder.
- Evaluate the renal collecting system when excretory urography is unsuccessful.

- Evaluate space-occupying lesions or congenital anomalies of the urinary system.
- Evaluate the structure and integrity of the renal collecting system.

INTERFERING FACTORS
Contraindications

Patients who are pregnant or suspected of being pregnant, unless the potential benefits of a procedure using radiation far outweigh the risk of radiation exposure to the fetus and mother.

Patients with conditions associated with adverse reactions to contrast medium (e.g., asthma, food allergies, or allergy to contrast medium). Although patients are asked specifically if they have a known allergy to iodine or shellfish (shellfish contain high levels of iodine), it has been well established that the reaction is not to iodine; an actual iodine allergy would be problematic because iodine is required for the production of thyroid hormones. In the case of shellfish, the reaction is to a muscle protein called *tropomyosin;* in the case of iodinated contrast medium, the reaction is to the noniodinated part of the contrast molecule. Patients with a known hypersensitivity to the medium may benefit from premedication with corticosteroids and diphenhydramine; the use of nonionic contrast or an alternative noncontrast imaging study, if available, may be considered for patients who have severe asthma or who have experienced moderate to severe reactions to ionic contrast medium.

Patients with conditions associated with preexisting renal insufficiency (e.g., chronic kidney disease, single kidney transplant, nephrectomy, diabetes, multiple myeloma, treatment with aminoglycosides and NSAIDs), *because iodinated contrast is nephrotoxic.*

Patients who are chronically dehydrated before the test, especially older adults and patients whose health is already compromised, *because of their risk of contrast-induced acute kidney injury.*

Patients with bleeding disorders, because the puncture site may not stop bleeding.

Factors that may alter the results of the study
- Gas or feces in the gastrointestinal tract resulting from inadequate cleansing or failure to restrict food intake before the study.
- Retained barium from a previous radiological procedure.
- Metallic objects (e.g., jewelry, body rings) within the examination field, which may inhibit organ visualization and cause unclear images.
- Inability of the patient to cooperate or remain still during the procedure, because movement can produce blurred or otherwise unclear images.

POTENTIAL MEDICAL DIAGNOSIS: CLINICAL SIGNIFICANCE OF RESULTS
Abnormal findings related to
- Congenital renal or urinary tract abnormalities
- Hydronephrosis
- Tumors
- Obstruction as a result of tumor, blood clot, stricture, or calculi
- Obstruction of ureteropelvic junction
- Perinephric abscess
- Perinephric inflammation or suppuration
- Polycystic kidney disease
- Prostatic enlargement
- Tumor of the kidneys or the collecting system

R

NURSING IMPLICATIONS

POTENTIAL NURSING PROBLEMS: ASSESSMENT & NURSING DIAGNOSIS

Problems	Signs and Symptoms
Infection *(related to stones, urinary stasis, invasive procedure, postoperative change in skin condition [incision])*	Fever; chills; changes in laboratory studies (WBC, C-reactive protein, urine culture); diaphoresis; increased heart rate; urine frequency and burning; cloudy, foul-smelling urine; red, indurated incision
Insufficient fluid volume *(related to vomiting, nausea)*	Dry mucous membranes, low blood pressure, increased heart rate, slow capillary refill, diminished skin turgor, diminished urine output
Pain *(related to stones, obstruction and/or anomalies, spasm)*	Self-report of pain in flank area, facial grimace, moaning, crying, abdominal guarding

BEFORE THE STUDY: PLANNING AND IMPLEMENTATION

Teaching the Patient What to Expect

▶ Inform the patient this procedure can assist in assessing the urinary tract.

▶ Explain that prior to the procedure, laboratory testing may be required to determine the possibility of bleeding risk (coagulation testing) or to assess for impaired kidney function (creatinine level and estimated glomerular filtration rate) if use of iodinated contrast medium is anticipated.

▶ Pregnancy is a general contraindication to procedures involving radiation. Explain to the female patient that she will be asked the date of her last menstrual period. Pregnancy testing may be performed to determine the possibility of pregnancy before exposure to radiation.

▶ Review the procedure with the patient. Address concerns about pain and explain that there may be moments of discomfort or pain experienced when the IV line or catheter is inserted to allow infusion of fluids such as saline, anesthetics, sedatives, contrast medium, medications used in the procedure, or emergency medications.

▶ Explain that contrast medium will be injected, by catheter, at a separate site from the IV line.

▶ Advise that a burning and flushing sensation may be felt throughout the body during injection of the contrast medium and that the patient may experience an urge to cough, flushing, nausea, or a salty or metallic taste.

▶ Inform the patient that if a local anesthetic is used, the patient may feel (1) some pressure in the kidney area as the catheter is introduced and contrast medium injected and (2) the urgency to void.

▶ Inform the patient that the procedure is performed in a special department, usually in a radiology or vascular suite, by a health-care provider (HCP), with support staff, and takes approximately 30 to 60 min.

▶ Instruct the patient to remove jewelry and other metallic objects from the area to be examined prior to the procedure.

▶ Baseline vital signs are recorded and monitored throughout the procedure. Protocols may vary among facilities.

▶ Explain that electrocardiographic electrodes are placed for cardiac monitoring to establish a baseline rhythm and identify any ventricular dysrhythmias.

R

- Positioning for this procedure is supine on the examination table in the lithotomy position.
- A kidney, ureter, and bladder (KUB) or plain image is taken to ensure that no barium or stool will obscure visualization of the urinary system. The patient may be asked to hold his or her breath to facilitate visualization.
- The patient is given a local anesthetic, and a cystoscopic examination is performed and the bladder is inspected.
- A catheter is inserted, and the renal pelvis is emptied by gravity. Contrast medium is introduced into the catheter. Inform the patient that the contrast medium may cause a temporary flushing of the face, a feeling of warmth, or nausea.
- X-ray images are taken and the results processed. Inform the patient that additional images may be necessary to visualize the area in question.
- Additional contrast medium is injected through the catheter to outline the ureters as the catheter is withdrawn.
- The catheter may be kept in place and attached to a gravity drainage unit until urinary flow has returned or is corrected.
- Additional x-ray images are taken 10 to 15 min after the catheter is removed to evaluate retention of the contrast medium, indicating urinary stasis.
- Explain to the patient that he or she will be monitored for complications related to the procedure (e.g., allergic reaction, anaphylaxis, bronchospasm).
- Explain that once the study is completed, the needle or catheter is removed, and a pressure dressing is applied over the puncture site.

Potential Nursing Actions

- Follow the facility's guidelines regarding the administration of prophylactic antibiotics, by medical direction, prior to a procedure that involves manipulation of the ureters.

Safety Considerations

- Anticoagulants, aspirin, and other salicylates should be discontinued by medical direction for the appropriate number of days prior to a procedure in which bleeding is a potential complication.

Avoiding Complications

- Establishing an IV site and injection of contrast medium are invasive procedures. Complications are rare but include risk for allergic reaction *(related to contrast reaction),* bleeding from the puncture site *(related to a bleeding disorder or the effects of natural products and medications with known anticoagulant, antiplatelet, or thrombolytic properties),* hematoma *(related to blood leakage into the tissue following needle insertion),* infection *(which might occur if bacteria from the skin surface are introduced at the puncture site),* hematuria *(related to insertion of cystoscope),* nerve injury *(which might occur if the needle strikes a nerve),* nephrotoxicity *(a deterioration of renal function associated with contrast administration),* sepsis *(related to bacterial contamination from infected urine),* or urinary tract infection *(related to insertion of cystoscope or catheter).* Monitor the patient for complications related to the procedure (e.g., allergic reaction, anaphylaxis, bronchospasm, infection, injury). Immediately report symptoms such as difficulty breathing, chest pain, fever, hyperpnea, hypertension, nausea, palpitations, pruritus, rash, tachycardia, urticaria, or vomiting to the appropriate HCP. Observe/assess the needle/catheter insertion site for bleeding, inflammation, or hematoma formation. Administer ordered antihistamines or prophylactic steroids if the patient has an allergic reaction.

Treatment Considerations

- Instruct the patient to resume usual diet, fluids, medications, and activity, as directed by the HCP. Kidney function should be assessed before metformin is resumed.
- Monitor vital signs and neurological status every 15 min for 1 hr, then every 2 hr for 4 hr, and then as ordered. Take temperature every 4 hr for 24 hr. Monitor intake and output at least every 8 hr. Compare with baseline values. Notify the HCP if temperature is elevated. Protocols may vary among facilities.

R

- Monitor for signs of sepsis and severe pain in the kidney area.
- Infection: Monitor and trend laboratory results, vital signs, surgical site for redness, induration, drainage, and urine characteristics (color, odor, blood). Administer ordered antibiotics and antipyretic.
- Maintain adequate hydration after the procedure and encourage drinking lots of fluids to prevent stasis and to prevent the buildup of bacteria.
- Insufficient Fluid Volume: Monitor and trend vital signs and laboratory studies (uric acid, BUN, Cr, electrolytes), intake and output, and urine color. Administer ordered parenteral fluids and encourage oral fluid intake. Administer ordered antiemetics.
- Pain: Assess pain character, location, duration, and intensity using an easily understood pain rating scale. Consider alternative measures for pain management (imagery, relaxation, music, etc.). Place in a position for comfort; knees to chest may be most effective. Administer ordered analgesics, parenteral fluids, and encourage an increase in oral fluids. Monitor and trend laboratory studies; BUN, Cr, WBC count, uric acid, calcium, and electrolytes. Strain urine.

- Explain the use of any ordered medications and the importance of adhering to the therapy regimen.
- Instruct the patient in the care and assessment of the site.
- Explain the importance of applying cold compresses to the puncture site as needed to reduce discomfort or edema.
- Provide information on significant adverse effects associated with the prescribed medication. Encourage a review of corresponding literature provided by a pharmacist.

Safety Considerations
- Advise diabetic patients to avoid all medications containing metformin for 48 hr following a procedure with iodinated contrast. Iodinated contrast can temporarily impair kidney function, and failure to withhold metformin may indirectly result in drug-induced lactic acidosis, a dangerous and sometimes fatal adverse effect of metformin (related to renal impairment that does not support sufficient excretion of metformin).

Follow-Up, Evaluation, and Desired Outcomes
- Correctly identifies symptoms of delayed allergic reaction or infection and whom to contact should they occur.

Rheumatoid Factor

SYNONYM/ACRONYM: RF, RA.

RATIONALE: To primarily assist in diagnosing rheumatoid arthritis.

PATIENT PREPARATION: There are no food, fluid, activity, or medication restrictions unless by medical direction.

NORMAL FINDINGS: (Method: Immunoturbidimetric) Less than 14 international units/mL. Elevated values may be detected in healthy adults 60 yr and older.

CRITICAL FINDINGS AND POTENTIAL INTERVENTIONS: N/A

OVERVIEW: (Study type: Blood collected in a gold-, red-, or red/gray-top tube; related body system: Immune and Musculoskeletal systems.) Rheumatoid arthritis (RA) is a chronic, systemic autoimmune disease that damages the synovium or membrane surrounding the joints. Collagen, the main fibrous protein in tendons, bone, and other types of connective tissue, is gradually destroyed, narrowing the joint space. As the disease progresses, a pannus or growth of thickened synovial tissue forms and permeates the bone and cartilage, leading to permanent damage and joint deformity. Inflammation caused by autoimmune responses can affect other organs and body systems. The American College of Rheumatology (ACR)'s current criteria focuses on earlier classification of newly presenting patients who have at least one swollen joint unrelated to another condition. The criteria includes four determinants:

1. Joint involvement (number and size of joints involved)
2. Serological test results (rheumatoid factor [RF] and/or anticitrullinated protein antibody [ACPA])
3. Indications of acute inflammation (C-reactive protein [CRP] and/or erythrocyte sedimentation rate [ESR])
4. Duration of symptoms (weeks)

Each determinant includes specific criteria with assigned values (e.g., duration of symptoms less than 6 wk = 0, duration of symptoms equal to or greater than 6 wk = 1). The scores from each determinant are added together. A score of 6 of 10 or greater for the score based algorithm defines the presence of RA. Patients with longstanding RA, whose condition is inactive, or whose prior history would have satisfied the previous classification criteria by having four of seven findings—morning stiffness, arthritis of three or more joint areas, arthritis of hand joints, symmetric arthritis, rheumatoid nodules, abnormal amounts of rheumatoid factor, and radiographic changes—should remain classified as having RA. The ACR favors the consideration of classification criteria rather than endorsement of *diagnostic* criteria for RA because of the difficulty in establishing a consistent set of criteria. The study of RA is complex, and it is believed that multiple genes may be involved in the manifestation of RA. The diagnosis of RA is made for patients on an individual basis by considering the ACR's classification criteria, in the presence of additional information unique to the patient, and his or her genetic predisposition, lifestyle, and environment. The study of RA is complex, and it is believed that multiple genes may be involved in the manifestation of RA. Individuals with RA harbor a macroglobulin-type antibody called *rheumatoid factor* in their blood. Patients with other diseases (e.g., systemic lupus erythematosus [SLE] and occasionally tuberculosis, chronic hepatitis, infectious mononucleosis, and subacute bacterial endocarditis) may also test positive for RF. RF antibodies

R

are usually immunoglobulin M (IgM) but may also be IgG or IgA. Women are two to three times more likely than men to develop RA. Although RA is most likely to affect people aged 35 to 50, it can affect all ages.

Other Serum Markers for RA: Studies show that detection of antibodies formed against citrullinated peptides is specific and sensitive in detecting RA in both early and established disease. Anti–cyclic citrullinated peptide (anti-CCP) assays have 96% specificity and 78% sensitivity for RA, compared to the traditional IgM RF marker with a specificity of 60% to 80% and sensitivity of 75% to 80% for RA. Anti-CCP antibodies are being used as a marker for erosive disease in RA, and the antibodies have been detected in healthy patients years before the onset of RA symptoms and diagnosed disease. Some studies have shown that as many as 40% of patients seronegative for RF are anti-CCP positive. The combined presence of RF and anti-CCP has a 99.5% specificity for RA.

INDICATIONS
Assist in the diagnosis of rheumatoid arthritis, especially when clinical diagnosis is difficult.

INTERFERING FACTORS
Factors that may alter the results of the study
- Older healthy patients may have higher values.
- Recent blood transfusion, multiple vaccinations or transfusions, or an inadequately activated complement may affect results.
- Serum with cryoglobulin or high lipid levels may cause a false-positive test and may require that the test be repeated after a fat-restriction diet.

POTENTIAL MEDICAL DIAGNOSIS: CLINICAL SIGNIFICANCE OF RESULTS:
Increased in
Pathophysiology is unclear, but RF is present in numerous conditions, including rheumatoid arthritis.

- Chronic hepatitis
- Chronic viral infections
- Cirrhosis
- Dermatomyositis
- Infectious mononucleosis
- Leishmaniasis
- Leprosy
- Malaria
- Rheumatoid arthritis
- Sarcoidosis
- Scleroderma
- Sjögren syndrome
- SLE
- Syphilis
- Tuberculosis
- Waldenström macroglobulinemia

Decreased in: N/A

R

NURSING IMPLICATIONS

POTENTIAL NURSING PROBLEMS: ASSESSMENT & NURSING DIAGNOSIS

Problems	Signs and Symptoms
Body image *(related to deformed joints secondary to immune system dysfunction)*	Negative self-remarks, expressions of feelings or concerns over visual physical changes, fear of rejection by others due to appearance

Problems	Signs and Symptoms
Mobility *(related to deformed joints secondary to immune system dysfunction, fatigue, pain)*	Unsteady gait, lack of coordination, difficult purposeful movement, inadequate range of motion

BEFORE THE STUDY: PLANNING AND IMPLEMENTATION

Teaching the Patient What to Expect
▶ Inform the patient this test can assist in diagnosing arthritic disorders.
▶ Explain that a blood sample is needed for the test.

AFTER THE STUDY: POTENTIAL NURSING ACTIONS

Treatment Considerations
▶ Be supportive of impaired activity related to anticipated chronic pain resulting from joint inflammation, impairment in mobility, musculoskeletal deformity, and loss of independence.
▶ Discuss the implications of abnormal test results on lifestyle.
▶ Provide information regarding the clinical implications of the test results.
▶ Provide information regarding access to counseling services.
▶ Body Image: Assess feelings related to body image changes associated with disease process. Negative feelings may be evidenced by refusal to discuss changes or participate in care or by withdrawal from social situations.

Determine the patient's expectations regarding appearance and influences of culture, religion, ethnicity, and gender on body image perceptions. Monitor verbalization of self-criticism and encourage participation in support groups.
▶ Mobility: Assess gait, muscle strength, weakness, coordination, physical endurance, and level of fatigue. Evaluate the ability to perform independent activities of daily living; safe, independent movement; and need for assistive device. Encourage safe self-care, and administer prescribed steroids.

Follow-Up, Evaluation, and Desired Outcomes
▶ Acknowledges contact information provided for the American College of Rheumatology (www.rheumatology.org) or Arthritis Foundation (www.arthritis .org).
▶ The patient and family state that taking anti-inflammatory medication prior to activity may improve mobility.
▶ The patient and family state the risks and benefits of steroid use.
▶ The patient demonstrates the proficient use of assistive devices to support mobility and decrease fatigue.

Rubella Testing

R

SYNONYM/ACRONYM: German measles serology.

RATIONALE: To assess for antibodies related to rubella immunity or for presence of rubella infection.

PATIENT PREPARATION: There are no food, fluid, activity, or medication restrictions unless by medical direction.

NORMAL FINDINGS: Method: Chemiluminescent immunoassay.

	IgM	Interpretation	IgG	Interpretation
Negative	0.9 index or less	No significant level of detectable antibody	Less than 8 units/ mL	No significant level of detectable antibody; indicative of nonimmunity
Indeterminate	0.91–1.09 index	Equivocal results; retest in 10–14 days	8–12 units/ mL	Equivocal results; retest in 10–14 days
Positive	1.1 index or greater	Antibody detected; indicative of recent immunization, current or recent infection	Greater than 12 units/ mL	Antibody detected; indicative of immunization, current or past infection

CRITICAL FINDINGS AND POTENTIAL INTERVENTIONS

A nonimmune status in pregnant patients may present significant health consequences for the developing fetus if the mother is exposed to an infected individual.

Timely notification to the requesting health-care provider (HCP) of any critical findings and related symptoms is a role expectation of the professional nurse. A listing of these findings varies among facilities.

OVERVIEW: (Study type: Blood collected in a gold-, red-, or red/gray-top tube; related body system: Immune and Reproductive systems.) Rubella, commonly known as *German measles*, is a communicable viral disease transmitted by contact with respiratory secretions and aerosolized droplets of the secretions. The incubation period is 14 to 21 days. This disease produces a pink, macular rash that disappears in 2 to 3 days. Rubella infection induces immunoglobulin (Ig) G and IgM antibody production. This test can determine current infection or immunity from past infection. Rubella serology is part of the TORCH (*t*oxoplasmosis, *o*ther [congenital syphilis and viruses], *r*ubella, cytomegalovirus, and *h*erpes simplex type 2) panel routinely performed on pregnant women. Fetal infection during the first trimester can affect all organs in the developing fetus and cause spontaneous abortion, fetal demise, or congenital defects. Up to 90% of infants born to mothers infected during the first trimester will develop a pattern of birth defects called *congenital rubella syndrome* (CRS). The rate of CRS decreases when infection occurs later in the gestational period. Ideally, the immune status of women of childbearing age should be ascertained before pregnancy, when vaccination can be administered to provide lifelong immunity. The presence of IgM antibodies indicates acute infection. The presence of IgG antibodies indicates current or past infection. Susceptibility to rubella is indicated by a negative reaction. Many laboratories use a qualitative assay that detects the presence of both IgM and IgG rubella antibodies. IgM- and IgG-specific enzyme immunoassays are also available to help distinguish acute infection from immune status. Either the rubella-combined or IgG-specific assay should be used in routine prenatal testing of maternal serum.

INDICATIONS

- Assist in the diagnosis of rubella infection.
- Determine presence of rubella antibodies.
- Determine susceptibility to rubella, particularly in pregnant women.
- Perform as part of routine prenatal serological testing.

INTERFERING FACTORS: N/A

POTENTIAL MEDICAL DIAGNOSIS: CLINICAL SIGNIFICANCE OF RESULTS
Positive findings in
- Rubella infection (past or present)

NURSING IMPLICATIONS

POTENTIAL NURSING PROBLEMS: ASSESSMENT & NURSING DIAGNOSIS

Problems	Signs and Symptoms
Infection *(related to exposure to viral organism from an infected individual)*	Fever and rash lasting 2 to 3 days, runny nose, headache, malaise
Grief *(related to loss of potential child, loss secondary to rubella viral infection)*	Crying, report of grief, expression of emotional shock, psychological distress, disturbed sleep, loss of appetite, detachment, withdrawal, anger, blame, despair

BEFORE THE STUDY: PLANNING AND IMPLEMENTATION

Teaching the Patient What to Expect
- Inform the patient this test can indicate rubella infection or immunity.
- Explain that a blood sample is needed for the test. Inform the patient that several tests may be necessary to confirm the diagnosis. Any individual positive result should be repeated in 7 to 14 days to monitor a change in detectable levels of antibody.

Potential Nursing Actions
- Teach good hygiene and emphasize that good hand hygiene be used by family members and visitors in the home when preventing exposure is a concern.

AFTER THE STUDY: POTENTIAL NURSING ACTIONS

Avoiding Complications
- **Vaccination Considerations:** Record the date of the last menstrual period and determine the possibility of pregnancy prior to administration of rubella vaccine to female rubella-nonimmune patients. Instruct patient not to become pregnant for 1 mo after being vaccinated with the rubella vaccine to protect any fetus from contracting the disease and having serious birth defects. Instruct the patient on birth control methods to prevent pregnancy, if appropriate. Delay rubella vaccination in pregnancy until after childbirth, and give immediately prior to discharge from the hospital.

R

Treatment Considerations
- Provide instruction in isolation precautions during time of communicability or contagion.
- Emphasize the need to return to have a convalescent blood sample taken in 7 to 14 days.
- Infection: Explain that those infected can expose others to the virus from 1 wk before the rash is present up to 2 wk after the rash is gone. Administer prescribed acetaminophen for headache and fever. Discuss fetal risk associated with infection during pregnancy: miscarriage or stillbirth. Teach good hygiene.
- Grief: Provide emotional support if results are positive and the patient is pregnant. Monitor for manifestation of grief: crying, loud grief vocalization. Assess for the stages of grief and evaluate coping strategies. Consider the cultural norm for grief expression, encourage sharing feelings,

and recommend grief support group. Encourage the family to seek counseling if concerned with pregnancy termination. Decisions regarding elective abortion should take place in the presence of both parents. Administer prescribed medication to offset the emotional impact of grief, and recognize the need to relive the loss.

Follow-Up, Evaluation, and Desired Outcomes
- Acknowledges contact information provided regarding vaccine-preventable diseases where indicated (e.g., rubella) for the Centers for Disease Control and Prevention (www.cdc.gov/vaccines/vpd/vaccines-diseases.html) and (www.cdc.gov/DiseasesConditions).
- Acknowledges information provided related to the risks and challenges of raising a developmentally challenged infant as well as alternative options such as pregnancy termination or adoption.

Rubeola Testing

SYNONYM/ACRONYM: Measles serology.

RATIONALE: To assess for a rubeola infection or immunity.

PATIENT PREPARATION: There are no food, fluid, activity, or medication restrictions unless by medical direction.

NORMAL FINDINGS: Method: Enzyme immunoassay.

	IgM	Interpretation	IgG	Interpretation
Negative	0.79 AU or less	No significant level of detectable antibody	0.89 index or less	No significant level of detectable antibody; indicative of nonimmunity
Indeterminate	0.8–1.2 AU	Equivocal results; retest in 10–14 days	0.9–1 index	Equivocal results; retest in 10–14 days

	IgM	Interpretation	IgG	Interpretation
Positive	1.3 AU or greater	Antibody detected; indicative of recent immunization, current or recent infection	1.1 index or greater	Antibody detected; indicative of immunization, current or past infection

CRITICAL FINDINGS AND POTENTIAL INTERVENTIONS: N/A

OVERVIEW: (**Study type:** Blood collected in a gold-, red-, or red/gray-top tube; **related body system:** Immune and Reproductive systems.) Measles is caused by a single-stranded ribonucleic acid (RNA) paramyxovirus that invades the respiratory tract and lymphoreticular tissues. It is transmitted by respiratory secretions and aerosolized droplets of the secretions. The incubation period is 10 to 11 days. Symptoms initially include conjunctivitis, cough, and fever. Koplik spots develop 4 to 5 days later, followed by papular eruptions, body rash, and lymphadenopathy. The presence of immunoglobulin (Ig) M antibodies indicates acute infection. The presence of IgG antibodies indicates current or past infection. Susceptibility to measles is indicated by a negative reaction. Many laboratories use a qualitative assay that detects the presence of both IgM and IgG rubeola antibodies. IgM- and IgG-specific enzyme immunoassays are also available to help distinguish acute infection from immune status.

INDICATIONS
• Determine resistance to or protection against measles virus.

• Differential diagnosis of viral infection, especially in pregnant women with a history of exposure to measles.

INTERFERING FACTORS: N/A

POTENTIAL MEDICAL DIAGNOSIS: CLINICAL SIGNIFICANCE OF RESULTS

Positive findings in
• Measles infection

NURSING IMPLICATIONS

BEFORE THE STUDY: PLANNING AND IMPLEMENTATION

Teaching the Patient What to Expect
▶ Inform the patient this test is to assess for measles.
▶ Explain that a blood sample is needed for the test. Inform the patient that several tests may be necessary to confirm the diagnosis. Any individual positive result should be repeated in 7 to 14 days to monitor a change in detectable levels of antibody.

Potential Nursing Actions
▶ Teach good hygiene and emphasize that good hand hygiene be used by family members and visitors in the home when preventing exposure is a concern.

R

AFTER THE STUDY: POTENTIAL
NURSING ACTIONS

Avoiding Complications

▶ **Vaccination Considerations:**
Record the date of the last menstrual
period and determine the possibility
of pregnancy prior to administration
of rubeola vaccine to female rubeola-
nonimmune patients. Instruct patient
not to become pregnant for 1 mo after
being vaccinated with the rubeola
vaccine to protect any fetus from
contracting the disease. The danger
of contracting measles while pregnant
include the possibilities of miscarriage,
stillbirth, or preterm delivery. Instruct
the patient on birth control methods
to prevent pregnancy, if appropriate. Delay rubeola vaccination in

pregnancy until after childbirth, and
give immediately prior to discharge
from the hospital.

Treatment Considerations

▶ Instruct the patient in isolation precautions during time of communicability or
contagion.

▶ Emphasize the need to return to have
a convalescent blood sample taken in
7 to 14 days.

**Follow-Up, Evaluation, and
Desired Outcomes**

▶ Acknowledges information provided
regarding vaccine-preventable diseases
where indicated (e.g., measles) for the
Centers for Disease Control and Prevention (www.cdc.gov/vaccines/vpd/
vaccines-diseases.html) and (www.cdc
.gov/DiseasesConditions).

R

Schirmer Tear Test

SYNONYM/ACRONYM: N/A

RATIONALE: To assess tear duct function.

PATIENT PREPARATION: There are no food, fluid, activity, or medication restrictions unless by medical direction.

NORMAL FINDINGS
- 10 mm of moisture on test strip after 5 min. It may be slightly less than 10 mm in older adult patients.

CRITICAL FINDINGS AND POTENTIAL INTERVENTIONS: N/A

OVERVIEW: (Study type: Sensory, ocular; related body system: Nervous system.) The tear film, secreted by the lacrimal, Krause, and Wolfring glands, covers the surface of the eye. Blinking spreads tears over the eye and moves them toward an opening in the lower eyelid known as the *punctum*. Tears drain through the punctum into the nasolacrimal duct and into the nose. The Schirmer tear test simultaneously tests both eyes to assess lacrimal gland function by determining the amount of moisture accumulated on standardized filter paper or strips held against the conjunctival sac of each eye. The Schirmer test measures both reflex and basic secretion of tears. The Schirmer II test measures basic tear secretion and is used to evaluate the accessory glands of Krause and Wolfring. The Schirmer test is performed by instilling a topical anesthetic before insertion of filter paper. The topical anesthetic inhibits reflex tearing of major lacrimal glands by the filter paper, allowing testing of the accessory glands. The Schirmer II test is performed by irritating the nostril with a cotton swab to stimulate tear production.

In many cases the discomfort caused by a tearing deficiency or related inflammation, also known as "dry eye," can be treated successfully either with over-the-counter eye drops or prescription eye drops. Other, more invasive resolutions, include the insertion of punctal plugs to help tears remain on the surface of the eye longer or by expression of the meibomian glands to release the oily meibum required to prevent rapid tear film evaporation. Both procedures can be completed during an office visit. Punctal plugs are small, sterile, biocompatible medical devices that are inserted into the puncta (drainage duct openings in the inner corners of the upper and lower eyelids) to prevent draining of tears from the eye. Temporary plugs are made of dissolvable collagen material and permanent plugs are usually made of silicone or acrylic material; the placement of the plug also determines the length of time the plug remains inside the duct and whether removal, if needed, would require a surgical procedure. Expression of the meibomian glands is required when the openings of the glands become occluded and a condition called evaporative dry eye develops. The procedure to unblock the meibomian glands, which are located along the edge of the eyelids near the base of the eyelashes, begins with application

S

of warm compresses to the eyelids, after which forceps are used to manually express any hardened substances obstructing the openings of the meibomian glands. Significant pressure must be applied to the eyelids and this procedure may be considered quite uncomfortable by the patient. There is an automated, in office treatment for meibomian gland expression; it is reported to produce good results with less discomfort but may not be covered by health insurance.

INDICATIONS

• Assess adequacy of tearing for contact lens comfort and for successful LASIK surgery.
• Assess suspected tearing deficiency.

INTERFERING FACTORS

Factors that may alter the results of the study
• Rubbing or squeezing the eyes may affect results.
• Clinical conditions such as pregnancy may temporarily result in dry eye due to hormonal fluctuations.

POTENTIAL MEDICAL DIAGNOSIS: CLINICAL SIGNIFICANCE OF RESULTS

Abnormal findings related to
• Tearing deficiency related to aging, dry eye syndrome, or Sjögren syndrome.
• Tearing deficiency secondary to leukemia, lupus erythemastosus, lymphoma, rheumatoid arthritis, or scleroderma.

S

NURSING IMPLICATIONS

BEFORE THE STUDY: PLANNING AND IMPLEMENTATION

Teaching the Patient What to Expect
▶ Inform the patient this procedure can assist in evaluating tear duct function.

▶ Review the procedure with the patient. Address concerns about pain and explain that some discomfort may be experienced after the test when the numbness wears off from anesthetic drops administered prior to the test.
▶ Explain that the test is performed by a health-care provider (HCP) and takes about 15 min to complete.
▶ Positioning for this procedure is in the seated position looking straight ahead, keeping the eyes open and unblinking.
▶ Topical anesthetic is instilled in each eye and provided time to work.
▶ A test strip is inserted into each eye, and the patient is asked to gently close both eyes for approximately 5 min.
▶ Explain that the test strips will then be removed and the strips measured for the amount of moisture present.

Potential Nursing Actions
▶ Instruct the patient to remove contact lenses or glasses.

AFTER THE STUDY: POTENTIAL NURSING ACTIONS

Avoiding Complications
▶ Corneal abrasion can be caused by the patient rubbing the eye before topical anesthetic has worn off. Instruct the patient to avoid rubbing the eyes for 30 min after the procedure. Assess for corneal abrasion caused by patient rubbing the eye before topical anesthetic has worn off.

Treatment Considerations
▶ If appropriate, instruct the patient not to reinsert contact lenses for 2 hr.
▶ Explain how to use any ordered medications, usually eyedrops intended to provide additional lubrication and/or treat an underlying inflammatory process. As appropriate, instruct the patient in significant adverse effects associated with the prescribed medication.
▶ Emphasize the importance of adhering to the therapy regimen.
▶ Encourage a review of corresponding literature provided by a pharmacist.
▶ Be supportive of pain related to decreased lacrimation or inflammation.
▶ Discuss the implications of abnormal test results on the lifestyle choices.

Follow-Up, Evaluation, and Desired Outcomes

▶ Acknowledges contact information provided for patient education on the topic of eye care, such as the American Academy of Ophthalmologists (www .aao.org) or American Optometric Association (www.aoa.org or www.allaboutvision.com).

Semen Analysis

SYNONYM/ACRONYM: N/A

RATIONALE: To assess for male infertility related to disorders such as obstruction, testicular failure, and atrophy.

PATIENT PREPARATION: There are no food, fluid, or medication restrictions unless by medical direction. Instruct the patient to refrain from any sexual activity for 3 days before specimen collection.

NORMAL FINDINGS: Method: Macroscopic and microscopic examination.

Test	Normal Result
Volume	2–5 mL
Color	White or opaque
Appearance	Viscous (pours in droplets, not clumps or strings)
Clotting and liquefaction	Complete in 15–20 min, rarely over 60 min
pH	7.2–8
Sperm count	Greater than 15 million/mL
Total sperm count	Greater than 39 million/ejaculate
Motility	At least 40% at 60 min
Vitality (membrane intact)	At least 58%
Morphology	Greater than 25%–30% normal oval-headed forms

The number of normal sperm is calculated by multiplying the total sperm count by the percentage of normal forms.

CRITICAL FINDINGS AND POTENTIAL INTERVENTIONS: N/A

OVERVIEW: (**Study type:** Body fluid, semen from ejaculate specimen collected in a clean, dry, glass container known to be free of detergent; **related body system:** Reproductive system. The specimen should be promptly transported to the laboratory for processing and analysis. The specimen container should be kept at body temperature [37°C] during transportation.) Semen analysis is a valid measure of overall male fertility. Semen contains a combination of elements produced by various parts of the male reproductive system. Spermatozoa are produced in the testes and account for only a small volume of seminal fluid. Fructose and other nutrients are provided by fluid produced in the seminal vesicles.

S

The prostate gland provides acid phosphatase and other enzymes required for coagulation and liquefaction of semen. Sperm motility depends on the presence of a sufficient level of ionized calcium. If the specimen has an abnormal appearance (e.g., bloody, oddly colored, turbid), the patient may have an infection. Specimens can be tested with a leukocyte esterase strip to detect the presence of white blood cells.

INDICATIONS

- Assist in the diagnosis of azoospermia and oligospermia.
- Evaluate infertility.
- Evaluate effectiveness of vasectomy.
- Evaluate the effectiveness of vasectomy reversal.
- Support or disprove sterility in paternity suit.

INTERFERING FACTORS

Factors that may alter the results of the study
- Drugs and other substances that may decrease sperm count include arsenic, azathioprine, cannabis, cimetidine, cocaine, cyclophosphamide, estrogens, ketoconazole, lead, methotrexate, methyltestosterone, nitrofurantoin, nitrogen mustard, procarbazine, sulfasalazine, and vincristine.
- Testicular radiation may decrease sperm counts.
- Cigarette smoking is associated with decreased production of semen.
- Caffeine consumption is associated with increased sperm density and number of abnormal forms.

Other considerations
- Delays in transporting the specimen and failure to keep the specimen warm during transportation are the most common reasons for specimen rejection.

POTENTIAL MEDICAL DIAGNOSIS: CLINICAL SIGNIFICANCE OF RESULTS

There is marked intraindividual variation in sperm count. Indications of suboptimal fertility should be investigated by serial analysis of two to three samples collected over several months. If abnormal results are obtained, additional testing may be requested.

Abnormality	Test Ordered	Normal Result
Decreased count	Fructose	Present (greater than 150 mg/dL)
Decreased motility with clumping	Male antisperm antibodies	Absent
Normal semen analysis with infertility	Female antisperm antibodies	Absent

Abnormal findings related to
- Hyperpyrexia *(unusual and abnormal elevation in body temperature may result in insufficient sperm production)*
- Infertility *(related to insufficient production of sperm)*
- Obstruction of ejaculatory system
- Orchitis *(insufficient sperm production usually related to viral infection, rarely bacterial infection)*
- Postvasectomy period *(related to obstruction of the vas deferens)*
- Primary and secondary testicular failure *(congenital, as in Klinefelter syndrome, or acquired via infection)*
- Testicular atrophy *(e.g., recovery from mumps)*
- Varicocele *(abnormal enlargement of the blood vessels in the scrotal area eventually damages testicular tissue and affects sperm production)*

S

NURSING IMPLICATIONS

BEFORE THE STUDY: PLANNING AND IMPLEMENTATION

Teaching the Patient What to Expect

▸ Inform the patient this test can assess for infertility.

▸ Explain that a semen sample is needed for the test.

▸ Review the procedure with the patient. Address concerns about pain and explain that there should be no discomfort during the procedure.

▸ The requesting health-care provider (HCP) usually provides the patient with instructions for specimen collection.

▸ Instruct the patient to bring the specimen to the laboratory within 30 to 60 min of collection and to keep the specimen warm (close to body temperature) during transportation.

Ejaculated Specimen

▸ Ideally, the specimen is obtained by masturbation in a private location close to the laboratory. In cases in which the patient expresses psychological or religious concerns about masturbation, the specimen can be obtained during coitus interruptus, through the use of a condom, or through postcoital collection of samples from the cervical canal and vagina of the patient's sexual partner. The patient should be warned about the possible loss of the sperm-rich portion of the sample if coitus interruptus is the collection approach. If a condom is used, the patient must be instructed to carefully wash and dry the condom completely before use to prevent contamination of the specimen with spermicides.

Cervical Vaginal Specimen

▸ The patient's partner will be assisted into the lithotomy position on the examination table. A speculum will be inserted and the specimen obtained by direct smear or aspiration of saline lavage.

Specimens Collected From Skin or Clothing

▸ Dried semen may be collected by sponging the skin with a gauze soaked in saline or by soaking the material in a saline solution.

AFTER THE STUDY: POTENTIAL NURSING ACTIONS

Treatment Considerations

▸ Provide a supportive, nonjudgmental environment when assisting through the process of fertility testing.

▸ Discuss the implications of abnormal test results on lifestyle choices.

▸ Provide information regarding the clinical implications of the test results.

Follow-Up, Evaluation, and Desired Outcomes

▸ Recognizes the value of seeking counseling and other support services related to infertility concerns.

Sialography

SYNONYM/ACRONYM: Ptyalogram, radiosialography, salivary gland studies.

RATIONALE: To assess parotid, submaxillary, sublingual, and submandibular ducts for structure, tumors, and inflammation related to pain, swelling, and tenderness.

PATIENT PREPARATION: There are no activity restrictions unless by medical direction. Computed tomography (CT) sialography studies performed without contrast usually do not require the patient to fast before the procedure. If iodinated contrast medium is scheduled to be used, instruct the patient to fast and restrict fluids, as ordered, prior to the procedure. Fasting may be ordered as a precaution against aspiration related to possible nausea and vomiting. The American Society of Anesthesiologists has fasting guidelines for risk levels according to patient status. More information can be located at www.asahq.org.

Note: If iodinated contrast medium is scheduled to be used in patients receiving metformin or drugs containing metformin for type 2 diabetes, the drug may be discontinued on the day of the test and continue to be withheld for 48 hr after the test.

NORMAL FINDINGS

• Normal salivary ducts with no indication of gland abnormalities.

CRITICAL FINDINGS AND POTENTIAL INTERVENTIONS: N/A

OVERVIEW: (Study type: Radiology, special/contrast; related body system: Digestive system [base of the tongue, mandible, parotid gland, submandibular gland, sublingual gland].) Sialography is the radiographic visualization of the salivary glands and ducts. These glands secrete saliva into the mouth, and there are three pairs of salivary glands: the parotid, the submandibular, and the sublingual. Sialography involves the introduction of a water-soluble contrast medium into the orifices of the salivary gland ducts with a small cannula, followed by a series of radiographic images. There are four imaging methods that can be used in the evaluation of the salivary glands:

• Ultrasound—noninvasive, cost effective, and provides results quickly; commonly used for assessment
• CT sialography—invasive, good visualization, good diagnostic tool, similar to the conventional sialography procedure; drawbacks associated with use of contrast and radiation
• MR sialography—noninvasive, rapid results, good visualization, good diagnostic tool; drawbacks associated with presence of pacemakers, implants, claustrophobia,

dental fillings, and so on, that can disqualify the patient or produce unclear images
• Conventional/fluoroscopic sialography (with or without digital subtraction)—invasive, allows therapeutic application to remove salivary stones or repair narrowing of ducts; drawbacks associated with use of contrast, radiation, and high failure rate due to difficulty achieving effective cannulation and lack of patient cooperation during the procedure

Conventional sialography is the method of choice when a definite diagnosis is required for pathology such as sialadenitis (inflammation of the salivary glands) or if the oral component of Sjögren syndrome is a concern.

INDICATIONS

• Evaluate the presence of calculi in the salivary glands.
• Evaluate the presence of tumors in the salivary glands.
• Evaluate narrowing of the salivary ducts.

INTERFERING FACTORS

Contraindications

⚜ Patients who are pregnant or suspected of being pregnant, unless the potential benefits of a procedure using radiation far outweigh the risk of radiation exposure to the fetus and mother.

⚜ Patients with conditions associated with adverse reactions to contrast medium (e.g., asthma, food allergies, or allergy to contrast medium). Although patients are asked specifically if they have a known allergy to iodine or shellfish (shellfish contain high levels of iodine), it has been well established that the reaction is not to iodine; an actual iodine allergy would be problematic because iodine is required for the production of thyroid hormones. In the case of shellfish, the reaction is to a muscle protein called *tropomyosin;* in the case of iodinated contrast medium, the reaction is to the noniodinated part of the contrast molecule. Patients with a known hypersensitivity to the medium may benefit from premedication with corticosteroids and diphenhydramine; the use of nonionic contrast or an alternative noncontrast imaging study, if available, may be considered for patients who have severe asthma or who have experienced moderate to severe reactions to ionic contrast medium.

⚜ Patients with conditions associated with preexisting renal insufficiency (e.g., chronic kidney disease, single kidney transplant, nephrectomy, diabetes, multiple myeloma, treatment with aminoglycosides and NSAIDs), *because iodinated contrast is nephrotoxic.*

⚜ Patients who are chronically dehydrated before the test, especially older adults and patients whose health is already compromised, *because of their risk of contrast-induced acute kidney injury.*

⚜ Patients with bleeding disorders *because the puncture site may not stop bleeding.*

POTENTIAL MEDICAL DIAGNOSIS: CLINICAL SIGNIFICANCE OF RESULTS

Abnormal findings related to
- Calculi
- Fistulas
- Mixed parotid tumors
- Sialectasia (dilation of a duct)
- Strictures of the ducts

NURSING IMPLICATIONS

BEFORE THE STUDY: PLANNING AND IMPLEMENTATION

Teaching the Patient What to Expect

▶ Inform the patient this procedure can assist in assessing duct glands in the neck and mouth.

▶ Pregnancy is a general contraindication to procedures involving radiation. Explain to the female patient that she will be asked the date of her last menstrual period. Pregnancy testing may be performed to determine the possibility of pregnancy before exposure to radiation.

▶ Review the procedure with the patient. Address concerns about pain and explain that there may be moments of discomfort or pain experienced when the IV line or catheter is inserted to allow infusion of fluids such as saline, anesthetics, sedatives, contrast medium, medications used in the procedure, or emergency medications.

▶ Instruct the patient to remove dentures or removable bridgework prior to examination.

▶ Explain that lemon juice may be given to dilate the salivary orifice, and a local anesthetic spray or liquid may be applied to the throat to ease with insertion of the cannula.

▶ Explain that the procedure is performed in a radiology department by a health-care provider (HCP) specializing in this procedure, with support staff, and takes approximately 15 to 30 min.

S

- Positioning for this procedure is in the supine position on an examination table. Topical anesthetic is instilled in the throat and allowed time to work.
- The salivary duct is located and dilated. Following insertion of the cannula, the contrast medium is injected, and a series of x-ray images is taken; a CT scan may also be performed. Delayed images may be taken to examine the ducts in cases of ductal obstruction. If lemon juice was given, additional images are taken to examine drainage of saliva from the ducts and glands into the mouth.
- Explain that the patient will be asked to inhale deeply and hold his or her breath while the x-ray images are taken, and then to exhale after the images are taken.
- Monitoring will be in place to observe for complications related to the procedure (e.g., allergic reaction, anaphylaxis, bronchospasm).
- Once the procedure is completed, the needle or cannula is removed.

Potential Nursing Actions

Make sure a written and informed consent has been signed prior to the procedure and before administering any medications.

- If iodinated contrast medium is scheduled to be used in patients receiving metformin or drugs containing metformin for type 2 diabetes, the drug may be discontinued on the day of the test and continue to be withheld for 48 hr after the test. Protocols may vary among facilities.

AFTER THE STUDY: POTENTIAL NURSING ACTIONS

Avoiding Complications

- Establishing an IV site and injection of contrast medium are invasive procedures. Complications are rare but include risk for allergic reaction *(related to contrast reaction)* or bleeding from the puncture site *(related to*

a bleeding disorder or the effects of natural products and medications with known anticoagulant, antiplatelet, or thrombolytic properties). Monitor the patient for complications related to the procedure (e.g., allergic reaction, anaphylaxis, bronchospasm, infection, injury). Immediately report symptoms such as difficulty breathing, chest pain, fever, hyperpnea, hypertension, nausea, palpitations, pruritus, rash, tachycardia, urticaria, or vomiting to the appropriate HCP. Observe/assess the needle/catheter insertion site for bleeding, inflammation, or hematoma formation. Administer ordered antihistamines or prophylactic steroids if the patient has an allergic reaction.

Treatment Considerations

- Instruct the patient to resume usual diet, fluids, medications, or activity, as directed by the HCP. Kidney function should be assessed before metformin is resumed.
- Provide instruction on the care and assessment of the needle insertion site.
- Explain that cold compresses can be applied to the puncture site as needed to reduce discomfort or edema.

Safety Considerations

- Advise diabetic patients to avoid all medications containing metformin for 48 hr following a procedure with iodinated contrast. Iodinated contrast can temporarily impair kidney function, and failure to withhold metformin may indirectly result in drug-induced lactic acidosis, a dangerous and sometimes fatal adverse effect of metformin (related to renal impairment that does not support sufficient excretion of metformin).

Follow-Up, Evaluation, and Desired Outcomes

- Acknowledges that further testing may be necessary to evaluate disease progression and treatment effectiveness.

Sigmoidoscopy

SYNONYM/ACRONYM: Anoscopy (anal canal), proctoscopy (anus and rectum), flexible fiberoptic sigmoidoscopy, flexible proctosigmoidoscopy, sigmoidoscopy (sigmoid colon).

RATIONALE: To visualize and assess the anus, rectum, and sigmoid colon to assist in diagnosing disorders such as cancer, inflammation, prolapse, and evaluate the effectiveness of medical and surgical therapeutic interventions.

PATIENT PREPARATION: There are no activity restrictions unless by medical direction. Instruct the patient to eat a low-residue diet for 3 days prior to the procedure. Only clear liquids should be consumed the evening before, and food and fluids should be restricted for 8 hr prior to the procedure. Protocols may vary among facilities. Note intake of oral iron preparations within 1 wk before the procedure because these cause black, sticky feces that are difficult to remove with bowel preparation. Ensure that this procedure is performed before an upper gastrointestinal (GI) study or barium swallow.

Regarding the patient's risk for bleeding, the patient should be instructed to avoid taking natural products and medications with known anticoagulant, antiplatelet, or thrombolytic properties or to reduce dosage, as ordered, prior to the procedure. Number of days to withhold medication is dependent on the type of anticoagulant. Note the last time and dose of medication taken.

NORMAL FINDINGS

• Normal mucosa of the anal canal, rectum, and sigmoid colon.

CRITICAL FINDINGS AND POTENTIAL INTERVENTIONS: N/A

OVERVIEW: (Study type: Endoscopy; related body system: Digestive system.) Sigmoidoscopy allows direct visualization of the mucosa of the anal canal (anoscopy), anus and rectum (proctoscopy), and distal sigmoid colon (sigmoidoscopy). The procedure can be performed using a rigid or flexible fiberoptic endoscope, but the flexible instrument is generally preferred. The endoscope is a multichannel device allowing visualization of the mucosal lining of the colon, instillation of air, removal of fluid and foreign objects, obtainment of tissue biopsy specimens, and use of a laser for the destruction of tissue and control of bleeding. The endoscope is advanced approximately 60 cm into the colon. This procedure is commonly used in patients with lower abdominal and perineal pain; changes in bowel habits; rectal prolapse during defecation; or passage of blood, mucus, or pus in the stool. Sigmoidoscopy can also be a therapeutic procedure, allowing removal of polyps or hemorrhoids or reduction of a volvulus. Biopsy specimens of suspicious sites may be obtained during the procedure.

INDICATIONS

• Confirm the diagnosis of diverticular disease.
• Confirm the diagnosis of Hirschsprung disease and colitis in children.

S

- Determine the cause of pain and rectal prolapse during defecation.
- Determine the cause of rectal itching, pain, or burning.
- Evaluate the cause of blood, pus, or mucus in the stool.
- Evaluate postoperative anastomosis of the colon.
- Examine the distal colon before barium enema (BE) x-ray to obtain improved visualization of the area, and after a BE when x-ray findings are inconclusive.
- Reduce volvulus of the sigmoid colon.
- Remove hemorrhoids by laser therapy.
- Screen for and excise polyps.
- Screen for colon cancer.

INTERFERING FACTORS
Contraindications

 Patients with bleeding disorders, especially disorders associated with uremia and cytotoxic chemotherapy.

 Patients with cardiac conditions or dysrhythmias.

 Patients with bowel perforation, acute peritonitis, ischemic bowel necrosis, toxic megacolon, diverticulitis, recent bowel surgery, advanced pregnancy, severe cardiac or pulmonary disease, recent myocardial infarction, known or suspected pulmonary embolus, large abdominal aortic or iliac aneurysm, or coagulation abnormality.

Factors that may alter the results of the study
- Strictures or other abnormalities preventing passage of the scope.
- Barium swallow or upper GI series within the preceding 48 hr.
- Severe lower GI bleeding or the presence of feces, barium, blood, or blood clots.

Other considerations
- Use of bowel preparations that include laxatives or enemas should be avoided in pregnant patients or patients with inflammatory bowel disease unless specifically directed by a health-care provider (HCP).

POTENTIAL MEDICAL DIAGNOSIS: CLINICAL SIGNIFICANCE OF RESULTS
Abnormal findings related to
- Anal fissure or fistula
- Anorectal abscess
- Benign lesions
- Bleeding sites
- Bowel infection or inflammation
- Crohn disease
- Diverticula
- Hypertrophic anal papillae
- Internal and external hemorrhoids
- Polyps
- Rectal prolapse
- Tumors
- Ulcerative colitis
- Vascular abnormalities

NURSING IMPLICATIONS

POTENTIAL NURSING PROBLEMS: ASSESSMENT & NURSING DIAGNOSIS

Problems	Signs and Symptoms
Altered fecal elimination (related to blockage, inflammation, infection)	Postoperative fecal diversion
Pain (related to abdominal distention, postoperative incision)	Self-report of pain, moaning, crying, restlessness, anxiety, increased heart rate, increased blood pressure, abdominal guarding

S

Teaching the Patient What to Expect

▶ Inform the patient this procedure can assist in evaluating the rectum and lower colon for disease.

▶ Explain that prior to the procedure, laboratory testing may be required to determine the possibility of bleeding risk (coagulation testing).

▶ Review the procedure with the patient. Address concerns about pain related to the procedure and explain that some pain may be experienced during the test, and there may be moments of discomfort.

▶ Explain that a sedative and/or analgesia will be administered to promote relaxation and reduce discomfort prior to insertion of the anoscope.

▶ Explain that the procedure is performed in a GI lab by an HCP specializing in this procedure, with support staff, and takes approximately 30 to 60 min.

▶ Advise that a laxative may be needed the day before the procedure, with cleansing enemas on the morning of the procedure, depending on the institution's policy.

▶ Advise that the urge to defecate may be experienced when the scope is passed. Explain that slow, deep breathing through the mouth may help alleviate the feeling.

▶ Explain that flatus may be expelled during and after the procedure owing to air that is injected into the scope to improve visualization.

▶ Two small-volume enemas will be administered 1 hr before the procedure.

▶ Baseline vital signs are recorded and continuously monitored throughout the procedure. Protocols may vary among facilities.

▶ Positioning for this study is on an examination table in the left lateral decubitus position or the knee-chest position with the buttocks draped and exposed. The table may be slightly tilted and the buttocks slightly extended beyond the edge of the table for optimal positioning.

▶ Explain that the HCP will perform a visual inspection of the perianal area and a digital rectal examination, possibly obtaining a fecal specimen for evaluation.

▶ The scope is gently manipulated to facilitate passage, and air may be insufflated through the scope to improve visualization. Suction and cotton swabs can be used to remove materials that hinder visualization.

▶ Explain to the patient that they will be asked to take deep breaths to aid in movement of the scope downward through the ascending colon to the cecum and into the terminal portion of the ileum.

▶ Once the examination is completed, the scope is gradually withdrawn. Photographs are obtained for future reference.

▶ Residual lubricant is cleansed from the anal area.

▶ Fecal or tissue samples and polyps are placed in properly labelled specimen containers and promptly transported to the laboratory for processing and analysis.

Potential Nursing Actions

◆ *Make sure a written and informed consent has been signed prior to the procedure and before administering any medications.*

Safety Considerations

▶ Anticoagulants, aspirin and other salicylates should be discontinued by medical direction for the appropriate number of days prior to a procedure where bleeding is a potential complication.

Avoiding Complications

▶ Complications of the procedure may include bleeding and cardiac dysrhythmias. Monitor for any rectal bleeding. Instruct the patient that any abdominal pain, tenderness, or distention; pain on defecation; or fever must be reported to the HCP immediately.

Treatment Considerations

▶ Instruct the patient to resume diet, medication, and activity, as directed by the HCP.

S

▶ Encourage the patient to drink several glasses of water to help replace fluid lost during test preparation.

▶ Monitor vital signs and neurological status every 15 min for 1 hr, then every 2 hr for 4 hr, and then as ordered by the HCP. Monitor temperature every 4 hr for 24 hr. Monitor intake and output at least every 8 hr. Compare with baseline values. Notify the HCP if temperature changes. Protocols may vary among facilities.

▶ Advise the patient to expect slight rectal bleeding for 2 days after removal of polyps or biopsy specimens, but heavy rectal bleeding must be immediately reported to the HCP.

▶ Explain that any bloating or flatulence is the result of air insufflation.

▶ Altered Fecal Elimination: Some patients will require surgery based on the results of this study and biopsy findings. Depending on the type of surgery, it may be necessary to implement ostomy care and engage an ostomy care nurse for assistance. Assess for active bowel sounds in all four quadrants, and keep NPO until bowel sound are active. Implement new dietary restrictions and administer ordered parenteral fluids until patient can take adequate fluids orally.

▶ Pain: Assess pain character, location, duration, and intensity using an easily understood pain rating scale. Place in a position of comfort and administer ordered pain medications. Consider alternative measures for pain management (imagery, relaxation, music, etc.). Assess and trend vital signs.

Follow-Up, Evaluation, and Desired Outcomes

▶ Recognizes colon cancer screening options and understands that decisions regarding the need for and frequency of occult blood testing, colonoscopy, or other cancer screening procedures may be made after consultation between the patient and HCP. Colonoscopy should be used to follow up abnormal findings obtained by any of the screening tests. The most current guidelines for colon cancer screening of the general population as well as of individuals with increased risk are available from the American Cancer Society (www.cancer.org), U.S. Preventive Services Task Force (www.uspreventiveservicestaskforce.org), and American College of Gastroenterology (http://gi.org). For additional information regarding screening guidelines, refer to the study titled "Colonoscopy."

▶ Teach the patient and family disease-specific pathophysiology.

Slit-Lamp Biomicroscopy

SYNONYM/ACRONYM: Slit-lamp examination.

RATIONALE: To detect abnormalities in the external and anterior eye structures to assist in diagnosing disorders such as corneal injury, hemorrhage, ulcers, and abrasion.

PATIENT PREPARATION: There are no food or fluid restrictions unless by medical direction. Instruct the patient to withhold eye medications (particularly miotic eye drops, which may constrict the pupil, preventing a clear view of the fundus, and mydriatic eyedrops in order to avoid instigation of an acute open-angle attack in patients with narrow-angle glaucoma) for at least 1 day prior to the procedure. Patients with blue or hazel eye color have the option of requesting dilating drops with a lower concentration than standard drops as blue or hazel eyes dilate faster than brown eyes and will remain dilated for a longer period of time. Ensure that the patient understands that he or she must refrain from driving until the pupils return to normal (about 4 hr) after the test and has made arrangements to have someone else be responsible for transportation after the test.

NORMAL FINDINGS
• Normal anterior tissues and structures of the eyes.

CRITICAL FINDINGS AND POTENTIAL INTERVENTIONS: N/A

OVERVIEW: (Study type: Sensory, ocular; related body system: Nervous system.) This noninvasive procedure is used to visualize the anterior portion of the eye and its parts, including the eyelids and eyelashes, sclera, conjunctiva, cornea, iris, lens, and anterior chamber, and to detect pathology of any of these areas of the eyes. The slit-lamp has a binocular microscope and light source that can be adjusted to examine the fluid, tissues, and structures of the eyes. For example, slit-lamp ophthalmoscopy can be performed using the microscope part of the slit-lamp and a special lens placed close to the eye to examine the retina, optic disc, choroid, and blood vessels in the back or fundus of the eye. Ophthalmoscopy is helpful in the identification of retinal detachment, diseases such as glaucoma that affect the movement of eye fluid, and diseases that affect the blood vessels in the eyes, such as hypertension and diabetes. Special attachments to the slit-lamp are used for special studies and more detailed views of specific areas. Dilating drops or mydriatics may be used to enlarge the pupil in order to allow the examiner to see the eye in greater detail. Mydriatics work either by temporarily paralyzing the muscle that makes the pupil smaller or by stimulating the iris dilator muscle.

INDICATIONS
• Detect conjunctival and corneal injuries by foreign bodies and determine if ocular penetration or anterior chamber hemorrhage is present.
• Detect corneal abrasions, ulcers, or abnormal curvatures (keratoconus).
• Detect deficiency in tear formation indicative of lacrimal dysfunction causing dry eye disease that can lead to corneal erosions or infection.
• Detect lens opacities indicative of cataract formation.
• Determine the presence of blepharitis, conjunctivitis, hordeolum, entropion, ectropion, trachoma, scleritis, and iritis.
• Evaluate the fit of contact lenses.

INTERFERING FACTORS
Contraindications

Patients with narrow-angle closure glaucoma if pupil dilation is performed; dilation can initiate a severe and sight-threatening open-angle attack.

Patients with allergies to mydriatics if pupil dilation using mydriatics is performed.

POTENTIAL MEDICAL DIAGNOSIS: CLINICAL SIGNIFICANCE OF RESULTS
Abnormal findings related to
• Blepharitis
• Conjunctivitis
• Corneal abrasions
• Corneal foreign bodies
• Corneal ulcers
• Diabetes
• Ectropion

S

- Entropion
- Glaucoma
- Hordeolum
- Iritis
- Keratoconus (abnormal curvatures)
- Lens opacities
- Scleritis
- Trachoma

NURSING IMPLICATIONS

BEFORE THE STUDY: PLANNING AND IMPLEMENTATION

Teaching the Patient What to Expect

▶ Inform the patient this procedure can assist in evaluating the structures of the eye.
▶ Review the procedure with the patient. Address concerns about pain and explain that mydriatics, if used, may cause blurred vision and sensitivity to light. Explain that there may also be a brief stinging sensation when the drop is put in the eye.
▶ Explain that a health-care provider (HCP) performs the test in a quiet, darkened room, and that to evaluate both eyes, the test can take up to 30 min (including time for the pupils to dilate before the test is actually performed).
▶ Positioning for this procedure is seated with placement of the chin in the chin rest with the forehead gently pressed against the support bar.
▶ Explain that if dilation is to be performed, mydriatic drops will be administered to each eye and repeated in 5 to 15 min.
▶ Once the procedure is ready to begin, the HCP places the slit-lamp in front of the patient's eyes in line with the examiner's eyes.
▶ The external structures of the eyes are inspected with the special bright light and microscope of the slit lamp.
▶ The light is then directed into the eyes to inspect the anterior fluids and structures and is adjusted for shape, intensity, and depth needed to visualize these areas.
▶ Magnification of the microscope is also adjusted to optimize visualization of the eye structures.
▶ Special attachments and procedures can also be used to obtain further diagnostic information about the eyes.
▶ These may include a camera to photograph specific parts, gonioscopy to determine anterior chamber closure, and a cobalt-blue filter to detect minute corneal scratches, breaks, and abrasions with corneal staining.

Potential Nursing Actions

▶ Instruct the patient to remove contact lenses or glasses unless the study is being done to check the fit and effectiveness of the contact lenses.

AFTER THE STUDY: POTENTIAL NURSING ACTIONS

Avoiding Complications

▶ Dilation can initiate a severe and sight-threatening open-angle attack in patients with narrow-angle glaucoma.

Treatment Considerations

▶ Instruct the patient to resume usual medications, as directed by the HCP.
▶ Remind the patient to wear dark glasses after the test until the pupils return to normal size.
▶ Review the implications of abnormal test results on the patient's lifestyle.
▶ Be supportive of impaired activity related to vision loss, anticipated loss of driving privileges, or the possibility of requiring corrective lenses (self-image).

Follow-Up, Evaluation, and Desired Outcomes

▶ Acknowledges contact information provided for patient education on the topic of eye care, such as the American Academy of Ophthalmologists (www.aao.org) or American Optometric Association (www.aoa.org or www.allaboutvision.com).

S

Sodium, Blood

SYNONYM/ACRONYM: Serum Na⁺.

RATIONALE: To assess electrolyte balance related to hydration levels and disorders such as diarrhea and vomiting and to monitor the effect of diuretic use.

PATIENT PREPARATION: There are no food, fluid, activity, or medication restrictions unless by medical direction.

NORMAL FINDINGS: Method: Ion-selective electrode.

Age	Conventional and SI Units
Cord	126–166 mEq/L or mmol/L
1–12 hr	124–156 mEq/L or mmol/L
12–48 hr	132–159 mEq/L or mmol/L
48–72 hr	139–162 mEq/L or mmol/L
Newborn	135–145 mEq/L or mmol/L
Child–adult–older adult	135–145 mEq/L or mmol/L

Anion Gap	Conventional and SI Units
Child or adult	8–16 mmol/L

Note: Older adults are at increased risk for both hypernatremia and hyponatremia. Diminished thirst, illness, and lack of mobility are common causes for hypernatremia in older adults. There are multiple causes of hyponatremia in older adults, but the most common factor may be related to the use of thiazide diuretics.

CRITICAL FINDINGS AND POTENTIAL INTERVENTIONS

• *Hyponatremia:* Less than 120 mEq/L or mmol/L (SI: Less than 120 mmol/L)
• *Hypernatremia:* Greater than 160 mEq/L or mmol/L (SI: Greater than 160 mmol/L).

Timely notification to the requesting health-care provider (HCP) of any critical findings and related symptoms is a role expectation of the professional nurse. A listing of these findings varies among facilities.

Consideration may be given to verification of critical findings before action is taken. Policies vary among facilities and may include requesting immediate recollection and retesting by the laboratory or retesting using a rapid point-of-care testing instrument at the bedside, if available.

Signs and symptoms of hyponatremia include confusion, irritability, convulsions, tachycardia, nausea, vomiting, and loss of consciousness. Possible interventions include maintenance of airway, monitoring for convulsions, fluid restriction, and performance of hourly neurological checks. Administration of saline for replacement requires close attention to serum and urine osmolality.

S

Signs and symptoms of hypernatremia include restlessness, intense thirst, weakness, swollen tongue, seizures, and coma. Possible interventions include treatment of the underlying cause of water loss or sodium excess, which includes sodium restriction and administration of diuretics combined with IV solutions of 5% dextrose in water (D_5W).

OVERVIEW: (**Study type:** Blood collected in a gold-, red-, red/gray-, or green-top [heparin] tube; related body system: Circulatory, Endocrine, and Urinary systems.) Electrolytes dissociate into electrically charged ions when dissolved. Cations, including sodium, carry a positive charge. Body fluids contain approximately equal numbers of anions and cations, although the nature of the ions and their mobility differs between the intracellular and extracellular compartments. Both types of ions affect the electrical and osmolar functions of the body. Electrolyte quantities and the balance among them are controlled by oxygen and carbon dioxide exchange in the lungs; absorption, secretion, and excretion of many substances by the kidneys; and secretion of regulatory hormones by the endocrine glands. Sodium is the most abundant extracellular cation that together with chloride and bicarbonate participate in a number of essential functions to include maintaining the osmotic pressure of extracellular fluid, regulating renal retention and excretion of water, maintaining acid-base balance, regulating potassium levels, stimulating neuromuscular reactions, and maintaining systemic blood pressure. *Hypernatremia* (elevated sodium level) occurs when there is excessive water loss or abnormal retention of sodium. *Hyponatremia* (low sodium level) occurs when there is inadequate sodium retention or inadequate intake.

The anion gap is a calculated value often reported from a set of electrolytes (sodium, potassium, chloride, and carbon dioxide) and is used most frequently as a clinical indicator of metabolic acidosis. The most common causes of an increased gap are lactic acidosis and ketoacidosis. The concept of estimating electrolyte disturbances in the extracellular fluid is based on the principle of electrical neutrality. The formula includes the major cation (sodium) and anions (chloride and bicarbonate) found in extracellular fluid. The anion gap is calculated as follows: anion gap = sodium – (chloride + HCO_3^-). Some laboratories may include potassium in the calculation of the anion gap. Calculations including potassium can be invalidated because minor amounts of hemolysis can contribute significant levels of potassium leaked into the serum as a result of cell rupture.

Because bicarbonate (HCO_3^-) is not directly measured on most chemistry analyzers, it is estimated by substitution of the total carbon dioxide (Tco_2) value in the calculation. The anion gap is also widely used as a laboratory quality-control measure because low gaps usually indicate a reagent, calibration, or instrument error.

INDICATIONS
- Determine whole-body stores of sodium, because the ion is predominantly extracellular.

- Monitor the effectiveness of drug therapy, especially diuretics, on serum sodium levels.

INTERFERING FACTORS
Factors that may alter the results of the study
- Drugs and other substances that may increase serum sodium levels include anabolic steroids, angiotensin, bicarbonate, cisplatin, corticotropin, cortisone, gamma globulin, and mannitol.
- Drugs and other substances that may decrease serum sodium levels include amphotericin B, bicarbonate, cathartics (excessive use), chlorpropamide, chlorthalidone, diuretics, ethacrynic acid, fluoxetine, furosemide, laxatives (excessive use), methyclothiazide, metolazone, nicardipine, quinethazone, theophylline (IV infusion), thiazides, and triamterene.
- Specimens should never be collected above an IV line because of the potential for dilution when the specimen and the IV solution combine in the collection container, falsely decreasing the result. There is also the potential of contaminating the sample with the substance of interest, if it is present in the IV solution, falsely increasing the result.

POTENTIAL MEDICAL DIAGNOSIS: CLINICAL SIGNIFICANCE OF RESULTS
Increased in
- Azotemia *(related to increased renal retention)*
- Burns *(hemoconcentration related to excessive loss of free water)*
- Cushing disease
- Dehydration
- Diabetes *(dehydration related to frequent urination)*
- Diarrhea *(related to water loss in excess of salt loss)*

- Excessive intake
- Excessive saline therapy *(related to administration of IV fluids)*
- Excessive sweating *(related to loss of free water, which can cause hemoconcentration)*
- Fever *(related to loss of free water through sweating)*
- Hyperaldosteronism *(related to excessive production of aldosterone, which increases renal absorption of sodium and increases blood levels)*
- Lactic acidosis *(related to diabetes)*
- Nasogastric feeding with inadequate fluid *(related to dehydration and hemoconcentration)*
- Vomiting *(related to dehydration)*

Decreased in
- Central nervous system disease
- Cystic fibrosis *(related to loss from chronic diarrhea; poor intestinal absorption)*
- Excessive antidiuretic hormone production *(related to excessive loss through renal excretion)*
- Excessive use of diuretics *(related to excessive loss through renal excretion; renal absorption is blocked)*
- Heart failure *(diminished renal blood flow due to reduced cardiac capacity decreases urinary excretion and increases blood sodium levels)*
- Hepatic failure *(hemodilution related to fluid retention)*
- Hypoproteinemia *(related to fluid retention)*
- Insufficient intake
- IV glucose infusion *(hypertonic glucose draws water into extracellular fluid and sodium is diluted)*
- Mineralocorticoid deficiency (Addison disease) *(related to inadequate production of aldosterone, which results in decreased absorption by the kidneys)*
- Nephrotic syndrome *(related to decreased ability of renal tubules to reabsorb sodium)*

S

NURSING IMPLICATIONS

POTENTIAL NURSING PROBLEMS: ASSESSMENT & NURSING DIAGNOSIS

Problems	Signs and Symptoms
Confusion *(related to sodium excess or deficit secondary to metabolic alterations, disease process, or burns)*	Disorganized thinking, restlessness, irritability, altered concentration and attention span, changeable mental function over the day, hallucinations
Diarrhea *(related to gastric irritation from diet or disease, stress, drug adverse effect, laxative misuse, malabsorption, alcohol misuse, chemotherapy, enteric infections)*	Abdominal pain, cramping, frequent stools that exceed three per day, watery stools, gastrointestinal (GI) urgency, hyperactive bowel sounds
Electrolyte imbalance: **Excess** *(related to excess fluid loss, watery diarrhea, inability to take oral fluids, excess perspiration, large-area burns, excess sodium intake)*	**Excess:** Furrowed tongue, dry mouth, headache, dry skin, seizures, coma, tachycardia, hypotension, vascular collapse, restlessness, increased urine output, weight gain, altered mental status
Deficit *(related to excess sodium loss through kidneys, diuretic use, adrenal insufficiency with altered cortisol and aldosterone production, vomiting and diarrhea, heart failure, chronic kidney disease, cirrhosis)*	**Deficit:** Muscle cramps, weakness, fatigue, confusion, anorexia, nausea, vomiting, abdominal cramps, diarrhea, headache, depression, personality changes, irritability, muscle twitching, coma, anxiety
Fluid volume *(related to an excess or deficit of sodium associated with electrolyte disturbance and related disease process)*	**Deficit:** Decreased urinary output, fatigue, sunken eyes, dark urine, decreased blood pressure, increased heart rate, altered mental status
	Excess: Edema, shortness of breath, increased weight, ascites, rales, rhonchi, diluted laboratory values

BEFORE THE STUDY: PLANNING AND IMPLEMENTATION

Teaching the Patient What to Expect
- Inform the patient this test can assist in evaluating electrolyte balance.
- Explain that a blood sample is needed for the test.

AFTER THE STUDY: POTENTIAL NURSING ACTIONS

Treatment Considerations
- Confusion: Collaborate with the HCP to treat the medical condition. Correlate confusion with the need to reverse altered electrolytes. Evaluate medications. Prevent falls and injury through appropriate use of postural support, bed alarm, or restraints. Consider pharmacological interventions.
- Diarrhea: Assess bowel sounds. Send ordered stool for culture and sensitivity. Assess for food intolerances that can irritate the GI tract and tolerance to dairy products. Check for a history of GI disease or surgery, ask about foreign travel, administer prescribed antidiarrheal, evaluate and replace lost fluids, and consider dietary bulk.

S

▶ Electrolyte Imbalance: Correlate sodium imbalance with disease process, nutritional intake, kidney function, and medications. Monitor electrocardiogram status and respiratory changes. Collaborate with the pharmacist and HCP for appropriate pharmacologic interventions and dietitian for dietary modifications. Reduce or increase intake of high-sodium foods and salts as required. Ensure medication dosage is adjusted to compensate for renal impairment. Be aware that renal dialysis may be necessary. If a deficit is present, avoid thiazide diuretics, and if an excess is present, use diuretics to increase sodium excretion. IV fluids may be used as a remedy for dehydration and an IV NACL infusion for low sodium.

▶ Fluid Volume: Evaluate the patient for signs and symptoms of dehydration. Decreased skin turgor, dry mouth, and multiple longitudinal furrows in the tongue are symptoms of dehydration. Dehydration is a significant and common finding in older adults and other patients in whom kidney function has deteriorated. Establish baseline assessment data. Monitor and trend daily weight, intake and output, urine characteristics, and respiratory status. Collaborate with the HCP regarding administration of IV fluids to support hydration. Monitor laboratory values that reflect alterations in fluid status: potassium, BUN, Cr, calcium, Hbg, Hct, and sodium. Administer ordered replacement electrolytes and adjust diuretics as appropriate.

Nutritional Considerations

▶ Provide education to those with low sodium levels that the major source of dietary sodium is found in table salt.

▶ Explain that foods such as milk and other dairy products are good sources of dietary sodium.

▶ Additional dietary sodium is available through the consumption of processed foods; some examples are baking mixes (pancakes or muffins), sauces (barbecue), butter, canned soups and sauces, dry soup mixes, frozen or microwave meals, ketchup, pickles, and snack foods (potato chips, pretzels).

▶ Patients on low-sodium diets should be advised to avoid beverages such as colas, ginger ale, sports drinks, lemon-lime sodas, and root beer.

▶ Explain that many over-the-counter medications, including antacids, laxatives, analgesics, sedatives, and antitussives, contain significant amounts of sodium.

▶ Emphasize the importance of reading all food, beverage, and medicine labels.

Follow-Up, Evaluation, and Desired Outcomes

▶ Acknowledges contact information provided for the U.S. Department of Agriculture's resource for nutrition (www.choosemyplate.gov).

▶ Successfully states the symptoms of both an excess and a deficit of sodium.

▶ Understands an altered sodium level can have a significant impact on cognitive function.

▶ Acknowledges the importance of fluid replacement with multiple diarrhea episodes.

Sodium, Urine

S

SYNONYM/ACRONYM: Urine Na⁺.

RATIONALE: To assist in evaluating for acute kidney injury, chronic kidney disease, acute oliguria, and to assist in the differential diagnosis of hyponatremia.

PATIENT PREPARATION: There are no food, fluid, activity, or medication restrictions unless by medical direction. Usually, a 24-hr urine collection is ordered.

As appropriate, provide the required urine collection container and specimen collection instructions.

NORMAL FINDINGS: Method: Ion-selective electrode.

Age	Conventional Units	SI Units (Conventional Units × 1)
6–10 yr		
Male	41–115 mEq/24 hr or mmol/24 hr	41–115 mmol/24 hr
Female	20–69 mEq/24 hr or mmol/24 hr	20–69 mmol/24 hr
10–14 yr		
Male	63–177 mEq/24 hr or mmol/24 hr	63–177 mmol/24 hr
Female	48–168 mEq/24 hr or mmol/24 hr	48–168 mmol/24 hr
Adult–older adult	51–287 mEq/24 hr or mmol/24 hr	51–287 mmol/24 hr

Values vary markedly depending on dietary intake and hydration state.

CRITICAL FINDINGS AND POTENTIAL INTERVENTIONS: N/A

OVERVIEW: (Study type: Urine from an unpreserved random or timed specimen collected in a clean plastic collection container; related body system: Endocrine and Urinary systems.) Sodium balance is dependent on a number of influences in addition to dietary intake, including aldosterone, renin, and atrial natriuretic hormone levels. Regulating electrolyte balance is a major function of the kidneys. In normally functioning kidneys, urine sodium levels increase when serum levels are high and decrease when serum levels are low to maintain homeostasis. Analyzing these urinary levels can provide important clues to the functioning of the kidneys and other major organs. There is diurnal variation in excretion of sodium, with values lower at night. Urine sodium tests usually involve timed urine collections over a 12- or 24-hr period. Measurement of random specimens may also be requested.

INDICATIONS
- Determine potential cause of renal calculi.
- Evaluate known or suspected endocrine disorder.
- Evaluate known or suspected kidney disease.
- Evaluate malabsorption disorders.

INTERFERING FACTORS
Factors that may alter the results of the study
- Drugs and other substances that may increase urine sodium levels include acetazolamide, acetylsalicylic acid, amiloride, ammonium chloride, azosemide, benzthiazide, bumetanide, calcitonin, chlorothiazide, clopamide, cyclothiazide, diapamide, dopamine, ethacrynic acid, furosemide, hydrocortisone, isosorbide, levodopa, mercurial diuretics, methyclothiazide, metolazone, polythiazide, quinethazone, spironolactone, sulfates, tetracycline, thiazides, torasemide, triamterene, trichlormethiazide, triflocin, verapamil, and vincristine.

S

- Drugs and other substances that may decrease urine sodium levels include aldosterone, anesthetics, angiotensin, corticosteroids, cortisone, etodolac, indomethacin, levarterenol, lithium, and propranolol.

Other considerations
- Sodium levels are subject to diurnal variation (output being lowest at night), which is why 24-hr collections are recommended.
- All urine voided for the timed collection period must be included in the collection or else falsely decreased values may be obtained. Compare output records with volume collected to verify that all voids were included in the collection.

POTENTIAL MEDICAL DIAGNOSIS: CLINICAL SIGNIFICANCE OF RESULTS
Increased in
- Adrenal failure *(inadequate production of aldosterone results in decreased renal sodium absorption)*
- Dehydration *(related to decreased water excretion, which results in higher concentration of the urine constituents)*
- Diabetes *(increased glucose levels result in hypertonic extracellular fluid; dehydration from excessive urination can cause hemoconcentration)*
- Diuretic therapy *(medication causes sodium to be lost by the kidneys)*
- Excessive intake
- Salt-losing nephritis *(related to diminished capacity of the kidneys to reabsorb sodium)*
- Syndrome of inappropriate antidiuretic hormone secretion *(related to increased reabsorption of water by the kidneys, which results in higher concentration of the urine constituents)*

Decreased in
- Adrenal hyperfunction, such as Cushing disease and hyperaldostronism *(overproduction of aldosterone and other corticosteroids stimulate renal absorption of sodium decreasing urine sodium levels)*
- Heart failure *(decreased renal blood flow related to diminished cardiac output)*
- Diarrhea *(related to decreased intestinal absorption; a decrease in blood levels will cause sodium to be retained by the kidneys and will lower urine sodium levels)*
- Excessive sweating *(excessive loss of sodium through sweat; sodium will be retained by the kidneys)*
- Extrarenal sodium loss with adequate hydration
- Insufficient intake
- Postoperative period (first 24 to 48 hr)
- Prerenal azotemia
- Sodium retention *(premenstrual)*

NURSING IMPLICATIONS

BEFORE THE STUDY: PLANNING AND IMPLEMENTATION

Teaching the Patient What to Expect
▸ Inform the patient this test can assist in evaluating kidney function.
▸ Explain that a urine sample is needed for the test. Information regarding specimen collection is presented with other general guidelines in Appendix A: Patient Preparation and Specimen Collection.

Potential Nursing Actions
▸ Include on the collection container's label urine total volume, test start and stop times/dates, and any medications that may interfere with test results.

S

AFTER THE STUDY: POTENTIAL NURSING ACTIONS

Treatment Considerations
- Instruct the patient to resume usual diet, fluids, medications, and activity, as directed by the health-care provider (HCP).

Nutritional Considerations
- Provide education to those with low sodium levels that the major source of dietary sodium is found in table salt.
- Explain that foods such as milk and other dairy products are also good sources of dietary sodium.
- Additional dietary sodium is available through the consumption of processed foods; some examples are baking mixes (pancakes or muffins), sauces (barbecue), butter, canned soups and sauces, dry soup mixes, frozen or microwave meals, ketchup, pickles, and snack foods (potato chips, pretzels).
- Patients on low-sodium diets should be advised to avoid beverages such as colas, ginger ale, sports drinks, lemon-lime sodas, and root beer.
- Explain that many over-the-counter medications, including antacids, laxatives, analgesics, sedatives, and antitussives, contain significant amounts of sodium.
- Emphasize the importance of reading all food, beverage, and medicine labels.

Follow-Up, Evaluation, and Desired Outcomes
- Acknowledges contact information provided for the U.S. Department of Agriculture's resource for nutrition (www.choosemyplate.gov).

Spondee Speech Recognition Threshold

SYNONYM/ACRONYM: SRT, speech reception threshold, speech recognition threshold.

RATIONALE: To evaluate for hearing loss related to speech discrepancies.

PATIENT PREPARATION: There are no food, fluid, activity, or medication restrictions unless by medical direction.

NORMAL FINDINGS
- Normal spondee threshold of about 6 to 10 dB (decibels) of the normal pure tone threshold with 50% of the words presented being correctly repeated at the appropriate intensity (see study titled "Audiometry, Hearing Loss")
- Normal speech recognition with 90% to 100% of the words presented being correctly repeated at an appropriate intensity.

CRITICAL FINDINGS AND POTENTIAL INTERVENTIONS: N/A

OVERVIEW: (Study type: Sensory, auditory; **related body system:** Nervous system.) This noninvasive speech audiometric procedure measures the degree of hearing loss for speech. The speech recognition threshold is the lowest hearing level at which speech can barely be recognized or understood. In this test, a number of spondaic words are presented to the patient at different intensities. Spondaic words, or *spondees,* are words containing two syllables that are equally accented or emphasized when they are spoken to the patient. The SRT is defined as the lowest

S

hearing level at which the patient correctly repeats 50% of a list of spondaic words. Examples are *airplane, hot dog, outside, ice cream,* and *baseball.*

INDICATIONS

- Determine appropriate gain during hearing aid selection.
- Determine the extent of hearing loss related to speech recognition, as evidenced by the faintest level at which spondee words are correctly repeated.
- Differentiate a real hearing loss from pseudohypoacusis.
- Verify pure tone results.

INTERFERING FACTORS

Factors that may alter the results of the study

- Unfamiliarity with the language in which the words are presented or with the words themselves will alter the results.
- Improper placement of the earphones and inconsistency in frequency of word presentation will affect results.

POTENTIAL MEDICAL DIAGNOSIS: CLINICAL SIGNIFICANCE OF RESULTS

Abnormal findings related to

- Conductive hearing loss
- Impacted cerumen
- Obstruction of external ear canal *(related to presence of a foreign body)*
- Otitis externa *(related to infection in ear canal)*
- Otitis media *(related to poor eustachian tube function or infection)*
- Otitis media serus *(related to fluid in middle ear due to allergies or a cold)*
- Otosclerosis
- High-frequency hearing loss *(normal hearing range is 20 Hz to 20,000 Hz; high-frequency range begins at 4,000 Hz)*

- Presbycusis *(related to gradual hearing loss experienced in advancing age, which occurs in the high-frequency range)*
- Noise induced *(related to exposure over long periods of time)*
- Sensorineural hearing loss (acoustic nerve impairment)
- Congenital damage or malformations of the inner ear
- Ménière disease
- Ototoxic drugs *(aminoglycosides, e.g., gentamicin or tobramycin; salicylates, e.g., aspirin)*
- Serious infections *(meningitis, measles, mumps, other viral infections, syphilis)*
- Trauma to the inner ear *(related to exposure to noise in excess of 90 dB or as a result of physical trauma)*
- Tumor *(e.g., acoustic neuroma, cerebellopontine angle tumor, meningioma)*
- Vascular disorders

NURSING IMPLICATIONS

BEFORE THE STUDY: PLANNING AND IMPLEMENTATION

Teaching the Patient What to Expect

- Inform the patient this procedure can assist in measuring hearing loss related to speech.
- Review the procedure with the patient. Address concerns about pain and explain that no discomfort will be experienced during the test.
- Ensure understanding of words and sounds in the language to be used for the test.
- Explain that a series of words that change from loud to soft tones will be presented using earphones, and then the patient will be asked to repeat the word. Each ear is tested separately.
- Explain that a health-care provider (HCP) performs the test, in a quiet, soundproof room, and that the evaluation takes 5 to 10 min.

S

- Positioning for this procedure is seated on a chair in a soundproof booth.
- Earphones are placed on the head and secured over the ears.
- The audiometer is set at 20 dB above the known pure tone threshold obtained from audiometry. The test represents hearing levels at speech frequencies of 500, 1,000, and 2,000 Hz.
- The spondee words are presented to the ear with the best auditory response using a speech audiometer. The intensity is decreased and then increased to the softest sound at which the patient is able to hear the words and respond correctly to 50% of them. The procedure is then repeated for the other ear.

Potential Nursing Actions
- Obtain a history of a known or suspected hearing loss, including type and cause; ear conditions with treatment regimens; ear surgery; and other tests and procedures to assess and diagnose hearing deficit.

AFTER THE STUDY: POTENTIAL NURSING ACTIONS

Treatment Considerations
- Be supportive of activity related to impaired hearing and perceived loss of independence.
- Discuss the implications of abnormal test results on lifestyle choices.

Follow-Up, Evaluation, and Desired Outcomes
- Acknowledges contact information provided for the American Speech-Language-Hearing Association (www.asha.org).

Stereotactic Biopsy, Breast

SYNONYM/ACRONYM: N/A

RATIONALE: To assess suspicious breast tissue for cancer.

PATIENT PREPARATION: There are no food, fluid, or activity restrictions unless by medical direction. The patient should be instructed not to wear deodorant, powder, lotion, or perfume under the arms or on the chest/breasts on the day of the procedure.

Regarding the patient's risk for bleeding, the patient should be instructed to avoid taking natural products and medications with known anticoagulant, antiplatelet, or thrombolytic properties or to reduce dosage, as ordered, prior to the procedure. Number of days to withhold medication is dependent on the type of anticoagulant. Note the last time and dose of medication taken. Protocols may vary among facilities.

NORMAL FINDINGS
- No abnormal cells or tissue.

CRITICAL FINDINGS AND POTENTIAL INTERVENTIONS
- Identification of malignancy.

Timely notification to the requesting health-care provider (HCP) of any critical findings and related symptoms is a role expectation of the professional nurse. A listing of these findings varies among facilities.

OVERVIEW: (Study type: Radiology, plain; related body system: Immune and Reproductive systems. Label the appropriate specimen containers with the corresponding patient demographics, initials of the person collecting the specimen, date and time of collection, and site location, especially right or left breast.) A stereotactic breast biopsy is helpful when a mammogram or ultrasound examination shows a mass, a cluster of microcalcifications (tiny calcium deposits that are closely grouped together), or an area of abnormal tissue change, usually with no lump being felt on a careful breast examination. A number of biopsy instruments and methods are utilized with x-ray guidance. They include large-core needle biopsy that is used to remove a generous portion of breast tissue for examination, fine-needle aspiration biopsy, or a vacuum-assisted needle biopsy device. An initial x-ray locates the abnormality, and two stereo views are obtained, each angled 15 degrees to either side of the initial image. The computer calculates how much the area of interest has changed with each image and determines the exact site in three-dimensional space. The sample of breast tissue is obtained and can indicate whether the breast mass is cancerous. A pathologist examines the tissue that was removed and makes a final diagnosis to allow for effective treatment.

INDICATIONS

• A mammogram showing a suspicious cluster of small calcium deposits.

• A mammogram showing a suspicious solid mass that cannot be felt on breast examination.
• Evidence of breast lesion by palpation, mammography, or ultrasound.
• New mass or area of calcium deposits present at a previous surgery site.
• Observable breast changes such as "peau d'orange" skin, scaly skin of the areola, drainage from the nipple, or ulceration of the skin.
• Patient preference for a nonsurgical method of lesion assessment.
• Structure of the breast tissue is distorted.

INTERFERING FACTORS

Contraindications

Patients undergoing biopsy who have bleeding disorders, because the site may not stop bleeding.

Factors that may alter the results of the study

• Metallic objects (e.g., jewelry, body rings) within the examination field, which may inhibit organ visualization and cause unclear images.
• Inability of the patient to cooperate or remain still during the procedure, because movement can produce blurred or otherwise unclear images.

POTENTIAL MEDICAL DIAGNOSIS: CLINICAL SIGNIFICANCE OF RESULTS

• Positive findings in cancer of the breast

NURSING IMPLICATIONS

BEFORE THE STUDY: PLANNING AND IMPLEMENTATION

Teaching the Patient What to Expect

▶ Inform the patient this procedure can assist in assessing breast health.
▶ Pregnancy is a general contraindication to procedures involving radiation.

S

Explain to the female patient that she will be asked the date of her last menstrual period. Pregnancy testing may be performed to determine the possibility of pregnancy before exposure to radiation.

▶ Review the procedure with the patient. Address concerns about pain and explain that there may be moments of discomfort or pain experienced when the IV line or catheter is inserted to allow infusion of fluids such as saline, anesthetics, sedatives, medications used in the procedure, or emergency medications.

▶ Explain that the procedure is performed in a special room for stereotactic biopsies, usually a mammography suite, by an HCP specializing in this procedure, with support staff, and takes approximately 30 to 60 min.

▶ Instruct the patient to remove jewelry and other metallic objects from the area of the procedure.

▶ Baseline vital signs and neurological status are recorded. Protocols may vary among facilities.

▶ The selected area is cleansed and covered with a sterile drape.

▶ Preliminary images are taken.

▶ A local anesthetic is injected at the computer-generated coordinates for the site of interest, and a small incision is made or a needle inserted.

▶ Positioning for the procedure is dependent upon the system being used. Some systems are designed with an opening in the table that, when the patient is in the prone position, allows the breast to hang freely through the opening to facilitate performance of the biopsy procedure from beneath the table, after mammography is completed.

▶ A second positioning option is a sitting position in an upright position.

▶ In either position, the breast to be examined is compressed and held in position by the equipment for imaging and biopsy.

▶ Tissue samples are obtained using a vacuum-assisted device that pulls tissue into a biopsy needle. Multiple tissue samples are obtained, and a final set of images is taken.

▶ Once the procedure is completed, the needle or catheter is removed and a pressure dressing is applied over the puncture site.

▶ Tissue samples are placed in properly labelled specimen containers, especially identifying laterality, and promptly transported to the laboratory for processing and analysis.

Potential Nursing Actions

※ *Make sure a written and informed consent has been signed prior to the procedure and before administering any medications.*

Safety Considerations

▶ Anticoagulants, aspirin, and other salicylates should be discontinued by medical direction for the appropriate number of days prior to a procedure in which bleeding is a potential complication.

AFTER THE STUDY: POTENTIAL NURSING ACTIONS

Avoiding Complications

▶ Establishing an IV site is an invasive procedures. Complications are rare but include risk for bleeding from the puncture site *(related to a bleeding disorder or the effects of natural products and medications with known anticoagulant, antiplatelet, or thrombolytic properties),* cardiac dysrhythmias, hematoma *(related to blood leakage into the tissue following needle insertion),* infection *(which might occur if bacteria from the skin surface is introduced at the puncture site),* nerve injury *(which might occur if the needle strikes a nerve),* or seeding of the biopsy tract. Monitor the patient for complications related to the procedure (e.g., infection, injury). Observe/assess the needle/catheter insertion site for bleeding, inflammation, or hematoma formation.

Treatment Considerations

▶ Instruct the patient to resume usual medications, as directed by the HCP.

▶ Explain the importance of reporting symptoms such as bleeding, fast heart rate, difficulty breathing, fever, or inflammation immediately to the HCP. Explain that some bruising may occur.

▶ Provide instruction on the care and assessment of the site.

S

Follow-Up, Evaluation, and Desired Outcomes

▶ Understands that decisions regarding the need for and frequency of breast self-examination, mammography, magnetic resonance imaging or ultrasound of the breast, or other cancer screening procedures should be made after consultation between the patient and HCP.

▶ Acknowledges that the most current guidelines for breast cancer screening of the general population as well as of individuals with increased risk are available from the American Cancer Society (www.cancer.org), American College of Obstetricians and Gynecologists (www.acog.org), and American College of Radiology (www.acr.org). Screening guidelines vary depending on the age and health history of those at average risk and those at high risk for breast cancer. Guidelines may not always agree between organizations; therefore, it is important for patients to participate in their health care, be informed, ask questions, and follow their HCP's recommendations regarding frequency and type of screening. For additional information regarding screening guidelines, refer to the study titled "Mammography."

Stress Testing: Exercise and Pharmacological

SYNONYM/ACRONYM: Exercise electrocardiogram, graded exercise tolerance test, cardiac stress testing, nuclear stress testing, stress testing, treadmill test.

RATIONALE: To assess cardiac function in relation to increased workload, evidenced by dysrhythmia or pain during exercise.

PATIENT PREPARATION: Instruct the patient to fast, restrict fluids (especially those containing caffeine), and abstain from the use of tobacco products for 4 to 6 hr prior to the procedure. Instruct the patient to withhold medications for 24 hr before the test, *as ordered* by the health-care provider (HCP). Protocols vary depending on the type of test, and in general, protocols may vary among facilities. The patient should be instructed to wear comfortable shoes and clothing for the exercise stress test.

NORMAL FINDINGS

• Normal heart rate during physical exercise. Heart rate and systolic blood pressure rise in direct proportion to workload and to metabolic oxygen demand, which is based on age and exercise protocol. Maximum heart rate for adults is estimated by subtracting the age in years from 220 (e.g., estimated maximum heart rate for a 45-year-old adult is 220 – 45, or 175 beats/min.

CRITICAL FINDINGS AND POTENTIAL INTERVENTIONS: N/A

OVERVIEW: (Study type: Electrophysiological; related body system: Circulatory system.) Understanding the stress test can be confusing until it becomes clear that there are two main types of stress testing (exercise and pharmacologic), each type of testing can be performed as a nonnuclear study or a nuclear study, and the protocols may differ depending on which drug

S

and/or radionuclide is used. In most cases, the goal of the cardiac stress test is to increase heart rate to a level just below (85%) a person's age-predicted maximum target heart rate, either through physical exercise or through the use of specific drugs whose effects increase heart rate in a simulation of physical exercise. The target heart rate can be calculated in a number of ways. One way is by subtracting the patient's age from 220 (theoretical maximum heart rate) and multiplying by 0.85 (85%). For example, the study target heart rate for a patient age 50 years would be

$$(220 - 50) \times 0.85 = 144.$$

The risks involved in the procedure are possible myocardial infarction (MI; 1 in 500) and death (1 in 10,000) in patients experiencing frequent angina episodes before the test. Although useful, this procedure is not as accurate as cardiac nuclear scans for diagnosing coronary artery disease (CAD). For additional information regarding screening guidelines for *atherosclerotic cardiovascular disease* (ASCVD), refer to the study titled "Cholesterol, Total and Fractions."

The exercise stress test is a noninvasive study to measure cardiac function during physical stress. Exercise electrocardiography is primarily useful in determining the extent of coronary artery occlusion by the heart's ability to meet the need for additional oxygen in response to the stress of exercising in a safe environment. The patient exercises on a treadmill or pedals a stationary bicycle to increase the heart

rate. Every 2 to 3 min, the speed and/or grade of the treadmill is increased to yield an increment of stress. The patient's electrocardiogram (ECG) and blood pressure are monitored during the test. The test proceeds until the patient reaches the target heart rate or experiences chest pain or fatigue. During exercise, areas of heart muscle supplied by normal arteries increase their blood supply to a greater extent than regions of the heart muscle supplied by stenosed coronary arteries. This discrepancy in blood flow becomes apparent in ECG readings, in pulse or blood pressure changes, in nonnuclear studies, and in adjunctive nuclear perfusion stress imaging as the injected radionuclide is delivered to the heart muscle. Comparison of early perfusion images with images taken after 3 to 4 hr redistribution (delayed images) enables quantifiable differentiation between normally perfused, healthy myocardium (which is normal at rest but ischemic on stress) and infarcted myocardium.

For patients unable to complete the exercise test, pharmacological stress testing can be done. Medications used to pharmacologically exercise the patient's heart include vasodilators such as regadenoson (Lexiscan), dipyridamole (Persantine) and adenosine, or dobutamine (which stimulates heart rate and pumping force). The medication can be administered orally or by IV injection and is administered before the radionuclide. Stress testing should be discontinued when maximum performance has been reached or if certain criteria occur as noted in the Contraindications section. The patient's ECG, pulse, and blood pressure are monitored during the exercise phase. The test proceeds until the stimulated exercise portion is completed, that is, when the medication has stimulated heart activity to its target. Then images are taken with a conventional gamma camera or with SPECT/CT during the stimulated portion to compare with the images taken at rest. If the pharmacological challenge is to be followed with nuclear perfusion imaging a radiotracer, such as thallium-201 chloride, technetium-99m (Tc-99) sestamibi, or Tc-99m tetrofosmin is injected, and images are taken with a conventional gamma camera or with SPECT/CT during the stimulated portion to compare with the images taken at rest.

INDICATIONS

- Detect dysrhythmias during exercising, as evidenced by ECG changes.
- Detect peripheral arterial disease (PAD), as evidenced by leg pain or cramping during exercising.
- Determine exercise-induced hypertension.
- Evaluate cardiac function after myocardial infarction or cardiac surgery to determine safe exercise levels for cardiac rehabilitation as well as work limitations.
- Evaluate effectiveness of medication regimens, such as antianginals or antidysrhythmics.
- Evaluate suspected CAD in the presence of chest pain and other symptoms.
- Screen for CAD in the absence of pain and other symptoms in patients at risk.

INTERFERING FACTORS
Contraindications
A variety of circumstances that may be considered absolute or relative depending on the facility's providers:

- Abnormal ECG changes causing symptoms *related to the possibility of stress-induced infarction.*
- Acute myocardial infarction (within 2 days) *related to the possibility of stress-induced reinfarction.*
- Acute myocarditis *related to low stress tolerance.*
- Aortic dissection *related to the possibility of stress-induced tears and rupture.*
- Chest pain *related to the possibility of stress-induced infarction.*
- Heart failure with symptoms (e.g., shortness of breath) *related to low stress tolerance.*
- Mental or physical (e.g., severe leg claudication) impairment that prevents the patient from performing the required exercise.
- Severe asthma.
- Significant hypertension or hypotension.
- Stenotic valvular disease with symptoms *related to low stress tolerance from having the heart work harder to pump blood through the narrow valve.*
- Very fast (tachydysrhythmia) or very slow (bradydysrhythmia) heart rate.

The following factors may impair interpretation of examination results because they create an artificial state that makes it difficult to determine true physiological function:

- Anxiety or panic attack.
- Drugs such as barbiturates, beta blockers, cardiac glycosides, calcium channel blockers, coronary vasodilators, and xanthines (e.g., caffeine, theophylline).

S

- High food intake or smoking before testing.
- Hypertension, hypoxia, left bundle branch block, and ventricular hypertrophy.
- Improper electrode placement.
- Potassium or calcium imbalance.
- Viagra should not be taken in combination with nitroglycerin or other nitrates 24 hr prior to the procedure because it may result in a dangerously low blood pressure.
- Wolff-Parkinson-White syndrome (anomalous atrioventricular excitation).

POTENTIAL MEDICAL DIAGNOSIS: CLINICAL SIGNIFICANCE OF RESULTS

Abnormal findings related to

- Activity intolerance related to oxygen supply and demand imbalance
- Bradycardia
- CAD
- Chest pain related to ischemia or inflammation
- Decreased cardiac output
- Dysrhythmias
- Hypertension
- PAD
- ST segment depression of 1 mm (considered a positive test), indicating myocardial ischemia
- Tachycardia

NURSING IMPLICATIONS

BEFORE THE STUDY: PLANNING AND IMPLEMENTATION

Teaching the Patient What to Expect

- Inform the patient this procedure can assist in assessing the heart's ability to respond to an increasing workload.
- Pregnancy is a general contraindication to procedures involving radiation. Explain to the female patient that she will be asked the date of her last menstrual period.

Pregnancy testing may be performed to determine the possibility of pregnancy before exposure to radiation if contrast is used.

- Review the procedure with the patient. Address concerns about pain related to the procedure and explain that some discomfort may be experienced during the stimulated portion of the test or when the IV line is inserted if contrast is used.
- If contrast is used, reassure the patient that the radionuclide poses no radioactive hazard and rarely produces adverse effects.
- Inform the patient that the procedure is performed in a special department by an HCP, and staff, specializing in this procedure and takes approximately 30 to 60 min.
- Emphasize to the patient the importance of reporting fatigue, pain, or shortness of breath before or during the procedure.
- To perform the procedure electrodes are placed in appropriate positions on the patient with a blood pressure cuff connected to a monitoring device. Baseline 12-lead ECG and vital signs are recorded. If the patient's oxygen consumption is to be continuously monitored, the patient is connected to a machine via a mouthpiece or to a pulse oximeter via a finger lead.
- Explain that the test will be terminated under specific conditions: presence of severe pain or fatigue; maximum heart rate under stress is attained; signs of ischemia are present; maximum effort has been achieved; or dyspnea, hypertension (systolic blood pressure greater than 200 mm Hg, diastolic blood pressure greater than 110 mm Hg, or both), tachycardia (greater than 200 beats/min minus person's age), new dysrhythmias, chest pain that begins or worsens, faintness, extreme dizziness, or confusion develops.

Types of Stress Tests

- *Treadmill or bicycle (nonnuclear):* The patient is assisted onto the treadmill or bicycle ergometer and is exercised to a calculated 80% to 85% of the maximum heart rate as determined by the protocol selected.

▶ *Treadmill or bicycle (nuclear thallium):* An IV line is inserted before the patient begins exercise. During thallium nuclear stress studies, the radionuclide is injected at peak exercise, after which the patient continues to exercise for a couple of minutes. The test is then terminated and followed by a scan. The patient is asked to return in 2 hrs for a resting scan.

▶ *Treadmill or bicycle (nuclear technetium):* An IV line is inserted, the technetium is administered, and a resting scan is taken before the patient begins exercise. The radionuclide is injected again at peak exercise, after which the patient continues to exercise for a couple of minutes. The test is then terminated and followed by a scan.

▶ *Pharmacological stress test (nonnuclear, e.g., dobutamine, a drug that stimulates heart rate and pumping force):* The patient is positioned on a table in the supine position, an IV line is inserted and dobutamine is administered, and a resting echocardiogram is taken (images will be taken throughout the test). The dobutamine causes the heart to react as if it were experiencing exercise. Sensations may include increased heart rate; a warm, flushed feeling; or mild headache. At peak "exercise," the test is terminated and a final echocardiogram is taken. Heart rate should return to normal in about 5 to 10 min after the IV is removed.

▶ *Pharmacological stress test (nuclear, e.g., persantine, a vasodilator, and the radionuclide thallium):* The patient is positioned on a table in the supine position, an IV line is inserted and the radionuclide is administered, and a resting scan is taken. Persantine is administered, and at peak "exercise," the test is terminated and followed by a scan.

▶ After the chosen stress test is completed, the patient will be allowed a 3- to 15-min rest period in a sitting position. During this period, the ECG, blood pressure, and heart rate monitoring is continued. The electrodes are removed and the skin cleansed of any remaining gel or ECG electrode adhesive. Accumulated ECG and vital sign data is interpreted, and test results are usually reported to the patient for nonnuclear exercise tests. Data or images collected by echocardiography, gamma cameras, or SPECT usually require review and interpretation by the cardiologist performing the study before the results are given to the patient.

Potential Nursing Actions

▶ Inquire if the patient has had a recent MI, any chest pain within the past 48 hr, or has a history of anginal attacks; if any of these have occurred, inform the HCP immediately because the stress test may be too risky and should be rescheduled in 4 to 6 wk.

▶ Evaluate for the presence of other risk factors, such as family history of heart disease, smoking, obesity, diet, lack of physical activity, hypertension, diabetes, previous MI, and previous vascular disease, which should be investigated. Understanding genetics assists in identifying those who may benefit from additional education, risk assessment, and counseling. Genetics is the study and identification of genes, genetic mutations, and inheritance. For example, genetics provides some insight into the likelihood of inheriting a medical condition such as CAD. Genomic studies evaluate the interaction of groups of genes. The combined activity or combined expression of groups of genes allows assumptions or predictions to be made. As an example, genomic studies measure the levels of activity in multiple genes to predict how they, along with environmental and lifestyle decisions, influence the development of type 2 diabetes, CAD, MI, or ischemic stroke.

✦ *Make sure a written and informed consent has been signed prior to the procedure and before administering any medications.*

S

Avoiding Complications

◗ MI. The patient should have been prescreened for history indicative of increased risk of MI/repeat MI. Emphasize to the patient the importance of reporting fatigue, pain, or shortness of breath after the procedure.

◗ Aminophylline can be used to reverse the effects of dipyridamole and regadenoson. Propranolol can be used to reverse the effects of dobutamine.

Treatment Considerations

◗ Teach the patient how to pace activities to better manage oxygen demand and improve gas exchange.

◗ Provide information on the pathophysiology of cardiac disease and physical limitations that are appropriate to the disease process.

◗ Provide resources to arrange for assistance that may be required at home until regular activity can be restored. Suggest strategies for the patient and family to bundle activities to place the least amount of stress on the heart.

◗ Discuss lifestyle changes that will improve cardiac health. Emphasize the importance of reporting chest pain as soon as it occurs to receive prompt medical attention.

Safety Considerations

◗ Breastfeeding patients should consult with the requesting HCP regarding alternate testing that does not involve radiation if contrast is used. In general, if a woman who is breastfeeding must have a nuclear scan, she should not breastfeed the infant for 72 hr after the scan, until the radionuclide has been eliminated. She should be instructed to express the milk in order to prevent cessation of milk production; the milk can be stored and used after the 3-day period.

◗ Refer to organizational policy for additional precautions that may include instructions on handwashing, toilet flushing, limited contact with others, and other aspects of nuclear medicine safety.

Nutritional Considerations

◗ Discuss ideal body weight and the purpose of and relationship between ideal weight and caloric intake to support cardiac health. Review ways to decrease intake of saturated fats and increase intake of polyunsaturated fats. Discuss limiting intake of refined processed sugar and sodium; discuss limiting cholesterol intake to less than 300 mg per day. Encourage the intake of fresh fruits and vegetables, unprocessed carbohydrates, poultry, and grains.

◗ Nutritional therapy is recommended for those with identified CAD risk, especially for those with elevated low-density lipoprotein cholesterol levels, other lipid disorders, diabetes, insulin resistance, or metabolic syndrome. Always consider cultural influences with dietary choices to ensure better adherence to a change in lifestyle. A variety of dietary patterns are beneficial for people with ASCVD. For additional information regarding nutritional guidelines, refer to the study titled "Cholesterol, Total and Fractions."

◗ Other changeable risk factors warranting education include strategies to encourage regular participation in moderate aerobic physical activity three to four times per week, eliminating tobacco use, and adhering to a heart-healthy diet.

◗ Those with elevated triglycerides should be advised to eliminate or reduce alcohol.

Follow-Up, Evaluation, and Desired Outcomes

◗ Acknowledges contact information provided for the American Heart Association (www.heart.org/HEARTORG), National Heart, Lung, and Blood Institute (www.nhlbi.nih.gov), and U.S. Department of Agriculture's resource for nutrition (www.choosemyplate .gov).

◗ Recognizes the importance and health benefits associated with attending cardiac rehabilitation support.

S

Synovial Fluid Analysis

SYNONYM/ACRONYM: Arthrocentesis, joint fluid analysis, knee fluid analysis.

RATIONALE: To identify the presence and assist in the management of joint disease related to disorders such as arthritis and gout.

PATIENT PREPARATION: Refer to the study titled "Arthroscopy" for additional and detailed information regarding patient preparation. Note that there are no fluid restrictions unless by medical direction. Fasting for at least 12 hr before the procedure is recommended if fluid glucose measurements are included in the analysis.

Regarding the patient's risk for bleeding, the patient should be instructed to avoid taking natural products and medications with known anticoagulant, antiplatelet, or thrombolytic properties or to reduce dosage, as ordered, prior to the procedure. Number of days to withhold medication is dependent on the type of anticoagulant. Note the last time and dose of medication taken. Protocols may vary among facilities.

NORMAL FINDINGS: Method: Macroscopic evaluation of appearance; spectrophotometry for glucose, lactic acid, protein, and uric acid; Gram stain, acid-fast stain, and culture for microbiology; microscopic examination of fluid for cell count and evaluation of crystals; ion-selective electrode for pH; nephelometry for RF and C3 complement; indirect fluorescence for ANAs.

Test	Normal Result
Color	Colorless to pale yellow
Clarity	Clear
Viscosity	High
ANA	Parallels serum level
C3	Parallels serum level
Glucose	Less than 10 mg/dL of blood level
Lactic acid	5–20 mg/dL
pH	7.2–7.4
Protein	Less than 3 g/dL
RF	Parallels serum level
Uric acid	Parallels serum level
Crystals	None present
RBC count	None
WBC count	Less than 200 cells/microL
Neutrophils	Less than 25%
WBC morphology	No abnormal cells or inclusions
Gram stain and culture	No organisms present
AFB smear and culture	No AFB present

AFB = acid-fast bacilli; ANA = antinuclear antibodies; C3 = complement;
RBC = red blood cell; RF = rheumatoid factor; WBC = white blood cell.

S

CRITICAL FINDINGS AND POTENTIAL INTERVENTIONS

• Positive culture findings in any sterile body fluid.

Timely notification to the requesting health-care provider (HCP) of any critical findings and related symptoms is a role expectation of the professional nurse. A listing of these findings varies among facilities.

OVERVIEW: (Study type: Body fluid; Synovial fluid collected in a red-top tube for antinuclear antibodies [ANAs], complement, crystal examination, protein, rheumatoid factor [RF], and uric acid; sterile [red-top] tube for microbiological testing; lavender-top [EDTA[tube for mucin clot/viscosity, complete blood count [CBC] and differential; gray-top [sodium fluoride (NaFl)] tube for glucose; green-top [heparin] tube for lactic acid and pH; **related body system:** Immune and Musculoskeletal systems.) Synovial fluid analysis is performed via arthrocentesis, an invasive procedure involving insertion of a needle into the joint space. Synovial effusions are associated with disorders or injuries involving the joints. The most commonly aspirated joint is the knee, although samples also can be obtained from the shoulder, hip, elbow, wrist, and ankle if clinically indicated. Joint disorders can be classified into five categories: noninflammatory, inflammatory, septic, crystal-induced, and hemorrhagic. The mucin clot test is used to correlate the qualitative assessment of synovial fluid viscosity with the presence of hyaluronic acid. The test is performed by mixing equal amounts of synovial fluid and 5% acetic acid solution on a glass slide and grading the ropiness of the subsequent clot as good, fair, or poor. Long, ropy strands are seen in normal synovial fluid.

INDICATIONS

• Administration of anti-inflammatory medications by injection.
• Assist in the diagnosis of arthritis.
• Assist in the evaluation of joint effusions.
• Assist in the diagnosis of joint infection.
• Differentiate gout from pseudogout.

INTERFERING FACTORS

• Blood in the sample from traumatic arthrocentesis may falsely elevate the RBC count.
• Undetected hypoglycemia or hyperglycemia may produce misleading glucose values.
• Refrigeration of the sample may result in an increase in monosodium urate crystals secondary to decreased solubility of uric acid; exposure of the sample to room air with a resultant loss of carbon dioxide and rise in pH encourages the formation of calcium pyrophosphate crystals.

POTENTIAL MEDICAL DIAGNOSIS: CLINICAL SIGNIFICANCE OF RESULTS

Fluid Values Increased In
• *Acute bacterial infection:* Elevated WBC count with marked predominance of neutrophils (greater than 90% neutrophils), positive Gram stain, positive cultures, possible presence of rice bodies, increased lactic acid (produced by bacteria), and complement levels paralleling those found in serum (may be elevated or decreased)
• *Gout:* Elevated WBC count with a predominance of neutrophils (90% neutrophils), presence

of monosodium urate crystals, increased uric acid, and complement levels paralleling those of serum (may be elevated or decreased)

- *Osteoarthritis, traumatic arthritis, degenerative joint disease:* Elevated WBC count with less than 25% neutrophils and the presence of cartilage cells
- *Pseudogout:* Presence of calcium pyrophosphate crystals
- *Rheumatoid arthritis:* Elevated WBC count with a predominance of neutrophils (greater than 70% neutrophils), presence of ragocyte cells and possibly rice bodies, presence of cholesterol crystals if effusion is chronic, increased protein, increased lactic acid, and presence of rheumatoid factor
- *Systemic lupus erythematosus (SLE):* Elevated WBC count with a predominance of neutrophils, presence of SLE cells, and presence of antinuclear antibodies
- *Trauma, joint tumors, or hemophilic arthritis:* Elevated RBC count, increased protein level, and presence of fat droplets (if trauma involved)
- *Tuberculous arthritis:* Elevated WBC count with a predominance of neutrophils (up to 90% neutrophils), possible presence of rice bodies, presence of cholesterol crystals if effusion is chronic, in some cases a positive culture and smear for acid-fast bacilli (results frequently negative), and lactic acid

Fluid Values Decreased in (Analytes in Parentheses Are Decreased)
- Acute bacterial arthritis (glucose and pH)
- Gout (glucose)
- Rheumatoid arthritis (glucose, pH, and complement)
- SLE (glucose, pH, and complement)
- Tuberculous arthritis (glucose and pH)

NURSING IMPLICATIONS

BEFORE THE STUDY: PLANNING AND IMPLEMENTATION

Teaching the Patient What to Expect
- Inform the patient this procedure can assist in assessing joint health.
- Explain that a synovial fluid sample is needed for the test. Refer to study titled "Arthroscopy" for additional detailed information pertaining to patient preparation and specimen collection procedure.
- Review the procedure with the patient. Address concerns about pain and explain that a sedative and/or analgesia will be administered to promote relaxation and reduce discomfort prior to needle insertion through the joint space.
- Explain that it may be necessary to remove hair from the site before the procedure.
- Explain that any discomfort with the needle insertion will be minimized with local anesthetics and systemic analgesics; the anesthetic injection may cause an initial stinging sensation. After the skin has been anesthetized, a large needle will be inserted through the joint space, and a "popping" sensation may be experienced as the needle penetrates the joint.
- Explain that the procedure is performed by an HCP specializing in this procedure. The procedure usually takes approximately 20 min to complete.
- Positioning for this procedure is in a comfortable sitting or supine position.
- Explain that clippers are used to remove hair from the site prior to the administration of general or local anesthesia. The site is cleansed with antiseptic solution and draped with sterile towels.
- Once the local anesthetic is administered, the needle is inserted at the

S

collection site and a syringe is used to remove fluid. Manual pressure may be applied to facilitate fluid removal.

▸ Explain that if medication is to be injected into the joint after the sample collection, the HCP will do so with gentle pressure.

▸ Explain that when the procedure is completed, the needle is withdrawn and direct pressure applied to the site for a few minutes. If there is no evidence of bleeding, a sterile dressing is applied to the site and an elastic bandage to the joint.

▸ Samples are placed in properly labelled specimen containers and promptly transported to the laboratory for processing and analysis. If bacterial culture and sensitivity tests are to be performed, any antibiotic therapy being received should be recorded on the specimen label.

Potential Nursing Actions

✦ *Make sure a written and informed consent has been signed prior to the procedure and before administering any medications.*

AFTER THE STUDY: POTENTIAL NURSING ACTIONS

Avoiding Complications

▸ The patient should be monitored for complications related to the procedure (allergic reaction, anaphylaxis, infection). Observe/assess puncture site for bleeding, bruising, inflammation, and

excessive drainage of synovial fluid approximately every 4 hr for 24 hr and daily thereafter for several days. Advise the patient to immediately report to the HCP elevated temperature, excessive pain, bleeding, swelling, or inability to move the joint.

Treatment Considerations

▸ Instruct the patient to resume usual diet and medications, as directed by the HCP.

▸ After local anesthesia, monitor vital signs and compare with baseline values. Protocols may vary among facilities.

▸ Monitor for pain and nausea. Administer ordered antiemetic and analgesic medications as needed.

▸ Explain the importance of applying an ice pack to the site for 24 to 48 hr.

▸ Administer ordered antibiotics and instruct the patient in the importance of completing the entire course of antibiotic therapy even if no symptoms are present.

▸ Be supportive of impaired activity related to anticipated chronic pain resulting from joint inflammation, impairment in mobility, musculoskeletal deformity, and loss of independence.

Follow-Up, Evaluation, and Desired Outcomes

▸ Acknowledges contact information provided for the American College of Rheumatology (www.rheumatology.org) or Arthritis Foundation (www.arthritis .org).

Syphilis Testing

SYNONYM/ACRONYM: Automated reagin testing (ART), fluorescent treponemal antibody testing (FTA-ABS), microhemagglutination–*Treponema pallidum* (MHA-TP), rapid plasma reagin (RPR), treponemal studies, Venereal Disease Research Laboratory (VDRL) testing.

RATIONALE: To indicate past or present syphilis infection.

PATIENT PREPARATION: There are no food, fluid, activity, or medication restrictions unless by medical direction.

NORMAL FINDINGS: Method: Dark-field microscopy, rapid plasma reagin, enzyme-linked immunosorbent assay (ELISA), microhemagglutination, fluorescence. Nonreactive or absence of treponemal organisms.

CRITICAL FINDINGS AND POTENTIAL INTERVENTIONS: N/A

OVERVIEW: (Study type: Blood collected in a gold-, red-, or red/gray-top tube; related body system: Immune and Reproductive systems.) Syphilis is a sexually transmitted infection (STI) with three stages. On average, symptoms start within 3 wk of infection but can appear as soon as 10 days or as late as 90 days after infection. The primary stage of syphilis is usually marked by the appearance of a single sore, called a *chancre*, at the site where the organism entered the body. The chancre is small and round in appearance, is firm, and is usually painless. The chancre lasts 3 to 6 wk and heals with or without treatment. If untreated, the infection progresses to the secondary stage as the chancre is healing or several weeks after the chancre has healed. The secondary stage is characterized by a skin rash and lesions of the mucous membranes. Other symptoms may include fever, swollen lymph glands, sore throat, patchy hair loss, headaches, weight loss, muscle aches, and fatigue. As with the primary stage, the signs and symptoms of secondary syphilis will resolve either with or without treatment. If untreated, the infection will progress to the latent or hidden stage in which the infection and ability to transmit infection is present even though the infected person is asymptomatic. The latent stage begins when the primary and secondary symptoms disappear, and it can last for

years. About 15% of people in the latent stage, who have not been treated, will develop late-stage syphilis, which can appear 10 to 20 yr after infection. Untreated disease at this stage can result in significant damage to the brain, nerves, eyes, heart, blood vessels, liver, bones, and joints—damage serious enough to cause death. Signs and symptoms of the late stage of syphilis include difficulty coordinating muscle movements, numbness, paralysis, blindness, and dementia.

There are numerous methods for detecting *T. pallidum,* the gram-negative spirochete bacterium known to cause syphilis. Syphilis serology is routinely ordered as part of a prenatal work-up and is required for evaluating donated blood units before release for transfusion. Selection of the proper testing method is important. ART, RPR, and VDRL testing have traditionally been used for screening purposes. These nontreponemal assays detect antibodies directed against lipoidal antigens from damaged host cells. FTA-ABS, MHA-TP, and *T. pallidum* by particle agglutination (TP-PA) are confirmatory methods for samples that screen positive or reactive. Some laboratories have begun using a reverse-screening approach. Highly automated, rapid-testing treponemal enzyme immunoassays (EIA) and chemiluminescent assays (CIA) detect antibodies directed against *T. pallidum* proteins.

S

These assays detect early primary infections as well as past treated infections. The problem with the EIAs and CIAs is that they are very sensitive but less specific; therefore, positive test results should be confirmed using a nontreponemal assay. If reverse screening is used, the Centers for Disease Control and Prevention (CDC) recommends (1) positive EIA/CIA be confirmed using the RPR, and reactive RPR test results should be reported as the endpoint titer of reactivity; (2) a positive EIA/CIA followed by a nonreactive RPR should be tested by a direct treponemal assay such as the TP-PA or FTA-ABS to ensure a false-positive result is not reported and acted upon. Cerebrospinal fluid should be tested only by the FTA-ABS method. Cord blood should not be submitted for testing by any of the aforementioned methods; instead, the mother's serum should be tested to establish whether the infant should be treated.

INDICATIONS

• Monitor effectiveness of treatment for syphilis.
• Screen for and confirm the presence of syphilis.

INTERFERING FACTORS

Other considerations

• Nontreponemal assays can produce false-positive results, which are associated with older age or conditions unrelated to syphilis, such as autoimmune disorders or injection drug use, and require confirmation by a treponemal test method.

POTENTIAL MEDICAL DIAGNOSIS: CLINICAL SIGNIFICANCE OF RESULTS:

Positive findings in

• Syphilis

False-Positive or False-Reactive Findings in Screening (RPR, VDRL) Tests

• Infectious:
 Bacterial endocarditis
 Chancroid
 Chickenpox
 HIV
 Infectious mononucleosis
 Leprosy
 Leptospirosis
 Lymphogranuloma venereum
 Malaria
 Measles
 Mumps
 Mycoplasma pneumoniae
 Pneumococcal pneumonia
 Psittacosis
 Relapsing fever
 Rickettsial disease
 Scarlet fever
 Trypanosomiasis
 Tuberculosis
 Vaccinia (live or attenuated)
 Viral hepatitis
• Noninfectious:
 Advanced cancer
 Advancing age
 Chronic liver disease
 Connective tissue diseases
 IV drug use
 Multiple blood transfusions
 Multiple myeloma and other immunological disorders
 Narcotic addiction
 Pregnancy

False-Positive or False-Reactive Findings in Confirmatory (FTA-ABS, MHA-TP) Tests

• Infectious:
 Infectious mononucleosis

Leprosy
Leptospirosis
Lyme disease
Malaria
Relapsing fever
• Noninfectious:
Systemic lupus erythematosus

*False-Positive Findings in
Confirmatory (TP-PA) Tests*
• Infectious:
Pinta
Yaws

Negative findings in: N/A

NURSING IMPLICATIONS

POTENTIAL NURSING PROBLEMS: ASSESSMENT & NURSING DIAGNOSIS

Problems	Signs and Symptoms
Infection	Rash on body; rash on the palms of the hands; rash on the soles of the feet; small, firm nodules on genitalia, anus, or mouth; lack of coordinated movement; paralysis; gradual blindness; numbness; dementia; internal organ damage (brain, nerves, eyes, heart, liver, bones, joints); death at end stage
Sexuality *(related to alterations in sexual role secondary to syphilis infection)*	Hesitancy to discuss sexual relationship with significant other

BEFORE THE STUDY: PLANNING AND IMPLEMENTATION

Teaching the Patient What to Expect
▶ Inform the patient this test can assist in diagnosing syphilis.
▶ Explain that a blood sample is needed for the test.

AFTER THE STUDY: POTENTIAL NURSING ACTIONS

Treatment Considerations
▶ Offer support those who may be the victim of sexual assault. Provide a nonjudgmental, nonthreatening atmosphere for a discussion during which risks of STIs are explained. It is also important to discuss problems the patient may experience (e.g., guilt, depression, anger).

▶ Explain that repeat testing may be needed at 3-mo intervals for 1 yr to monitor treatment effectiveness.
▶ Infection: Assess for signs and symptoms of syphilis (rash, sores, neurological changes, organ damage). Make sure the patient understands that the infection is sexually transmitted through direct contact with syphilis sores located in genitalia, vagina, anus, inside the rectum, and mouth. Discuss the risk of disease transmission and proper prophylaxis. Reinforce the importance of strict adherence to the treatment regimen. Explain the importance of identifying sexual partners who are at risk and notify them. Administer ordered antibiotic.
▶ Sexuality: Facilitate a discussion of realistic changes to sexual intimacy

S

associated with syphilis infection. Provide a relaxed atmosphere in which to discuss sexuality concerns and contact information for a support group.

Follow-Up, Evaluation, and Desired Outcomes

▶ Understands that positive findings must be reported to local health department

officials, who will ask questions regarding sexual partners.

▶ Acknowledges information provided regarding vaccine-preventable diseases if indicated (e.g., STIs such as hepatitis B and human papillomavirus) from the CDC (www.cdc.gov/vaccines/vpd/vaccines-diseases.html).

S

Testosterone, Total and Free

SYNONYM/ACRONYM: N/A

RATIONALE: To evaluate testosterone to assist in identification of disorders related to early puberty, late puberty, and infertility while assessing gonadal and adrenal function.

PATIENT PREPARATION: There are no food, fluid, activity, or medication restrictions unless by medical direction.

NORMAL FINDINGS: Method: HPLC/tandem MS for total and immunochemiluminometric assay (ICMA) for free testosterone.

Total Testosterone

Age	Conventional Units	SI Units (Conventional Units × 0.0347)
Newborn		
Male	75–400 ng/dL	2.6–13.9 nmol/L
Female	16–44 ng/dL	0.56–1.53 nmol/L
1–5 mo		
Male	Less than 300 ng/dL	Less than 10.41 nmol/L
Female	Less than 20 ng/dL	Less than 0.69 nmol/L
6–11 mo		
Male	Less than 40 ng/dL	Less than 1.39 nmol/L
Female	Less than 9 ng/dL	Less than 0.31 nmol/L
1–5 yr		
Male and female	Less than 20 ng/dL	Less than 0.69 nmol/L
6–7 yr		
Male	Less than 20 ng/dL	Less than 0.69 nmol/L
Female	Less than 10 ng/dL	Less than 0.35 nmol/L
8–10 yr		
Male	2–25 ng/dL	0.07–0.87 nmol/L
Female	1–30 ng/dL	0.04–1 nmol/L
11–12 yr		
Male	Less than 350 ng/dL	Less than 12.1 nmol/L
Female	Less than 50 ng/dL	Less than 1.74 nmol/L
13–15 yr		
Male	15–500 ng/dL	0.52–17.35 nmol/L
Female	Less than 50 ng/dL	Less than 1.74 nmol/L
Adult		
Male	241–827 ng/dL	8.36–28.7 nmol/L
Female	15–70 ng/dL	0.52–2.43 nmol/L
Older adult		
Male	300–720 ng/dL	10.41–24.98
Female	5–32 ng/dL	0.17–1.11

Post menopausal levels are about half the normal adult level for females; levels in women who are pregnant are three to four times the normal adult level for females who are not pregnant.

T

Free Testosterone

Age	Conventional Units	SI Units (Conventional Units × 3.47)
1–12 yr		
Male and female	Less than 2 pg/mL	Less than 6.94 pmol/L
12–14 yr		
Male	Less than 60 pg/mL	Less than 208 pmol/L
Female	Less than 2 pg/mL	Less than 6.94 pmol/L
14–18 yr		
Male	4–100 pg/mL	13.88–347 pmol/L
Female	Less than 10 pg/mL	Less than 34.7 pmol/L
Adult		
Male	50–224 pg/mL	173.5–777.28 pmol/L
Female	1–8.5 pg/mL	3.47–29.5 pmol/L
Older adult		
Male	5–75 pg/mL	17.35–260.25 pmol/L
Female	1–8.5 pg/mL	3.47–29.5 pmol/L

CRITICAL FINDINGS AND POTENTIAL INTERVENTIONS: N/A

OVERVIEW: (Study type: Blood collected in a red-, red/gray-, or green-top [heparin] tube; related body system: Endocrine and Reproductive systems.) Testosterone is the major androgen responsible for sexual differentiation. In males, testosterone is made by the Leydig cells in the testicles and is responsible for spermatogenesis and the development of secondary sex characteristics. In females, the ovary and adrenal gland secrete small amounts of this hormone; however, most of the testosterone in females comes from the metabolism of androstenedione. Testosterone levels have a slight diurnal variation with the highest levels occurring around 0800 and lowest levels around 2000. Measurements of total testosterone levels are used most often in evaluating suspected hormone imbalances. Free testosterone is the active form of the hormone.

It is used in conjunction with total testosterone to evaluate hormone levels in conditions known to alter the effectiveness of testosterone-binding protein, also called *sex hormone–binding globulin,* or SHBG. Alterations in the affinity of SHBG to bind free testosterone are known to occur with obesity, liver disease, and hyperthyroidism. In males, a testicular, adrenal, or pituitary tumor can cause an overabundance of testosterone, triggering precocious puberty. In females, adrenal tumors, hyperplasia, and medications can cause an overabundance of this hormone, resulting in masculinization or hirsutism.

INDICATIONS
- Assist in the diagnosis of hypergonadism.
- Assist in the diagnosis of male sexual precocity before age 10.

T

- Distinguish between primary and secondary hypogonadism.
- Evaluate hirsutism.
- Evaluate male infertility.

INTERFERING FACTORS
Factors that may alter the results of the study
- Drugs and other substances that may increase testosterone levels include barbiturates, bromocriptine, cimetidine, flutamide, gonadotropin, levonorgestrel, mifepristone, moclobemide, nafarelin (males), nilutamide, oral contraceptives, rifampin, and tamoxifen.
- Drugs and other substances that may decrease testosterone levels include cyclophosphamide, cyproterone, danazol, dexamethasone, diethylstilbestrol, digoxin, D-Trp-6-LHRH, fenoldopam, goserelin, ketoconazole, leuprolide, magnesium sulfate, medroxyprogesterone, methylprednisone, oral contraceptives, pravastatin, prednisone, pyridoglutethimide, spironolactone, tetracycline, and thioridazine.

POTENTIAL MEDICAL DIAGNOSIS: CLINICAL SIGNIFICANCE OF RESULTS
Increased in
- Adrenal hyperplasia *(oversecretion of the androgen precursor dehydroepiandrosterone [DHEA])*
- Adrenocortical tumors *(oversecretion of the androgen precursor DHEA)*
- Hirsutism *(any condition that results in increased production of testosterone or its precursors)*
- Hyperthyroidism *(high thyroxine levels increase the production of sex hormone–binding protein, which increases measured levels of total testosterone)*

- Idiopathic sexual precocity *(related to stimulation of testosterone production by elevated levels of luteinizing hormone)*
- Polycystic ovaries *(high estrogen levels increase the production of sex hormone–binding protein, which increases measured levels of total testosterone)*
- Syndrome of androgen resistance
- Testicular or extragonadal tumors *(related to excessive secretion of testosterone)*
- Trophoblastic tumors during pregnancy
- Virilizing ovarian tumors

Decreased in
- Anovulation
- Cryptorchidism *(related to dysfunctional testes)*
- Delayed puberty
- Down syndrome *(related to diminished or dysfunctional testes)*
- Excessive alcohol intake *(alcohol inhibits secretion of testosterone)*
- Hepatic insufficiency *(related to decreased binding protein and reflects decreased measured levels of total testosterone)*
- Impotence *(decreased testosterone levels can result in impotence)*
- Klinefelter syndrome *(chromosome abnormality XXY associated with testicular failure)*
- Malnutrition
- Myotonic dystrophy *(related to testicular atrophy)*
- Orchiectomy *(testosterone production occurs in the testes)*
- Primary and secondary hypogonadism
- Primary and secondary hypopituitarism
- Uremia

T

NURSING IMPLICATIONS

POTENTIAL NURSING PROBLEMS: ASSESSMENT & NURSING DIAGNOSIS

Problems	Signs and Symptoms
Body image *(related to altered male sexual development secondary to lack of testosterone)*	Negative verbalization of physical appearance and lack of male attributes, preoccupation with lack of physical body changes, distress and refusal to talk about appearance, negative verbalization about physical appearance
Sexuality *(related to insufficient testosterone level)*	Delayed puberty, poor development of muscle mass, minimal body hair, insufficient penile and testicle growth, gynecomastia (breast development), arms and legs grow faster than the body trunk, erectile dysfunction, infertility, osteoporosis

BEFORE THE STUDY: PLANNING AND IMPLEMENTATION

Teaching the Patient What to Expect
▶ Inform the patient this test can assist with evaluating hormone levels.
▶ Explain that a blood sample is needed for the test.

AFTER THE STUDY: POTENTIAL NURSING ACTIONS

Treatment Considerations
▶ Body Image: Assess the patient's perception of physical appearance. Note the frequency of negative comments about lack of male attributes associated with physical appearance. Assist in the identification of positive coping strategies to address feelings of inadequacy. Provide reassurance that physical appearance may change with testosterone therapy, and provide a referral to local support groups.
▶ Sexuality: Explain the importance of testosterone replacement therapy; administer prescribed testosterone replacement medication.

Follow-Up, Evaluation, and Desired Outcomes
▶ Understands that the lack of development of male attributes is associated with inadequate testosterone and that hormonal therapy may support male attribute development.
▶ Agrees to counseling associated with concerns related to erectile dysfunction and intimacy.

Thyroglobulin

SYNONYM/ACRONYM: Tg.

RATIONALE: To evaluate thyroid gland function related to disorders such as tumor, inflammation, structural damage, and cancer.

PATIENT PREPARATION: There are no food, fluid, activity, or medication restrictions unless by medical direction.

NORMAL FINDINGS: Method: Chemiluminescent enzyme immunoassay.

Age	Conventional Units	SI Units (Conventional Units × 1)
6 mo–3 yr	7–50 ng/mL	7–50 mcg/L
4–7 yr	4–40 ng/mL	4–40 mcg/L
8–17 yr	0.8–27 ng/mL	0.8–27 mcg/L
Adult–older adult	0.5–40 ng/mL	0.5–40 mcg/L

CRITICAL FINDINGS AND POTENTIAL INTERVENTIONS: N/A

OVERVIEW: (**Study type:** Blood collected in a gold-, red-, or red/gray-top tube; **related body system:** Endocrine system.) Thyroglobulin is an iodinated glycoprotein secreted by follicular epithelial cells of the thyroid gland. It is the storage form of the thyroid hormones thyroxine (T_4) and triiodothyronine (T_3). When thyroid hormones are released into the bloodstream, they split from thyroglobulin in response to thyroid-stimulating hormone. Values greater than 55 ng/mL are indicative of tumor recurrence in patients who are athyrotic.

INDICATIONS
- Assist in the diagnosis of subacute thyroiditis.
- Assist in the diagnosis of suspected disorders of excess thyroid hormone.
- Manage differentiated or metastatic cancer of the thyroid.
- Monitor response to treatment of goiter.
- Monitor T_4 therapy in patients with solitary nodules.

INTERFERING FACTORS
Factors that may alter the results of the study
- Drugs and other substances that may decrease thyroglobulin levels include neomycin and T_4.
- Autoantibodies to thyroglobulin can cause decreased values.

Other considerations
- Recent thyroid surgery or needle biopsy can interfere with test results.

POTENTIAL MEDICAL DIAGNOSIS: CLINICAL SIGNIFICANCE OF RESULTS
Increased in
Thyroglobulin is secreted by normal, abnormal, and cancerous thyroid tissue cells.

- Differentiated thyroid cancer
- Graves disease (untreated) *(autoimmune destruction of thyroid tissue cells)*
- Surgery or irradiation of the thyroid *(elevated levels indicate residual or disseminated cancer)*
- T_4-binding globulin deficiency
- Thyroiditis *(related to leakage from inflamed, damaged thyroid tissue cells)*
- Thyrotoxicosis

Decreased in
- Administration of thyroid hormone *(feedback loop suppresses production)*
- Congenital athyrosis (neonates) *(related to insufficient synthesis)*
- Thyrotoxicosis factitia

NURSING IMPLICATIONS

BEFORE THE STUDY: PLANNING AND IMPLEMENTATION

Teaching the Patient What to Expect
▸ Inform the patient this test can assist in assessing the thyroid gland.
▸ Explain that a blood sample is needed for the test.

T

Thyroid-Binding Inhibitory Immunoglobulins

SYNONYM/ACRONYM: Thyrotropin receptor antibodies, thyrotropin-binding inhibitory immunoglobulin, TBII, TRAb (TSH receptor antibodies).

RATIONALE: To assist in diagnosing Graves disease related to thyroid function.

PATIENT PREPARATION: There are no food, fluid, activity, or medication restrictions unless by medical direction.

NORMAL FINDINGS: Method: Radioreceptor assay. Less than 17% of basal activity.

CRITICAL FINDINGS AND POTENTIAL INTERVENTIONS: N/A

OVERVIEW: (Study type: Blood collected in a red-top tube; **related body system:** Endocrine system.) There are two functional types of thyroid receptor immunoglobulins: *thyroid-stimulating immunoglobulin* (TSI) and *thyroid-binding inhibitory immunoglobulin* (TBII). TSI reacts with the receptors, activates intracellular enzymes, and promotes epithelial cell activity that operates outside the feedback regulation for thyroid-stimulating hormone (TSH), resulting in continuous production of thyroid hormones (see study titled "Thyroid-Stimulating Immunoglobulins"); TBII blocks the action of TSH and is believed to cause certain types of hyperthyroidism. These antibodies were formerly known as *long-acting thyroid stimulators*. High levels in pregnancy may have some predictive value for neonatal thyrotoxicosis: A positive result indicates that the antibodies are stimulating (TSI); a negative result indicates that the antibodies are blocking (TBII). TBII testing measures thyroid receptor immunoglobulin levels in the evaluation of thyroid disease.

INDICATIONS
• Evaluate suspected acute toxic goiter.
• Investigate suspected neonatal thyroid disease secondary to maternal thyroid disease.
• Monitor hyperthyroid patients at risk for relapse or remission.

INTERFERING FACTORS
Factors that may alter the results of the study
• Lithium may cause false-positive results.

POTENTIAL MEDICAL DIAGNOSIS: CLINICAL SIGNIFICANCE OF RESULTS
Increased in
Evidenced by antibodies that block the action of TSH and result in hyperthyroid conditions.

T

- Graves disease
- Hyperthyroidism (various forms)
- Maternal thyroid disease
- Neonatal thyroid disease
- Toxic goiter

Decreased in: N/A

NURSING IMPLICATIONS

BEFORE THE STUDY: PLANNING AND IMPLEMENTATION

Teaching the Patient What to Expect
▶ Inform the patient this test can assist in evaluating thyroid function.

▶ Explain that a blood sample is needed for the test.

AFTER THE STUDY: POTENTIAL NURSING ACTIONS

Treatment Considerations
▶ Answer any questions or address any concerns voiced by the patient or family.

Follow-Up, Evaluation, and Desired Outcomes
▶ Understands that depending on the results of this study, additional testing may be performed to monitor disease progression and determine the need for a change in therapy.

Thyroid Scan

SYNONYM/ACRONYM: Iodine thyroid scan, technetium thyroid scan, thyroid scintiscan.

RATIONALE: To assess thyroid gland size, structure, function, and shape toward diagnosing disorders such as tumor, inflammation, cancer, and bleeding.

PATIENT PREPARATION: There are no activity or medication restrictions unless by medical direction. Instruct the patient to fast for 8 to 12 hr prior to the procedure. Protocols may vary among facilities. Ensure that this procedure is performed before other radiographic procedures using iodinated contrast medium.

NORMAL FINDINGS

- Normal size, contour, position, and function of the thyroid gland with homogeneous uptake of the radionuclide.

CRITICAL FINDINGS AND POTENTIAL INTERVENTIONS: N/A

OVERVIEW: (**Study type:** Nuclear scan; **related body system:** Endocrine system.) The thyroid scan is a nuclear medicine study performed to assess thyroid size, shape, position, and function. It is useful for evaluating thyroid nodules, multinodular goiter, and thyroiditis; assisting in the differential diagnosis of masses in the neck, base of the tongue, and mediastinum; and ruling out possible ectopic thyroid tissue in these areas. Thyroid scanning is performed after oral administration of radioactive iodine-123 (I-123) or I-131 or IV injection of technetium-99m (Tc-99m). Increased or decreased uptake by the thyroid gland and surrounding area and tissue is noted: Areas of increased radionuclide uptake ("hot spots") are caused by hyperfunctioning thyroid nodules, which are usually

T

nonmalignant; areas of decreased uptake ("cold spots") are caused by hypofunctioning nodules, which are more likely to be malignant. Ultrasound imaging may be used to determine if the cold spot is a solid, semicystic lesion or a pure cyst (cysts are rarely cancerous). To determine whether the cold spot depicts a malignant tumor, however, a biopsy must be performed.

INDICATIONS
- Assess palpable nodules and differentiate between a benign tumor or cyst and a malignant tumor.
- Assess the presence of a thyroid nodule or enlarged thyroid gland.
- Detect benign or malignant thyroid tumors.
- Detect causes of neck or substernal masses.
- Detect forms of thyroiditis (e.g., acute, chronic, Hashimoto disease).
- Detect thyroid dysfunction.
- Differentiate between Graves disease and Plummer disease, both of which cause hyperthyroidism.
- Evaluate thyroid function in hyperthyroidism and hypothyroidism (analysis combined with interpretation of laboratory tests, thyroid function panel including thyroxine and triiodothyronine, and thyroid uptake tests).

INTERFERING FACTORS
Contraindications

⬥ Patients who are pregnant or suspected of being pregnant, unless the potential benefits of a procedure using radiation far outweigh the risk of radiation exposure to the fetus and mother.

Factors that may alter the results of the study
- Ingestion of foods containing iodine (iodized salt) or medications

containing iodine (cough syrup, potassium iodide, vitamins, Lugol solution, thyroid replacement medications), which can decrease the uptake of the radionuclide.
- Antihistamines, antithyroid medications (propylthiouracil), corticosteroids, isoniazid, nitrates, sulfonamides, thyroid hormones, and warfarin, which can decrease the uptake of the radionuclide.
- Increased uptake of iodine in persons with an iodine-deficient diet or who are on phenothiazine therapy.
- Vomiting and severe diarrhea, which can affect absorption of orally administered radionuclide.
- Gastroenteritis, which can interfere with absorption of orally administered radionuclide.
- Metallic objects (e.g., jewelry, body rings) within the examination field, other nuclear scans done within the previous 24 to 48 hr, or iodinated contrast from a previous radiological procedure, which may inhibit organ visualization and cause unclear images.
- Improper injection of the radionuclide that allows the tracer to seep deep into the muscle tissue can produce erroneous hot spots.
- Inability of the patient to cooperate or remain still during the procedure because movement can produce blurred or otherwise unclear images.

POTENTIAL MEDICAL DIAGNOSIS: CLINICAL SIGNIFICANCE OF RESULTS
Abnormal findings related to
- Adenoma
- Cysts
- Fibrosis
- Goiter
- Graves disease (diffusely enlarged, hyperfunctioning gland)
- Hematoma
- Metastasis

T

- Plummer disease (nodular hyper-functioning gland)
- Thyroiditis (Hashimoto disease)
- Thyrotoxicosis
- Tumors, benign or malignant

NURSING IMPLICATIONS

BEFORE THE STUDY: PLANNING AND IMPLEMENTATION

Teaching the Patient What to Expect

▶ Inform the patient this procedure can assist in evaluating the thyroid glands' structure and function.
▶ Pregnancy is a general contraindication to procedures involving radiation. Explain to the female patient that she will be asked the date of her last menstrual period and pregnancy testing may be performed to determine the possibility of pregnancy before she is exposed to radiation.
▶ Review the procedure with the patient. Address concerns about pain and explain that there may be moments of discomfort or pain experienced when the IV line is inserted to allow infusion of fluids such as saline, anesthetics, sedatives, radionuclides, medications used in the procedure, or emergency medications.
▶ Explain that the procedure is performed in a nuclear medicine department by a health-care provider (HCP) specializing in this procedure, with support staff, and takes 30 to 60 min.
▶ Tc-99m pertechnetate is injected IV 20 min before scanning.
▶ If oral radioactive nuclide is used instead, I-123 will be administered 24 hr before scanning.
▶ Reassure the patient that the radionuclide poses no radioactive hazard and rarely produces adverse effects.
▶ Instruct the patient to remove jewelry and other metallic objects from the area to be examined prior to the procedure.
▶ Baseline vital signs and neurological status are recorded. Protocols may vary among facilities.

▶ Positioning for this procedure is in a supine position on a flat table to obtain images of the neck area.
▶ Explain that once the study is completed, the needle or catheter is removed and a pressure dressing applied over the puncture site.

Potential Nursing Actions
◈ *Make sure a written and informed consent has been signed prior to the procedure and before administering any medications.*
▶ Ensure thyroid blood tests are completed prior to this procedure.

AFTER THE STUDY: POTENTIAL NURSING ACTIONS

Avoiding Complications
▶ Establishing an IV site and injection of radionuclides are invasive procedures. Complications are rare but include risk for allergic reaction *(related to contrast reaction),* hematoma *(related to blood leakage into the tissue following needle insertion),* bleeding from the puncture site *(related to a bleeding disorder or the effects of natural products and medications with known anticoagulant, antiplatelet, or thrombolytic properties),* or infection *(which might occur if bacteria from the skin surface is introduced at the puncture site).* Monitor the patient for complications related to the procedure (e.g., allergic reaction, anaphylaxis, bronchospasm). Immediately report symptoms such as fast heart rate, difficulty breathing, skin rash, itching, or chest pain to the appropriate HCP. Observe/assess the needle/catheter insertion site for bleeding, inflammation, or hematoma formation.

Treatment Considerations
▶ Explain that the radionuclide is eliminated from the body within 6 to 24 hr. Advise the patient to drink increased amounts of fluids for 24 to 48 hr to eliminate the radionuclide from the body, unless contraindicated.
▶ Instruct the patient to resume usual diet, fluids, medications, and activity as directed by the HCP.
▶ Administer ordered antiemetics as needed.

◆ Instruct the patient in the care and assessment of the injection site.
◆ Explain that application of cold compresses to the puncture site may reduce discomfort or edema.

Safety Considerations
◆ The patient who is breastfeeding should consult with the requesting HCP regarding alternate testing that does not involve radiation. In general, if a woman who is breastfeeding must have a nuclear scan, she should not breastfeed the infant for 72 hr after the scan, until the radionuclide has been eliminated. She should be instructed to express the milk in order to prevent cessation of milk production; the milk can be stored and used after the 3-day period.
◆ Refer to organizational policy for additional precautions that may include instructions on handwashing, toilet flushing, limited contact with others, and other aspects of nuclear medicine safety.

Follow-Up, Evaluation, and Desired Outcomes
◆ Understands that depending on the results of this study, additional testing may be performed to monitor disease progression and determine the need for a change in therapy.

Thyroid-Stimulating Hormone

SYNONYM/ACRONYM: Thyrotropin, TSH.

RATIONALE: To evaluate thyroid gland function related to the primary cause of hypothyroidism and assess for congenital disorders, tumor, and inflammation.

PATIENT PREPARATION: There are no food, fluid, activity, or medication restrictions unless by medical direction.

NORMAL FINDINGS: Method: Immunoassay.

Age	Conventional Units	SI Units (Conventional Units × 1)
Neonates–3 days	Less than 40 micro-international units/mL	Less than 40 milli-international units/L
2 wk–5 mo	1.7–9.1 micro-international units/mL	1.7–9.1 milli-international units/L
6 mo–1 yr	0.7–6.4 micro-international units/mL	0.7–6.4 milli-international units/L
2 yr–19 yr	0.5–4.5 micro-international units/mL	0.5–4.5 milli-international units/L
Greater than 20 yr	0.4–4.2 micro-international units/mL	0.4–4.2 milli-international units/L
Pregnancy		
First trimester	0.3–2.7 micro-international units/mL	0.3–2.7 milli-international units/L
Second trimester	0.5–2.7 micro-international units/mL	0.5–2.7 milli-international units/L
Third trimester	0.4–2.9 micro-international units/mL	0.4–2.9 milli-international units/L

CRITICAL FINDINGS AND POTENTIAL INTERVENTIONS: N/A

OVERVIEW: (Study type: Blood collected in a gold-red- or tiger-top tube; for a neonate, use filter paper; related body system: Endocrine system.) Thyroid-stimulating hormone (TSH) is produced by the pituitary gland in response to stimulation by thyrotropin-releasing hormone (TRH), a hypothalamic-releasing factor. TRH regulates the release and circulating levels of thyroid hormones in response to variables such as cold, stress, and increased metabolic need. Thyroid and pituitary function can be evaluated by TSH measurement. TSH exhibits diurnal variation, peaking between midnight and 0400 and troughing between 1700 and 1800. TSH values are high at birth but reach adult levels in the first week of life. Elevated TSH levels combined with decreased thyroxine (T_4) levels indicate hypothyroidism and thyroid gland dysfunction. In general, decreased TSH and T_4 levels indicate secondary congenital hypothyroidism and pituitary hypothalamic dysfunction. A normal TSH level and a depressed T_4 level may indicate (1) hypothyroidism owing to a congenital defect in T_4-binding globulin or (2) transient congenital hypothyroidism owing to hypoxia or prematurity. Early diagnosis and treatment in the neonate are crucial for the prevention of congenital hypothyroidism (cretinism).

INDICATIONS
• Assist in the diagnosis of congenital hypothyroidism.
• Assist in the diagnosis of hypothyroidism or hyperthyroidism or suspected pituitary or hypothalamic dysfunction.

• Differentiate functional euthyroidism from true hypothyroidism in debilitated individuals.

INTERFERING FACTORS
Factors that may alter the results of the study
• Drugs and other substances that may increase TSH levels include amiodarone, benserazide, erythrosine, flunarizine (males), iobenzamic acid, iodides, lithium, methimazole, metoclopramide, morphine, propranolol, radiographic medium, TRH, and valproic acid.
• Drugs and other substances that may decrease TSH levels include acetylsalicylic acid, amiodarone, anabolic steroids, carbamazepine, corticosteroids, glucocorticoids, hydrocortisone, interferon-alfa-2b, iodamide, levodopa (in hypothyroidism), levothyroxine, methergoline, nifedipine, T_4, and triiodothyronine (T_3).

Other considerations
• Failure to let the filter paper sample dry may affect test results.

POTENTIAL MEDICAL DIAGNOSIS: CLINICAL SIGNIFICANCE OF RESULTS
Increased in
A decrease in thyroid hormone levels activates the feedback loop to increase production of TSH.

• Congenital hypothyroidism in the neonate (filter paper test)
• Ectopic TSH-producing tumors (lung, breast)
• Primary hypothyroidism *(related to a dysfunctional thyroid gland)*
• Secondary hyperthyroidism owing to pituitary hyperactivity
• Thyroid hormone resistance
• Thyroiditis (Hashimoto autoimmune disease)

Decreased in
An increase in thyroid hormone levels activates the feedback loop to decrease production of TSH.

T

- Excessive thyroid hormone replacement
- Graves disease
- Primary hyperthyroidism
- Secondary hypothyroidism *(related to pituitary involvement*

that decreases production of TSH)
- Tertiary hypothyroidism *(related to hypothalamic involvement that decreases production of TRH)*

NURSING IMPLICATIONS

POTENTIAL NURSING PROBLEMS: ASSESSMENT & NURSING DIAGNOSIS

Problems	Signs and Symptoms
Altered thought processes *(related to decreased cardiac output and impaired cerebral perfusion secondary to a deficit of thyroid hormone)*	Altered memory, mental impairment, decreased concentration, depression, inaccurate environmental perception, inappropriate thinking, memory deficits
Decreased cardiac output *(related to a deficit of thyroid hormone)*	Bradycardia, lethargy, hypotension, decreased thyroid hormone levels, fatigue, activity intolerance, poor peripheral perfusion, cool skin, shortness of breath
Nutrition *(related to slow metabolism)*	Decreased appetite with weight gain; selection of high-calorie, high-sodium foods; sedentary lifestyle; caloric intake greater than metabolic needs; constipation; decreased activity

BEFORE THE STUDY: PLANNING AND IMPLEMENTATION

Teaching the Patient What to Expect
▶ Inform the patient this test can assist in evaluating thyroid function.
▶ Explain that a blood sample is needed for the test.

Filter Paper Test (Neonate)
▶ A kit is obtained to complete the testing.
▶ The heel is cleansed with antiseptic.
▶ A heel stick is performed by gently squeezing the infant's heel and touching the filter paper to the puncture site. Gauze is used to completely dry the stick area.
▶ When collecting samples for newborn screening, it is important to apply each blood drop to the correct side of the filter paper card and fill each circle with a single application of blood. Overfilling

or underfilling the circles will cause the specimen card to be rejected by the testing facility.
▶ Testing facility regulations usually require the specimen cards to be submitted within 24 hr of collection.
▶ Additional information is required on newborn screening cards and may vary by testing facility.
▶ Newborn screening cards should be allowed to air dry for several hours on a level, nonabsorbent, unenclosed area. If multiple patients are tested, do not stack cards.

AFTER THE STUDY: POTENTIAL NURSING ACTIONS

Treatment Considerations
▶ Altered Thought Process: Minimize apprehension and dread. Collaborate with the health-care provider (HCP) to manage medical problem

T

associated with decreased cerebral perfusion. Promote comprehension and understanding of current events. Provide a modified environment that promotes safety. Monitor the ability to provide self-care (activities of daily living), monitor injury risk (violence, fall risk, self-harm risk), and administer ordered thyroid hormone replacement medication.

▶ Decreased Cardiac Output: Assess and trend vital signs. Monitor and trend thyroid laboratory studies: TSH, T3, T4, and radioactive iodine uptake. Assess cardiac status indicators: peripheral pulses; skin color; skin temperature; dry, scaly skin; and periorbital edema. Administer ordered thyroid hormone replacement medication. Facilitate measures to improve patient warmth: blankets, warm clothing and liquids, and warmer environment. Pace activity and schedule rest periods to manage fatigue. Use pulse oximetry to monitor oxygen saturation. Assess respiratory status checking for crackles and

increased respiratory rate, and monitor for fluid overload.

Nutritional Considerations

▶ Teach the patient to avoid foods with high sodium, saturated fat, and cholesterol content; teach the patient to eat a diet high in protein and low in calories to promote weight loss; encourage the patient to eat small, frequent meals to prevent overeating and enhance weight management; encourage the consumption of high-fiber foods such as fruits and vegetables with the skins and whole-grain breads to improve gastric motility; monitor daily weight; accurately assess appetite and measure caloric intake over a 24-hr period; arrange consult with a registered dietitian.

Follow-Up, Evaluation, and Desired Outcomes

▶ Understands that depending on the results of this study, additional testing may be performed to monitor disease progression and determine the need for a change in therapy.

Thyroid-Stimulating Immunoglobulins

SYNONYM/ACRONYM: Thyrotropin receptor antibodies, thyroid-stimulating immunoglobulins, TRAb (TSH receptor antibodies).

RATIONALE: To differentiate between antibodies that stimulate or inhibit thyroid hormone production related to disorders such as Graves disease.

PATIENT PREPARATION: There are no food, fluid, activity, or medication restrictions unless by medical direction.

NORMAL FINDINGS: Method: Animal cell transfection with luciferase marker. Less than 130% of basal activity.

CRITICAL FINDINGS AND POTENTIAL INTERVENTIONS: N/A

OVERVIEW: (Study type: Blood collected in a red-top tube; **related body system:** Endocrine system.) There are two functional types of thyroid receptor immunoglobulins: *thyroid-stimulating immunoglobulin* (TSI) and *thyroid-binding inhibitory immunoglobulin* (TBII). TSI reacts with the receptors, activates intracellular enzymes, and promotes epithelial cell

T

activity that operates outside the feedback regulation for thyroid-stimulating hormone (TSH); TBII blocks the action of TSH and is believed to cause certain types of hyperthyroidism (see study titled "Thyroid-Binding Inhibitory Immunoglobulin"). These antibodies were formerly known as *long-acting thyroid stimulators.* High levels in pregnancy may have some predictive value for neonatal thyrotoxicosis: A positive result indicates that the antibodies are stimulating (TSI); a negative result indicates that the antibodies are blocking (TBII). TSI testing measures thyroid receptor immunoglobulin levels in the evaluation of thyroid disease.

INDICATIONS
- Follow-up to positive TBII assay in differentiating antibody stimulation from neutral or suppressing activity.
- Monitor hyperthyroid patients at risk for relapse or remission.

INTERFERING FACTORS
Factors that may alter the results of the study
- Lithium may cause false-positive TBII results.

POTENTIAL MEDICAL DIAGNOSIS: CLINICAL SIGNIFICANCE OF RESULTS
Increased in
- Graves disease *(this form of hyperthyroidism has an autoimmune component; the antibodies stimulate release of thyroid hormones outside the feedback loop that regulates TSH levels)*

Decreased in: N/A

NURSING IMPLICATIONS

BEFORE THE STUDY: PLANNING AND IMPLEMENTATION
Teaching the Patient What to Expect
- Inform the patient this test can assist in assessing thyroid gland function.
- Explain that a blood sample is needed for the test.

AFTER THE STUDY: POTENTIAL NURSING ACTIONS
Treatment Considerations
- Answer any questions or address any concerns voiced by the patient or family.
Follow-Up, Evaluation, and Desired Outcomes
- Understands that depending on the results of this study, additional testing may be performed to monitor disease progression and determine the need for a change in therapy.

Thyroxine-Binding Globulin

SYNONYM/ACRONYM: TBG.

RATIONALE: To evaluate thyroid hormone levels related to deficiency or excess to assist in diagnosing disorders such as hyperthyroidism and hypothyroidism.

PATIENT PREPARATION: There are no food, fluid, activity, or medication restrictions unless by medical direction.

NORMAL FINDINGS: Method: Immunochemiluminometric assay (ICMA).

Age	Conventional Units	SI Units (Conventional Units × 10)
0–1 wk	3–8 mg/dL	30–80 mg/L
1–12 mo	1.6–3.6 mg/dL	16–36 mg/L
14–19 yr	1.2–2.5 mg/dL	12–25 mg/L
Greater than 20 yr	1.3–3.3 mg/dL	13–33 mg/L
Pregnancy, third trimester	4.7–5.9 mg/dL	47–59 mg/L
Oral contraceptives	1.5–5.5 mg/dL	15–55 mg/L

CRITICAL FINDINGS AND POTENTIAL INTERVENTIONS: N/A

OVERVIEW: (Study type: Blood collected in a gold-, red-, or red/gray-top tube; **related body system:** Endocrine system.) Thyroxine-binding globulin (TBG) is the predominant transport protein for the thyroid hormones thyroxine (T_4) and triiodothyronine (T_3). T_4-binding prealbumin and T_4-binding albumin are the other transport proteins. Conditions that affect TBG levels and binding capacity also affect free T_3 and free T_4 levels.

INDICATIONS
- Differentiate elevated T_4 due to hyperthyroidism from increased TBG binding in euthyroid patients.
- Evaluate hypothyroid patients.
- Identify deficiency or excess of TBG due to hereditary abnormality.

INTERFERING FACTORS
Factors that may alter the results of the study
- Drugs and other substances that may increase TBG levels include estrogens, oral contraceptives, perphenazine, and tamoxifen.
- Drugs and other substances that may decrease TBG levels include anabolic steroids, androgens, asparaginase, corticosteroids, corticotropin, danazol, phenytoin, and propranolol.

POTENTIAL MEDICAL DIAGNOSIS: CLINICAL SIGNIFICANCE OF RESULTS
Increased in
- Acute intermittent porphyria *(pathophysiology is unclear)*
- Estrogen therapy *(TBG is increased in the presence of exogenous or endogenous estrogens)*
- Genetically high TBG (rare)
- Hyperthyroidism *(related to increased levels of total thyroxine available for binding)*
- Infectious hepatitis and other liver diseases *(pathophysiology is unclear)*
- Neonates
- Pregnancy *(TBG is increased in the presence of exogenous or endogenous estrogens)*

Decreased in
- Acromegaly
- Chronic hepatic disease *(related to general decrease in protein synthesis)*
- Genetically low TBG
- Major illness *(related to general decrease in protein synthesis)*
- Marked hypoproteinemia, malnutrition *(related to general decrease in protein synthesis)*
- Nephrotic syndrome *(related to general increase in protein loss)*
- Ovarian hypofunction *(TBG is decreased in the absence of estrogens)*

T

- Surgical stress *(related to general decrease in protein synthesis)*
- Testosterone-producing tumors *(TBG is decreased in the presence of testosterone)*

◗ Explain that a blood sample is needed for the test.

AFTER THE STUDY: POTENTIAL NURSING ACTIONS

Treatment Considerations
◗ Answer any questions or address any concerns voiced by the patient or family.

Follow-Up, Evaluation, and Desired Outcomes
◗ Understands that depending on the results of this study, additional testing may be performed to monitor disease progression and determine the need for a change in therapy.

NURSING IMPLICATIONS

BEFORE THE STUDY: PLANNING AND IMPLEMENTATION

Teaching the Patient What to Expect
◗ Inform the patient this test can assist in assessing thyroid gland function.

Thyroxine, Total and Free

SYNONYM/ACRONYM: T_4, FT_4.

RATIONALE: T_4 is a complementary laboratory test in evaluating thyroid hormone levels, a screening test for newborns to detect thyroid dysfunction, and a tool to evaluate the effectiveness of therapeutic thyroid therapy. FT_4 is a reflex test for thyroid function to assist in diagnosing hyperthyroidism and hypothyroidism in the presence of an abnormal TSH level.

PATIENT PREPARATION: There are no food, fluid, activity, or medication restrictions unless by medical direction.

NORMAL FINDINGS: Method: Immunoassay.

T_4		
Age	**Conventional Units**	**SI Units (Conventional Units × 12.9)**
Cord blood	6.6–17.5 mcg/dL	85–226 nmol/L
Newborn	5.4–22.6 mcg/dL	70–292 nmol/L
1 mo–23 mo	5.4–16.6 mcg/dL	70–214 nmol/L
2–6 yr	5.3–15 mcg/dL	68–194 nmol/L
7–11 yr	5.7–14.1 mcg/dL	74–182 nmol/L
12–19 yr	4.7–14.6 mcg/dL	61–188 nmol/L
Adult	5.5–12.5 mcg/dL	71–161 nmol/L
Pregnant female	5.5–16 mcg/dL	71–206 nmol/L
Over 60 yr	5–10.7 mcg/dL	64–138 nmol/L

T

FT$_4$

Age	Conventional Units	SI Units (Conventional Units × 12.9)
Newborn	0.8–2.8 ng/dL	10–36 pmol/L
1–12 mo	0.8–2 ng/dL	10–26 pmol/L
1–18 yr	0.8–1.7 ng/dL	10–22 pmol/L
Adult–older adult	0.8–1.5 ng/dL	10–19 pmol/L
Pregnancy	0.7–1.4 ng/dL	9–18 pmol/L

CRITICAL FINDINGS AND POTENTIAL INTERVENTIONS

- T$_4$: *Hypothyroidism:* Less than 2 mcg/dL (SI: Less than 26 nmol/L)
- T$_4$: *Hyperthyroidism:* Greater than 20 mcg/dL (Greater than 258 nmol/L).

Timely notification to the requesting health-care provider (HCP) of any critical findings and related symptoms is a role expectation of the professional nurse. A listing of these findings varies among facilities.

Consideration may be given to verification of critical findings before action is taken. Policies vary among facilities and may include requesting immediate recollection and retesting by the laboratory.

At levels less than 2 mcg/dL (SI: less than 26 nmol/L), the patient is at risk for myxedema coma. Signs and symptoms of severe hypothyroidism include hypothermia, hypotension, bradycardia, hypoventilation, lethargy, and coma. Possible interventions include airway support, hourly monitoring for neurological function and blood pressure, and administration of intravenous thyroid hormone.

At levels greater than 20 mcg/dL (greater than 258 nmol/L), the patient is at risk for thyroid storm. Signs and symptoms of severe hyperthyroidism include hyperthermia, diaphoresis, vomiting, dehydration, and shock. Possible interventions include supportive treatment for shock, fluid and electrolyte replacement for dehydration, and administration of antithyroid drugs (propylthiouracil and Lugol solution).

OVERVIEW: (**Study type:** Blood collected in a gold-, red-, red/gray-, or green-top [heparin] tube; **related body system:** Endocrine system.) Thyroxine (T$_4$) is a hormone produced and secreted by the thyroid gland. Most T$_4$ in the serum (99.97%) is bound to thyroxine-binding globulin (TBG), prealbumin, and albumin. The remainder (0.03%) circulates as unbound or free T$_4$, which is the physiologically active form. Levels of free T$_4$ are proportional to levels of total T$_4$. The advantage of measuring free T$_4$ instead of total T$_4$ is that, unlike total T$_4$ measurements, free T$_4$ levels are not affected by fluctuations in TBG levels; as a result, free T$_4$ levels are considered the most accurate indicator of T$_4$ and its thyrometabolic activity. Untreated deficiency of T$_4$ in newborns can result in untreatable, severe intellectual deficits and growth impairment. Neonatal screening for hypothyroidism is mandatory in all 50 states. Measurement of free T$_4$ is recommended during treatment for hyperthyroidism until symptoms have abated and levels have decreased into the normal range.

T

INDICATIONS

General

- Evaluate signs of hypothyroidism or hyperthyroidism.
- Monitor response to therapy for hypothyroidism or hyperthyroidism.

T_4

- Evaluate thyroid response to protein deficiency associated with severe illnesses.
- Neonatal screening for congenital hypothyroidism.

INTERFERING FACTORS

T_4

- Drugs and other substances that may increase T_4 levels include amiodarone, amphetamines, corticosteroids, ether, fluorouracil, glucocorticoids, halofenate, insulin, iobenzamic acid, iopanoic acid, iopodate, levarterenol, levodopa, levothyroxine, opiates, oral contraceptives, phenothiazine, and prostaglandins.
- Drugs and other substances that may decrease T_4 levels include acetylsalicylic acid, aminoglutethimide, aminosalicylic acid, amiodarone, anabolic steroids, anticonvulsants, asparaginase, barbiturates, carbimazole, chlorpromazine, chlorpropamide, cholestyramine, clofibrate, cobalt, colestipol, corticotropin, cortisone, cotrimoxazole, cytostatic therapy, danazol, dehydroepiandrosterone, dexamethasone, diazepam, diazo dyes (e.g., Evans blue), ethionamide, fenclofenac, halofenate, interferon alfa-2b, iron, isotretinoin, liothyronine, lithium, lovastatin, methimazole, methylthiouracil, mitotane, norethindrone, penicillamine, penicillin, phenylbutazone, potassium iodide, propylthiouracil, reserpine, salicylate, sodium nitroprusside, sulfonylureas, tolbutamide, and triiodothyronine (T_3).

FT_4

- Drugs and other substances that may increase free T_4 levels include acetylsalicylic acid, amiodarone, halofenate, heparin, iopanoic acid, levothyroxine, methimazole, and radiographic medium.
- Drugs and other substances that may decrease free T_4 levels include amiodarone, anabolic steroids, asparaginase, methadone, methimazole, oral contraceptives, and phenylbutazone.

POTENTIAL MEDICAL DIAGNOSIS: CLINICAL SIGNIFICANCE OF RESULTS
Increased in

General

- Hyperthyroidism *(thyroxine is produced independently of stimulation by TSH)*

T_4

- Acute mental health illnesses *(pathophysiology is unknown, although there is a relationship between thyroid hormone levels and certain types of mental illness)*
- Excessive intake of iodine *(iodine is rapidly taken up by the body to form thyroxine)*
- Hepatitis *(related to decreased production of TBG by damaged liver cells)*
- Obesity
- Thyrotoxicosis due to Graves disease *(thyroxine is produced independently of stimulation by TSH)*
- Thyrotoxicosis factitia *(laboratory tests do not distinguish between endogenous and exogenous sources)*

FT_4

- Hypothyroidism treated with T_4 *(laboratory tests do not distinguish between endogenous and exogenous sources)*

Decreased in

General
- **Hypothyroidism** *(thyroid hormones are not produced in sufficient quantities regardless of TSH levels)*

T$_4$
- **Decreased TBG** *(nephrotic syndrome, liver disease, gastrointestinal protein loss, malnutrition)*
- **Panhypopituitarism** *(dysfunctional pituitary gland does not secrete enough thyrotropin to stimulate the thyroid to produce thyroxine)*
- Strenuous exercise

FT$_4$
- Pregnancy (late)

NURSING IMPLICATIONS

BEFORE THE STUDY: PLANNING AND IMPLEMENTATION

Teaching the Patient What to Expect
- Inform the patient this test can assist in assessing thyroid gland function.
- Explain that a blood sample is needed for the test.

AFTER THE STUDY: POTENTIAL NURSING ACTIONS

Treatment Considerations
- Teach about the relationship between the development of goiter and exophthalmos and hyperthyroidism.
- Teach how to identify the symptoms that may indicate a thyroid storm.
- Teach how to identify symptoms that would indicate hypothyroidism.
- Altered thought processes can occur with inadequate thyroid function and associated decreased cardiac output and cerebral perfusion. One goal would be to collaborate with the HCP to manage the medical problem associated with decreased cerebral perfusion. Interventions would be to provide a modified environment that promotes safety, monitor the ability to provide self-care, fall and injury risk, and ensure administration of (violence, fall risk, self-harm risk); administer prescribed thyroid hormone replacement medication.
- Thyroid alterations can cause changes in physical appearance, such as goiter and exophthalmos, resulting in body image disturbances. Assess the patient's perception of physical changes and note the frequency of negative comments related to changed physical state. Assist in the identification of positive coping strategies to address changed physical appearance.
- Inadequate thyroid can be associated with decreased cardiac output. Monitor and trend vital signs, thyroid laboratory studies (TSH, T3, T4, radioactive iodine uptake), cardiac status indicators peripheral pulses, skin color, skin temperature, dry scaly skin, periorbital edema, respiratory rate, oxygen saturation, and breath sounds for fluid overload. Administer prescribed thyroid hormone replacement medication.
- Elevated body temperature can occur due to an emotionally labile event that could precipitate a thyroid storm or crisis. Ensure the patient's immediate environment remains cool. Encourage the use of light bedding and lightweight clothing to prevent overheating, increase fluid intake to offset insensible fluid loss, encourage bathing with tepid water for comfort and promotion of cooling. Administer prescribed antithyroid therapy.

Follow-Up, Evaluation, and Desired Outcomes
- Demonstrates proficiency in selecting clothing that will assist in remaining cool and prevent overheating.
- Demonstrates proficiency in the self-administration of thyroid or antithyroid medication correctly as prescribed.
- Displays acceptance of changed appearance and refrains from negative self-comments.
- Adheres to recommended medication regime.

Toxoplasma Testing

SYNONYM/ACRONYM: Toxoplasmosis serology, toxoplasmosis titer; may be requested as part of TORCH panel.

RATIONALE: To assess for a past or present toxoplasmosis infection and to assess for the presence of antibodies.

PATIENT PREPARATION: There are no food, fluid, activity, or medication restrictions unless by medical direction.

NORMAL FINDINGS: Method: Chemiluminescent immunoassay.

	IgM and IgG	Interpretation
Negative	0.89 index or less	No significant level of detectable antibody
Indeterminate	0.9–1 index	Equivocal results; retest in 10–14 days
Positive	1.1 index or greater	Antibody detected; indicative of recent immunization, current or recent infection

CRITICAL FINDINGS AND POTENTIAL INTERVENTIONS: N/A

OVERVIEW: (**Study type:** Blood collected in a gold-, red-, or red/gray-top tube; **related body system:** Immune system.) Toxoplasmosis is a severe, generalized granulomatous central nervous system disease caused by the protozoan *Toxoplasma gondii*. The disease is more common in warm, humid climates at lower altitudes. Domestic and related cats are the only known definitive hosts for oocysts of *T. gondii*. Intermediate hosts become infected by ingesting the oocysts, which then transform into the tachyzoite form. Tachyzoites migrate to neural and muscle tissue and develop into tissue cysts. Transmission to humans occurs by ingesting undercooked meat of infected animals, handling contaminated matter such as cat litter, drinking contaminated water, receiving a blood product transfusion or organ transplant from an infected donor, or across the placenta from mother to fetus. Immunoglobulin M (IgM) antibodies develop approximately 5 days after infection and can remain elevated for 3 wk to several months. Immunoglobulin G (IgG) antibodies develop 1 to 2 wk after infection and can remain elevated for months or years. Healthy patients who become infected may not exhibit any symptoms, or if symptoms are present, they may be vague and common to other conditions. Some patients may develop lesions in the eye, which can inflame the retina and form scars upon resolution. Successive reactivation of the inflammation can lead to progressive loss of vision. *T. gondii* serology is part of the TORCH (*t*oxoplasmosis, *o*ther [congenital syphilis and viruses], *r*ubella, *c*ytomegalovirus, and *h*erpes simplex type 2) panel routinely performed on pregnant women. Fetal infection during the first trimester can cause spontaneous abortion or congenital defects such as microcephaly, microphthalmia, hydranencephaly, and hydrocephalus. Immunocompromised individuals are also at high risk for serious complications if infected. While most healthy people recover without treatment, pregnant women, newborns, infants, and immunocompromised patients receive effective treatment until the worst symptoms have passed and the infection resolves. However, the location of the parasite makes it difficult to completely eradicate with medications. The presence of IgM antibodies indicates acute or congenital infection; the presence of IgG antibodies indicates current or past infection.

INDICATIONS

- Assist in establishing a diagnosis of toxoplasmosis.
- Document past exposure or immunity.
- Serological screening during pregnancy.

INTERFERING FACTORS: N/A

POTENTIAL MEDICAL DIAGNOSIS: CLINICAL SIGNIFICANCE OF RESULTS
Positive findings in
- *Toxoplasma* infection

NURSING IMPLICATIONS

BEFORE THE STUDY: PLANNING AND IMPLEMENTATION

Teaching the Patient What to Expect
- Inform the patient this test can assist in assessing for toxoplasmosis infection.
- Explain that a blood sample is needed for the test.
- Explain that several tests may be necessary to confirm the diagnosis.
- Explain that any individual positive result should be repeated in 3 wk to monitor a change in detectable level of antibody.

AFTER THE STUDY: POTENTIAL NURSING ACTIONS

Treatment Considerations
- If eye lesions are present, explain that an ophthalmologist may need to be consulted. Administer ordered medications to patients who are HIV positive or are immunosuppressed.
- Explain the use of isolation precautions during time of communicability or contagion.
- Provide emotional support if results are positive and the patient is pregnant and/or immunocompromised.
- Emphasize the need to return to have a convalescent blood sample taken in 3 wk.

Follow-Up, Evaluation, and Desired Outcomes
- Recognizes the importance of making lifestyle changes to support the health of self and family.

Triglycerides

T

SYNONYM/ACRONYM: Trigs, TG.

RATIONALE: To evaluate triglyceride (TG) levels to assess cardiovascular disease risk and evaluate the effectiveness of therapeutic interventions.

PATIENT PREPARATION: There are no activity or medication restrictions unless by medical direction. Instruct the patient to fast for 12 hr before specimen collection; fasting is required prior to measurement of TG levels. Ideally, the patient should be on a stable diet for 3 wk and avoid alcohol consumption for 3 days before specimen collection; alcohol increases TG levels. Protocols may vary among facilities.

NORMAL FINDINGS: Method: Spectrophotometry.

Classification	Conventional Units	SI Units (Conventional Units × 0.0113)
Normal	Less than 150 mg/dL	Less than 1.7 mmol/L
Borderline high	150–199 mg/dL	1.7–2.2 mmol/L
High	200–499 mg/dL	2.2–5.6 mmol/L
Very high	Greater than 500 mg/dL	Greater than 5.6 mmol/L

CRITICAL FINDINGS AND POTENTIAL INTERVENTIONS: N/A

OVERVIEW: (**Study type:** Blood collected in a gold-, red-, red/ gray-, or green-top [heparin] tube; **related body system:** Circulatory system.) Fat or adipose is an important source of energy. TGs are a combination of three fatty acids and one glycerol molecule. Much of the fatty acids used in various metabolic processes come from dietary sources. However, the body also generates fatty acids, from available glucose and amino acids, that are converted into glycogen or stored energy by the liver. Beyond TG, total cholesterol, high-density lipoprotein (HDL), and low-density lipoprotein (LDL) cholesterol values, other important risk factors must be considered. For additional information regarding screening guidelines for *atherosclerotic cardiovascular disease* (ASCVD), refer to the study titled "Cholesterol, Total and Fractions." Evidence-based risk factors include age, sex, ethnicity, total cholesterol, HDLC, LDLC, blood pressure, blood-pressure treatment status, diabetes, and current use of tobacco products. TG levels vary by age, sex, weight, and ethnicity:

Levels increase with age.
Levels are higher in men than in women (among women, those who take oral contraceptives have levels that are 20 to 40 mg/dL higher than those who do not).
Levels are higher in overweight and obese people than in those with normal weight.
Levels in African Americans are approximately 10 to 20 mg/dL lower than in people of European descent.

INDICATIONS
- Evaluate known or suspected disorders associated with altered TG levels.
- Identify hyperlipoproteinemia (hyperlipidemia) in patients with a family history of the disorder.
- Monitor the response to drugs known to alter TG levels.
- Screen adults who are either over 40 yr or obese to estimate the risk for atherosclerotic cardiovascular disease.

INTERFERING FACTORS
Factors that may alter the results of the study
- Drugs and other substances that may increase TG levels include acetylsalicylic acid, atenolol, bisoprolol, beta blockers, bendroflumethiazide,

cholestyramine, conjugated estrogens, cyclosporine, estrogen/progestin therapy, estropipate, ethynodiol, etretinate, furosemide, glucocorticoids, hydrochlorothiazide, isotretinoin, labetalol, levonorgestrel, medroxyprogesterone, mepindolol, methyclothiazide, metoprolol, miconazole, mirtazapine, nadolol, nafarelin, oral contraceptives, oxprenolol, pindolol, prazosin, propranolol, tamoxifen, thiazides, ticlopidine, timolol, and tretinoin.

- Drugs and other substances that may decrease TG levels include anabolic steroids, ascorbic acid, beclobrate, bezafibrate, captopril, carvedilol, celiprolol, chenodiol, cholestyramine, cilazapril, ciprofibrate, clofibrate, colestipol, danazol, doxazosin, enalapril, eptastatin (type IIb only), fenofibrate, flaxseed oil, fluvastatin, gemfibrozil, halofenate, insulin, levonorgestrel, levothyroxine, lifibrol, lovastatin, medroxyprogesterone, metformin, niacin, niceritrol, Norplant, pentoxifylline, pindolol, pravastatin, prazosin, probucol, simvastatin, and verapamil.

POTENTIAL MEDICAL DIAGNOSIS: CLINICAL SIGNIFICANCE OF RESULTS
Increased in
- Acute myocardial infarction (AMI) *(elevated TG is identified as an independent risk factor in the development of coronary artery disease [CAD])*
- Alcohol misuse *(related to decreased breakdown of fats in the liver and increased blood levels)*
- Anorexia nervosa *(compensatory increase secondary to starvation)*
- Chronic ischemic heart disease *(elevated TG is identified as an independent risk factor in the development of CAD)*

- Cirrhosis *(increased TG blood levels related to decreased breakdown of fats in the liver)*
- Glycogen storage disease *(G6PD deficiency, e.g., von Gierke disease, results in hepatic overproduction of very-low-density lipoprotein [VLDL] cholesterol, the TG-rich lipoprotein)*
- Gout *(TG is frequently elevated in patients with gout, possibly related to alterations in apolipoprotein E genotypes)*
- Hyperlipoproteinemia *(related to increase in transport proteins)*
- Hypertension *(associated with elevated TG, which is identified as an independent risk factor in the development of CAD)*
- Hypothyroidism *(significant relationship between elevated TG and decreased metabolism)*
- Impaired glucose tolerance *(increase in insulin stimulates production of TG by liver)*
- Metabolic syndrome *(syndrome consisting of obesity, high blood pressure, and insulin resistance)*
- Nephrotic syndrome *(related to absence or insufficient levels of lipoprotein lipase to remove circulating TG and to decreased catabolism of TG-rich VLDL lipoproteins)*
- Obesity *(significant and complex relationship between obesity and elevated TG)*
- Pancreatitis *(acute and chronic; related to effects on insulin production)*
- Pregnancy *(increased demand for production of hormones related to pregnancy)*
- Chronic kidney disease *(related to diabetes; elevated insulin levels stimulate production of TG by liver)*
- Respiratory distress syndrome *(related to artificial lung surfactant used for therapy)*

T

- **Stress** *(related to poor diet; effect of hormones secreted under stressful situations that affect glucose levels)*
- **Werner's syndrome** *(clinical features resemble metabolic syndrome)*

Decreased in

- **End-stage liver disease** *(related to cessation of liver function that results in decreased production of TG and TG transport proteins)*

- **Hyperthyroidism** *(related to increased catabolism of VLDL transport proteins and general increase in metabolism)*
- **Hypolipoproteinemia and abetalipoproteinemia** *(related to decrease in transport proteins)*
- **Intestinal lymphangiectasia**
- **Malabsorption disorders** *(inadequate supply from dietary sources)*
- **Malnutrition** *(inadequate supply from dietary sources)*

NURSING IMPLICATIONS

POTENTIAL NURSING PROBLEMS: ASSESSMENT & NURSING DIAGNOSIS

Problems	Signs and Symptoms
Nutrition *(related to excess caloric intake with large amounts of dietary sodium and fat; cultural lifestyle; overeating associated with anxiety, depression, compulsive disorder; genetics; inadequate or unhealthy food resources)*	Observable obesity, high fat or sodium food selections, high BMI, high consumption of ethnic foods, sedentary lifestyle, dietary religious beliefs and food selections, binge eating, diet high in refined sugar, repetitive dieting and failure
Tissue perfusion *(related to hypovolemia, decreased hemoglobin, interrupted arterial flow, interrupted venous flow)*	Hypotension, dizziness, cool extremities, pallor, capillary refill greater than 3 sec in fingers and toes, weak pedal pulses, altered level of consciousness, altered sensation

BEFORE THE STUDY: PLANNING AND IMPLEMENTATION

Teaching the Patient What to Expect

▸ Inform the patient this test can assist in monitoring and evaluating lipid levels.
▸ Explain that a blood sample is needed for the test.

Potential Nursing Actions

▸ Evaluate for the presence of other risk factors, such as family history of heart disease, smoking, obesity, diet, lack of physical activity, hypertension, diabetes, previous myocardial infarction, and previous vascular disease, which should be investigated.
▸ Explain that understanding genetics assists in identifying those who may benefit from additional education, risk assessment, and counseling.

AFTER THE STUDY: POTENTIAL NURSING ACTIONS

Treatment Considerations

▸ Tissue Perfusion: Monitor blood pressure; assess for dizziness, capillary refill, pedal pulses, numbness, tingling, hyperesthesia, hypoesthesia, and extremities for deep venous thrombosis. Monitor skin temperature, color, and warmth. Instruct in careful use of heat and cold on affected areas and the use of a foot cradle to keep pressure off of affected body parts.

Nutritional Considerations
▶ Discuss ideal body weight and the purpose of and relationship between ideal weight and caloric intake to support cardiac health. Review ways to decrease intake of saturated fats and increase intake of polyunsaturated fats. Discuss limiting intake of refined processed sugar and sodium; discuss limiting cholesterol intake to less than 300 mg per day. Encourage the intake of fresh fruits and vegetables, unprocessed carbohydrates, poultry, and grains.
▶ *Sensitivity to Social and Cultural Issues:* Numerous studies point to the prevalence of excess body weight in American children and adolescents. Findings from the 2015-2016 National Health and Nutrition Examination Survey (NHANES), regarding the prevalence of obesity in younger members of the population, estimate that obesity is present in 13.9% of the population ages 2-5 yr, 18.4% ages 6 to 11 yr, and 20.6% ages 12-19 yr. The medical, social, and emotional consequences of excess body weight are significant. Special attention should be given to instructing the pediatric patient and caregiver regarding health risks and weight management education.
▶ Nutritional therapy is recommended for those with identified CAD risk, especially for those with elevated LDL cholesterol levels, other lipid disorders, diabetes, insulin resistance, or metabolic syndrome. Always consider cultural influences with dietary choices to ensure better adherence to a change in lifestyle. A variety of dietary patterns are beneficial for people with ASCVD. For additional information regarding nutritional guidelines, refer to the study titled "Cholesterol, Total and Fractions."
▶ Other changeable risk factors warranting education include strategies to encourage regular participation in moderate aerobic physical activity three to four times per week, eliminating tobacco use, and adhering to a heart-healthy diet.
▶ Those with elevated triglycerides should be advised to eliminate or reduce alcohol.

Follow-Up, Evaluation, and Desired Outcomes
▶ Acknowledges contact information provided for the American Heart Association (www.heart.org/HEARTORG), National Heart, Lung, and Blood Institute (www.nhlbi.nih.gov), and U.S. Department of Agriculture's resource for nutrition (www.choosemyplate.gov).

Triiodothyronine, Total and Free

SYNONYM/ACRONYM: T_3 and FT_3.

RATIONALE: To assist in evaluating thyroid function primarily related to diagnosing hyperthyroidism and monitoring the effectiveness of therapeutic interventions.

PATIENT PREPARATION: There are no food, fluid, activity, or medication restrictions unless by medical direction.

NORMAL FINDINGS: Method: Immunoassay.

T

T_3

Age	Conventional Units	SI Units (Conventional Units × 0.0154)
Cord blood	14–86 ng/dL	0.22–1.32 nmol/L
1–3 days	100–292 ng/dL	1.54–4.5 nmol/L
4–30 days	62–243 ng/dL	0.96–3.74 nmol/L
1–12 mo	105–245 ng/dL	1.62–3.77 nmol/L
1–5 yr	105–269 ng/dL	1.62–4.14 nmol/L
6–10 yr	94–241 ng/dL	1.45–3.71 nmol/L
16–20 yr	80–210 ng/dL	1.23–3.23 nmol/L
Adult	70–204 ng/dL	1.08–3.14 nmol/L
Older adult	40–181 ng/dL	0.62–2.79 nmol/L
Pregnant woman (last 4 mo gestation)	116–247 ng/dL	1.79–3.8 nmol/L

FT_3

Age	Conventional Units	SI Units (Conventional Units × 1.54)
0–3 days	2–7.9 pg/mL	3.1–12.2 pmol/L
4–30 days	2–5.2 pg/mL	3.1–8 pmol/L
1–23 mo	1.6–6.4 pg/mL	2.5–9.9 pmol/L
2–6 yr	2–6 pg/mL	3.1–9.2 pmol/L
7–17 yr	2.9–5.1 pg/mL	4.5–7.8 pmol/L
Adults and older adults	2.6–4.8 pg/mL	4–7.4 pmol/L
Pregnant women (4–9 mo gestation)	2–3.4 pg/mL	3.1–5.2 pmol/L

CRITICAL FINDINGS AND POTENTIAL INTERVENTIONS: N/A

OVERVIEW: (Study type: Blood collected in a gold-, red-, or red/gray-top tube; **related body system:** Endocrine system.) Unlike the thyroid hormone thyroxine (T_4), most T_3 is converted enzymatically from T_4 in the tissues rather than being produced directly by the thyroid gland (see study titled "Thyroxine, Total and Free"). Approximately one-third of T_4 is converted to T_3. Most T_3 in the serum (99.97%) is bound to thyroxine-binding globulin (TBG), prealbumin, and albumin. The remainder (0.03%) circulates as unbound or free T_3, which is the physiologically active form. Levels of free T_3 are proportional to levels of total T_3. The advantage of measuring free T_3 instead of total T_3 is that, unlike total T_3 measurements, free T_3 levels are not affected by fluctuations in TBG levels. T_3 is four to five times more biologically potent than T_4. This hormone, along with T_4, is responsible for maintaining a euthyroid state. Free T_3 measurements are rarely required, but they are indicated in the diagnosis of T_3 toxicosis and when certain drugs are being administered that interfere with the conversion of T_4 to T_3.

INDICATIONS

- General: Adjunctive aid to thyroid-stimulating hormone (TSH) and free T_4 assessment.
- FT_3: Assist in the diagnosis of T_3 toxicosis.

INTERFERING FACTORS

Factors that may alter the results of the study

T_3

- Drugs and other substances that may increase total T_3 levels include amiodarone, amphetamine, clofibrate, fluorouracil, halofenate, insulin, levothyroxine, methadone, opiates, oral contraceptives, phenothiazine, phenytoin, prostaglandins, and T_3.
- Drugs and other substances that may decrease total T_3 levels include acetylsalicylic acid, amiodarone, anabolic steroids, asparaginase, carbamazepine, cholestyramine, clomiphene, colestipol, dexamethasone, fenclofenac, furosemide, glucocorticoids, hydrocortisone, interferon alfa-2b, iobenzamic acid, iopanoic acid, ipodate, isotretinoin, lithium, methimazole, netilmicin, oral contraceptives, penicillamine, phenylbutazone, phenytoin, potassium iodide, prednisone, propranolol, propylthiouracil, radiographic medium, sodium ipodate, salicylate, sulfonylureas, and tyropanoic acid.

FT_3

- Drugs and other substances that may increase free T_3 include acetylsalicylic acid, amiodarone, and levothyroxine.
- Drugs and other substances that may decrease free T_3 include amiodarone, methimazole, phenytoin, propranolol, and radiographic medium.

POTENTIAL MEDICAL DIAGNOSIS: CLINICAL SIGNIFICANCE OF RESULTS

Increased in

T_3

- Conditions with increased TBG *(e.g., pregnancy and estrogen therapy)*
- Early thyroid failure
- Hyperthyroidism *(triiodothyronine is produced independently of stimulation by TSH)*
- Iodine-deficiency goiter
- T_3 toxicosis
- Thyrotoxicosis factitia *(laboratory tests do not distinguish between endogenous and exogenous sources)*
- Treated hyperthyroidism

FT_3

- High altitude
- Hyperthyroidism *(triiodothyronine is produced independently of stimulation by TSH)*
- T_3 toxicosis

Decreased in

T_3

- Acute and subacute nonthyroidal disease *(pathophysiology is unclear)*
- Conditions with decreased TBG *(TBG is the major transport protein)*
- Hypothyroidism *(thyroid hormones are not produced in sufficient quantities regardless of TSH levels)*
- Malnutrition *(related to insufficient protein sources to form albumin and TBG)*

FT_3

- Hypothyroidism *(thyroid hormones are not produced in sufficient quantities regardless of TSH levels)*
- Malnutrition *(related to protein or iodine deficiency; iodine is needed for thyroid hormone synthesis and proteins are needed for transport)*
- Nonthyroidal chronic diseases
- Pregnancy (late)

T

NURSING IMPLICATIONS

Treatment Considerations
▶ Answer any questions or address any concerns voiced by the patient or family.

BEFORE THE STUDY: PLANNING AND IMPLEMENTATION

Teaching the Patient What to Expect
▶ Inform the patient this test can assist in assessing thyroid gland function.
▶ Explain that a blood sample is needed for the test.

Follow-Up, Evaluation, and Desired Outcomes
▶ Understands that depending on the results of this study, additional testing may be performed to monitor disease progression and determine the need for a change in therapy.

Troponins I and T

SYNONYM/ACRONYM: Cardiac troponin, cardiac troponin I (cTnI), cardiac troponin T (cTnT).

RATIONALE: To assist in evaluating myocardial muscle damage related to disorders such as myocardial infarction (MI).

PATIENT PREPARATION: There are no food, fluid, activity, or medication restrictions unless by medical direction.

NORMAL FINDINGS: Method: Enzyme immunoassay.

Troponin I	Conventional Units	SI Units (Conventional Units × 1)
Adult	Less than 0.05 ng/mL	Less than 0.05 mcg/L
Troponin T	Less than 0.01 ng/mL	Less than 0.01 mcg/L

Normal values can vary significantly due to differences in test kit reagents and instrumentation. The testing laboratory should be consulted for comparison of results to the corresponding reference range.

CRITICAL FINDINGS AND POTENTIAL INTERVENTIONS: N/A

OVERVIEW: (**Study type:** Blood collected in a gold-, red-, red/gray-, or green-top [heparin] tube; **related body system:** Circulatory system. Serial sampling is highly recommended. Care must be taken to use the same type of collection container if serial measurements are to be taken.) Troponin is a complex of three contractile proteins that regulate the interaction of actin and myosin. Troponin C is the calcium-binding subunit; it does not have a cardiac muscle–specific subunit. Troponin I and troponin T, however, do have cardiac muscle–specific subunits. They are detectable a few hours to 7 days after the onset of symptoms of myocardial damage. Troponin I is thought to be a more specific marker than troponin T of cardiac damage. Cardiac troponin I begins to rise 2 to 6 hr after MI. It has a biphasic peak: It initially peaks at 15 to 24 hr after MI and then exhibits a lower peak

T

after 60 to 80 hr. Cardiac troponin T levels rise 2 to 6 hr after MI and remain elevated. Both proteins return to the reference range 7 days after MI. For additional information regarding screening guidelines for *atherosclerotic cardiovascular disease* (ASCVD), refer to the study titled "Cholesterol, Total and Fractions."

Timing for Appearance and Resolution of Serum/Plasma Cardiac Markers in Acute MI

Cardiac Marker	Appearance (hr)	Peak (hr)	Resolution (d)
CK (total)	4–6	24	2–3
CK-MB	4–6	15–20	2–3
LDH	12	24–48	10–14
Myoglobin	1–3	4–12	1
Troponin I	2–6	15–20	5–7

CK = creatine kinase; CK-MB = creatine kinase MB fraction; LDH = lactate dehydrogenase.

INDICATIONS

• Assist in establishing a diagnosis of MI.
• Evaluate myocardial cell damage.

INTERFERING FACTORS: N/A

POTENTIAL MEDICAL DIAGNOSIS: CLINICAL SIGNIFICANCE OF RESULTS

Increased in

Conditions that result in cardiac tissue damage; troponin is released from damaged tissue into the circulation.

• Acute MI
• Minor myocardial damage
• Myocardial damage after coronary artery bypass graft surgery or percutaneous transluminal coronary angioplasty
• Unstable angina pectoris

Decreased in: N/A

NURSING IMPLICATIONS

POTENTIAL NURSING PROBLEMS: ASSESSMENT & NURSING DIAGNOSIS

Problems	Signs and Symptoms
Cardiac output *(prolonged myocardial ischemia, acute MI, reduced cardiac muscle contractility, rupture papillary muscle, mitral insufficiency)*	Weak peripheral pulses; slow capillary refill; decreased urinary output; cool, clammy skin; tachypnea; dyspnea; altered level of consciousness; abnormal heart sounds; fatigue; hypoxia; loud holosystolic murmur; electrocardiogram (ECG) changes; increased jugular venous distention
Pain *(related to myocardial ischemia, MI)*	Reports of chest pain, new onset of angina, shortness of breath, pallor, weakness, diaphoresis, palpitations, nausea, vomiting, epigastric pain or discomfort, increased blood pressure, increased heart rate

T

Teaching the Patient What to Expect

▶ Inform the patient this test can assist in evaluating heart damage.
▶ Explain that a blood sample is needed for the test.

Potential Nursing Actions

▶ Evaluate for the presence of other risk factors, such as family history of heart disease, smoking, obesity, diet, lack of physical activity, hypertension, diabetes, previous MI, and previous vascular disease, which should be investigated.
▶ Explain that understanding genetics assists in identifying patients and family members who may benefit from additional education, risk assessment, and counseling. Genetics is the study and identification of genes, genetic mutations, and inheritance. For example, genetics provides some insight into the likelihood of inheriting a medical condition such as CAD. Genomic studies evaluate the interaction of groups of genes. The combined activity or combined expression of groups of genes allows assumptions or predictions to be made. As an example, genomic studies measure the levels of activity in multiple genes to predict how they, along with environmental and lifestyle decisions, influence the development of type 2 diabetes, CAD, MI, or ischemic stroke.

Treatment Considerations

▶ Cardiac Output: Assess peripheral pulses and capillary refill, respiratory rate, breath sounds, orthopnea, skin color and temperature, and level of consciousness. Monitor blood pressure and check for orthostatic changes and urinary output. Use pulse oximetry to monitor oxygenation and monitor ECG. Administer ordered inotropic and peripheral vasodilator medications, nitrates, and oxygen.
▶ Teach the patient and family to report chest pain as soon as it starts.

▶ Pain: Assess pain characteristics: duration and onset (minimal exertion, sleep, or rest), squeezing pressure, and location in substernal back neck or jaw. Identify pain relief modalities that have worked in the past. Monitor and trend cardiac biomarkers (CK-MB, troponin, myoglobin). Collaborate with ancillary departments to complete ordered echocardiography, exercise stress testing, or pharmacological stress testing. Administer ordered pain medication, anticoagulants, antiplatelets, beta blockers, calcium channel blockers, ACE inhibitors, Angiotensin II Receptor Blockers (ARBs), and thrombolytic drugs. Monitor and trend vital signs and administer prescribed oxygen.

Nutritional Considerations

▶ Discuss ideal body weight and the purpose of and relationship between ideal weight and caloric intake to support cardiac health. Review ways to decrease intake of saturated fats and increase intake of polyunsaturated fats. Discuss limiting intake of refined processed sugar and sodium; discuss limiting cholesterol intake to less than 300 mg per day. Encourage the intake of fresh fruits and vegetables, unprocessed carbohydrates, poultry, and grains.
▶ Nutritional therapy is recommended for those with identified CAD risk, especially for those with elevated low-density lipoprotein cholesterol levels, other lipid disorders, diabetes, insulin resistance, or metabolic syndrome. Always consider cultural influences with dietary choices to ensure better adherence to a change in lifestyle. A variety of dietary patterns are beneficial for people with ASCVD. For additional information regarding nutritional guidelines, refer to the study titled "Cholesterol, Total and Fractions."
▶ Other changeable risk factors warranting education include strategies to encourage regular participation in moderate aerobic physical activity three to four times per week, eliminating tobacco use, and adhering to a heart-healthy diet.

T

▶ Those with elevated triglycerides should be advised to eliminate or reduce alcohol.

Follow-Up, Evaluation, and Desired Outcomes
▶ Acknowledges contact information provided for the American Heart Association (www.heart.org/HEARTORG),

National Heart, Lung, and Blood Institute (www.nhlbi.nih.gov), and U.S. Department of Agriculture's resource for nutrition (www.choosemyplate.gov).
▶ Understands risk factors for CAD, necessary lifestyle changes (diet, smoking, alcohol use), the importance of weight management, and reportable signs and symptoms of heart attack.

Tuberculosis: Skin and Blood Tests

SYNONYM/ACRONYM: TST, TB tine test, PPD, Mantoux skin test, QuantiFERON-TB Gold blood test (QFT-G), QuantiFERON-TB Gold In-Tube test (QFT-GIT), T-SPOT.TB test (T-SPOT).

RATIONALE: To evaluate for current or past tuberculin infection or exposure.

PATIENT PREPARATION: There are no food, fluid, activity, or medication restrictions unless by medical direction.

NORMAL FINDINGS: Method: Intradermal skin test, enzyme-linked immunosorbent assay (ELISA) blood test for QuantiFERON assays, enzyme-linked ImmunoSpot (ELISPOT) for T-SPOT.TB test. Negative.

CRITICAL FINDINGS AND POTENTIAL INTERVENTIONS
• Positive results

Timely notification to the requesting health-care provider (HCP) of any critical findings and related symptoms is a role expectation of the professional nurse. A listing of these findings varies among facilities.

OVERVIEW: (**Study type:** Blood collected in a green-top [LiHep] tube [QuantiFERON-TB Gold and T-SPOT.TB blood tests], whole blood collected in each of three special [nil, antigen, and mitogen] specimen containers [Quanti FERON-TB Gold In-Tube test]; **related body system:** Immune and Respiratory systems.) Routine screening for tuberculosis (TB) has not been needed for some time because, until recently, the disease had largely been eradicated. Recommendations for the timing of initial and subsequent

screening may vary according to state laws, practitioners' guidelines, and specific circumstances (foreign adoptions or immigration from areas where TB is endemic or in high-risk environments such as health-care or congregated settings). Children and adults are screened on the basis of a risk assessment. For example, the American Academy of Pediatrics recommends identifying individuals at highest risk by means of a questionnaire before testing, and adults who either work or reside in a high-risk environment

T

are required to submit to annual Mantoux testing or chest x-ray (for individuals with a previously positive Mantoux test or individuals from other countries who have received the Bacillus Calmette–Guérin [BCG] vaccine). Tuberculin skin tests are done to determine past or present exposure to TB. The multipuncture or tine test is no longer used as a screening technique and has been largely replaced by the more definitive Mantoux test using Aplisol or Tubersol, purified protein derivatives (PPDs) of the mycobacterial cell wall, administered by intradermal injection. The Mantoux test is the test of choice in symptomatic patients. It is also used in some settings as a screening test. A negative result is judged if there is no sign of redness or induration at the site of the injection or if the zone of redness and induration is less than 5 mm in diameter. TB skin tests are classified in three categories depending on the measured diameter (in millimeters) of the induration and the person's risk of being infected or of progressing to developing TB if infected.

1. A positive result evidenced by an area of erythema and induration at the injection site greater than 5 mm is considered to be positive in persons infected with HIV, persons who have been in recent contact with an individual who has TB, persons with chest x-ray findings consistent with a previous TB infection, persons who have received transplanted organs, or persons who are immunosuppressed from other causes.

2. A positive result evidenced by an area of erythema and induration at the injection site greater than 10 mm is considered to be positive in persons who have immigrated or are foreign adoptees from a country with a high prevalence of TB within the past 5 yr; persons who misuse drugs by injection; persons who work in mycobacteriology laboratories; persons who work or live in highly congregated settings; children less than 4 yr of age; any person with a clinical condition whose immune system is immature, suppressed, or otherwise compromised; and any younger person (infant through adolescent) who has been exposed to adults in a high-risk group.

3. A positive result evidenced by an area of erythema and induration at the injection site greater than 15 mm is considered to be positive in any person.

A positive result does not distinguish between active and dormant infection. A positive response to the Mantoux test is followed up with chest radiography and bacteriological sputum testing to confirm diagnosis. The QuantiFERON-TB Gold (QFT-G), QuantiFERON-TB Gold In-Tube (QFT-GIT), and T-SPOT TB interferon-gamma release blood tests, also known as *interferon-gamma release assays* (IGRAs), are approved by the U.S. Food and Drug Administration for all applications in which the TB skin test is used. The blood tests are procedures in which T lymphocytes from the patient, either in whole blood or harvested from whole blood, are incubated with a reagent cocktail of peptides that simulate two or three proteins made only by *Mycobacterium tuberculosis*. These proteins are not found in the blood of previously vaccinated individuals or individuals who do not have TB. The blood test offers the advantage of eliminating many of the false reactions encountered with skin testing, only a single patient visit is required, and results can be available within 24 hr. Results obtained by the QFT-G test are not affected by BCG vaccination. The blood tests and skin tests are approved as indirect tests for *M. tuberculosis*, and the Centers for Disease Control and Prevention (CDC) recommends their use in conjunction with risk assessment, chest x-ray, and other appropriate medical and diagnostic evaluations.

INDICATIONS

- Evaluate cough, weight loss, fatigue, hemoptysis, and abnormal x-rays to determine if the cause of symptoms is TB.
- Evaluate known or suspected exposure to TB, with or without symptoms, to determine if TB is present.
- Evaluate patients with medical conditions placing them at risk for TB (e.g., AIDS, lymphoma, diabetes).
- Screen populations at risk for developing TB (e.g., health-care workers, residents of long-term care facilities, correctional facility personnel, prison inmates, and residents of the inner city living in poor hygienic conditions).

INTERFERING FACTORS

Factors that may alter the results of the study

General

- Each of the blood and skin tests evaluate different facets of the immune response and use different methodologies and reagents;

interpretations may not be interchangeable.

Skin Test

- Drugs such as immunosuppressive drugs or steroids can alter results.
- Diseases such as hematological cancers or sarcoidosis can alter results.
- Recent or present bacterial, fungal, or viral infections may affect results. False-positive results may be caused by the presence of nontuberculous mycobacteria or by serial testing.
- False-negative results can occur if sensitized T cells are temporarily decreased. False-negative results also can occur in the presence of bacterial infections, immunological deficiencies, immunosuppressive agents, live-virus vaccinations (e.g., measles, mumps, varicella, rubella), malnutrition, old age, overwhelming TB, kidney disease, and active viral infections (e.g., chickenpox, measles, mumps).
- Improper storage of the tuberculin solution (e.g., with respect to temperature, exposure to light, and stability on opening) may affect the results.
- Improper technique when performing the intradermal injection (e.g., injecting into subcutaneous tissue) may cause false-negative results.
- Incorrect amount or dilution of antigen injected or delayed injection after drawing the antigen up into the syringe may affect the results.
- Incorrect reading of the measurement of response or timing of the reading may interfere with results.
- It is not known whether the test has teratogenic effects or reproductive implications; the test should be administered to pregnant women only when clearly indicated.
- The test should not be administered to a patient with a previously positive tuberculin skin test

T

because of the danger of severe reaction, including vesiculation, ulceration, and necrosis.

- The test does not distinguish between current and past infection.

Blood Test
- The performance of these blood tests has not been evaluated in large studies with patients who have impaired or altered immune function, have or are highly likely to develop TB, are younger than 17, are pregnant, or have diseases other than TB. These individuals are either immunosuppressed, immunocompromised, or have immature immune function and may not produce sufficient numbers of T lymphocytes for accurate results. The testing laboratory should be consulted for interpretation of results or limitations for use with patients in these categories.

- False-negative results are possible due to exposure or infection prior to development of detectable immune response.
- False-positive results are possible due to some cross-reactivity to some strains of environmental mycobacteria.
- False-negative results are possible due to exposure or infection prior to development of detectable immune response.

POTENTIAL MEDICAL DIAGNOSIS: CLINICAL SIGNIFICANCE OF RESULTS
Positive findings in
- Pulmonary TB

NURSING IMPLICATIONS

POTENTIAL NURSING PROBLEMS: ASSESSMENT & NURSING DIAGNOSIS

Problems	Signs and Symptoms
Breathing *(related to productive cough, fatigue, inflammation)*	Tachypnea, dyspnea, orthopnea, change in the rate and depth of respirations, retractions, nasal flare, use of accessory muscles
Infection *(related to exposure to M. tuberculosis)*	Productive cough of bloody sputum, fever with temperature spikes, positive acid-fast bacilli (AFB) smear, fatigue, night sweats, weight loss, chills, lack of appetite
Nutrition *(related to poor appetite secondary to M. tuberculosis infection)*	Unintended weight loss; pale, dry skin; dry mucous membranes; documented inadequate caloric intake; subcutaneous tissue loss; hair pulls out easily; self-report of no appetite

BEFORE THE STUDY: PLANNING AND IMPLEMENTATION

Teaching the Patient What to Expect
- Inform the patient this test can assess for a tuberculin infection or exposure.
- Explain that a blood sample is needed for the QuantiFERON-TB Gold and T-SPOT.TB tests.

Skin Test
- Before beginning the test, ensure there is no current active TB and there is no history of a previously positive skin test.
- Explain that the procedure takes approximately 5 min.
- The test should not be administered if there is a skin rash or other eruptions at the test site.

▶ Address concerns about pain and explain that a moderate amount of pain may be experienced when the intradermal injection is performed.

▶ Emphasize the importance of not scratching or disturbing the area after the injection and before the reading.

▶ Ensure that epinephrine hydrochloride solution (1:1,000) is available in the event of anaphylaxis.

▶ The skin site should be cleansed on the lower anterior forearm with alcohol swabs and allow to air-dry.

Mantoux (Intradermal) Test

▶ A PPD or old tuberculin in a tuberculin syringe is prepared with a short, 26-gauge needle attached.

▶ The appropriate dilution and amount is prepared by qualified and trained personnel. The most commonly used intermediate strength is 5 tuberculin units in 0.1 mL or a first strength usually used for children (1 tuberculin unit in 0.1 mL).

▶ Appropriately trained personnel injects the preparation intradermally at the prepared site as soon as it is drawn up into the syringe. When properly injected, a bleb or wheal 6 to 10 mm in diameter is formed within the layers of the skin.

▶ The site is recorded and the patient reminded to return in 48 to 72 hr to have the test read.

▶ At the time of the reading, a plastic ruler is used to measure the diameter of the largest indurated area. The area is palpated for thickening of the tissue; a positive result is indicated by a reaction of 5 mm or more with erythema and edema. To ensure accuracy, the reading is performed by specially trained personnel in a room with sufficient light.

Potential Nursing Actions

▶ Obtain a history of TB or TB exposure, signs and symptoms indicating possible TB, and other skin tests or vaccinations and sensitivities.

AFTER THE STUDY: POTENTIAL NURSING ACTIONS

Treatment Considerations

▶ Be supportive of perceived loss of independence and fear of shortened life expectancy. Discuss the implications of abnormal test results on the patient's lifestyle.

▶ Discuss the implications of abnormal test results on lifestyle choices.

▶ Explain the clinical implications of the test results.

▶ Inform the patient that the effects from a positive response at the skin testing site can remain for 1 wk.

▶ Explain that a positive result may place one at risk for infection related to impaired primary defenses, impaired gas exchange related to decrease in effective lung surface, and intolerance to activity related to an imbalance between oxygen supply and demand.

▶ Breathing: Assess and trend respiratory rate and effort. Monitor for retractions, nasal flare, and use of accessory muscles. Evaluate cough effectiveness and auscultate lungs for adventitious breath sounds. Monitor pulse oximetry and administer ordered oxygen therapy, prepare for possible mechanical intubation. Encourage oral fluids, cough and deep breathing, and pace activities.

▶ Infection: Send ordered sputum specimen for culture. Consider inducing a sputum specimen if the patient is unable to provide one through cough. Place the patient in isolation (negative airflow) until AFB results are obtained. Administer prescribed medications. Instruct the patient regarding the proper way to cover the mouth when coughing or sneezing and to frequently wash hands, especially after coming into contact with contaminated sputum. Explain the importance of visitors wearing masks. Explain that all confirmed TB cases are reported to the department of health.

Nutritional Considerations

▶ Encourage a high-calorie, high-protein diet and an increased intake of oral fluids. Perform a daily weight and obtain an accurate nutritional history. Assess attitude toward eating, promote a dietary consult to evaluate current eating habits and best method of nutritional supplementation. Monitor nutritional laboratory values (albumin), assess swallowing ability, and encourage cultural home foods. Provide a pleasant environment for eating; alter

T

food seasoning to enhance flavor; provide parenteral or enteral nutrition as prescribed.

Follow-Up, Evaluation, and Desired Outcomes
▶ Acknowledges the risk of transmission and proper prophylaxis, and agrees to adhere to the treatment regimen.
▶ Aware that positive findings must be reported to local health department

officials, who will question him or her regarding other persons who may have been exposed through contact. Educate the patient regarding access to counseling services.
▶ Understands that those who receive skin testing must return and have the test results read within the specified timeframe of 48 to 72 hr after injection.

Tuning Fork Tests

SYNONYM/ACRONYM: Bing test, Rinne test, Schwabach test, Weber test.

RATIONALE: To assess for and determine type of hearing loss.

PATIENT PREPARATION: There are no food, fluid, activity, or medication restrictions unless by medical direction.

NORMAL FINDINGS
• Normal air and bone conduction in both ears; no evidence of hearing loss
• Bing Test: Pulsating sound that gets louder and softer when the opening to the ear canal is alternately opened and closed (*Note:* This result, observed in patients with normal hearing, is also observed in patients with sensorineural hearing loss.)
• Rinne Test: Longer and louder tone heard by air conduction than by bone conduction (*Note:* This result, observed in patients with normal hearing, is also observed in patients with sensorineural hearing loss.)
• Schwabach Test: Same tone loudness heard equally long by the examiner and the patient
• Weber Test: Same tone loudness heard equally in both ears.

CRITICAL FINDINGS AND POTENTIAL INTERVENTIONS: N/A

OVERVIEW: (Study type: Sensory, auditory; **related body system:** Nervous system.) These noninvasive assessment procedures are done to distinguish conduction hearing loss from sensorineural hearing loss. They may be performed as part of the physical assessment examination and followed by hearing loss audiometry for confirmation of questionable results. The tuning fork tests described in this study are named for the four German otologists who described their use. Tuning fork tests are used less frequently by audiologists in favor of more sophisticated electronic methods, but presentation of the tuning fork test methodology is useful to illustrate the principles involved in electronic test methods.

A tuning fork is a bipronged metallic device that emits a clear tone at a particular pitch when it is set into vibration by holding

T

the stem in the hand and striking one of the prongs or tines against a firm surface. The Bing test samples for conductive hearing loss by intermittently occluding and unblocking the opening of the ear canal while holding a vibrating tuning fork to the mastoid process behind the ear. The occlusion effect is absent in patients with conductive hearing loss and is present in patients with normal hearing or with sensorineural hearing loss. The Rinne test compares the patient's own hearing by bone conduction to his or her hearing by air conduction to determine whether hearing loss, if detected, is conductive or sensorineural. The Schwabach test compares the patient's level of bone conduction hearing to that of a presumed normal-hearing examiner. The Weber test has been modified by many audiologists for use with electronic equipment. When the test is administered, the patient is asked to tell the examiner the location of the tone heard (left ear, right ear, both ears, or midline) in order to determine whether the hearing loss is conductive, sensorineural, or mixed.

INDICATIONS
- Evaluate type of hearing loss (conductive or sensorineural).
- Screen for hearing loss as part of a routine physical examination and to determine the need for referral to an audiologist.

INTERFERING FACTORS

Factors that may alter the results of the study
- Poor technique in striking the tuning fork or incorrect placement can cause inaccurate results.

- Inability of the patient to understand how to identify responses or unwillingness of the patient to cooperate during the test can cause inaccurate results.
- Hearing loss in the examiner can affect results in those tests that utilize hearing comparisons between patient and examiner.
- Recent ear infection or cold can cause inaccurate results.
- Exposure to very loud noises (in the general or work environment) on the day previous to the test may cause inaccurate results.

POTENTIAL MEDICAL DIAGNOSIS: CLINICAL SIGNIFICANCE OF RESULTS
Abnormal findings related to
- Conduction hearing loss related to or evidenced by:
  Impacted cerumen
  Obstruction of external ear canal *(presence of a foreign body)*
  Otitis externa *(infection in ear canal)*
  Otitis media *(poor eustachian tube function or infection)*
  Otitis media serous *(fluid in middle ear due to allergies or a cold)*
  Otosclerosis
  Bing Test: No change in the loudness of the sound
  Rinne Test: Tone louder or detected for a longer time than the air-conducted tone
  Schwabach Test: Prolonged duration of tone when compared to that heard by the examiner
  Weber Test: Lateralization of tone to one ear, indicating loss of hearing on that side (i.e., tone is heard in the poorer ear)
- Sensorineural hearing loss related to or evidenced by:
  Congenital damage or malformations of the inner ear
  Ménière disease
  Ototoxic drugs *(aminoglycosides, e.g., gentamicin or tobramycin; salicylates, e.g., aspirin)*
  Presbycusis *(gradual hearing loss experienced in advancing age)*

T

Serious infections (*meningitis, measles, mumps, other viral, syphilis*)

Trauma to the inner ear (*related to exposure to noise in excess of 90 dB or as a result of physical trauma*)

Tumor (*e.g., acoustic neuroma, cerebellopontine angle tumor, meningioma*)

Vascular disorders

Bing Test: Pulsating sound that gets louder and softer when the opening to the ear canal is alternately opened and closed

Rinne Test: Tone heard louder by air conduction

Schwabach Test: Shortened duration of tone when compared to that heard by the examiner

Weber Test: Lateralization of tone to one ear indicating loss of hearing on the other side (i.e., tone is heard in the better ear)

NURSING IMPLICATIONS

BEFORE THE STUDY: PLANNING AND IMPLEMENTATION

Teaching the Patient What to Expect

▶ Inform the patient this procedure can assist in assessing for hearing loss.

▶ Review the procedure with the patient. Address concerns about pain and explain that no discomfort will be experienced during the test.

▶ Explain that a health-care provider (HCP) performs the test in a quiet, darkened room, and that to evaluate both ears, the test can take 5 to 10 min.

▶ Positioning for the procedure is comfortably seated in a quiet environment facing the examiner. A tuning fork of 1,024 Hz is used because it tests within the range of human speech (400 to 5,000 Hz).

▶ *Bing Test:* This procedure is completed by tapping the tuning fork handle against the hand to start a light vibration.

▶ The handle is held to the mastoid process behind the ear while alternately opening and closing the ear canal with a finger.

▶ The patient is asked to report a change in loudness or softness in sound.

▶ The results are recorded as a positive Bing if the patient reports a pulsating change in sound or a negative Bing if no change in loudness is detected.

▶ *Rinne Test:* The tuning fork handle is tapped against the hand to start a light vibration.

▶ The patient is asked to mask the ear not being tested by moving a finger in and out of the ear canal of that ear.

▶ Explain that the base of the vibrating tuning fork is held between with the thumb and forefinger of the tester's dominant hand and placed in contact with the mastoid process (bone conduction).

▶ Explain to the patient that he or she will be asked to report when the sound is no longer heard.

▶ Explain that this process is repeated with placement of the same vibrating tuning fork in front of the ear canal (air conduction) without touching the external part of the ear.

▶ Advise the patient that he or she will be asked which of the two has the loudest or longest tone. The same procedure is repeated with the other ear.

▶ Results are recorded as Rinne positive if air conduction is heard longer and Rinne negative if bone conduction is heard longer.

▶ *Schwabach Test:* The tuning fork handle is tapped against the hand to start a light vibration.

▶ Explain that the base of the tuning fork is held against one side of the mastoid process and the patient will be asked if the tone is heard.

▶ Explain to the patient that he or she will be asked to mask the ear not being tested by moving a finger in and out of the ear canal of that ear.

▶ The examiner places the tuning fork against the same side of his or her own mastoid process and listens for the tone.

▶ The tuning fork is alternated on the same side between the patient and

examiner until the sound is no longer heard, noting whether the sound ceased to be heard by both the patient and the examiner at the same point in time.
▶ The procedure is repeated on the other ear.
▶ If the patient hears the tone for a longer or shorter time, the difference is counted and noted in seconds.
▶ *Weber Test:* The tuning fork handle is tapped against the hand to start a light vibration.
▶ Explain that the base of the vibrating tuning fork is held with the thumb and forefinger of the dominant hand and placed on the middle of the forehead or at the vertex of the head.
▶ Explain to the patient that he or she will be asked to determine if the sound is heard better and longer on one side than the other.
▶ The results are recorded as Weber right or left. If sound is heard equally, it is recorded as Weber negative.

Potential Nursing Actions
▶ Obtain a history of the patient's known or suspected hearing loss, including type and cause; ear conditions with treatment regimens; ear surgery; and other tests and procedures to assess and diagnose auditory deficit.
▶ Ensure that the external auditory canal is clear of impacted cerumen.

AFTER THE STUDY: POTENTIAL NURSING ACTIONS

Treatment Considerations
▶ Discuss the implications of abnormal test results on lifestyle choices.
▶ Provide education related to the clinical implications of the test results.
▶ Instruct the patient in the use, cleaning, and storage of a hearing aid.

Follow-Up, Evaluation, and Desired Outcomes
▶ Acknowledges contact information provided for the American Speech-Language-Hearing Association (www.asha.org).

Ultrasound, Arterial Doppler, Carotid Studies

SYNONYM/ACRONYM: Carotid Doppler, carotid ultrasound, arterial ultrasound, cerebrovascular ultrasound.

RATIONALE: To visualize and assess blood flow through the carotid arteries toward evaluating risk for stroke related to atherosclerosis.

PATIENT PREPARATION: There are no food or medication restrictions unless by medical direction. Some protocols may require the patient to restrict nicotine and caffeine for 1 to 2 hr before the procedure in order to avoid vasoconstriction or vasodilation.

NORMAL FINDINGS
- Normal blood flow through the carotid arteries with no evidence of occlusion or narrowing.

CRITICAL FINDINGS AND POTENTIAL INTERVENTIONS: N/A

OVERVIEW: (Study type: Ultrasound; related body system: Circulatory system.) Ultrasound (US) procedures are diagnostic, noninvasive, and relatively inexpensive. They take a short time to complete, do not use radiation, and cause no harm to the patient. High-frequency sound waves of various intensities are delivered by a transducer, a flashlight-shaped device, pressed against the skin. The waves are bounced back off internal anatomical structures and fluids, converted to electrical energy, amplified by the transducer, and displayed as images on a monitor.

Different types of transducers and imaging systems are sometimes used in clinical settings. Conventional US systems assume that sound waves pass through tissue at a constant speed. Advances in technology have led to the development of "smart" transducers that can compensate for tissue aberrations in technically difficult patients. Other advancements in imaging systems include three-dimensional and Doppler US. Color Doppler US uses color to indicate the velocity and direction of blood flow. Power Doppler is a more sensitive Doppler variation, capable of providing detailed images of blood flow; a limitation of power Doppler is that it cannot provide information regarding the direction of blood flow. Spectral Doppler provides data from blood flow measurements in formats other than color—for example, it can convert the measurements into a graph representing distance of blood flow against time or as a unique sound heard with every heartbeat.

Using the duplex scanning method, carotid US records sound waves to obtain information about the carotid arteries. The amplitude and waveform of the carotid pulse are measured, resulting in a two-dimensional image of the artery. Carotid arterial sites used for the studies include the common carotid, external carotid, and internal carotid. Blood flow direction, velocity, and the presence of flow disturbances can be readily assessed. The sound waves that hit the moving red blood cells and are reflected back to the transducer correspond to the velocity of the blood flow through the vessel. Color Doppler US can be used with the duplex method whereby red and blue are assigned to represent the direction of blood flow, and the intensity of the color is an indication of velocity. The result is the visualization of the artery to assist in the diagnosis (i.e., presence, amount, location) of plaque causing vessel stenosis or atherosclerotic occlusion affecting the flow of blood to the brain. Depending on the degree of stenosis causing a reduction in vessel diameter, additional testing can be performed to determine the effect of stenosis on the hemodynamic status of the artery.

The combined information obtained from carotid US and ankle-brachial index (ABI) provides significant support for predicting coronary artery disease. ABI is a noninvasive, simple comparison of blood pressure measurements in the arms and legs and can be used to detect peripheral arterial disease (PAD). A Doppler stethoscope is used to obtain the systolic pressure in either the dorsalis pedis or the posterior tibial artery. This ankle pressure is then divided by the highest brachial systolic pressure acquired after taking the blood pressure in both of the patient's arms. This index should be greater than 1 with a range of 0.85 to 1.4. When the index falls below 0.5, blood flow impairment is considered significant. Patients should be scheduled for a vascular consult for an abnormal ABI. Patients with diabetes or kidney disease, and some older adult patients, may have a falsely elevated ABI due to calcifications of the vessels in the ankle causing an increased systolic pressure. The ABI test approaches 95% accuracy in detecting PAD. However, a normal ABI value does not absolutely rule out the possibility of PAD for some individuals, and additional tests should be done to evaluate symptoms.

INDICATIONS
- Assist in the diagnosis of carotid artery occlusive disease, as evidenced by visualization of blood flow disruption.
- Detect irregularities in the structure of the carotid arteries.
- Detect plaque or stenosis of the carotid artery, as evidenced by turbulent blood flow or changes in Doppler signals indicating occlusion.

INTERFERING FACTORS
Factors that may alter the results of the study
- Attenuation of the sound waves by bony structures, which can impair clear imaging of the vessels.
- Incorrect placement of the transducer over the desired test site; quality of the US study is very dependent on the skill of the ultrasonographer.
- Metallic objects (e.g., jewelry, body rings) within the examination field, which may inhibit organ visualization and cause unclear images.
- Patients who are technically difficult and who present challenges in obtaining reliable results (e.g., who are obese; have reduced rib spaces; present with fatty liver; have postoperative incisions, bandages, or dressings; have significant scarring in the area of interest). Aberrations in tissue composition may attenuate the sound waves and alter findings.

U

POTENTIAL MEDICAL DIAGNOSIS: CLINICAL SIGNIFICANCE OF RESULTS
Abnormal findings related to
- Arterial aneurysm
- Carotid artery occlusive disease (atherosclerosis)
- Plaque or stenosis of carotid artery
- Reduction in vessel diameter of more than 16%, indicating stenosis
- Tumor

NURSING IMPLICATIONS

POTENTIAL NURSING PROBLEMS: ASSESSMENT & NURSING DIAGNOSIS

Problems	Signs and Symptoms
Inadequate cerebral tissue perfusion *(related to infarct, hemorrhage, mass, edema, infection, plaque, atrophy)*	Diminished or altered level of consciousness, aphasia that can be expressive or receptive, loss of sensory functionality, slurred speech, difficulty swallowing, difficulty in completing a learned activity or in recognizing familiar objects (apraxia, agnosia), motor function deficits, spatial neglect, facial droop and/or varying degrees of flaccid extremities
Inadequate self-care *(related to loss of cognitive or motor function)*	Unable to complete the activities of daily living without assistance (eating, bathing, dressing, toileting)
Mobility *(related to altered muscular function secondary to cerebral injury)*	Loss of sensation, weakness on one side, uncoordinated movement, difficulty understanding and following instructions, spatial neglect

BEFORE THE STUDY: PLANNING AND IMPLEMENTATION

Teaching the Patient What to Expect
- Inform the patient this procedure can assist in assessing the carotid arteries in the neck.
- Review the procedure with the patient. Address concerns about pain related to the procedure and explain that no pain or discomfort should be experienced during the test.
- Explain that the procedure is performed in a US department by a health-care provider (HCP) who specializes in this procedure, with support staff, and takes approximately 30 to 60 min.
- Advise the patient that he or she will be asked to remove jewelry and other metallic objects from the area to be examined.
- Positioning for this procedure is in the supine position on an examination table; other positions may be used during the examination.
- Explain to the patient that he or she will be draped and that the neck will be exposed.
- Explain that conductive gel is applied to the skin, and a Doppler transducer is moved over the skin to obtain images of the area of interest.
- Advise the patient to breathe normally during the examination. Explain that if necessary, the patient may be asked to inhale deeply and hold his or her breath for better organ visualization.
- Once the study is completed, the gel is cleansed from the skin.

Potential Nursing Actions
- Evaluate for the presence of other risk factors, such as family history of heart disease, smoking, obesity, diet, lack of

physical activity, hypertension, diabetes, previous myocardial infarction (MI), and previous vascular disease, which should be investigated.

▶ Understanding genetics assists in identifying those who may benefit from additional education, risk assessment, and counseling.

AFTER THE STUDY: POTENTIAL NURSING ACTIONS

Treatment Considerations

▶ Instruct the patient to resume usual diet, fluids, and medications, as directed by the HCP.

▶ Inadequate Cerebral Tissue Perfusion: Complete a baseline neurological assessment for ongoing comparison to evaluate improvement or deterioration. Monitor and trend vital signs. Prepare for and facilitate complementary diagnostic studies: magnetic resonance imaging, positron emission tomography, US, or subtraction angiography. Elevate the head of the bed and maintain a quiet, restful environment. Administer ordered antiplatelet, anticoagulant, or thrombolytic medication. Administer ordered antihypertensive, steroids, diuretic, calcium channel blocker, or antiseizure medications.

▶ Inadequate Self-Care: Assess self-care deficits, identify areas where the patient can provide own care, and encourage participation. Evaluate the families' ability to assist with self-care needs, facilitate home health evaluation, and provide assistive devices to support self-care (commode, special utensils). Collaborate with a dietician and design a diet to altered swallowing ability (thick liquids, puree, small bites etc.); remind the patient to chew and swallow slowly.

▶ Mobility: Assess current functional level. Facilitate physical therapy evaluation and treatment, including active or passive range of motion to maintain muscle strength. Encourage the appropriate use of assistive devices (walker, cane) and provide assistance with activities to decrease fall risk (gait belt). Assess the skin for alterations in integrity (pressure ulcers), and teach proper turning and assisting techniques.

▶ Be supportive of fear of shortened life expectancy and perceived loss of independent function.

▶ Provide teaching and information regarding the clinical implications of the test results.

Nutritional Considerations

▶ Discuss ideal body weight and the purpose and relationship between ideal weight and caloric intake to support cardiac health.

▶ Encourage consultation with a registered dietitian to learn how to plan and prepare healthy meals for the entire family.

▶ Nutritional therapy is recommended for the patient identified to be at risk for developing CAD or for individuals who have specific risk factors and/or existing medical conditions (e.g., elevated low-density lipoprotein cholesterol levels, other lipid disorders, diabetes, insulin resistance, or metabolic syndrome).

▶ Other changeable risk factors warranting patient education include strategies to encourage patients, especially those who are overweight and with high blood pressure, to safely decrease sodium intake, achieve a normal weight, ensure regular participation of moderate aerobic physical activity three to four times per week, eliminate tobacco use, and adhere to a heart-healthy diet. If triglycerides are elevated, the patient should be advised to eliminate or reduce alcohol. Always consider cultural influences with dietary choices to ensure better adherence to a change in lifestyle. A variety of dietary patterns are beneficial for people with CAD.

Follow-Up, Evaluation, and Desired Outcomes

▶ Acknowledges contact information provided for the American Heart Association (www.heart.org/HEARTORG), National Heart, Lung, and Blood Institute (www.nhlbi.nih.gov), and U.S. Department of Agriculture's resource for nutrition (www.choosemyplate.gov).

▶ Understands the importance of adhering to the therapy regimen, including the significant adverse effects associated with the prescribed medication and the value of reviewing corresponding literature provided by a pharmacist.

U

Ultrasound, Arterial Doppler, Lower and Upper Extremity Studies

SYNONYM/ACRONYM: Doppler, arterial ultrasound, duplex scan.

RATIONALE: To visualize and assess blood flow through the arteries of the upper and lower extremities toward diagnosing disorders such as occlusion and aneurysm and to evaluate for the presence of plaque and stenosis. This procedure can also be used to assess the effectiveness of therapeutic interventions such as arterial graphs and blood flow to transplanted organs.

PATIENT PREPARATION: There are no food or medication restrictions unless by medical direction. Some protocols may require the patient to restrict nicotine and caffeine for 1 to 2 hr before the procedure in order to avoid vasoconstriction or vasodilation.

NORMAL FINDINGS
- Normal blood flow through the lower extremity arteries with no evidence of vessel occlusion or narrowing
- Normal arterial systolic and diastolic Doppler signals
- Normal reduction in systolic blood pressure (i.e., less than 20 mm Hg) when compared to a normal extremity
- Normal ABI (greater than 0.85).

CRITICAL FINDINGS AND POTENTIAL INTERVENTIONS: N/A

OVERVIEW: (Study type: Ultrasound; **related body system:** Circulatory system.) Ultrasound (US) procedures are diagnostic, noninvasive, and relatively inexpensive. They take a short time to complete, do not use radiation, and cause no harm to the patient. High-frequency sound waves of various intensities are delivered by a transducer, a flashlight-shaped device, pressed against the skin. The waves are bounced back off internal anatomical structures and fluids, converted to electrical energy, amplified by the transducer, and displayed as images on a monitor. Color Doppler US can be used with the duplex method whereby red and blue are assigned to represent the direction of blood flow, and the intensity of the color is an indication of velocity. Using the duplex scanning method, arterial leg US records sound waves to obtain information about the arteries of the lower extremities from the common femoral arteries and their branches as they extend into the calf area. The amplitude and waveform of the pulses are measured, resulting in a two-dimensional image of the artery. Blood flow direction, velocity, and the presence of flow disturbances can be readily assessed, and for diagnostic studies, the technique is done bilaterally. The sound waves hit the moving red blood cells and are reflected back to the transducer corresponding to the velocity of the blood flow through the vessel. The result is the visualization of the artery to assist in the diagnosis (i.e., presence, amount, and location) of plaque causing vessel stenosis or occlusion and to help determine the cause of claudication. Arterial reconstruction and graft condition and patency can also be evaluated.

In arterial Doppler studies, arteriosclerotic disease of the peripheral vessels can be detected by slowly deflating blood pressure cuffs that are placed on an extremity such as the calf, ankle, or upper extremity. The systolic pressure of the various arteries of the extremities can be measured. The Doppler transducer can detect the first sign of blood flow through the cuffed artery, even the most minimal blood flow, as evidenced by a swishing noise. There is normally a reduction in systolic blood pressure from the arteries of the arms to the arteries of the legs; a reduction exceeding 20 mm Hg is indicative of occlusive disease (deep vein thrombosis) proximal to the area being tested. This procedure may also be used to monitor the patency of a graft, status of previous corrective surgery, vascular status of the blood flow to a transplanted organ, blood flow to a mass, or the extent of vascular trauma.

The ankle-brachial index (ABI) can also be assessed during this study. This noninvasive, simple comparison of blood pressure measurements in the arms and legs can be used to detect peripheral arterial disease (PAD). A Doppler stethoscope is used to obtain the systolic pressure in either the dorsalis pedis or the posterior tibial artery. This ankle pressure is then divided by the highest brachial systolic pressure acquired after taking the blood pressure in both of the patient's arms. This index should be greater than 1 with a range of 0.85 to 1.4. When the index falls below 0.5, blood flow impairment is considered significant. Patients should be scheduled for a vascular consult for an abnormal ABI. Patients with diabetes or kidney disease, and some older adult patients, may have a falsely elevated ABI due to calcifications of the vessels in the ankle causing an increased systolic pressure. The ABI test approaches 95% accuracy in detecting PAD. However, a normal ABI value does not absolutely rule out the possibility of PAD for some individuals, and additional tests should be done to evaluate symptoms.

INDICATIONS

- Aid in the diagnosis of small or large vessel PAD.
- Aid in the diagnosis of spastic arterial disease, such as Raynaud's phenomenon.
- Assist in the diagnosis of aneurysm, pseudoaneurysm, hematoma, arteriovenous malformation, or hemangioma.
- Assist in the diagnosis of ischemia, arterial calcification, or plaques, as evidenced by visualization of blood flow disruption. For additional information regarding screening guidelines for *atherosclerotic cardiovascular disease* (ASCVD), refer to the study titled "Cholesterol, Total and Fractions."
- Detect irregularities in the structure of the arteries.
- Detect plaque or stenosis of the lower extremity artery, as evidenced by turbulent blood flow or changes in Doppler signals indicating occlusion.
- Determine the patency of a vascular graft, stent, or previous surgery.
- Evaluate possible arterial trauma.

U

INTERFERING FACTORS

Factors that may alter the results of the study

- Attenuation of the sound waves by bony structures, which can impair clear imaging of the vessels.
- Incorrect placement of the transducer over the desired test site; quality of the US study is very dependent on the skill of the ultrasonographer.
- Cold extremities, resulting in vasoconstriction, which can cause inaccurate measurements.
- Occlusion proximal to the site being studied, which would affect blood flow to the area.
- Cigarette smoking, because nicotine can cause constriction of the peripheral vessels.
- Metallic objects (e.g., jewelry, body rings) within the examination field, which may inhibit organ visualization and cause unclear images.
- Patients who are technically difficult and who present challenges in obtaining reliable results (e.g., who are obese; have reduced rib spaces; present with fatty liver; have postoperative incisions, bandages, or dressings; have significant scarring in the area of interest). Aberrations in tissue composition may attenuate the sound waves and alter findings.

Other considerations

- An abnormally large leg, making direct examination difficult.

POTENTIAL MEDICAL DIAGNOSIS: CLINICAL SIGNIFICANCE OF RESULTS

Abnormal findings related to

- ABI less than 0.85, indicating significant arterial occlusive disease within the extremity
- Aneurysm
- Arterial calcification or plaques
- Embolic arterial occlusion
- Graft diameter reduction
- Hemangioma
- Hematoma
- Ischemia
- PAD
- Pseudoaneurysm
- Reduction in vessel diameter of more than 16%, indicating stenosis
- Spastic arterial occlusive disease, such as Raynaud phenomenon

NURSING IMPLICATIONS

BEFORE THE STUDY: PLANNING AND IMPLEMENTATION

Teaching the Patient What to Expect

- Inform the patient this procedure can assist in assessing blood flow to the upper and lower extremities.
- Review the procedure with the patient. Address concerns about pain related to the procedure and explain that no pain or discomfort should be experienced during the test.
- Explain that the procedure is performed in a US department by a health-care provider (HCP) who specializes in this procedure, with support staff, and takes approximately 30 to 60 min.
- Advise the patient that he or she will be asked to remove jewelry and other metallic objects from the area to be examined.
- Explain that positioning for this procedure is in the supine position on an examination table; other positions may be used during the examination.
- Explain to the patient that he or she will be draped and the area of interest exposed.
- Blood pressure cuffs are placed on the thigh, calf, and ankle.
- Conductive gel is applied to the skin over the area distal to each of the cuffs to promote the passage of sound waves as a Doppler transducer is moved over the skin to obtain images of the area of interest.

U

- Explain that the thigh cuff is inflated to a level above the patient's systolic pressure found in the normal extremity.
- Explain that the pressure in cuff is slowly released, and when the swishing sound of blood flow is heard, it is recorded at the highest point along the artery at which it is audible.
- The test is repeated at the calf and then the ankle.
- Once the study is completed, the gel is removed from the skin.

Potential Nursing Actions
- Report the presence of a lesion that is open or draining; maintain clean, dry dressing for the ulcer; protect the limb from trauma.

AFTER THE STUDY: POTENTIAL NURSING ACTIONS

Treatment Considerations
- Provide education regarding the clinical implications of the test results.
- Instruct the patient to continue diet, fluids, and medications, as directed by the HCP.
- Pain can be present due to ischemia, inflammation or obstruction. Assess pain character, location, duration, intensity and use an easily understood pain rating scale. Place the patient in a position of comfort. Administer ordered pain medications and consider alternative measures for pain management (imagery, relaxation, music, etc.). Use caution when moving extremities.
- Mobility challenges can be present due to ischemia, inflammation, or obstruction. Immobilize affected extremity as ordered. Facilitate the use of assistive devices, and administer ordered medications (analgesics, steroids, antibiotics). Monitor and trend diagnostic study results, circulation, and sensation, and encourage ambulation when appropriate. Institute fall risk protocols.

Nutritional Considerations
- Discuss ideal body weight and the purpose of and relationship between ideal weight and caloric intake to support cardiac health. Review ways to decrease intake of saturated fats and increase intake of polyunsaturated fats. Discuss limiting intake of refined processed sugar and sodium; discuss limiting cholesterol intake to less than 300 mg per day. Encourage the intake of fresh fruits and vegetables, unprocessed carbohydrates, poultry, and grains.
- Nutritional therapy is recommended for those with identified CAD risk, especially for those with elevated low-density lipoprotein cholesterol levels, other lipid disorders, diabetes, insulin resistance, or metabolic syndrome. Always consider cultural influences with dietary choices to ensure better adherence to a change in lifestyle. A variety of dietary patterns are beneficial for people with ASCVD. For additional information regarding nutritional guidelines, refer to the study titled "Cholesterol, Total and Fractions."
- Other changeable risk factors warranting education include strategies to encourage regular participation in moderate aerobic physical activity three to four times per week, eliminating tobacco use, and adhering to a heart-healthy diet.
- Those with elevated triglycerides should be advised to eliminate or reduce alcohol.
- Patients on low-sodium diets should be advised to avoid beverages such as colas, ginger ale, sports drinks, lemon-lime sodas, and root beer.
- Many over-the-counter medications, including antacids, laxatives, analgesics, sedatives, and antitussives, contain significant amounts of sodium.
- Emphasize the importance of reading all food, beverage, and medicine labels.

Follow-Up, Evaluation, and Desired Outcomes
- Understands the importance of decreasing fall risk by adhering to fall risk protocols.
- Recognizes the value of working with the health-care team to discuss treatment options and expected outcomes.

U

Ultrasound, A-scan

SYNONYM/ACRONYM: Amplitude modulation scan, A-scan ultrasound biometry.

RATIONALE: To assess for ocular tissue abnormality and to determine the power of the intraocular lens required for replacement in cataract surgery.

PATIENT PREPARATION: There are no food, fluid, activity, or medication restrictions unless by medical direction.

NORMAL FINDINGS
• Normal homogeneous ocular tissue.

CRITICAL FINDINGS AND POTENTIAL INTERVENTIONS: N/A

OVERVIEW: (**Study type:** Ultrasound; **related body system:** Nervous system.) Diagnostic techniques such as A-scan ultrasonography can be used to identify abnormal tissue. The A-scan employs a single-beam, linear sound wave to detect abnormalities by returning an echo when interference disrupts its straight path. When the sound wave is directed at lens vitreous, the normal homogeneous tissue does not return an echo; an opaque lens with a cataract will produce an echo. The returning waves produced by abnormal tissue are received by a microfilm that converts the sound energy into electrical impulses that are amplified and displayed on an oscilloscope as an ultrasonogram or echogram. The A-scan echo can be used to indicate the position of the cornea and retina. The A-scan is most commonly used to measure the axial length of the eye. This measurement is used to determine the power requirement for an intraocular lens used to replace the abnormal, opaque lens of the eye removed in cataract surgery. There are two different methods

currently in use. The applanation method involves placement of an ultrasound (US) probe directly on the cornea. The immersion technique is more popular because it does not require direct contact and compression of the cornea. The immersion technique protects the cornea by placement of a fluid layer between the eye and the US probe. The accuracy of the immersion technique is thought to be greater than applanation because no corneal compression is caused by the immersion method. Therefore, the measured axial length achieved by immersion is closer to the true axial length of the cornea.

INDICATIONS
• Determination of power requirement for replacement intraocular lens in cataract surgery.

INTERFERING FACTORS
Factors that may alter the results of the study
• Rubbing or squeezing the eyes may affect results.
• Improper placement of the probe tip to the surface of the eye may produce inaccurate results.

U

POTENTIAL MEDICAL DIAGNOSIS: CLINICAL SIGNIFICANCE OF RESULTS

Abnormal findings related to

• Cataract

NURSING IMPLICATIONS

BEFORE THE STUDY: PLANNING AND IMPLEMENTATION

Teaching the Patient What to Expect

▶ Inform the patient this procedure determines the strength of the lens that will be replaced during cataract surgery.

▶ Review the procedure with the patient. Address concerns about pain and explain that some discomfort may be experienced after the test when the numbness wears off from the anesthetic drops administered prior to the test.

▶ Explain that a health-care provider (HCP) performs the test in a quiet, darkened room and that evaluation of the eye upon which surgery is to be performed can take up 10 min.

▶ Explain to the patient that he or she will be comfortably seated for the procedure and instructed to look straight ahead, keeping the eyes open and unblinking.

▶ Explain that a topical anesthetic is instilled in each eye and given time to work.

▶ Explain that the chin is placed in a chin rest and the forehead gently pressed against the support bar. Once the US probe is properly positioned on the surgical eye, a reading is automatically taken.

▶ Multiple measurements may be taken to ensure that a consistent and accurate reading has been achieved. Variability between serial measurements is unavoidable using the applanation technique.

Potential Nursing Actions

▶ Investigate the patient's history of known or suspected vision loss; changes in visual acuity, including type and cause; use of glasses or contact lenses; eye conditions with treatment regimens; eye surgery; and other tests and procedures to assess and diagnose visual deficit.

▶ Advise the patient that he or she will be asked to remove contact lenses or glasses, as appropriate.

AFTER THE STUDY: POTENTIAL NURSING ACTIONS

Treatment Considerations

▶ Reassure the patient regarding concerns related to potential impending cataract surgery.

▶ Be supportive of impaired activity related to vision loss, anticipated loss of driving privileges, or the possibility of requiring corrective lenses (self-image).

Follow-Up, Evaluation, and Desired Outcomes

▶ Acknowledges that some temporary or permanent lifestyle changes may be required depending on procedure results. Additional testing may be performed to monitor disease progression and determine the need for a change in therapy.

Ultrasound, Biophysical Profile, Obstetric

SYNONYM/ACRONYM: BPP ultrasound, fetal age sonogram, gestational age sonogram, OB sonography, pregnancy ultrasound, pregnancy echo, pregnant uterus ultrasonography.

RATIONALE: To visualize and assess the fetus in utero to monitor fetal health related to growth, congenital abnormalities, distress, and demise. Also used

U

to identify gender and multiple pregnancy and to obtain amniotic fluid for analysis.

PATIENT PREPARATION: There are no food, fluid, activity, or medication restrictions unless by medical direction. There should be 24 hr between administration of barium and this test.

NORMAL FINDINGS

- Normal age, size, viability, position, and functional capacities of the fetus.
- Normal placenta size, position, and structure; adequate volume of amniotic fluid.
- Biophysical profile (BPP) score of 8 to 10 is considered normal. Each of the fetal movements evaluated in the BPP is related to oxygen-dependent activities that originate from the central nervous system. Their presence is assumed to indicate normal brain function and absence of systemic hypoxia.

CRITICAL FINDINGS AND POTENTIAL INTERVENTIONS

- Abruptio placentae
- BPP score between 0 and 2 is abnormal and indicates the need for assessment and decisions regarding early or immediate delivery.
- Ectopic pregnancy
- Fetal death
- Placenta previa

Timely notification to the requesting health-care provider (HCP) of any critical findings and related symptoms is a role expectation of the professional nurse. A listing of these findings varies among facilities.

OVERVIEW: (Study type: Ultrasound; related body system: Reproductive system.) Ultrasound (US) procedures are diagnostic, noninvasive, and relatively inexpensive. They take a short time to complete, do not use radiation, and cause no harm to the patient. High-frequency sound waves of various intensities are delivered by a transducer, a flashlight-shaped device, pressed against the skin. The waves are bounced back off internal anatomical structures and fluids, converted to electrical energy, amplified by the transducer, and displayed as images on a monitor to visualize the fetus and placenta. US is often used as a diagnostic and therapeutic tool for guiding minimally invasive procedures such as needle biopsies and fluid aspiration (amniocentesis). The contraindications and complications for biopsy and fluid aspiration are discussed in detail in the individual studies. This procedure is done by a transabdominal or transvaginal approach, depending on when the procedure is performed (first trimester [transabdominal or transvaginal or combination] vs. second or third trimester [transabdominal]). It is the safest method of examination to evaluate the uterus and determine fetal size, growth, and position; fetal structural abnormalities; ectopic pregnancy; placenta position and amount of amniotic fluid; and multiple gestation.

Obstetric US is used to secure different types of information regarding the fetus and placenta, varying with the trimester during which the procedure is done. This procedure may also include a nonstress test (NST) in combination with Doppler monitoring of amniotic fluid volume, fetal heart, gross fetal movements, fetal muscle tone, and fetal respiratory movements to detect high-risk pregnancy. The procedure is indicated as a guide for amniocentesis, cordocentesis, fetoscopy, aspiration of multiple oocytes for in vitro fertilization, and other intrauterine interventional procedures.

The BPP considers five antepartum parameters measured to predict fetal wellness. The BPP is indicated in women with high-risk pregnancies to identify a fetus in distress or in jeopardy of demise. It includes fetal heart rate (FHR) measurement, fetal breathing movements, fetal body movements, fetal muscle tone, and amniotic fluid volume. Each of the five parameters is assigned a score of either 0 or 2, allowing a maximum or perfect score of 10. The NST is an external US monitoring of FHR performed either as part of the BPP or when one or more of the US procedures have abnormal results. The NST is interpreted as either reactive or nonreactive.

BPP Parameter	Normal: Score = 2	Abnormal: Score = 0
Fetal heart rate reactivity	Two or more movement-associated FHR accelerations of 15 or more beats/min above baseline, lasting 15 sec, in a 20-min interval	One or no movement-associated FHR accelerations of 15 or more beats/min above baseline in a 20-min interval
Fetal breathing movements	One or more breathing movements lasting 20–60 sec in a 30-min interval	Absent or no breathing movements lasting longer than 19 sec in a 30-min interval
Fetal body movements	Two or more discrete body or limb movements in a 30-min interval	Less than two discrete body or limb movements in a 30-min interval
Fetal muscle tone	One or more episodes of active limb extension and return to flexion (to include opening and closing of hand)	Absent movement, slow extension with partial return to flexion, partial opening of hand
Amniotic fluid volume	One or more pockets of fluid that are 2 cm or more in the vertical axis	No pockets of fluid or no pocket measuring at least 2 cm in the vertical axis

A contraction stress test (CST, or oxytocin challenge test) may be requested in the event of an abnormal fetal heart rate in the BPP or NST. The CST is used to assess the fetus's ability to tolerate low oxygen levels as experienced during labor contractions. The CST includes external FHR monitoring by US and measurement of oxytocin (Pitocin)-induced uterine contractions. Pressure changes during contractions are monitored on an external tocodynamometer. Results of the two tests are interpreted as negative or positive. A negative or normal finding is no late decelerations of FHR during three induced contractions over a 10-min period.

A positive or abnormal finding is identified when frequent contractions of 90 sec or more occur and FHR decelerates beyond the time of the contractions. The amniotic fluid index is another application of US used to estimate amniotic fluid volume. The abdomen is divided into four quadrants using the umbilicus to delineate upper and lower halves and linea nigra to delineate the left and right halves. The numbered score is determined by adding the sum in centimeters of fluid in pockets seen in each of the four quadrants. The score is interpreted in relation to gestational age. The median index is considered normal between 8 and 12 cm. Oligohydramnios (too little amniotic fluid) is associated with an index between 5 and 6 cm, and polyhydramnios (too much amniotic fluid) with an index between 18 and 22 cm.

INDICATIONS

- Detect blighted ovum (missed abortion), as evidenced by empty gestational sac.
- Detect fetal death, as evidenced by absence of movement and fetal heart tones.
- Detect fetal position before birth, such as breech or transverse presentations.
- Detect tubal and other forms of ectopic pregnancy.
- Determine and confirm pregnancy or multiple gestation by determining the number of gestational sacs in the first trimester.
- Determine cause of bleeding, such as placenta previa or abruptio placentae.
- Determine fetal effects of Rh incompatibility due to maternal sensitization.

- Determine fetal gestational age by uterine size and measurements of crown-rump length, biparietal diameter, fetal extremities, head, and other parts of the anatomy at key phases of fetal development.
- Determine fetal heart and body movements and detect high-risk pregnancy by monitoring fetal heart and respiratory movements in combination with Doppler US or real-time grayscale scanning.
- Determine fetal structural anomalies, usually at the 20th week of gestation or later.
- Determine the placental size, location, and site of implantation.
- Differentiate a tumor (hydatidiform mole) from a normal pregnancy.
- Guide the needle during amniocentesis and fetal transfusion.
- Measure fetal gestational age and evaluate umbilical artery, uterine artery, and fetal aorta by Doppler examination to determine fetal intrauterine growth retardation.
- Monitor placental growth and amniotic fluid volume.

INTERFERING FACTORS
Factors that may alter the results of the study

- Attenuation of the sound waves by bony structures, which can impair clear imaging in the area of interest.
- Incorrect placement of the transducer over the desired test site; quality of the US study is very dependent on the skill of the ultrasonographer.
- Retained air, barium, or gas from a previous radiological procedure may block the transmission of sound waves.
- Dehydration, which can cause failure to demonstrate the boundaries between organs and tissue structures.
- Insufficiently full bladder, which fails to push the bowel from the

U

pelvis and the uterus from the symphysis pubis, thereby prohibiting clear imaging of the pelvic organs in transabdominal imaging.

- Patients who are technically difficult and who present challenges in obtaining reliable results (e.g., who are obese; have reduced rib spaces; present with fatty liver; have postoperative incisions, bandages, or dressings; have significant scarring in the area of interest). Aberrations in tissue composition may attenuate the sound waves and alter findings.

- Metallic objects (e.g., jewelry, body rings) within the examination field, which may inhibit organ visualization and cause unclear images.

- Inability of the patient to cooperate or remain still during the procedure, because movement can produce blurred or otherwise unclear images.

Other considerations

- Patients with latex allergy; use of the vaginal probe requires the probe to be covered with a condom-like sac, usually made from latex. Latex-free covers are available.

- Absence of activity in a particular parameter of the BPP may be related to fetal sleep pattern; gestational age less than 33 wk or greater than 42 wk; maternal ingestion of glucose, nicotine, or alcohol; maternal administration of magnesium or medications; artificial or premature rupture of membranes; and/or labor.

POTENTIAL MEDICAL DIAGNOSIS: CLINICAL SIGNIFICANCE OF RESULTS
Abnormal findings related to

- Abruptio placentae
- Cardiac abnormalities
- Ectopic pregnancy
- Fetal death
- Fetal deformities (organs or skeleton)

- Fetal hydrops (nonimmune)
- Fetal intestinal atresia
- Fetal malpresentation (breech, transverse)
- Hydrocephalus
- Myelomeningocele
- Multiple pregnancy
- Placenta previa
- Renal or skeletal defects
- BPP score between 4 and 6 is considered equivocal. Gestational age is important in determining intervals for retesting and/or a decision to deliver.

NURSING IMPLICATIONS

BEFORE THE STUDY: PLANNING AND IMPLEMENTATION

Teaching the Patient What to Expect

▶ Inform the patient this procedure can assess fetal health.

▶ Review the procedure with the patient. Address concerns about pain related to the procedure and explain that there may be moments of discomfort.

▶ Explain that the procedure is performed in a US department, usually by an HCP specializing in this procedure, and takes approximately 30 to 60 min.

▶ Advise the patient having a transvaginal approach that a sterile latex- or sheath-covered probe will be inserted into the vagina. Patients receiving transvaginal US only do not need to have a full bladder.

▶ Advise the patient having a transabdominal US to drink three to four glasses of fluid 90 min before the procedure, and not to void, because the procedure requires a full bladder.

▶ Explain that the patient will be asked to remove jewelry and other metallic objects from the area to be examined prior to the procedure.

▶ Positioning for this procedure is in the supine position on an examination table. The right- or left-side-up position may be used to allow gravity to reposition the liver, gas, and fluid to facilitate better organ visualization.

U

▶ Explain to the patient that she will be draped with the abdominal area exposed for the procedure.

▶ *Transabdominal Approach:* Conductive gel is applied to the skin, and a transducer is moved over the skin while the bladder is distended to obtain images of the area of interest.

▶ *Transvaginal Approach:* A lubricated, covered probe is inserted into the vagina and moved to different levels to obtain images.

▶ Advise the patient that she will be asked to breathe normally during the examination. If necessary for better organ visualization, she will be asked to inhale deeply and hold her breath.

▶ Once the study is completed, the gel is removed from the skin.

Potential Nursing Actions
▶ Record the date of the last menstrual period.
▶ Obtain a history of menstrual dates, previous pregnancy, and treatment received for high-risk pregnancy.

AFTER THE STUDY: POTENTIAL NURSING ACTIONS

Treatment Considerations
▶ Provide education related to the clinical implications of the test results.

▶ Provide a nonjudgmental, nonthreatening atmosphere for discussing the risks and difficulties of delivering and raising a developmentally challenged infant and for exploring other options (termination of pregnancy or adoption).

▶ Decisions regarding elective abortion should take place in the presence of both parents.

▶ Discuss problems the mother and father may experience (guilt, depression, anger) if fetal abnormalities are detected.

▶ Explain that there are numerous tests for fetal genetic testing associated with inherited diseases and congenital abnormalities. The tests can be performed from amniotic fluid by methods that include polymerase chain reaction, microarray, and cell culture with karyotyping comparison.

Follow-Up, Evaluation, and Desired Outcomes
▶ Acknowledges the importance of seeking counseling if concerned with pregnancy termination and of seeking genetic counseling if a chromosomal abnormality is determined.
▶ Understands that depending on the results of this procedure, additional testing may be performed.

Ultrasound Studies, Various Sites
(Abdomen, Bladder, Breast, Pelvis, Prostate, Scrotum, Thyroid and Parathyroid Glands)

SYNONYM/ACRONYM: Sonography, ultrasound.

RATIONALE: To visualize and assess solid organs of the abdominal area (including the aorta, bile ducts, bladder, gallbladder, kidneys, liver, pancreas, spleen, and other large abdominal blood vessels), breast, pelvis, prostate, scrotum, thyroid and parathyroid glands. Ultrasound (US) can be used to provide guidance in the performance of biopsies and assist in diagnosing disorders such as aneurysm, cancer, infections, fluid collections, masses, and obstructions. US can also be used to evaluate therapeutic interventions such as organ transplants.

PATIENT PREPARATION: There are no food, fluid, activity, or medication restrictions unless by medical direction for US bladder, breast, kidneys, pelvis, prostate,

U

scrotal, thyroid and parathyroid glands. Note any recent procedures that can interfere with abdominal US test results (e.g., surgery, biopsy, barium studies, colonoscopy, endoscopic retrograde cholangiopancreatography). Ensure that interfering studies were performed at least 24 hr before this test or can be rescheduled after this procedure.

- US Abdomen, Liver and Biliary System, Pancreas, Spleen: Instruct the patient to fast and restrict fluids for 8 hr prior to the procedure; instruct the caregiver of a pediatric patient to have the patient fast and restrict fluids for 8 hr prior to the procedure or as ordered. Patients may be asked to eat a low- or fat-free diet the night before the procedure. Food restrictions help ensure reduction of bowel gas, which can interfere with the transmission of US waves. Protocols may vary among facilities.
- US Bladder: If required, instruct the patient receiving transabdominal US bladder/pelvis to drink three to four glasses of fluid 90 min before the procedure, and not to void, because the procedure requires a full bladder.
- US Breast: Instruct the patient not to apply lotions, deodorant, bath powder, or other substances to the chest and breast area before the examination.
- US Prostate: Inform the patient that a small-volume enema will be administered prior to the procedure to help remove gas or feces that could interfere with the rectal probe; after the enema, a sterile latex- or sheath-covered probe will be inserted into the rectum.

NORMAL FINDINGS
- Normal anatomic structures, size, position, and shape; includes associated structures and blood flow/rate.
- No evidence of congenital anomalies, cysts, nodules, or tumors.
- Normal subcutaneous, mammary, and retromammary layers of tissue in both breasts; no evidence of pathological lesions (cyst or tumor) in either breast.
- Absence of renal calculi, cysts, hydronephrosis, obstruction, or tumor.
- Normal patency of the cystic and common bile ducts.
- Uniform echo patterns throughout the thyroid and parathyroid glands.

CRITICAL FINDINGS AND POTENTIAL INTERVENTIONS
- Abscess
- Adnexal torsion
- Aortic aneurysm measuring 5 cm or more in diameter
- Appendicitis
- Infection
- Testicular torsion
- Tumor with significant mass effect

Timely notification to the requesting health-care provider (HCP) of any critical findings and related symptoms is a role expectation of the professional nurse. A listing of these findings varies among facilities.

OVERVIEW: (Study type: Ultrasound; related body system: Digestive, Endocrine, Reproductive, and Urinary systems.) US procedures are diagnostic, noninvasive, and relatively inexpensive. They take a short time to complete, do not use radiation, and cause no harm to the patient. High-frequency sound waves of various intensities are delivered by a transducer, a flashlight-shaped

U

device, pressed against the skin. The waves are bounced back off internal anatomical structures and fluids, converted to electrical energy, amplified by the transducer, and displayed as images on a monitor. US is often used as a diagnostic and therapeutic tool for guiding minimally invasive procedures such as needle biopsies and fluid aspiration (paracentesis). The contraindications and complications for biopsy and fluid aspiration are discussed in detail in the individual related studies.

Different types of transducers and imaging systems are sometimes used in clinical settings. Conventional US systems assume that sound waves pass through tissue at a constant speed. Advances in technology have led to the development of "smart" transducers that can compensate for tissue aberrations in technically difficult patients. Other advancements in imaging systems include three-dimensional and Doppler US. Color Doppler US uses color to indicate the velocity and direction of blood flow. Power Doppler is a more sensitive Doppler variation, capable of providing detailed images of blood flow; a limitation of power Doppler is that it cannot provide information regarding the direction of blood flow. Spectral Doppler provides data from blood flow measurements in formats other than color—for example, it can convert the measurements into a graph representing distance of blood flow against time or as a unique sound heard with every heartbeat.

Abdominal Area
Abdominal US is valuable in determining aortic aneurysms, determining the internal components of organ masses (solid versus cystic), and evaluating other abdominal diseases, ascites, and abdominal obstruction. Abdominal US can be performed on the same day as a radionuclide scan or other radiological procedure and is especially valuable in patients who have hypersensitivity to contrast medium or are pregnant. US is also widely used for pediatric patients to help diagnose appendicitis and for infants to assign cause for recurrent vomiting.

To visualize and assess the solid organs of the abdomen, including the aorta, bile ducts, gallbladder, kidneys, pancreas, spleen, and other large abdominal blood vessels. This study is used to perform biopsies and assist in diagnosing disorders such as aortic aneurysm, infections, fluid collections, masses, and obstructions. This procedure can also be used to evaluate therapeutic interventions such as organ transplants.

Bladder
To visualize and assess the bladder toward diagnosing disorders such as retention, obstruction, distention, cancer, infection, bleeding, and inflammation.

Bladder US evaluates the structure and position of the contents of the bladder and identifies disorders of the bladder, such as masses or lesions. The methods for imaging may include the transrectal, transurethral, and transvaginal approaches. The examination is helpful for monitoring a patient's response to therapy for bladder disease. Bladder images can be included in other US studies such as the kidneys, ureters, bladder, urethra, and gonads in diagnosing renal/neurological disorders.

U

The bladder scan is another noninvasive US study commonly used to assess postvoid residual. Advantages of the bladder scan over other studies, such as cystometry, is that the study can be performed at the bedside and does not require the patient to be catheterized, thereby eliminating the possibility of the patient developing a catheter-related urinary tract infection (UTI). The patient's gynecological history should be obtained prior to using the scanner in order to select the proper setting. The scanners have settings for male, female, and child, but scanning a female patient who has had a hysterectomy and is without a uterus should be performed using the settings for a male patient. This test is not usually performed on pregnant women. Normal findings are less than 30 to 50 mL.

Breasts

When used in conjunction with mammography and clinical examination, breast US is indispensable in the diagnosis and management of benign and malignant processes. Both breasts are usually examined during this procedure. Images displayed on a monitor can determine the presence of palpable and nonpalpable masses; size and structure of the mass can also be evaluated. This procedure is useful in patients with an abnormal mass on a mammogram, because it can determine whether the abnormality is cystic or solid; that is, it can differentiate between a palpable, fluid-filled cyst and a palpable, solid breast lesion (benign or malignant). It is especially useful in patients with dense breast tissue and in those with silicone prostheses, because

the US beam easily penetrates in these situations, allowing routine examination that cannot be performed with x-ray mammography. The procedure can be done as an adjunct to mammography, or it can be done in place of mammography in patients who refuse x-ray exposure or in whom it is contraindicated (e.g., pregnant women, women less than 25 yr *related to increased breast tissue density that produces unclear images*).

Knowledge of genetics assists in identifying those who may benefit from additional education, risk assessment, and counseling. Genetics is the study and identification of genes, genetic mutations, and inheritance. For example, genetics provides some insight into the likelihood of inheriting a condition associated with a type of cancer such as breast cancer. Genomic studies evaluate the interaction of groups of genes. The combined activity or combined expression of groups of genes allows assumptions or predictions to be made. As an example, genomic studies measure the levels of activity in multiple genes to predict how they influence the development and growth of a tumor. Further information regarding inheritance of genes can be found in the study titled "Genetic Testing."

Kidneys

Renal US is used to evaluate the structure, size, and position of the kidneys and to identify renal system disorders. It is valuable for determining the internal components of renal masses (solid versus cystic) and for evaluating other renal diseases, renal parenchyma, perirenal tissues, and obstruction. Renal US can be performed on the same day as a radionuclide scan or other radiological procedure and is especially valuable in patients who are in acute kidney injury, chronic kidney disease, or end-stage renal disease; have hypersensitivity to contrast medium; have a kidney that did not visualize on intravenous pyelography (IVP); or are pregnant. It does not rely on renal function or the injection of contrast medium to obtain a diagnosis. The procedure is indicated for evaluation after a kidney transplant and is used as a guide for biopsy and other interventional procedures, abscess drainage, and nephrostomy tube placement. Renal US may be the diagnostic examination of choice because no radiation is used and, in most cases, the accuracy is sufficient to make the diagnosis without further imaging procedures.

Liver

Hepatobiliary US is used to evaluate the structure, size, and position of the liver and gallbladder in the right upper quadrant (RUQ) of the abdomen. The biliary tract, which includes the liver, gallbladder and bile ducts, collects, stores, concentrates, and transports bile to the intestines to aid in digestion. This procedure allows visualization of the gallbladder and bile ducts when the patient may have impaired liver function, and it is especially helpful when done on patients in whom gallstones cannot be visualized with oral or IV radiological studies. Liver US can be done in combination with a nuclear scan to obtain information about liver function and density differences in the liver.

Pancreas

Pancreatic US is used to determine the size, shape, and position of the pancreas; determine the presence of masses or other abnormalities of the pancreas; and examine the surrounding viscera. Pancreatic US is usually done in combination with computed tomography (CT) or magnetic resonance imaging (MRI) of the pancreas.

Pelvis

Gynecologic US is used to determine the presence, size, and structure of masses and cysts and determine the position of an intrauterine contraceptive device (IUD); evaluate postmenopausal bleeding; and examine other abnormalities of the uterus, ovaries, fallopian tubes, and vagina. This procedure can also be useful in evaluating ovulation and fallopian tube function related to fertility issues. This procedure is done by a transabdominal or transvaginal approach. The transabdominal approach provides a view of the pelvic organs posterior to the bladder. It requires a full bladder, thereby allowing a window for transmission of the US waves, pushing the uterus away from the pubic symphysis, pushing the bowel out of the pelvis, and acting as a reference for comparison in the evaluation of the internal structures of a mass or cyst being examined. The transvaginal approach focuses on the female reproductive organs and is often used to monitor ovulation over a period of days in patients undergoing fertility assessment. This approach is also used in patients who are obese or in patients with retroversion of the uterus because the sound waves are better able to reach the organ from the vaginal site. Transvaginal images are significantly more accurate compared to anterior transabdominal images in identifying paracervical, endometrial, and ovarian pathology, and the transvaginal approach does not require a full bladder.

Prostate

Prostate US is used to evaluate the structure, size, and position of the contents of the prostate (e.g., masses). This procedure can evaluate abnormal pathology in prostate tissue, the seminal vesicles, and surrounding perirectal tissue. Prostate US aids in the diagnosis of prostatic cancer by evaluating palpable nodules as a complement to a digital rectal examination (DRE) or in response to an elevated prostrate-specific antigen (PSA) level. The DRE is a simple procedure used to examine, by palpation, the lower rectum and prostate gland. It is performed by the health-care provider (HCP), who inserts a lubricated, gloved finger into the rectum while the patient is properly positioned. Prostate US can also be used to stage cancer and to assist in radiation seed placement. Micturition disorders can also be evaluated by this procedure. The examination is helpful in monitoring patient response to therapy for prostatic disease.

Scrotum

Scrotal US is used to evaluate the structure, size, and position of the contents of the scrotum and for the evaluation of disorders of the scrotum. It is valuable in determining the internal components of masses (solid versus cystic) and for the evaluation of the testicle, extratesticular and intrascrotal tissues, benign and malignant tumors, and other scrotal pathology. Scrotal US can be performed

before or after a radionuclide scan for further clarification of a testicular mass. Extratesticular lesions such as hydrocele, hematocele (blood in the scrotum), and pyocele (pus in the scrotum) can be identified, as can cryptorchidism (undescended testicles).

Spleen

Spleen US is used to evaluate the structure, size, and position of the spleen. This test is valuable for determining the internal components of splenic masses (solid versus cystic) and evaluating other splenic pathology, splenic trauma, and left upper quadrant perisplenic tissues. It can be performed to supplement a radionuclide scan or CT. It is especially valuable in patients who have chronic kidney disease or an acute kidney injury, are hypersensitive to contrast medium, or are pregnant, because it does not rely on adequate kidney function or the injection of contrast medium to obtain a diagnosis.

Thyroid and Parathyroid Glands

Thyroid and parathyroid US is used to determine the position, size, shape, weight, and presence of masses of the thyroid gland; enlargement of the parathyroid glands; and other abnormalities of the thyroid and parathyroid glands and surrounding tissues. The primary purpose of this procedure is to determine whether a nodule is a fluid-filled cyst (usually benign) or a solid tumor (possibly malignant). This procedure is useful in evaluating the glands' response to medical treatment or assessing the remaining tissue after surgical resection. US is clearly the procedure of choice when examining the glands of pregnant patients. This procedure is usually done in combination with nuclear

U

medicine imaging procedures and CT of the neck. Despite the advantages of the procedure, in some cases it may not detect small nodules and lesions (less than 1 cm), leading to false-negative findings.

INDICATIONS

Abdominal Area

- Determine the patency and function of abdominal blood vessels, including the abdominal aorta; vena cava; and portal, splenic, renal, and superior and inferior mesenteric veins.
- Detect and measure an abdominal aortic aneurysm.
- Monitor abdominal aortic aneurysm expansion to prevent rupture.
- Determine changes within small aortic aneurysms pre- and postsurgery.
- Evaluate abdominal ascites.
- Evaluate size, shape, and pathology of intra-abdominal organs.

Bladder

- Assess residual urine after voiding to diagnose urinary tract obstruction causing overdistention.
- Detect tumor of the bladder wall or pelvis, as evidenced by distorted position or changes in bladder contour.
- Determine end-stage malignancy of the bladder caused by extension of a primary tumor of the ovary or other pelvic organ.
- Evaluate the cause of UTI, urine retention, and flank pain.
- Evaluate hematuria, urinary frequency, dysuria, and suprapubic pain.
- Measure urinary bladder volume by transurethral or transvaginal approach.

Breasts

- Detect tiny tumors in combination with mammography for diagnostic validation.

- Determine the presence of nonpalpable abnormalities viewed on mammography of dense breast tissue and monitor changes in these abnormalities.
- Differentiate among types of breast masses (e.g., cyst, solid tumor, other lesions) in dense breast tissue.
- Evaluate palpable masses in young (less than age 25), pregnant, and lactating patients.
- Guide interventional procedures such as cyst aspiration, large-needle core biopsy, fine-needle aspiration biopsy, abscess drainage, presurgical localization, and galactography.
- Identify an abscess in a patient with mastitis.

Kidneys

- Aid in the diagnosis of the effect (e.g., decrease in size) of chronic glomerulonephritis or chronic kidney disease on the kidneys.
- Detect an accumulation of fluid in the kidney caused by backflow of urine, hemorrhage, or perirenal fluid.
- Detect masses and differentiate between cysts or solid tumors, *as evidenced by specific waveform patterns or absence of sound waves.*
- Determine the presence and location of renal or ureteral calculi and obstruction.
- Determine the size, shape, and position of a nonfunctioning kidney to identify the cause.
- Evaluate or plan therapy for renal tumors.
- Evaluate renal transplantation for changes in kidney size.
- Locate the site of and guide percutaneous renal biopsy, aspiration needle insertion, or nephrostomy tube insertion.
- Monitor kidney development in children when renal disease has been diagnosed.
- Provide the location and size of renal masses in patients who are

U

unable to undergo IVP because of poor renal function or an allergy to iodinated contrast medium.

Liver and Biliary System

- Detect cysts, polyps, hematoma, abscesses, hemangioma, adenoma, metastatic disease, hepatitis, or solid tumor of the liver or gallbladder, *as evidenced by echoes specific to tissue density and sharply or poorly defined masses.*
- Detect gallstones or inflammation when oral cholecystography is inconclusive.
- Detect hepatic lesions, as evidenced by density differences and echo-pattern changes.
- Determine the cause of unexplained hepatomegaly and abnormal liver function tests.
- Determine cause of unexplained RUQ pain.
- Determine patency and diameter of the hepatic duct for dilation or obstruction.
- Differentiate between obstructive and nonobstructive jaundice by determining the cause.
- Evaluate response to therapy for tumor, *as evidenced by a decrease in size of the organ.*
- Guide biopsy or tube placement.
- Guide catheter placement into the gallbladder for stone dissolution and gallbladder fragmentation.

Pancreas

- Detect anatomic abnormalities as a consequence of pancreatitis.
- Detect pancreatic cancer, *as evidenced by a poorly defined mass or a mass in the head of the pancreas that obstructs the pancreatic duct.*
- Detect pancreatitis, *as evidenced by pancreatic enlargement with increased echoes.*
- Detect pseudocysts, *as evidenced by a well-defined mass with absence of echoes from the interior.*

- Monitor therapeutic response to tumor treatment.
- Provide guidance for percutaneous aspiration and fine-needle biopsy of the pancreas.

Pelvis

- Detect and monitor the treatment of pelvic inflammatory disease (PID) when done in combination with other laboratory tests.
- Detect bleeding into the pelvis resulting from trauma to the area or ascites associated with tumor metastasis.
- Detect masses in the pelvis and differentiate them from cysts or solid tumors, *as evidenced by differences in sound-wave patterns.*
- Detect pelvic abscess or peritonitis caused by a ruptured appendix or diverticulitis.
- Detect the presence of ovarian cysts and malignancy and determine the type, if possible, *as evidenced by size, outline, and change in position of other pelvic organs.*
- Evaluate the effectiveness of tumor therapy, *as evidenced by a reduction in mass size.*
- Evaluate suspected fibroid tumor or bladder tumor.
- Evaluate the thickness of the uterine wall.
- Monitor placement and location of an IUD.
- Monitor follicular size associated with fertility studies or to remove follicles for in vitro transplantation.

Prostate

- Aid in the diagnosis of micturition disorders.
- Aid in prostate cancer diagnosis.
- Assess prostatic calcifications.
- Assist in guided needle biopsy of a suspected tumor.
- Assist in radiation seed placement.
- Determine prostatic cancer staging.
- Detect prostatitis.

U

Scrotum
- Aid in the diagnosis of a chronic inflammatory condition such as epididymitis.
- Aid in the diagnosis of a mass and differentiate between a cyst and a solid tumor, *as evidenced by specific waveform patterns or the absence of sound waves respectively.*
- Aid in the diagnosis of scrotal or testicular size, abnormality, or pathology.
- Aid in the diagnosis of testicular torsion and associated testicular infarction.
- Assist guided needle biopsy of a suspected testicle tumor.
- Determine the cause of chronic scrotal swelling or pain.
- Determine the presence of a hydrocele, pyocele, spermatocele, or hernia before surgery.
- Evaluate the effectiveness of treatment for testicular infections.
- Locate an undescended testicle.

Spleen
- Detect the presence of a subphrenic abscess after splenectomy.
- Detect splenic masses; differentiate between cysts or solid tumors (in combination with CT), *as evidenced by specific waveform patterns or absence of sound waves respectively,* and determine whether they are intrasplenic or extrasplenic.
- Determine late-stage sickle cell disease, *as evidenced by decreased spleen size and presence of echoes.*
- Determine the presence of splenomegaly and assess the size and volume of the spleen in these cases, *as evidenced by increased echoes and visibility of the spleen.*
- Differentiate spleen trauma from blood or fluid accumulation between the splenic capsule and parenchyma.
- Evaluate the effect of medical or surgical therapy on the progression or resolution of splenic disease.

- Evaluate the extent of abdominal trauma and spleen involvement, including enlargement or rupture, after a recent trauma.
- Evaluate the spleen before splenectomy performed for thrombocytopenic purpura.

Thyroid and Parathyroid Glands
- Assist in determining the presence of a tumor, *as evidenced by an irregular border and shadowing at the distal edge, peripheral echoes, or high- and low-amplitude echoes, depending on the density of the tumor mass,* and diagnosing tumor type (e.g., benign, adenoma, cancer).
- Assist in diagnosing the presence of a cyst, *as evidenced by a smoothly outlined, echo-free amplitude except at the far borders of the mass.*
- Assist in diagnosis in the presence of a parathyroid enlargement indicating a tumor or hyperplasia, *as evidenced by an echo pattern of lower amplitude than that for a thyroid tumor.*
- Determine the need for surgical biopsy of a tumor or fine-needle biopsy of a cyst.
- Differentiate among a nodule, solid tumor, or fluid-filled cyst.
- Evaluate the effect of a therapeutic regimen for a thyroid mass or Graves disease by determining the size and weight of the gland.
- Evaluate thyroid abnormalities during pregnancy (mother or baby).

INTERFERING FACTORS
Contraindications

 The contraindications and complications for biopsy and fluid aspiration are discussed in detail in the individual related biopsy and body fluid analysis studies.

Factors that may alter the results of the study
- Attenuation of the sound waves by bony structures, which can impair

clear imaging of the upper abdominal structures.

- Incorrect placement of the transducer over the desired test site; quality of the US study is very dependent on the skill of the ultrasonographer.
- Retained air, barium, or gas from a previous radiological procedure may block the transmission of sound waves.
- Gas or feces in the gastrointestinal (GI) tract resulting from inadequate cleansing or failure to restrict food intake before the study.
- Metallic objects (e.g., jewelry, body rings) within the examination field, which may inhibit organ visualization and cause unclear images.
- Patients who are technically difficult and who present challenges in obtaining reliable results (e.g., who are obese; have reduced rib spaces; present with fatty liver; have postoperative incisions, bandages, or dressings; have significant scarring in the area of interest). Aberrations in tissue composition may attenuate the sound waves and alter findings.

POTENTIAL MEDICAL DIAGNOSIS: CLINICAL SIGNIFICANCE OF RESULTS
Abnormal findings related to

General

Identification of abnormal findings is assisted by comparison of parameters such as size, shape, symmetry, and location; for example, areas of altered echo patterns in either an expected or unexpected location may indicate enlargement of an organ or the presence of blood or other fluids, tumors, or cysts. Comparison by type of abnormal findings may also assist in evaluating areas of altered patterns; for example, small round or oval areas with well-defined borders and clear central areas can differentiate a fluid-filled cyst from a solid tumor.

- Abscess
- Calculi
- Cancer
- Congenital anomalies, such as absent, ectopic, duplicate, or malplacement of organs
- Cysts
- Hematoma
- Infarction
- Infection
- Obstructions
- Tumor (benign or malignant)

Abdominal Area
- Ascitic fluid
- Aortic aneurysm greater than 4 cm

Bladder
- Bladder diverticulum
- Cystitis
- Ureterocele

Breasts
- Fibroadenoma
- Focal fibrosis
- Galactocele
- Hamartoma (fibroadenolipoma)
- Papilloma
- Phyllodes tumor
- Radial scar

Kidneys
- Acute glomerulonephritis
- Acute pyelonephritis
- Chronic kidney disease
- Hydronephrosis
- Polycystic kidney
- Rejection of kidney transplant
- Ureteral obstruction

Liver and Biliary System
- Cirrhosis
- Hepatocellular disease, adenoma
- Hepatomegaly

Pancreas
- Acute pancreatitis
- Pseudocysts

Pelvis
- Adnexal torsion
- Appendicitis
- Endometrioma

- Fibroids (leiomyoma)
- Peritonitis
- PID

Prostate
- Benign prostatic hyperplasia
- Micturition disorders
- Prostatitis

Scrotum
- Epididymal cyst
- Epididymitis
- Hydrocele
- Microlithiasis
- Orchitis
- Pyocele
- Scrotal hernia
- Spermatocele
- Testicular torsion

- Tunica albuginea cyst
- Undescended testicle (cryptorchidism)
- Varicocele

Spleen
- Accessory or ectopic spleen
- Lymphatic disease; lymph node enlargement
- Splenic calcifications
- Splenic trauma
- Splenomegaly

Thyroid and Parathyroid Glands
- Glandular enlargement
- Goiter
- Graves disease
- Parathyroid hyperplasia

NURSING IMPLICATIONS

POTENTIAL NURSING PROBLEMS: ASSESSMENT & NURSING DIAGNOSIS

Problems	Signs and Symptoms
Bladder, Kidney: Pain *(related to spasm, obstruction, infection, cyst, tumor, inflammation)*	Self-report of bladder pain, report of bladder spasms, moaning, crying, restlessness, anxiety, increased heart rate, increased blood pressure
Bladder, Kidney: Infection *(related to obstruction, cyst, inflammation, tumor)*	Positive culture, fever, chills, elevated temperature, elevated WBC, flank pain, hematuria, urinary frequency
Bladder, Kidney: Insufficient fluid volume (water) *(related to nausea, vomiting, pain)*	Elevated heart rate; low blood pressure; cool, clammy skin; poor urine output (less than 30 mL/hr); confusion; restlessness; agitation; capillary refill delay; hemoconcentration; dehydration
Breast: Body image *(related to self-deprecation secondary to breast removal)*	Stated loss or fear of intimacy, stated dissatisfaction with appearance, refusal to view postoperative site, crying, anger, grief, anxiety
Breast: Sexuality *(related to loss of breast and perceived change in desirability)*	Stated loss or fear of loss of attractiveness, sexual intimacy, desirability; fear of rejection or repulsion by sexual partner; stated loss of sexual partner secondary to breast removal
Prostate, Scrotal: Body image *(related to self-deprecation secondary to testicular removal)*	Stated loss or fear of intimacy, stated dissatisfaction with appearance, refusal to view postoperative site, crying, anger, grief, anxiety

U

Problems	Signs and Symptoms
Prostate, Scrotal: Sexuality *(related to concerns regarding inability to perform, sexual limitations secondary to disease process)*	Verbalization of concerns, fear of impotence or occasional impotence, social isolation, fear of infertility, fear of loss of intimacy

BEFORE THE STUDY: PLANNING AND IMPLEMENTATION

Teaching the Patient What to Expect

General

▶ Inform the patient this procedure can assist in assessing the organ or site of interest.

▶ Review the procedure with the patient. Address concerns about pain. Explain that there may be moments of discomfort experienced during the test.

▶ Explain that the procedure is performed in an US department, by an HCP specializing in this procedure, with support staff, and takes approximately 30 to 60 min.

Pediatric Considerations: Preparing children for an abdominal US depends on the age of the child. Encourage parents to be truthful about what the child may experience during the procedure and to use words that they know their child will understand. Toddlers and preschool-age children have a short attention span, so the best time to talk about the test is right before the procedure. The child should be assured that he or she will be allowed to bring a favorite comfort item into the examination room and, if appropriate, that a parent will be with the child during the procedure. Provide older children with information about the test, and allow them to participate in as many decisions as possible (e.g., choice of clothes to wear to the appointment) in order to reduce anxiety and encourage cooperation. If the child will be asked to maintain a certain position for the test, encourage the child to practice the required position, provide a CD that demonstrates the procedure, and teach strategies to

remain calm, such as deep breathing, humming, or counting to himself or herself.

▶ Advise the patient that he or she will be asked to remove jewelry and other metallic objects in the area to be examined.

▶ Positioning for an ultrasound of the abdominal area, bladder, breast, kidneys, liver and biliary system, pancreas, pelvis, or spleen is in the supine position on an examination table.

▶ Explain that the right- or left-side-up positions may be used to allow gravity to facilitate better organ visualization and in some studies to reposition the organ of interest or to displace gas and fluid.

Bladder

▶ Instruct the patient who is to be examined for residual urine volume to empty the bladder; repeat the procedure and calculate the volume.

Pelvis

▶ Instruct the female patient that a latex or sterile sheath-covered probe will be inserted into the vagina for the transvaginal approach.

▶ **Transvaginal Approach:** Patients receiving transvaginal US only do not need to have a full bladder. Explain that a covered and lubricated probe will be inserted into the vagina and moved to different levels. Images will be obtained and recorded.

Prostate

▶ Explain that positioning for this procedure is on an examination table, lying knee to chest on the left side. Other positions may be used during the examination.

▶ Explain to the patient that he will be draped with the rectal areas exposed for the procedure.

U

▶ The rectal probe will be covered with a lubricated condom and inserted into the rectum.

▶ Explain that there may be a feeling of slight pressure as the transducer is inserted.

▶ Water may be introduced through the sheath surrounding the transducer.

Scrotal

▶ Explain to the patient that he will be draped with the abdomen/pelvic area exposed for the procedure.

▶ Once the patient is draped and area exposed, penis will be lifted and gently taped to the lower part of the abdomen. The scrotum will be elevated with rolled towel or sponge for immobilization.

Thyroid and Parathyroid Glands

▶ Explain that positioning for this procedure is in the supine position on an examination table. However, other positions may be used during the examination.

▶ Explain that the neck will be hyperextended with a pillow placed under the shoulders to maintain a comfortable position. (An alternative method of imaging includes the use of a bag filled with water or gel placed over the neck area.)

General

▶ Explain to the patient that he or she will be draped and the area of interest will be exposed.

▶ A conductive gel is applied to the skin, and a Doppler transducer is moved over the skin to obtain images of the area of interest.

▶ Explain that it is important to breathe normally during the examination. However, it may be necessary to inhale deeply and hold the breath for better organ visualization.

▶ Once the study is completed, the gel is removed from the skin.

Potential Nursing Actions

▶ US Pelvis and and Prostate: Ensure the use of equipment containing latex is avoided if the patient has a history of allergic reaction to latex.

AFTER THE STUDY: POTENTIAL NURSING ACTIONS

Treatment Considerations

General

▶ Do not allow the patient to eat or drink until the gag reflex returns due to aspiration risk.

▶ Anxiety is a normal human reaction to a situation that may have unknown life-changing results. Review strategies that can be used to manage anxiety. Some of these are imagery, music, and relaxation techniques. Provide detailed explanations related to the purpose of all diagnostic studies in clear, age-appropriate, and culturally appropriate terms.

▶ Both grief over probable diagnosis and concerns related to possible death are human responses to poor diagnostic results and prognosis. Consider facilitating the support of a spiritual advisor and the cultural aspects of grieving in planning care. Ensure clear easy-to-understand information related to disease and treatment options.

▶ Lack of knowledge related to a new diagnosis is a normal human response. Assess for clear understanding of information provided that is related to disease process and treatment options. Ensure the use of language that is age, culture, and literacy-appropriate. Move from simple to complex concepts when teaching and consider the learning style of those involved (patient, family, significant others) when selecting teaching methods.

▶ Adequate nutrition can become a challenge when faced with physical and emotional events such as anxiety, pain, and grief. Complete a culturally appropriate nutritional assessment and institute evaluative assessments such as a daily weight and intake and output. Administer ordered IV fluids with supplements such as electrolytes. Depending on the disease process, it may be necessary to keep the patient NPO, as ordered, with nasogastric tube to low suction. Monitor and trend specific laboratory studies: lipase, amylase, albumin, total protein, electrolytes, glucose, calcium, iron, and folic acid.

U

Facilitate a dietary consult and administer ordered dietary supplements.

Bladder, Kidney

▶ *Infection:* Monitor and trend laboratory studies: BUN, Cr, WBC, Hgb, Hct, electrolytes; and urine cultures. Monitor for results of complementary diagnostic studies: KUB, CT, MRI, and IVP. Administer ordered antibiotics, increase oral fluid intake, administer ordered parenteral fluids, and monitor and trend temperature.

▶ *Pain:* Assess pain character, location, duration, and intensity. Use an easily understood pain rating scale. Administer ordered pain medications and consider alternative measures for pain management: imagery, relaxation, music. Encourage oral fluids if not contraindicated and administer ordered parenteral fluids. Monitor voiding patterns (urgency, frequency, incontinence) and for the presence of hematuria. Strain urine, monitor and trend laboratory and diagnostic studies (BUN, Cr, electrolytes, WBC count, KUB, IVP).

▶ *Fluid Deficit:* Assess skin turgor and perform a daily weight. Monitor and trend laboratory studies: BUN, Cr, Hgb, Hct, and electrolytes. Monitor and trend blood pressure, heart rate, temperature, and assess capillary refill. Administer ordered parenteral fluids and encourage oral fluids. Institute strict intake and output and monitor for fluid overload. When stones are present, encourage the intake of milk and milk products while discouraging intake of beer, chocolate, tea, and tomatoes.

Breast

▶ *Body Image:* Provide assurance that feelings of distress related to body image changes are normal. Facilitate the grieving process for the lost breast; consider the cultural aspects of body image and incorporate them into the plan of care. Ensure privacy to explore personal grief. Listen. Support positive coping strategies and encourage viewing surgical site, as sometimes the imagined is worse than the real.

▶ *Sexuality:* Allow for verbalization of concerns related to a changed sense of attractiveness and desirability associated with breast removal. Encourage open communication with sexual partner and provide information on prosthetic appliances and reconstruction. Provide emotional support and assure the patient that these fears are normal.

Prostate, Scrotal

▶ *Body Image:* Facilitate the grieving process for the lost scrotum and assure the patient that feelings of distress are normal. Incorporate the cultural aspects of loss into the plan of care. Ensure privacy to explore personal grief.

▶ *Sexuality:* Assess feeling about sexual performance and identify concerns regarding incontinence during sexual performance. Address concerns regarding deteriorating libido secondary to disease process. Facilitate consultation regarding fertility concerns and consider sperm banking.

▶ Instruct the patient to resume usual diet and fluids if previously restricted and as directed by the HCP.

Nutritional Considerations

▶ US Prostate: There is growing evidence that inflammation and oxidation play key roles in the development of numerous diseases, including prostate cancer. Research also indicates that diets containing dried beans, fresh fruits and vegetables, nuts, spices, whole grains, and smaller amounts of red meats can increase the amount of protective antioxidants. Regular exercise, especially in combination with a healthy diet, can bring about changes in the body's metabolism that decrease inflammation and oxidation.

Follow-Up, Evaluation, and Desired Outcomes

▶ Correctly states the pathophysiology related to the specific disease process.

▶ Understands that depending on the results of this procedure, additional testing may be performed to monitor disease progression and determine the need for a change in therapy.

▶ Those with body image changes agree to seek psychological counseling to address intimacy concerns.

U

- Those with kidney disease agree to avoid foods that facilitate stone formation (tea, beer, chocolate) when diagnosed with stones.
- Those with pancreatic disease recognize that the consumption of alcohol can exacerbate the pain due to pancreatic stimulation.

Breast Cancer
- Understands that decisions regarding the need for and frequency of breast self-examination, mammography, MRI or US of the breast, or other cancer screening procedures should be made after consultation between the patient and HCP. Acknowledges that the most current guidelines for breast cancer screening of the general population as well as of individuals with increased risk are available from the American Cancer Society (ACS) (www.cancer.org), the American College of Obstetricians and Gynecologists (www.acog.org), and the American College of Radiology (www.acr.org). Screening guidelines vary depending on the age and health history of those at average risk and those at high risk for breast cancer. Guidelines may not always agree between organizations; therefore, it is important for patients to participate in their health care, be informed, ask questions, and follow

their HCP's recommendations regarding frequency and type of screening. For additional information regarding screening guidelines, refer to the study titled "Mammography."
- *Pelvis:* Acknowledges contact information provided for the ACS (www.cancer.org).

Prostate Cancer
- Understands that decisions regarding the need for and frequency of routine PSA testing or other prostate cancer screening procedures should be made after consultation between the patient and HCP. Recommendations made by various medical associations and national health organizations regarding prostate cancer screening are moving away from routine PSA screening and toward informed decision making. The most current guidelines for prostate cancer screening of the general population as well as of individuals with increased risk are available from the ACS (www.cancer.org) and the American Urological Association (www.auanet.org). Counsel the patient, as appropriate, that sexual dysfunction related to altered body function, drugs, or radiation may occur. For additional information regarding screening guidelines, refer to the study titled "Prostate-Specific Antigen."

Ultrasound, Venous Doppler, Extremity Studies

SYNONYM/ACRONYM: Vascular ultrasound, venous duplex, venous sonogram, venous ultrasound.

RATIONALE: To assess venous blood flow in the upper and lower extremities toward diagnosing disorders such as deep vein thrombosis, venous insufficiency, causation of pulmonary embolism, varicose veins, and monitor the effects of therapeutic interventions.

PATIENT PREPARATION: There are no food or medication restrictions unless by medical direction. Some protocols may require the patient to restrict nicotine and caffeine for 1 to 2 hr before the procedure in order to avoid vasoconstriction or vasodilation. Ensure that interfering studies (e.g., surgery, biopsy, barium studies, colonoscopy, endoscopic retrograde cholangiopancreatography) were performed at least 24 hr before this test or can be rescheduled after this procedure.

NORMAL FINDINGS

• Normal Doppler venous signal that occurs spontaneously with the patient's respiration
• Normal blood flow through the veins of the extremities with no evidence of vessel occlusion.

CRITICAL FINDINGS AND POTENTIAL INTERVENTIONS

• DVT
• Pulmonary embolism (PE)

Timely notification to the requesting health-care provider (HCP) of any critical findings and related symptoms is a role expectation of the professional nurse. A listing of these findings varies among facilities.

OVERVIEW: (Study type: Ultrasound; **related body system:** Circulatory system.) Ultrasound (US) procedures are diagnostic, noninvasive, and relatively inexpensive. They take a short time to complete, do not use radiation, and cause no harm to the patient. High-frequency sound waves of various intensities are delivered by a transducer, a flashlight-shaped device, pressed against the skin. The waves are bounced back off internal anatomical structures and fluids, converted to electrical energy, amplified by the transducer, and displayed as images on a monitor. US is often used as a diagnostic and therapeutic tool for guiding minimally invasive procedures such as needle biopsies and fluid aspiration. The contraindications and complications for biopsy and fluid aspiration are discussed in detail in the individual studies.

US procedures are used to obtain information about the patency of the venous vasculature in the upper and lower extremities to identify narrowing or occlusions of the veins or arteries. In venous Doppler studies, the Doppler identifies moving red blood cells (RBCs) within the vein. The US beam is directed at the vein and through the Doppler transducer, and the RBCs reflect the beam back to the transducer. The reflected sound waves or echoes are transformed by a computer into scans, graphs, or audible sounds. Blood flow direction, velocity, and the presence of flow disturbances can be readily assessed. The velocity of the blood flow is transformed as a "swishing" noise, audible through the audio speaker. If the vein is occluded, no swishing sound is heard. For diagnostic studies, the procedure is done bilaterally. The sound emitted by the equipment corresponds to the velocity of the blood flow through the vessel occurring with spontaneous respirations. Changes in these sounds during respirations indicate the possibility of abnormal venous flow secondary to occlusive disease; the absence of sound indicates complete obstruction. Compression with a transducer augments a vessel for evaluation of thrombosis. Noncompressibility of the vessel indicates a thrombosis. Plethysmography may be performed to determine the filling

U

time of calf veins to diagnose thrombotic disorder of a major vein and to identify incompetent valves in the venous system. An additional method used to evaluate incompetent valves is the Valsalva technique combined with venous duplex imaging.

The ankle-brachial index (ABI) can also be assessed during this study. This noninvasive, simple comparison of blood pressure measurements in the arms and legs can be used to detect peripheral arterial disease (PAD). A Doppler stethoscope is used to obtain the systolic pressure in either the dorsalis pedis or the posterior tibial artery. This ankle pressure is then divided by the highest brachial systolic pressure acquired after taking the blood pressure in both of the patient's arms. This index should be greater than 1 with a range of 0.85 to 1.4. When the index falls below 0.5, blood flow impairment is considered significant. Patients should be scheduled for a vascular consult for an abnormal ABI. Patients with diabetes or kidney disease, and some older adult patients, may have a falsely elevated ABI due to calcifications of the vessels in the ankle causing an increased systolic pressure. The ABI test approaches 95% accuracy in detecting PAD. However, a normal ABI value does not absolutely rule out the possibility of PAD for some individuals, and additional tests should be done to evaluate symptoms.

INDICATIONS
- Aid in the diagnosis of venous occlusion secondary to thrombosis or thrombophlebitis.
- Aid in the diagnosis of superficial thrombosis or deep vein thrombosis (DVT) leading to venous occlusion or obstruction, as evidenced by absence of venous flow, especially upon augmentation of the extremity; variations in flow during respirations; or failure of the veins to compress completely when the extremity is compressed.
- Detect chronic venous insufficiency, as evidenced by reverse blood flow indicating incompetent valves.
- Determine if further diagnostic procedures are needed to make or confirm a diagnosis.
- Determine the source of emboli when PE is suspected or diagnosed.
- Determine venous damage after trauma to the site.
- Differentiate between primary and secondary varicose veins.
- Evaluate the patency of the venous system in patients with a swollen, painful leg.
- Evaluate peripheral vascular disease (PVD).
- Monitor the effectiveness of therapeutic interventions.

INTERFERING FACTORS
- Patients with an open or draining lesion.

Factors that may alter the results of the study
- Attenuation of the sound waves by bony structures, which can impair clear imaging of the vessels.
- Incorrect placement of the transducer over the desired test site; quality of the US study is very dependent on the skill of the ultrasonographer.
- Metallic objects (e.g., jewelry, body rings) within the examination field, which may inhibit organ visualization and cause unclear images.
- Patients who are technically difficult and who present challenges in obtaining reliable results (e.g., who

U

are obese; have reduced rib spaces; present with fatty liver; have post-operative incisions, bandages, or dressings; have significant scarring in the area of interest). Aberrations in tissue composition may attenuate the sound waves and alter findings.

Other considerations
- Cigarette smoking, because nicotine can cause constriction of the peripheral vessels.
- Cold extremities, resulting in vasoconstriction that can cause inaccurate measurements.
- Occlusion proximal to the site being studied, which would affect blood flow to the area.

- An abnormally large or swollen leg, making sonic penetration difficult.

POTENTIAL MEDICAL DIAGNOSIS: CLINICAL SIGNIFICANCE OF RESULTS

Abnormal findings related to
- Chronic venous insufficiency
- Primary varicose veins
- PE
- PVD
- Recannulization in the area of an old thrombus
- Secondary varicose veins
- Superficial thrombosis or DVT
- Venous narrowing or occlusion secondary to thrombosis or thrombophlebitis
- Venous trauma

NURSING IMPLICATIONS

POTENTIAL NURSING PROBLEMS: ASSESSMENT & NURSING DIAGNOSIS

Problems	Signs and Symptoms
Inadequate tissue perfusion *(related to obstruction, insufficiency, thrombus, stenosis, trauma)*	Pain, tenderness, warmth, edema, palpable vein, pedal pulse greater than 3 sec, cool extremities
Mobility *(related to pain, stenosis, obstruction, inflammation, insufficiency, thrombus, trauma)*	Inability to meet physical demands associated with activities of daily living, ineffective range of motion, pain

BEFORE THE STUDY: PLANNING AND IMPLEMENTATION

Teaching the Patient What to Expect
- Inform the patient this procedure can assist in assessing the veins.
- Review the procedure with the patient. Address concerns about pain related to the procedure and explain that no pain or discomfort should be experienced during the test.
- Explain that the procedure is performed in a US department by a health-care provider (HCP) who specializes in this procedure, with support staff, and takes approximately 30 to 60 min.
- Advise the patient that they will be instructed to remove jewelry and other

metallic objects from the area to be examined.
- Explain that positioning for this procedure is in the supine position on an examination table; other positions may be used during the examination.
- Explain to the patient that he or she will be draped and the area of interest exposed.
- Explain that a conductive gel is applied to the skin, and a transducer is moved over the area to obtain images of the area of interest.
- Waveforms are visualized and recorded with variations in respirations.
- Images with and without compression are performed proximally or distally to an obstruction to obtain

U

information about a venous occlusion or obstruction.

▶ The procedure can be performed for both arms and legs to obtain bilateral blood flow determination.

▶ Advise the patient that the transducer will not be placed where there is evidence of venous stasis or ulcer.

▶ Advise the patient he or she will be asked to breathe normally during the examination. If necessary for better organ visualization, the patient will be asked to take a deep breath and hold it.

▶ Once the study is completed, the gel is cleansed from the skin.

Potential Nursing Actions

▶ Report the presence of a lesion that is open or draining; maintain clean, dry dressing for the ulcer; protect the limb from trauma.

AFTER THE STUDY: POTENTIAL NURSING ACTIONS

Treatment Considerations

▶ Instruct the patient to resume usual fluids, as directed by the HCP.

▶ Inadequate Tissue Perfusion: Manage pain with the administration of ordered narcotics or other prescribed pain medication (NSAIDs). Assess site (DVT)

for degree of warmth, redness, edema and trend. Review diagnostic study results (impedance plethysmography, US). Enforce bedrest, elevate affected limb, apply ordered moist heat packs to the affected limb, and encourage oral fluids to decrease blood viscosity.

▶ Mobility: Immobilize affected extremity as ordered. Facilitate the use of assistive devices, and administer ordered medications (analgesics, steroids, antibiotics). Monitor and trend diagnostic study results, circulation, and sensation, and encourage ambulation when appropriate. Institute fall risk protocols.

▶ Anxiety is a normal human response to a situation that has unknown consequences. Allow the patient to verbalize concerns; explain pathophysiology related to disease process, including therapeutic options.

▶ Provide education regarding the clinical implications of the test results.

Follow-Up, Evaluation, and Desired Outcomes

▶ Understands the importance of decreasing fall risk by adhering to fall risk protocols.

▶ Recognizes the value of working with the health-care team to discuss treatment options and expected outcomes.

Upper Gastrointestinal and Small Bowel Series

SYNONYM/ACRONYM: Gastric radiography, stomach series, small bowel study, upper GI series, UGI.

RATIONALE: To assess the esophagus, stomach, and small bowel for disorders related to obstruction, perforation, weight loss, swallowing, pain, cancer, reflux disease, ulcers, and structural anomalies.

PATIENT PREPARATION: There are no activity restrictions unless by medical direction. Instruct the patient to fast and restrict fluids for 8 hr, or as ordered, prior to the procedure. **Pediatric Considerations:** The fasting period prior to the time of the examination depends on the child's age. General guidelines are that the patient should not eat for the period of time between normal meals: newborn, 2 to 3 hr; infants to 4 yr, 3 to 4 hr; 5 yr through adolescence, 6 to 8 hr. Fasting may be ordered as a precaution against aspiration related to possible nausea and vomiting. The American Society of Anesthesiologists has fasting guidelines for risk levels according to patient status. More information can be located at www.asahq.org.

Note: If iodinated contrast medium is scheduled to be used in patients receiving metformin or drugs containing metformin for type 2 diabetes, the drug may be discontinued on the day of the test and continue to be withheld for 48 hr after the test.

Regarding the patient's risk for bleeding, the patient should be instructed to avoid taking natural products and medications with known anticoagulant, antiplatelet, or thrombolytic properties or to reduce dosage, as ordered, prior to the procedure. Number of days to withhold medication is dependent on the type of anticoagulant. Note the last time and dose of medication taken. Protocols may vary among facilities.

Ensure that this procedure is performed before a barium swallow and after IVP or CT of the abdomen or pelvis.

NORMAL FINDINGS

- Normal size, shape, position, and functioning of the esophagus, stomach, and small bowel.

CRITICAL FINDINGS AND POTENTIAL INTERVENTIONS

- Foreign body
- Perforated bowel
- Tumor with significant mass effect

Timely notification to the requesting health-care provider (HCP) of any critical findings and related symptoms is a role expectation of the professional nurse. A listing of these findings varies among facilities.

OVERVIEW: (Study type: X-ray, special/contrast; related body system: Digestive system.) The upper gastrointestinal (GI) series is a radiological examination of the esophagus, stomach, and small intestine after ingestion of barium sulfate, which is a milkshake-like, radiopaque substance. A combination of x-ray and fluoroscopy techniques are used to record the study. Air or gas may be instilled to provide double contrast and better visualization of the lumen of the esophagus, stomach, and duodenum. If perforation or obstruction is suspected, a water-soluble iodinated contrast medium is used. This test is especially useful in the evaluation of patients experiencing dysphagia, regurgitation, gastroesophageal reflux (GER), epigastric pain, hematemesis, melena, and unexplained weight loss. This test is also used to evaluate the results of gastric surgery, especially when an anastomotic leak is suspected. When a small bowel series is included, the test detects disorders of the jejunum and ileum. The patient's position is changed during the examination to allow visualization of the various structures and their function. Images of the swallowed contrast medium as it moves through the digestive system are visualized on a fluoroscopic screen, recorded, and stored electronically for review. Drugs such as glucagon may be given during an upper GI series to relax the GI tract; drugs such as metoclopramide (Reglan) may be given to accelerate the passage of the barium through the stomach and small intestine.

U

When the small bowel series is performed separately, the patient may be asked to drink several glasses of barium, or enteroclysis may be used to instill the barium. With enteroclysis, a catheter is passed through the nose or mouth and advanced past the pylorus and into the duodenum. Barium, followed by methylcellulose solution, is instilled via the catheter directly into the small bowel.

Pediatrics: An upper GI series is usually done in the pediatric population to diagnose the cause of recurrent GI signs (bleeding) and symptoms. The etiology is often related to age. In infants, recurrent symptoms such as vomiting after feeding, poor feeding, poor weight gain, and abdominal pain (evidenced by frequent crying during or after a feeding) may trigger an investigation. The most common causes of upper or lower GI bleeding in infants up to 1 mo include allergies to milk proteins, anorectal fissures, bacterial enteritis, coagulopathy, esophagitis, Hirschsprung disease, intussusception, peptic ulcer, stenosis, varices, or Meckel diverticulum. Children between 2 to 23 mo are most commonly diagnosed with allergies to milk proteins, anorectal fissures, esophagitis caused by gastroesophageal reflux (GER), gastritis, intussusception, Meckel diverticulum, NSAID-induced ulcer, and ingested foreign body. Pediatric patients 24 mo and older are most commonly diagnosed with esophageal varices, Mallory-Weiss tears, peptic ulcer, related to *Helicobacter pylori* infection or peptic ulcer secondary to some other type of systemic disease (e.g., Crohn disease or inflammatory bowel disease [IBD]). Other abnormal findings in this age group include IBD, polyps, malignancy, sepsis, and Meckel diverticulum.

INDICATIONS
- Determine the cause of regurgitation or epigastric pain.
- Determine the presence of tumors, ulcers, diverticula, obstruction, foreign body, and hiatal hernia.
- Evaluate suspected GER, inflammatory process, congenital anomaly, motility disorder, or structural change.
- Evaluate unexplained weight loss or anemia.
- Identify and locate the origin of hematemesis.

INTERFERING FACTORS
Contraindications

❂ Patients who are pregnant or suspected of being pregnant, unless the potential benefits of a procedure using radiation far outweigh the risk of radiation exposure to the fetus and mother.

❂ Patients suspected of having upper GI perforation, unless water-soluble iodinated contrast medium, such as Gastrografin, is used.

❂ Patients with conditions associated with adverse reactions to contrast medium (e.g., asthma, food allergies, or allergy to contrast medium). Although patients are asked specifically if they have a known allergy to iodine or shellfish (shellfish contain high levels of iodine), it has been well established that the reaction is not to iodine; an actual iodine allergy would be problematic because iodine is required for the production of thyroid hormones. In the case of shellfish, the reaction is to a muscle protein called *tropomyosin;* in the case of iodinated contrast medium, the reaction is to the noniodinated part of the contrast molecule. Patients with a known hypersensitivity to the medium may benefit from pre-medication with corticosteroids and diphenhydramine; the use of nonionic contrast or an alternative noncontrast imaging study, if available, may be considered for patients who have severe asthma or who have experienced moderate to severe reactions to ionic contrast medium.

✸ Conditions associated with preexisting renal insufficiency (e.g., chronic kidney disease, single kidney transplant, nephrectomy, diabetes, multiple myeloma, treatment with aminoglycosides and NSAIDs), *because iodinated contrast is nephrotoxic.*

✸ Patients who are chronically dehydrated before the test, especially older adults and patients whose health is already compromised, *because of their risk of contrast-induced acute kidney injury.*

✸ Patients with an intestinal obstruction, *because the barium or water from the enema may make the condition worse.*

Factors that may alter the results of the study
- Patients with swallowing problems may aspirate the barium, which could interfere with the procedure and cause patient complications.
- Possible constipation or partial bowel obstruction caused by retained barium in the small bowel or colon may affect test results.

- Metallic objects (e.g., jewelry, body rings) within the examination field, which may inhibit organ visualization and cause unclear images.
- Inability of the patient to cooperate or remain still during the procedure, because movement can produce blurred or otherwise unclear images.

Other considerations
- This procedure should be done after a kidney x-ray (intravenous pyelography) or computed tomography of the abdomen or pelvis.

POTENTIAL MEDICAL DIAGNOSIS: CLINICAL SIGNIFICANCE OF RESULTS
Abnormal findings related to
- Achalasia
- Cancer of the esophagus
- Chalasis
- Congenital abnormalities
- Duodenal cancer, and ulcers
- Esophageal diverticula, motility disorders, ulcers, varices, and inflammation
- Foreign body
- Gastric cancer or tumors, and ulcers
- Gastritis
- Hiatal hernia
- Perforation of the esophagus, stomach, or small bowel
- Polyps
- Small bowel tumors
- Strictures

NURSING IMPLICATIONS

POTENTIAL NURSING PROBLEMS: ASSESSMENT & NURSING DIAGNOSIS

Problems	Signs and Symptoms
Altered GI elimination *(related to obstruction, tumor, stricture, congenital abnormality)*	Variances in bowel sounds between high-pitched and absent sounds, crampy abdominal pain, nausea, vomiting, odorous emesis (fecal smell and appearance), constipation or diarrhea

U

(table continues on page 1178)

Problems	Signs and Symptoms
Insufficient fluid volume *(related to NPO status, nausea, vomiting, fluid shift to peritoneal area secondary to obstruction)*	Altered electrolytes; increased heart rate; decreased blood pressure; dry skin and mucous membranes; poor skin turgor; dark-colored urine; hemoconcentration; cool, clammy skin; poor urine output (less than 30 mL/hr); confusion; restlessness; agitation; capillary refill delay
Pain *(related to obstruction, tumor, stricture, congenital abnormality)*	Self-report of abdominal pain; crying, moaning, groaning; increased heart rate and blood pressure; facial grimace

BEFORE THE STUDY: PLANNING AND IMPLEMENTATION

Teaching the Patient What to Expect

▶ Inform the patient this procedure can assist in assessing the esophagus, stomach, and small intestine.

▶ Explain that prior to the procedure, laboratory testing may be required to determine the possibility of bleeding risk (coagulation testing) or to assess for impaired kidney function (creatinine level and estimated glomerular filtration rate) if use of iodinated contrast medium is anticipated.

▶ Pregnancy is a general contraindication to procedures involving radiation. Explain to the female patient that she will be asked the date of her last menstrual period. Pregnancy testing may be performed to determine the possibility of pregnancy before exposure to radiation.

▶ Review the procedure with the patient. Address concerns about pain and explain that there may be moments of discomfort or pain experienced when the IV line or catheter is inserted to allow infusion of fluids such as saline, anesthetics, sedatives, contrast medium, medications used in the procedure, or emergency medications.

▶ Explain to the patient that he or she will be asked to drink a milkshake-like solution that has an unpleasant chalky taste.

▶ Explain that if used, contrast medium will be injected by catheter at a separate site from the IV line.

▶ Advise that a burning and flushing sensation may be felt throughout the body during injection of the contrast medium and they may experience an urge to cough, flushing, nausea, or a salty or metallic taste.

▶ Explain that the procedure is usually performed in a radiology department by an HCP, with support staff, and takes approximately 30 to 60 min.

▶ Instruct the patient to remove jewelry and other metallic objects from the area to be examined prior to the procedure.

▶ Baseline vital signs and neurological status are assessed and recorded. Protocols may vary among facilities.

Pediatric Considerations

▶ Preparing children for an upper GI examination depends on the age of the child. Encourage parents to be truthful about unpleasant sensations the child may experience during the procedure and to use words that they know their child will understand. Toddlers and preschool-age children have a short attention span, so the best time to talk about the test is right before the procedure. The child should be assured that he or she will be allowed to bring a favorite comfort item into the examination room, and if appropriate, that a parent will be with the child during the procedure.

Upper GI Series

▶ Positioning for this procedure is on the x-ray table in a supine position, or standing in front of a fluoroscopy screen.

▶ Advise the patient that he or she will be asked to take several swallows of the barium mixture through a straw while images are taken of the pharyngeal

U

motion. An effervescent contrast medium may also be administered to introduce air into the stomach. **Pediatric Considerations:** For infants, barium contrast may be mixed with a small amount of the infant's feeding to take in a bottle. If the patient is unable to drink the barium, a thin, flexible tube may be placed through his or her nose to get the barium into the esophagus.

Small Bowel Series

▶ If the small bowel is to be examined after the upper GI series, the patient will be instructed to drink an additional glass of barium while the small intestine is observed for passage of barium. Images are taken at 30- to 60-min intervals until the barium reaches the ileocecal valve. This process can last up to 5 hr, with follow-up images taken at 24 hr.

Potential Nursing Actions

* *Make sure a written and informed consent has been signed prior to the procedure and before administering any medications.*

▶ If iodinated contrast medium is scheduled to be used in patients receiving metformin or drugs containing metformin for type 2 diabetes, the drug may be discontinued on the day of the test and continue to be withheld for 48 hr after the test. Protocols may vary among facilities.

Safety Considerations

▶ Anticoagulants, aspirin, and other salicylates should be discontinued by medical direction for the appropriate number of days prior to a procedure where bleeding is a potential complication.

AFTER THE STUDY: POTENTIAL NURSING ACTIONS

Avoiding Complications

▶ Establishing an IV site and injection of contrast medium are invasive procedures. Complications are rare but include risk for allergic reaction *(related to contrast reaction),* aspiration of the barium, bleeding from the puncture site *(related to a bleeding disorder or the effects of natural products and medications with known anticoagulant,*

antiplatelet, or thrombolytic properties), significant diarrhea *(related to use of Gastrografin),* hematoma *(related to blood leakage into the tissue following needle insertion),* infection *(which might occur if bacteria from the skin surface is introduced at the puncture site),* nerve injury *(which might occur if the needle strikes a nerve),* nephrotoxicity *(a deterioration of renal function associated with contrast administration),* or partial bowel obstruction caused by thickened or congealed barium. Monitor the patient for complications related to the procedure (e.g., allergic reaction, anaphylaxis, bronchospasm, infection, injury). Immediately report symptoms such as difficulty breathing, chest pain, fever, hyperpnea, hypertension, nausea, palpitations, pruritus, rash, tachycardia, urticaria, or vomiting to the appropriate HCP. Observe/assess the needle/catheter insertion site for bleeding, inflammation, or hematoma formation. Administer ordered antihistamines or prophylactic steroids if the patient has an allergic reaction.

Treatment Considerations

▶ Instruct the patient to resume usual diet, fluids, medications, or activity, as directed by the HCP. Kidney function should be assessed before metformin is resumed.

▶ Instruct the patient to take a mild laxative and increase fluid intake (4 glasses) to aid in the elimination of barium unless contraindicated. **Pediatric Considerations:** Instruct the parents of pediatric patients to hydrate the child with electrolyte fluid post barium enema. **Older Adult Considerations:** Chronic dehydration can also result in frequent bouts of constipation. Therefore, after the procedure, older adult patients should be encouraged to hydrate with fluids containing electrolytes (e.g., Gatorade, Gatorade low calorie for patients with diabetes, or Pedialyte) and to use a mild laxative daily until the stool is back to normal color.

▶ Explain that the stool will be white or light in color for 2 to 3 days. If the patient is unable to eliminate the barium, or if the stool does not return

U

to normal color, the patient should notify the HCP.

▶ Altered GI Elimination: Enforce a nothing by mouth order (NPO). Facilitate gastric decompression as appropriate (nasogastric tube with intermittent suction). Administer ordered antiemetics, analgesics, and antibiotics. Assess the color and odor of any emesis (fecal odor or appearance). Assess the abdomen for bowel sounds, pain, tenderness, and distention. Administer ordered parenteral fluids. Prepare for ordered surgery; monitor and trend appropriate laboratory values and diagnostic studies (complete blood count, arterial blood gases, electrolytes, GI studies), and intake and output.

▶ Insufficient Fluid Volume: Monitor and trend laboratory studies: BUN, Cr, Hgb, Hct, and electrolytes. Monitor and trend blood pressure, heart rate, temperature, capillary refill, and skin turgor. Administer ordered parenteral fluids and replacement electrolytes. Perform a strict intake and output and monitor for fluid overload. Administer ordered antiemetics, analgesics, and antibiotics.

▶ Pain: Assess pain character, location, duration, and intensity and use an easily understood pain rating scale. Consider alternative measures for pain management (imagery, relaxation, music, etc.). Assess and trend vital signs. Facilitate a calm, quiet environment and place in a position of comfort. Administer ordered antiemetics, analgesics, and antibiotics.

Safety Considerations
▶ Advise patients with diabetes to avoid all medications containing metformin for 48 hr following a procedure with iodinated contrast. Iodinated contrast can temporarily impair kidney function, and failure to withhold metformin may indirectly result in drug-induced lactic acidosis, a dangerous and sometimes fatal adverse effect of metformin (related to renal impairment that does not support sufficient excretion of metformin).

Follow-Up, Evaluation, and Desired Outcomes
▶ Understands the medical and surgical options associated with the disease process.

Urea Nitrogen, Blood

SYNONYM/ACRONYM: BUN.

RATIONALE: To assist in assessing for kidney function toward diagnosing disorders such as kidney disease and dehydration. Also used in monitoring the effectiveness of therapeutic interventions such as hemodialysis.

PATIENT PREPARATION: There are no food, fluid, activity, or medication restrictions unless by medical direction.

NORMAL FINDINGS: Method: Spectrophotometry.

Age	Conventional Units	SI Units (Conventional Units × 0.357)
Newborn–3 yr	5–17 mg/dL	1.8–6.1 mmol/L
4–13 yr	7–17 mg/dL	2.5–6.1 mmol/L
14 yr–adult	8–21 mg/dL	2.9–7.5 mmol/L
Adult older than 90 yr	10–31 mg/dL	3.6–11.1 mmol/L

CRITICAL FINDINGS AND POTENTIAL INTERVENTIONS

Adults
- Greater than 100 mg/dL (SI: Greater than 35.7 mmol/L) (nondialysis patients)

Children
- Greater than 55 mg/dL (SI: Greater than 19.6 mmol/L) (nondialysis patients)

Timely notification to the requesting health-care provider (HCP) of any critical findings and related symptoms is a role expectation of the professional nurse. A listing of these findings varies among facilities.

Consideration may be given to verification of critical findings before action is taken. Policies vary among facilities and may include requesting immediate recollection and retesting by the laboratory or retesting using a rapid point-of-care testing instrument at the bedside, if available.

A patient with a grossly elevated BUN may have signs and symptoms including acidemia, agitation, confusion, fatigue, nausea, vomiting, and coma. Possible interventions include treatment of the cause, administration of IV bicarbonate, a low-protein diet, hemodialysis, and caution with respect to prescribing and continuing nephrotoxic medications.

OVERVIEW: (Study type: Blood collected in a gold-, red-, red/gray-, or green-top [heparin] tube; **related body system:** Urinary system.) Unlike fats and carbohydrates, protein cannot be stored by the body. The amino acids and nitrogen used to make proteins are either obtained from dietary sources or from the normal turnover of aging cells in the body. Urea is a nonprotein nitrogen (NPN) compound formed in the liver from ammonia and excreted by the kidneys as an end product of protein metabolism. Other NPN compounds excreted by the kidneys include uric acid and creatinine. Blood urea nitrogen (BUN) levels reflect the balance between the amount of nitrogen ingested and excreted which is a representation of overall protein metabolism. BUN and creatinine values are commonly evaluated together. The normal BUN/creatinine ratio is 15:1 to 24:1 (e.g., if a patient has a BUN of 15 mg/dL, the creatinine should be approximately 0.6 to 1 mg/dL). BUN is used in the following calculation to estimate serum osmolality: $(2 \times Na^+) + (glucose/18) + (BUN/2.8)$.

INDICATIONS
- Assess nutritional support.
- Evaluate hemodialysis therapy.
- Evaluate hydration.
- Evaluate liver function.
- Evaluate patients with lymphoma after chemotherapy (tumor lysis).
- Evaluate kidney function.
- Monitor the effects of drugs known to be nephrotoxic or hepatotoxic.

INTERFERING FACTORS
Factors that may alter the results of the study
- Drugs and other substances that may increase BUN levels include acetaminophen, alanine, alkaline antacids, amphotericin B, antimony compounds, arsenicals, bacitracin, bismuth subsalicylate, capreomycin, cephalosporins, chloral hydrate, chloramphenicol,

U

chlorthalidone, colistimethate, colistin, cotrimoxazole, dexamethasone, dextran, diclofenac, doxycycline, ethylene glycol, gentamicin, guanethidine, guanoxan, ibuprofen, ifosfamide, ipodate, kanamycin, mephenesin, metolazone, mitomycin, neomycin, phosphorus, plicamycin, tertatolol, tetracycline, triamterene, triethylenemelamine, viomycin, and vitamin D.

- Drugs and other substances that may decrease BUN levels include chloramphenicol, fluorides, and streptomycin.

POTENTIAL MEDICAL DIAGNOSIS: CLINICAL SIGNIFICANCE OF RESULTS
Increased in
- Acute kidney injury *(related to decreased renal excretion)*
- Chronic glomerulonephritis *(related to decreased renal excretion)*
- Decreased renal perfusion *(reflects decreased renal excretion and increased blood levels)*
- Diabetes *(related to decreased renal excretion)*
- Excessive protein ingestion *(related to increased protein metabolism)*
- GI bleeding *(excessive blood protein in the GI tract and increased protein metabolism)*
- Heart failure *(related to decreased blood flow to the kidneys, decreased renal excretion, and accumulation in circulating blood)*
- Hyperalimentation *(related to increased protein metabolism)*
- Hypovolemia *(related to decreased blood flow to the kidneys, decreased renal excretion, and accumulation in circulating blood)*

- Ketoacidosis *(dehydration from ketoacidosis correlates with decreased renal excretion of urea nitrogen)*
- Muscle wasting from starvation *(related to increased protein metabolism)*
- Tumors *(related to increased protein metabolism or to decreased renal excretion)*
- Nephrotoxic drugs *(related to decreased renal excretion and accumulation in circulating blood)*
- Pyelonephritis *(related to decreased renal excretion)*
- Shock *(related to decreased blood flow to the kidneys, decreased renal excretion, and accumulation in circulating blood)*
- Urinary tract obstruction *(related to decreased renal excretion and accumulation in circulating blood)*

Decreased in
- Inadequate dietary protein *(urea nitrogen is a by-product of protein metabolism; less available protein is reflected in decreased BUN levels)*
- Low-protein/high-carbohydrate diet *(urea nitrogen is a by-product of protein metabolism; less available protein is reflected in decreased BUN levels)*
- Malabsorption syndromes *(urea nitrogen is a by-product of protein metabolism; less available protein is reflected in decreased BUN levels)*
- Pregnancy
- Severe liver disease *(BUN is synthesized in the liver, so liver damage results in decreased levels)*

NURSING IMPLICATIONS

POTENTIAL NURSING PROBLEMS: ASSESSMENT & NURSING DIAGNOSIS

Problems	Signs and Symptoms
Cardiac output *(related to excess fluid volume, pericarditis, electrolyte imbalance, toxin accumulation, dysrhythmias, altered cardiac muscle contractility secondary to heart failure)*	Weak peripheral pulses; slow capillary refill; decreased urinary output; cool, clammy skin; tachypnea; dyspnea; altered level of consciousness; abnormal heart sounds; fatigue; hypoxia; loud holosystolic murmur; electrocardiogram (ECG) changes; increased jugular vein distention (JVD)
Fluid volume (water) *(related to excess fluid and sodium intake, compromised kidney function)*	**Excess:** Edema, shortness of breath, increased weight, ascites, rales, rhonchi, and diluted laboratory values, distended neck veins, tachycardia, restlessness, presence of S3 heart sound
Infection *(related to uremia and decreased immune response, venous catheters, Foley catheters, endotracheal tubes)*	Temperature, elevated white cell count, cloudy urine, sediment in urine, blood in urine
Kidney function *(related to renal ischemia associated with shock, sepsis, hypovolemia; postoperative injury; trauma; nephrotoxic drugs [aminoglycoside, heavy metals, radiographic contrast]; renal vascular occlusion; hemolytic transfusion reaction; decreased cardiac output; tubular necrosis; obstruction; tumor; medications [NSAIDs, ACE inhibitors, immunosuppressants, antineoplastics, antifungals])*	Increased BUN, increased creatinine (Cr), decreased Cr clearance, increased urine specific gravity (greater than 1.029), hematuria, proteinuria, decreased urine output less than 400 mL/day (with adequate intake and no fluid loss), weight gain, elevated potassium, elevated phosphate, decreased calcium, decreased sodium, increased magnesium, metabolic acidosis, decreased hemoglobin (Hgb) and hematocrit (Hct)

BEFORE THE STUDY: PLANNING AND IMPLEMENTATION

Teaching the Patient What to Expect
▶ Inform the patient this test can assist in assessing kidney function.

AFTER THE STUDY: POTENTIAL NURSING ACTIONS

Treatment Considerations
▶ Cardiac Output: Assess peripheral pulses and capillary refill. Monitor blood pressure and check for orthostatic

U

changes. Assess respiratory rate, breath sounds, and orthopnea, level of consciousness, skin color and temperature. Monitor urinary output, pulse oximetry and oxygenation, ECG and third heart sound, which is indicative of heart failure or pericarditis. Administer ordered inotropic and peripheral vasodilator medications, nitrates, oxygen, sodium bicarbonate, glucose, insulin drip, potassium excretion resin, or calcium salt.

- Fluid Volume: Record daily weight and monitor trends, and perform an accurate intake and output. Monitor laboratory values that reflect alterations in fluid status: potassium, BUN, Cr, calcium, Hgb, Hct, and sodium. Manage underlying cause of fluid alteration. Monitor urine characteristics, respiratory status, pulse oximetry, oxygenation, heart rate and blood pressure. Assess for symptoms of fluid overload such as JVD, shortness of breath, dyspnea, and crackles. Provide low-sodium diet. Administer ordered diuretic and antihypertensive. Elevate feet when sitting, administer ordered oxygen, and elevate the head of the bed. Prepare for hemodialysis as appropriate. Limit fluids as appropriate.

- Infection: Monitor urinary output and assess urine color, odor, presence of blood. Monitor and trend temperature and white cell count and obtain urine for culture and sensitivity. Administer ordered antibiotics. Avoid long-term indwelling catheters. Encourage frequent personal and oral hygiene with the use of encourage use of gentle soaps. Assist in preventing skin breakdown. Use meticulous care and sterile technique in provision of care for peripheral or venous catheters.

- Kidney function: Monitor, record, and trend intake and output, urine specific gravity, BUN, Cr, sodium, potassium,

magnesium, pH, urinalysis, Hgb, and Hct. Assess and monitor for edema, JVD, hypertension, adventitious breath sounds, and impaired gas exchange. Use pulse oximetry; administer ordered oxygen, diuretics, appropriate fluids, antibiotics (consider renal function); and facilitate ordered hemodialysis.

Nutritional Considerations

- Greater than 100 nitrogen balance is commonly used as a nutritional assessment tool to indicate protein change. In healthy individuals, protein anabolism and catabolism are in equilibrium. During various disease states, nutritional intake decreases, resulting in a negative balance. During recovery from illness and with proper nutritional support, the nitrogen balance becomes positive. BUN is an important analyte to measure during administration of total parenteral nutrition (TPN). Educate the patient, as appropriate, in dietary adjustments required to maintain proper nitrogen balance. Inform the patient that the requesting HCP may prescribe TPN as part of the treatment plan.

- An elevated BUN can be caused by a high-protein diet or dehydration. Unless medically restricted, a healthy diet should be consumed daily. Acknowledges contact information provided for the U.S. Department of Agriculture's resource for nutrition (www.choosemyplate.gov). Fluid consumption should include six to eight 8-oz glasses of water or water-containing fluid per day.

Follow-Up, Evaluation, and Desired Outcomes

- Understands that depending on the results of this procedure, additional testing may be necessary to monitor disease progression and determine the need for a change in therapy.

Urea Nitrogen, Urine

SYNONYM/ACRONYM: N/A

RATIONALE: To assess kidney function related to the progression of disorders such as diabetes, liver disease, and kidney disease.

PATIENT PREPARATION: There are no food, fluid, activity, or medication restrictions unless by medical direction. Usually, a 24-hr urine collection is ordered. As appropriate, provide the required urine collection container and specimen collection instructions.

NORMAL FINDINGS: Method: Spectrophotometry.

Conventional Units	SI Units (Conventional Units × 35.7)
12–20 g/24 hr	428–714 mmol/24 hr

CRITICAL FINDINGS AND POTENTIAL INTERVENTIONS: N/A

OVERVIEW: (**Study type:** Urine, from an unpreserved random or timed specimen collected in a clean plastic collection container; **related body system:** Urinary system.) Urea is a nonprotein nitrogen compound formed in the liver from ammonia as an end product of protein metabolism. Urea diffuses freely into extracellular and intracellular fluid and is ultimately excreted by the kidneys. Urine urea nitrogen levels reflect the balance between the production and excretion of urea.

INDICATIONS
- Evaluate kidney disease.
- Predict the impact that other conditions, such as diabetes and liver disease, will have on the kidneys.

INTERFERING FACTORS
Factors that may alter the results of the study
- Drugs and other substances that may increase urine urea nitrogen levels include alanine and glycine.

- Drugs and other substances that may decrease urine urea nitrogen levels include furosemide, growth hormone, insulin, and testosterone.

Other considerations
- All urine voided for the timed collection period must be included in the collection or else falsely decreased values may be obtained. Compare output records with volume collected to verify that all voids were included in the collection.

POTENTIAL MEDICAL DIAGNOSIS: CLINICAL SIGNIFICANCE OF RESULTS
Increased in
- Diabetes *(related to increased protein metabolism)*
- Hyperthyroidism
- Increased dietary protein *(related to increased protein metabolism)*
- Postoperative period

Decreased in
- Kidney disease *(related to decreased renal excretion)*
- Liver disease *(BUN is synthesized in the liver, so liver damage results in decreased levels)*

U

- Low-protein/high-carbohydrate diet *(urea nitrogen is a by-product of protein metabolism; less available protein is reflected in decreased BUN levels)*
- Normal-growing pediatric patients *(increased demand for protein; less available protein is reflected in decreased BUN levels)*
- Pregnancy *(increased demand for protein; less available protein is reflected in decreased BUN levels)*
- Toxemia *(related to hypertension and decreased renal excretion)*

NURSING IMPLICATIONS

BEFORE THE STUDY: PLANNING AND IMPLEMENTATION

Teaching the Patient What to Expect
▶ Inform the patient this test can assist in assessing kidney function.
▶ Explain that a urine sample is needed for the test. Information regarding specimen collection is presented with other general guidelines in Appendix A: Patient Preparation and Specimen Collection.

Potential Nursing Actions
▶ Include on the collection container's label urine total volume, test start and stop times/dates, and any medications that may interfere with test results.

AFTER THE STUDY: POTENTIAL NURSING ACTIONS

Treatment Considerations
▶ Monitor kidney function. Monitor and trend urine specific gravity, BUN, Cr, sodium, potassium, magnesium, pH, urinalysis, Hgb, and Hct. Assess and monitor for edema, jugular vein distention, hypertension, adventitious breath sounds, and impaired gas exchange.

Nutritional Considerations
▶ An elevated BUN can be caused by a high-protein diet or dehydration. Acknowledges contact information provided for the U.S. Department of Agriculture's resource for nutrition (www.choosemyplate.gov). Fluid consumption should include six to eight 8-oz glasses of water or water containing fluid per day.

Follow-Up, Evaluation, and Desired Outcomes
▶ Understands that depending on the results of this procedure, additional testing may be necessary to monitor disease progression and determine the need for a change in therapy.

Urethrography, Retrograde

SYNONYM/ACRONYM: Pyelography, retrograde.

RATIONALE: To assess urethral patency in order to evaluate the success of surgical interventions on patients who have urethral structures or other anomalies that interfere with urination.

PATIENT PREPARATION: There are no food, fluid, or activity restrictions unless by medical direction.

Note: If iodinated contrast medium is scheduled to be used in patients receiving metformin or drugs containing metformin for type 2 diabetes, the drug may be discontinued on the day of the test and continue to be withheld for 48 hr after the test.

U

Regarding the patient's risk for bleeding, the patient should be instructed to avoid taking natural products and medications with known anticoagulant, antiplatelet, or thrombolytic properties or to reduce dosage, as ordered, prior to the procedure. Number of days to withhold medication is dependent on the type of anticoagulant. Note the last time and dose of medication taken. Protocols may vary among facilities.

Ensure that this procedure is performed before an upper gastrointestinal study or barium swallow.

NORMAL FINDINGS

- Normal size, shape, and course of the membranous, bulbar, and penile portions of the urethra in male patients
- If the prostatic portion can be visualized, it also should appear normal.

CRITICAL FINDINGS AND POTENTIAL INTERVENTIONS: N/A

OVERVIEW: (Study type: X-ray, special/contrast; related body system: Urinary system.) Retrograde urethrography uses contrast medium, either injected or instilled via a catheter into the urethra, to visualize the membranous, bulbar, and penile portions, particularly after surgical repair of the urethra to assess the success of the surgery in male patients. The posterior portion of the urethra is visualized better when the procedure is performed with voiding cystourethrography. In women, it may be performed after surgical repair of the urethra to assess the success of the surgery and to assess structural abnormalities in conjunction with an evaluation for voiding dysfunction.

INDICATIONS

- Aid in the diagnosis of urethral strictures, lacerations, diverticula, and congenital anomalies.

INTERFERING FACTORS

Contraindications

Patients who are pregnant or suspected of being pregnant, unless the potential benefits of a procedure using radiation far outweigh the risk of radiation exposure to the fetus and mother.

Patients with conditions associated with adverse reactions to contrast medium (e.g., asthma, food allergies, or allergy to contrast medium). Although patients are asked specifically if they have a known allergy to iodine or shellfish (shellfish contain high levels of iodine), it has been well established that the reaction is not to iodine; an actual iodine allergy would be problematic because iodine is required for the production of thyroid hormones. In the case of shellfish, the reaction is to a muscle protein called *tropomyosin;* in the case of iodinated contrast medium, the reaction is to the noniodinated part of the contrast molecule. Patients with a known hypersensitivity to the medium may benefit from premedication with corticosteroids and diphenhydramine; the use of nonionic contrast or an alternative noncontrast imaging study, if available, may be considered for patients who have severe asthma or who have experienced moderate to severe reactions to ionic contrast medium.

Patients with conditions associated with preexisting renal insufficiency (e.g., chronic kidney disease, single kidney transplant, nephrectomy, diabetes, multiple myeloma, treatment with aminoglycosides and NSAIDs), *because iodinated contrast is nephrotoxic.*

U

✦ Patients who are chronically dehydrated before the test, especially older adults and patients whose health is already compromised, *because of their risk of contrast-induced acute kidney injury.*

✦ Patients with bleeding disorders, *because the puncture site may not stop bleeding.*

Factors that may alter the results of the study

• Metallic objects (e.g., jewelry, body rings) within the examination field, which may inhibit organ visualization and cause unclear images.

• Inability of the patient to cooperate or remain still during the procedure, because movement can produce blurred or otherwise unclear images.

POTENTIAL MEDICAL DIAGNOSIS: CLINICAL SIGNIFICANCE OF RESULTS
Abnormal findings related to

• Congenital anomalies, such as urethral valves and perineal hypospadias

• False passages in the urethra *related to failed catheterization event*

• Prostatic enlargement

• Tumors of the urethra

• Urethral calculi

• Urethral diverticula

• Urethral fistulas

• Urethral strictures indicated by a narrowing and lacerations

NURSING IMPLICATIONS

BEFORE THE STUDY: PLANNING AND IMPLEMENTATION

Teaching the Patient What to Expect

▶ Inform the patient this procedure can assist in assessing the urethral patency.

▶ Explain that prior to the procedure, laboratory testing may be required to determine the possibility of bleeding risk (coagulation testing) or to assess for impaired kidney function (creatinine level and estimated glomerular filtration rate) if use of iodinated contrast medium is anticipated.

▶ Pregnancy is a general contraindication to procedures involving radiation. Explain to the female patient that she will be asked the date of her last menstrual period. Pregnancy testing may be performed to determine the possibility of pregnancy before exposure to radiation.

▶ Review the procedure with the patient. Address concerns about pain and explain that there may be moments of discomfort or pain experienced when the IV line or catheter is inserted to allow infusion of fluids such as saline, anesthetics, sedatives, contrast medium, medications used in the procedure, or emergency medications.

▶ Explain that contrast medium will be injected, by catheter, at a separate site from the IV line.

▶ Advise that a burning and flushing sensation may be felt throughout the body during injection of the contrast medium and the patient may experience an urge to cough, flushing, nausea, or a salty or metallic taste.

▶ Explain that the procedure is performed in a cystoscopy room by a health-care provider (HCP), with support staff, and takes approximately 30 min.

▶ Instruct the patient to remove jewelry and other metallic objects from the area to be examined prior to the procedure.

▶ Baseline vital signs are obtained and recorded.

▶ Positioning for this procedure is on the table in a supine position.

▶ Explain that a single plain film is taken of the bladder and urethra prior to the administration of contrast.

▶ Next, a catheter filled with contrast medium to eliminate air pockets is inserted until the balloon reaches the meatus. Inform the patient that some pressure may be experienced when the catheter is inserted and contrast medium is instilled.

▶ Explain that after three-fourths of the contrast medium is injected, another image is taken while the remainder of the contrast medium is injected.

▶ Advise female patients that the procedure may be done using a double balloon to occlude the bladder neck from above and below the external meatus.

Potential Nursing Actions

✦ *Make sure a written and informed consent has been signed prior to the procedure and before administering any medications.*

▶ If iodinated contrast medium is scheduled to be used in patients receiving metformin or drugs containing metformin for type 2 diabetes, the drug may be discontinued on the day of the test and continue to be withheld for 48 hr after the test. Protocols may vary among facilities.

Safety Considerations

▶ Anticoagulants, aspirin, and other salicylates should be discontinued by medical direction for the appropriate number of days prior to a procedure where bleeding is a potential complication.

AFTER THE STUDY: POTENTIAL NURSING ACTIONS

Avoiding Complications

▶ Establishing an IV site and injection of contrast medium are invasive procedures. Complications are rare but include risk for allergic reaction *(related to contrast reaction),* bleeding from the puncture site *(related to a bleeding disorder or the effects of natural products and medications with known anticoagulant, antiplatelet, or thrombolytic properties),* hematoma *(related to blood leakage into the tissue following needle insertion),* infection *(which might occur if bacteria from the skin surface is introduced at the puncture site),* nerve injury *(which*

might occur if the needle strikes a nerve), nephrotoxicity *(a deterioration of renal function associated with contrast administration),* severe pain in the kidney area, or sepsis. Monitor the patient for complications related to the procedure (e.g., allergic reaction, anaphylaxis, bronchospasm, infection, injury). Immediately report symptoms such as difficulty breathing, chest pain, fever, hyperpnea, hypertension, nausea, palpitations, pruritus, rash, tachycardia, urticaria, or vomiting to the appropriate HCP. Observe/assess the needle/catheter insertion site for bleeding, inflammation, or hematoma formation. Administer ordered antihistamines or prophylactic steroids if the patient has an allergic reaction.

Treatment Considerations

▶ Instruct the patient to resume usual diet, fluids, medications, or activity, as directed by the HCP. Kidney function should be assessed before metformin is resumed.

▶ Monitor vital and neurological signs every 15 min until they return to preprocedure levels.

▶ Monitor fluid intake and urinary output for 24 hr after the procedure. Decreased urine output may indicate impending kidney injury.

Safety Considerations

▶ Advise patients with diabetes to avoid all medications containing metformin for 48 hr following a procedure with iodinated contrast. Iodinated contrast can temporarily impair kidney function, and failure to withhold metformin may indirectly result in drug-induced lactic acidosis, a dangerous and sometimes fatal adverse effect of metformin *(related to renal impairment that does not support sufficient excretion of metformin).*

Follow-Up, Evaluation, and Desired Outcomes

▶ Acknowledges the importance of drinking plenty of fluids to prevent stasis and to prevent the buildup of bacteria.

U

Uric Acid, Blood

SYNONYM/ACRONYM: Urate.

RATIONALE: To monitor uric acid levels during treatment for gout and evaluation of tissue destruction, liver damage, renal function, and monitor the effectiveness of therapeutic interventions.

PATIENT PREPARATION: There are no food, fluid, activity, or medication restrictions unless by medical direction.

NORMAL FINDINGS: Method: Spectrophotometry.

Age	Conventional Units	SI Units (Conventional Units × 0.059)
1–30 days		
Male	1.3–4.9 mg/dL	0.08–0.29 mmol/L
Female	1.4–6.2 mg/dL	0.08–0.37 mmol/L
1–3 mo		
Male	1.4–5.3 mg/dL	0.08–0.31 mmol/L
Female	1.4–5.8 mg/dL	0.08–0.34 mmol/L
4–12 mo		
Male	1.5–6.4 mg/dL	0.09–0.38 mmol/L
Female	1.4–6.2 mg/dL	0.08–0.37 mmol/L
1–3 yr		
Male and female	1.8–5 mg/dL	0.11–0.3 mmol/L
4–6 yr		
Male and female	2.2–4.7 mg/dL	0.13–0.28 mmol/L
7–9 yr		
Male and female	2–5 mg/dL	0.12–0.3 mmol/L
10–12 yr		
Male and female	2.3–5.9 mg/dL	0.14–0.35 mmol/L
13–15 yr		
Male	3.1–7 mg/dL	0.18–0.41 mmol/L
Female	2.3–6.4 mg/dL	0.14–0.38 mmol/L
16–18 yr		
Male	2.1–7.6 mg/dL	0.12–0.45 mmol/L
Female	2.4–6.6 mg/dL	0.14–0.39 mmol/L
19 yr–Adult		
Male	4–8 mg/dL	0.24—0.47 mmol/L
Female	2.5–7 mg/dL	0.15–0.41 mmol/L
Adult older than 60 yr		
Male	4.2–8.2 mg/dL	0.25–0.48 mmol/L
Female	3.5–7.3 mg/dL	0.21–0.43 mmol/L

Therapeutic target for patients with gout: Less than 6 mg/dL (SI: Less than 0.4 mmol/L).

U

CRITICAL FINDINGS AND POTENTIAL INTERVENTIONS

Adults

• Greater than 13 mg/dL (SI: Greater than 0.8 mmol/L)

Children

• Greater than 12 mg/dL (SI: Greater than 0.7 mmol/L)

Timely notification to the requesting health-care provider (HCP) of any critical findings and related symptoms is a role expectation of the professional nurse. A listing of these findings varies among facilities.

Symptoms of acute renal dysfunction and/or chronic kidney disease associated with hyperuricemia include altered mental status, nausea and vomiting, fluid overload, pericarditis, and seizures. Prophylactic measures against the development of hyperuricemia should be undertaken before initiation of chemotherapy. Possible interventions include discontinuing medications that increase serum urate levels or produce acidic urine (e.g., thiazides and salicylates); administration of fluids with sodium bicarbonate as an additive to IV solutions to promote hydration and alkalinization of the urine to a pH greater than 7; administration of allopurinol 1 to 2 days before chemotherapy; monitoring of serum electrolyte, uric acid, phosphorus, calcium, and creatinine levels; and monitoring for ureteral obstruction by urate calculi using computed tomography or ultrasound studies. Possible interventions for advanced renal insufficiency and subsequent chronic kidney disease may include peritoneal dialysis or hemodialysis.

OVERVIEW: (Study type: Blood collected in a gold-, red-, red/gray-, or green-top [heparin] tube; related body system: Multisystem (metabolic disorders) and Urinary system. *Note:* Rasburicase will rapidly decrease uric acid in specimens left at room temperature. If patients are receiving this medication, collect the blood sample in a prechilled green-top [heparin] tube and transport in an ice slurry.) Uric acid is the end product of purine metabolism. Purines are important constituents of nucleic acids; purine turnover occurs continuously in the body, producing substantial amounts of uric acid even in the absence of purine intake from dietary sources such as organ meats (e.g., liver, thymus gland and/or pancreas [sweetbreads], kidney), legumes, and yeasts. Uric acid is filtered, absorbed, and secreted by the kidneys and is a common constituent of urine. Serum urate levels are affected by the amount of uric acid produced and by the efficiency of renal excretion. Values can vary based on diet, gender, body size, level of exercise, level of stress, and regularity in consumption of alcohol. Elevated uric acid levels can indicate conditions of critical cellular injury or destruction; hyperuricemia has an association with gout, hypertension, hypertriglyceridemia, kidney stones, obesity, myocardial infarct, renal disease, and diabetes. Rasburicase is a medication used in the treatment and prevention of acute hyperuricemia related to tumor lysis syndrome in children and for leukemias and lymphomas related

U

to the toxic effects of chemotherapy. Rasburicase is a recombinant form of uricase oxidase, an enzyme that converts uric acid to allantoin, a much more soluble and effectively excreted substance than uric acid.

INDICATIONS

- Assist in the diagnosis of gout when there is a family history (autosomal dominant genetic disorder) or signs and symptoms of gout, indicated by elevated uric acid levels.
- Determine the cause of known or suspected renal calculi.
- Evaluate the extent of tissue destruction in infection, starvation, excessive exercise, malignancies, chemotherapy, or radiation therapy.
- Evaluate possible liver damage in eclampsia, indicated by elevated uric acid levels.
- Monitor the effects of drugs known to alter uric acid levels, either as a adverse effect or as a therapeutic effect.

INTERFERING FACTORS

Factors that may alter the results of the study

- Drugs and other substances that may increase uric acid levels include acetylsalicylic acid (low doses), aminothiadiazole, anabolic steroids, antineoplastic drugs, atenolol, azathioprine, chlorambucil, chlorthalidone, cisplatin, corn oil, cyclosporine, cyclothiazide, cytarabine, diapamide, diuretics, ethacrynic acid, ethambutol, ethoxzolamide, flumethiazide, hydrochlorothiazide, hydroflumethiazide, ibufenac, ibuprofen, levarterenol, mefruside, mercaptopurine, methicillin, methotrexate, methyclothiazide, mitomycin, morinamide, polythiazide, prednisone, pyrazinamide, quinethazone, salicylate,

spironolactone, tacrolimus, theophylline, thiazide diuretics, thioguanine, thiotepa, triamterene, trichlormethiazide, vincristine, and warfarin.
- Drugs and other substances that may decrease uric acid levels include allopurinol, aspirin (high doses), azathioprine, benzbromaron, canola oil, chlorothiazide (given IV), chlorpromazine, chlorprothixene, clofibrate, corticosteroids, corticotropin, coumarin, dicumarol, enalapril, fenofibrate, guaifenesin, iodipamide, iodopyracet, iopanoic acid, ipodate, lisinopril, mefenamic acid, methotrexate, oxyphenbutazone, phenolsulfonphthalein, probenecid, radiographic medium, rasburicase, seclazone, sulfinpyrazone, and verapamil.
- Rasburicase will rapidly decrease uric acid in specimens left at room temperature. Specimens must be collected in prechilled tubes, transported in an ice slurry, and tested within 4 hr of collection.

POTENTIAL MEDICAL DIAGNOSIS: CLINICAL SIGNIFICANCE OF RESULTS

Increased in

Conditions that result in high cellular turnover release nucleic acids into circulation, which are converted to uric acid by the liver.

- Acute tissue destruction as a result of starvation or excessive exercise *(related to cellular destruction)*
- Alcohol misuse
- Chemotherapy and radiation therapy *(related to high cellular turnover)*
- Chronic lead toxicity *(cellular destruction related to hemolysis)*
- Diabetes *(decreased renal excretion results in increased blood levels)*
- Down syndrome
- Eclampsia

- Excessive dietary purines *(purines are nucleic acid bases converted to uric acid by the liver)*
- Glucose-6-phosphate dehydrogenase deficiency *(cellular destruction related to hemolysis)*
- Gout *(usually related to excess dietary intake)*
- Heart failure *(related to cellular destruction)*
- Hyperparathyroidism
- Hypertension *(related to effects on renal excretion)*
- Hypoparathyroidism *(related to disturbances in calcium and phosphorus homeostasis)*
- Lactic acidosis *(cellular destruction related to shock)*
- Lead poisoning *(cellular destruction related to hemolysis)*
- Lesch-Nyhan syndrome *(related to disorder of uric acid metabolism)*
- Multiple myeloma *(related to high cell turnover)*

- Pernicious anemia *(cellular destruction related to hemolysis)*
- Polycystic kidney disease *(related to decreased renal excretion, which results in increased blood levels)*
- Polycythemia *(related to increased cellular destruction)*
- Psoriasis
- Sickle cell anemia *(cellular destruction related to hemolysis)*
- Tumors *(related to high cell turnover)*
- Type III hyperlipidemia

Decreased in
- Fanconi syndrome *(related to increased renal excretion)*
- Low-purine diet *(related to insufficient nutrients for liver to synthesize uric acid)*
- Severe liver disease *(uric acid synthesis occurs in the liver)*
- Wilson disease *(affects normal liver function and is related to impaired tubular absorption)*

NURSING IMPLICATIONS

POTENTIAL NURSING PROBLEMS: ASSESSMENT & NURSING DIAGNOSIS

Problems	Signs and Symptoms
Electrolytes *(related to compromised excretion, kidney function)*	Increased blood urea nitrogen, increased creatinine, decreased sodium, increased urine specific gravity, increased potassium, decreased calcium, increased magnesium, increased phosphorus, altered uric acid
Fluid volume (water) *(related to decreased glomerular filtration or the presence of the diuretic stage of kidney disease)*	**Excess:** Edema, shortness of breath, increased weight, ascites, rales, rhonchi, and diluted laboratory values **Deficit:** Decreased urinary output, fatigue, sunken eyes, dark urine, decreased blood pressure, increased heart rate, and altered mental status
Nutrition *(related to altered taste, decreased food intake, nausea, vomiting)*	Poor nutrition with inadequate caloric intake; progressive weight loss; decreasing muscle mass; thin, weak, and apathetic; poor skin turgor with breakdown; difficulty healing; anemic; decreased respiratory and cardiac status

U

Teaching the Patient What to Expect
▶ Inform the patient this test can assist in diagnosing gout and assessing kidney function.

Treatment Considerations
▶ Electrolytes: Monitor laboratory values (electrolytes). Administer ordered IV infusions and medications to correct altered electrolytes. Collaborate with HCP in consideration of dialysis as appropriate to maintain homeostasis; monitor uric acid levels.
▶ Fluid Volume: Establish baseline assessment data. Manage underlying cause of fluid alteration. Record accurate intake and output. Monitor urine characteristics and respiratory status. Collaborate to adjust oral and IV fluids to provide optimal hydration status.
▶ Nutrition: Assess nutritional requirements and seek consultation with a registered dietitian. Consider implementing a calorie count. Correlate baseline nutritional intake with medical status. Consider individual and cultural food preferences. Collaborate with HCP, pharmacist, and clinical dietitian in consideration of enteral and parenteral nutrition.

Safety Considerations
▶ Confusion can occur due to altered fluid and electrolytes as well as renal or hepatic disease. Correlate confusion with the need to reverse altered electrolytes and evaluate medications. Prevent falls and injury through appropriate use of postural support, bed alarm, or restraints. Consider pharmacological interventions.

Nutritional Considerations
▶ Increased uric acid levels may be associated with the formation of kidney stones. Educate the patient, if appropriate, on the importance of drinking a sufficient amount of water when kidney stones are suspected.
▶ Increased uric acid levels may be associated with gout. Nutritional therapy may be appropriate for some patients identified as having gout. Educate the patient that foods high in oxalic acid include caffeinated beverages, raw blackberries, gooseberries, plums, whole-wheat bread, beets, carrots, beans, rhubarb, spinach, dry cocoa, and Ovaltine. Some fish, including anchovies, sardines, herring, mussels, codfish, scallops, trout, and haddock, are high in purines. Meats, such as bacon, goose, turkey, veal, venison, and organ meats (hearts, kidneys, liver, oxtail, spleen, sweetbreads, and ox/ cow lungs), are high in purines. Foods high in purines should be restricted. In other cases, the requesting HCP may not prescribe a low-purine or purine-restricted diet for treatment of gout because medications can control the condition easily and effectively.

Follow-Up, Evaluation, and Desired Outcomes
▶ Acknowledges the value of lifestyle alterations that may improve health.

Uric Acid, Urine

SYNONYM/ACRONYM: Urine urate.

RATIONALE: To assist in confirming a diagnosis of gout, assess renal function, evaluate for kidney stones, and monitor the effectiveness of therapeutic interventions.

PATIENT PREPARATION: There are no food, fluid, activity, or medication restrictions unless by medical direction. Usually, a 24-hr urine collection is ordered. As appropriate, provide the required urine collection container and specimen collection instructions.

NORMAL FINDINGS: Method: Spectrophotometry.

Gender	Conventional Units	SI Units (Conventional Units × 0.0059)
Male	250–800 mg/24 hr	1.48–4.72 mmol/24 hr
Female	250–750 mg/24 hr	1.48–4.43 mmol/24 hr

Values reflect average purine diet.

CRITICAL FINDINGS AND POTENTIAL INTERVENTIONS: N/A

OVERVIEW: (Study type: Urine, from a random or timed specimen collected in a clean plastic, unrefrigerated collection container; related body system: Urinary system. Sodium hydroxide preservative may be recommended to prevent precipitation of urates.) Uric acid is the end product of purine metabolism. Purines are important constituents of nucleic acids; purine turnover occurs continuously in the body, producing substantial amounts of uric acid even in the absence of purine intake from dietary sources such as organ meats (e.g., liver, thymus gland and/or pancreas [sweetbreads], kidney), legumes, and yeasts. Uric acid is filtered, absorbed, and secreted by the kidneys and is a common constituent of urine. The ratio of 24-hr urine uric acid to creatinine can be used as a test for detection of Lesch-Nyhan syndrome, a disorder of uric acid metabolism associated with absence of the enzyme hypoxanthine-guanine phosphoribosyltransferase. The ratio in healthy patients is reported to range from 0.21 to 0.59. Patients with partial or complete enzyme deficiency can have ratios from 2 to 5. Uric acid levels are also used to assist in the diagnosis of gout and kidney stones.

INDICATIONS
- Compare urine and serum uric acid levels to provide an index of renal function.
- Detect enzyme deficiencies and metabolic disturbances that affect the body's production of uric acid.
- Monitor the response to therapy with uricosuric drugs.
- Monitor urinary effects of disorders that cause hyperuricemia.

INTERFERING FACTORS
Factors that may alter the results of the study
- Drugs and other substances that may increase urine uric acid levels include ampicillin, ascorbic acid, azapropazone, benzbromarone, chlorpromazine, chlorprothixene, corticotropin, coumarin, dicumarol, ethyl biscoumacetate, iodipamide, iodopyracet, iopanoic acid, ipodate, mannose, mercaptopurine, methotrexate, niacinamide, nifedipine, phenolsulfonphthalein, phenylbutazone, probenecid, salicylates (long-term, large doses), seclazone, sulfinpyrazone, and verapamil.

U

- Drugs and other substances that may decrease urine uric acid levels include acetazolamide, allopurinol, angiotensin, benzbromarone, bumetanide, chlorothiazide, chlorthalidone, ethacrynic acid, ethambutol, ethoxzolamide, hydrochlorothiazide, levarterenol, niacin, pyrazinoic acid, and thiazide diuretics.

Other considerations

- All urine voided for the timed collection period must be included in the collection or else falsely decreased values may be obtained. Compare output records with volume collected to verify that all voids were included in the collection.

POTENTIAL MEDICAL DIAGNOSIS: CLINICAL SIGNIFICANCE OF RESULTS

Increased in

- Disorders associated with impaired renal tubular absorption, such as Fanconi syndrome and Wilson disease

- Disorders of purine metabolism
- Excessive dietary intake of purines
- Gout
- Neoplastic disorders, such as leukemia, lymphosarcoma, and multiple myeloma *(related to increased cell turnover)*
- Pernicious anemia *(related to increased cell turnover)*
- Polycythemia vera *(related to increased cell turnover)*
- Renal calculus formation *(related to increased urinary excretion)*
- Sickle cell anemia *(related to increased cell turnover)*

Decreased in

- Chronic alcohol ingestion *(related to decreased excretion)*
- Hypertension *(related to decreased excretion)*
- Severe kidney damage *(possibly resulting from chronic glomerulonephritis, collagen disorders, diabetic glomerulosclerosis, lactic acidosis, ketoacidosis, or alcohol misuse)*

NURSING IMPLICATIONS

POTENTIAL NURSING PROBLEMS: ASSESSMENT & NURSING DIAGNOSIS

Problems	Signs and Symptoms
Electrolytes *(related to compromised excretion)*	Increased blood urea nitrogen, increased creatinine, decreased sodium, increased urine specific gravity, increased potassium, decreased calcium, increased magnesium, increased phosphorus, altered uric acid
Fluid volume (water) *(related to decreased glomerular filtration or the presence of the diuretic stage of kidney disease)*	**Excess:** Edema, shortness of breath, increased weight, ascites, rales, rhonchi, and diluted laboratory values **Deficit:** Decreased urinary output, fatigue, sunken eyes, dark urine, decreased blood pressure, increased heart rate, and altered mental status
Skin *(related to altered fluid and nutritional status and associated inactivity)*	Decreased skin turgor, dry mouth, furrowed tongue, dry lips, jaundice

U

Teaching the Patient What to Expect

▶ Inform the patient this test can assist in diagnosing gout and kidney disease.

▶ Explain that a urine sample is needed for the test. Information regarding specimen collection is presented with other general guidelines in Appendix A: Patient Preparation and Specimen Collection.

Potential Nursing Actions

▶ Include on the collection container's label urine total volume, test start and stop times/dates, and any medications that may interfere with test results.

Avoiding Complications

▶ Increased uric acid levels may be associated with the formation of kidney stones. Educate the patient, if appropriate, on the importance of drinking a sufficient amount of water when kidney stones are suspected.

Treatment Considerations

▶ Electrolytes: Monitor laboratory values (electrolytes). Administer ordered IV infusions and medications to correct altered electrolytes. Collaborate with health-care provider (HCP) in consideration of dialysis as appropriate to maintain homeostasis; monitor uric acid levels.

▶ Fluid Volume: Establish baseline assessment data. Manage underlying cause of fluid alteration. Record accurate intake and output. Monitor urine characteristics and respiratory status. Collaborate to adjust oral and IV fluids to provide optimal hydration status.

▶ Nutrition: Assess nutritional requirements and seek consultation with a registered dietitian. Consider implementing a calorie count. Correlate baseline nutritional intake with medical status. Consider individual and cultural food preferences. Collaborate with HCP, pharmacist, and clinical dietitian in consideration of enteral and parenteral nutrition.

▶ Skin: Maintain mucous membrane and skin integrity; provide oral care; reposition every 2 hr or more frequent as needed.

Safety Considerations

▶ Confusion can occur due to altered fluid and electrolytes as well as renal or hepatic disease. Correlate confusion with the need to reverse altered electrolytes and evaluate medications. Prevent falls and injury through appropriate use of postural support, bed alarm, or restraints. Consider pharmacological interventions.

Nutritional Considerations

▶ Increased uric acid levels may be associated with gout. Nutritional therapy may be appropriate for some patients identified as having gout. Educate the patient that foods high in oxalic acid include caffeinated beverages, raw blackberries, gooseberries, plums, whole-wheat bread, beets, carrots, beans, rhubarb, spinach, dry cocoa, and Ovaltine. Some fish, including anchovies, sardines, herring, mussels, codfish, scallops, trout and haddock, are high in purines. Meats, such as bacon, goose, turkey, veal, venison, and organ meats (hearts, kidneys, liver, oxtail, spleen, sweetbreads, and ox/cow lungs), are high in purines. Foods high in purines should be restricted. In other cases, the requesting HCP may not prescribe a low-purine or purine-restricted diet for treatment of gout because medications can control the condition easily and effectively.

Follow-Up, Evaluation, and Desired Outcomes

▶ Acknowledges the value of lifestyle alterations that may improve health.

U

Urinalysis

SYNONYM/ACRONYM: UA.

RATIONALE: To screen urine for multiple markers to assist in diagnosing disorders such as kidney and liver disease as well as to assess hydration status.

PATIENT PREPARATION: There are no food, fluid, activity, or medication restrictions unless by medical direction. As appropriate, provide the required urine collection container and specimen collection instructions.

NORMAL FINDINGS: Method: Macroscopic evaluation by dipstick and microscopic examination. Urinalysis comprises a battery of tests including a description of the color and appearance of urine; measurement of specific gravity and pH; and semiquantitative measurement of protein, glucose, ketones, urobilinogen, bilirubin, hemoglobin (Hgb), nitrites, and leukocyte esterase. Urine sediment may also be examined for the presence of crystals, casts, renal epithelial cells, transitional epithelial cells, squamous epithelial cells, white blood cells (WBCs), red blood cells (RBCs), bacteria, yeast, sperm, and any other substances excreted in the urine that may have clinical significance. Examination of urine sediment is performed microscopically under high power, and results are reported as the number seen per high-power field (hpf). The color of normal urine ranges from light yellow to deep amber. The color depends on the patient's state of hydration (more concentrated samples are darker in color), diet, medication regimen, and exposure to other substances that may contribute to unusual color or odor. The appearance of normal urine is clear. Cloudiness is sometimes attributable to the presence of amorphous phosphates or urates as well as blood, WBCs, fat, or bacteria.

Dipstick

pH	4.5–8
Protein	Less than 20 mg/dL
Glucose	Negative
Ketones	Negative
Hemoglobin	Negative
Bilirubin	Negative
Urobilinogen	Up to 1 mg/dL
Nitrite	Negative
Leukocyte esterase	Negative
Specific gravity	1.005–1.03

Microscopic Examination

RBCs	Less than 5/hpf
WBCs	Less than 5/hpf
Renal cells	None seen
Transitional cells	None seen

U

Squamous cells	Rare; usually no clinical significance
Casts	Rare hyaline; otherwise, none seen
Crystals in acid urine	Uric acid, calcium oxalate, amorphous urates
Crystals in alkaline urine	Triple phosphate, calcium phosphate, ammonium biurate, calcium carbonate, amorphous phosphates
Bacteria, yeast, parasites	None seen

CRITICAL FINDINGS AND POTENTIAL INTERVENTIONS

Possible critical findings are the presence of uric acid, cystine, leucine, or tyrosine crystals.

The combination of grossly elevated urine glucose and ketones is also considered significant.

Timely notification to the requesting health-care provider (HCP) of any critical findings and related symptoms is a role expectation of the professional nurse. A listing of these findings varies among facilities.

OVERVIEW: (**Study type:** Urine, from an unpreserved, random specimen collected in a clean plastic collection container; **related body system:** Urinary system.) Routine urinalysis, one of the most widely ordered laboratory procedures, is used for basic screening purposes. It is a group of tests that evaluate the kidneys' ability to selectively excrete and reabsorb substances while maintaining proper water balance. The results can provide valuable information regarding the overall health of the patient and the patient's response to disease and treatment. The urine dipstick has a number of pads on it to indicate various biochemical markers. Urine pH is an indication of the kidneys' ability to help maintain balanced hydrogen ion concentration in the blood. Specific gravity is a reflection of the concentration ability of the kidneys. Urine protein is the most common indicator of kidney disease, although there are conditions that can cause benign proteinuria. Glucose is used as an indicator of diabetes. The presence of ketones indicates impaired carbohydrate metabolism. Hemoglobin indicates the presence of blood, which is associated with kidney disease. Bilirubin is used to assist in the detection of liver disorders. Urobilinogen indicates hepatic or hematopoietic conditions. Nitrites and leukocytes are used to test for bacteriuria and other sources of urinary tract infections (UTIs). Most laboratories have established criteria for the microscopic examination of urine based on patient population (e.g., pediatric, oncology, urology), unusual appearance, and biochemical reactions.

INDICATIONS

- Determine the presence of a genitourinary infection or abnormality.
- Monitor the effects of physical or emotional stress.
- Monitor fluid imbalances or treatment for fluid imbalances.
- Monitor the response to drug therapy and evaluate undesired reactions to drugs that may impair renal function.
- Provide screening as part of a general physical examination, especially on admission to a health-care facility or before surgery.

INTERFERING FACTORS

Factors that may alter the results of the study

- Certain foods, such as onion, garlic, and asparagus, contain substances that may give urine an unusual odor. An ammonia-like odor may be produced by the presence of bacteria. Urine with a maple syrup–like odor may indicate a congenital metabolic defect (maple syrup urine disease).
- The various biochemical strips are subject to interference that may produce false-positive or false-negative results. Consult the laboratory for specific information regarding limitations of the method in use and a listing of interfering drugs.
- The dipstick method for protein detection is mostly sensitive to the presence of albumin; light-chain or Bence Jones proteins may not be detected by this method. Alkaline pH may produce false-positive protein results.
- Large amounts of ketones or ascorbic acid may produce false-negative or decreased color development on the glucose pad. Contamination of the collection container or specimen with chlorine, sodium hypochlorite, or peroxide may cause false-positive glucose results.
- False-positive ketone results may be produced in the presence of ascorbic acid, levodopa metabolites, valproic acid, phenazopyridine, phenylketones, or phthaleins.
- The Hgb pad may detect myoglobin, intact RBCs, and free Hgb. Contamination of the collection container or specimen with sodium hypochlorite or iodine may cause false-positive Hgb results. Negative or decreased Hgb results may occur in the presence of formalin, elevated protein, nitrite, ascorbic acid, or high specific gravity.
- False-negative nitrite results are common. Negative or decreased results may be seen in the presence of ascorbic acid and high specific gravity. Other causes of false-negative values relate to the amount of time the urine was in the bladder before voiding or the presence of pathogenic organisms that do not reduce nitrates to nitrites.
- False-positive leukocyte esterase reactions result from specimens contaminated by vaginal secretions. The presence of high glucose, protein, or ascorbic acid concentrations may cause false-negative results. Specimens with high specific gravity may also produce false-negative results. Patients with neutropenia (e.g., oncology patients) may also have false-negative results because they do not produce enough WBCs to exceed the sensitivity of the biochemical reaction.
- Specimens that cannot be delivered to the laboratory or tested within 1 hr should be refrigerated or should have a preservative added that is recommended by the laboratory. Specimens collected more than 2 hr before submission may be rejected for analysis.
- Because changes in the urine specimen occur over time, prompt and proper specimen processing, storage, and analysis are important to achieve accurate results. Changes that may occur over time include:
  Production of a stronger odor and an increase in pH (bacteria in the urine break urea down to ammonia)
  A decrease in clarity (as bacterial growth proceeds or precipitates form)
  A decrease in bilirubin and urobilinogen (oxidation to biliverdin and urobilin)
  A decrease in ketones (lost through volatilization)
  Decreased glucose (consumed by bacteria)
  An increase in bacteria (growth over time)
  Disintegration of casts, WBCs, and RBCs
  An increase in nitrite (overgrowth of bacteria)

POTENTIAL MEDICAL DIAGNOSIS: CLINICAL SIGNIFICANCE OF RESULTS

Unusual Color

Color	Presence Of
Deep yellow	Riboflavin
Orange	Bilirubin, chrysophanic acid (e.g., rhubarb), phenazopyridine, santonin
Pink	Beet pigment, Hgb, myoglobin, porphyrin, rhubarb
Red	Beet pigment, Hgb, myoglobin, porphyrin, uroerythrin
Green	Oxidized bilirubin, Clorets (breath mint)
Blue	Diagnex, indican, methylene blue
Brown	Bilirubin, hematin, methemoglobin, metronidazole, nitrofurantoin, metabolites of rhubarb, senna
Black	Homogentisic acid, melanin
Smoky	RBCs

Test	Increased In	Decreased In
pH	Ingestion of citrus fruits	Ingestion of cranberries
	Vegetarian diets	High-protein diets
	Metabolic and respiratory alkalosis	Metabolic or respiratory acidosis
Protein	Benign proteinuria owing to stress, physical exercise, exposure to cold, or standing	N/A
	Diabetic nephropathy	
	Glomerulonephritis	
	Nephrosis	
	Toxemia of pregnancy	
Glucose	Diabetes	N/A
Ketones	Diabetes	N/A
	Fasting	
	Fever	
	High-protein diets	
	Isopropanol intoxication	
	Postanesthesia period	
	Starvation	
	Vomiting	
Hgb	Diseases of the bladder	N/A
	Exercise (march hemoglobinuria)	
	Glomerulonephritis	
	Hemolytic anemia or other causes of hemolysis (e.g., drugs, parasites, transfusion reaction)	
	Malignancy	

(table continues on page 1202)

U

Test	Increased In	Decreased In
	Menstruation	
	Paroxysmal cold hemoglobinuria	
	Paroxysmal nocturnal hemoglobinuria	
	Pyelonephritis	
	Snake or spider bites	
	Trauma	
	Tuberculosis	
	Urinary tract infections	
	Urolithiasis	
Urobilinogen	Cirrhosis	Antibiotic therapy (suppresses normal intestinal flora)
	Heart failure	
	Hemolytic anemia	Obstruction of the bile duct
	Hepatitis	
	Infectious mononucleosis	
	Malaria	
	Pernicious anemia	
Bilirubin	Cirrhosis	N/A
	Hepatic tumor	
	Hepatitis	
Nitrites	Presence of nitrite-forming bacteria (e.g., *Citrobacter, Enterobacter, Escherichia coli, Klebsiella, Proteus, Pseudomonas, Salmonella,* and some species of *Staphylococcus*)	N/A
Leukocyte esterase	Bacterial infection	N/A
	Calculus formation	
	Fungal or parasitic infection	
	Glomerulonephritis	
	Interstitial nephritis	
	Tumor	
Specific gravity	Adrenal insufficiency	Diuresis
	Dehydration	Excess IV fluids
	Diabetes	Excess hydration
	Diarrhea	Hypothermia
	Fever	Impaired renal concentrating ability
	Heart failure	
	Proteinuria	
	Sweating	
	Vomiting	
	Water restriction	
	X-ray dyes	

U

Formed Elements in Urine Sediment

Cellular Elements

- Clue cells (cell wall of the bacteria causes adhesion to epithelial cells) are present in nonspecific vaginitis caused by *Gardnerella vaginitis, Mobiluncus curtisii,* and *M. mulieris.*
- RBCs are present in glomerulonephritis, lupus nephritis, focal glomerulonephritis, calculus, malignancy, infection, tuberculosis, infarction, renal vein thrombosis, trauma, hydronephrosis, polycystic kidney, urinary tract disease, prostatitis, pyelonephritis, appendicitis, salpingitis, diverticulitis, gout, scurvy, subacute bacterial endocarditis, infectious mononucleosis, hemoglobinopathies, coagulation disorders, heart failure, and malaria.
- Renal cells that have absorbed cholesterol and triglycerides are also known as *oval fat bodies.*
- Renal cells come from the lining of the collecting ducts, and increased numbers indicate acute tubular damage, as seen in acute tubular necrosis, pyelonephritis, malignant nephrosclerosis, acute glomerulonephritis, acute drug or substance (salicylate, lead, or ethylene glycol) intoxication, or chemotherapy, resulting in desquamation, urolithiasis, and kidney transplant rejection.
- Squamous cells line the vagina and distal portion of the urethra. The presence of normal squamous epithelial cells in female urine is generally of no clinical significance. Abnormal cells with enlarged nuclei indicate the need for cytological studies to rule out malignancy.
- Transitional cells line the renal pelvis, ureter, bladder, and proximal portion of the urethra. Increased numbers are seen with infection, trauma, and malignancy.
- WBCs are present in acute UTI, tubulointerstitial nephritis, lupus nephritis, pyelonephritis, kidney transplant rejection, fever, and strenuous exercise.

Casts

- Granular casts are formed from protein or by the decomposition of cellular elements. They may be seen in kidney disease, viral infections, or lead intoxication.
- Large numbers of hyaline casts may be seen in kidney diseases, hypertension, heart failure, or nephrotic syndrome and in more benign conditions such as fever, exposure to cold temperatures, exercise, or diuretic use.
- RBC casts may be found in acute glomerulonephritis, lupus nephritis, and subacute bacterial endocarditis.
- Waxy casts are seen in chronic kidney disease or conditions such as kidney transplant rejection, in which there is renal stasis.
- WBC casts may be seen in lupus nephritis, acute glomerulonephritis, interstitial nephritis, and acute pyelonephritis.

Crystals

- Crystals found in freshly voided urine have more clinical significance than crystals seen in a urine sample that has been standing for more than 2 to 4 hr.
- Calcium oxalate crystals are found in ethylene glycol poisoning, urolithiasis, high dietary intake of oxalates, and Crohn disease.

U

- Cystine crystals are seen in patients with cystinosis or cystinuria.
- Leucine or tyrosine crystals may be seen in patients with severe liver disease.
- Large numbers of uric acid crystals are seen in patients with urolithiasis, gout, high dietary intake of

foods rich in purines, or who are receiving chemotherapy (see study titled "Uric Acid, Urine").

Yeast
- Yeast cells, usually *Candida albicans,* may be seen in diabetes and vaginal moniliasis.

NURSING IMPLICATIONS

POTENTIAL NURSING PROBLEMS: ASSESSMENT & NURSING DIAGNOSIS

Problems	Signs and Symptoms
Confusion *(related to an alteration in fluid and electrolytes secondary to hepatic disease and encephalopathy, acute alcohol consumption, hepatic metabolic insufficiency)*	Disorganized thinking; restlessness; irritability; altered concentration and attention span; changeable mental function over the day; hallucinations; inability to follow directions; disoriented to person, place, time, and purpose; inappropriate affect
Fluid volume (water) *(related to hypovolemia associated with body fluid shifts to third space, body fluid loss, reduced oral intake; increased perspiration; diaphoresis; gastrointestinal [GI] tract loss from vomiting, diarrhea; overly aggressive diuresis)*	**Deficit:** Decreased urinary output, fatigue, sunken eyes, dark urine, decreased blood pressure, increased heart rate, and altered mental status
Kidney function *(related to renal ischemia associated with shock, sepsis, hypovolemia; postoperative injury; trauma; nephrotoxic drugs [aminoglycoside, heavy metals, radiographic contrast]; renal vascular occlusion; hemolytic transfusion reaction; decreased cardiac output; tubular necrosis; obstruction; tumor; medications [NSAIDs, angiotensin-converting enzyme, immunosuppressants, antineoplastics, antifungals])*	Increased BUN, increased Cr, decreased Cr clearance, increased urine specific gravity (greater than 1.029), hematuria, proteinuria, decreased urine output less than 400 mL/day (with adequate intake and no fluid loss), weight gain, elevated potassium, elevated phosphate, decreased calcium, decreased sodium, increased magnesium, metabolic acidosis, decreased Hgb/Hct

BEFORE THE STUDY: PLANNING AND IMPLEMENTATION

Teaching the Patient What to Expect
- Inform the patient this test can assist in assessing for disease, infection,

and inflammation and evaluate for dehydration.
- Explain that a urine sample is needed for the test. If a catheterized specimen is to be collected, explain this procedure to the patient, and obtain a catheterization tray.

U

Information regarding specimen collection is presented with other general guidelines in Appendix A: Patient Preparation and Specimen Collection.

Potential Nursing Actions

Include on the collection container's label the specimen collection type (e.g. clean catch, catheter), date and time of collection, and any medications that may interfere with test results.

Promptly transport the specimen to the laboratory for processing and analysis.

AFTER THE STUDY: POTENTIAL NURSING ACTIONS

Avoiding Complications

Instruct the patient to report symptoms such as pain related to tissue inflammation, pain or irritation during void, bladder spasms, or alterations in urinary elimination.

Observe/assess for signs of inflammation if the specimen is obtained by suprapubic aspiration.

Treatment Considerations

Fluid Volume: Establish baseline assessment data. Manage underlying cause of fluid alteration. Record accurate intake and output. Monitor urine characteristics and respiratory status. Collaborate to adjust oral and IV fluids to provide optimal hydration status.

Monitor laboratory values that reflect alterations in fluid status; potassium, BUN, Cr, calcium, Hgb, and Hct.

Kidney Function: Monitor, record, and trend intake and output and daily weight. Monitor and trend urine specific gravity, BUN, Cr, sodium, potassium, magnesium, pH, urinalysis, and Hgb/Hct. Assess and monitor for edema, jugular vein distention, hypertension, adventitious breath sounds, and impaired gas exchange. Administer prescribed oxygen, fluids, diuretics; consider renal function with antibiotic administration. Facilitate ordered hemodialysis.

Safety Considerations

Confusion can occur due to altered fluid and electrolytes, acute alcohol consumption, as well as renal or hepatic disease. Correlate confusion with the need to reverse altered electrolytes and evaluate medications. Prevent falls and injury through appropriate use of postural support, bed alarm, or restraints. Consider pharmacological interventions.

Follow-Up, Evaluation, and Desired Outcomes

Understands the importance of completing prescribed medications such as antibiotic therapy even if symptoms are no longer present.

Uterine Fibroid Embolization

SYNONYM/ACRONYM: UFE; uterine artery embolization.

RATIONALE: A less invasive modality used to assist in treating fibroid tumors found in the uterine lining, heavy menstrual bleeding, and pelvic pain.

PATIENT PREPARATION: There are no activity restrictions unless by medical direction. Instruct the patient to fast and restrict fluids for 8 hr, or as ordered, prior to the procedure. Fasting may be ordered as a precaution against aspiration related to possible nausea and vomiting. The American Society of Anesthesiologists has fasting guidelines for risk levels according to patient status. More information can be located at www.asahq.org.

Note: If iodinated contrast medium is scheduled to be used in patients receiving metformin or drugs containing metformin for type 2 diabetes, the

U

drug may be discontinued on the day of the test and continue to be withheld for 48 hr after the test.

Regarding the patient's risk for bleeding, the patient should be instructed to avoid taking natural products and medications with known anticoagulant, antiplatelet, or thrombolytic properties or to reduce dosage, as ordered, prior to the procedure. Number of days to withhold medication is dependent on the type of anticoagulant. Note the last time and dose of medication taken.

Patients on beta blockers before the surgical procedure should be instructed to take their medication as ordered during the perioperative period. Protocols may vary among facilities.

NORMAL FINDINGS
- Decrease in uterine bleeding
- Decrease of pelvic pain or fullness.

CRITICAL FINDINGS AND POTENTIAL INTERVENTIONS: N/A

OVERVIEW: (Study type: X-ray Special/Contrast; **related body system:** Reproductive system.) Uterine fibroid embolization (UFE) is a way of treating fibroid tumors of the uterus. Fibroid tumors, also known as *myomas,* are masses of fibrous and muscle tissue in the uterine wall that are benign but that may cause heavy menstrual bleeding, pain in the pelvic region, or pressure on the bladder or bowel. Using angiographic methods, a catheter is placed in each of the two uterine arteries, and small particles are injected to block the arterial branches that supply blood to the fibroids. The fibroid tissue dies, the mass shrinks, and the symptoms are relieved. This procedure, which is done under local anesthesia, is less invasive than open surgery done to remove uterine fibroids. Because the effects of uterine fibroid embolization on fertility are not yet known, the ideal candidate is a premenopausal woman with symptoms from fibroid tumors who no longer wishes to become pregnant. This technique is an alternative for women who do not want to receive blood transfusions or do not wish to receive general anesthesia. This procedure may be used to halt severe bleeding following childbirth or caused by gynecological tumors.

INDICATIONS
- Treatment for anemia from chronic blood loss.
- Treatment of fibroid tumors and tumor vascularity, for both single and multiple tumors.
- Treatment of tumors in lieu of surgical resection.

INTERFERING FACTORS
Contraindications

Patients who are pregnant or suspected of being pregnant, unless the potential benefits of a procedure using radiation far outweigh the risk of radiation exposure to the fetus and mother.

Patients with conditions associated with adverse reactions to contrast medium (e.g., asthma, food allergies, or allergy to contrast medium). Although patients are asked specifically if they have a known allergy to iodine or shellfish (shellfish contain high levels of iodine), it has been well established that the reaction is not to iodine; an actual iodine allergy would be problematic because iodine is required for the production of thyroid hormones. In the case of shellfish, the reaction is to a muscle protein called *tropomyosin;* in the case of iodinated contrast medium, the reaction is to the noniodinated part of the contrast molecule. Patients with a known hypersensitivity to the medium may benefit from premedication with corticosteroids and diphenhydramine; the use of nonionic contrast or an alternative noncontrast imaging study, if available, may be considered for patients who have severe asthma or who have experienced moderate to severe reactions to ionic contrast medium.

✸ Patients with conditions associated with preexisting renal insufficiency (e.g., chronic kidney disease, single kidney transplant, nephrectomy, diabetes, multiple myeloma, treatment with aminoglycosides and NSAIDs), *because iodinated contrast is nephrotoxic.*

✸ Patients who are chronically dehydrated before the test, especially older adults and patients whose health is already compromised, *because of their risk of contrast-induced acute kidney injury.*

✸ Patients with bleeding disorders, *because the puncture site may not stop bleeding.*

✸ Patients in whom cancer is a possibility or who have inflammation or infection in the pelvis.

Factors that may alter the results of the study
- Gas or feces in the gastrointestinal tract resulting from inadequate cleansing or failure to restrict food intake before the study.
- Retained barium from a previous radiological procedure.
- Metallic objects (e.g., jewelry, body rings) within the examination field, which may inhibit organ visualization and cause unclear images.

Other considerations
- A small percentage of women may pass a small piece of fibroid tissue

after the procedure. Women with this problem may require a procedure called a D & C (dilatation and curettage).
- Some women may experience menopause shortly after the procedure.

POTENTIAL MEDICAL DIAGNOSIS: CLINICAL SIGNIFICANCE OF RESULTS

Abnormal findings related to
- No reduction in size of fibroid

NURSING IMPLICATIONS

BEFORE THE STUDY: PLANNING AND IMPLEMENTATION

Teaching the Patient What to Expect
▶ Inform the patient this procedure can assist in assessing and treating the uterus.
▶ Review the procedure with the patient.
▶ Address concerns about pain and explain that there may be moments of discomfort and some pain experienced during the test.
▶ Explain that a sedative and/or anesthetic may be administered before the procedure to promote relaxation.
▶ Explain that the procedure is performed in a radiology or vascular department by a health-care provider (HCP), with support staff, and takes approximately 30 to 120 min.
▶ Advise the patient that prior to the procedure, laboratory testing may be required to determine the possibility of bleeding risk (coagulation testing) or to assess for impaired kidney function (creatinine level and estimated glomerular filtration rate) if use of iodinated contrast medium is anticipated.
▶ Pregnancy is a general contraindication to procedures involving radiation. Explain to the female patient that she will be asked the date of her last menstrual period and pregnancy testing may be performed to determine the possibility of pregnancy before she is exposed to radiation.
▶ Explain that an IV line may be inserted to allow infusion of fluids such as

U

saline, anesthetics, sedatives, or emergency medications. Explain that the contrast medium will be injected, by catheter, at a separate site from the IV line.

▶ Inform the patient that a burning and flushing sensation may be felt throughout the body during injection of the contrast medium and they may experience an urge to cough, flushing, nausea, or a salty or metallic taste.

▶ Instruct the patient to remove jewelry and other metallic objects from the area to be examined prior to the procedure.

▶ Baseline vital signs and neurological status are completed and recorded. Protocols may vary among facilities.

▶ Explain that electrocardiographic electrodes are placed for cardiac monitoring, establish baseline rhythm, and to determine the presence of any ventricular dysrhythmias.

▶ Using a pen, mark the site of the patient's peripheral pulses before angiography; this allows for quicker and more consistent assessment of the pulses after the procedure.

▶ Positioning for this procedure is in the supine position on an examination table. The selected areas are cleansed and covered with a sterile drape.

▶ Explain that once the contrast medium is injected, a rapid series of images is taken during and after the filling of the vessels to be examined. Delayed images may be taken to examine the vessels after a time and to monitor the venous phase of the procedure.

▶ Advise the patient that she will be asked to inhale deeply and hold her breath while the x-ray images are taken, and then asked to exhale after the images are taken.

▶ Advise the patient to take slow, deep breaths if nausea occurs during the procedure. An ordered antiemetic drug can be administered as needed. An emesis basin can be ready for use.

▶ Explain that particles are injected through the catheter to block the blood flow to the fibroids. The particles include polyvinyl alcohol, gelatin sponge (Gelfoam), and micospheres.

▶ Once the needle or catheter is removed, a pressure dressing is applied over the puncture site.

Potential Nursing Actions

✦ *Make sure a written and informed consent has been signed prior to the procedure and before administering any medications.*

▶ If iodinated contrast medium is scheduled to be used in patients receiving metformin or drugs containing metformin for type 2 diabetes, the drug may be discontinued on the day of the test and continue to be withheld for 48 hr after the test. Protocols may vary among facilities.

Safety Considerations

▶ Anticoagulants, aspirin, and other salicylates should be discontinued by medical direction for the appropriate number of days prior to a procedure where bleeding is a potential complication.

AFTER THE STUDY: POTENTIAL NURSING ACTIONS

Avoiding Complications

▶ Establishing an IV site and injection of contrast medium are invasive procedures. Complications are rare but include risk for allergic reaction *(related to contrast reaction);* bleeding from the puncture site *(related to a bleeding disorder or the effects of natural products and medications with known anticoagulant, antiplatelet, or thrombolytic properties);* blood clot formation *(related to thrombus formation on the tip of the catheter sheath surface or in the lumen of the catheter; the use of a heparinized saline flush during the procedure decreases the risk of emboli);* cardiac dysrhythmias; detachment of small pieces of fibroid tissue during UFE, which will pass, but a D & C may be required to verify that all material is removed to prevent further bleeding or infection; the occurrence of menopause following UFE, which is generally experienced in women older than 45 yr of age; hematoma *(related to blood leakage into the tissue following needle insertion);* infection *(which might occur if bacteria from the skin surface is introduced at the puncture site);* nerve injury *(which might occur if the needle strikes a nerve);* neph-rotoxicity *(a deterioration of renal function associated with contrast administration);* or tissue damage *(related to extravasation, leaking of contrast into the tissues).* Monitor the patient for complications related to the procedure (e.g., allergic reaction, anaphylaxis, bronchospasm, infection, injury). Immediately report symptoms such as difficulty breathing, chest pain, fever, hyperpnea, hypertension, nausea, palpitations, pruritus, rash, tachycardia, urticaria, or vomiting to the appropriate HCP. Observe/assess the needle/catheter insertion site for bleeding, inflammation, or hematoma formation. Administer ordered antihistamines or prophylactic steroids if the patient has an allergic reaction.

Treatment Considerations

▶ Instruct the patient to resume usual diet, fluids, medications, or activity, as directed by the HCP. Kidney function should be assessed before metformin is resumed.

▶ Monitor vital signs and neurological status every 15 min for 1 hr, then every 2 hr for 4 hr, and then as ordered by the HCP. Take temperature every 4 hr for 24 hr. Monitor intake and output at least every 8 hr. Compare with baseline values. Protocols may vary among facilities.

▶ Inform the patient that she may experience pelvic cramps for several days after the procedure and possible mild nausea and fever.

▶ Assess extremities for signs of ischemia or absence of distal pulse caused by a catheter-induced thrombus.

▶ Instruct the patient in the care and assessment of the injection site.

▶ Instruct the patient to apply cold compresses to the puncture site as needed, to reduce discomfort or edema.

Safety Considerations

▶ Advise diabetic patients to avoid all medications containing metformin for 48 hr following a procedure with iodinated contrast. Iodinated contrast can temporarily impair kidney function, and failure to withhold metformin may indirectly result in drug-induced lactic acidosis, a dangerous and sometimes fatal adverse effect of metformin (related to renal impairment that does not support sufficient excretion of metformin).

Follow-Up, Evaluation, and Desired Outcomes

▶ Acknowledges the importance of adhering to the therapy regimen.

▶ Understands the significant adverse effects associated with the prescribed medication and agrees to review corresponding literature provided by a pharmacist.

U

Vanillylmandelic Acid, Urine

SYNONYM/ACRONYM: VMA.

RATIONALE: To assist in the diagnosis and follow up treatment of pheochromo-cytoma, neuroblastoma, and ganglioblastoma. This test can also be useful in evaluation and follow-up of hypertension.

PATIENT PREPARATION: There are no fluid restrictions unless by medical direction. Instruct the patient to abstain from smoking tobacco for 24 hr before testing. Usually, a 24-hr urine collection is ordered. As appropriate, provide the required urine collection container and specimen collection instructions. Inform the patient of the following dietary, medication, and activity restrictions in preparation for the test (protocols may vary among facilities):

The patient should not consume foods high in amines (bananas, avocados, beer, aged cheese, chocolate, cocoa, coffee, fava beans, grains, tea, vanilla, walnuts, and red wine) for 48 hr before testing.

The patient should not consume foods or fluids high in caffeine (coffee, tea, cocoa, and chocolate) for 48 hr before testing.

The patient should not consume any foods or fluids containing vanilla or licorice.

The patient should avoid self-prescribed medications (especially aspirin) and prescribed medications (especially pyridoxine, levodopa, amoxicillin, carbidopa, reserpine, and disulfiram) for 2 wk before testing and as directed.

The patient should avoid excessive exercise and stress during the 24-hr collection of urine.

NORMAL FINDINGS: Method: High-pressure liquid chromatography.

Age	Conventional Units	SI Units (Conventional Units × 5.05)
3–6 yr	Less than 2.6 mg/24 hr	Less than 13 micromol/24 hr
7–10 yr	Less than 3.2 mg/24 hr	Less than 16 micromol/24 hr
11–16 yr	Less than 5.2 mg/24 hr	Less than 26 micromol/24 hr
17–83 yr	Less than 6.5 mg/24 hr	Less than 33 micromol/24 hr

CRITICAL FINDINGS AND POTENTIAL INTERVENTIONS: N/A

OVERVIEW: (Study type: Urine, from a timed specimen collected in a clean plastic collection container with 6N hydrochloric acid as a preservative; **related body system:** Endocrine system.) Vanillyl-mandelic acid (VMA) is a major metabolite of epinephrine and norepinephrine. It is elevated in conditions that also are marked by over production of catecholamines. Creatinine is usually measured simultaneously to ensure adequate collection and to calculate an excretion ratio of metabolite to creatinine.

INDICATIONS
- Assist in the diagnosis of neuroblastoma, ganglioneuroma, or pheochromocytoma.
- Evaluate hypertension of unknown cause.

INTERFERING FACTORS

Factors that may alter the results of the study

- Drugs and other substances that may increase VMA levels include ajmaline, chlorpromazine, glucagon, guaifenesin, guanethidine, isoproterenol, methyldopa, nitroglycerin, oxytetracycline, phenazopyridine, phenolsulfonphthalein, prochlorperazine, rauwolfia, reserpine, and sulfobromophthalein.
- Drugs and other substances that may decrease VMA levels include brofaromine, guanethidine, guanfacine, imipramine, isocarboxazid, methyldopa, monoamine oxidase inhibitors, morphine, nialamide (in patients with schizophrenia), and reserpine.
- Stress, hypoglycemia, hyperthyroidism, strenuous exercise, smoking, and drugs can produce elevated VMA.
- All urine voided for the timed collection period must be included in the collection or else falsely decreased values may be obtained. Compare output records with volume collected to verify that all voids were included in the collection.

POTENTIAL MEDICAL DIAGNOSIS: CLINICAL SIGNIFICANCE OF RESULTS

Increased in

Catecholamine-secreting tumors will cause an increase in VMA.

- Ganglioneuroma
- Hypertension secondary to pheochromocytoma
- Neuroblastoma
- Pheochromocytoma

Decreased in: N/A

NURSING IMPLICATIONS

BEFORE THE STUDY: PLANNING AND IMPLEMENTATION

Teaching the Patient What to Expect

◗ Inform the patient this test can assist in evaluating or the presence of endocrine tumors
◗ Explain that a urine sample is needed for the test. Information regarding specimen collection is presented with other general guidelines in Appendix A: Patient Preparation and Specimen Collection.

Potential Nursing Actions

◗ Include on the collection container's label urine total volume, test start and stop times/dates, and any medications that may interfere with test results.

AFTER THE STUDY: POTENTIAL NURSING ACTIONS

Treatment Considerations

◗ Instruct the patient to resume usual diet, fluids, medications, and activity, as directed by the health-care provider (HCP).
◗ Over-the-counter medications should be taken only under the advice of the patient's HCP.

Follow-Up, Evaluation, and Desired Outcomes

◗ Understands that depending on the results of this procedure, additional testing may be performed to evaluate disease progression and determine the need for a change in therapy.

Varicella Testing

SYNONYM/ACRONYM: Varicella-zoster antibodies, chickenpox, VZ.

RATIONALE: To assist in diagnosing chickenpox or shingles related to a varicella-zoster infection and to assess for immunity.

V

PATIENT PREPARATION: There are no food, fluid, activity, or medication restrictions unless by medical direction.

NORMAL FINDINGS: Method: Enzyme immunoassay.

	IgM and IgG	Interpretation
Negative	0.89 index or less	No significant level of detectable antibody
Indeterminate	0.9–1 index	Equivocal results; retest in 10–14 days
Positive	1.1 index or greater	Antibody detected; indicative of recent immunization, current or recent infection

CRITICAL FINDINGS AND POTENTIAL INTERVENTIONS: N/A

OVERVIEW: (**Study type:** Blood collected in a gold-, red-, or red/gray-top tube; **related body system:** Immune and Reproductive systems.) Varicella-zoster is a double-stranded DNA herpes virus that is responsible for two clinical syndromes: chickenpox and shingles. The incubation period for varicella infection is 2 to 3 wk, and it is highly contagious for about 2 wk beginning 2 days before a rash develops. It is transmitted via respiratory secretions and by direct contact with the secretions inside. Painful eruptions appear on the skin and mucus membranes. The primary exposure to the highly contagious virus usually occurs in susceptible school-age children. Adults without prior exposure and who become infected may have severe complications, including pneumonia. Neonatal infection from the mother is possible if exposure occurs during the last 3 wk of gestation. The second syndrome, shingles, results when the presumably latent virus is reactivated and produces painful skin eruptions along nerve tracks. In both syndromes, the presence of immunoglobulin (Ig) M antibodies indicates acute infection and the presence of IgG antibodies indicates current or past infection. A reactive varicella antibody result indicates immunity but does not protect an individual from shingles. There are also polymerase chain reaction methods that can detect varicella-zoster DNA in various specimen types.

INDICATIONS
• Determine susceptibility or immunity to chickenpox.

INTERFERING FACTORS: N/A

POTENTIAL MEDICAL DIAGNOSIS: CLINICAL SIGNIFICANCE OF RESULTS
Positive findings in
• Varicella infection

Negative findings in: N/A

NURSING IMPLICATIONS

POTENTIAL NURSING PROBLEMS: ASSESSMENT & NURSING DIAGNOSIS

Problems	Signs and Symptoms
Infection *(related to exposure to Varicella zoster)*	Headache, fever, malaise, blister rash, chills, nausea, pain and tingling at area of rash before appearance, itching, open sores, loss of appetite
Fluid volume (water) *(related to inadequate fluid intake secondary to nausea and altered appetite associated with varicella infection)*	Hypotension, decreased cardiac output, decreased urinary output, dry skin/mucous membranes, poor skin turgor, sunken eyeballs, increased urine specific gravity, hemoconcentration
Pain *(related to altered nerve root function secondary to viral infection)*	Pain that is burning, stabbing, tearing
Skin *(related to itching secondary to varicella infection)*	Scratching with open sores, drainage from open sores

BEFORE THE STUDY: PLANNING AND IMPLEMENTATION

Teaching the Patient What to Expect

- Inform the patient this test can assist in assessing for a viral infection or immunity.
- Explain that a blood sample is needed for the test.
- Explain that several tests may be necessary to confirm the diagnosis. Any individual positive result should be repeated in 7 to 14 days to monitor a change in detectable levels of antibody.

AFTER THE STUDY: POTENTIAL NURSING ACTIONS

Treatment Considerations

- **Vaccination Considerations:** Record the date of last menstrual period and determine the possibility of pregnancy prior to administration of varicella vaccine to female varicella-nonimmune patients. Instruct patient not to become pregnant for 1 mo after being vaccinated with the varicella vaccine to protect any fetus from contracting the disease and having serious birth defects. Instruct on birth control methods to prevent pregnancy, if appropriate.

- Instruct the patient in isolation precautions during the time of communicability or contagion.
- Provide emotional support if results are positive and the patient is pregnant. Provide teaching and information regarding the clinical implications of the test results, as appropriate.
- Discuss the implications of abnormal test results on lifestyle choices.
- Provide education regarding access to counseling services.
- Infection: Encourage vaccination of all at-risk family members or friends. Administer ordered antiviral medication. Monitor and trend white blood cell count and temperature. Decrease exposure to noninfected individuals by limiting visitors and practicing vigilant handwashing. Keep infected individuals at home and prevent exposure to others from cough or touching infected fluids.
- Fluid Volume: Monitor intake and output, daily weight, and assess for symptoms of dehydration: dry skin, dry mucous membranes, poor skin turgor, or sunken eyeballs. Monitor and trend vital signs and for symptoms of poor cardiac output (rapid, weak, thready pulse). Collaborate with health-care

V

provider (HCP) on administration of IV fluids to support hydration. Monitor laboratory values that reflect alterations in fluid status: potassium, BUN, Cr, calcium, Hgb, Hct, and sodium. Monitor urine characteristics and respiratory status and establish baseline assessment data. Manage underlying cause of fluid alteration and collaborate with HCP to adjust oral and IV fluids to provide optimal hydration status. Administer replacement electrolytes as ordered.

▶ Pain: Inform the patient with shingles about access to pain management. Keep clothing or bedding from touching the affected area. Use a foot cradle as appropriate and assess and monitor the location, duration, and characteristics of pain. Explain the importance of pain medication and administer as prescribed. Teach how to apply antipruritic lotion (e.g., calamine) and discuss

the application of wet compresses to decrease itching. Consider the use of distraction and relaxation techniques as a pain management modality.

▶ Skin: Teach how to decrease the itch-scratch cycle; use warm water and pat dry rather than rub. Administer prescribed antipruritic creams or lotion.

Follow-Up, Evaluation, and Desired Outcomes

▶ Understands the importance of returning to have a convalescent blood sample taken in 7 to 14 days. Provide information regarding vaccine-preventable diseases where indicated (e.g., varicella).

▶ Acknowledges contact information provided for the Centers for Disease Control and Prevention (www.cdc.gov/vaccines/vpd/vaccines-diseases.html and www.cdc.gov/DiseasesConditions).

Venography, Lower Extremity Studies

SYNONYM/ACRONYM: Lower limb venography, phlebography, venogram.

RATIONALE: To visualize and assess the venous vasculature in the lower extremities related to diagnosis of deep vein thrombosis (DVT) and congenital anomalies.

PATIENT PREPARATION: There are no activity restrictions unless by medical direction. Instruct the patient to fast and restrict fluids for 8 hr, or as ordered, prior to the procedure. Fasting may be ordered as a precaution against aspiration related to possible nausea and vomiting. The American Society of Anesthesiologists has fasting guidelines for risk levels according to patient status. More information can be located at www.asahq.org.

Note: If iodinated contrast medium is scheduled to be used in patients receiving metformin or drugs containing metformin for type 2 diabetes, the drug may be discontinued on the day of the test and continue to be withheld for 48 hr after the test.

Regarding the patient's risk for bleeding, the patient should be instructed to avoid taking natural products and medications with known anticoagulant, antiplatelet, or thrombolytic properties or to reduce dosage, as ordered, prior to the procedure. Number of days to withhold medication is dependent on the type of anticoagulant. Note the last time and dose of medication taken. Protocols may vary among facilities.

NORMAL FINDINGS: No obstruction to flow and no filling defects after injection of radiopaque contrast medium; steady opacification of superficial and deep vasculature with no filling defects.

CRITICAL FINDINGS AND POTENTIAL INTERVENTIONS
- DVT
- Pulmonary embolism (PE)

Timely notification to the requesting health-care provider (HCP) of any critical findings and related symptoms is a role expectation of the professional nurse. A listing of these findings varies among facilities.

OVERVIEW: (Study type: X-ray, Special/Contrast; related body system: Circulatory system.) Venography allows x-ray visualization of the venous vasculature system of the extremities after injection of an iodinated contrast medium. Lower extremity studies identify and locate thrombi within the venous system of the lower limbs. After injection of the contrast medium, x-ray images are taken at timed intervals. Usually both extremities are studied, and the unaffected side is used for comparison with the side suspected of having DVT or other venous abnormalities, such as congenital malformations or incompetent valves. Thrombus formation usually occurs in the deep calf veins and at the venous junction and its valves. If DVT is not treated, it can lead to femoral and iliac venous occlusion, or the thrombus can become an embolus, causing a pulmonary embolism. Venography is accurate for identifying thrombi in veins below the knee.

INDICATIONS
- Assess deep vein valvular competence.
- Confirm a diagnosis of DVT.
- Determine the cause of extremity swelling or pain.
- Determine the source of emboli when PE is suspected or diagnosed.
- Distinguish clot formation from venous obstruction.
- Evaluate congenital venous malformations.
- Locate a vein for arterial bypass graft surgery.

INTERFERING FACTORS
Contraindications

Patients who are pregnant or suspected of being pregnant, unless the potential benefits of a procedure using radiation far outweigh the risk of radiation exposure to the fetus and mother.

Patients with conditions associated with adverse reactions to contrast medium (e.g., asthma, food allergies, or allergy to contrast medium). Although patients are asked specifically if they have a known allergy to iodine or shellfish (shellfish contain high levels of iodine), it has been well established that the reaction is not to iodine; an actual iodine allergy would be problematic because iodine is required for the production of thyroid hormones. In the case of shellfish, the reaction is to a muscle protein called *tropomyosin;* in the case of iodinated contrast medium, the reaction is to the noniodinated part of the contrast molecule. Patients with a known hypersensitivity to the medium may benefit from premedication with corticosteroids and diphenhydramine; the use of nonionic contrast or an alternative noncontrast imaging study, if available, may be considered for patients who have severe asthma or who have experienced moderate to severe reactions to ionic contrast medium.

Patients with conditions associated with preexisting renal insufficiency (e.g., chronic kidney disease, single kidney transplant, nephrectomy, diabetes, multiple myeloma, treatment with aminoglycosides and

NSAIDs), *because iodinated contrast is nephrotoxic.*

✦ Patients who are chronically dehydrated before the test, especially older adults and patients whose health is already compromised, *because of their risk of contrast-induced acute kidney injury.*

✦ Patients with bleeding disorders, because the puncture site may not stop bleeding.

✦ Patients with severe edema of the legs in whom venous access is not possible.

Factors that may alter the results of the study

• Movement of the leg being tested, excessive tourniquet constriction, insufficient injection of contrast medium, and delay between injection and the x-ray.

• Severe edema of the legs, making venous access impossible.

• Metallic objects (e.g., jewelry, body rings) within the examination field, which may inhibit organ visualization and cause unclear images.

• Inability of the patient to cooperate or remain still during the procedure, because movement can produce blurred or otherwise unclear images.

POTENTIAL MEDICAL DIAGNOSIS: CLINICAL SIGNIFICANCE OF RESULTS

Abnormal findings related to

• Deep vein valvular incompetence
• DVT
• PE
• Venous obstruction

NURSING IMPLICATIONS

BEFORE THE STUDY: PLANNING AND IMPLEMENTATION

Teaching the Patient What to Expect

♦ Inform the patient this procedure can assist in assessing the veins in the lower extremities.

♦ Explain that prior to the procedure, laboratory testing may be required to determine the possibility of bleeding risk (coagulation testing) or to assess for impaired kidney function (creatinine level and estimated glomerular filtration rate) if use of iodinated contrast medium is anticipated.

♦ Pregnancy is a general contraindication to procedures involving radiation. Explain to the female patient that she will be asked the date of her last menstrual period. Pregnancy testing may be performed to determine the possibility of pregnancy before exposure to radiation.

♦ Review the procedure with the patient. Address concerns about pain and explain that there may be moments of discomfort or pain experienced when the IV line or catheter is inserted to allow infusion of fluids such as saline, anesthetics, sedatives, contrast medium, medications used in the procedure, or emergency medications.

♦ Explain that contrast medium will be injected, by catheter, at a separate site from the IV line.

♦ Advise that a burning and flushing sensation may be felt throughout the body during injection of the contrast medium and they may experience an urge to cough, flushing, nausea, or a salty or metallic taste.

♦ Explain that the procedure is usually performed in a radiology or vascular suite by an HCP, with support staff, and takes approximately 30 to 60 min.

♦ Instruct the patient to remove jewelry and other metallic objects from the area of examination.

♦ Baseline vital signs are recorded and monitored throughout the procedure. Protocols may vary among facilities.

♦ Explain that electrocardiographic electrodes are placed for cardiac monitoring to establish a baseline rhythm and identify any ventricular dysrhythmias.

♦ Explain that peripheral pulses are marked with a pen before the venography, allowing for a quicker and more consistent assessment of the pulses after the procedure.

♦ Positioning for this procedure is in the supine position on an examination table. The selected area is cleansed and covered with a sterile drape.

▶ A local anesthetic is injected at the site, and a small incision is made or a needle inserted.

▶ Explain that contrast medium is injected, and a rapid series of images is taken during and after the filling of the vessels to be examined.

▶ Advise the patient that he or she will be instructed to inhale deeply, hold the breath while the x-ray images are taken, and then exhale.

▶ Advise taking slow, deep breaths if nausea occurs during the procedure. An ordered antiemetic drug can be administered as needed. An emesis basin can be ready for use.

▶ Explain to the patient that he or she will be monitored for complications related to the procedure (e.g., allergic reaction, anaphylaxis, bronchospasm).

▶ Explain that once the study is completed, the needle or catheter is removed, and a pressure dressing is applied over the puncture site.

Potential Nursing Actions

❖ *Make sure a written and informed consent has been signed prior to the procedure and before administering any medications.*

▶ If iodinated contrast medium is scheduled to be used in patients receiving metformin or drugs containing metformin for type 2 diabetes, the drug may be discontinued on the day of the test and continue to be withheld for 48 hr after the test. Protocols may vary among facilities

Safety Considerations

▶ Anticoagulants, aspirin, and other salicylates should be discontinued by medical direction for the appropriate number of days prior to a procedure where bleeding is a potential complication.

AFTER THE STUDY: POTENTIAL NURSING ACTIONS

Avoiding Complications

▶ Establishing an IV site and injection of contrast medium are invasive procedures. Complications are rare but include risk for allergic reaction *(related*

to contrast reaction), bleeding from the puncture site *(related to a bleeding disorder or the effects of natural products and medications with known anticoagulant, antiplatelet, or thrombolytic properties),* cellulitis or pain *(related to infiltration at the injection site),* hematoma *(related to blood leakage into the tissue following needle insertion),* infection *(which might occur if bacteria from the skin surface is introduced at the puncture site),* nerve injury *(which might occur if the needle strikes a nerve),* nephrotoxicity *(a deterioration of renal function associated with contrast administration),* venous thrombophlebitis *(that is caused by contrast),* or venous embolism *(related to dislodgement of a deep-vein clot).* Monitor the patient for complications related to the procedure (e.g., allergic reaction, anaphylaxis, bronchospasm, infection, injury). Immediately report symptoms such as difficulty breathing, chest pain, fever, hyperpnea, hypertension, nausea, palpitations, pruritus, rash, tachycardia, urticaria, or vomiting to the appropriate HCP. Observe/assess the needle/catheter insertion site for bleeding, inflammation, or hematoma formation. Administer ordered antihistamines or prophylactic steroids if the patient has an allergic reaction.

Treatment Considerations

▶ Instruct the patient to resume diet, fluids, and medications, as directed by the HCP. Kidney function should be assessed before metformin is resumed.

▶ Monitor vital signs and neurological status every 15 min for 1 hr, then every 2 hr for 4 hr, and then as ordered by the HCP. Take temperature every 4 hr for 24 hr. Monitor intake and output at least every 8 hr. Compare with baseline values. Notify the HCP if temperature is elevated. Protocols may vary among facilities.

▶ Instruct the patient to maintain bedrest for 4 to 6 hr after the procedure or as ordered.

▶ Provide instructions on the care and assessment of the procedure site.

▶ Explain the value of applying cold compresses to the puncture site as needed to reduce discomfort or edema.

Safety Considerations

▶ Advise diabetic patients to avoid all medications containing metformin for 48 hr following a procedure with iodinated contrast. Iodinated contrast can temporarily impair kidney function, and failure to withhold metformin may indirectly result in drug-induced lactic acidosis, a dangerous and sometimes fatal adverse effect of metformin (related to renal impairment that does not support sufficient excretion of metformin).

Follow-Up, Evaluation, and Desired Outcomes

▶ Understands that depending on the results of this procedure, additional testing may be needed to monitor disease progression and determine the need for a change in therapy. Evaluate test results in relation to the patient's symptoms and other tests performed.

Vertebroplasty

SYNONYM/ACRONYM: None.

RATIONALE: A minimally invasive procedure to treat the spine for disorders such as tumor, lesions, osteoporosis, and vertebral compression.

PATIENT PREPARATION: There are no activity restrictions unless by medical direction. Instruct the patient to fast and restrict fluids for 8 hr, or as ordered, prior to the procedure. Fasting may be ordered as a precaution against aspiration related to possible nausea and vomiting. The American Society of Anesthesiologists has fasting guidelines for risk levels according to patient status. More information can be located at www.asahq.org.

Note: If iodinated contrast medium is scheduled to be used in patients receiving metformin or drugs containing metformin for type 2 diabetes, the drug may be discontinued on the day of the test and continue to be withheld for 48 hr after the test.

Regarding the patient's risk for bleeding, the patient should be instructed to avoid taking natural products and medications with known anticoagulant, antiplatelet, or thrombolytic properties or to reduce dosage, as ordered, prior to the procedure. Number of days to withhold medication is dependent on the type of anticoagulant. Note the last time and dose of medication taken. Protocols may vary among facilities.

NORMAL FINDINGS

• Improvement in the ability to ambulate without pain
• Relief of back pain.

CRITICAL FINDINGS AND POTENTIAL INTERVENTIONS: N/A

OVERVIEW: (Study type: X-ray, plain; **related body system:** Musculoskeletal system.) Vertebroplasty is a minimally invasive, nonsurgical therapy used to repair a broken vertebra and to provide relief of pain related to vertebral compression in the spine that has been weakened by osteoporosis or tumoral lesions. Osteoporosis affects over 10 million women in the United States and accounts for over 700,000 vertebral fractures per year. This procedure is usually successful at alleviating the pain caused by a compression fracture less than 6 mo in duration with pain directly referable to the location of the fracture. Secondary benefits may include vertebra stabilization and reduction of the risk of further compression. Vertebroplasty involves the injection of an orthopedic cement mixture through a needle into a fracture site. The cement hardens, stabilizes the bone preventing further collapse, and reduces the pain caused by bone rubbing against bone. The injection is visualized with guidance from radiological imaging or fluoroscopy; a small amount of contrast (with or without iodine) may be used to provide imaged guidance for the injection of the cement. Vertebroplasty may be the preferred procedure when patients are older adults or too frail to tolerate open spinal surgery or if bones are too weak for surgical repair. Patients with a malignant tumor may benefit from vertebroplasty. Other possible applications include in younger patients whose osteoporosis is caused by long-term steroid use or a metabolic disorder. This procedure is recommended after basic treatments such as bedrest and orthopedic braces have failed or when pain medication has been ineffective or caused the patient medical problems, including stomach ulcers.

INDICATIONS

- Assist in the detection of nonmalignant tumors before surgical resection.
- Repair of compression spinal fractures of varying ages. Fractures older than 6 mo will respond but at a slower rate. Fractures less than 4 wk old should be given a chance to heal without intervention unless they are associated with disabling pain or hospitalization.
- Repair of spinal problems due to tumors.

INTERFERING FACTORS
Contraindications

Patients who are pregnant or suspected of being pregnant, unless the potential benefits of a procedure using radiation far outweigh the risk of radiation exposure to the fetus and mother.

Patients with conditions associated with adverse reactions to vertebroplasty cement.

Patients with conditions associated with adverse reactions to contrast medium (e.g., asthma, food allergies, or allergy to contrast medium). Although patients are asked specifically if they have a known allergy to iodine or shellfish (shellfish contain high levels of iodine), it has been well established that the reaction is not to iodine; an actual iodine allergy would be problematic because iodine is required for the production of thyroid hormones. In the case of shellfish, the reaction is to a muscle protein called *tropomyosin;* in the case of iodinated contrast medium, the reaction is to the noniodinated part of the contrast molecule. Patients with a known hypersensitivity to the medium may benefit from premedication with corticosteroids and diphenhydramine; the use of nonionic contrast or an alternative noncontrast imaging study, if available, may be considered for patients who have severe asthma or who have experienced moderate to severe reactions to ionic contrast medium.

Patients with conditions associated with preexisting renal insufficiency (e.g., chronic kidney disease, single kidney transplant, nephrectomy, diabetes, multiple myeloma, treatment with aminoglycosides and NSAIDs), *because iodinated contrast is nephrotoxic.*

◈ Patients who are chronically dehydrated before the test, especially older adults and patients whose health is already compromised, *because of their risk of contrast-induced acute kidney injury.*

◈ Patients with bleeding disorders receiving an arterial or venous puncture, *because the site may not stop bleeding.*

◈ Patients with pain that is primarily radicular in nature.

◈ Patients with pain that is improving or that has been present and unchanged for years.

◈ Patients who have undergone imaging procedures that suggest no fracture is present or that the fracture is remote from the patient's pain.

Factors that may alter the results of the study
• Gas or feces in the gastrointestinal tract resulting from inadequate cleansing or failure to restrict food intake before the study.
• Retained barium from a previous radiological procedure.
• Metallic objects (e.g., jewelry, body rings) within the examination field, which may inhibit organ visualization and cause unclear images.
• Inability of the patient to cooperate or remain still during the procedure, because movement can produce blurred or otherwise unclear images.

POTENTIAL MEDICAL DIAGNOSIS: CLINICAL SIGNIFICANCE OF RESULTS
Abnormal findings related to
• Failure to reduce the patient's pain
• Failure to improve the patient's mobility

NURSING IMPLICATIONS

BEFORE THE STUDY: PLANNING AND IMPLEMENTATION

Teaching the Patient What to Expect
▶ Inform the patient this procedure can assist in improving spinal cord function.
▶ Explain that prior to the procedure, laboratory testing may be required to determine the possibility of bleeding risk (coagulation testing) or to assess for impaired kidney function (creatinine level and estimated glomerular filtration rate) if use of iodinated contrast medium is anticipated.
▶ Pregnancy is a general contraindication to procedures involving radiation. Explain to the female patient that she will be asked the date of her last menstrual period. Pregnancy testing may be performed to determine the possibility of pregnancy before exposure to radiation.
▶ Review the procedure with the patient. Address concerns about pain and explain that there may be moments of discomfort or pain experienced when the IV line or catheter is inserted to allow infusion of fluids such as saline, anesthetics, sedatives, contrast medium, medications used in the procedure, or emergency medications.
▶ Explain that contrast medium, if ordered, may be used to verify placement of the vertebroplasty cement and will be injected, by catheter, at a separate site from the IV line.
▶ Advise that a burning and flushing sensation may be felt throughout the body during injection of the contrast medium, and the patient may experience an urge to cough, flushing, nausea, or a salty or metallic taste.
▶ Inform the patient that the procedure is usually performed in the radiology department by a health-care provider (HCP), with support staff, and takes approximately 30 to 90 min.
▶ Instruct the patient to remove jewelry and other metallic objects from the area of examination.

▶ **Older Adult Considerations:** Older adult patients present with a variety of concerns when undergoing diagnostic procedures. Level of cooperation and fall risk may be complicated by underlying problems such as visual and hearing impairment, joint and muscle stiffness, physical weakness, mental confusion, and the effects of medications. A fall injury can be avoided by providing assistance getting on and off the x-ray table. Older adult patients are often chronically dehydrated; anticipating the effects of hypovolemia and orthostasis can also help prevent falls.

▶ Baseline vital signs are recorded and monitored throughout the procedure. Protocols may vary among facilities.

▶ Explain that electrocardiographic electrodes are placed for cardiac monitoring and to establish a baseline rhythm and determine the presence of ventricular dysrhythmias.

▶ Positioning for the procedure is in the prone position on an examination table. The selected area is cleansed and covered with a sterile drape.

▶ Explain that a local anesthetic is injected at the site, and a small incision made or a needle inserted under fluoroscopy.

▶ Explain that orthopedic cement is injected through the needle into the fracture.

▶ Advise the patient he or she will be asked to inhale deeply, hold the breath while the images are taken, and then exhale.

▶ Advise taking slow, deep breaths if nausea occurs during the procedure. An ordered antiemetic drug can be administered as needed. An emesis basin can be ready for use.

▶ Explain to the patient he or she will be monitored for complications related to the procedure (e.g., allergic reaction, anaphylaxis, bronchospasm).

▶ Explain that once the study is completed, the needle or catheter is removed, and a pressure dressing is applied over the puncture site.

Potential Nursing Actions

 Make sure a written and informed consent has been signed prior to

the procedure and before administering any medications.

▶ If iodinated contrast medium is scheduled to be used in patients receiving metformin or drugs containing metformin for type 2 diabetes, the drug may be discontinued on the day of the test and continue to be withheld for 48 hr after the test. Protocols may vary among facilities.

Safety Considerations

▶ Anticoagulants, aspirin, and other salicylates should be discontinued by medical direction for the appropriate number of days prior to a procedure where bleeding is a potential complication.

AFTER THE STUDY: POTENTIAL NURSING ACTIONS

Avoiding Complications

▶ Establishing an IV site and injection of contrast medium are invasive procedures. Complications are rare but include risk for allergic reaction *(related to cement or contrast reaction)*, cardiac dysrhythmias, hematoma *(related to blood leakage into the tissue following needle insertion)*, bleeding from the puncture site *(related to a bleeding disorder or the effects of natural products and medications with known anticoagulant, antiplatelet, or thrombolytic properties)*, or infection *(which might occur if bacteria from the skin surface is introduced at the puncture site)*. Other complications related to the use of the cement include soft tissue damage and nerve impingement *(related to extravasation of cement)*, embolism to the lungs *(related to a blood clot or cement leakage)*, and respiratory and cardiac failure. Risk for complications increases when more than one vertebra is treated at the same time. Monitor the patient for complications related to the procedure (e.g., allergic reaction, anaphylaxis, bronchospasm, infection, injury). Immediately report symptoms such as difficulty breathing, chest pain, fever, hyperpnea, hypertension, nausea, palpitations, pruritus, rash, tachycardia, urticaria, or vomiting to the appropriate HCP. Observe/assess the needle/catheter insertion site for bleeding, inflammation, or hematoma formation. Administer ordered antihistamines or prophylactic steroids if the patient has an allergic reaction.

Treatment Considerations

▶ Instruct the patient to resume diet, fluids, and medications, as directed by the HCP. Kidney function should be assessed before metformin is resumed.

▶ Monitor vital signs and neurological status every 15 min for 1 hr, then every 2 hr for 4 hr, and then as ordered by the HCP. Take temperature every 4 hr for 24 hr. Monitor intake and output at least every 8 hr. Compare with baseline values. Notify the HCP if temperature is elevated. Protocols may vary among facilities.

▶ Instruct the patient to maintain bedrest for 4 to 6 hr after the procedure or as ordered.

▶ Provide instruction on the care and assessment of the procedure site.

▶ Explain the value of applying cold compresses to the puncture site as needed to reduce discomfort or edema.

Safety Considerations

▶ Advise diabetic patients to avoid all medications containing metformin for 48 hr following a procedure with iodinated contrast. Iodinated contrast can temporarily impair kidney function, and failure to withhold metformin may indirectly result in drug-induced lactic acidosis, a dangerous and sometimes fatal adverse effect of metformin (related to renal impairment that does not support sufficient excretion of metformin).

Follow-Up, Evaluation, and Desired Outcomes

▶ Understands that depending on the results of this procedure, additional testing may be needed to monitor disease progression and determine the need for a change in therapy. Evaluate test results in relation to the patient's symptoms and other tests performed.

▶ Acknowledges contact information provided for the National Osteoporosis Foundation (www.nof.org), National Institutes of Health (www.nih.gov), and Centers for Disease Control and Prevention (www.cdc.gov).

Visual Fields Test

SYNONYM/ACRONYM: Perimetry, VF.

RATIONALE: To assess visual field function related to the retina, optic nerve, and optic pathways to assist in diagnosing visual loss disorders such as brain tumors, macular degeneration, and diabetes.

PATIENT PREPARATION: There are no food, fluid, activity, or medication restrictions unless by medical direction.

NORMAL FINDINGS

• Normal central vision field extends in a circle approximately 25 to 30 degrees on all sides of central fixation and out 60 degrees superiorly (upward), 60 degrees medially (nasally), 75 degrees inferiorly (downward), and 90 degrees temporally (laterally). There is a normal physiological blind spot, 12° to 15° degrees temporal to the central fixation point and approximately 1.5 degrees below the horizontal meridian, which is approximately 7.5 degrees high and 5.5 degrees wide. The patient should be able to see the test object throughout the entire central vision field except within the physiological blind spot.

CRITICAL FINDINGS AND POTENTIAL INTERVENTIONS: N/A

OVERVIEW: (Study type: Sensory, ocular; related body system: Nervous system.) The visual field (VF) is the area within which objects can be seen by the eye as it fixes on a central point. The central field is an area extending 25 degrees surrounding the fixation point. The peripheral field is the remainder of the area within which objects can be viewed. This test evaluates the central VF, except within the physiological blind spot, through systematic movement of the test object across a tangent screen. It tests the function of the retina, optic nerve, and optic pathways. VF testing may be performed manually by the examiner (confrontation VF examination) or by using partially or fully automated equipment (tangent screen, Goldman, Humphrey VF examination). In the manual VF test, the patient is asked to cover one eye and fix his or her gaze on the examiner. The examiner moves his or her hand out of the patient's VF and then gradually brings it back into the patient's VF. The patient signals the examiner when the hand comes back into view. The test is repeated on the other eye. The manual test is frequently used for screening because it is quick and simple. Tangent screen or Goldman testing is an automated method commonly used to create a map of the patient's VF.

INDICATIONS

- Detect field vision loss and evaluate its progression or regression.

INTERFERING FACTORS

Factors that may alter the results of the study

- A patient who is uncooperative or a patient with severe vision loss who has difficulty seeing even a large vision screen may have test results that are invalid.
- Assess and make note of the patient's cooperation and reliability as good, fair, or poor, because it is difficult to evaluate factors such as general health, fatigue, or reaction time that affect test performance.

POTENTIAL MEDICAL DIAGNOSIS: CLINICAL SIGNIFICANCE OF RESULTS

Abnormal findings related to

- Amblyopia
- Blepharochalasis
- Blurred vision
- Brain injury
- Brain tumors
- Cerebrovascular accidents
- Choroidal nevus
- Diabetes with ophthalmic manifestations (For additional information regarding screening guidelines and management of diabetes, refer to the study titled "Glucose.")
- Glaucoma
- Headache
- Macular degeneration
- Macular drusen
- Nystagmus
- Optic neuritis or neuropathy
- Ptosis of eyelid
- Retinal detachment, hole, or tear
- Retinal exudates or hemorrhage
- Retinal occlusion of the artery or vein
- Retinitis pigmentosa
- Rheumatoid arthritis
- Stroke
- Subjective visual disturbance
- Use of high-risk medications
- VF defect
- Vitreous traction syndrome

V

NURSING IMPLICATIONS

BEFORE THE STUDY: PLANNING AND IMPLEMENTATION

Teaching the Patient What to Expect

▶ Inform the patient this procedure assesses visual field function and vision loss.

▶ Review the procedure with the patient. Address concerns about pain and explain that no discomfort will be experienced during the test.

▶ Explain that visual acuity with and without corrective lenses will be measured prior to testing.

▶ Inform the patient that a health-care provider (HCP) performs the test in a quiet, darkened room and that to evaluate both eyes, the test can take up 30 min.

▶ Explain that positioning for this procedure is seated 3 ft away from the tangent screen with the eye being tested directly in line with the central fixation tangent, usually a white disk, on the screen. The eye that is not being tested is covered.

▶ Advise the patient that he or she will be asked to place his or her chin in the chin rest and gently press the forehead against the support bar.

▶ Repositioning may occur, as appropriate, to ensure the eye to be tested is properly aligned in front of the VF testing equipment.

▶ Advise the patient that while he or she stares at the disk on the screen, the examiner moves an object toward the visual field and the patient is asked to signal the examiner when the object enters the visual field.

▶ Responses are recorded, and a map of the VF, including areas of visual defect, can be drawn on paper manually or by a computer.

Potential Nursing Actions

▶ Investigate history of the patient's concerns related to known or suspected vision loss; changes in visual acuity, including type and cause; use of glasses or contact lenses; eye conditions with treatment regimens; eye surgery; and other tests and procedures to assess and diagnose visual deficit.

▶ Advise wearing corrective lenses if appropriate and if worn to correct for distance vision.

AFTER THE STUDY: POTENTIAL NURSING ACTIONS

Avoiding Complications

▶ Emphasize, as appropriate, that good management of glucose levels delays the onset and slows the progression of diabetic retinopathy, nephropathy, and neuropathy.

▶ Explain that unmanaged diabetes can cause multiple health issues, including diabetic kidney disease, amputation of limbs, and ultimately in death.

Treatment Considerations

▶ Encourage the family to recognize and be supportive of impaired activity related to vision loss, anticipated loss of driving privileges, or the possibility of requiring corrective lenses (self-image).

▶ Provide education in the use of any ordered medications and explain the importance of adhering to the therapy regimen.

▶ Provide instruction on the significant adverse effects associated with the prescribed medication and encourage a review of corresponding literature provided by a pharmacist.

Nutritional Considerations

▶ Abnormal findings may be associated with diabetes. There is no "diabetic diet"; however, many meal-planning approaches with nutritional goals are endorsed by the American Diabetes Association (ADA). Patients who adhere to dietary recommendations report a better general feeling of health, better weight management, better management of glucose and lipid values, and improved use of insulin. Instruct the patient, as appropriate, in nutritional management of diabetes. A variety of dietary patterns are beneficial for people with diabetes. Encourage consultation with a registered dietitian who is a certified diabetes educator.

Follow-Up, Evaluation, and Desired Outcomes
- Acknowledges contact information provided for the following:
- Patient education on the topic of eye care: American Academy of Ophthalmologists (www.aao.org) and American Optometric Association (AOA) (www.aoa.org or www.allaboutvision .com). The AOA's recommendations for the frequency of eye examinations can be accessed at www.aoa .org.
- Diseases affecting vision: American Macular Degeneration Foundation (www.macular.org), American Heart Association (www.heart.org/ HEARTORG), ADA (www.diabetes .org), National Heart, Lung, and Blood Institute (www.nhlbi.nih.gov).

Vitamin Studies

SYNONYM/ACRONYM: Vitamin A: retinol, carotene; Vitamin B_1: thiamine; Vitamin B_6: pyroxidine, P-5'-P, pyridoxyl-5-phosphate; Vitamin B_{12}: cyanocobalamin; Vitamin C: ascorbic acid; Vitamin D: cholecalciferol, vitamin D 25-hydroxy, vitamin D 1,25-dihydroxy; Vitamin E: alpha-tocopherol; Vitamin K: phylloquinone, phytonadione.

RATIONALE: To assess vitamin deficiency or toxicity to assist in diagnosing nutritional disorders such as malabsorption; disorders that affect vision, skin, and bones; and other diseases.

PATIENT PREPARATION: There are no activity or medication restrictions unless by medical direction. Patient should fast overnight for 12 hr prior to specimen collection for vitamins A, B_6, E, and K and should not consume alcohol for 24 hr prior to specimen collection for vitamins A, E, and K.

NORMAL FINDINGS: Method: High-performance liquid chromatography: vitamins A, B_1, B_6, C, D, E and K; Immunochemiluminescent assay: vitamin B_{12}.

Age	Conventional Units	SI Units
Vitamin A		*(Conventional Units × 0.0349)*
Birth–1 yr	14–52 mcg/dL	0.49–1.81 micromol/L
1–6 yr	20–43 mcg/dL	0.7–1.5 micromol/L
7–12 yr	26–49 mcg/dL	0.91–1.71 micromol/L
13–19 yr	26–72 mcg/dL	0.91–2.51 micromol/L
Adult	30–120 mcg/dL	1.05–4.19 micromol/L
Vitamin B_1		*(Conventional Units × 29.6)*
	0.21–1 mcg/dL	6.2–30 nmol/L
Vitamin B_6		*(Conventional Units × 4.046)*
	5–30 ng/mL	20–121 nmol/L
Vitamin B_{12}		*(Conventional Units × 0.7378)*
Newborn–10 yr	160–1,300 pg/mL	118–959 pmol/L
11–17 yr	260–900 pg/mL	192–664 pmol/L
Adult	200–1,100 pg/mL	148–812 pmol/L

(table continues on page 1226)

V

Age	Conventional Units	SI Units
Vitamin C		*(Conventional Units × 56.78)*
	0.6–1.9 mg/dL	34.1–107.9 micromol/L
Vitamin D		*(Conventional Units × 2.496)*
25-hydroxy		
Deficient	Less than 20 ng/mL	Less than 49.9 nmol/L
Insufficient	20–30 ng/mL	49.9–74.9 nmol/L
Optimal	30–100 ng/mL	74.9–249.6 nmol/L
Possible Toxicity	Greater than 150 ng/mL	Greater than 374.4 nmol/L
Vitamin D		*(Conventional Units × 2.6)*
1,25-dihydroxy		
Adult	18–72 pg/mL	47–187 pmol/L
Vitamin E		*(Conventional Units × 2.322)*
Newborn	1–3.5 mg/L	2.3–8.1 micromol/L
Neonate	2.5–3.7 mg/L	5.8–8.6 micromol/L
2–5 mo	2–6 mg/L	4.6–13.9 micromol/L
6–12 mo	3.5–8 mg/L	8.1–18.6 micromol/L
1–6 yr	3–9 mg/L	7–20.9 micromol/L
7–12 yr	4–9 mg/L	9.3–20.9 micromol/L
13–19 yr	6–10 mg/L	13.9–23.2 micromol/L
Adult	5–18 mg/L	11.6–41.8 micromol/L
Vitamin K		*(Conventional Units × 2.22)*
	0.13–1.19 ng/mL	0.29–2.64 nmol/L

Vitamin B_1, vitamin B_6, vitamin B_{12}, and vitamin C levels tend to decrease in older adults.

CRITICAL FINDINGS AND POTENTIAL INTERVENTIONS

Timely notification to the requesting health-care provider (HCP) of any critical findings and related symptoms is a role expectation of the professional nurse. A listing of these findings varies among facilities.

Vitamin toxicity can be as significant as problems brought about by vitamin deficiencies. The potential for toxicity is especially important to consider with respect to fat-soluble vitamins (A, D, E, and K), which are not eliminated from the body as quickly as water-soluble vitamins and can accumulate in the body. Most cases of toxicity are brought about by oversupplementing and can be avoided by consulting a registered dietitian for recommended daily dietary and supplemental allowances. Signs and symptoms of vitamin A toxicity may include headache, blurred vision, bone pain, joint pain, dry skin, and loss of appetite. Signs and symptoms of vitamin D toxicity include nausea, loss of appetite, vomiting, polyuria, muscle weakness, and constipation. Excessive supplementation of vitamin E (greater than 60 times the recommended dietary allowance over a period of 1 yr or longer) can result in excessive bleeding, delayed healing of wounds, and depression. The naturally occurring forms vitamins K_1 and K_2 do not cause toxicity. Signs and symptoms of vitamin K_3 toxicity include bleeding and jaundice. Possible interventions include withholding the source.

OVERVIEW: (Study type: Blood collected in a gold-, red/gray-, green- [sodium or lithium heparin], light green-, green/green gray-, lavender- [EDTA], or pink- [K_2 EDTA] top tube for **vitamin A;** green- [sodium or lithium heparin], light green-, green/green gray-, lavender- [EDTA], or pink- [K_2 EDTA] top tube for **vitamin B_1;** green-, green/green gray-, red-top tube protected from light at all times for **vitamin B_6;** gold-, red-, red/gray-, light green-, green/green gray-top tube protected from light at all times for **vitamin B_{12};** green- [sodium or lithium heparin] top tube protected from light at all times for **vitamin C;** gold-, red-, red/gray-, green- [lithium heparin], or lavender- [EDTA] top tube for **vitamin D 1,25 dihydroxy;** gold- or red/gray-top tube for **vitamin D 25 hydroxy;** gold-, red/gray-, green- [sodium or lithium heparin], lavender- [EDTA], or pink- [K_2 EDTA] top tube for **vitamin E;** and gold-, red-, red/gray-, lavender- [EDTA], or pink- [K_2 EDTA] top tube protected from light at all times for **vitamin K;** related body system: vitamins contribute to multisystem effects.)

Vitamin assays are used in the measurement of nutritional status. Low levels indicate inadequate oral intake, poor nutritional status, or malabsorption problems. High levels indicate excessive intake, vitamin intoxication, or absorption problems. Vitamin A is a fat-soluble nutrient that promotes normal vision and prevents night blindness; contributes to growth of bone, teeth, and soft tissues; supports thyroxine formation; maintains epithelial cell membranes, skin, and mucous membranes; and acts against infection. Vitamins B_1, B_6, and C are water soluble. Vitamin B_1 acts as an enzyme and plays an important role in the Krebs cycle of cellular metabolism. Vitamin B_6 is important in heme synthesis and functions as a coenzyme in amino acid metabolism and glycogenolysis. It includes pyridoxine, pyridoxal, and pyridoxamine. Vitamin C promotes collagen synthesis, maintains capillary strength, facilitates release of iron from ferritin to form hemoglobin, and functions in the stress response.

Vitamin B_{12} has a ringed crystalline structure that surrounds an atom of cobalt. It is essential in DNA synthesis, hematopoiesis, and central nervous system (CNS) integrity. It is derived solely from dietary intake. Animal products are the richest source of vitamin B_{12}. Its absorption depends on the presence of intrinsic factor. Circumstances that may result in a deficiency of this vitamin include the presence of stomach or intestinal disease as well as insufficient dietary intake of foods containing vitamin B_{12}. A significant increase in red blood cells (RBCs) means corpuscular volume may be an important indicator of vitamin B_{12} deficiency.

Vitamin D is a group of interrelated sterols that have hormonal activity in multiple organs and tissues of the body, including the kidneys, liver, skin, and bones. There are two metabolically active forms of vitamin D: vitamin D 25-hydroxy and vitamin D 1,25-dihydroxy. Ergocalciferol (vitamin D_2) is formed when ergosterol in plants is exposed to sunlight. Ergocalciferol is absorbed by the stomach and intestine when orally ingested. Cholecalciferol (vitamin D_3) is formed when the skin is exposed to sunlight or ultraviolet light. Vitamins D_2 and D_3 enter the bloodstream after absorption. Vitamin D_3 is converted to vitamin D 25-hydroxy by the liver and is the major circulating form of the vitamin. Vitamin D_2 is converted to vitamin D 1,25-dihydroxy (calcitriol) by the kidneys and is the more biologically active form. Vitamin D acts with parathyroid hormone and calcitonin to regulate calcium metabolism and osteoblast function. The effects of vitamin D deficiency have been studied for many years, and continued research indicates a link between vitamin D deficiency and the development of diseases such as heart failure, stroke, hypertension, cancer, autism, multiple sclerosis, type 2 diabetes, systemic lupus erythematosus, depression, and immune function. The amount of vitamin D_3 produced by exposure of the skin to ultraviolet radiation depends on the intensity of the radiation as well as the duration of exposure. The use of lotions containing sun block significantly decreases production of vitamin D_3.

Vitamin E is a collection of powerful, fat-soluble antioxidants. Alpha-tocopherol appears to be the most plentiful and important form of eight vitamin E antioxidants; there are four tocopherols (alpha-, beta-, gamma-, and delta-) and four tocotrienols (alpha-, beta-, gamma-, and delta-). Antioxidants limit the production of free radicals by preventing the oxidation of unsaturated fatty acids. Free radicals are unstable chemical compounds that contain unshared electrons. They combine rapidly with oxygen during normal metabolic processes in the body when food is converted into energy or when they are taken into the body by environmental exposure from sources such as ultraviolet radiation, air pollution, or secondhand smoke. Vitamin E reserves in lung tissue provide a barrier against air pollution and protect RBC membrane integrity from oxidation. Oxidation of fatty acids in RBC membranes can result in irreversible membrane damage and hemolysis. For many years, scientists have been investigating whether vitamin E might play a role in the amelioration or prevention of chronic and degenerative diseases associated with damage caused by free radicals. Clinical trials, in general, have not provided consistent evidence to support the function of vitamin E as a defense against cardiovascular disease, cataracts, macular degeneration, cancer, and cognitive decline. Studies are currently in progress to further evaluate the potential protective properties of vitamin E. The use of vitamin E as a dietary supplement remains controversial. Current guidelines state that nutrition needs be met through healthy dietary intake. Because vitamin E is found in a wide variety of foods, a deficiency secondary to inadequate dietary intake is rare. There is research to support the potential interaction between vitamin E and other medications, most notably anticoagulant and antiplatelet drugs. Overuse of supplementary vitamin E has been associated, in some studies, with increased risk of hemorrhagic stroke.

Vitamin K is one of the fat-soluble vitamins. It is essential for the formation of prothrombin; factors VII, IX, and X; and proteins C and S. Vitamin K also works with vitamin D in synthesizing bone protein and regulating calcium levels. Vitamin K levels are not often requested, but vitamin K is often prescribed as a medication. Approximately one-half of the body's vitamin K is produced by intestinal bacteria; the other half is obtained from dietary sources. There are three forms of vitamin K: vitamin K_1, or phylloquinone, which is found in foods; vitamin K_2, or menaquinone, which is synthesized by intestinal bacteria; and vitamin K_3, or menadione, which is the synthetic, water-soluble, pharmaceutical form of the vitamin. Vitamin K_3 is two to three times more potent than the naturally occurring forms.

INDICATIONS

Vitamin A
- Assist in the diagnosis of night blindness.
- Evaluate skin disorders.
- Investigate suspected vitamin A deficiency.

Vitamin B_1
- Investigate suspected beriberi.
- Monitor the effects of chronic alcohol misuse.

Vitamin B_6
- Investigate suspected malabsorption or malnutrition.
- Investigate suspected vitamin B_6 deficiency.

Vitamin B_{12}
- Assist in the diagnosis of CNS disorders.
- Assist in the diagnosis of megaloblastic anemia.

- Evaluate alcohol misuse.
- Evaluate malabsorption syndromes.

Vitamin C
- Investigate suspected metabolic or malabsorptive disorders.
- Investigate suspected scurvy.

Vitamin D
- Differential diagnosis of disorders of calcium and phosphorus metabolism.
- Evaluate deficiency or suspected toxicity.
- Investigate bone diseases.
- Investigate malabsorption.

Vitamin E
- Evaluate neuromuscular disorders in premature infants and adults.
- Evaluate patients with malabsorption disorders.
- Evaluate suspected hemolytic anemia in premature infants and adults.
- Monitor patients on long-term parenteral nutrition.

Vitamin K
- Evaluate bleeding of unknown cause (e.g., frequent nosebleeds, bruising).

INTERFERING FACTORS
Factors that may alter the results of the study

General
- Various diseases may affect vitamin levels (see Potential Medical Diagnoses section).
- Long-term hyperalimentation may result in decreased vitamin levels.
- Exposure of some specimens to light or temperature variations decreases vitamin levels, resulting in a falsely low results.

Vitamin A
- Drugs and other substances that may increase vitamin A levels include alcohol (moderate intake), oral contraceptives, and probucol.

V

- Drugs and other substances that may decrease vitamin A levels include alcohol (chronic intake, alcohol misuse), allopurinol, cholestyramine, colestipol, mineral oil, and neomycin.

Vitamin B₁

- Drugs and other substances that may decrease vitamin B₁ levels include glibenclamide, isoniazid, and valproic acid.
- Diets high in freshwater fish and tea, which are thiamine antagonists, may cause decreased vitamin B₁ levels.

Vitamin B₆

- Drugs and other substances that may decrease vitamin B₆ levels include amiodarone, anticonvulsants, cycloserine, disulfiram, ethanol, hydralazine, isoniazid, levodopa, oral contraceptives, penicillamine, pyrazinoic acid, and theophylline.

Vitamin B₁₂

- Drugs that may increase vitamin B₁₂ levels include chloral hydrate.
- Drugs that may decrease vitamin B₁₂ levels include alcohol, aminosalicylic acid, anticonvulsants, ascorbic acid, cholestyramine, cimetidine, colchicine, metformin, neomycin, oral contraceptives, ranitidine, and triamterene.
- Hemolysis or exposure of the specimen to light invalidates vitamin B₁₂ results.
- Specimen collection soon after blood transfusion can falsely increase vitamin B₁₂ levels.

Vitamin C

- Drugs and other substances that may decrease vitamin C levels include acetylsalicylic acid, barbiturates, estrogens, heavy metals, oral contraceptives, nitrosamines, and paraldehyde.
- Chronic tobacco smoking decreases vitamin C levels.

Vitamin D

- Drugs and other substances that may increase vitamin D levels include cholestyramine, orlistat (a medication for weight loss), and phenytoin.

Vitamin E

- Drugs that may increase vitamin E levels include anticonvulsants (in women).
- Drugs that may decrease vitamin E levels include anticonvulsants (in men).

Vitamin K

- Drugs and substances that may decrease vitamin K levels include antibiotics, cholestyramine, coumarin, mineral oil, and warfarin.

POTENTIAL MEDICAL DIAGNOSIS: CLINICAL SIGNIFICANCE OF RESULTS
Increased in

Vitamin A

- Chronic kidney disease
- Idiopathic hypercalcemia in infants
- Vitamin A toxicity

Vitamin B₁

- NA

Vitamin B₆

- NA

Vitamin B₁₂

Increases are noted in a number of conditions; pathophysiology is unclear.

- Chronic granulocytic leukemia
- Chronic kidney disease
- Chronic obstructive pulmonary disease
- Diabetes
- Leukocytosis
- Liver cell damage (hepatitis, cirrhosis) *(stores in damaged hepatocytes are released into circulation; synthesis of transport proteins is diminished by liver damage)*
- Obesity
- Polycythemia vera

- Protein malnutrition *(lack of transport proteins increases circulating levels)*
- Severe heart failure
- Some cancer

Vitamin D
- Endogenous vitamin D intoxication *(in conditions such as sarcoidosis, cat scratch disease, and some lymphomas, extrarenal conversion of 25-hydroxy to 1,25-dihydroxy vitamin D occurs with a corresponding abnormal elevation of calcium)*
- Exogenous vitamin D intoxication

Vitamin E
- Obstructive liver disease *(related to malabsorption associated with obstructive liver disease)*
- Vitamin E intoxication *(related to excessive intake)*

Vitamin K
- Excessive administration of vitamin K

Decreased in

Vitamin A
- Abetalipoproteinemia *(related to poor absorption)*
- Carcinoid syndrome *(related to poor absorption)*
- Chronic infections *(vitamin A deficiency decreases ability to fight infection)*
- Cystic fibrosis *(related to poor absorption)*
- Disseminated tuberculosis *(related to poor absorption)*
- Hypothyroidism *(condition decreases ability of beta carotene to convert to vitamin A)*
- Infantile blindness *(related to dietary deficiency)*
- Liver, gastrointestinal, or pancreatic disease *(related to malabsorption or poor absorption)*
- Night blindness *(related to chronic dietary deficiency or lack of absorption)*

- Protein malnutrition *(related to dietary deficiency)*
- Sterility and teratogenesis *(related to dietary deficiency)*
- Zinc deficiency *(zinc is required for generation of vitamin A transport proteins)*

Vitamin B₁
- Alcohol misuse *(related to dietary deficiency)*
- Carcinoid syndrome *(related to dietary deficiency or lack of absorption)*
- Hartnup disease *(related to dietary deficiency)*
- Pellagra *(related to dietary deficiency)*

Vitamin B₆
(This vitamin is involved in many essential functions, such as nucleic acid synthesis, enzyme activation, antibody production, electrolyte balance, and RBC formation; deficiencies result in a variety of conditions.)

- Alcohol misuse *(related to dietary deficiency)*
- Asthma
- Carpal tunnel syndrome
- Gestational diabetes
- Kidney dialysis
- Lactation *(related to dietary deficiency and/or increased demand)*
- Malabsorption
- Malnutrition
- Neonatal seizures
- Normal pregnancies *(related to dietary deficiency and/or increased demand)*
- Occupational exposure to hydrazine compounds *(enzymatic pathways are altered by hydralazines in a manner that increases excretion of vitamin B₆)*
- Pellagra *(related to dietary deficiency)*
- Pre-eclamptic edema
- Uremia

V

Vitamin B$_{12}$

- Abnormalities of cobalamin transport or metabolism
- Bacterial overgrowth *(vitamin is consumed and utilized by the bacteria)*
- Crohn disease *(related to poor absorption)*
- Dietary deficiency *(related to insufficient intake, e.g., in vegetarians)*
- *Diphyllobothrium* (fish tapeworm) infestation *(vitamin is consumed and utilized by the parasite)*
- Gastric or small intestine surgery *(related to dietary deficiency or poor absorption)*
- Hypochlorhydria *(related to ineffective digestion resulting in poor absorption)*
- Inflammatory bowel disease *(related to dietary deficiency or poor absorption)*
- Intestinal malabsorption
- Intrinsic factor deficiency *(required for proper vitamin B$_{12}$ absorption)*
- Late pregnancy *(related to dietary deficiency or poor absorption)*
- Pernicious anemia *(related to dietary deficiency or poor absorption)*

Vitamin C

- Alcohol misuse *(related to dietary deficiency)*
- Anemia *(related to dietary deficiency)*
- Cancer *(related to dietary deficiency or lack of absorption)*
- Hemodialysis *(vitamin C is lost during the treatment)*
- Hyperthyroidism *(related to dietary deficiency and/or increased demand)*
- Kidney dialysis *(vitamin C is lost during the treatment)*
- Malabsorption
- Pregnancy *(related to dietary deficiency and/or increased demand)*
- Rheumatoid disease
- Scurvy *(related to dietary deficiency or lack of absorption)*

Vitamin D

- Bowel resection *(related to lack of absorption)*
- Celiac disease *(related to lack of absorption)*
- Inflammatory bowel disease *(related to lack of absorption)*
- Malabsorption *(related to lack of absorption)*
- Osteomalacia *(related to dietary insufficiency)*
- Pancreatic insufficiency *(lack of digestive enzymes to metabolize fat-soluble vitamin D; malabsorption)*
- Rickets *(related to dietary insufficiency)*
- Thyrotoxicosis *(possibly related to increased calcium loss through sweat, urine, or feces with corresponding decrease in vitamin D levels)*

Vitamin E

- Abetalipoproteinemia *(rare inherited disorder of fat metabolism evidenced by poor absorption of fat and fat-soluble vitamin E)*
- Hemolytic anemia *(related to deficiency of vitamin E, an important antioxidant that protects RBC membranes from weakening)*
- Malabsorption disorders, such as biliary atresia, cirrhosis, cystic fibrosis, chronic pancreatitis, pancreatic cancer, and chronic cholestasis

Vitamin K

- Antibiotic therapy *(related to decreased intestinal flora)*
- Chronic fat malabsorption *(related to lack of digestive enzymes and poor absorption)*
- Cystic fibrosis *(related to lack of digestive enzymes and poor absorption)*
- Diarrhea (in infants) *(related to increased loss in feces)*
- Gastrointestinal disease *(related to malabsorption)*
- Hemorrhagic disease of the newborn *(newborns normally have low levels of vitamin K; neonates at*

risk are those who are not given a prophylactic vitamin K shot at birth or those receiving nutrition strictly from breast milk, which has less vitamin K than cow's milk)

- Hypoprothrombinemia *(related to insufficient levels of prothrombin, a vitamin K–dependent protein)*

- Liver disease *(interferes with storage of vitamin K)*
- Obstructive jaundice *(related to insufficient levels of bile salts required for absorption of vitamin K)*
- Pancreatic disease *(related to insufficient levels of enzymes to metabolize vitamin K)*

NURSING IMPLICATIONS

POTENTIAL NURSING PROBLEMS: ASSESSMENT & NURSING DIAGNOSIS

Problems	Signs and Symptoms	Interventions
Body image *(related to deformities, e.g., associated with rickets or bone loss from osteoporosis and vitamin D insufficiency)*	Visible physical deformity, presence of kyphosis or lordosis, verbalized negative feelings about appearance, altered social interactions with others due to embarrassment about appearance	Acknowledge the patient's emotional distress, encourage a positive attitude, coordinate meetings with a support group within the community
Nutrition *(related to lack of specific vitamin-rich foods in the diet)*	Failure to select vitamin-rich foods specific to address the deficiency, difficulty in opening food containers and feeding self	Determine the patient's ability to select vitamin D–rich foods, discuss the efficacy of increasing exposure to sunlight, collaborate with the HCP in determining the need for vitamin D supplements
Self-care *(related to physical deformity, pain, and limited range of motion)*	Difficulty fastening clothing, difficulty performing personal hygiene, unable to maintain appropriate appearance, difficulty with independent mobility	Reinforce self-care techniques as taught by occupational therapy, ensure the patient has adequate time to perform self-care, encourage use of assistive devices to maintain independence

BEFORE THE STUDY: PLANNING AND IMPLEMENTATION

Teaching the Patient What to Expect

▶ Inform the patient this test can assist in diagnosing a vitamin toxicity or deficiency.

▶ Explain that a blood sample is needed for the test.

AFTER THE STUDY: POTENTIAL NURSING ACTIONS

Treatment Considerations

▶ Body Image: Some vitamin deficiencies can be linked to physical changes that cause emotional distress. Acknowledge the patient's emotional distress and encourage a positive attitude. Coordinate meetings

V

with a support group within the community.

- Self-Care: Reinforce self-care techniques as taught by occupational therapy; ensure the patient has adequate time to perform self-care; encourage use of assistive devices to maintain independence.

Nutritional Considerations

General

- Determine the patient's ability to select appropriate vitamin-rich foods, and collaborate with the HCP in determining the need for vitamin supplements. All supplements and dietary choices should be used appropriately in relation to the patient's clinical condition or health concerns.

Vitamin A

- Explain to those with a deficiency that the main dietary source of vitamin A is carotene, a yellow pigment noticeable in most fruits and vegetables, most specifically in carrots, sweet potatoes, squash, apricots, and cantaloupe. It is also present in spinach, collards, broccoli, and cabbage. This vitamin is fairly stable at most cooking temperatures, but it is destroyed easily by light and oxidation.

Vitamin B_1

- Vitamin B_1 is the most stable with respect to the effects of environmental factors. Educate the patient with vitamin B_1 deficiency that the main dietary sources of vitamin B_1 are meats, coffee, peanuts, and legumes. The body is also capable of making some vitamin B_1 by converting the amino acid tryptophan to niacin.

Vitamin B_6

- Explain to those with vitamin B_6 deficiency that the main dietary sources of vitamin B_6 include meats (especially beef and pork), whole grains, wheat germ, legumes (beans, peas, lentils), potatoes, oatmeal, and bananas. As with other water-soluble vitamins, it is best preserved by rapid cooking, although it is relatively stable at most cooking temperatures (except frying) and when exposed to acidic foods. This vitamin is destroyed rapidly by light and alkalis.

Vitamin B_{12}

- Advise the patient with vitamin B_{12} deficiency in the use of vitamin supplements. Explain that the best dietary sources of vitamin B_{12} are meats, fish, poultry, eggs, and milk.

Vitamin C

- Educate those with vitamin C deficiency that citrus fruits are excellent dietary sources of vitamin C. Other good sources are green and red peppers, tomatoes, white potatoes, cabbage, broccoli, chard, kale, turnip greens, asparagus, berries, melons, pineapple, and guava. Vitamin C is destroyed by exposure to air, light, heat, or alkalis. Boiling water before cooking eliminates dissolved oxygen that destroys vitamin C in the process of boiling. Vegetables should be crisp and cooked as quickly as possible.

Vitamin D

- Advise those with vitamin D deficiency that foods high in calcium and vitamin D should be included in the diet. Explain that vitamin D is also synthesized by the body, in the skin, and is activated by sunlight. Examples of foods rich in calcium and vitamin D are yogurt, cheese, cottage cheese, canned sardines with bones, flounder, salmon, dried figs, and dark green leafy vegetables such as spinach and broccoli. Processed foods with added calcium, such as breads and cereals, can also be included. Avoiding red meat and high-fat foods that bind calcium in the intestine can reduce loss. The excess use of alcohol, salt, or caffeine can also decrease absorption. Explain that vitamin D is also synthesized by the body, in the skin, and is activated by sunlight. Daily recommendations for calcium and vitamin D intake are based on age. Calcium and vitamin D supplements may be used if dietary intake is insufficient.

Vitamin E

- Educate those with a vitamin E deficiency that the main dietary sources of vitamin E are vegetable oils (including olive oil), whole grains, fortified cereals, wheat germ, nuts, seeds, soy products, milk (fat-free or low-fat milk and milk products), eggs, seafood, meats, fish, fruits, and vegetables, especially legumes and green leafy vegetables. Vitamin E is fairly stable at most cooking temperatures (except frying) and when exposed to acidic foods.

Vitamin K

- Advise those with a vitamin K deficiency that the main dietary sources of vitamin K are broccoli, cabbage, cauliflower, kale, spinach, leaf lettuce, watercress, parsley, and other raw green leafy vegetables, pork, liver, soybeans, mayonnaise, and vegetable oils.

Follow-Up, Evaluation, and Desired Outcomes

General

- Acknowledges contact information provided for the U.S. Department of Agriculture's resource for nutrition (www.choosemyplate.gov).
- Those with a specific vitamin deficiency recognize the value of dietary sources of these vitamins and will consider asking a registered dietitian to assist in the development of a diet plan to meet specific needs.

Vitamin D

- The patient with vitamin D deficiency acknowledges contact information provided for the National Osteoporosis Foundation (www.nof.org), National Institutes of Health (www.nih.gov), and Centers for Disease Control and Prevention (www.cdc.gov).

Vitamin K

- Acknowledges the importance of reporting bleeding from any areas of the skin or mucous membranes.
- Acknowledges the importance of taking precautions against bleeding or bruising, including the use of a soft bristle toothbrush, use of an electric razor, avoidance of constipation, avoidance of aspirin products, and avoidance of intramuscular injections.

V

WBC Count, Blood Smear and Differential

SYNONYM/ACRONYM: WBC with diff, leukocyte count, white cell count.

RATIONALE: To evaluate viral and bacterial infections and to assist in diagnosing and monitoring leukemic disorders.

PATIENT PREPARATION: There are no food, fluid, activity, or medication restrictions unless by medical direction.

NORMAL FINDINGS: Method: Automated, computerized, multichannel analyzers. Many analyzers can determine a five- or six-part WBC differential. The six-part automated white blood cell (WBC) differential identifies and enumerates neutrophils, lymphocytes, monocytes, eosinophils, basophils, and immature granulocytes (IG), where IG represents the combined enumeration of promyelocytes, metamyelocytes, and myelocytes as both an absolute number and a percentage. The five-part WBC differential includes all but the immature granulocyte parameters.

WBC Count and Differential

Age	Conventional Units WBC × 10³/microL	Neutrophils (Absolute and %)	Lymphocytes (Absolute and %)	Monocytes (Absolute and %)	Eosinophils (Absolute and %)	Basophils (Absolute and %)
Birth	9.1–30.1	(5.5–18.3) 24%–58%	(2.8–9.3) 26%–56%	(0.5–1.7) 7%–13%	(0.02–0.7) 0%–8%	(0.1–0.2) 0%–2.5%
1–23 mo	6.1–17.5	(1.9–5.4) 21%–67%	(3.7–10.7) 20%–64%	(0.3–0.8) 4%–11%	(0.2–0.5) 0%–3.3%	(0–0.1) 0%–1%
2–10 yr	4.5–13.5	(2.4–7.3) 30%–77%	(1.7–5.1) 14%–50%	(0.2–0.6) 4%–9%	(0.1–0.3) 0%–5.8%	(0–0.1) 0%–1%
11 yr–older adult	4.5–11.1	(2.7–6.5) 40%–75%	(1.5–3.7) 12%–44%	(0.2–0.4) 4%–9%	(0.05–0.5) 0%–5.5%	(0–0.1) 0%–1%

*SI Units (conventional units × 1 or WBC count × 10⁹/L).

WBC Count and Differential

Age	Immature Granulocytes (Absolute) (10³/microL)	Immature Granulocyte Fraction (IGF) (%)
Birth–9 yr	0–0.03	0%–0.4%
10 yr–older adult	0–0.09	0%–0.9%

CRITICAL FINDINGS AND POTENTIAL INTERVENTIONS
- Total WBC count of less than 2×10^3/microL (SI: Less than 2×10^9/L)
- Absolute neutrophil count of less than 0.5×10^3/microL (SI: Less than 0.5×10^9/L)
- Total WBC count of greater than 30×10^3/microL (SI: Greater than 30×10^9/L)

Timely notification to the requesting health-care provider (HCP) of any critical findings and related symptoms is a role expectation of the professional nurse. A listing of these findings varies among facilities.

Consideration may be given to verifying the critical findings before action is taken. Policies vary among facilities and may include requesting immediate recollection and retesting by the laboratory.

The presence of abnormal cells, other morphological characteristics, or cellular inclusions may signify a potentially life-threatening or serious health condition and should be investigated. Examples are hypersegmented neutrophils, agranular neutrophils, blasts or other immature cells, Auer rods, Döhle bodies, marked toxic granulation, and plasma cells.

OVERVIEW: (Study type: Blood from a lavender-top [EDTA] tube; related body system: Circulatory/Hematopoietic and Immune systems. The specimen should be mixed gently by inverting the tube 10 times. The specimen should be analyzed within 24 hr when stored at room temperature or within 48 hr if stored at refrigerated temperature. If it is anticipated the specimen will not be analyzed within 24 hr, two blood smears should be made immediately after the venipuncture and submitted with the blood sample. Smears made from specimens older than 24 hr may contain an unacceptable number of misleading artifactual abnormalities of the WBCs, such as necrobiotic WBCs.) WBCs constitute the body's primary defense system against foreign organisms, tissues, and other substances. The life span of a normal WBC is 13 to 20 days. Old WBCs are destroyed by the lymphatic system and excreted in the feces. Reference values for WBC counts vary significantly with age. WBC counts vary diurnally, with counts being lowest in the morning and highest in the late afternoon. Other variables such as stress and high levels of activity or physical exercise can trigger transient increases of 2×10^3/microL to 5×10^3/microL. The main WBC types are neutrophils (band and segmented neutrophils), eosinophils, basophils, monocytes, and lymphocytes. WBCs are produced in the bone marrow. B-cell lymphocytes remain in the bone marrow to mature. T-cell lymphocytes migrate to and mature in the thymus. The WBC count can be performed alone with the differential cell count or as part of the complete blood count (CBC). The WBC differential can be performed by an automated instrument or manually on a slide prepared from a stained peripheral blood sample. Automated instruments provide excellent, reliable information, but the accuracy of the WBC count can be affected by the presence of circulating nucleated red blood cells (RBCs), clumped platelets, fibrin strands, cold agglutinins, cryoglobulins, intracellular parasitic organisms, or other significant blood cell inclusions and may not be identified in the interpretation of an automated blood count. The decision to report a manual or automated differential is based on specific criteria established by the laboratory. The criteria are designed to identify findings that warrant further investigation or confirmation by manual review. An increased WBC count is termed *leukocytosis,* and a decreased WBC count is termed *leukopenia.* A total WBC count indicates the degree of response to a pathological process, but a more complete evaluation for specific diagnoses for any one disorder is provided by the differential count. The WBCs in the count and differential are reported as an *absolute value* and as a percentage. The relative percentages of cell types are arrived at by basing the enumeration of each cell type on a 100-cell count. The absolute value is obtained by multiplying the relative percentage value of each cell type by the total WBC count. For example, on a CBC report, with a total WBC of 9 × 10^3/microL and WBC differential with 92% segmented neutrophils, 1% band neutrophils, 5% lymphocytes, and 1% monocytes the absolute values are calculated as follows: 92/100 × 9 = 8.3 segs, 1/100 × 9 = 0.09 bands, 5/100 × 9 = 0.45 lymphs, 1/100 × 9 = 0.1 monos for a total of 9 WBC count. The absolute neutrophil count (ANC) for this patient would be 9 × (0.92 + 0.01) = 8.4.

The ANC reflects the number of segmented and band type neutrophils in the total WBC count. It is used as an indicator of immune status because it reflects the type and number of WBC available to rapidly respond to an infection. Neutropenia is a decrease below normal in the number of neutrophils. ANC = Total WBC × [(Segs/100) + (Bands/100)] or total WBC × (% Segs + % Bands). The normal value varies with age but in general mild neutropenia is less than 1.5, moderate neutropenia is between 0.5 and 1, and severe neutropenia is less than 0.5. The ANC is helpful when managing patients receiving chemotherapy. It can drive decisions to place a hospitalized patient in isolation in order to protect the patient from exposure to infectious agents. Patients who are aware of their ANC can also make informed decisions in taking actions to avoid exposure to crowds, avoid touching things in public places that may carry germs, or avoid friends and family who may be sick.

Acute leukocytosis is initially accompanied by changes in the WBC count population, followed by changes within the individual WBCs. Leukocytosis usually occurs by way of increase in a single WBC family rather than a proportional increase in all cell types. Toxic granulation and vacuolation are commonly seen in leukocytosis accompanied by a *shift to the left,* or increase in the percentage of immature neutrophils to mature segmented neutrophils. An increased number or percentage of immature granulocytes, reflected by a shift to the left, represents production of WBCs and is useful as an indicator of infection. Immature neutrophils are called *bands* and can represent 3% to 5% of total circulating neutrophils in healthy individuals. *Bandemia* is defined by the presence of greater than 6% to 10% band neutrophils in the total neutrophil cell population. These changes in the white cell population are most commonly associated with an infectious process, usually bacterial, but they can occur in healthy individuals who are under stress (in response to epinephrine production), such as women in childbirth and very young infants. The WBC count and differential of a woman in labor or of an actively crying infant may show an overall increase in WBCs with a shift to the left. Before initiating any kind of intervention, it is important to determine whether an increased WBC count is the result of a normal condition involving physiological stress or a pathological process. The use of multiple specimen types may confuse the interpretation of results in infants. Multiple samples from the same collection site (i.e., capillary versus venous) may be necessary to obtain an accurate assessment of the WBC picture in these young patients.

Neutrophils are normally found as the predominant WBC type in the circulating blood. Also called *polymorphonuclear cells,* they are the body's first line of defense through the process of phagocytosis. They also contain enzymes and pyogenes, which combat foreign invaders.

Lymphocytes are agranular, mononuclear blood cells that are smaller than granulocytes. They are found in the next highest percentage in normal circulation. Lymphocytes are classified as B cells and T cells. Both types are formed in the bone marrow, but B cells mature in the bone marrow and T cells mature in the thymus. Lymphocytes play a major role in the body's natural defense system. B cells differentiate into immunoglobulin-synthesizing plasma cells. T cells function as cellular mediators of immunity and comprise helper/inducer (CD4) lymphocytes, delayed hypersensitivity lymphocytes, cytotoxic (CD8 or CD4) lymphocytes, and suppressor (CD8) lymphocytes.

Monocytes are mononuclear cells similar to lymphocytes, but they are related more closely to granulocytes in terms of their function. They are formed in the bone marrow from the same cells as those that produce neutrophils. The major function of monocytes is phagocytosis. Monocytes stay in the peripheral blood for about 70 hr, after which they migrate into the tissues and become macrophages.

The function of eosinophils is phagocytosis of antigen-antibody complexes. They become active in the later stages of inflammation. Eosinophils respond to allergic and parasitic diseases: They have granules that contain histamine used to kill foreign cells in the body and proteolytic enzymes that damage parasitic worms (see study titled "Eosinophil Count").

Basophils are found in small numbers in the circulating blood. They have a phagocytic function and, similar to eosinophils, contain numerous specific granules. Basophilic granules contain heparin, histamines, and serotonin. Basophils may also be found in tissue and as such are classified as mast cells. Basophilia is noted in conditions such as leukemia, Hodgkin disease, polycythemia vera, ulcerative colitis, nephrosis, and chronic hypersensitivity states.

INDICATIONS

- Assist in confirming suspected bone marrow depression.
- Assist in determining the cause of an elevated WBC count (e.g., infection, inflammatory process).
- Detect hematological disorder, tumor, or immunological abnormality.
- Determine the presence of a hereditary hematological abnormality.
- Monitor the effects of physical or emotional stress.
- Monitor the progression of non-hematological disorders, such as chronic obstructive pulmonary disease, malabsorption syndromes, cancer, and kidney disease.
- Monitor the response to drugs or chemotherapy and evaluate undesired reactions to drugs that may cause blood dyscrasias.
- Provide screening as part of a CBC in a general physical examination, especially on admission to a healthcare facility or before surgery.

INTERFERING FACTORS

Factors that may alter the results of the study

- Drugs and other substances that may decrease the overall WBC count include acetylsalicylic acid, aminosalicylic acid, ampicillin, amsacrine, antazoline, anticonvulsants, antineoplastic drugs (therapeutic intent), antipyrine, barbiturates, busulfan, carmustine, chlorambucil, chloramphenicol, chlordane, chlorophenothane, chlorpromazine, chlorthalidone, cisplatin, colchicine, colistimethate, cycloheximide, cyclophosphamide, cytarabine, dacarbazine, dactinomycin, diazepam, diethylpropion, digitalis, dipyridamole, dipyrone, fumagillin, glaucarubin, glucosulfone, hexachlorobenzene, hydroxychloroquine, iothiouracil, iproniazid, lincomycin, local anesthetics, mefenamic acid, meprobamate, mercaptopurine, methotrexate, methylpromazine, mitomycin, paramethadione, parathion, penicillin, phenacemide, phenothiazine, pipamazine, prednisone (by Coulter S method), primaquine, procainamide, procarbazine, prochlorperazine, promethazine, pyrazolones, pyrimethamine, quinacrine, quinines, radioactive compounds, razoxane, ristocetin, sulfa drugs, tamoxifen, tetracycline, thenalidine, thioridazine, tolazamide, tolazoline, tolbutamide, trimethadione, and urethane.
- A significant decrease in basophil count occurs rapidly after IV injection of propanidid and thiopental.
- A significant decrease in lymphocyte count occurs rapidly after administration of corticotropin, mechlorethamine, methysergide, and x-ray therapy; and after megadoses of niacin, pyridoxine, and thiamine.
- Drugs and other substances that may increase the overall WBC count include amphetamine, amphotericin B, chloramphenicol, chloroform (normal response to anesthesia), colchicine (leukocytosis follows leukopenia), corticotropin, erythromycin, ether (normal

response to anesthesia), isoflurane (normal response to anesthesia), niacinamide, phenylbutazone, prednisone, and quinine.

- Drug allergies may have a significant effect on eosinophil count and may affect the overall WBC count. Refer to the study titled "Eosinophil Count" for a detailed listing of interfering drugs.
- The WBC count may vary depending on the patient's position, decreasing when the patient is recumbent owing to hemodilution and increasing when the patient rises owing to hemoconcentration.
- Venous stasis can falsely elevate results; the tourniquet should not be left on the arm for longer than 60 sec.
- The presence of nucleated RBCs or giant or clumped platelets affects the automated WBC, requiring a manual correction of the WBC count.
- Patients with cold agglutinins or monoclonal gammopathies may have a falsely decreased WBC count as a result of cell clumping.

Other considerations
- Care should be taken in evaluating the CBC during the first few hours after transfusion.
- Failure to fill the tube sufficiently (i.e., tube less than three-quarters full) may yield inadequate sample volume for automated analyzers and may be reason for specimen rejection.
- Hemolyzed or clotted specimens should be rejected for analysis.

POTENTIAL MEDICAL DIAGNOSIS: CLINICAL SIGNIFICANCE OF RESULTS
Increased in

Leukocytosis
- Normal physiological and environmental conditions:
  Early infancy *(increases are believed to be related to the physiological stress of*

birth and metabolic demands of rapid development)*
  Emotional stress *(related to secretion of epinephrine)*
  Exposure to extreme heat or cold *(related to physiological stress)*
  Pregnancy and labor *(WBC counts may be modestly elevated due to increased neutrophils into the third trimester and during labor, returning to normal within a week postpartum)*
  Strenuous exercise *(related to epinephrine secretion; increases are short in duration, minutes to hours)*
  Ultraviolet light *(related to physiological stress and possible inflammatory response)*
- Pathological conditions:
  Acute hemolysis, especially due to splenectomy or transfusion reactions *(related to leukocyte response to remove lysed RBC fragments)*
  All types of infections *(related to an inflammatory or infectious response)*
  Anemias *(bone marrow disorders affecting RBC production may result in elevated WBC count)*
  Appendicitis
  Collagen disorders *(related to an inflammatory or infectious response)*
  Cushing disease *(related to overproduction of cortisol, a corticosteroid, which stimulates WBC production)*
  Inflammatory disorders *(related to an inflammatory or infectious response)*
  Leukemias and other malignancies *(related to bone marrow disorders that result in abnormal WBC production)*
  Parasitic infestations *(related to an inflammatory or infectious response)*
  Polycythemia vera *(myeloproliferative bone marrow disorder causing an increase in all cell lines)*

Decreased in

Leukopenia
- Normal physiological conditions:
  Diurnal rhythms (lowest in the morning)
- Pathological conditions:
  Alcohol misuse *(related to WBC changes associated with nutritional deficiencies of vitamin B_{12} or folate)*

Anemias *(related to WBC changes associated with nutritional deficiencies of vitamin B$_{12}$ or folate, especially in megaloblastic anemias)*

Bone marrow depression *(related to decreased production)*

Malaria *(related to hypersplenism)*

Malnutrition *(related to WBC changes associated with nutritional deficiencies of vitamin B$_{12}$ or folate)*

Radiation *(related to physical cell destruction due to toxic effects of radiation)*

Rheumatoid arthritis *(related to adverse effect of medications used to treat the condition)*

Systemic lupus erythematosus (SLE) and other autoimmune disorders *(related to adverse effect of drugs used to treat the condition)*

Toxic and antineoplastic drugs *(related to bone marrow suppression)*

Very low birth weight neonates *(related to bone marrow activity being diverted to develop RBCs in response to hypoxia)*

Viral infections *(leukopenia, lymphocytopenia, and abnormal lymphocytes may be present in the early stages of viral infections)*

Neutrophils Increased (Neutrophilia)

- Acute hemolysis
- Acute hemorrhage
- Extremes in temperature
- Infectious diseases
- Inflammatory conditions (rheumatic fever, gout, rheumatoid arthritis, vasculitis, myositis)
- Malignancies
- Metabolic disorders (uremia, eclampsia, diabetic ketoacidosis, thyroid storm, Cushing syndrome)
- Myelocytic leukemia
- Physiological stress (e.g., allergies, asthma, exercise, childbirth, surgery)
- Tissue necrosis (burns, crushing injuries, abscesses, myocardial infarction)
- Tissue poisoning with toxins and venoms

Neutrophils Decreased (Neutropenia)

- Acromegaly
- Addison disease
- Anaphylaxis
- Anorexia nervosa, starvation, malnutrition
- Bone marrow depression (viruses, toxic chemicals, overwhelming infection, radiation, Gaucher disease)
- Disseminated SLE
- Thyrotoxicosis
- Viral infection (mononucleosis, hepatitis, influenza)
- Vitamin B$_{12}$ or folate deficiency

Lymphocytes Increased (Lymphocytosis)

- Addison disease
- Felty syndrome
- Infections (viral, e.g., cytomegalovirus, hepatitis, HIV, infectious mononucleosis, rubella, varicella; or bacterial, e.g., tuberculosis, whooping cough)
- Lymphocytic leukemia
- Lymphomas
- Lymphosarcoma
- Myeloma
- Rickets
- Thyrotoxicosis
- Ulcerative colitis
- Waldenström macroglobulinemia

Lymphocytes Decreased (Lymphopenia)

- Antineoplastic drugs
- Aplastic anemia
- Bone marrow failure
- Burns
- Gaucher disease
- Hemolytic disease of the newborn
- High doses of adrenocorticosteroids
- Hodgkin disease
- Hypersplenism
- Immunodeficiency diseases
- Infections
- Malnutrition
- Pernicious anemia

W

W

- Pneumonia
- Radiation
- Rheumatic fever
- Septicemia
- Thrombocytopenic purpura
- Toxic chemical exposure
- Transfusion reaction

Monocytes Increased (Monocytosis)
- Cancers
- Cirrhosis
- Collagen diseases

- Gaucher disease
- Hemolytic anemias
- Hodgkin disease
- Infections
- Lymphomas
- Monocytic leukemia
- Polycythemia vera
- Radiation
- Sarcoidosis
- SLE
- Thrombocytopenic purpura
- Ulcerative colitis

NURSING IMPLICATIONS

POTENTIAL NURSING PROBLEMS: ASSESSMENT & NURSING DIAGNOSIS

Problems	Signs and Symptoms
Fever (related to increased basal metabolic rate, infection)	Elevated temperature; flushed, warm skin; diaphoresis; skin warm to touch; tachycardia; tachypnea; seizures; convulsions
Fluid volume (water) (related to metabolic imbalances associated with disease process, insensible fluid loss, excessive diaphoresis)	**Deficit:** Decreased urinary output, fatigue, sunken eyes, dark urine, decreased blood pressure, increased heart rate, and altered mental status
Infection (related to metabolic or endocrine dysfunction, chronic debilitating illness, cirrhosis, trauma, vectors, decreased tissue perfusion, presence of gram-positive or gram-negative organisms)	Temperature, increased heart rate, increased blood pressure, shaking, chills, mottled skin, lethargy, fatigue, swelling, edema, pain, localized pressure, diaphoresis, night sweats, confusion, vomiting, nausea, headache

BEFORE THE STUDY: PLANNING AND IMPLEMENTATION

Teaching the Patient What to Expect
- Inform the patient this test can assist in assessing for infection or monitoring conditions that affect the white blood cells (e.g., leukemia).
- Explain that a blood sample is needed for the test.

AFTER THE STUDY: POTENTIAL NURSING ACTIONS

Treatment Considerations
- Fever: Frequently assess and trend the temperature. Ensure the patient's

immediate environment remains cool. Encourage the use of light bedding and lightweight clothing to prevent overheating. Increase fluid intake to offset insensible fluid loss. Encourage bathing with tepid water for comfort and promotion of cooling. Administer ordered antipyretics.
- Fluid Volume: Record daily weight and monitor trends including an accurate intake and output. Collaborate with HCP for administration of IV fluids to support hydration and encourage oral fluids to maximize hydration. Monitor laboratory values that reflect alterations in fluid status: potassium, BUN, Cr, calcium, Hgb, and Hct. Manage

underlying cause of fluid loss. Monitor urine characteristics and respiratory status. Administer ordered replacement electrolytes.

▶ Infection: Promote good hygiene and assist with hygiene when needed. Administer prescribed antibiotics, antipyretics, and IV fluids. Monitor vital signs and trend temperatures. Adhere to standard precautions, isolate as appropriate, obtain ordered cultures, encourage use of lightweight clothing and bedding. Monitor and trend indicators of infection: WBC count, C-reactive protein.

Nutritional Considerations

▶ Infection, fever, sepsis, and trauma can result in an impaired nutritional status. Malnutrition can occur for many reasons, including fatigue, lack of appetite, and gastrointestinal distress.

▶ Adequate intake of vitamins A and C, and zinc are also important for regenerating body stores depleted by the effort exerted in fighting infections. Provide information regarding the importance of following the prescribed diet including specific vitamin or mineral rich food sources.

▶ Explain that the main dietary source of vitamin A comes from carotene, a yellow pigment noticeable in most fruits and vegetables, especially carrots, sweet potatoes, squash, apricots, and cantaloupe. It is also present in spinach, collards, broccoli, and cabbage. This vitamin is fairly stable at most cooking temperatures, but it is destroyed easily by light and oxidation.

▶ Explain that citrus fruits are excellent dietary sources of vitamin C. Other good sources are green and red peppers, tomatoes, white potatoes, cabbage, broccoli, chard, kale, turnip greens, asparagus, berries, melons, pineapple, and guava. Vitamin C is destroyed by exposure to air, light, heat, or alkalis. Boiling water before cooking eliminates dissolved oxygen that destroys vitamin C in the process of boiling. Vegetables should be crisp and cooked as quickly as possible.

▶ Topical or oral supplementation may be ordered for patients with zinc deficiency. Dietary sources high in zinc include shellfish, red meat, wheat germ, nuts, and processed foods such as canned pork and beans and canned chili. Patients should be informed that phytates (from whole grains, coffee, cocoa, or tea) bind zinc and prevent it from being absorbed. Decreases in zinc also can be induced by increased intake of iron, copper, or manganese. Vitamin and mineral supplements with a greater than 3:1 iron/zinc ratio inhibit zinc absorption.

Follow-Up, Evaluation, and Desired Outcomes

▶ Acknowledges contact information provided for the U.S. Department of Agriculture's resource for nutrition (www.choosemyplate.gov).

▶ Recognizes the importance of compliance with follow-up laboratory tests to manage disease process.

▶ Adheres to the request to increase fluid intake to offset fluid loss and prevent dehydration.

West Nile Virus Testing

SYNONYM/ACRONYM: N/A

RATIONALE: To assist in the diagnosis of West Nile virus (WNV) infection.

PATIENT PREPARATION: There are no food, fluid, activity, or medication restrictions unless by medical direction.

NORMAL FINDINGS: (Method: Enzyme immunoassay [EIA] is generally used for clinical specimens, and nucleic acid testing [NAT] is generally used for testing specimens from potential donors of blood products, cellular therapy, or solid organ transplants.) Normal findings for EIA/ELISA (IgG & IgM): no antibody detected; for NAT viral RNA: nonreactive.

CRITICAL FINDINGS AND POTENTIAL INTERVENTIONS: N/A

OVERVIEW: (Study type: Blood collected in a red-top tube or CSF collected in a sterile plastic container; related body system: Immune system.) The WNV, a single-stranded RNA virus, is classified as a flavivirus. Prior to 1999, the virus was primarily found in Africa; since then, it is found worldwide throughout Australia, North America, Europe, the Middle East, South America, and West Asia. WNV is one of three types of arbovirus capable of transmitting encephalitis and other febrile type diseases in North America via an arthropod vector: *Togaviridae, Flaviviridae,* and *Bunyaviridae.* The primary mode of this arboviral transmission to humans is mosquito bite. Many mosquito species (notably Culex) can serve as the disease vector; birds serve as the reservoir hosts (mainly crows, sparrows, and blue jays). WNV is not transmitted directly from human to human, by handling infected birds (dead or alive), from exposure to an infected equine, or by eating meat from infected birds or animals. Horses and humans are classified as "dead" hosts because, when infected, they do not produce a sufficient viral load to transmit virus when bitten by an uninfected mosquito vector. WNV can cause severe illness or death in horses; a vaccine has been developed for horses. There are rare reports of transmission by an infected person via blood product,

tissue, or solid organ transplant; for that reason, all human products are tested for WNV prior to transfusion or transplantation. Although the majority of babies born to infected mothers do not contract the disease or suffer any associated congenital abnormalities, there are rare cases of known transmission from mother to baby during pregnancy and breast feeding.

The incubation period for WNV disease is from 2 to 14 days but can extend beyond that range in immunocompromised patients. About 80% of WNV infections are subclinical or asymptomatic, but of those who develop symptoms, the onset is described as an acute systemic febrile illness that can rapidly escalate into life-threatening sequelae that could include viral meningitis, an acute flaccid paralysis that is indistinguishable from poliovirus-associated poliomyelitis, or a severe encephalitis. Conditions that present like radiculopathy and Guillain-Barré syndrome have also been associated with WNV infection and can be distinguished from WNV acute flaccid paralysis by clinical signs and symptoms and electrophysiologic studies. However, in most cases, the symptoms are non–life threatening and nonspecific: headache, lethargy, weakness, aching muscles and bones, gastrointestinal discomfort, and/or skin rash. Symptoms may last for a period of days or persist for weeks or months. Therapy is supportive, and there is no commercially available human vaccine at this time. WNV infection is a significant infectious disease, and the first human clinical trial for a vaccine, sponsored by the National Institutes of Health, was initiated in 2015 at Duke University.

Assays for immunoglobulin G (IgG) and immunoglobulin M (IgM) antibodies to WNV assist in differentiating recent infection from prior exposure in the general population. Cerebrospinal fluid (CSF) specimens are used to document central nervous system (CNS) infection by WNV. WNV IgM antibodies appear the earliest and are soon followed by development of IgG antibodies. Presence of antibodies is detectable within 3 to 10 days after reported onset of symptoms and remain in circulation for approximately 30 to 90 days. If results from the IgM-specific or from both assays are positive, recent infection is suspected. Absence of detectable antibody within 10 days of onset does not rule out infection, and testing should be repeated within a short period of time. If the IgM-specific test results are negative and the IgG-specific antibody test results are positive, past infection is indicated. WNV testing is not widely available in routine clinical laboratories. Testing may be sent to a referral laboratory for enzyme immunoassay (EIA) and enzyme-linked immunosorbent assay (ELISA) or to a public health testing facility for a more specific and quantitative confirmatory analysis known as *plaque reduction*

neutralization testing (PRNT), depending on the situation. Aliquots of all specimens should be sequestered for a specified period of time after collection; protocols vary by facility. Positive results obtained by EIA/ELISA testing should be confirmed by neutralizing antibody testing on both acute and convalescent serum specimens that have been collected 2 to 3 weeks apart. PRNTs can also confirm acute infection by demonstrating a fourfold or greater increase in PRNT antibody titer between acute and convalescent serum samples. Other testing methods for WNV disease include viral cultures on blood or body fluid (to detect viral RNA [ribonucleic acid]), immunohistochemistry using formalin-fixed tissue (to detect viral antigen), and reverse transcriptase polymerase chain reaction on serum, CSF, and tissue specimens (to detect viral RNA).

INDICATIONS

- Assist in the diagnosis of WNV.
- Assist in the differential diagnosis of other arboviral causes of encephalitis (e.g., Eastern equine, La Crosse, Powassan, St. Louis encephalitis, and Western equine).

INTERFERING FACTORS

Factors that may alter the results of the study

False-positive results may be obtained in the presence of cross-reacting antibodies produced by other members of the *Flaviviridae* family, such as the St. Louis encephalitis virus.

POTENTIAL MEDICAL DIAGNOSIS: CLINICAL SIGNIFICANCE OF RESULTS

Positive findings in

- WNV infection

W

NURSING IMPLICATIONS

BEFORE THE STUDY: PLANNING AND IMPLEMENTATION

Teaching the Patient What to Expect

▶ Inform the patient this test can indicate the presence of WNV infection.
▶ Explain that a blood or CSF sample is needed for the test.
▶ Inform the patient/caregiver that the CSF specimen collection will be performed by a health-care provider (HCP) trained to perform the procedure and takes approximately 20 min. The procedure for lumbar puncture is described in the study titled "Cerebrospinal Fluid Analysis."

AFTER THE STUDY: POTENTIAL NURSING ACTIONS

Treatment Considerations

▶ Explain that positive findings must be reported to local health department officials.
▶ Recognize anxiety related to test results, and provide emotional support if results are positive.
▶ Provide education related to the clinical implications of the test results.
▶ If the patient is pregnant, explain that risk of transmission from mother to

fetus is believed to be very low. However, it is believed that transmission may be passed to the baby through breast milk. All patients and breastfeeding mothers should be advised to take precautions against exposure to mosquito bites by wearing protective clothing and insect repellent, especially during peak times of insect activity (at dawn and dusk, July through October). Effective repellents include those containing diethyltoluamide (DEET), picaridin, and lemon eucalyptus oil.
▶ Additional prevention strategies also include the elimination of mosquito breeding grounds, as can be found in sources of standing water (drinking stations for pets, flower pots, bird baths, water barrels, children's wading pools or gym sets, etc.).

Follow-Up, Evaluation, and Desired Outcomes

▶ Understands the importance of adhering to HCP referral regarding further testing and treatment.
▶ Recognizes the importance of returning to have a convalescent blood sample taken in 7 to 14 days.
▶ Acknowledges contact information provided for the Centers for Disease Control and Prevention (www.cdc.gov/westnile/resources/pdfs/wnvFactsheet_508.pdf and www.cdc.gov/DiseasesConditions/az/w.html).

White Blood Cell Scan

SYNONYM/ACRONYM: Infection scintigraphy, inflammatory scan, labelled autologous leukocytes, labelled leukocyte scan, WBC imaging.

RATIONALE: To assist in identification of abscess, infection, and inflammation of the bone, bowel, wound, and skin.

PATIENT PREPARATION: There are no food, fluid, activity, or medication restrictions unless by medical direction. No other radionuclide tests should be scheduled within 24 to 48 hr before this procedure.

W

NORMAL FINDINGS

- No focal localization of the radionuclide, along with some slight localization of the radionuclide within the reticuloendothelial system (liver, spleen, and bone marrow).

CRITICAL FINDINGS AND POTENTIAL INTERVENTIONS: N/A

OVERVIEW: (Study type: Nuclear scan; **related body system:** Immune system.) Because white blood cells (WBCs) naturally accumulate in areas of inflammation, the WBC scan uses radiolabelled WBCs to help determine the site of an acute infection or confirm the presence or absence of infection or inflammation at a suspected site. A gamma camera detects the radiation emitted from the injected radionuclide, and a representative image of the radionuclide distribution is obtained and recorded or stored electronically. Because of its better image resolution and greater specificity for acute infections, the WBC scan has replaced scanning with gallium-67 citrate (Ga-67). Some chronic infections associated with pulmonary disease, however, may be better imaged with Ga-67. The WBC scan is especially helpful in detecting postoperative infection sites and in documenting lack of residual infection after a course of therapy.

INDICATIONS

- Aid in the diagnosis of infectious or inflammatory diseases.
- Differentiate infectious from noninfectious process.
- Evaluate the effects of treatment.
- Evaluate inflammatory bowel disease (IBD).
- Evaluate patients with fever of unknown origin.

- Evaluate postsurgical sites and wound infections.
- Evaluate suspected infection of an orthopedic prosthesis.
- Evaluate suspected osteomyelitis.

INTERFERING FACTORS
Contraindications

✧ Patients who are pregnant or suspected of being pregnant, unless the potential benefits of a procedure using radiation far outweigh the risk of radiation exposure to the fetus and mother.

Factors that may alter the results of the study
- Lesions smaller than 1 to 2 cm, which may not be detectable.
- A distended bladder, which may obscure pelvic detail.
- False-negative images may be a result of hemodialysis, hyperglycemia, hyperalimentation, steroid therapy, and antibiotic therapy.
- The presence of multiple myeloma or thyroid cancer can result in a false-negative scan for bone abnormalities.
- Metallic objects (e.g., jewelry, body rings) within the examination field, other nuclear scans done within the previous 24 to 48 hr, or Ga-67 scans within 4 wk before the procedure, which may inhibit organ visualization and cause unclear images.
- Improper injection of the radionuclide that allows the tracer to seep deep into the muscle tissue can produce erroneous hot spots.

W

- Inability of the patient to cooperate or remain still during the procedure, because movement can produce blurred or otherwise unclear images.

Other considerations
- Patients with a low WBC count may need donor WBCs to complete the radionuclide labelling process; otherwise, Ga-67 scanning should be performed instead.

POTENTIAL MEDICAL DIAGNOSIS: CLINICAL SIGNIFICANCE OF RESULTS
Abnormal findings related to
- Abscess
- Arthritis
- Infection
- Inflammation
- IBD
- Osteomyelitis

NURSING IMPLICATIONS

BEFORE THE STUDY: PLANNING AND IMPLEMENTATION

Teaching the Patient What to Expect
- Inform the patient this test can assist in assessing for the presence of infection or inflammation.
- Pregnancy is a general contraindication to procedures involving radiation. Explain to the female patient that she will be asked the date of her last menstrual period. Pregnancy testing may be performed to determine the possibility of pregnancy before exposure to radiation.
- Review the procedure with the patient. Address concerns about pain and explain that some pain or discomfort may be experienced when a 50- to 80-mL sample of blood will be drawn on the day of the test. The WBCs will be labelled in vitro with radionuclide.
- Explain that an IV line will be inserted to allow infusion of the labelled WBCs and other fluids such as saline, anesthetics, sedatives, medications

used in the procedure, or emergency medications; some discomfort may be experienced.
- Explain that the procedure is performed in a nuclear medicine department by a health-care provider (HCP). Images are recorded 1 to 6 hr postinjection depending on the radionuclide used.
- Advise that delayed images may be needed 24 hr later and that they may leave the department and return later to undergo delayed imaging.
- Reassure the patient that the radionuclide poses no radioactive hazard and rarely produces adverse effects.
- Instruct the patient to remove jewelry and other metallic objects from the area to be examined.
- Baseline vital signs and neurological status are assessed before the procedure. Protocols may vary among facilities.
- Positioning for the procedure is in a supine position on a flat table with foam wedges to help maintain position and immobilization.
- IV radionuclide-labelled autologous WBCs are administered.
- Explain that once the study is completed, the needle or catheter is removed and a pressure dressing applied over the puncture site.
- Explain that if abdominal abscess or infection is suspected, laxatives or enemas may be ordered before delayed imaging.

Potential Nursing Actions
- *Make sure a written and informed consent has been signed prior to the procedure and before administering any medications.*

AFTER THE STUDY: POTENTIAL NURSING ACTIONS

Avoiding Complications
- Establishing an IV site and injection of radionuclides are invasive procedures. Complications are rare but include risk for allergic reaction *(related to contrast reaction)*, hematoma *(related to blood leakage into the tissue following needle insertion)*, bleeding from the puncture site *(related to a bleeding disorder or the effects of natural products and*

medications with known anticoagulant, antiplatelet, or thrombolytic properties), or infection *(which might occur if bacteria from the skin surface is introduced at the puncture site)*. Monitor the patient for complications related to the procedure (e.g., allergic reaction, anaphylaxis, bronchospasm). Immediately report symptoms such as fast heart rate, difficulty breathing, skin rash, itching, or chest pain to the appropriate HCP. Observe/assess the needle/catheter insertion site for bleeding, inflammation, or hematoma formation.

Treatment Considerations
▶ Explain that the radionuclide is eliminated from the body within 6 to 24 hr. Advise the patient to drink increased amounts of fluids for 24 to 48 hr to eliminate the radionuclide from the body, unless contraindicated.
▶ Provide support for perceived loss of independent function.
▶ Discuss the implications of abnormal test results on lifestyle choices.
▶ Provide education related to the clinical implications of the test results.
▶ Instruct the patient to resume usual medication and activity, as directed by the HCP.
▶ Provide education in the care and assessment of the injection site.

▶ Explain that application of cold compresses to the puncture site may reduce discomfort or edema.

Safety Considerations
▶ The patient who is breastfeeding should consult with the requesting HCP regarding alternate testing that does not involve radiation. In general, if a woman who is breastfeeding must have a nuclear scan, she should not breastfeed the infant for 72 hr after the scan, until the radionuclide has been eliminated. She should be instructed to express the milk in order to prevent cessation of milk production; the milk can be stored and used after the 3-day period.
▶ No other radionuclide tests should be scheduled for 24 to 48 hr after this procedure.
▶ Refer to organizational policy for additional precautions that may include instructions on handwashing, toilet flushing, limited contact with others, and other aspects of nuclear medicine safety.

Follow-Up, Evaluation, and Desired Outcomes
▶ Understands that depending on the results of this procedure, additional testing may be necessary to monitor disease progression and determine the need for a change in therapy.

Zinc

SYNONYM/ACRONYM: Zn.

RATIONALE: To assist in assessing for zinc deficiency or toxicity, monitor therapeutic interventions, and assist in diagnosing disorders related to healing and immune function.

PATIENT PREPARATION: There are no food, fluid, activity, or medication restrictions unless by medical direction.

NORMAL FINDINGS: Method: Atomic absorption spectrophotometry.

Age	Conventional Units	SI Units (Conventional Units × 0.153)
Newborn–6 mo	26–141 mcg/dL	4–21.6 micromol/L
6–11 mo	29–131 mcg/dL	4.4–20 micromol/L
1–4 yr	31–115 mcg/dL	4.7–17.6 micromol/L
4–5 yr	48–119 mcg/dL	7.3–18.2 micromol/L
6–9 yr	48–129 mcg/dL	7.3–19.7 micromol/L
10–13 yr	25–148 mcg/dL	3.8–22.6 micromol/L
14–17 yr	46–130 mcg/dL	7–19.9 micromol/L
Adult	70–120 mcg/dL	10.7–18.4 micromol/L

CRITICAL FINDINGS AND POTENTIAL INTERVENTIONS: N/A

OVERVIEW: (**Study type:** Blood collected in a trace element-free, royal blue-top tube; **related body system:** Multisystem.) Zinc is found in all body tissues, but the highest concentrations are found in the eye, bone, and male reproductive organs. Zinc is involved in RNA and DNA synthesis and is essential in the process of tissue repair. It is also required for the formation of collagen and the production of active vitamin A (for the visual pigment rhodopsin). Zinc also functions as a chelating agent to protect the body from lead and cadmium poisoning. Zinc is absorbed from the small intestine. Its absorption and excretion seem to be through the same sites as those for iron and copper. The body does not store zinc as it does copper and iron. Untreated zinc deficiency in infants may result in a condition called *acrodermatitis enteropathica*. Symptoms include delayed growth, diarrhea, impaired wound healing, and frequent infections. Adolescents and adults with zinc deficiency exhibit similar adverse effects on growth, sexual development, and immune function, as well as altered taste and smell, emotional instability, impaired adaptation to darkness, impaired night vision, tremors, and a bullous, pustular rash over the extremities.

INDICATIONS

- Assist in confirming acrodermatitis enteropathica.
- Evaluate nutritional deficiency.
- Evaluate possible toxicity.
- Monitor replacement therapy in individuals with identified deficiencies.
- Monitor therapy of individuals with Wilson disease.

INTERFERING FACTORS
Factors that may alter the results of the study
- Drugs and other substances that may increase zinc levels include auranofin, chlorthalidone, corticotropin, oral contraceptives, and penicillamine.
- Drugs and other substances that may decrease zinc levels include anticonvulsants, cisplatin, citrates, corticosteroids, estrogens, interferon, oral contraceptives, and prednisone.

POTENTIAL MEDICAL DIAGNOSIS: CLINICAL SIGNIFICANCE OF RESULTS
Increased in
Zinc is contained in and secreted by numerous types of cells in the body. Damaged cells release zinc into circulation and increase blood levels.

- **Anemia** *(related to competitive relationship with copper; copper deficiency is associated with decreased production of red blood cells)*

Decreased in
This trace metal is an essential component of enzymes that participate in protein and carbohydrate metabolism. It is involved in DNA replication, insulin storage, carbon dioxide gas exchange, cellular immunity and healing, promotion of body growth, and sexual maturity. Deficiencies result in a variety of conditions.

- **Acrodermatitis enteropathica** *(congenital abnormality that affects zinc uptake and results in zinc deficiency)*
- AIDS
- Acute infections
- Acute stress
- Burns
- Cirrhosis
- Conditions that decrease albumin *(related to lack of available transport proteins)*

- Diabetes
- Long-term total parenteral nutrition
- Malabsorption
- Myocardial infarction
- Nephrotic syndrome
- Nutritional deficiency
- Pregnancy *(related to increased uptake by fetus; related to excessive levels of iron and folic acid prescribed during pregnancy and which interfere with absorption)*
- Pulmonary tuberculosis

NURSING IMPLICATIONS

BEFORE THE STUDY: PLANNING AND IMPLEMENTATION
Teaching the Patient What to Expect
- Inform the patient this test can assist in evaluating for disorders associated with abnormal zinc levels and monitor response to therapy.
- Explain that a blood sample is needed for the test.

AFTER THE STUDY: POTENTIAL NURSING ACTIONS
Treatment Considerations
- Provide education regarding access to nutritional counseling services.

Nutritional Considerations
- Topical or oral supplementation may be ordered for patients with zinc deficiency. Dietary sources high in zinc include shellfish, red meat, wheat germ, nuts, and processed foods such as canned pork and beans and canned chili.
- Patients should be informed that phytates (from whole grains, coffee, cocoa, or tea) bind zinc and prevent it from being absorbed.
- Decreases in zinc also can be induced by increased intake of iron, copper, or manganese.
- Vitamin and mineral supplements with a greater than 3:1 iron/zinc ratio inhibit zinc absorption.

Follow-Up, Evaluation, and Desired Outcomes

▶ Understands that depending on the results of this procedure, additional testing may be necessary to monitor disease progression and determine the need for a change in therapy.

▶ Acknowledges contact information provided for the U.S. Department of Agriculture's resource for nutrition (www.choosemyplate.gov).

INTRODUCTION: *The checklist is a basic template for all sites and types of studies; detailed information is found in the individual studies and Appendix A, Patient Preparation and Specimen Collection.*

PRETEST: *Preparation begins with good communication, active listening, timely education, and organization.*

1	Obtain/review a history of the patient's health concerns, symptoms, surgical procedures, and results of previously performed studies.	Y	N	N/A
2	Obtain/review a history of known allergens, especially allergies to latex, anesthetics, contrast medium, sedatives, and other medications.	Y	N	N/A
3	Obtain/review a list of the patient's current medications, including over-the-counter medications, dietary supplements, anticoagulants, aspirin, and other salicylates. Some may be discontinued by medical direction prior to a study. Note the last time and dose of medications taken.	Y	N	N/A
4	Note any current medications, allergies, therapies, or other procedures that might affect study results.	Y	N	N/A
5	Introduce yourself and positively identify the patient using two person-specific identifiers before services, treatments, or procedures are performed. Explain that the ID process is a safety measure, and it applies to each patient encounter.	Y	N	N/A
6	Explain how the procedure will aid in evaluation and assessment of the patient's clinical condition.	Y	N	N/A
7	Inform the patient of any instructions regarding pretesting diet, fluid, medication, or activity.	Y	N	N/A
8	Review the details of the procedure with the patient, including but not limited to a description of the procedure, what part of the body will be evaluated, whether or not the procedure is invasive, where it will take place, how long it will take, and who will be involved.	Y	N	N/A
9	Demonstrate sensitivity to cultural issues as well as concern for modesty.	Y	N	N/A
10	Address concerns about pain and explain that there may be some discomfort during the venipuncture, IV insertion, or procedure itself.	Y	N	N/A
11	Explain that sedation may be ordered for patients who are unable to cooperate (due to fear of medical procedures, combativeness, cognitive impairment, etc., or for pediatric patients).	Y	N	N/A

(continues on page 1256)

| 12 | *Ensure informed, written consent has been signed and documented prior to the procedure and before administering any medications related to the procedure.* | Y | N | N/A |
| 13 | Notify the individual who is performing a study in which bleeding is a known complication if the patient is taking aspirin or prescribed or natural anticoagulants. | Y | N | N/A |

Diagnostic Specifics

14	Consider whether scheduling conflicts exist. Check history of recent procedures, and consult with the laboratory or imaging department regarding potential interferences.	Y	N	N/A
15	Record the date of the last menstrual period. Pregnancy testing may be indicated before exposure to radiation.	Y	N	N/A
16	Consider complications regarding the use of iodinated contrast medium in patients with *preexisting renal insufficiency* (BUN, Cr, GFR with notification of abnormal results to the radiologist prior to study); patients who are *taking metformin for type 2 diabetes* (metformin should be discontinued on the day of the test and may continue to be withheld for 48 hours after the test); and patients who have a *sensitivity to contrast* (administer ordered premedication of corticosteroids and diphenhydramine).	Y	N	N/A
17	Instruct the patient to remove jewelry and other metallic objects from the area to be examined before going to the procedure location.	Y	N	N/A

Pediatric Considerations

| 18 | Be aware of general guidelines for pretest fasting: birth to 6 mo—3 hours; 7 mo to 2 yr—4 hr; 3 yr and older—6 hr. | Y | N | N/A |
| 19 | Consider the age of the child; use words the child will understand to give instructions. Encourage parents to be truthful about what the child may experience or must do. | Y | N | N/A |

INTRATEST: *These may be performed by health-care providers (HCPs) in other departments.*

20	Positively identify the patient.	Y	N	N/A
21	Review and ensure the patient followed all pretesting instructions regarding food, fluids, medications, activity, etc.	Y	N	N/A
22	Verify informed, written consent has been signed and documented prior to the procedure and before administering any medications related to the procedure.	Y	N	N/A
23	Communicate known allergies; avoid the use of allergenic materials if possible.	Y	N	N/A

CHK

24	Labelling of containers should be completed *after* specimen collection and should include patient demographics, initials of the person collecting the specimen, date and time of collection, and laterality.	Y	N	N/A

Diagnostic Specifics

25	Ensure that emergency medical equipment and medications are readily available in case of complications (e.g., bleeding, allergic reaction).	Y	N	N/A
26	Insert the IV for administration of ordered contrast, radionuclides, fluids, or medications. Ensure patency.	Y	N	N/A
27	Administer ordered medications: sedatives, anesthetics, or (for patients with a history of allergic reaction) prophylactic steroids or antihistamines.	Y	N	N/A
28	Instruct the patient to void prior to the procedure (unless a full bladder is needed) and to change into the robe, gown, and foot coverings.	Y	N	N/A
29	Clip hair from the area immediately before the procedure per organizational policy or standards of practice.	Y	N	N/A
30	Record baseline vital signs and assess neurological status.	Y	N	N/A
31	Monitor the patient for complications during the procedure (e.g., allergic reaction, anaphylaxis, bronchospasm, bleeding).	Y	N	N/A

POSTTEST: *The patient should be monitored for any related complications, be provided the opportunity to ask questions or express concerns, and be provided education regarding his or her health care.*

32	Observe the needle/catheter insertion site for bleeding, hematoma, inflammation; apply direct pressure with dry gauze and secure with an adhesive bandage.	Y	N	N/A
33	Transport specimens promptly to the laboratory for processing and analysis.	Y	N	N/A
34	Inform the patient that the requesting HCP will discuss the results with him or her.	Y	N	N/A
35	Instruct the patient to resume usual diet, fluids, medications, and activity as directed by the HCP (ensure gag reflex has returned).	Y	N	N/A
36	Complete postprocedural vital signs, assessments (venipuncture site, diagnostic study site), and neurological checks in relation to the procedure performed.	Y	N	N/A
37	Monitor the patient for related postprocedure complications (e.g., allergic reaction, anaphylaxis, bronchospasm, bleeding).	Y	N	N/A
38	Compare current findings with previous results. Evaluate test results in relation to the patient's symptoms and other tests performed.	Y	N	N/A

(continues on page 1258)

39	Provide timely notification of a critical finding and related symptoms. The notification process should include A. Read back to the caller of patient's name, one other patient-specific identifier, critical finding, name of the person giving the report, time and date of the report, name of the person receiving the report. B. Similar documentation is made when handing off communication to the requesting HCP.	Y	N	N/A
40	Review policy regarding any delay in a timely report of a critical finding. Actions may require completion of a notification form with review by risk management personnel.	Y	N	N/A
41	Provide a compassionate, reassuring environment. Recognize patient/family anxiety related to study results, and support coping strategies.	Y	N	N/A
42	Encourage questions, verbalization of concerns; provide answers and support.	Y	N	N/A
43	Provide teaching and information regarding the clinical implications of results.	Y	N	N/A
44	Explain any posttest restrictions (e.g., breastfeeding and nuclear medicine tests).			
45	Reinforce information given by the patient's HCP regarding further testing, treatment, or referral to another HCP.	Y	N	N/A
46	Explain that additional testing may be performed to evaluate or monitor progression of the disease process and determine the need for a change in therapy. Be prepared to educate the patient regarding access to the appropriate counseling services.	Y	N	N/A
47	Discuss the implications of abnormal results on the patient's lifestyle and explain the patient/family role in successfully achieving expected patient outcomes.	Y	N	N/A

CHK

Student Name _____   **Date** _____

Instructor Name _____   **Date** _____

Patient Preparation and Specimen Collection

COMMUNICATION AND PATIENT SAFETY

Successful encounters with patients begin with a professional, respectful, and compassionate approach.

- Positive communications should begin by addressing the patient using proper titles such as Ms., Mrs., or Mr.; the inappropriate use of terms of endearment is a common patient complaint.
- Health-care providers (HCPs) should always introduce and identify themselves to the patient before explaining the upcoming laboratory or diagnostic study. An example is to say, "Good morning. My name is Lilli and I will be your nurse today."
- Always conclude the conversation by asking if there are any questions before leaving the room.
- If you have a concern about a patient's level of understanding with the conversation, ask the individual to repeat what you have just explained so you can confirm that there are no issues.

Teach the patient what to expect.

Statement of the purpose of the study.

- The level of detail provided to patients about the test purpose depends on numerous factors and should be individualized appropriately in each setting. After the introduction, explain in easily understandable age-, culture-, and gender-appropriate terms about the study that is to be performed. Ask the patient to discuss his or her health concerns to give you a sense of how to begin the discussion. General information to communicate should include study type (e.g., blood, x-ray, MRI, urine, etc.) and the purpose or common use of the test (e.g., to assist in the diagnosis of diabetes, to assess the function of the kidneys, to identify the presence of findings that would either confirm a condition or confirm the absence of a health problem).

Description of the procedure and associated safety practices.

- Describe the procedure, what part of the body will be evaluated, whether or not the procedure is invasive, where the procedure will take place, and who will participate in performing the study.
- It is a good idea to explain to the patient that gloves will be worn by the HCPs throughout the procedure. Many institutions require hand washing at the beginning and end of each specimen collection encounter and between each patient. This explanation should help the patient understand that the use of gloves is standard practice established for everyone's safety and protection.
- Inquire about and document the patient's known allergies.
- Explain that it is essential the patient be positively and properly identified at each and every encounter before care, treatment, or services are provided. Patients may become concerned that they are asked to repeat their personal identification information. They may misinterpret this safety practice as incompetence, lack of communication, or lack of interest.

APP

- Typically, two patient-specific identifiers are used and may vary between inpatient and outpatient areas. Chosen identifiers may include full name, medical record number, or date of birth.

Addressing the need for informed consent.

- Some procedures may require informed, written consent as described in the facility's policy and procedure manual. What does informed (written) consent mean? Who is responsible for obtaining a consent?
- The exact definition and implementation of informed consent varies among states and individual health-care facilities in the United States. Best practices suggest a team approach. However, the concept of *informed consent* is generally based on the underlying moral and legal premises of patient autonomy found in a health-care facility's Bill of Patient's Rights and specific clinical policies. The U.S. Department of Health and Human Services describes informed consent to mean that if treatment is needed, the requesting HCP must provide that individual with the information needed to make the decision to agree with or decline the specified treatment plan. While many common patient-HCP interactions involve an implied voluntary consent, some specific procedures require *informed, written consent.* The list of tests and treatments requiring consent varies among facilities and may change with advances in clinical practice and technology. Generally, informed written consent is required for invasive procedures, tests, or treatments with significant risks, benefits, and alternatives. Once the requesting HCP has provided information to the patient, the informed patient's written consent must then be obtained and documented by the person designated in the facility's policy. The consent must be signed after the patient has been informed and before the procedure or administration of any medications that would affect his or her ability to make an important decision. There are a few legal exceptions to obtaining an informed (written) consent. Most commonly, they occur when there is a medical emergency that would result in death if not addressed immediately or in the case of mental incompetence in which an individual is unable to give or refuse consent and there is no surrogate (legal guardian or health-care proxy). *Patient assault* and *patient battery* are the legal terms put forth regarding the failure to obtain consent (as required by a facility's policies) before performing a test or procedure or allowing a deviation from the consented test or procedure to occur (unless an additional consent is appropriately obtained).
- Make sure a written and informed consent has been signed for the requested study and properly documented prior to the procedure and prior to administering any medications and according to your facility's requirements (Figure A–1).

Description of the sensations, including discomfort and pain, that may be experienced during specimen collection or a diagnostic procedure.

- Address concerns about pain related to the procedure, and suggest breathing or visualization techniques to promote relaxation.
- For pediatric patients, a doll may be used to "show" the procedure.
- Explain that where appropriate, sedative or anesthetizing agents may be used to assist in allaying anxiety the patient may experience related to anticipation of pain associated with the procedure.

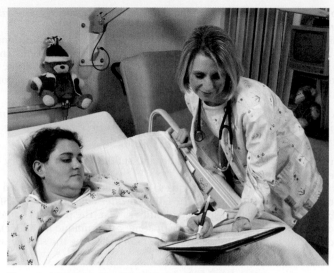

Figure A–1 Obtaining an informed and signed consent.

- Sedation and anesthesia are used to facilitate the completion of selected studies. Conscious or monitored sedation uses medication to promote relaxation and minimize pain while at the same time allowing the patient to remain conscious enough to communicate with the HCP. This approach is used to prevent pain and injury during a procedure.
- General anesthesia is medication given to cause a type of coma in which the patient is without consciousness or awareness and is protected from experiencing any pain associated with the procedure. However, with this type of sedation, the patient is also left without any protective reflexes.

General instruction regarding pretesting preparations.

- Explain pretesting diet, fluid, medication, or activity instructions and why strict adherence to the instructions is required to obtain accurate results.
- Fasting means no caloric intake for 8 or more hours.
- Failure to follow dietary, fluid, medication, activity, or other restrictions before the blood test or diagnostic procedure may cause the procedure to be canceled or repeated.
- *The practice of an overnight fast before a laboratory test is a general recommendation.*
- Reference ranges are often based on fasting populations to provide some level of standardization for comparison.
- Some test results are dramatically affected by foods, and fasting is a pretest requirement.
- The presence of lipids in the blood also may interfere with the test method; fasting eliminates this potential source of error, especially if the patient already has elevated lipid levels.
- The laboratory should always be consulted if there is a question whether fasting is a requirement or a recommendation.

- *The practice of an overnight fast before a diagnostic test is a general recommendation.*
- Dietary restrictions are usually related either to avoiding complications (e.g., aspiration), as with the use of anesthesia or other medications known to cause nausea and vomiting, or to avoiding factors that may alter the results of the study (e.g., undigested food that obscures visualization of the area of interest).

Specific patient preparation instructions and specimen collection techniques vary by site, study required, and level of invasiveness. The following guidelines should be implemented for all studies.

- Orders should be completed accurately and submitted per laboratory or diagnostic procedural policy.
- Positive patient identification extends to all specimens collected from the patient. Specimens should always be labelled, *after collection* per CLSI standards, with two patient-specific identifiers (e.g., the patient's name, date of birth, medical record number, or some other unique identifier), date collected, time collected, initials of the person collecting the sample, and laterality, if applicable (e.g., biopsies).

Recognition of anxiety related to test results.

- Provide a compassionate, reassuring environment.
- Encourage the patient to ask questions and verbalize concerns.
- Offer contact information for nationally recognized Web sites.

Results notification.

- Timely notification of a critical finding for laboratory or diagnostic studies is a role expectation of the professional nurse.
- Follow the facility's procedure for reporting and documenting critical findings.

Pediatric considerations for a laboratory or diagnostic study.

- Preparing children depends on the age of the child. Encourage parents to be truthful about unpleasant sensations (cramping, pressure, pinching, etc.) the child may experience during the procedure and to use words that they know their child will understand. Toddlers and preschool-age children have a very short attention span, so the best time to talk about the test is right before the procedure. The child should be assured that he or she will be allowed to bring a favorite comfort item into the examination room, and if appropriate, that a parent will be with the child during the procedure.
- Explain to parents and caregivers that special equipment (balloon-tip catheters to assist with retention of barium during a barium enema, foam wedges used to hold a limb in place during a nuclear scan, etc.) may be needed to assist with a successful study.
- Postprocedural recovery interventions, such as achieving adequate hydration, require close attention. The parents or caregivers must receive education to help them address specific needs and to be watchful for indications of a developing problem because pediatric patients cannot do so for themselves.

Older adult considerations for a laboratory or diagnostic study.

- Older adult patients present with a variety of concerns when undergoing diagnostic procedures. Level of cooperation and fall risk may be complicated by underlying problems such as visual and hearing impairment, joint and muscle stiffness, physical weakness, mental confusion, and the effects of medications.
- A fall injury can be avoided by providing assistance getting on and off the examination table and getting on and off the toilet before and at the end of the examination.
- Older adult patients are often chronically dehydrated; anticipating the effects of hypovolemia and orthostasis can also help prevent falls.
- Older patients who are small in size compared to other adults also may receive a higher radiation dose than necessary if settings are not adjusted for their size.
- Special equipment (balloon-tip catheters to assist with retention of barium during a barium enema, foam wedges used to hold a limb in place during a nuclear scan, etc.) may be needed to assist with a successful study.
- Postprocedural recovery interventions, such as achieving adequate hydration, require close attention.
- Many older patients wish to maintain their independence. Their caregivers must receive education to help them address specific needs and to be watchful for indications of a developing problem; the limits of an older adult patient's physical and intellectual abilities may be an obstacle to independently carrying out the proper postprocedural care.

BLOOD SPECIMENS

Most laboratory tests that require a blood specimen use venous blood. Arterial blood specimens are usually collected for specific tests such as blood gas analysis.

- *Venous blood* can be collected directly from the vein or by way of capillary puncture.
  Venous blood also can be obtained from vascular access devices, such as:
  1. Saline locks
  2. Central venous (triple-lumen subclavian, implanted venous access port, Groshong) catheters.
- *Capillary blood can be obtained from the fingertips or earlobes of adults and small children and from the heels of infants.*
  The circumstances in which the capillary method is selected over direct venipuncture include cases in which:
  1. The patient has poor veins.
  2. The patient has small veins.
  3. The patient has a limited number of available veins.
  4. The patient has significant anxiety about the venipuncture procedure.
- *Fetal blood samples can be obtained, when warranted, by a qualified HCP from the scalp or from the umbilical cord.*
- *Arterial blood can be collected from the radial, brachial, or femoral artery if blood gas analysis is requested.*

APP

In addition to guidelines presented in previous section, when collecting and handling blood specimens:

- Stress can cause variations in some test results. A sleeping patient should be gently awakened and allowed the opportunity to become oriented before collection site selection.
- Comatose or unconscious patients should be greeted in the same gentle manner because, although they are unable to respond, they may be capable of hearing and understanding.
- Anticipate instances in which patient cooperation may be an issue. Enlist a second person to assist with specimen collection to ensure a safe, quality collection experience for all involved.
- Gloves and any other additional personal protective equipment indicated by the patient's condition should always be worn during the specimen collection process.
- The facility's specific standard precautions policy should be consulted for further details.
- Often, several blood specimens are collected together. Ensure the blood specimens are collected in the correct order to protect the integrity of the studies. *Always follow your facility's protocol for order of draw.* Generally:
  1. Blood culture tube (yellow) or bottle.
  2. Sodium citrate (blue); coagulation studies. *Note:*
     A. When using a butterfly and the blue-top tube is the first tube drawn, a nonadditive red-top or coagulation discard tube should be collected first and discarded.
     B. The amount of blood in the discard tube needs to be sufficient to fill the winged collection set tubing's "dead space" or fill one-quarter of the discard tube.
     C. The blue-top tube to be used for testing must be completely filled to ensure the proper ratio of blood to additive in the test specimen blue-top tube.
  3. Serum—plain, additive, gel (red, SST); most chemistries, drug levels, and serologies.
  4. Heparin—additive or gel (light or dark green); most chemistries.
  5. EDTA—additive or gel (lavender, pink, pearl white); hematology blood counts, blood bank, molecular studies.
  6. Sodium fluoride/potassium oxalate—antiglycolytic inhibitor (gray); glucose studies, tolerance tests.
- Localized activity such as the application of a tourniquet or clenching the hand to assist in visualizing the vein can cause variations in some test results. It is important to be aware of affected studies before specimen collection.
  - Hemoconcentration may cause variations in some test results. *The tourniquet should never be left in place for longer than 1 min.*
  - Previous puncture sites should be avoided when accessing a blood vessel by any means to reduce the potential for infection.
  - Blood specimens should never be collected above an IV line because of the potential for dilution when the specimen and the IV solution combine in the collection container, falsely decreasing the result. It is also possible that substances in the IV solution could contaminate the specimen and result in falsely elevated test results.

APP

- Changes in posture from supine to erect or long-term maintenance of a supine posture causes variations in some test results. It is important to be aware of this effect when results are interpreted and compared with previous values.
- Collection times for therapeutic drug (peak and trough) or other specific monitoring (e.g., chemotherapy, glucose, insulin, or potassium) should be documented carefully in relation to the time of medication administration. It is essential that this information be communicated clearly and accurately to avoid misunderstanding of the dose time in relation to the collection time. Miscommunication between the individual administering the medication and the individual collecting the specimen is the most frequent cause of subtherapeutic levels, toxic levels, and misleading information used in the calculation of future therapies.
- The laboratory should be consulted regarding minimum specimen collection requirements when multiple tube types or samples are required. Factors that invalidate estimation of blood volume include conditions such as anemia, polycythemia, dehydration, and overhydration.
- The laboratory should be consulted regarding the preferred container/specimen type before sample collection.
  - In many cases when a blood sample is required, serum is the specimen type of choice.
  - Plasma may be frequently substituted, however. Specimen processing is more rapid for plasma samples than for serum samples because the anticoagulated sample does not need to clot before centrifugation. Plasma samples also require less centrifugation time to achieve adequate separation.
  - Consultation regarding collection containers is also important because some laboratory methods are optimized for a specific specimen type (serum versus plasma).
  - Preservatives present in collection containers, such as sodium fluoride, may exhibit a chemical interference with test reagents that can cause underestimation or overestimation of measured values.
  - Other preservatives, such as EDTA, can block the analyte of interest in the sample (e.g., calcium) from participating in the test reaction, invalidating test results.
  - It is possible that some high-throughput, robotic equipment systems require specific and standardized collection containers.
- Prompt and proper specimen processing, storage, and analysis are essential to achieve accurate results. Results that are evaluated outside the entire context of the preparatory, collection, and handling process may be interpreted erroneously if consideration is not given to these general guidelines in addition to the collection guidelines.
  - Specimens collected in containers with solid or liquid preservatives or with gel separators should be mixed by inverting the tube 10 times immediately after the tube has been filled.
  - Specimens should be mixed and handled gently to avoid hemolysis.
- Specimens should always be transported to the laboratory as quickly as possible after collection.
- Once the draws are completed, tell the patient that a report of the results will be made available to the requesting HCP, who will discuss the results with the patient.

APP

Special Considerations Regarding Multiple Venipunctures in the Pediatric and Older Adult Populations

- *Two venipuncture-related concerns that are especially important pertain to the selection of specimen collection materials and the volume of specimen required.*

1. Iatrogenic anemia is a significant concern for hospitalized infants.
2. Anemia from chronic blood sampling can be an issue for older adults who may also suffer malnutrition, dehydration, and diminished hematopoietic system response.

- The use of Microtainers allows for specimen collection from capillary sites.
- Many vacuum tubes, including blood culture tubes, are available in pediatric sizes to reduce collection volume.
- Advances in the technology of laboratory equipment has dramatically reduced, to microsamples, the amount of specimen required for testing.

There have been other changes in equipment used specifically to address specimen collection issues in the pediatric and older adult populations.

- The use of butterfly needles or winged infusion sets has become very popular with older adults who believe "they hurt less and are smaller than" conventional needles. This is a patient perception; butterfly and vacutainer holder needles are available in the same sizes.
- The skin of pediatric and older adult patients is very delicate, and traditionally tape is used to hold the bandage in place after the venipuncture. Many patients cannot even tolerate paper tape that is made with less adhesive.
- A self-adhesive wrap is now commonly used instead of tape; a section of the wrap is placed over the bandage and then the roll of adhesive is wrapped several times around the bandage.
- The wrap sticks to itself instead of to the skin, very effectively holds the bandage in place, comes in a wide array of colors, and is very popular with patients.
- The venipuncture site can also be dressed using a bandage over-wrapped with gauze and held in place by tape, without touching the skin. *This approach is safer for pediatric and older adult patients who may forget to remove the self-adhesive wrap in a timely fashion. Excessive tension and compression to the skin can result in unintended injury.*

Capillary Puncture: Assess the selected area. It should be free of lesions and calluses, there should be no edema, and the site should feel warm. If the site feels cool or appears pale or cyanotic, warm compresses can be applied over 3 to 5 min to dilate the capillaries. For fingersticks, the central, fleshy, distal portions of the third or fourth fingers are the preferred collection sites (Figure A–2, Capillary puncture of the finger). For neonatal heel sticks, the medial and lateral surfaces of the plantar area are preferred to avoid direct puncture of the heel bone, which could result in osteomyelitis (Figure A–3, Capillary puncture of the heel).

Venipuncture of Arm: Assess the arm for visibly accessible veins. The selected area should not be burned or scarred, have a tattoo, or have hematoma present. Even after the tourniquet is applied, not all patients have a prominent median

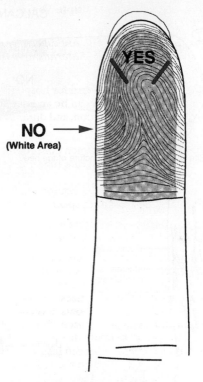

Figure A–2 Site selection. Capillary puncture of the finger.

cubital, cephalic, or basilic vein. Both arms should be observed because some patients have accessible veins in one arm and not the other. The median cubital vein in the antecubital fossa is the preferred venipuncture site. The patient may be able to provide the best information regarding venous access if he or she has had previous venipuncture experience. Alternative techniques to increase visibility of veins may include warming the arm, allowing the arm to dangle downward for a minute or two, tapping the antecubital area with the index finger, or massaging the arm upward from wrist to elbow. The condition of the vein also should be assessed before venipuncture. Sclerotic (hard, scarred) veins or veins in which phlebitis previously occurred should be avoided. Arms with a functioning hemodialysis access site should not be used. The arm on the affected side of a mastectomy should be avoided. In the case of a double mastectomy, the requesting HCP should be consulted before specimen collection.

Venipuncture of Hand and Wrist: If no veins in the arms are available, hands and wrists should be examined as described for the arm (Figure A-4,

APP

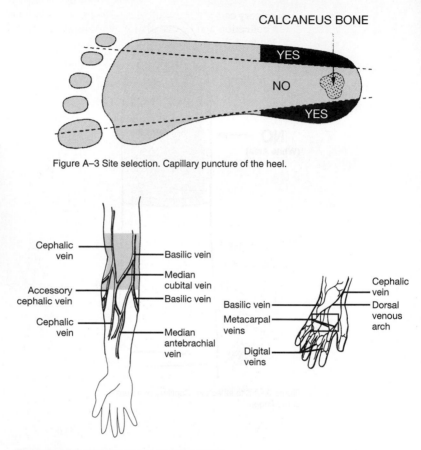

Figure A–3 Site selection. Capillary puncture of the heel.

Figure A–4 Site selection. Venipuncture arm/hand.

Venipuncture arm/hand). Consideration should be given to the venipuncture equipment selected because the veins in these areas are much smaller. Pediatric-sized collection containers and needles with a larger gauge may be more appropriate.

Venipuncture of Legs and Feet: The veins in the legs and feet can be accessed as with sites located on the arm, hand, or wrist. These extremities should be used only on the approval of the requesting HCP because veins in these locations are more prone to infection and formation of blood clots, especially in patients with diabetes, cardiac disease, and bleeding disorders.

Radial Arterial Puncture: The radial artery is the artery of choice for obtaining arterial blood gas specimens because it is close to the surface of the wrist and does not require a deep puncture (Figure A–5, Arterial arm/hand). Its easy access also allows for more effective compression after the needle has been removed. The nearby ulnar artery can provide sufficient collateral circulation to the hand during specimen collection and postcollection compression. See also Figure A-6, Allen test and Figure A-7, Arterial puncture.

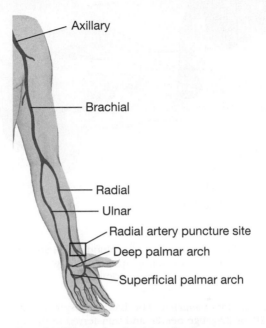

Figure A–5 Site selection. Arterial arm/hand.

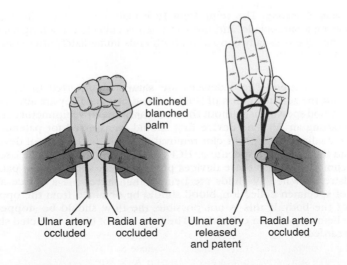

Figure A–6 Allen test.

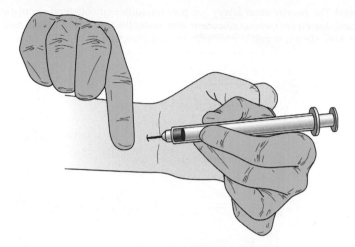

Figure A–7 Arterial puncture.

Percutaneous Umbilical Cord Sampling: The blood is aspirated from the umbilical cord under the guidance of ultrasonography and using a 20- or 22-gauge spinal needle inserted through the mother's abdomen.

Postnatal Umbilical Cord Sampling: The blood is aspirated from the umbilical cord using a 20- or 22-gauge needle and transferred to the appropriate collection container.

Fetal Scalp Sampling: The requesting HCP makes a puncture in the fetal scalp using a microblade, and the specimen is collected in a long capillary tube. The tube is usually capped on both ends immediately after specimen collection.

Locks and Catheters: These devices are sometimes inserted to provide a means for the administration of fluids or medications. They are also used to obtain blood specimens without the need for frequent venipuncture (Figure A–8, Starting an IV). The device first should be assessed for patency. The need for saline irrigation or clot removal depends on the type of device in use and the institution-specific or HCP-specific protocols in effect. Use sterile technique because these devices provide direct access to the patient's bloodstream. When IV fluids are being administered via a device at the time of specimen collection, blood should be obtained from the opposite side of the body. If this is not possible, the flow should be stopped for 5 min before specimen collection. The first 5 mL of blood collected should be discarded.

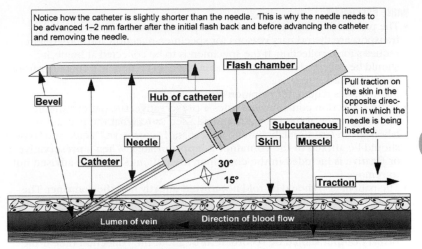

Notice how the catheter is slightly shorter than the needle. This is why the needle needs to be advanced 1–2 mm farther after the initial flash back and before advancing the catheter and removing the needle.

Figure A–8 Site selection. Starting an IV.

Complications Associated with Invasive Punctures of the Skin

- Pain is commonly associated with needles, and although pain experienced during a needle puncture is usually mild, on a rare occasion the needle may strike a nerve, causing severe and lasting pain.
- Hematoma results when blood leaks into the tissue during or after a needle puncture, as evidenced by pain, bruising, and/or swelling at the puncture site. The swelling can cause temporary or permanent injury by compressing the surrounding nerves. Hematomas occur more often in older adult or frail patients or in those with vessels that are difficult to access.
- Prolonged bleeding is a complication that occurs with patients who are taking blood thinners, such as aspirin or warfarin, or who have coagulopathies, such as hemophilia.
- Once the needle has been removed, bleeding or bruising can be prevented by applying direct pressure to the puncture site with gauze for a minute or two. The site should then be observed/assessed for bleeding or bruising. If no further action is required, the site can be covered by the gauze and an adhesive bandage or paper tape.
- Some patients experience a vasovagal reaction during the needle puncture procedure, evidenced by sweating (diaphoresis), low blood pressure (hypotension), fainting (syncope), or near fainting (near syncope). The potential for a fall injury is a significant concern related to vasovagal reactions.
- Other, more unusual complications of needle puncture include cellulitis, phlebitis, seizures, inadvertent arterial puncture during a venipuncture, and sepsis.
- Sepsis can be caused by introduction of bacteria from the surface of the skin into the blood as the result of improper cleansing of the puncture site.
- Immunocompromised patients are at higher risk for developing sepsis as a complication of venipuncture.

URINE SPECIMENS

- The patient should be informed that improper collection, storage, and transport are the primary reasons for specimen rejection and subsequent requests for recollection. If the specimen is to be collected at home, it should be collected in a clean plastic container (preferably a container from the testing laboratory).
- Many studies require refrigeration after collection.
- If the collection container includes a preservative, the patient should be made aware of the contents and advised as to what the precaution labels mean (caution labels such as "caustic," "corrosive," "acid," and "base" should be affixed to the container as appropriate). When a preservative or fixative is included in the container, the patient should be advised not to remove it.
- The patient also should be told not to void directly into the container. The patient should be given a collection device, if indicated, and instructed to void into the collection device.
- The specimen should be carefully transferred into the collection container. Urinary output should be recorded throughout the collection time if the specimen is being collected over a specified time interval. Some laboratories provide preprinted collection instructions tailored to their methods. The specimen should be transported promptly to the laboratory after collection.

Random: These samples are used mainly for routine screening and can be collected at any time of the day. The patient should be instructed to void either directly into the collection container (if there is no preservative) or into a collection device for transfer into the specimen container.

First Morning: Urine on rising in the morning is very concentrated. These specimens are indicated when screening for substances that may not be detectable in a more dilute random sample. These specimens are also necessary for testing conditions such as orthostatic proteinuria, in which levels vary with changes in posture.

Second Void: In some cases, it is desirable to test freshly produced urine to evaluate the patient's current status, as with glucose and ketones. Explain to the patient that he or she should first void and then drink a glass of water. The patient should be instructed to wait 30 min and then void either directly into the collection container or into a collection device for transfer into the collection container.

Clean Catch: These midstream specimens are generally used for microbiological or cytological studies. They also may be requested for routine urinalysis to provide a specimen that is least contaminated with urethral cells, microorganisms, mucus, or other substances that may affect the interpretation of results. Instruct the male patient first to wash hands thoroughly, then cleanse the meatus, void a small amount into the toilet, and void either directly into the specimen container or into a collection device for transfer into the specimen container. Instruct the female patient first to wash hands thoroughly, and then to cleanse the labia from front to back. While keeping the labia separated, the patient should void a small amount into the toilet, and then, without interrupting the urine stream, void either directly into the specimen container or into a collection device for transfer into the specimen container.

Catheterized Random or Clean Catch: "Straight catheterization" is indicated when the patient is unable to void, when the patient is unable to prepare properly for clean-catch specimen collection, or when the patient has an indwelling catheter in place from which a urine sample may be obtained. Before collecting a specimen from the catheter, observe the drainage tube to ensure that it is empty, and then clamp the tube distal to the collection port 15 min before specimen collection. Cleanse the port with an antiseptic swab such as 70% alcohol and allow the port to dry. Use a needle and syringe (sterile if indicated) to withdraw the required amount of specimen (Figure A-9, Urine collection from an indwelling catheter). Unclamp the tube.

Timed: To quantify substances in urine, 24-hr urine collections are used. They are also used to measure substances whose level of excretion varies over time. The use of preservatives and the handling of specimens during the timed collection may be subject to variability among laboratories. The testing laboratory should be consulted regarding specific instructions before starting the test. Many times, the specimen must be refrigerated or kept on ice throughout the entire collection period. Explain to the patient that it is crucial for *all* urine to be included in the collection. Urinary output should be recorded throughout the collection time if the specimen is being collected

APP

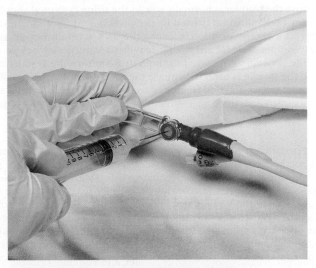

Figure A–9 Urine collection from an indwelling catheter.

over a specified time interval. The test should begin between 0600 and 0800 if possible. Instruct the patient to collect the first void of the day and discard it. The start time of the collection period begins at the time the first voided specimen was discarded and should be recorded along with the date on the collection container. Urine from all subsequent voidings should be collected and transferred into the collection container. The patient should be instructed to void at the same time the following morning and to add this last voiding to the container. This is the end time of the collection and should be recorded along with the date on the container. For patients who are in the hospital, the urinary output should be compared with the volume measured in the completed collection container. Discrepancies between the two volumes indicate that a collection might have been discarded. A creatinine level often is requested along with the study of interest to evaluate the completeness of the collection.

Catheterized Timed: Instructions for this type of collection are basically the same as those for timed specimen collection. The test should begin by changing the tubing and drainage bag. If a preservative is required, it can be placed directly in the drainage bag, or the specimen can be removed at frequent intervals (every 2 hr) and transferred to the collection container to which the preservative has been added. The drainage bag must be kept on ice or emptied periodically into the collection container during the entire collection period if indicated by the testing laboratory. The tubing should be monitored throughout the collection period to ensure continued drainage.

Suprapubic Aspiration: This procedure is performed by inserting a needle directly into the bladder (Figure A-10, Suprapubic aspiration of a urine specimen). Because the bladder is normally sterile, the urine collected should also be free from any contamination caused by the presence of microorganisms. Place the patient in a supine position. Cleanse the area with antiseptic and drape with sterile drapes. A local anesthetic may be administered before insertion of the needle. A needle is inserted through the skin into the bladder. A syringe attached to the needle is used to aspirate the urine sample. The needle is then removed and a sterile dressing is applied to the site. Place the sterile sample in a sterile specimen container. The site must be observed for signs of inflammation or infection.

Pediatric: Specimen collection can be achieved by any of the previously described methods using collection devices specifically designed for pediatric patients. Appropriately cleanse the genital area and allow the area to dry. For a random collection, remove the covering of the adhesive strips on the collector bag and apply over the genital area (Figure A-11, Pediatric urine collection). Diaper the child. When the specimen is obtained, place the entire collection bag in the specimen container (use a sterile container as appropriate for the requested study). Some laboratories may have specific preferences for the submission of urine specimens for culture. Consult the laboratory before collection to avoid specimen rejection.

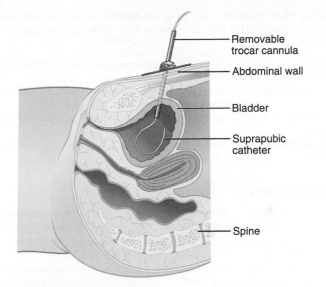

- Removable trocar cannula
- Abdominal wall
- Bladder
- Suprapubic catheter
- Spine

Figure A–10 Suprapubic aspiration of a urine specimen.

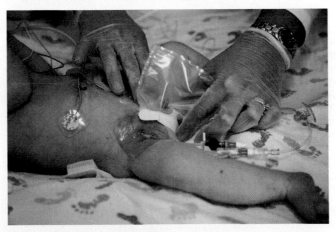

Figure A–11 Pediatric urine collection.

DIAGNOSTIC IMAGING TESTS

Imaging technology has exploded since its introduction in the early 1900s. The four most commonly used imaging modalities include radiography, nuclear medicine, magnetic resonance imaging (MRI), and ultrasound (US). The current menu of diagnostic studies can quickly become confusing, especially since some involve radiation and some do not, imaging using combined modalities is becoming more common, and most modalities can be ordered either with or without contrast. The use of contrast may introduce additional nursing implications.

- Radiography—detection of x-ray emissions generated by external exposure to radiation emitting equipment
- Nuclear medicine—detection of gamma ray emissions generated from radio-isotopes administered internally to the patient
- MRI—detection of radiowaves generated by external exposure to a magnetic field
- US—detection of sound waves generated by a transducer, applied externally to the skin

APP

Imaging Study Types		
	Ordered without contrast	**Ordered with contrast: Contrast commonly used**
Radiography (involves radioactivity provided by an external source in the form of x-ray emissions)		
Plain X-ray	Yes	Iodine or barium based
Fluoroscopy	Yes	Iodine, barium, air; various others by examination or procedure type
Angiography	N/A	Iodine based
Computed Tomography (CT)	Yes	Iodine or barium based
Mammography	Yes	Iodine based
Nuclear Medicine (involves radioactivity emitted from an internal source in the form of gamma ray emissions)		
Nuclear Scans and Positron Emission Tomography (PET) Scans	Contrast is not used in these types of studies unless in combination with CT or other modalities	
MRI		
MRI Scans	Yes	Gadolinium based
US		
US Studies	Yes	Microbubbles of perfluorocarbon or nitrogen gas

Contrast Agents

Contrast medium is used to enhance the radio-density or radio-opaqueness of the target site. It does this by blocking the x-ray or radio wave emissions from passing through anatomical areas of various densities. Radiolucency refers to greater passage of x-ray or radio wave emissions through various densities. The opacity of an area being visualized is determined both by its density and also by the chemical properties of the elements of which it is made. Bone is the densest tissue in the body and contains a lot of calcium. Calcium has a relatively high atomic number (protons). As an example, of the common elements that make up the solids and liquids in our body, the atomic number of calcium is 20, oxygen is 8, carbon is 6, and hydrogen is 1. It is not a coincidence that materials used as contrast agents in diagnostic imaging have relatively high atomic numbers compared to the elements that comprise our body fluids and tissues; for example, iodine is 53, barium is 56, gallium is 31.

Oral Contrast Medium for X-ray and CT Imaging	Rectal Contrast Medium for X-ray and CT Imaging	IV Contrast Medium for X-ray and CT Imaging	IV Contrast Medium for MRI Imaging	IV Contrast Medium for US
Barium based	Barium based	Iodine based	Gadolinium based	Microbubble
Target Site				
GI tract	GI tract	Internal organs, GI tract, arteries and veins, soft tissue, breast tissue, brain tissue	Specific site of interest	

Radiography

Radiography is a general term to describe types of studies that use x-ray emissions to look inside the body. This technology is the cornerstone of diagnostic imaging. Radiography is based on the absorption of x-rays as they pass through areas of the body composed of material having different densities. X-rays readily pass through air, water, body fluids, fat, and soft tissue and are termed *radiolucent;* they pass through the exposed area to the film. The images are developed respectively in shades from black to gray. Bone tissue is relatively dense and absorbs x-rays. The effect is termed *radiopaque;* the bones block radiation from reacting with the x-ray detectors so their images are white; the image created by the bones is essentially the shadow cast from the areas of undeveloped x-ray media.

Uses of radiography include obtaining static internal structural images to diagnose disease, structural damage, or abnormalities; identifying foreign objects; verification of surgical marker placement; planning of radiation therapy regimens. The chest x-ray is the most common radiograph.

Fluoroscopy

Images produced by this technique are generated in similar fashion to the plain x-ray, but the technology uses a continuous stream of x-rays, at a lower dose, to create a "moving picture."

Uses of fluoroscopy include evaluation of specific areas of the body; evaluation of functional organs during a procedure (e.g., barium enema); guidance during insertion and manipulation of catheters, placement of devices (e.g., stents) or implants, and injections into joints or the spine; angiography; identification and location of foreign bodies; and numerous other applications.

Angiography

Angiography involves injection of contrast into the area of interest allowing for x-ray visualization of organ or vessel structure and function. Angiography should be performed after other studies using contrast to avoid the additive effect of visualizing residual contrast medium; consult the appropriate imaging department.

Uses of angiography include diagnostic and therapeutic applications related to blood vessels and the major associated organ systems (e.g., circulatory, brain). Examples are narrowing or blockage of blood vessels; identification of areas of inflammation or bleeding; and insertion of devices like stents or guide wires for catheterization.

Computed Tomography

CT without contrast is a relatively painless, fast, and accurate noninvasive diagnostic tool. CT uses a motorized x-ray source as opposed to a static source, as with the plain x-ray. The rotation of the x-ray tube around the patient creates detailed cross-sectional images of internal organs, bones, soft tissue and blood vessels, including the identification of internal bleeding. CT becomes invasive when contrast is introduced via a catheter.

Images can be immediately reviewed on multiple planes and in a three-dimensional format in the imaging department, stored in the facility's PACS (picture archiving communication system), or copied to an electronic storage device and given to the patient. CT should be performed after other studies using contrast to avoid the additive effect of visualizing residual contrast medium; consult the appropriate imaging department.

Uses of CT are extensive and are not limited to but include rapid assessment or internal injuries due to trauma; diagnosis of bone and soft tissue diseases; identification and location of tumors, thrombosis, or infection; guide surgical procedures, collection of biopsy samples; and monitor response to therapeutic regimens.

Nuclear Medicine

	Radiopharmaceuticals commonly used	Route of tracer administration	Target site
Nuclear Medicine (involves radioactivity in the form of gamma ray emissions)			
Nuclear Scans	C^{14}, Ga^{67}, I^{123}, I^{124}, I^{131}, In^{111}, Tc^{99}, Tl^{201}	IV, orally, inhalation	Determined by the site of interest
PET	F^{18}	IV	Varies but includes brain, heart, pelvis

Nuclear medicine studies use radioactive tracers that can be injected into a blood vessel (e.g., hepatobiliary scan), inhaled (e.g., lung scan), or swallowed (e.g., C-14 urea breath test) to obtain information on disease processes. Radioactive tracers emit gamma ray energy that can be detected by a conventional gamma camera or SPECT/CT camera, and then used to create computerized images.

Nuclear medicine studies can involve multiple images taken over a specified period of time, after a radionuclide is administered. Imaging intervals vary by study. Each image takes about 20 minutes; serial images may be taken in a single day or over a period of 2 to 3 days. Previous nuclear medicine scans completed within 24 to 48 hr may interfere with the current study due to the measurement of residual tracer in addition to tracer from the current study. The plasma half-life of medical radionuclides is usually short with complete clearance from the blood within 24 to 48 hr. Exceptions include Gallium-67 (78 hr), Indium-111 (2.8 days), Iodine-124 (4.2 days), Iodine-131 (8 days), and Thallium-201 (73 hr).

Pretest dietary considerations vary by procedure. Some procedures have no dietary considerations (e.g., thyroid scan). Patients may need to be NPO for 8 hr before the procedure (e.g., Meckel's diverticulum scan), NPO for 8 hr before the procedure but given a special meal in the nuclear medicine department on the day of the scan (e.g., a gastric emptying study), or in other cases patients may be instructed to follow a low carbohydrate diet in the 24 hr prior to the study and be NPO for 8 hr before the study (e.g., PET scan). Individual studies should be reviewed for specific information.

Uses of nuclear medicine applications are extensive and apply to diagnostic imaging as well as planning and implementing therapeutic regimens.

- Treatments using internal exposure to radiation include brachytherapy (irradiation of areas inside a patient, such as implanted radioactive seeds) or teletherapy treatments (noninvasive, serial radiation treatments).
- Alpha radioimmunotherapy or targeted alpha therapy (TAT) is a developing area of study in which a monoclonal antibody is labelled with an alpha-emitting radioisotope. The radioisotope targets cancer at the cellular level for destruction.

PET scans are a relatively new and specialized group of nuclear medicine studies that can evaluate organ and tissue function in addition to location and structure.

- PET uses radiotracers to map organ and tissue function (blood flow, glucose metabolism, oxygen use) and documents findings with the use of imaging equipment that detects the presence of the radioactive emissions. Technology is now available to simultaneously combine or superimpose the information collected in the PET scan with a CT or MRI study. Evaluation of cellular body changes allows for early recognition of disease onset even before it is noted through other forms of examination.
- PET scans can be used to identify cancer, discern whether the cancer has spread or returned, and evaluate the effectiveness of cancer treatment; it can also be used to evaluate cardiac health, cardiac muscle blood flow, damage caused by heart attack, and the potential benefit of invasive procedures such as angioplasty or surgery such as coronary artery bypass graft.
- PET scans can map heart and brain function and identify tumors and causes of memory disorders, seizures, or central nervous disorders.
- FDA approved PET radiopharmaceuticals include: F–18 sodium fluoride (bone imaging), Rb-82 rubidium chloride (cardiovascular assessment for MI), F-18 fluorodeoxyglucose (cardiovascular, neurologic, oncology applications), and N-13 ammonia (cardiovascular assessment of blood flow).

APP

Magnetic Resonance Imaging

MRI uses magnetic and radio waves to evaluate areas of soft tissue area of interest for diagnosis of disease and evaluation of the effectiveness of therapeutic interventions. MRI is considered to be a safer alternative than studies involving radiation, such as radiography and CT; the number of MRI studies performed is not limited as with x-ray or CT. However, with MRI, the extremely powerful magnet can inactivate, move, or shift metallic objects inside a patient. Use of an MRI screening tool is recommended to obtain accurate information and foster patient safety. Any questions related to MRI compatibility with the materials used in a patient device should be verified with the manufacturer.

Patients with extreme cases of claustrophobia may require sedation before completing the study. Patients on mechanical ventilators may need to be bagged during MRI. Ear plugs may need to be provided to dampen the loud noises made by the MRI equipment.

In specific situations where gadolinium-based contrast agent (GBCA) will be administered, the risk versus benefit must be evaluated. GBCAs cross the placental barrier, enter the fetal circulation, and pass via the fetal urinary system into the amniotic fluid. Although no definite adverse effects of GBCA administration on the human fetus have been documented, the potential bioeffects of fetal GBCA exposure are not well understood. GBCA administration should therefore be avoided during pregnancy unless no suitable alternative imaging is possible and the benefits of contrast administration outweigh the potential risk to the fetus. The use of GBCAs should also be avoided in patients with kidney dysfunction unless the benefits of the studies outweigh the risks and if essential diagnostic information is not available using non-contrast-enhanced diagnostic studies.

Uses of MRI are extensive and provide especially excellent soft-tissue imaging.

Ultrasound

Ultrasound is a fast, inexpensive, noninvasive way to visualize images with the use of high-frequency sound waves instigated by a transducer. The sound waves bounce off anatomical structures and fluids to provide diagnostic information without the use of radiation.

• Procedures such as endoscopy, surgery, biopsy, barium studies, colonoscopy, and endoscopic retrograde cholangiopancreatography can interfere with US results. US should be performed after other studies using contrast to avoid the additive effect of visualizing residual contrast medium; consult the appropriate imaging department

Uses for US include assessment of organ perfusion; identification of thrombosis, structural abnormalities of an organ, and tumor; indication of inflammation; response to therapeutic regimens.

Radiation Safety
• The goal for diagnostic studies and medical treatments using radioisotopes or imaging equipment that emits radiation is to prevent unnecessary exposure of staff and patient while meeting clinical diagnostic goals.
• The three most common types of radioactive emissions are alpha, beta, and gamma. Alpha rays are relatively harmless because they do not travel far

from the source and do not penetrate most materials. Beta rays can travel several feet from the source, have a lot of energy, and are very small; they can penetrate clothing and skin, making them somewhat more dangerous. Gamma rays have the most energy and are able to penetrate most forms of matter (e.g., air, liquids, solids); they represent a highly dangerous type of exposure that can produce extreme damage.

- Radiation exposure can be external or internal. External exposure can occur either using well-controlled technology to perform diagnostic studies or negligently through inadequate time, distance, and shielding from the radiation source. Internal exposure occurs purposefully through diagnostic or therapeutic means. It can also take place unknowingly with the inhalation of radioactive gas, ingestion of contaminated food or fluids, and absorption of radiation through exposure to contaminated urine, emesis, or other body fluids. The best way to control exposure is to follow the facility's radiation safety policies and procedures.

Pediatric Imaging Radiation risk is higher in young patients because they have more rapidly dividing cells than adults, and radiation damage occurs during cell division. Therefore, the younger the patient, the more radiation-sensitive the patient is. The Image Gently Campaign is an initiative of the Alliance for Radiation Safety in Pediatric Imaging. Information on the Image Gently Campaign can be found at the Alliance for Radiation Safety in Pediatric Imaging (www.image-gently.org/). The campaign goal is to change practice by increasing awareness of the opportunities to promote radiation protection in the imaging of children. Three unique considerations in pediatric imaging are as follows:

- Children are considerably more sensitive to radiation than adults, which is evidenced in epidemiologic studies of exposed populations.
- Children have a longer life expectancy than adults, resulting in a larger window of opportunity for showing radiation damage.
- Children may receive a higher radiation dose than necessary if settings are not adjusted for their small size.

Older Adult Imaging
- Some older adults may receive a higher radiation dose than necessary if settings are not adjusted for their small size.

Risks are associated with the use of contrast media, especially iodinated contrast mediums. Pediatric patients have immature or incompletely developed organ and immune systems that do not tolerate the rigors of diagnostic testing as well as adults. Older adults are also potentially less able to tolerate some procedures because their systems are weakened by the natural aging process and interactions that may occur due to the presence of complex multisystem diseases.

- Care should be taken if iodinated contrast medium is scheduled to be used in patients with preexisting renal insufficiency (e.g., chronic kidney disease, single kidney transplant, nephrectomy, diabetes, multiple myeloma, treatment with aminoglycosides and NSAIDs) because iodinated contrast is nephrotoxic. Consideration should also be given to patients who are chronically dehydrated before the test, especially older adults and patients whose health is already compromised, because of their risk of contrast-induced acute kidney injury.

- If iodinated contrast medium is scheduled to be used in patients receiving metformin or medications containing metformin for type 2 diabetes, the drug may be discontinued on the day of the test and continue to be withheld for 48 hr after the test. Failure to withhold metformin may indirectly result in drug-induced lactic acidosis, a dangerous and sometimes fatal side effect of metformin *(related to renal impairment that does not support sufficient excretion of metformin).*

Laboratory Critical Findings

Study	Critical Finding (Conventional Units [CU])	Conversion Factor	Critical Finding (SI)
Therapeutic Drugs			
Analgesic and Antipyretic Drugs			
Acetaminophen	Greater than 200 mcg/mL (4 hr post-ingestion)	SI = CU × 6.62	Greater than 1,324 micromol/L (4 hr post-ingestion)
Acetylsalicylic acid	Greater than 40 mg/dL	SI = CU × 0.073	Greater than 2.9 mmol/L
Anticonvulsant Drugs			
Carbamazepine	Greater than 20 mcg/mL	SI = CU × 4.23	Greater than 85 micromol/L
Ethosuximide	Greater than 200 mcg/mL	SI = CU × 7.08	Greater than 1,416 micromol/L
Lamotrigine	Greater than 20 mcg/mL	SI = CU × 3.9	Greater than 78 micromol/L
Phenobarbital	Greater than 60 mcg/mL	SI = CU × 4.31	Greater than 259 micromol/L
Phenytoin	Greater than 40 mcg/mL	SI = CU × 3.96	Greater than 158 micromol/L
Primidone	Greater than 15 mcg/mL	SI = CU × 4.58	Greater than 69 micromol/L
Valproic Acid	Greater than 200 mcg/mL	SI = CU × 6.93	Greater than 1,386 micromol/L
Antidepressant Drugs (Cyclic)			
Amitriptyline	Greater than 500 ng/mL	SI = CU × 3.6	Greater than 1,800 nmol/L
Nortriptyline	Greater than 500 ng/mL	SI = CU × 3.8	Greater than 1,900 nmol/L
Protriptyline	Greater than 500 ng/mL	SI = CU × 3.8	Greater than 1,900 nmol/L
Doxepin	Greater than 500 ng/mL	SI = CU × 3.58	Greater than 1,790 nmol/L
Imipramine	Greater than 500 ng/mL	SI = CU × 3.57	Greater than 1,785 nmol/L
Antidysrhythmic Drugs			
Amiodarone	Greater than 2.5 mcg/mL	SI = CU × 1.55	Greater than 3.9 micromol/L
Digoxin	Greater than 2.5 ng/mL	SI = CU × 1.28	Greater than 3.2 nmol/L

(table continues on page 1284)

APP

Study	Critical Finding (Conventional Units [CU])	Conversion Factor	Critical Finding (SI)
Disopyramide	Greater than 7 mcg/mL	SI = CU × 2.95	Greater than 20.6 micromol/L
Flecainide	Greater than 1 mcg/mL	SI = CU × 2.41	Greater than 2.41 micromol/L
Lidocaine	Greater than 6 mcg/mL	SI = CU × 4.27	Greater than 25.6 micromol/L
Procainamide	Greater than 10 mcg/mL	SI = CU × 4.25	Greater than 42.5 micromol/L
N-Acetyl Procainamide	Greater than 40 mcg/mL	SI = CU × 4.25	Greater than 170 micromol/L
Quinidine	Greater than 6 mcg/mL	SI = CU × 3.08	Greater than 18.5 micromol/L
Antimicrobial Drugs			
Aminoglycosides: Amikacin	Greater than 10 mcg/mL	SI = CU × 1.71	Greater than 17.1 micromol/L
Aminoglycosides: Gentamicin	Peak greater than 12 mcg/mL, trough greater than 2 mcg/mL	SI = CU × 2.09	Peak greater than 25.1 micromol/L, trough greater than 4.2 micromol/L
Aminoglycosides: Tobramycin	Peak greater than 12 mcg/mL, trough greater than 2 mcg/mL	SI = CU × 2.09	Peak greater than 25.1 micromol/L, trough greater than 4.2 micromol/L
Tricyclic Glycopeptide: Vancomycin	Trough greater than 30 mcg/mL	SI = CU × 0.69	Trough greater than 20.7 micromol/L
Antipsychotic Drugs and Antimanic Drugs			
Haloperidol	Greater than 42 ng/mL	SI = CU × 2.66	Greater than 112 nmol/L
Lithium	Greater than 2 mEq/L	SI = CU × 1	Greater than 2 mmol/L
Immunosuppressants			
Cyclosporine	Greater than 500 mcg/mL	SI = CU × 0.832	Greater than 416 nmol/L
Everolimus	Greater than 15 ng/mL	SI = CU × 1.04	Greater than 15.6 mcg/L
Methotrexate	Greater than or equal to 5 micromol/L	SI = CU × 1	Greater than or equal to 5 micromol/L
Sirolimus	Greater than 25 ng/mL	SI = CU × 1.1	Greater than 28 mcg/L
Tacrolimus	Greater than 25 ng/mL	SI = CU × 1.24	Greater than 31 mcg/L

Study	Critical Finding (Conventional Units [CU])	Conversion Factor	Critical Finding (SI)
Drug Screen			
Alcohol	80 to 400 mg/dL		
Amphetamine	Greater than 200 ng/mL		
Cocaine	Greater than 1,000 ng/mL		
Heroin and morphine	Greater than 200 ng/mL		
PCP	Greater than 100 ng/mL		
Alphabetical Listing			
Amniotic Fluid Analysis: Lecithin/ Sphingomyelin Ratio	An L/S ratio less than 1.5:1 is predictive of respiratory distress syndrome at the time of delivery		
Bilirubin and Bilirubin Fractions	*Adults and Children:* Total bilirubin greater than 15 mg/dL; *Newborns:* Total bilirubin greater than 13 mg/dL	SI = CU × 17.1	*Adults and Children:* Total bilirubin greater than 257 micromol/L; *Newborns:* Total bilirubin greater than 222 micromol/L
Biopsies	Assessment of clear margins after tissue excision; classification or grading of tumor; identification of malignancy	N/A	
Biopsy, Chorionic Villus	Identification of abnormalities in chorionic villus tissue	N/A	
Bioterrorism and Public Health Safety Concerns: Testing for Infectious Agents	Positive findings of suspected bacterial or viral organisms	N/A	

(table continues on page 1286)

Study	Critical Finding (Conventional Units [CU])	Conversion Factor	Critical Finding (SI)
	or toxins by Gram stain, culture, serology, immunochemical testing, PCR, or any other method. Lists of specific organisms may vary by facility; specific organisms are required to be reported to local, state, and national departments of health	N/A	
Bladder cancer markers	Positive findings may be an indication for expedited confirmatory procedures as ordered	N/A	
Bleeding Time	Greater than 14 min	N/A	
Blood Gases	*Adults and Children:* pH less than 7.2 or greater than 7.6; HCO_3 less than 10 or greater than 40 mmol/L; Pco_2 less than 20 or greater than 67 mm Hg; *Adults and Children:* Po_2 less than 45 mm Hg; *Newborns:* Po_2 less than 37 mm Hg or greater than 92 mm Hg	pH SI = CU × 1; HCO_3 SI = CU × 1; pCO_2 SI = CU × 0.133; pO_2 SI = CU × 0.133	*Adults and Children:* pH less than 7.2 or greater than 7.6; HCO_3 less than 10 or greater than 40 mmol/L; Pco_2 less than 2.7 or greater than 8.9 kPa; *Adults and Children:* Po_2 less than 6 kPa; *Newborns:* Po_2 less than 4.9 or greater than 12.2 kPa

Study	Critical Finding (Conventional Units [CU])	Conversion Factor	Critical Finding (SI)
Blood Typing, Antibody Screen, and Crossmatch	Note and immediately report to the health-care provider any signs and symptoms associated with a blood transfusion reaction	N/A	
Calcium, Blood Total	Less than 7 mg/dL or greater than 12 mg/dL	SI = CU × 0.25	Less than 1.8 or greater than 3 mmol/L
Calcium, Ionized (see Calcium Total and Ionized)	Less than 3.2 mg/dL or greater than 6.2 mg/dL	SI = CU × 0.25	Less than 0.8 or greater than 1.6 mmol/L
Carbon Dioxide	Less than 15 mEq/L or mmol/L; greater than 40 mEq/L or mmol/L	SI = CU × 1	Less than 15 mmol/L or greater than 40 mmol/L
Carbon Monoxide	30%–40%: Dizziness, muscle weakness, vision problems, confusion, increased heart rate, increased breathing rate; 50%–60%: Loss of consciousness, coma; greater than 60%: Death	N/A	
Cerebrospinal Fluid Analysis	Positive Gram stain, India ink preparation, or culture; presence of malignant cells or blasts; elevated WBC count; *Adults:* Glucose less	Glucose SI = CU × 0.0555	Positive Gram stain, India ink preparation, or culture; presence of malignant cells or blasts; elevated WBC count; *Adults:* Glucose less

(table continues on page 1288)

APP

Study	Critical Finding (Conventional Units [CU])	Conversion Factor	Critical Finding (SI)
	than 37 mg/dL or greater than 440 mg/dL; *Children:* Less than 31 mg/dL or greater than 440 mg/dL		than 2.1 mmol/L or greater than 24.4 mmol/L; *Children:* Less than 1.7 mmol/L or greater than 24.4 mmol/L
Chloride, Blood	Less than 80 mEq/L or mmol/L; greater than 115 mEq/L or mmol/L	SI = CU × 1	Less than 80 mmol/L; greater than 115 mmol/L
Chloride, Sweat	Greater than 60 mEq/L or mmol/L considered diagnostic of cystic fibrosis	SI = CU × 1	Greater than 60 mmol/L considered diagnostic of cystic fibrosis
Creatinine, Blood	*Adults:* Potential critical value is greater than 7.4 mg/dL (nondialysis patient); *Children:* Potential critical value is greater than 3.8 mg/dL (nondialysis patient)	SI = CU × 88.4	*Adults:* Potential critical value is greater than 654.2 micromol/L (nondialysis patient); *Children:* Potential critical value is greater than 336 micromol/L (nondialysis patient)
Creatinine Clearance, Urine (see "Creatinine, Urine, and Creatinine Clearance, Urine")	Degree of impairment—marked: Less than 28 mL/min/1.73 m²	SI = CU × 0.0167	Degree of impairment—marked: Less than 0.5 mL/s/1.73 m²
Cultures	Positive for acid-fast bacillus *Mycobacterium, Campylobacter, Clostridium difficile, Corynebacterium diphtheriae, Escherichia coli O157:H7,*	N/A	

Study	Critical Finding (Conventional Units [CU])	Conversion Factor	Critical Finding (SI)
	influenza, *Legionella*, *Listeria*, methicillin-resistant *Staphylococcus aureus*, respiratory syncytial virus, rotavirus, *Salmonella*, *Shigella*, vancomycin-resistant enterococcus, varicella, *Vibrio*, and *Yersinia*. Positive findings of bacterial or viral organisms in any sterile body fluid such as amniotic fluid, blood, pericardial fluid, peritoneal fluid, pleural fluid. Lists of specific organisms may vary by facility; specific organisms are required to be reported to local, state, and national departments of health		
Cytology, Sputum and Urine	Identification of malignancy	N/A	
Fibrinogen	Less than 80 mg/dL; greater than 800 mg/dL	SI = CU × 0.0294	Less than 2.4 micomol/L; greater than 23.5 micromol/L

(table continues on page 1290)

APP

Study	Critical Finding (Conventional Units [CU])	Conversion Factor	Critical Finding (SI)
Glucose	*Adults and Children:* Less than 40 mg/dL; greater than 400 mg/dL; *Newborns:* Less than 32 mg/dL; greater than 328 mg/dL	SI = CU × 0.0555	*Adults and Children:* Less than 2.22 mmol/L; greater than 22.2 mmol/L; *Newborns:* Less than 1.8 mmol/L; greater than 18.2 mmol/L
Gram Stain	Any positive results in blood, cerebrospinal fluid, or any body cavity fluid	N/A	
Hematocrit (see Hemoglobin and Hematocrit)	*Adults and Children:* Less than 19.8% or greater than 60%; *Newborns:* Less than 28.5% or greater than 66.9%	SI = CU × 0.01	*Adults and Children:* Less than 0.2 volume fraction or greater than 0.6 volume fraction; *Newborns:* Less than 0.28 volume fraction or greater than 0.67 volume fraction
Hemoglobin (see Hemoglobin and Hematocrit)	*Adults and Children:* Less than 6.6 g/dL or greater than 20 g/dL; *Newborns:* Less than 9.5 g/dL or greater than 22.3 g/dL	SI = CU × 10	*Adults and Children:* Less than 66 g/L or greater than 200 g/L; *Newborns:* Less than 95 g/L or greater than 223 g/L
Iron (see Iron Studies)	Serious toxicity: Greater than 400 mcg/dL; lethal: greater than 1,000 mcg/dL	SI = CU × 0.179	Serious toxicity: Greater than 71.6 micromol/L; lethal: greater than 179 micromol/L
Ketones, Blood and Urine	Strongly positive test results for ketones	N/A	

Study	Critical Finding (Conventional Units [CU])	Conversion Factor	Critical Finding (SI)
Lactic Acid	*Adults:* Greater than 31 mg/dL; *Children:* Greater than 37 mg/dL	SI = CU × 0.111	*Adults:* Greater than 3.4 mmol/L; *Children:* Greater than 4.1 mmol/L
Lead	Levels equal to or greater than 5 mcg/dL indicate exposure above the reference level. Levels equal to or greater than 45 mcg/dL require chelation therapy. Levels greater than 70 mcg/dL may cause severe brain damage and result in death.	SI = CU × 0.0483	Levels equal to or greater than 0.24 micromol/L indicate exposure above the reference level. Levels equal to or greater than 2.2 micromol/L require chelation therapy. Levels greater than 3.3 micromol/L may cause severe brain damage and result in death.
Magnesium, Blood	*Adults:* Less than 1.2 mg/dL; greater than 4.9 mg/dL; *Children:* Less than 1.2 mg/dL; greater than 4.3 mg/dL	SI = CU × 0.4114	*Adults:* Less than 0.5 mmol/L; greater than 2 mmol/L; *Children:* Less than 0.5 mmol/L; greater than 1.8 mmol/L
Methemoglobin (see Hemoglobin Electrophoresis and Abnormal Hemoglobins)	Signs of central nervous system depression can occur at levels greater than 45%; death may occur at levels greater than 70%	N/A	
Osmolality, Blood	Less than 265 mOsm/kg; greater than 320 mOsm/kg	SI = CU × 1	Less than 265 mmol/kg; greater than 320 mmol/kg
Partial Thromboplastin Time (PTT)	*Adults and Children:* Greater than 70 sec	N/A	

(table continues on page 1292)

APP

Study	Critical Finding (Conventional Units [CU])	Conversion Factor	Critical Finding (SI)
Pericardial Fluid Analysis	Positive culture findings in any sterile body fluid	N/A	
Peritoneal Fluid Analysis	Positive culture findings in any sterile body fluid	N/A	
Phosphorus, Blood	*Adults:* Less than 1 mg/dL; greater than 8.9 mg/dL; *Children:* Less than 1.3 mg/dL; greater than 8.9 mg/dL	SI = CU × 0.323	*Adults:* Less than 0.3 mmol/L; greater than 2.9 mmol/L; *Children:* Less than 0.4 mmol/L; greater than 2.9 mmol/L
Platelet Count	Less than 30×10^3/microL; greater than $1,000 \times 10^3$/microL	SI = CU × 1	Less than 30×10^9/L; greater than $1,000 \times 10^9$/L
Pleural Fluid Analysis	Positive culture findings in any sterile body fluid	N/A	
Potassium, Blood	*Adults and Children:* Less than 2.5 mEq/L or mmol/L; greater than 6.2 mEq/L or mmol/L; *Newborns:* Less than 2.8 mEq/L or mmol/L; greater than 7.6 mEq/L or mmol/L	SI = CU × 1	*Adults and Children:* Less than 2.5 mmol/L; greater than 6.2 mmol/L; *Newborns:* Less than 2.8 mmol/L; greater than 7.6 mmol/L
Prothrombin Time and International Normalized Ratio	PT greater than 27 sec; INR greater than 5	N/A	
Pseudocholinesterase and Dibucaine Number	A positive result indicates that the patient is at risk for prolonged or unrecoverable apnea related to the inability to metabolize succinylcholine	N/A	

Study	Critical Finding (Conventional Units [CU])	Conversion Factor	Critical Finding (SI)
RBC Morphology and Inclusions (see RBC count, Indices, Morphology, and Inclusions)	The presence of abnormal cells, other morphological characteristics, or cellular inclusions may signify a potentially life-threatening or serious health condition and should be investigated. Examples are the presence of sickle cells, moderate numbers of spherocytes, marked schistocytosis, oval macrocytes, basophilic stippling, nucleated RBCs (if the patient is not an infant), or malarial organisms	N/A	
Rubella Testing	A nonimmune status in pregnant patients may present significant health consequences for the developing fetus if the mother is exposed to an infected individual	N/A	

(table continues on page 1294)

Study	Critical Finding (Conventional Units [CU])	Conversion Factor	Critical Finding (SI)
Sodium, Blood	Less than 120 mEq/L or mmol/L; greater than 160 mEq/L or mmol/L	SI = CU × 1	Less than 120 mmol/L; greater than 160 mmol/L
Synovial Fluid Analysis	Positive culture findings in any sterile body fluid	N/A	
Thyroxine, Total	Less than 2 mcg/dL; greater than 20 mcg/dL	SI = CU × 12.9	Less than 26 nmol/L; greater than 258 nmol/L
Tuberculin Skin Tests	Positive results	N/A	
Urea Nitrogen, Blood	*Adults:* Greater than 100 mg/dL (nondialysis patients); *Children:* Greater than 55 mg/dL (nondialysis patients)	SI = CU × 0.357	*Adults:* Greater than 35.7 mmol/L (nondialysis patients); *Children:* Greater than 19.6 mmol/L (nondialysis patients)
Uric Acid, Blood	*Adults:* Greater than 13 mg/dL; *Children:* Greater than 12 mg/dL	SI = CU × 0.059	*Adults:* Greater than 0.8 mmol/L; *Children:* Greater than 0.7 mmol/L
Urinalysis	Presence of uric acid, cystine, leucine, or tyrosine crystals; the combination of grossly elevated urine glucose and ketones is also considered significant	N/A	
Vitamins A, D, E, K (see Vitamin Studies)	Vitamin toxicity can be as significant as problems brought about by vitamin deficiencies. The potential for toxicity	N/A	

Study	Critical Finding (Conventional Units [CU])	Conversion Factor	Critical Finding (SI)
	is especially important to consider with respect to fat-soluble vitamins, which are not eliminated from the body as quickly as water-soluble vitamins and can accumulate in the body		
WBC Count and Differential	Less than 2×10^3/microL; greater than 30×10^3/microL; absolute neutrophil count less than 0.5×10^3/microL	$SI = CU \times 1$	Less than 2×10^9/L; greater than 30×10^9/L; absolute neutrophil count less than 0.5×10^9/L

Diagnostic Critical Findings

Study	Critical Finding
Angiography, Various Sites (Abdomen)	Abscess; aneurysm
Angiography, Various Sites (Adrenal glands)	Adrenal disease
Angiography, Various Sites (Carotid artery)	Stroke
Angiography, Various Sites (Lungs)	Pulmonary embolism
Cardiac Catheterization	Aneurysm; aortic dissection
Chest X-Ray	Foreign body; malposition of tube, line, or postoperative device (pacemaker); pneumonia; pneumoperitoneum; pneumothorax; spine fracture
Computed Tomography, Various Sites (Abdomen)	Abscess; acute gastrointestinal (GI) bleed; aortic aneurysm; appendicitis; aortic dissection; bowel perforation; bowel obstruction; mesenteric torsion; tumor with significant mass effect; visceral injury (significant solid organ laceration)
Computed Tomography, Various Sites (Angiography)	Brain or spinal cord ischemia; emboli; hemorrhage; leaking aortic aneurysm; occlusion; tumor with significant mass effect
Computed Tomography, Various Sites (Brain and Head)	Abscess; acute hemorrhage; aneurysm; infarction; infection; tumor with significant mass effect
Computed Tomography, Various Sites (Chest)	Aortic aneurysm; aortic dissection; pneumothorax; pulmonary embolism
Computed Tomography, Various Sites (Pelvis)	Ectopic pregnancy; tumor with significant mass effect
Computed Tomography, Various Sites (Spine)	Cord compression; fracture; tumor with significant mass effect
Computed Tomography, Various Sites (Spleen)	Abscess; hemorrhage; laceration
Ductography	Ductal cancer in situ (DSIS); invasive breast cancer
Echocardiography	Aneurysm; infection; obstruction; tumor with significant mass effect
Echocardiography, Transesophageal	Aneurysm; aortic dissection

Study	Critical Finding
Electrocardiogram	*Adult:* Acute changes in ST elevation may indicate acute myocardial infarction or pericarditis; asystole; heart block, second and third degree with bradycardia less than 60 beats per min; pulseless electrical activity; pulseless ventricular tachycardia; PVCs greater than three in a row, pauses greater than 3 sec, or identified blocks; unstable tachycardia; ventricular fibrillation
Electrocardiogram	*Pediatric:* Asystole; bradycardia less than 60 beats per minute; pulseless electrical activity; pulseless ventricular tachycardia; supraventricular tachycardia; ventricular fibrillation
Electroencephalography	Abscess; brain death; head injury; hemorrhage; intracranial hemorrhage
Esophagogastroduodenoscopy	Presence and location of acute GI bleed
Fundoscopy	Detached retina
Gastrointestinal Blood Loss Scan	Acute GI bleed
Intraocular pressure	Increased IOP in the presence of sudden pain, sudden change in vision; a partially dilated, nonreactive pupil and firm globe implies acute angle-closure glaucoma, which is an ocular emergency requiring immediate attention to avoid permanent vision loss
Kidney, Ureter, and Bladder Study	Bowel obstruction; ischemic bowel; visceral injury
Laparoscopy, Abdominal	Appendicitis
Laparoscopy, Gynecologic	Ectopic pregnancy; foreign body; tumor with significant mass effect
Liver and Spleen Scan	Visceral injury
Lung Scans (Perfusion and Ventilation studies)	Pulmonary embolism
Magnetic Resonance Imaging, Various Sites (Angiography)	Aortic aneurysm; aortic dissection; occlusion; tumor with significant mass effect; vertebral artery dissection
Magnetic Resonance Imaging, Various Sites (Abdomen)	Acute GI bleed; aortic aneurysm; infection; tumor with significant mass effect
Magnetic Resonance Imaging, Various Sites (Brain)	Abscess; cerebral aneurysm; cerebral infarct; hydrocephalus; skull fracture or contusion; tumor with significant mass effect

(table continues on page 1298)

Study	Critical Finding
Magnetic Resonance Imaging, Various Sites (Chest)	Aortic aneurysm; aortic dissection; tumor with significant mass effect
Magnetic Resonance Imaging, Various Sites (Venography)	Cerebral embolus; occlusion; pulmonary embolus; tumor with significant mass effect
Plethysmography	Deep vein thrombosis
Positron Emission Tomography, Various Sites (Brain)	Aneurysm; cerebrovascular accident; tumor with significant mass effect
Ultrasound, Various Sites (Abdomen)	Aneurysm 5 cm or greater
Ultrasound, Biophysical Profile, Obstetric	Abruptio placentae; adnexal torsion; biophysical profile score between 0 and 2 is abnormal and indicates the need for assessment and decisions regarding early or immediate delivery; ectopic pregnancy; fetal death; placenta previa
Ultrasound, Various Sites (Pelvis; Gynecologic, Nonobstetric)	Abscess; adnexal torsion; appendicitis; infection; tumor with significant mass effect
Ultrasound, Various Sites (Scrotal)	Testicular torsion
Ultrasound, Venous Doppler, Extremity Studies	Deep vein thrombosis; pulmonary embolism
Upper GI and Small Bowel Series	Foreign body; perforated bowel; tumor with significant mass effect
Venography, Lower Extremity Studies	Deep vein thrombosis; pulmonary embolism

Bibliography

AABB. (2017, October). Circular of information for the use of human blood and blood components. Retrieved from www.aabb.org/tm/coi/Documents/coi1017.pdf

AABB. (2017). Technical manual (19th ed.). Bethesda, MD: American Association of Blood Banks

Abdominal ultrasound. (2018, January 6). Retrieved from https://www.mayoclinic.org/tests-procedures/abdominal-ultrasound/about/pac-20392738

Abell, T., Camilleri, M., Donohoe, K., et al. (2008). Consensus recommendations for gastric emptying scintigraphy: A joint report of the American Neurogastroenterology and Motility Society and the Society of Nuclear Medicine. *Am J Gastroenterol* 103(3):753–763

ACR–SPR practice parameter for the performance of gastrointestinal scintigraphy. (2015). Retrieved from https://www.acr.org/-/media/ACR/Files/Practice-Parameters/GI-Scint.pdf

Adekanle, D., Adeyemo, O., Adeniyi, A., et al. (2014, June 15). Serum magnesium levels in healthy pregnant and pre-eclamptic patients—A cross-section study. Retrieved from https://file.scirp.org/pdf/pdf/OJOG_2014062609124624.pdf

Aetna Clinical Policy Bulletins. (2017, September 21). Urea breath testing for *H. pylori* infection. Retrieved from www.aetna.com/cpb/medical/data/100_199/0177.html

Aetna Clinical Policy Bulletins. (2017, August 8). T-wave alternans. Retrieved from www.aetna.com/cpb/medical/data/500_599/0579.html

Aging effect on laboratory values. (2018). Retrieved from www.clinlabnavigator.com/aging-effect-on-laboratory-values.html

Ahmed, S., Jayawarna, C., & Jude, E. (2006, November). Post lumbar puncture headache: Diagnosis and management. Retrieved from https://www.ncbi.nlm.nih.gov/pmc/articles/PMC2660496

Alamria, H., Almoghairia, A., Alghamdib, A., et al. (2012, January). Efficacy of a single dose intravenous heparin in reducing sheath-thrombus formation during diagnostic angiography: A randomized controlled trial. Retrieved from www.sciencedirect.com/science/article/pii/S1016731511002065

Alder, A., & Carlton, C. (2012). Introduction to radiologic sciences and patient care (5th ed.). St. Louis, MO: Elsevier Saunders

Aletaha, D., Neogi, T., Silman, A., et al. (2010, September). 2010 Rheumatoid arthritis classification criteria: An American College of Rheumatology/European League against rheumatism collaborative initiative. Retrieved from https://www.rheumatology.org/Portals/0/Files/2010_revised_criteria_classification_ra.pdf

Alexander, D. (2017, November 14). Pseudocholinesterase deficiency. Retrieved from https://emedicine.medscape.com/article/247019-overview

American Academy of Audiology. (2011, September). Childhood hearing screening guidelines. Retrieved from https://www.cdc.gov/ncbddd/hearingloss/documents/AAA_Childhood%20Hearing%20Guidelines_2011.pdf

American Academy of Pediatrics. (2015, November 21). Thrush and other Candida infections. Retrieved from www.healthychildren.org/English/health-issues/conditions/infections/Pages/Thrush-and-Other-Candida-Infections.aspx

American Association of Clinical Endocrinologists and American College of Endocrinology. (2017). Guidelines for management of dyslipidemia and prevention of cardiovascular disease. Retrieved from https://www.aace.com/files/lipid-guidelines.pdf

American Cancer Society. (2018, February 5). Bone cancer: Early detection, diagnosis, and staging. Retrieved from https://www.cancer.org/cancer/bone-cancer/detection-diagnosis-staging/how-diagnosed.html

American Cancer Society. (2017, August 22). Colorectal cancer screening tests. Retrieved from https://www.cancer.org/cancer/colon-rectal-cancer/detection-diagnosis-staging/screening-tests-used.html

American Cancer Society. (2017, July 7). Guidelines for the early detection of cancer. Retrieved from https://www.cancer.org/healthy/find-cancer-early/cancer-screening-guidelines/american-cancer-society-guidelines-for-the-early-detection-of-cancer.html

American Cancer Society. (2016, February 22). How is chronic myeloid leukemia staged? Retrieved from https://www.cancer.org/cancer/chronic-myeloid-leukemia/detection-diagnosis-staging/staging.html

American Cancer Society. (2016, April 14). American Cancer Society recommendations for prostate cancer early detection. Retrieved from https://www.cancer.org/cancer/prostate-cancer/early-detection/acs-recommendations.html

American Cancer Society. (2016, May 20). What's new in research and treatment of melanoma skin cancer? Retrieved from https://www.cancer.org/cancer/melanoma-skin-cancer/about/new-research.html

American Cancer Society. (2016, January 26). Breast cancer in men diagnosing, treatment. Retrieved from https://www.cancer.org/content/dam/CRC/PDF/Public/8586.00.pdf

American Cancer Society. (2016, December 9). Guidelines for the prevention and early detection of cervical cancer. Retrieved from https://www.cancer.org/cancer/cervical-cancer/prevention-and-early-detection/cervical-cancer-screening-guidelines.html

American Clinical Neurophysiology Society. (2001–2018). Guidelines. Retrieved from https://www.acns.org/practice/guidelines

American College of Medical Genetics and Genomics. (2016, June). Noninvasive prenatal screening of fetal aneuploidy, 2016 update: A position statement of the American College of Medical Genetics and Genomics. Retrieved from https://www.acmg.net/docs/NIPS_AOP.pdf

American College of Obstetricians and Gynecologists. (2017, June 25). ACOG releases updated guidance on gestational diabetes. Retrieved from https://www.obgproject.com/2017/06/25/acog-releases-updated-guidance-gestational-diabetes

American College of Obstetricians and Gynecologists. (2016, May). ACOG issues new prenatal testing guidelines. Retrieved from https://prenatalinformation.org/2016/04/29/acog-issues-new-prenatal-testing-guidelines

American College of Obstetricians and Gynecologists. (2017, July). Breast cancer risk assessment and screening in average-risk women. Retrieved from https://www.acog.org/Clinical-Guidance-and-Publications/Practice-Bulletins/Committee-on-Practice-Bulletins-Gynecology/Breast-Cancer-Risk-Assessment-and-Screening-in-Average-Risk-Women

American College of Obstetricians and Gynecologists. (2017, April). Carrier screening. Retrieved from https://www.acog.org/Patients/FAQs/Carrier-Screening

American College of Obstetricians and Gynecologists. (2015, September). Cell-free DNA screening for fetal aneuploidy. Retrieved from https://www.acog.org/Clinical-Guidance-and-Publications/Committee-Opinions/Committee-on-Genetics/Cell-free-DNA-Screening-for-Fetal-Aneuploidy

American College of Obstetricians and Gynecologists. (2017, July). Loop electrosurgical excision procedure (LEEP). Retrieved from https://www.acog.org/Patients/FAQs/Loop-Electrosurgical-Excision-Procedure-LEEP

American College of Obstetricians and Gynecologists. (2013, September). New guidelines for cervical cancer screening. Retrieved from https://www.acog.org/-/media/For-Patients/pfs004.pdf?dmc=1&ts;=201803 27T1819045756

American College of Obstetricians and Gynecologists. (2016, March 1). Ob-Gyns release revised recommendations on screening and testing for genetic disorders. Retrieved from https://www.acog.org/About-ACOG/News-Room/News-Releases/2016/Ob-Gyns-Release-Revised-Recommendations-on-Screening-and-Testing-for-Genetic-Disorders

American College of Obstetricians and Gynecologists. (2017, July). Prenatal genetic screening tests. Retrieved from https://www.acog.org/Patients/FAQs/Prenatal-Genetic-Screening-Tests

American College of Obstetricians and Gynecologists. (2013, November). Special tests for monitoring fetal health. Retrieved from https://www.acog.org/Patients/FAQs/Special-Tests-for-Monitoring-Fetal-Health#contraction

American College of Obstetricians and Gynecologists. (2006, Reaffirmed 2010). Committee Opinion Number 348. Umbilical cord blood gas and acid base analysis. *Obstet Gynecol,* 108(5):1319–1322

American College of Radiology. (2017). ACR Manual on contrast media. Retrieved from https://www.acr.org/-/media/ACR/Files/Clinical-Resources/Contrast_Media.pdf

American College of Rheumatology. (2017, March). Fibromyalgia. Retrieved from https://www.rheumatology.org/I-Am-A/Patient-Caregiver/Diseases-Conditions/Fibromyalgia

American College of Rheumatology. (1997). 1997 Update of the 1982 American College of Rheumatology Revised Criteria for Classification of Systemic Lupus Erythematosus Retrieved from https://www.rheumatology.org/Portals/0/Files/1997%20Update%20of%201982%20Revised.pdf

American College of Rheumatology. (2010). The 2010 ACR-EULAR classification criteria for rheumatoid arthritis. Retrieved from https://www.eular.org/myUploadData/files/RA%20Class%20Slides%20ACR_Web.pdf

American Diabetes Association. (2009, December 29). American Diabetes Association's new clinical practice recommendations promote A1C as diagnostic test for diabetes. Retrieved from www.diabetes.org/newsroom/press-releases/2009/cpr-2010-a1c-diagnostic-tool.html

American Diabetes Association. (2016, November 21). Diagnosing diabetes and learning about prediabetes. Retrieved from www.diabetes.org/diabetes-basics/diagnosis

American Diabetes Association. (2018, January). Standards of medical care in diabetes—2018. Retrieved from https://diabetesed.net/wp-content/uploads/2017/12/2018-ADA-Standards-of-Care.pdf

American Diabetes Association. (n.d.) What can I eat? Retrieved from www.diabetes.org/food-and-fitness/food/what-can-i-eat

American Heart Association. (2017, May). Classes of heart failure. Retrieved from https://www.heart.org/en/health-topics/heart-failure/what-is-heart-failure/classes-of-heart-failure#.WrqfdogbOXJ

American Heart Association. (2018, February 20). Symptoms and diagnosis of PAD. Retrieved from https://www.heart.org/en/health-topics/peripheral-artery-disease/symptoms-and-diagnosis-of-pad#.WrqfsogbOXJ

American Liver Foundation. (2017). Liver disease diets. Retrieved from https://www.liverfoundation.org/for-patients/about-the-liver/health-wellness/nutrition

American Liver Foundation. (2017). Primary biliary cholangitis. Retrieved from https://www.liverfoundation.org/for-patients/about-the-liver/diseases-of-the-liver/primary-biliary-cholangitis

American Society of Anesthesiologists. (2017, March). Practice guidelines for preoperative fasting and the use of pharmacologic agents to reduce the risk of pulmonary aspiration: Application to healthy patients undergoing elective procedures: An updated report by the American Society of Anesthesiologists Committee on Standards and Practice Parameters. Retrieved from http://anesthesiology.pubs.asahq.org/article.aspx?articleid=2596245

American Society of Anesthesiologists Task Force on Perioperative Transesophageal Echocardiography. (2010, May). Practice guidelines for perioperative transesophageal echocardiography. Anesthesiology 5(112):1084–1096. doi: 10.1097/ALN.0b013e3181c51e90

American Society for Clinical Pathology, Twenty Things Physicians and Patients Should Question. (2016, September 14). Retrieved from http://www.choosingwisely.org/societies/american-society-for-clinical-pathology/

American Society of Health-System Pharmacists. (2016). AHFS drug information 2016. Bethesda, MD: American Society of Health-System Pharmacists

American Society of Nuclear Cardiology. (2009, January 16). Imaging guidelines for nuclear cardiology procedures. Retrieved from https://www.asnc.org/files/Stress%20Protocols%20and%20Tracers%202009.pdf

American Stroke Association. (2015, March 10). Anti-clotting agents explained. Retrieved from www.strokeassociation.org/STROKEORG/LifeAfterStroke/HealthyLivingAfterStroke/ManagingMedicines/Anti-Clotting-Agents-Explained_UCM_310452_Article.jsp#.WrqiZIgbOXJ

American Urological Association. (2013). PSA testing for the pretreatment staging and posttreatment management of prostate cancer: 2013 revision of 2009 best practice statement. Retrieved from https://www.auanet.org/Documents/education/clinical-guidance/PSA-Archive.pdf

Amjad, M., Moudgal, V., & Faisal, M. (2013). Laboratory methods for diagnosis and management of hepatitis C virus infection. *Lab Medicine,* 44(4):292–299. doi: 10.1309/LMASOYD8BRS0GC9

Amniotic fluid and the biophysical profile. (2007, December 14). Retrieved from www.gynob.com/biopamfl.htm

Analytes and their cutoffs. (2017, March 17). Retrieved from https://www.samhsa.gov/workplace/drug-testing

Andary, M., Oleszek, J., & Maurelus, K. (2017, October 6). Guillain-Barré syndrome workup. Retrieved from http://emedicine.medscape.com/article/315632-workup

Andersen-Berry, A. (2015, December 31). Neonatal sepsis. Retrieved from http://emedicine.medscape.com/article/978352-overview

Anderson, J. (2017, April 12). Celiac disease genetic testing. Determine your risk of developing celiac disease. Retrieved from https://www.verywell.com/celiac-disease-genetic-testing-562695

Anemia: Oral iron supplementation. (2014, September 9). Retrieved from http://my.clevelandclinic.org/health/diseases_conditions/hic_Anemia/hic_oral_iron_supplementation

Armstrong, D. (2009, September). Metformin therapy and lactic acidosis risk.https://www.arinursing.org/pdf/m_Metformin_Therapy_and_Lactic_Acidosis_Risk.pdf

Association for Radiologic and Imaging Nursing. (2015). Orientation manual for radiologic and imaging nursing (2nd ed.). Herndon, VA: Association for Radiologic and Imaging Nursing

ARUP Laboratories. (2018). Test directory. Retrieved from https://www.aruplab.com/testing

Athena Diagnostics. (2018). Test directory. Retrieved from http://www.athenadiagnostics.com/view-full-catalog

Azevado, E. (2015, October 9). Breast imaging in nipple discharge evaluation. Retrieved from https://emedicine.medscape.com/article/347305-overview

Baron, J., Cheng, X., Bazari, H., et al. (2015, January). Enhanced creatinine and estimated glomerular filtration rate reporting to facilitate detection of acute kidney injury. *Am J Clin Pathol,* 143:42–49. doi:10.1309/AJCP05XBCOPHTLGO

Beckman Coulter. (n.d.). Prostate health index (phi). Retrieved from https://www.beckmancoulter.com/en/products/immunoassay/phi

Berkow, R., & Beers, M. (2000). The Merck manual of geriatrics (3rd ed.): App I, Laboratory values. Hoboken, NJ: Wiley

Bernstein, M., & Munoz, N. (2014). Nutrition for the older adult (2nd ed.). Sudbury, MA: Jones & Bartlett

Bhimji, S. (2016, December 10). Vascular access in cardiac catheterization and intervention. Retrieved from https://emedicine.medscape.com/article/1894124-overview

Billing and coding guidelines for radiopharmaceutical agents (RAD-026). (2011, June 1). Retrieved from https://downloads.cms.gov/medicare-coverage-database/lcd_attachments/31361_1/L31361_RAD026_CBG_060111.pdf

Bishop, J. (2017, September 21). Diagnostic ambiguity in *C. difficile.* Retrieved from https://www.mlo-online.com/diagnostic-ambiguity-c.difficile

Bishop, M., Fody, E., & Schoeff, L. (2013). Clinical chemistry techniques, principles, correlations (7th ed.). Philadelphia, PA: Lippincott Williams & Wilkins

Bowlcn, L., & Cain, T. (2017, July 26). Nuclear medicine bone scan. Retrieved from https://www.insideradiology.com.au/nuclear-medicine-bone-scan

Burtis, C., Ashwood, E., & Bruns, D. (2011). Tietz textbook of clinical chemistry and molecular diagnostics (5th ed.). Philadelphia, PA: WB Saunders

Butterfield, S. (2016, August). Explaining Sepsis-3. Retrieved from https://acphospitalist.org/archives/2016/08/q-a-sepsis-3.htm

Cain, T. (2017, July 26). Nuclear medicine. Retrieved from https://www.insideradiology.com.au/nuclear-medicine

Cancer staging. (2015, March 9). Retrieved from https://www.cancer.gov/about-cancer/diagnosis-staging/staging

Cardiac computed tomography (multidetector CT, or MDCT). (2016, September 19). Retrieved from https://www.heart.org/en/health-topics/heart-attack/diagnosing-a-heart-attack/cardiac-computed-tomography-multidetector-ct-or-mdct#.WrrGQ4gbOXI

Cardona, R. (2016, February 24). Myocardial perfusion SPECT. Retrieved from https://emedicine.medscape.com/article/2114292-overview

Carlton, R., & McKenna Alder, A. (2012). Principles of radiographic imaging: An art and a science (5th ed.). Clifton Park, NY: Delmar Thomson

Carotid endarterectomy. (2018). Retrieved from https://surgery.ucsf.edu/conditions–procedures/carotid-endarterectomy.aspx

C. difficile infection. (2016, June 18). Retrieved from https://www.mayoclinic.org/diseases-conditions/c-difficile/symptoms-causes/syc-20351691

Cell-free fetal DNA. (2017, February 15). Retrieved from https://labtestsonline.org/tests/cell-free-fetal-dna

Centers for Disease Control and Prevention. (2017, October). Adult immunization schedules. Retrieved from https://www.cdc.gov/vaccines/schedules/hcp/adult.html

Centers for Disease Control and Prevention. (2015, September 1). Anthrax basics. Retrieved from https://www.cdc.gov/anthrax/basics

Centers for Disease Control and Prevention. (2018, January 4). Bioterrorism agents/diseases. Retrieved from https://emergency.cdc.gov/agent/agentlist.asp

Centers for Disease Control and Prevention. (2017, October). Birth–18 years & "catch-up" immunization schedules. Retrieved from https://www.cdc.gov/vaccines/schedules/hcp/child-adolescent.html

Centers for Disease Control and Prevention. (2018, January 29). Childhood obesity facts. Retrieved from https://www.cdc.gov/healthyschools/obesity/facts.htm

Centers for Disease Control and Prevention. (2017, December 12). Diagnostic tests for Zika virus. Retrieved from https://www.cdc.gov/zika/hc-providers/types-of-tests.html

Centers for Disease Control and Prevention. (2017, June 7). Facts about botulism. Retrieved from https://www.cdc.gov/botulism/general.html

Centers for Disease Control and Prevention. (2017, January 10). Food safety. Retrieved from https://www.cdc.gov/foodsafety/diseases/clostridium-perfringens.html

Centers for Disease Control and Prevention. Frequently asked questions about *Clostridium difficile* for healthcare providers. (2012, March 6). Retrieved from https://www.cdc.gov/hai/organisms/cdiff/cdiff_faqs_hcp.html

Centers for Disease Control and Prevention. (n.d.). Frequently asked questions (FAQ) about plague. Retrieved from www.bt.cdc.gov/agent/plague/faq.asp

Centers for Disease Control and Prevention. (2017, July 24). Guidance for US laboratories testing for Zika virus infection. Retrieved from www.bt.cdc.gov/agent/plague/faq.asp

Centers for Disease Control and Prevention. (2015, August 17). Interferon-gamma release assays (IGRAs)—Blood tests for TB infection. Retrieved from https://www.cdc.gov/tb/publications/factsheets/testing/igra.htm

BIB

Centers for Disease Control and Prevention. (2010, March 19). Investigational heptavalent botulinum antitoxin (HBAT) to replace licensed botulinum antitoxin AB and investigational botulinum antitoxin E. Retrieved from www .cdc.gov/mmwr/preview/mmwrhtml/ mm5910a4.htm

Centers for Disease Control and Prevention. (2016, September 27). Key facts about tularemia. Retrieved from https:// www.cdc.gov/Tularemia/

Centers for Disease Control and Prevention. (2017, May 17). Lead: What do parents need to know to protect their children? Retrieved from https://www .cdc.gov/nceh/lead/acclpp/blood_lead_ levels.htm

Centers for Disease Control and Prevention. Prion diseases. (2015, February 5). https://www.cdc.gov/prions/

Centers for Disease Control and Prevention. (2015, November 18). Ricin: Diagnosis & laboratory guidance for clinicians. Retrieved from https:// emergency.cdc.gov/agent/ricin/index .asp

Centers for Disease Control and Prevention. (2017, October 5). Rotavirus vaccination: What everyone should know. Retrieved from https://www.cdc.gov/ vaccines/vpd/rotavirus/public/index .html

Centers for Disease Control and Prevention. (2017, July 12). Smallpox disease overview. Retrieved from https://www .cdc.gov/smallpox

Centers for Disease Control and Prevention. (2017, December 8). Specimen selection. Retrieved from https:// www.cdc.gov/laboratory/specimen-submission/index.html

Centers for Disease Control and Prevention. Summary of notifiable infectious diseases and conditions—United States, 2014. (2016, October 16). Retrieved from https://www.cdc.gov/ mmwr/volumes/63/wr/mm6354a1 .htm?sBcid

Centers for Disease Control and Prevention. (2013, May 10). Testing for HCV infection: An update of guidance for clinicians and laboratorians. Retrieved from https://www.cdc.gov/mmwr/ preview/mmwrhtml/mm6218a5.htm

Centers for Disease Control and Prevention. (2016, May 11). Tuberculin skin testing. Retrieved from https://www .cdc.gov/tb/publications/factsheets/ testing/skintesting.htm

Centers for Disease Control and Prevention. (2018, February 9). Types of Zika virus tests. Retrieved from https://www.cdc .gov/zika/laboratories/types-of-tests.html

Centers for Disease Control and Prevention. (2017, January 10). Vaccine information statements. Retrieved from https://www.cdc.gov/vaccines/hcp/ vis/current-vis.html

Centers for Disease Control and Prevention. (2014, January 29). Viral hemorrhagic fevers. Retrieved from https:// www.cdc.gov/vhf/index.html

Ceramides levels significantly and independently linked to coronary artery disease risk. (2017, May). Retrieved from https://www.aacc.org/publications/ cln/articles/2017/may/ceramides-levels-significantly-and-independently-linked-to-coronary-artery-disease-risk

Chamberlain, N. (2017, November 6). Infectious mononucleosis. Retrieved from https://www.atsu.edu/faculty/ chamberlain/website/lectures/lecture/ mono.htm

Chawla, J. (2016, December 19). Anal sphincter electromyography and sphincter function profiles, contraindications. Retrieved from https://emedicine.medscape.com/ article/1948316-overview#aw2aab6b2b3

Children's Hospital of Philadelphia. (n.d.). Gastric emptying exam. Retrieved from www.chop.edu/service/radiology/ diagnostic-imaging/nuclear-medicine/ liquid-solid-gastric-emptying-exam.html

Chisti, M. (2017, August 5). Protein S deficiency workup. Retrieved from https://emedicine.medscape.com/ article/205582-workup

Chrousos, G. (2017, April). Hyperaldosteronism workup. Retrieved from https://emedicine.medscape.com/ article/920713-workup

Chua, W., Tan, L., Kamaraj, R., Chiong, E., Liang, S., & Esuvaranathan, K. (2010). The use of NMP22 and urine cytology for the surveillance of patients with superficial bladder cancer. Retrieved from http://ispub.com/IJU/6/2/7375

Cleveland Clinic. (1995–2018). Carotid stenting. Retrieved from https://my.clevelandclinic.org/health/treatments/16850-carotid-stenting

Cleveland Clinic. (1995–2018). MIBG scan. Retrieved from https://my.clevelandclinic.org/health/diagnostics/17226-mibg-scan

Clinical and Laboratory Standards Institute. (2009). Sweat testing: Sample collection and quantitative chloride analysis; approved guideline (3rd ed.). Wayne, PA: Clinical and Laboratory Standards Institute

Clinical Laboratory Reference. (2018–2019). Table of critical limits. Retrieved from https://www.clr-online.com/CLR_2018-19_Tableofcriticallimits.pdf

Coakley, F., Gould, R., Hess, C., Hope, M., Laros, R., & Thiet, M. (n.d.). Guidelines for the use of CT and MRI during pregnancy and lactation. Retrieved from https://radiology.ucsf.edu/patient-care/patient-safety/ct-mri-pregnancy

Computed tomography (CT). (n.d.). Retrieved from https://www.nibib.nih.gov/science-education/science-topics/computed-tomography-ct

Computed tomography. (2018). Retrieved from https://www.radiologyinfo.org/en/submenu.cfm?pg=ctscan

Conditions which may contraindicate the use of IV iodinated contrast. (2018, January 23). Retrieved from https://www.fda.gov/MedicalDevices/ProductsandMedicalProcedures/InVitroDiagnostics/ucm301431.htm

Conray-iothalamate meglumine injection. (2017, March 13). Retrieved from https://dailymed.nlm.nih.gov/dailymed/drugInfo.cfm?setid=1292abfc-496f-4df7-9a08-72072953e1f1

Contrast materials. (2017, February 21). Retrieved from https://www.radiologyinfo.org/en/info.cfm?pg=safety-contrast

Cordocentesis: Percutaneous umbilical blood sampling (PUBS). (2016, September 2). Retrieved from http://americanpregnancy.org/prenatal-testing/cordocentesis

Cornforth, T. (2017, August 7). Hysteroscopy FAQ. Retrieved from https://www.verywell.com/hysteroscopy-faqs-3521073

C-peptide. (2014, June 18). Retrieved from https://labtestsonline.org/tests/c-peptide

Cuker, A. (2017, July 18). Protein C deficiency. Retrieved from https://emedicine.medscape.com/article/205470-treatment

Currie, S., Hadjivassiliou, M., Craven, I., Griffiths, P., & Hoggard, N. (2013, March 29). Magnetic resonance spectroscopy of the brain. *Postgrad Med J,* 89(1048): 94–106

Davidson, M., London, M., & Ladewig, P. (2011). Olds' maternal-newborn nursing and women's health across the lifespan (9th ed.). Upper Saddle River, NJ: Prentice Hall

Dawood, A. (2016, August 4). Percutaneous transhepatic cholangiography. Retrieved from https://emedicine.medscape.com/article/1828033-overview

de Oliveira, W., Ade, S., Figueiredo, R., & Rios, D. (2015, February 6). Inflammation and poor response to treatment with erythropoietin in chronic kidney disease. Retrieved from http://www.jbn.org.br/details/1759/en-US

Denshaw-Burke, M. (2017, November 14). Methemoglobinemia. Retrieved from https://emedicine.medscape.com/article/204178-overview

Department of Health and Human Services. (2018, March 27). Guidelines for the use of antiretroviral agents in adults and adolescents living with HIV. Retrieved from https://aidsinfo.nih.gov/guidelines/html/1/adult-and-adolescent-arv/0

Deshpande, P. (2017, December 8). Breast milk jaundice. Retrieved from https://emedicine.medscape.com/article/973629-overview

Dhir, V., & Pinto, B. (2014, March). Antiphospholipid syndrome: A review. Retrieved from http://medind.nic.in/jaw/t14/i1/jawt14i1p19.pdf

Diabetes tests & diagnosis. (2016, November). Retrieved from https://www.niddk.nih.gov/health-information/diabetes/overview/tests-diagnosis

Diaper rash. (2018, March 5). Retrieved from https://medlineplus.gov/ency/article/000964.htm

DiPiro, J., Talbert, R., Yee, G., Matzke, G., Wells, B., & Posey, L. (2011). Pharmacotherapy: A pathophysiologic approach (8th ed.). New York, NY: McGraw-Hill Disorders of neuromuscular transmission. (2016, September). Retrieved from https://www.merckmanuals.com/professional/neurologic-disorders/peripheral-nervous-system-and-motor-unit-disorders/disorders-of-neuromuscular-transmission

Doherty, C., & Forbes, R. (2014, May). Diagnostic lumbar puncture. Retrieved from https://www.ncbi.nlm.nih.gov/pmc/articles/PMC4113153

Dooley, W. (2017, May 3). Ductoscopy. Retrieved from https://www.uptodate.com/contents/ductoscopy

Dorresteyn Stevens, C. (2010). Clinical immunology and serology: A laboratory perspective (3rd ed). Philadelphia, PA: FA Davis

Down syndrome facts. (2018). Retrieved from https://www.ndss.org/about-down-syndrome/down-syndrome-facts/

Driver, C. (2018, February 7). Fibromylagia. Retrieved from https://www.medicinenet.com/fibromyalgia_quiz/quiz.htm

Ductogram/galactogram: Imaging the breast ducts. (n.d.). Retrieved from www.imaginis.com/mammography/ductogram-galactogram-imaging-the-breast-ducts

Dugdale, D. (2016, July 22). Lactose tolerance tests. Retrieved from https://medlineplus.gov/ency/article/003500.htm

Dumping syndrome. (2013, September). Retrieved from https://www.niddk.nih.gov/health-information/digestive-diseases/dumping-syndrome

Dvorak, R., Brown, R., & Corbett, J. (2011, August 19). Interpretation of SPECT/CT myocardial perfusion images: Common artifacts and quality control techniques. Retrieved from https://pubs.rsna.org/doi/pdf/10.1148/rg.317115090

D-xylose absorption test. (2016, February 17). Retrieved from https://www.healthline.com/health/d-xylose-absorption

Eckel, R., Jakicic, J., Ard, J., et al. (2013). 2013 AHA/ACC guideline on lifestyle management to reduce cardiovascular risk: A report of the American College of Cardiology/American Heart Association Task Force on Practice Guidelines. Retrieved from http://circ.ahajournals.org/content/early/2013/11/11/01.cir.0000437740.48606.d1.full.pdf

Ejection fraction heart failure measurement. (2017, October 13). Retrieved from www.heart.org/HEARTORG/Conditions/HeartFailure/SymptomsDiagnosisofHeartFailure/Ejection-Fraction-Heart-Failure-Measurement_UCM_306339_Article.jsp#.W4gDvsInYri

Estimated average glucose (eAG). (2011, April 1). Retrieved from https://www.diabetesselfmanagement.com/diabetes-resources/definitions/estimated-average-glucose-eag

Estimating breast cancer risk. (2015, September 29). Retrieved from https://ww5.komen.org/BreastCancer/GailAssessmentModel.html

Evans, J. (2015, November 6). Hyperglycosylated hCG: A unique human implantation and invasion factor. Retrieved from https://onlinelibrary.wiley.com/doi/full/10.1111/aji.12459

Fei, C. (2015, March 26). Iron deficiency anemia: A guide to oral iron supplements. Retrieved from https://www.clinicalcorrelations.org/?p=8405

First trimester screening. (2017, February 2). Retrieved from https://labtestsonline.org/tests/first-trimester-screening

Fleming, S., Thompson, M., Stevens, R., et al. (2011, March 19). Normal ranges of heart rate and respiratory rate in children from birth to 18 years of age: A systematic review of observational studies. *Lancet, 377*(9770): 1011–1018. doi: 10.1016/S0140-6736(10)62226-X

Fluoroscopy procedure. (n.d.). Retrieved from https://www.hopkinsmedicine.org/healthlibrary/test_procedures/orthopaedic/fluoroscopy_procedure_92,p07662

Foods with vitamin K. (2016). Retrieved from www.coumadin.bmscustomerconnect.com/servlet/servlet.FileDownload?file=00Pi000000bxvTFEAY

Frank, E., Long, B., & Smith, B. (2012). Merrill's atlas of radiographic positions and radiologic procedures (12th ed.). St. Louis, MO: Mosby

Freedman, J. (2017, April 13). Acute angle-closure glaucoma in emergency medicine. Retrieved from https://emedicine.medscape.com/ article/798811-overview

Galactography. (n.d.). Retrieved from https://xranm.com/services/ womens-imaging/galactography

Galactography (ductography). (2016, March 16). Retrieved from https:// www.radiologyinfo.org/en/info .cfm?pg=galactogram

Gamma cameras. (n.d.). Retrieved from http://www.radioactivity.eu.com/site/ pages/Gamma_Camera.htm

Gandelman, G. (2012, June 18). Percutaneous transluminal coronary angioplasty (PTCA). Retrieved from https://medlineplus.gov/ency/ anatomyvideos/000096.htm

Gastric emptying scan. (2013, September). Retrieved from https://www .uwmedicine.org/services/radiology/ Documents/Articles/Gastric-Emptying- Scan.pdf

Gastric emptying study, Children's Hospital of Pittsburgh. (n.d.). Retrieved from www.chp.edu/our-services/ gastroenterology/patient-procedures/ gastric-emptying-study

Gearhart, P., Sehdev, H., & Ritchie, W. (2015, December 30). Ultrasonography in biophysical profile. Retrieved from https://emedicine.medscape.com/ article/405454-overview

Gebel, E. (2011, April). Back to basics: Blood glucose. Retrieved from www .diabetesforecast.org/2011/apr/back-to- basics-blood-glucose.html

Genetic testing. (2018, February 19). Retrieved from https://www .breastcancer.org/symptoms/testing/ genetic

Genetics home reference. (2018, March 27). Retrieved from https://ghr.nlm.nih.gov/ chromosome

George, J. (2011). Nursing theories: The base for professional nursing practice (6th ed.). Upper Saddle River, NJ: Pearson Education

Gershman, G., & Thomson, M. (2011). Practical pediatric gastrointestinal endoscopy (2nd ed.). Hoboken, NJ: Wiley

Ghobrial, I. (2012, December). Are you sure this is Waldenström macroglobulinemia? Retrieved from www.iwmf .com/sites/default/files/docs/wm_ ghobrial_Dec2012.pdf

Gill, B. (2016, April 25). Urodynamic studies for urinary incontinence. Retrieved from https://emedicine.medscape .com/article/1988665-overview

Goergen, S. (2017, July 26). Iodine-containing contrast medium. Retrieved from https://www.insideradiology.com.au/ iodine-containing-contrast-medium

Goff, D., Lloyd-Jones, D., Bennett, G., et al. (2013). 2013 ACC/AHA guideline on the assessment of cardiovascular risk: A report of the American College of Cardiology/American Heart Association Task Force on Practice Guidelines. Retrieved from http://circ.ahajournals .org/content/early/2013/11/11/01 .cir.0000437741.48606.98.full.pdf

Goldberg, J. (2015, May 22). Fundamentals of critical care: Hemodynamics, monitoring, shock. Retrieved from https://www.slideshare .net/kowalskij225/1502-reading- hemodynamics-monitoring-goldberg

Goldenberg, W. (2016, December 8). Myasthenia gravis. Retrieved from https://emedicine.medscape.com/ article/793136-overview

Goolsby, M. J., & Grubbs, L. (2015). Advanced assessment: Interpreting findings and formulating differential diagnoses (3rd ed.). Philadelphia, PA: FA Davis

Graff, L. (1983). A handbook of urinalysis. Philadelphia, PA: Lippincott Williams & Wilkins

Greer, J., Foerster, J., Rodgers, G., et al. (Eds.). (2008). Wintrobe's clinical hematology (12th ed.). Philadelphia, PA: Lippincott Williams & Wilkins

Griffing, G., Odeke, S., & Nagelberg, S. (2018, February 13). Addison disease workup. Retrieved from https://emedicine.medscape.com/ article/116467-workup

Grimmer, T., Riemenschneider, M., Förstl, H., et al. (2009, June 1). Beta amyloid in Alzheimer's disease: Increased deposition in brain is reflected in reduced concentration in cerebrospinal fluid. *Biol Psychiatry, 65*(11):927–934

BIB

Guidelines for the use of antiretroviral agents in adults and adolescents living with HIV. (2017, October 17). Retrieved from https://www.aidsinfo.nih.gov/Guidelines/HTML/1/adult-and-adolescent-treatment-guidelines/10/initiating-antiretroviral-therapy-in-treatment-naive-patients

Gulanick, M., & Meyers J., (2014). Nursing care plans nursing diagnosis and intervention (8th ed.). St. Louis, MO: Mosby

Gunnerson, K. (2017, March 6). Lactic acidosis. Retrieved from https://emedicine.medscape.com/article/167027-overview

Hales, C., Carroll, M., Fryar, C., and Ogden, C. (2017, October). Prevalence of obesity among adults and youth: United States, 2015–2016. Retrieved from https://www.cdc.gov/nchs/data/databriefs/db288.pdf

Hansen, T. (2017, December 28). Neonatal jaundice workup. Retrieved from https://emedicine.medscape.com/article/974786-workup

Harmening, D. (2008). Clinical hematology and fundamentals of hemostasis (5th ed.). Philadelphia, PA: FA Davis

Healthline Editorial Team. (2015, December). Treatment of preterm labor: Magnesium sulfate. Retrieved from https://www.healthline.com/health/pregnancy/preterm-labor-magnesium-sulfate

Heller, G., & Hendel, R. (2010). Nuclear cardiology: Practical applications. (2nd ed.). New York, NY: McGraw-Hill

Hemodynamic measurement terminology. (n.d.). Retrieved from www.rnceus.com/hemo/term.htm

Hemoglobin A1C. (2015, September 4). Retrieved from https://labtestsonline.org/tests/hemoglobin-a1c

Hendrich, E. (2017, March 29). Bone mineral density scan (bone densitometry or DXA scan). Retrieved from https://www.insideradiology.com.au/bone-mineral-density-scan

Hilliard, N. (2008, March 29). Drug–radiopharmaceutical interactions. Retrieved from http://nuclearpharmacy.uams.edu/wp-content/uploads/sites/61/2017/10/Interactions.pdf

Hoeltke, L. (2012). The complete textbook of phlebotomy (4th ed). Albany, NY: Delmar Thomson Learning

Hoover, K., & Park, I. (2011, February 11). Reverse sequence syphilis screening. An overview by CDC. Retrieved from https://www.cdc.gov/std/syphilis/syphilis-webinar-slides.pdf

Hopfer Deglin, J., & Hazard Vallerand, A. (2016, May 25). Davis's drug guide for nurses (15th ed.). Philadelphia, PA: FA Davis

Human chorionic gonadotropin (HCG): The pregnancy hormone. (2017, August 22). Retrieved from http://americanpregnancy.org/while-pregnant/hcg-levels

HPV vaccine information for young women. (2017, January 3). Retrieved from https://www.cdc.gov/std/hpv/stdfact-hpv-vaccine-young-women.htm

Hypertension and the AGT gene. (2018). Retrieved from https://www.gbhealthwatch.com/GND-Hypertension-AGT.php

Image gently. (2014). Retrieved from https://www.imagegently.org/About-Us/The-Alliance

Imaginis Corporation. (2008, December). History of medical diagnosis and diagnostic imaging. Retrieved from www.imaginis.com/faq/history-of-medical-diagnosis-and-diagnostic-imaging

Imaginis Corporation. (2010, August). Information about intravenous and oral contrast used in CT. Retrieved from www.imaginis.com/ct-scan/information-about-intravenous-and-oral-contrast-used-in-ct

Important information to know when you are taking: Warfarin (Coumadin) and vitamin K. (2012, September 5). Retrieved from https://www.cc.nih.gov/ccc/patient_education/drug_nutrient/coumadin1.pdf

Inoue, S. (2017, December 20). Leukocytosis. Retrieved from https://emedicine.medscape.com/article/956278-overview

Inside track: CLSI releases venipuncture guides. (2017, June 2). Retrieved from www.clpmag.com/2017/06/inside-track-clsi-releases-venipuncture-guides

Interpretations of decreased visual acuity. (n.d.). Retrieved from https://fpnotebook.com/eye/sx/DcrsdVslActy.htm

Iodine allergy and contrast administration. (2018). Retrieved from https://radiology.ucsf.edu/patient-care/patient-safety/contrast/iodine-allergy

Ishi, K. (2013, August 14). PET approaches for diagnosis of dementia. Retrieved from www.ajnr.org/content/early/2013/08/14/ajnr.A3695.full.pdf

Isotopes used in medicine. (n.d.). Retrieved from https://www.radiochemistry.org/nuclearmedicine/radioisotopes/ex_iso_medicine.htm

Jaskowski, T., Martins, T., Litwin, C., & Hill, H. (1999, January). Comparison of three different methods for measuring classical pathway complement activity. Retrieved from https://www.ncbi.nlm.nih.gov/pmc/articles/PMC95674

Jensen, M., Ryan, D., Apovian, C., et al. (2013). 2013 AHA/ACC/TOS guideline for the management of overweight and obesity in adults: A report of the American College of Cardiology/American Heart Association Task Force on Practice Guidelines and the Obesity Society. Retrieved from http://circ.ahajournals.org/content/early/2013/11/11/01.cir.0000437739.71477.ee

Johnson, K., & Sexton, D. (2017, April). Lumbar puncture: Technique, indications, contraindications, and complications in adults. Retrieved from https://www.uptodate.com/contents/lumbar-puncture-technique-indications-contraindications-and-complications-in-adults

Jones, A., Trzeciak, S., & Kline, J. (2010, May 1). The Sequential Organ Failure Assessment score for predicting outcome in patients with severe sepsis and evidence of hypoperfusion at the time of emergency department presentation. Retrieved from https://www.ncbi.nlm.nih.gov/pmc/articles/PMC2703722

Kalyoussef, S. (2017, July 10). Pediatric candidiasis treatment and management. Retrieved from https://emedicine.medscape.com/article/962300-overview

Karesh, S. (n.d.). Radiopharmaceuticals in nuclear medicine. Retrieved from https://nucmedtutorials.files.wordpress.com/2016/12/radioimmunotherapy-in-nhl1.pdf

Kaushansky, K., Lichtman, M., Prchal, J., et al. (2015). Williams hematology (9th ed.). New York, NY: McGraw-Hill

Kawamura, D., & Lunsford, B. (2012). Diagnostic medical sonography—Abdomen and superficial structures (3rd ed.). Baltimore, MD: Lippincott Williams & Wilkins

Khoury, N. (2017, September 21). Optimizing *C. difficile* testing in a large system lab by integrating inpatient and outpatient needs. Retrieved from https://www.mlo-online.com/optimizing-c.difficile-testing-large-system-lab-integrating-inpatient-outpatient-needs

Kimball, S. (2015, July 30). Speech audiometry. Retrieved from https://emedicine.medscape.com/article/1822315-overview

Korczowska, I. (2014, September 18). Rheumatoid arthritis susceptibility genes: An overview. Retrieved from https://www.ncbi.nlm.nih.gov/pmc/articles/PMC4133460

Krywko, D., and Shunkwiler, S. (2017, May 1). Kleihauer betke test. Retrieved from https://www.ncbi.nlm.nih.gov/books/NBK430876/

LabCorp. (2018). Test menu. Retrieved from https://www.labcorp.com/test-menu/search

Laboratory testing for the diagnosis of HIV infection: Updated recommendations. (2014, June 27). Retrieved from https://stacks.cdc.gov/view/cdc/23447

Lappas, B. (2013, April 26). Umbilical cord blood gas analysis. Retrieved from https://www.med.unc.edu/pedclerk/schedules/clerkship-at-unc/newborn-nursery/UmbilicalCordBloodGasAnalysis.pdf

Larkin, B., & Zimmank, R. (2015, October). Interpreting arterial blood gases Ssuccessfully. Retrieved from https://www.aorn.org/websitedata/cearticle/pdf_file/cea15542-0001.pdf

Lee, J., & Kim, N. (2015, January). Diagnosis of *Helicobacter pylori* by invasive test: Histology. Retrieved from https://www.ncbi.nlm.nih.gov/pmc/articles/PMC4293485

LeMone, P., Burke, K., & Baldoff, G. (2011). Medical surgical nursing: Critical thinking in patient care (5th ed.). Upper Saddle River, NJ: Pearson

Levels of ceramides in the blood help predict cardiovascular events. (2017, March 9). Retrieved from

https://www.acc.org/about-acc/
press-releases/2017/03/09/14/24/
levels-of-ceramides-in-the-blood-help-
predict-cardiovascular-events

Levison, M. (2016, July). Hantavirus
infection. Retrieved from https://
www.merckmanuals.com/
professional/infectious-diseases/
arboviridae-arenaviridae-and-filoviridae/
hantavirus-infection

Lewis, S., Ruff Dirksen, S., Heitkemper, M.,
Bucher, L., & Camera, I. (2010). Medical
surgical nursing assessment and management of clinical problems (8th ed.).
St. Louis, MO: Mosby

Lutz, C., & Przytulski, K. (2014). Nutrition
and diet therapy (6th ed.). Philadelphia,
PA: FA Davis

Marburg and Ebola virus infections.
(2016). Retrieved from https://
www.merckmanuals.com/
professional/infectious-diseases/
arboviridae-arenaviridae-and-filoviridae/
marburg-and-ebola-virus-infections

Marks, J. (n.d.). Gastroparesis. Retrieved
from https://www.medicinenet.com/
gastroparesis/article.htm#how_is_
gastroparesis_diagnosed

Martin, F., & Clark, J. (2011). Introduction
to audiology (11th ed.). Boston, MA:
Allyn & Bacon

Matching and compatibility. (n.d.).
Retrieved from http://ucdmc.ucdavis.
edu/transplant/livingdonation/donor_
compatible.html

Mawuenyega, K., Sigurdson, W., Ovod, V.,
et al. (2010, December 9). Decreased
clearance of CNS β-amyloid in Alzheimer's disease. *Science,* 330(6012):1774

Mayo Clinic. (2015, October 8).
Cordocentesis. Retrieved from
https://www.mayoclinic.org/
tests-procedures/percutaneous-
umbilical-blood-sampling/about/
pac-20393638

Mayo Clinic. (2018). Test ID: CERAM.
Ceramides, plasma. Retrieved from
https://www.mayomedicallaboratories
.com/test-catalog/Clinical+and+
Interpretive/65054

Mayo Clinic. (2018, January 11). Lymphocytosis. Retrieved from https://
www.mayoclinic.org/symptoms/
lymphocytosis/basics/definition/
sym-20050660

Mayo Clinic. (2018, March 9). Gastric
esophageal reflux disease (GERD).
Retrieved from https://www
.mayoclinic.org/diseases-conditions/
gerd/symptoms-causes/syc-20361940

McCall, R., & Tankersly, C. (2015). Phlebotomy essentials (6th ed.). Philadelphia,
PA: Lippincott Williams & Wilkins

McDonald, M. and Ziessman, H. (2016,
May 1). Gastrointestinal bleeding
scintigraphy. Retrieved from http://
appliedradiology.com/articles/
gastrointestinal-bleeding-scintigraphy

McPherson, R., & Pincus, M. (2011). Hen-
ry's clinical diagnosis and management
by laboratory methods (22nd ed.).
Philadelphia, PA: WB Saunders

Mehta, L., & Thomas, S. (2012, April 27).
The role of PET in dementia diagnosis
and treatment. Retrieved from http://
appliedradiology.com/articles/the-
role-of-pet-in-dementia-diagnosis-and-
treatment

Meeusen, J. (2017, February 2). A new lipid
to assess heart disease risk. Retrieved
from http://laboratory-manager
.advanceweb.com/a-new-lipid-to-assess-
heart-disease-risk

Mente, K., O'Donnell, J., Jones, S., et. al.
(2017). Fluorodeoxyglucose positron
emission tomography (FDG-PET)
correlation of histopathology and
MRI in prion disease. *Alzheimer Dis
Assoc Disord,* 31(1):1–7. doi: 10.1097/
WAD.0000000000000188

Merck manual: Professional version
(2018). Retrieved from https://www
.merckmanuals.com/professional

Metformin. (2018, January). Retrieved
from https://www.drugs.com/pro/
metformin.html

Mialich, M., Sicchieri, J., & Jordao, A. (2014,
January 8). Analysis of body composition: A critical review of the use of
bioelectrical impedance analysis. *IJCN,*
2(1):1–10. doi: 10.12691/ijcn-2-1–1

Milner, Q. J. W., & Mathews, G. R. (2012).
An assessment of the accuracy of pulse
oximeters. *Anaesthesia,* 67: 396–401.
doi: 10.1111/j.1365-2044.2011.07021.x

Moda, F., Gambetti, P., Notari, S., et al.
(2014, August 7). Prions in the urine of
patients with variant Creutzfeldt–Jakob
disease. *N Engl J Med,* 371:530–539.
doi: 10.1056/NEJMoa1404401

Monson, K., & Schoenstadt, A. (2017, January 27). Metformin and contrast medium. Retrieved from http://diabetes.emedtv.com/metformin/metformin-and-contrast-medium.html

Moore, N., & Lyerly, D. (2017, September 21). Overdiagnosis of *C. difficile* infection (CDI) and the importance of toxin detection. Retrieved from https://www.mlo-online.com/overdiagnosis-c.difficile-infection-cdi-importance-toxin-detection

Morris, S., & Wylie-Rosett, J. (2010). Medical nutrition therapy: A key to diabetes management and prevention. *Clin Diabetes, 28*(1):12–18. doi: https://doi.org/10.2337/diaclin.28.1.12

Mukhtar, F., & Pelletier, J. (2017, November 10). Acute hemolytic transfusion reaction. Retrieved from www.pathologyoutlines.com/topic/transfusionmedacutehemolytic.html

Myasthenia Gravis Foundation of America. (2010). Informational materials. Retrieved from www.myasthenia.org/LivingwithMG/InformationalMaterials.aspx

Myocardial perfusion imaging (MPI) test. (2016, September 16). Retrieved from https://www.heart.org/en/health-topics/heart-attack/diagnosing-a-heart-attack/myocardial-perfusion-imaging-mpi-test#.WrlWfYgbOXI

Nadalo, L. (2016, July 22). Carotid artery stenosis imaging. Retrieved from https://emedicine.medscape.com/article/417524-overview

Nandurkar, D. (2017, July 26). MIBG scan. Retrieved from https://www.insideradiology.com.au/mibg-scan

National Comprehensive Cancer Network. (2016, January). NCCN guidelines for patients: Breast cancer. Retrieved from https://www.nccn.org/patients/guidelines/stage_0_breast/index.html#6

National Heart, Lung, and Blood Institute. (2018, March 5). Pulmonary function tests. Retrieved from https://medlineplus.gov/ency/article/003853.htm

National Institute of Neurological Disorders and Stroke. (2017, May 19). Myasthenia gravis fact sheet. Retrieved from https://www.ninds.nih.gov/Disorders/Patient-Caregiver-Education/Fact-Sheets/Myasthenia-Gravis-Fact-Sheet

National Institutes of Health. (2015, June). Bone mass measurement: What the numbers mean. Retrieved from https://www.bones.nih.gov/health-info/bone/bone-health/bone-mass-measurement-what-numbers-mean

National Institutes of Health. (n.d.). Strengthening knowledge and understanding of dietary supplements. Retrieved from https://ods.od.nih.gov/factsheets/list-all

National Institutes of Health. (2018, March 5). Uroflowmetry. Retrieved from https://medlineplus.gov/ency/article/003325.htm

National Kidney and Urologic Diseases Information Clearinghouse. (2015, October). Diabetes insipidus. Retrieved from https://www.niddk.nih.gov/health-information/kidney-disease/diabetes-insipidus

National Kidney and Urologic Diseases Information Clearinghouse. (2014, February). Urodynamic testing. Retrieved from https://www.niddk.nih.gov/health-information/diagnostic-tests/urodynamic-testing

National Prion Disease Pathology Surveillance Center. (2017). Human prion diseases. Retrieved from http://case.edu/medicine/pathology/divisions/prion-center/human-prion-diseases

Nayar, R., & Wilbur, D. (2017, July 11). The Bethesda System for reporting cervical cytology: A historical perspective. Retrieved from https://www.karger.com/Article/FullText/477556

New CLSI venipuncture guidelines. (2017). Retrieved from https://www.acacert.com/files/ACAreerSummer_Fall2017.pdf

New York State Department of Health. (n.d.). Newborn screening: Information for health professionals. Retrieved from https://www.wadsworth.org/programs/newborn/screening/providers

Newborn screening. (2014). Retrieved from http://newbornscreening.info

Nicastri, D., & Weiser, T. (2012). Rigid bronchoscopy: Indications and techniques. Retrieved from https://www.optechtcs.com/article/S1522-2942(12)00052-9/pdf

Nuchal translucency test. (2018, March 5). Retrieved from https://medlineplus. gov/ency/article/007561.htm

Orru, C., Groveman, B., Hughson, A., Zanusso, G., Coulthart, M., & Caughey, B. (2015, January 20). Rapid and sensitive RT-QuIC detection of human Creutzfeldt-Jacob disease using cerebrospinal fluid. *mBio,* 6(1):e02451-14. doi: 10.1128/mBio.02451-14

Osteoporosis. (n.d.). Retrieved from www .stritch.luc.edu/lumen/MedEd/hmps/ Family%20Medicine-Osteoporosis.htm

Osto, E., Fallo, F., Pelizzo, M., et al. (2012, August 27). Coronary microvascular dysfunction induced by primary hyperparathyroidism is restored after parathyroidectomy. Retrieved from http://circ.ahajournals.org/ content/126/9/1031

Ototoxic medications. (2018). Retrieved from https://nvrc.org/wp-content/ uploads/2010/12/Drugs-that-Cause-HL .pdf

Pai, A. (2014, January 15). Protein C. Retrie ved from https://emedicine.medscape .com/article/2085992-overview

Pammi, M. (2017, March 31). Epidemiology and risk factors for Candida infection in neonates. Retrieved from https://www .uptodate.com/contents/epidemiology- and-risk-factors-for-candida-infection-in- neonates

PDR staff (Ed.). (2011, February 1). PDR for nonprescription drugs, dietary supplements, and herbs 2011 (32nd ed.). Montvale, NJ: PDR

Peart, O. (2015, March 9). Lange Q&A: Mammography examination (3rd ed.). New York, NY: McGraw-Hill

Peripheral vascular disease (PVD)/ peripheral artery disease (PAD). (2017). Retrieved from https:// stanfordhealthcare.org/medical- conditions/blood-heart-circulation/ peripheral-vascular-disease.html

PET/CT scan for patients with diabetes. (2018). Retrieved from https://www .uwmedicine.org/health-library/ pages/pet-ct-fdg-scan-for-patients-with- diabetes.aspx

Petri, M., Orbai, A., Alarcón, G., et al. (2012, August). Derivation and validation of systemic lupus international collaborating clinics classification criteria for systemic lupus erythematosus. *Arthritis Rheum,* 64(8):2677-2686. doi: 10.1002/art.34473

Petrosky, E., Bocchini, J., Hariri, S., et al. (2015, March 27). Use of 9-valent human papillomavirus (HPV) vaccine: Updated HPV vaccination recommendations of the advisory committee on immunization practices. Retrieved from https://www .cdc.gov/mmwr/preview/mmwrhtml/ mm6411a3.htm

Pham, H. (2015, November 15). Allergic and anaphylactic transfusion reaction. Retrieved from www .pathologyoutlines.com/topic/ transfusionmedallergic.html

Pham, H. (2017, November 16). Febrile nonhemolytic transfusion reaction. Retrieved from www .pathologyoutlines.com/topic/ transfusionmedfebrilenonhemolytic .html

Pinson, R. (2016, February). Sepsis is still confusing: Part 1 of 2: Diagnostic criteria are often misapplied. Retrieved from https://acphospitalist .org/archives/2016/02/coding-sepsis- confusing-part-1.htm

Polycythemia vera facts. (2015, April). Retrieved from https://www.lls.org/ sites/default/files/file_assets/FS13_ PolycythemiaVera_FactSheet_ final5.1.15.pdf

Post lumbar puncture headaches. (2014, March 31). Retrieved from http://rebelem.com/ post-lumbar-puncture-headaches/

Positron emission tomography— Computed tomography (PET/CT). (2017, January 23). Retrieved from https://www.radiologyinfo.org/en/info .cfm?PG=pet

Posthauer, M. (2011, June 24). Albumin and pre-albumin: Are they markers of nutritional status in wound management? Retrieved from https://www .woundsource.com/blog/albumin- and-pre-albumin-are-they-markers- nutritional-status-wound-management

Prion diseases. (n.d.). Retrieved from https://www.hopkinsmedicine .org/healthlibrary/conditions/ adult/nervous_system_disorders/ prion_diseases_134,56

Prostate MRI and MRI-targeted biopsy in patients with prior negative biopsy. (2016). Retrieved from http://auanet.org/guidelines/prostate-mri-and-mri-targeted-biopsy

PSA testing for the pretreatment staging and posttreatment management of prostate cancer: 2013 revision of 2009 best practice statement. (2013). Retrieved from https://www.auanet.org/common/pdf/education/clinical-guidance/Prostate-Specific-Antigen.pdf

Puchalski, A., & Chopra, I. (2014, March 1). Radioiodine treatment of differentiated thyroid cancer despite history of "iodine allergy." Retrieved from https://www.ncbi.nlm.nih.gov/pmc/articles/PMC3965283

Pulse. (2018, Mar 5). Retrieved from https://medlineplus.gov/ency/article/003399.htm

Pursley, D. (2015). Teaching acid-base interpretation: What is the best approach? Retrieved from http://academics.otc.edu/media/uploads/sites/8/2015/11/Teaching-acid-base-interpretation-handout.pdf

Quick sepsis related organ failure assessment. (n.d.). Retrieved from www.qsofa.org

Quest Diagnostics. (2000–2017). Test menu. Retrieved from www.questdiagnostics.com/testcenter/BUOrderInfo.action

Quinley, E. (2010). Immunohematology principles and practice (3rd ed.). Philadelphia, PA: Lippincott Williams & Wilkins

RadiologyInfo. (2018). Retrieved from www.radiologyinfo.org

Radionuclide ventriculography or radionuclide angiography (MUGA Scan). (2015, July). Retrieved from https://www.heart.org/en/health-topics/heart-attack/diagnosing-a-heart-attack/radionuclide-ventriculography-or-radionuclide-angiography-muga-scan#.WrKhPugbOXI

Radiopharmaceuticals. (2014, January 29). Retrieved from https://www.slideshare.net/hikikomorijcv18/list-of-radiopharmaceuticals-used-in-nuclear-medicine

Red Cross statement on Zika virus screening. (2016, August 29). Retrieved from https://www.redcross.org/news/press-release/Red-Cross-Statement-on-Zika-Virus-Screening

Reducing surgical site infection: Preoperative hair removal. (2014, March 21). Retrieved from www.open.hqsc.govt.nz/infections/news-and-events/news/1419

Reichel, W., Gallo, J., Busby-Whitehead, J., Rabins, P., Sillman, R., & Murphy, J. (2009). Reichel's care of the elderly: Clinical aspects of aging (6th ed.). New York, NY: Cambridge University Press

Renuart, A., Mistry, R., Avery, R., et al. (2011, July). Reference range for cerebrospinal fluid protein concentration in children and adolescents. Retrieved from https://jamanetwork.com/journals/jamapediatrics/fullarticle/1107544

Rinella, D. (2016, September 12). Lactate and sepsis: 10 things you need to know to save lives. Retrieved from https://www.ems1.com/mobile-healthcare/articles/125327048-Lactate-and-Sepsis-10-things-you-need-to-know-to-save-lives

Rodgers, S. G. (2008). Medical-surgical nursing care plans. Clifton Park, NY: Thomson Delmar Learning.

Rojas-Moreno, C., & Regunath, H. (2016, January 15). Procalcitonin in sepsis. Retrieved from http://medicine2.missouri.edu/jahm/procalcitonin-in-sepsis

Rotavirus. (2018, January 4). Retrieved from https://www.mayoclinic.org/diseases-conditions/rotavirus/symptoms-causes/syc-20351300

Ryan, K., Ray, C., Ahmad, N., Drew, W., & Plorde, J. (2010). Sherris medical microbiology (5th ed.). Columbus, OH: McGraw-Hill.

Schilling-McCann, J. A. (2010). Lippincott manual of nursing practice (9th ed.). Philadelphia, PA: Lippincott Williams & Wilkins

Schreiber, D., & Nix, D. (2018, January 8). Natriuretic peptides in congestive heart failure. Retrieved from https://emedicine.medscape.com/article/761722-overview

Second trimester maternal serum screening. (2017, February 3). Retrieved from https://labtestsonline.org/tests/maternal-serum-screening-second-trimester

Seeram, E. (2008). Computed tomography: Physical principles, clinical application, and quality control (3rd ed.). Philadelphia, PA: WB Saunders

Select normal pediatric laboratory values. (n.d.). Retrieved from http://wps.prenhall.com/wps/media/objects/354/362846/London%20App.%20B.pdf

Selvin, E., Francis, L., Ballantyne, C., et al. (2011, April). Nontraditional markers of glycemia. *Diabetes Care,* 34:960–967

Senthilnayagam, B., Kumar, T., Sukumaran, J., Jeya M., & Ramesh Rao, K. (2012, February 15). Automated measurement of immature granulocytes: Performance characteristics and utility in routine clinical practice. Retrieved from https://www.ncbi.nlm.nih.gov/pmc/articles/PMC3289863

Sequential Organ Failure Assessment (SOFA) score. (n.d.). Retrieved from https://www.mdcalc.com/sequential-organ-failure-assessment-sofa-score

Sequential (sepsis related) Organ Failure Assessment (SOFA) score. (n.d.). Retrieved from https://www.acphospitalist.org/archives/2016/03/acph-201603-coding-sepsis-confusing-part-2_t1.pdf

Sexually transmitted diseases. (2017, November 20). Retrieved from https://www.cdc.gov/std/general/default.htm

Shackett, P. (2008). Nuclear medicine technology: Procedures and quick reference. Philadelphia, PA: Lippincott Williams & Wilkins

Shah, A., McHargue, C., Yee, J,. & Rushakoff, R. (2016). Intravenous contrast in patients with diabetes on metformin: New common sense guidelines. *Endocr Pract,* 22(4):502–505.

Shea, M. (2017, September). Stress testing. Retrieved from www.merckmanuals.com/professional/cardiovascular_disorders/cardiovascular_tests_and_procedures/stress_testing.html

Short, M., & Domagalski, J. (2013, January 15). Iron deficiency anemia: Evaluation and management. Retrieved from https://www.aafp.org/afp/2013/0115/p98.html

Sialogram complications. (2018, February 28). Retrieved from https://medicine.uiowa.edu/iowaprotocols/sialogram-complications

Singer, M., Deutschman, C., Seymour, C., et al. (2016, February 23). The Third International Consensus Definitions for Sepsis and Septic Shock (Sepsis-3). Retrieved from https://jamanetwork.com/journals/jama/fullarticle/2492881

Singh, J., Singh, A., Saag, K., et al. (2015). American College of Rheumatology guideline for the treatment of rheumatoid arthritis. Retrieved from https://www.rheumatology.org/Portals/0/Files/ACR%202015%20RA%20Guideline.pdf

Single photon emission computed tomography (SPECT). (2015, July). Retrieved from www.heart.org/HEARTORG/Conditions/HeartAttack/SymptomsDiagnosisofHeartAttack/Single-Photon-Emission-Computed-Tomography-SPECT_UCM_446358_Article.jsp#.WrIW54gbOXI

Skaane, P., Bandos, A., Gullien, R., et al. (2013, April). Comparison of digital mammography alone and digital mammography plus tomosynthesis in a population-based screening program of medical care in diabetes—2012. *Radiology,* 267(1):47–56. doi: 10.1148/radiol.12121373

Smith, A. (2013, September). Jaundice in the breastfed baby. Retrieved from https://www.breastfeedingbasics.com/articles/jaundice-in-the-breastfed-baby

Smith, R., Shearer, E., Hildebrand, M., & Van Camp, G. (2017, July 27). Deafness and hearing loss overview. Retrieved from https://www.ncbi.nlm.nih.gov/books/NBK1434

Society of Nuclear Medicine. (2001). Procedure guidelines for C-14 urea breath test. Retrieved from http://interactive.snm.org/docs/pg_ch07_0403.pdf

Soldin, S., Brugnara, C., & Wong, E. (Eds.). (2003). Pediatric reference ranges (4th ed.). Washington, DC: AACC Press

Sommers, M. S. (2015). Diseases and disorders: A nursing therapeutics manual (5th ed.). Philadelphia, PA: FA Davis

Soo, G., & Cain, T. (2017, July 26). SPECT-CT scan. Retrieved from https://www.insideradiology.com.au/spect-ct-scan

Stone, N., Robinson, J., Lichtenstein, A., et al. (2013). 2013 ACC/AHA guideline on the treatment of blood cholesterol to reduce atherosclerotic cardiovascular risk in adults: A report of the American College of Cardiology/American Heart Association Task Force on Practice Guidelines. Retrieved from http://circ.ahajournals.org/content/early/2013/11/11/01.cir.0000437738.63853.7a

Stool DNA test. (2018). Retrieved from www.ccalliance.org/screening/stool-dna.html

Stowasser, M., Taylor, P., Pimenta, E., Ahmed, A., & Gordon, R. (2010, May). Laboratory investigation of primary aldosteronism. *Clin Biochem Rev,* 31(2):39–56. Retrieved from https://www.ncbi.nlm.nih.gov/pmc/articles/PMC2874431

Strasinger, S., & Dilorenzo, M. (2014). Urinalysis and body fluids (6th ed.). Philadelphia, PA: FA Davis

Street, T. (2014, March 16). Rheumatoid factor. Retrieved from https://emedicine.medscape.com/article/2087091-overview

Swaminathan, A. (2014, May 28). IV contrast myths. Retrieved from www.emdocs.net/iv-contrast-myths

Swearingen, P. L. (2008). All-in-one care planning resource: Medical-surgical, pediatric, maternity, and psychiatric nursing care plans (2nd ed.). St. Louis, MO: Mosby

Tang, Q., Liu, M., Ma, Z., Guo, X., Kuang, T., & Yang, Y. (2013, September 12). Noninvasive evaluation of hemodynamics in pulmonary hypertension by a septal angle measured by computed tomography pulmonary angiography: Comparison with right-heart catheterization and association with N-terminal pro-B-type natriuretic peptide. *Exp Ther Med,* 6:1350–1358

Target heart rates. (2018, January 4). Retrieved from https://healthyforgood.heart.org/move-more/articles/target-heart-rates#.V0iBQfkrI-U

TechneScan PYP. (2017, May). Retrieved from https://www.drugs.com/pro/technescan-pyp.html

Technetium TC 99M medronate. (2017, October). Retrieved from https://www.drugs.com/pro/technetium-tc-99m-medronate.html

Technetium TC 99M sestamibi. (2017, November). Retrieved from https://www.drugs.com/pro/technetium-tc-99m-sestamibi.html

Thompson, G. (2013). Understanding anatomy and physiology: A visual, auditory, interactive approach. Philadelphia, PA: FA Davis

Thrombocytopenia—drug induced. (2017, June 16). Retrieved from http://pennstatehershey.adam.com/content.aspx?productId=117&pid=1&gid=000556

Thyroid diseases. (2018, March 6). Retrieved from https://medlineplus.gov/thyroiddiseases.html

Torres, L., Dutton, A., & Linn-Watson, T. (2012, December 21). Torres' patient care in imaging technology (8th ed.). Philadelphia, PA: Lippincott Williams & Wilkins

Transcutaneous bilirubin measurement. (n.d.). Retrieved from www.newbornwhocc.org/pdf/tran.pdf

Transfusion-related acute lung injury. (2018, January 4). Retrieved from https://transfusion.com.au/adverse_transfusion_reactions/TRALI

Transudate or exudate. (2018). Retrieved from https://www.exeterlaboratory.com/test/transudate-or-exudate

Type, degree, and configuration of hearing loss. (2015). Retrieved from www.asha.org/uploadedFiles/AIS-Hearing-Loss-Types-Degree-Configuration.pdf

Ultrasound—prostate. (2016, March 17). Retrieved from https://www.radiologyinfo.org/en/info.cfm?pg=us-prostate

UCSF Memory and Aging Center. (2016). Tests for prion disease. http://memory.ucsf.edu/cjd/overview/tests

University of Iowa Department of Pathology. (2015, August 21). Allergen, (IgE) ImmunoCAP. Retrieved from https://www.healthcare.uiowa.edu/path_handbook/handbook/test2658.html

Understanding the 2013 AHA lipid guidelines. (2013, November 24). Retrieved from https://cardiologydoc.wordpress.com/2013/11/24/understanding-the-2013-aha-lipid-guidelines

Urden, L., Stacy, K., & Lough, M. (2013). Critical care nursing: Diagnosis and management (7th ed). St. Louis, MO: Mosby

Uroflowmetry. (2017, January 30). Retrieved from http://uoflphysiciansse3.adam.com/content.aspx?productId=117&pid=1&gid=003325

U.S. Department of Health and Human Services. (2014, August 11). What are my health care rights and responsibilities? Retrieved from https://www.hhs.gov/answers/health-care/what-are-my-health-care-rights/index.html

U.S. Food and Drug Administration. (2016, March). Donor screening recommendations to reduce the risk of transmission of Zika virus by human cells, tissues, and cellular and tissue-based products. Retrieved from https://www.fda.gov/downloads/biologicsbloodvaccines/guidancecomplianceregulatoryinformation/guidances/tissue/ucm488582.pdf

U.S. Food and Drug Administration. (2017, October 5). FDA approves first test for screening Zika virus in blood donations. Retrieved from https://www.fda.gov/downloads/BiologicsBloodVaccines/GuidanceComplianceRegulatoryInformation/Guidances/Blood/UCM518213.pdf

U.S. Food and Drug Administration. (2017, December 19). FDA drug safety communication: FDA warns that gadolinium-based contrast agents (GBCAs) are retained in the body; requires new class warnings. Retrieved from https://www.fda.gov/Drugs/DrugSafety/ucm589213.htm

U.S. Food and Drug Administration. (2009, September 24). Radiation emitting products/procedures. Retrieved from https://www.fda.gov/downloads/radiation-emittingproducts/radiationemittingproductsandprocedures/ucm183653.pdf

U.S. Food and Drug Administration. (2017, December 9). Radiography. Retrieved from https://www.fda.gov/Radiation-EmittingProducts/RadiationEmittingProductsandProcedures/MedicalImaging/MedicalX-Rays/ucm175028.htm

U.S. Food and Drug Administration. (2016, August). Revised recommendations for reducing the risk of Zika virus transmission by blood and blood components. Retrieved from https://www.fda.gov/downloads/BiologicsBloodVaccines/GuidanceComplianceRegulatoryInformation/Guidances/Blood/UCM518213.pdf

U.S. Preventive Services Task Force. (2014, January). New cervical cancer screening recommendations. Retrieved from https://www.uspreventiveservicestaskforce.org/Page/Name/us-preventive-services-task-force-issues-new-cervical-cancer-screening-recommendations

Vancomycin. (2017, December 18). Retrieved from file:///C:/FAD%20References%20Handbook/8e/Vancomycin%20-%20DrugBank.html

Vascular dysfunction, atherosclerosis, and vascular calcification. (2010). Retrieved from https://www.kidney.org/sites/default/files/12-10-0210_LBA_Vascular_bklt_LowRes.pdf

Venes, D., Fenton, B., & Patwell, J. (Eds.). (2017, January 31). Taber's cyclopedic medical dictionary (23rd ed.). Philadelphia, PA: FA Davis

Vitamin K content of common foods. (n.d.). Retrieved from https://www.med.unc.edu/im/files/patient-education-handouts/nutrition-and-diet-files/Vitamin%20K%20%20Content%20of%20Common%20Foods.pdf

Virk, M., & Sandler, G. (2013, September 12). Rh immunoprophylaxis for women with a serologic weak D phenotype. *Lab Medicine, 46*(3):190–194

Voiding cystourethrogram. (2018, March 4). Retrieved from https://medlineplus.gov/ency/article/003784.htm

Wang, J., Wang, X., Goa, X., & Vortmeyer, A. (2015, December 30). Prion diseases and their Prpsc-based molecular diagnostics. *J Neurol Neurosci, 6*(4):1–11

Weber, E., Vilensky, J., & Fog, A. (2013). Practical radiology: A symptom-based approach. Philadelphia, PA: FA Davis

What causes neural tube defects? (2017, September 1). Retrieved from https://www.nichd.nih.gov/health/topics/ntds/conditioninfo/causes

Wilkinson, J., & Barcus, L. (2017). Nursing diagnosis handbook (11th ed.). Saddle River, NJ: Prentice Hall

Willey, J., Sherwood, L., & Woolverton, C. (2013). Prescott's microbiology (9th ed.). Columbus, OH: McGraw-Hill

Wilson, D., & Hockenberry, M. (2011). Wong's clinical manual of pediatric nursing (8th ed.). St. Louis, MO: Mosby

World Health Organization. (2011). Pulse oximetry training manual. Retrieved from www.who.int/patientsafety/safesurgery/pulse_oximetry/who_ps_pulse_oxymetry_training_manual_en.pdf?ua=1

World Health Organization. (2018). Genes and human diseases. Retrieved from www.who.int/genomics/public/geneticdiseases/en/index2.html

World Health Organization. (2010). Laboratory manual for the examination and processing of human semen (5th ed.). Retrieved from http://apps.who.int/iris/bitstream/handle/10665/44261/9789241547789_eng.pdf;jsessionid=0147B92C3883F79D27FDB036DDD2D625?sequence=1

World Nuclear Association. (2017, December). Radioisotopes in medicine. Retrieved from www.world-nuclear.org/information-library/non-power-nuclear-applications/radioisotopes-research/radioisotopes-in-medicine.aspx

Wu, A. (Ed.). (2006). Tietz clinical guide to laboratory tests (4th ed.). St. Louis, MO: WB Saunders

Xavier, N., & Carmichael, K. (2013). When the A1c is unreliable. *Consultant'* 53(10):728

Yanko, J. (2012, July). Stroke and PCI: Best practice in the cardiac cath lab. Retrieved from https://www.cathlabdigest.com/articles/Stroke-PCI-Best-Practice-Cardiac-Cath-Lab

Yates, A. (2018, January 9). Prenatal screening and testing for hemoglobinopathy. Retrieved from https://www.uptodate.com/contents/prenatal-screening-and-testing-for-hemoglobinopathy

Yeomans, E., Hauth, J., Gilstrap, L., & Strickland, D. (1985). Umbilical cord pH, PCO_2, and bicarbonate following uncomplicated term vaginal deliveries. *Am J Obstet Gynecol* 151(6):798–800

Young, D. (2000). Effects of drugs on clinical laboratory tests (5th ed.). Washington, DC: AACC Press

Young, D., & Friedman, R. (2001). Effects of disease on clinical laboratory tests (4th ed.). Washington, DC: AACC Press

Zimmerman, B. (2016, June 17). Preoperative clipping: Identifying the best tools and practices for infection prevention. Retrieved from https://www.beckershospitalreview.com/quality/pre-operative-clipping-identifying-the-best-tools-and-practices-for-infection-prevention.html

BIB

Index

IND

IND

IND

IND

IND

IND

IND

IND

IND

IND

IND

IND

IND

IND

IND

IND

IND

IND

IND

IND

IND

IND

IND

IND

IND

IND

IND

IND

IND

IND

IND

IND

IND

IND

IND

IND

Commonly Requested Organ or Disease-Oriented Profiles and American Medical Association (AMA) Defined Panels

ANEMIA PROFILE
- Complete blood count (CBC with red blood cell [RBC] indices)
- Erythrocyte sedimentation rate (ESR)
- Ferritin (Ferr)
- Folate (Fol)
- Iron (microcytic anemia) (Fe)
- Reticulocyte count (Retic)
- Total iron-binding capacity (TIBC)
- Vitamin B_{12} (B_{12})

RHEUMATOID ARTHRITIS PROFILE
- C-reactive protein (CRP)
- Cyclic citrullinated peptide (CCP), antibodies
- Erythrocyte sedimentation rate (ESR)
- Rheumatoid factor (RF)

BASIC METABOLIC PANEL (BMP)—AMA DEFINED
- Blood urea nitrogen (BUN)
- Calcium, total or ionized (Ca or Ca^{++})
- Carbon dioxide (CO_2)
- Chloride (Cl)
- Creatinine (Cr)
- Glucose (Gluc)
- Potassium (K)
- Sodium (Na)

BONE-JOINT PROFILE
- Albumin (ALB)
- Alkaline phosphatase (ALKP)
- Calcium, total (Ca)
- Osteocalcin
- Phosphorus (Phos)
- Protein, total (TP)
- Rheumatoid factor (RF)
- Uric acid (UA)

CARDIAC INJURY PROFILE
- Creatine kinase (CK) and isoenzymes (CK-MB)
- Myoglobin
- Troponin

CARDIAC RISK PROFILE
- Complete blood count (CBC)
- Comprehensive metabolic panel (CMP)
- C reactive protein (CRP)
- Homocysteine
- Lipoprotein (a)
- Lipid panel

COMA PROFILE
- Acetaminophen
- Ammonia (NH_3)
- Basic metabolic panel (with anion gap) (BMP)
- Blood gases (arterial) (ABG)
- Carbon dioxide (CO_2)
- Chloride (Cl)
- Drugs of abuse screen/toxicology screen (Tox screen)
- Ethanol (ETOH)
- Glucose (Gluc)
- Lactic acid
- Osmolality (Osmo)
- Potassium (K)
- Salicylate (SA)
- Sodium (Na)

COMPREHENSIVE METABOLIC PANEL (CMP)—AMA DEFINED
- Alanine aminotransferase (ALT)
- Albumin (Alb)
- Alkaline phosphatase (ALKP)
- Aspartate aminotransferase (AST)
- Bilirubin, total (TBil)
- Blood urea nitrogen (BUN)
- Calcium, total or ionized (Ca or Ca^{++})
- Carbon dioxide (CO_2)
- Chloride (Cl)
- Creatinine (Cr)
- Glucose (Gluc)
- Potassium (K)
- Protein, total (TP)
- Sodium (Na)

DIABETES PROFILE
- Basic metabolic panel (BMP)
- Hemoglobin A_1C (A_1C)
- Lipid panel

ELECTROLYTES—AMA DEFINED
- Carbon dioxide (CO_2)
- Chloride (Cl)